ENDOSCOPIC INTERPRETATION

Normal and Pathologic Appearances of the Gastrointestinal Tract

ENDOSCOPIC INTERPRETATION

NORMAL AND PATHOLOGIC APPEARANCES OF THE GASTROINTESTINAL TRACT

Michael O. Blackstone, M.D.
Clinical Associate Professor of Medicine
Director of Gastrointestinal Endoscopy
Pritzker School of Medicine
University of Chicago
Chicago, Illinois

Raven Press ■ New York

Raven Press, 1140 Avenue of the Americas, New York, New York 10036

Library of Congress Cataloging in Publication Data

Blackstone, Michael O.
Endoscopic interpretation.

Includes index.
1. Endoscope and endoscopy. 2. Gastrointestinal system—Diseases—Diagnosis. I. Title.
RC804.E6B63 1984 616.3'307545 80-5832
ISBN 0-89004-789-8

Printed in Hong Kong by Mandarin Offset International Ltd.

To my parents

Who, in the words of my father, taught me the most important lesson of all—"Lasting success . . . doesn't just happen; it comes through hard work."

PREFACE

Developments in instrumentation during the past ten years have made the flexible fiberoptic examination of the upper gastrointestinal tract, colon, and terminal ileum routine. One result has been a shift away from radiology toward endoscopy as a primary tool for gastrointestinal diagnosis. An even more dramatic effect, coupled with improvements in instrumentation, has been the rise in the use of electrosurgical and other endoscopic techniques for therapy. Already this has had a profound effect on the management of colonic polyps, the large majority of which can now be excised immediately upon detection. In the future, the therapy of other common conditions such as biliary calculus disease, bleeding from esophageal varices, and peptic ulcer disease may be radically changed with an even greater utilization of therapeutic endoscopy.

It is not surprising that with the introduction of therapeutic procedures, the recent endoscopic literature, including books on endoscopy, has concentrated on technique, with less emphasis given to the interpretation of visual data, which is the basis of endoscopic diagnosis. Yet it is precisely because the newer instruments have increased both the range of the examination and the clarity of the visual image that the examiner is now presented with an increasingly wide variety of appearances. These must be accurately described, but also interpreted in terms of the symptoms or conditions which prompted the endoscopic examination, the expected histology, the prospects for treatment, and any possible need for endoscopic follow-up. If this interpretation is improperly done, there is a very real danger of reaching incorrect management decisions.

Endoscopic Interpretation is the result of my strong belief that there is a need for a book which is devoted almost exclusively to an analysis of endoscopic appearances through which a reader may acquire a point of view about a given appearance based on the best information currently available. For appearances one regards as normal, this entails an understanding of the range of normal for a given anatomic segment, including the variations which are of uncertain pathologic significance. For true pathologic appearances, there must be an indication of the best way to establish a diagnosis, as in the case of a suspected malignancy either by histologic or cytologic means, as well as the limitation of these modalities regarding a given appearance. Finally, in cases where one is dealing with appearances of questionable or unknown significance, as in the case of nonspecific gastric erythema (such as that following gastric surgery) or duodenitis, there must be an awareness concerning the limits of our knowledge about such appearances, particularly with respect to their unpredictable response to treatment.

Endoscopic Interpretation is intended for both experienced examiners, who will find the book helpful in dealing with unfamiliar appearances, and the trainee. Much of the material for this volume is drawn from a bimonthly teaching conference in endoscopy. At this conference, basic appearances and their variations are presented, with discussions focusing on: (a) the spatial orientation of an appearance and the technique that best demonstrates it; (b) the characteristics of the appearance itself, i.e., color, form, consistency, etc.; (c) the role of histology and/or cytology in demonstrating the nature of the appearance; and (d) the relationship, if any, of the endoscopic appearance to the clinical presentation of the patient, especially when the appearance is of questionable significance. The book itself has a comparable format. It is organized into five sections, four of which deal with a specific anatomic segment. Each of these sections begins with a chapter on orientation, technique of examination, and normal appearance, followed immediately by a chapter dealing with the variations of normal appearance of uncertain significance. These initial two chapters are followed by others dealing with the appearances of common inflammatory and neoplastic conditions, and finally, postsurgical and uncommon appearances that pertain to the segment. The remaining section which concerns upper gastrointestinal bleeding is organized somewhat differently in that the first two chapters concern orientation first to upper gastrointestinal bleeding and endoscopy in general, then take up the specific technical and interpretive problems presented by the bleeding patient. Rather than an arrangement of subsequent chapters around appearances, the organization is based on location of the bleeding site, which is more pertinent to the realities of examining a bleeding patient. The commentary provided by the author concerning a given topic is presented both to provide a prospective and to stimulate discussion with colleagues. The reader is encouraged to review critically the sources listed as well as the author's experience which forms the basis for the author's viewpoint. In this regard, the author will feel particularly well served if, frequently, the reader is challenged by a different experience or interpretation of a source to develop his own viewpoint. Whatever conclusions the reader arrives at, it is hoped they will always reflect a critical attitude, especially when dealing with appearances which have an uncertain significance.

Developing a critical attitude about the interpretation of endoscopic findings has always been one of the author's major concerns. Central to this has been a belief in the need to encourage the use of simple, descriptive and precise terms when referring to appearances, e.g., gastric "erythema" (rather than "gastritis") or "large folds" (rather than "edematous" or "swollen" rugae), in order to avoid descriptive adjectives which assume a histologic appearance that may not be present, thus adding to the general confusion about these appearances. The use of pathologic terms, in the book, to describe an appearance has been restricted to only those cases (e.g., "ulcer" or "malignancy") where the endoscopic appearance truly represents a specific lesion.

Another matter concerning terminology has been the need to define a given term as it is used in describing a finding for a particular anatomic segment. An appearance termed "erosion" will, in the esophagus, be a manifestation of chronic esophageal reflux and will not disappear from examination to examination as would be expected of gastric "erosions" which are the result of acute mucosal injury from a gastrotoxin (alcohol or aspirin) and would disappear after its discontinuation. Such terms are therefore redefined as they pertain to specific anatomic segments.

It is now almost fifteen years since I first viewed gastric mucosa through an endoscope. The fascination with endoscopic appearances and their variability remains. It is hoped that through this book my enthusiasm about endoscopic appearances will also become the reader's.

Michael O. Blackstone
Chicago, Illinois

CONTENTS

Section 4. Upper Gastrointestinal Bleeding

Section 5. The Colon and Terminal Ileum

ACKNOWLEDGMENTS

The help of many individuals who were indispensable in the actual preparation of this book must be acknowledged. However, even before the writing began I already owed much. Firstly, I must mention my own endoscopy teachers: Dr. Charles Gerson who along with teaching fundamental techniques first instilled in me the need to maintain a critical attitude about endoscopic findings and their relevance to clinical problems; and Dr. B. H. Gerald Rogers who first introduced me to the complexities and frustrations, as well as the ultimate satisfaction, of colonoscopy.

For me, as important a "teacher" of endoscopy as those who taught techniques is our superb gastrointestinal pathologist Dr. Robert H. Riddell. It was he more than any other who helped me come to understand the histologic basis of endoscopic appearances, as well as the problems and possibilities for interpretation from endoscopic biopsy specimens. One might wish that every endoscopist could enjoy the kind of close working relationship with a pathologist which it has been my pleasure to have had over the past eight years.

Also serving as my "teachers" were the three outstanding Visiting Fellows from the Aichi Cancer Center, Nagoya, Japan: Drs. Hiroshi Mizuno, Akira Matsuura, and especially Yoshiaki Ito, who stayed the longest and greatly enlarged our understanding of "early" gastric cancer.

I must also acknowledge the efforts of my colleagues in the Gastroenterology Section to help me better understand the endoscopic findings related to their areas of clinical specialization, with a special debt to Drs. Charles S. Winans in the field of esophageal disorders, Bernard Levin in the area of gastrointestinal cancer, and Alfred L. Baker in the realm of liver disease.

I must also thank Dr. Irwin H. Rosenberg for initiating this book and Dr. Joseph B. Kirsner for all his support and encouragement and especially for his perspective on the past 40 years of endoscopic practice as contained in his Introduction to this book.

Additional thanks are due to my colleagues in our Section who perform endoscopy in our Unit: Drs. B. H. Gerald Rogers, G. Jeelani Dhar, Charles S. Winans, Michael D. Sitrin, Stephan B. Hanauer and Stephen B. Hanauer, F. Deutsch who devote tireless effort in photodocumenting important case material.

Mr. Leroy Cockerham, until recently the cytotechnician for our GI Exfoliative Cytology Unit, is given special thanks for introducing me to the realities of performing and interpreting cytologic specimens as well as for providing other indispensable assistance over the years.

As great a debt as any I owe is to the Fellows in Gastroenterology for whom a biweekly teaching conference was begun and from which many of the concepts presented in this book derive. The Fellows were my endoscopy students, but as is true in all areas of education the students with their probing and insightful questioning lead the teacher toward an even greater understanding of his subject.

Although the writing of this book could not have occurred without the many who have taught me, the writing itself would not have been possible without the support of several key individuals: my tireless secretary, Mrs. Birdie Gold who singlehandedly typed the entire first draft of the manuscript; Dr. Diana Schneider, Executive Editor at Raven Press, who provided continuing support during all stages of the project; my unbelievably patient Production Editors, Ms. Mary Rogers and Ms. Marianne Milton; and my typist, Ms. Joan Hives, for her understanding and seemingly inexhaustible skill at incorporating numerous changes and other "scribblings" in the margin into the final form of the manuscript. Without her, it is doubtful whether this project could have been concluded. To my Medical Illustrator, Ms. Kathy Hirsch, I must acknowledge both my gratitude and unceasing amazement at her ability to translate the most inchoate artistic ideas into beautiful diagrams. I thank Drs. Rose Codini and Julia Dyer Jones for their special contribution at the beginning of this project, without which it is difficult to conceive how it would have gotten started.

Finally, to my family, my wife Barbara and my children Charles and Elissa, words are insufficient to express my appreciation for their understanding and sacrifice over the past 3 years.

INTRODUCTION

All Sciences are connected; they lend each other material aid, as parts of one great whole.

Roger Bacon (1220–1292)

In 1930, while a medical student and four years before Dr. Schindler arrived at the University of Chicago, I read a charming book by George S. Chappell entitled ***Through the Alimentary Canal with Gun and Camera—A Fascinating Trip to the Interior*** (F. A. Stokes, New York, 1930). Little could Mr. Chappell realize or could I then possibly imagine the prophetic implications of the book's title. For we indeed traverse the human alimentary tract with "gun" (endoscope) and camera; and the wondrous nature of this journey continues to excite us today as then.

Rarely in the history of medicine has a new technology so influenced a major specialty as has gastrointestinal endoscopy influenced gastroenterology. Within less than 50 years, endoscopy has reoriented diagnostic approaches to numerous clinical problems, facilitated ingenious therapeutic developments, permitted new physiological studies, and modified long-held concepts of gastrointestinal disease—events hardly to be anticipated by Adolf Kussmaul, the first to introduce a rigid gastroscope into a patient during the 1860s or by Rudolf Schindler during the 1930s at the University of Chicago. Here Dr. Schindler, assisted by Mrs. Schindler, with gentleness and skill demonstrated with his semiflexible optical gastroscope the clinical usefulness of endoscopic examinations of the stomach. Here too, physicians and scientists from everywhere observed and studied the revolutionary new diagnostic method and made initial attempts to correlate endoscopic observations with clinical and roentgenic findings. In retrospect, many of the gastroscopic interpretations then, in the absence of objective evidence from biopsies and cytologic examination, were subjective descriptions, reflecting primarily the experience of the master endoscopist. Nevertheless, I recall vividly the anticipation and the challenge of each examination, the wonderment at observing in living color the interior of the human stomach, and the animated discussions of the changes observed.

These activities predictably led in 1941 to the formation of the American Gastroscopic Club (the forerunner of the American Society for Gastrointestinal Endoscopy) with Dr Schindler its first President and myself its first Secretary-Treasurer. Those early days were dominated by the desire to establish the endoscopic method as a valid diagnostic tool. Pioneers such as Edward Benedict of Boston, John Fitzgibbon of Portland, Herman Moersch of the Mayo Clinic, and Walter L. Palmer and Marie Ortmayer of Chicago, among others, played major supportive roles in this effort. On the assumption that gastroscopy would be securely absorbed by gastroenterology, the original bylaws of the organization even included a mechanism for its dissolution after 20 years! Meetings were devoted to reports of new clinical experiences and to descriptions of technical advances, including the flexible rubber tip, which increased the ease of the examination and reduced the number of complications.

During the early 1950s, the initial development of gastric photography, the addition of a biopsy channel to the semiflexible gastroscope, and the application of exfoliative cytology of the stomach added a degree of objectivity to gastroscopic observations, though subjective interpretations continued to dominate the field. The pivotal development of fiberoptics and fiberoptic endoscopy during the late 1950s revolutionized gastrointestinal endoscopy, catalyzed the development of better instruments, especially by the Japanese, and enormously increased the diagnostic applicability of the method. At the University of Chicago, these developments led to a significant collaboration with endoscopists from the Aichi Cancer Center under the direction of Dr. T. Kasugai in Nagoya, Japan, beginning in 1968, a relationship which continues to this day. The earlier studies with Schindler had focused on the differentiation of benign and malignant gastric ulcers and on gastritis. Subsequent observations with our Japanese colleagues crystallized diagnostic criteria for the differentiation of benign and malignant gastric lesions and facilitated recognition of a subgroup of patients with "early" gastric cancer. We are greatly indebted to the Japanese endoscopists and technicians for these contributions and for their outstanding technical accomplishments.

Subsequent progress in fiberoptics, bending capability, wide-angle viewing, channel size, and biopsy capacity led to the development of instruments with bite diameters in some cases as small as 8 mm, which permitted the relatively comfortable and altogether revealing examination of not only the esophagus, stomach, and proximal duodenum but also the colon and terminal ileum. Intubation of the papilla of Vater, first accomplished through a duodenoscope in 1968, allowed for radiographic studies of the pancreatic and biliary ductal systems. Endoscopic inspection of the small intestine (jejunoileoscopy) became possible during the early 1970s although it was not yet utilized as a routine clinical procedure; fiberoptic laparoscopy, bronchoscopy, and cystoscopy now are standard procedures. Television cameras, furthermore, transmit endoscopic pictures to monitors for viewing by multiple observers simultaneously. We appear to have exhausted the potential for further developments in endoscopic instrumentation, but in all likelihood, additional endoscopic marvels are yet to come.

This spectacular technical progress now has brought gastrointestinal endoscopy from the period of technologic development to the present era of therapeutic endoscopy. It has provided greatly needed objectivity to therapeutic trials in regard to peptic ulcer and has facilitated such remarkable accomplishments as the identification of vascular malformations and other bleeding sites, electrosurgical laser-directed coagulation of bleeding gastric and duodenal ulcers, the removal of stones from the common bile duct, catheter drainage of obstructed bile ducts, duodenoscopic sphincterotomy, endoscopically guided sonar disintegration of common duct stones, sclerotherapy of esophageal and gastric varices, the removal of foreign bodies from the esophagus, stomach, and the small bowel, and the relatively safe removal of polyps from the colon and rectum by diathermy snare without abdominal operation. On the basis of such developments, even more amazing therapeutic accomplishments can be expected in the future, including the direct targeting of medication to disease sites and endoscopically facilitated gastrostomy at the bedside of seriously ill patients who are unable to swallow.

One of the truly major advances of endoscopy has been as an effective method of cancer detection in asymptomatic patients. A spectacular example of this new resource is in patients with positive Hemoccult tests. By endoscopy, 8 to 10% of these individuals are found to have a cancer, the majority in the curable Dukes A and B category. Another increasingly important area of screening is in patients with ulcerative colitis (or Crohn's colitis) of 10 years' or more duration; in these patients colonoscopic biopsies may reveal severe dysplasia, which is an index of increased vulnerability to colorectal cancer, or severe dysplasia may be seen with associated masses, an almost certain indication of the presence of a malignant bowel tumor. Endoscopic cancer screening opportunities in the upper gastrointestinal tract include the examination of: (a) patients with esophageal stricture and Barrett's esophagus; (b) those with previous gastric surgery after 15 years or longer; (c) patients with pernicious anemia, atrophic gastritis, or gastric polyps; and (d) patients with previously treated squamous cell cancer of the mouth, now recognized as being at especially high risk of esophageal cancer (300/100,000). In all of these areas, gastrointestinal endoscopy has revolutionized effective cancer surveillance, and its potential in this area is not yet fully developed.

Far exceeding even the most expansive expectations of its founders, gastrointestinal endoscopy has become an indispensable part of gastroenterology and a resource of the clinician, teacher, and investigator. In the words of a recent President of the American Society for Gastrointestinal Endoscopy, gastrointestinal endoscopy has become "a specialty within a specialty," a full partner with radiology in gastrointestinal diagnosis, and a respected companion to pathology in the study of gastrointestinal disease.

This saga of success is not without its limitations, however; there are concerns that are well known to those in leadership roles. Are there now too many endoscopists; are too many procedures undertaken; are we training technicians rather than gastroenterologic endoscopists? Are endoscopic findings overinterpreted, leading to unjustified therapy, even unnecessary surgery? With all the technical accomplishments, the examiner remains the most important component of the procedure. Everyone agrees that the gastrointestinal endoscopist must maintain a critical and thoughtful attitude, minimizing overinterpretation of uncertain endoscopic findings.

A prime example is diagnosing erythema (esophageal, gastric, duodenal, postsurgical), for which a symptom complex, natural history, therapeutic response, and pathogenetic mechanism, if any, have not been established. The potential for the endoscopist to do harm by suggesting a significance to such findings is considerable. The misery wrought by additional surgery in patients who already have undergone an ulcer operation and who are left with nonspecific symptoms and gastric mucosal erythema erroneously diagnosed as "alkaline reflux gastritis" is well known to experienced physicians. Other clinical uncertainties of doubtful significance also come to mind: the normal mammilations on gastric folds and prolapse of the gastric mucosa. Thus despite the improved diagnostic capabilities of modern endoscopic instruments, interpretation and evaluation of the observed changes remain critically significant requirements of the endoscopic examination.

It is in this area of thoughtful interpretation of findings and critical study of the total evidence, including the accompanying biopsy and cytologic material, that Dr. Michael Blackstone's monograph makes its most important contribution to the endoscopic literature. Dr. Blackstone, a superbly trained and experienced endoscopist and clinician, since 1974 has maintained the Schindler endoscopy tradition at the University of Chicago—questioning and reviewing as well as generating new concepts of endoscopically demonstrated findings.

This monograph, encompassing five sections and forty-eight chapters, is a comprehensive assembly of essential endoscopic information on the gastrointestinal tract from the esophagus to the colon. In contrast to the usual format, each section includes detailed descriptions of the normal appearances of each digestive organ, variations from the normal, and uncommon endoscopic appearances. This book is further distinguished from publications that emphasize the "doing" of endoscopy in that it emphasizes the "thinking" about endoscopy, an intellectual approach in the best tradition of the Schindler–University of Chicago endoscopy heritage.

Endoscopic Interpretation, in effect, is a "road map" of the comprehensive diagnostic resources of the endoscopic method. It will be a valuable guide for physicians and surgeons interested in digestive problems as well as for endoscopists and gastroenterologists. For, in the words of Henry David Thoreau (1817–1862) in Walden, "To know that we know what we know and that which we do not know, that is true knowledge."

Joseph B. Kirsner, M.D., Ph.D.
Louis Block Distinguished Service
Professor of Medicine
The University of Chicago

Section 1

THE ESOPHAGUS

1

THE ESOPHAGUS—ENDOSCOPIC ORIENTATION, TECHNIQUE OF EXAMINATION, AND NORMAL APPEARANCE

ENDOSCOPIC ORIENTATION

The raw data of endoscopy are the visual images viewed by the examiner in the instrument's eyepiece. Yet little has been written concerning these images in relation to actual points on the distal (objective) lens where the image is formed.[1] The utility of such information is considerable. It would enable the examiner to orient an image to structures which are always identified and have a fixed anatomic relationship, e.g., with the gastric angulus, which denotes the lesser curvature of the stomach. Such orientation would allow determination of the location of a structure with regard to its anterior-posterior, medial-lateral, or left-sided/right-sided positions, rather than only in relation to the depth of insertion or to the portion of the visual field. In addition, full orientation of an endoscopic appearance would provide a correlation with radiologic and surgical findings. Finally, it would heighten the examiner's understanding of visual cues, essential for both effective as well as safe endoscopy.

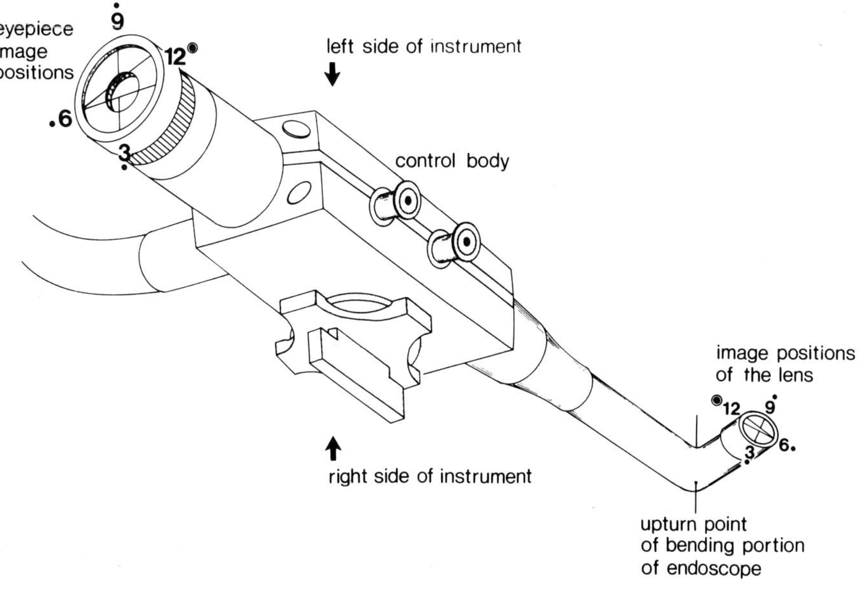

FIG. 1-1. Eyepiece image positions in relation to those of the lens.

Eyepiece Image in Relation to Positions on the Distal Lens

The sophisticated, distal (objective) lens system, part of all current-day instruments, allows for the image formed to be transmitted faithfully to the eyepiece.[2] An additional feature of the distal lens is its relationship to the upward deflecting ("upturn") point of the endoscope's bending portion (Fig. 1-1). An object placed in the midline across from the lens at the point at which the lens is closest to the "upturn" point causes a visual image to be formed by the distal lens system; this is transmitted through the fiberoptic image bundle and displayed in the eyepiece at its 12 o'clock (image) position. The position of the distal objective lens which "sees" the object whose visual image forms in the 12 o'clock position we refer to as the 12 o'clock image position of the lens; the side immediately opposite this, which would "see" an object whose eyepiece visual image would be at 6 o'clock, is referred to as the 6 o'clock image position.

With the 6 o'clock and 12 o'clock image positions of the eyepiece visual image stated to be in the midline, we may refer to the portion of the visual field to the left or right of the midline (with the instrument hand-held). One may speak about the 9 o'clock image position of the visual field as its most leftward portion and the 3 o'clock image position as its most rightward. The same relations hold for the distal lens system in that objects displayed at the corresponding 9 and 3 o'clock positions are ultimately found in these same locations in the visual image seen by the examiner in the eyepiece.

Hypopharynx

The visual image-distal lens relationships discussed in the preceding section have direct application in orienting the examiner to the hypopharynx. As the instrument is introduced into the hypopharynx, ideally in its midline, with its bending portion deflected up and with the patient lying on his left side, the 9 o'clock image position of the lens (Fig. 1-2a) views the left-hand side (left vocal cord, left side of posterior cricoid cartilage, left pyriform sinus), and the 3 o'clock image position views the corresponding structures of the right side. The 12 o'clock image position is closest to the anterior structures of the glottis and views these especially when, inadvertently or purposely, additional upward deflection of the tip is provided (Fig. 1-2b); the 6 o'clock image position views the posterior hypopharynx especially with a slight downward deflection of the tip. With an understanding of these relationships, the endoscopic orientation for the structures of the glottis and the hypopharynx becomes apparent (Fig. 1-2c).

Esophagus

The posterior hyopharynx and the esophagus are a continuous tube separated only by the cricopharyngeus, so that the relationships which were established in the posterior pharynx are maintained.

The 12 o'clock lens image position still "sees" the anterior wall, the 6 o'clock position the posterior wall, the 9 o'clock position the left wall, and the 3 o'clock position the right wall (Fig. 1-3b). These relations help us understand why cardiac pulsations which are transmitted directly to the anterior wall are seen in the 12 o'clock lens position (Fig. 1-3a), extrinsic compression in the mid-esophagus from the aorta on the left posterior aspect of the esophagus in the 9 to 12 o'clock position (Fig. 1-3b panel), and in the distal esophagus as it traverses to the right of the esophagus and posterior to it in the 3 to 6 o'clock position (Fig. 1-3c).

TECHNIQUE OF EXAMINATION

Endoscopic appearances cannot be divorced from the examination itself because: (a) the quality of the image depends to a great extent on the way in which the procedure is performed; and (b) biopsy and brushing cytology, which are easily performed as part of the examination, provide critical information concerning the nature of any appearance, giving us a greater understanding of the finding than if there were only visual characteristics by which to make judgments.

Our discussion of the technique for examination therefore includes the following: (a) preparation of the patient including premedication; (b) choice of instrument; (c) method of examination, including intubation of the hypopharynx; and finally (d) biopsy and cytology techniques.

Preparation of the Patient

The examination of the esophagus, unless obstruction is present, is generally performed as part of a full examination of the upper gastrointestinal tract and goes as far as

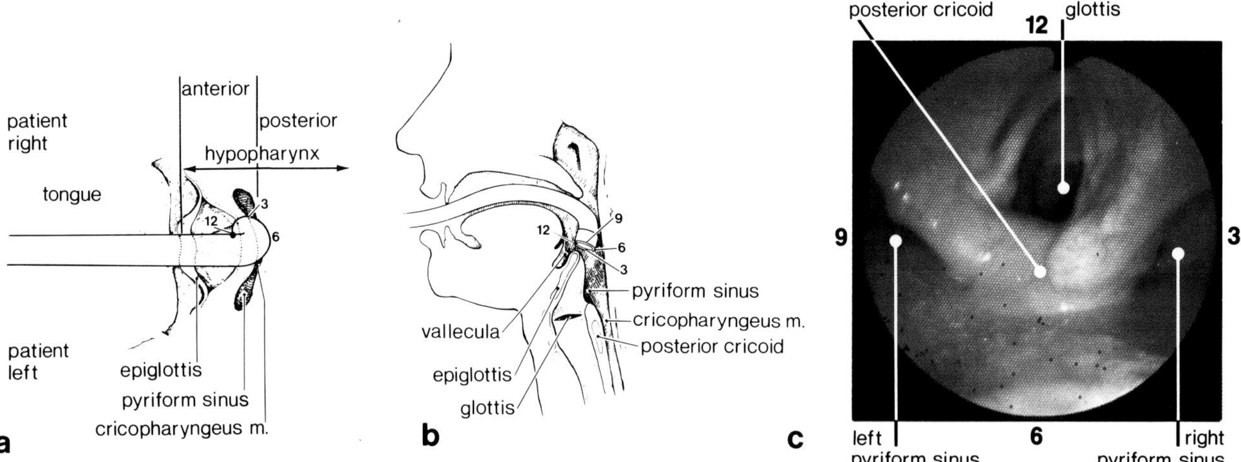

FIG. 1-2. Structures of the glottis and posterior hypopharynx in relation to the lens image positions.

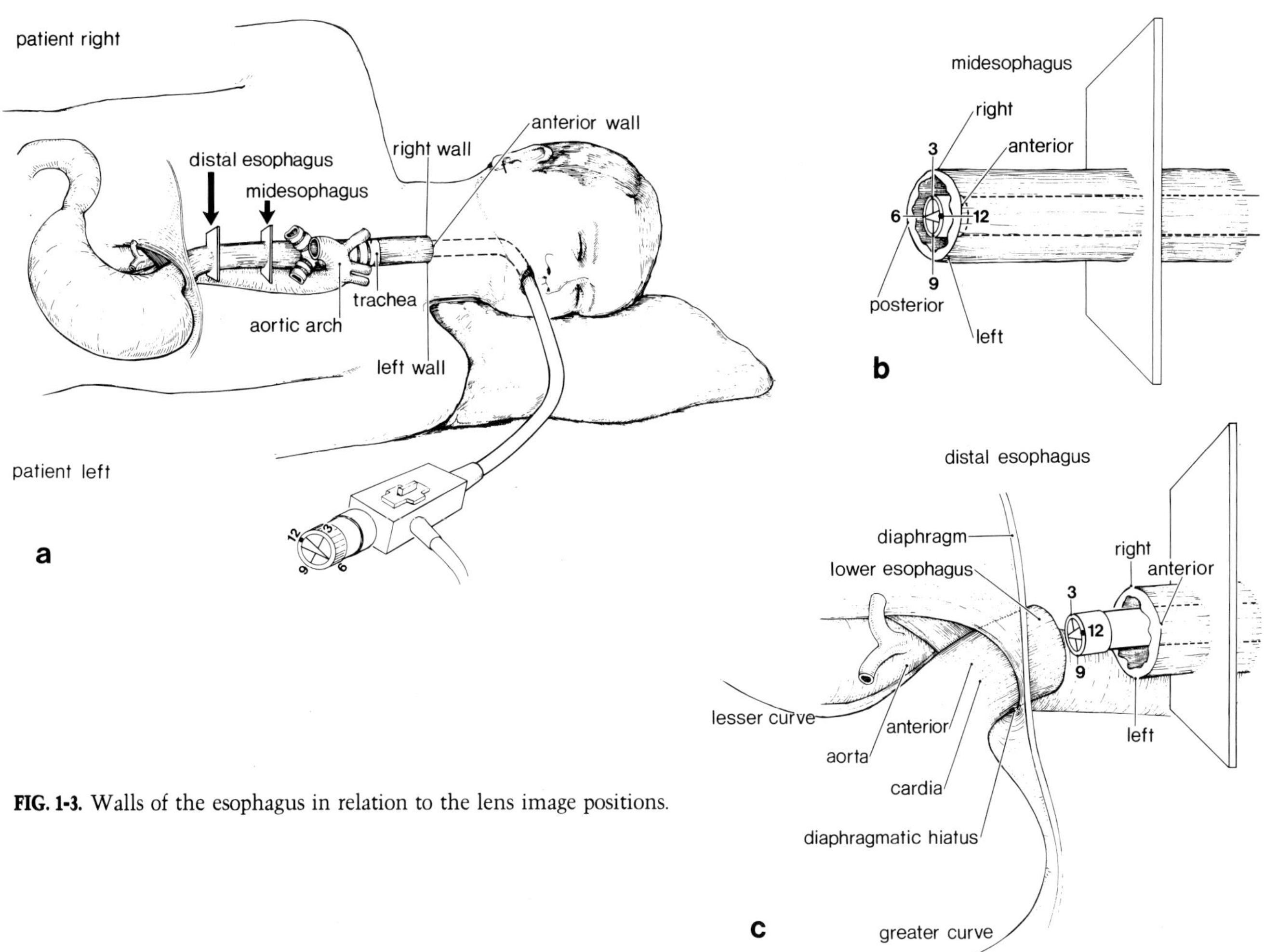

FIG. 1-3. Walls of the esophagus in relation to the lens image positions.

the third portion of the duodenum. Therefore the discussion of the preparation of the patient really concerns that procedure rather than esophagoscopy, which in current practice is rarely performed alone.

We find that the best preparation of the patient—but one which tends to be neglected—is a full explanation of the procedure to the patient, especially concerning what will be experienced with regard to gagging during intubation of the hypopharynx. In addition, the patient is instructed to have nothing by mouth, including antacids, for at least 6 hr, and preferably 12 hr, prior to the procedure.

In our Unit, baseline laboratory studies (complete blood count, platelet count, prothrombin time, partial thromboplastin time, electrocardiogram) are reviewed; the consent form is checked; and an initial set of vital signs (blood pressure, pulse rate, respiratory rate) are obtained prior to the administration of premedication.

Like others, we have the patient swallow 80 mg simethicone in a 30 cc solution; this preparation appears to reduce foam and bubbles which may obscure the visual field.[2] After this, we administer a topical pharyngeal anesthetic (2% Viscous Xylocaine, or Cetacaine or Hurricaine spray), which appears to promote better patient toleration of the procedure.[3]

The actual parenteral medications employed by endoscopists vary greatly. In the United States intravenous diazepam (Valium) is probably the most widely used. This is administered generally to the point of slurred speech, which occurs generally after a total dose of 10 to 20 mg,[4] although some patients, especially those who already take Valium, may require an additional 10 mg. It is doubtful whether more than 30 mg Valium will be effective (if not already at a lower dose), and therefore it is unwise to exceed 30 mg in any patient.

Many endoscopists administer meperidine (Demerol 0.5 to 1 mg/kg body weight) 30 min prior to the procedure, although the benefit of this is uncertain.[5] Similarly, many administer atropine (0.4 to 0.6 mg) along with the Demerol. Although this may decrease somewhat the amount of oral secretion and gastric motility during endoscopy, it does not appear to improve either the patient's tolerance for the examination or the endoscopist's performance.[6]

Choice of Instrument

The endoscope one would use to examine the esophagus, as well as the stomach and duodenum, is a "forward-viewing"-type instrument in which the objective lens is placed on the instrument's tip—in contrast to the "side-viewing" type of instrument where the lens is adjacent to the tip; the latter endoscope is used to examine specifically the stomach or duodenum (see Chapter 24).

Forward-viewing endoscopes are of varying caliber. There are standard or adult caliber endoscopes (12 to 13 mm), intermediate caliber endoscopes (11 mm), and pediatric or small caliber endoscopes (8.8 to 9.8 mm). In the past, the advantage of the adult over the pediatric instrument was the larger biopsy channel (2.5 mm), which accommodated a forceps having an "open bite" diameter of 9 mm and a central bayonet for a deeper bite.[7] The pediatric type had a biopsy channel of only 1.8 mm, accommodating forceps which had a smaller open bite diameter (5 mm) and no central bayonet, with the disadvantage that smaller samples would be obtained from any lesion. Another disadvantage of these instruments was the decreased illumination from the smaller light guides of the pediatric instruments in comparison to the adult instrument. The advantages of the larger biopsy forceps and the increased illumination of the adult instrument were offset by the difficulties encountered in intubating elderly patients, especially those in whom the lumen of the posterior hypopharynx was compromised by cervical spine lordosis; this is a frequent finding in these patients, in whom the effective diameter of the lumen posterior hypopharynx (between the cricoid cartilage and spine) is 13 mm or less, making intubation difficult if not impossible.

The newer generation of intermediate and pediatric size instruments now provides illumination which is equal to if not greater than that of adult instruments of the past. Furthermore, the trend is toward small instruments with large biopsy channels—as in the recently introduced Olympus G1F-XQ (Olympus Corporation of America, New Hyde Park, New York), in which a 9.8-mm (small caliber) instrument has a standard 2.8-mm biopsy channel. One expects that a newer generation of intermediate endoscopes may have a biopsy diameter of 3.5 mm which could accommodate a "jumbo" biopsy forceps with their capability for even deeper sampling than from the standard (2.5 mm) forceps.[7]

It is best to employ a pediatric-type instrument for elderly patients and others in whom difficult intubation is anticipated because of deformity, scarring, mechanical obstruction, etc.[8] Large instruments are reserved for cases where the examination seeks to establish a tissue diagnosis, in which case the depth and adequacy of biopsy are of prime importance.

Method of Examination

Intubation of the Hypopharynx

Most examiners place the patient in the left lateral recumbent position with the head bent forward so that the chin comes close to the chest wall, giving the posterior hypopharynx its greatest potential width (between the cricoid cartilage and posterior wall). Just prior to starting, the endoscopist makes a quick check of: (a) the eyepiece focus, (b) the air/water injection, (c) the suction, and (d) the tip controls to avoid intubating the patient with a defective instrument. In addition, we always check the up-down deflection of the tip and ensure that the tip enters the mouth in the midline. The tip is in a neutral position as it enters the mouth, but the examiner deflects upward to anticipate the sharp angle made by the base of the tongue, which now being closest to the upturn point is seen in the 12 o'clock image position (Fig. 1-4). Some endoscopists simply advance "blindly" to the point where resistance is encountered and then ask the patient to swallow. At the end of the swallow, with the cricopharyngeus relaxed, the endoscope is forcefully advanced into the esophagus. In most cases intubation will be successful with the "blind technique." Even when it is not, if a large-caliber (11 to 12 mm) instrument has been used its size protects against inadvertent entry across the glottis into the trachea. However, with the newer, narrow-caliber (9 to 11 mm) instruments, which have an extremely flexible bending portion, the tip may enter the anterior hypopharynx where intu-

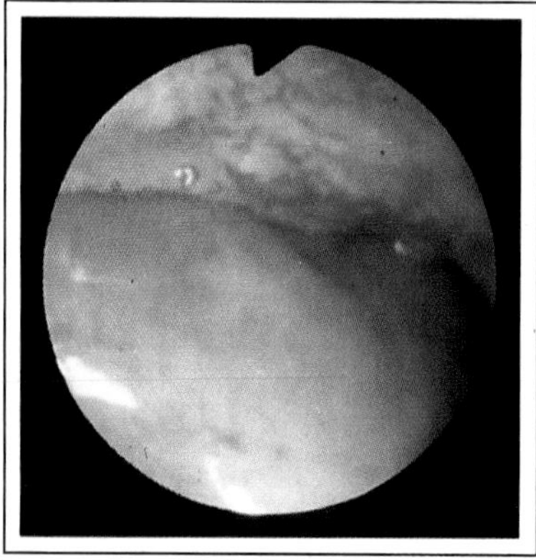

FIG. 1-4.

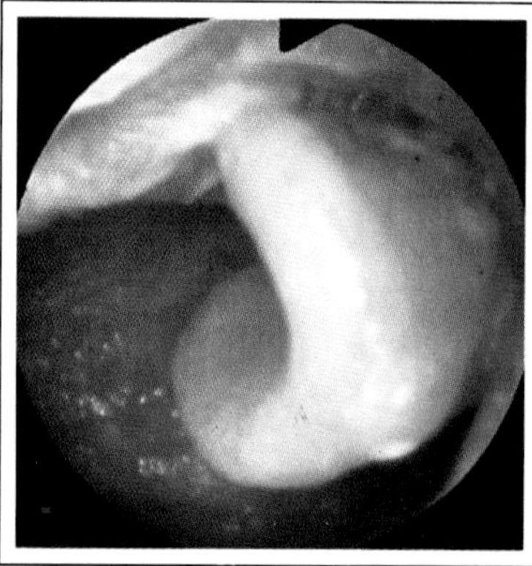

FIG. 1-5.

FIG. 1-4. Base of the tongue. Anterior (12 o'clock) to the endoscope tip, it is recognized by its pink, corrugated surface.

FIG. 1-5. Epiglottis. With intubation, the endoscope tip has rotated counterclockwise, resulting in the anterior epiglottis being viewed in the right (3 o'clock) position, along with the vallecula.

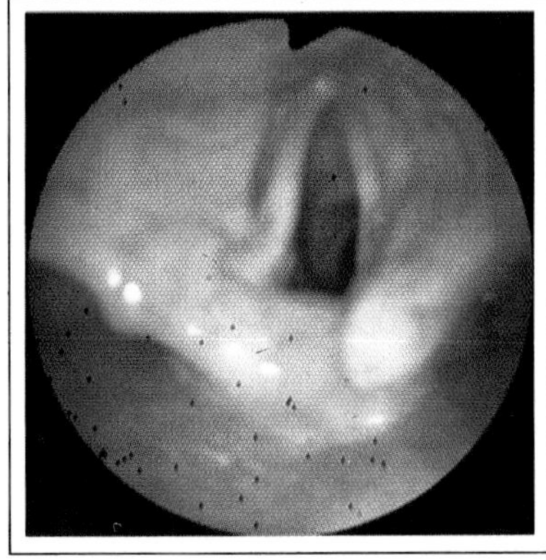

FIG. 1-6.

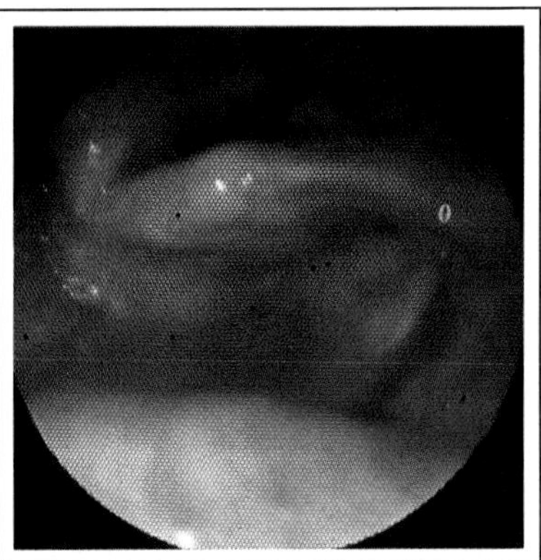

FIG. 1-7.

FIG. 1-6. Glottis and adjacent structures. The vocal cords run toward the anterior (12 o'clock) position, and the commissure of the posterior cricoid cartilage is seen at 6 o'clock. The left and right pyriform sinuses are at 9 and 3 o'clock, respectively.

FIG. 1-7. Posterior hypopharynx. The posterior commissure of the cricoid cartilage and glottis is anterior, with the right pyriform sinus at 3 o'clock. Lordosis of the cervical spine causes the convexity of the posterior wall at 6 o'clock.

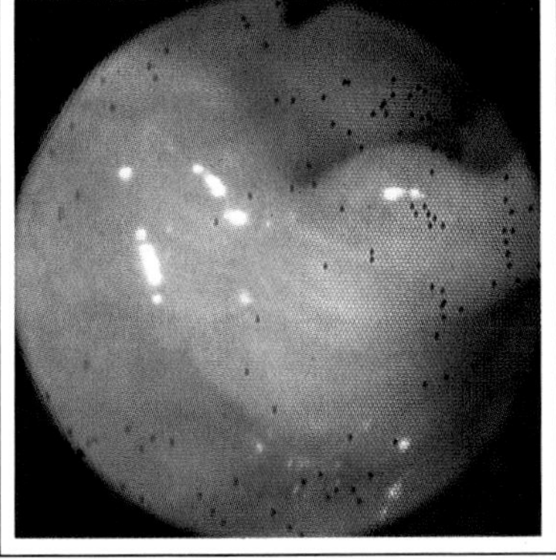

FIG. 1-8.

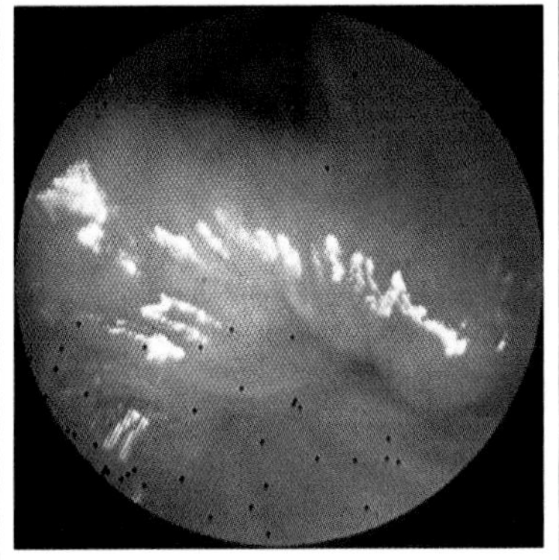

FIG. 1-9.

FIG. 1-8. Posterior hypopharynx bisected by the cricoid cartilage.

FIG. 1-9. Cricopharyngeus. This has been located by way of the right pyriform sinus.

bation of the glottis is possible, thus making "blind" intubation with these instruments undesirable. Another disadvantage of blind intubation with instruments of this caliber, with their shorter bending length, is to miss the opportunity of performing a survey examination of the glottal structures and finding significant lesions from time to time.

For a "directed" rather than a "blind" intubation, the endoscopist simply follows the base of the tongue (Fig. 1-4), past the vallecula and epiglottis (Fig. 1-5), down to the glottal structures (Fig. 1-6). Because these are anterior, they are closest to the upturn point of the bending section and are seen in the 12 o'clock position. The cricoid cartilage, which divides the anterior from the posterior hypopharynx, is seen toward 6 o'clock (Fig. 1-6). Continued downward tip deflection allows entry into the posterior hypopharynx (Fig. 1-7). Because the cricoid cartilage often bisects the posterior hypopharynx (Fig. 1-8), especially in elderly patients, there is often some compromise in the lumen of the posterior hypopharynx due to increased cervical spine lordosis (Fig. 1-7). Rather than continue with the midline, the examiner deflects to either the left (9 o'clock) or the right (3 o'clock) position in order to enter the posterior hypopharynx by way of the left or right pyriform sinus (Fig. 1-9). Once this has been performed, deflection in the opposite direction will then return the tip into the midline where the cricopharyngeus is expected.

The cricopharyngeus itself is recognized as a confluence of several folds to a central point (Fig. 1-10). There is only a slight elevation of any side of this point, which is no more than 2 to 3 mm thick. The cricopharyngeus is said to be in the midline, but it is frequently found just to the left of center. Once the posterior hypopharynx is entered, returning the tip to the midline if deflection was required to enter generally brings the cricopharyngeus into view. Should it not be found, then simply having the patient swallow and applying force "blindly" with the tip secure in the midline of the hypopharynx will enable advancement to the esophagus.

If the posterior hypopharynx is not entered because the tip is deflected laterally or posteriorly, a "J" position may result, with the examiner seeing the endoscope enter the hypopharynx (Fig. 1-11). At this point, the tip is placed in a neutral position and the endoscope withdrawn for several centimeters; re-establishment of the midline position is attempted so that the cricoid cartilage can be viewed directly and the posterior hypopharynx just behind it completely viewed and entered.

In many cases failure to traverse the cricopharyngeus is caused by the level of the cricopharyngeus in the distal posterior hypopharynx not being reached. Most often the reason for this is excessive compromise of the hypopharynx by cervical spine lordosis. Occasionally, pathologic change of the cricopharyngeus is seen as either the loss of rosette,

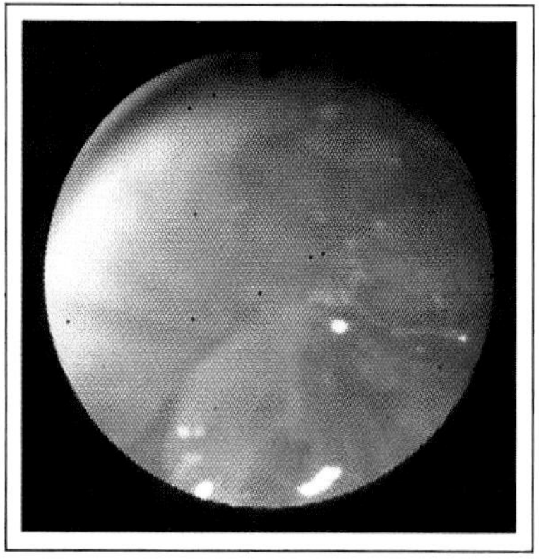

FIG. 1-10.

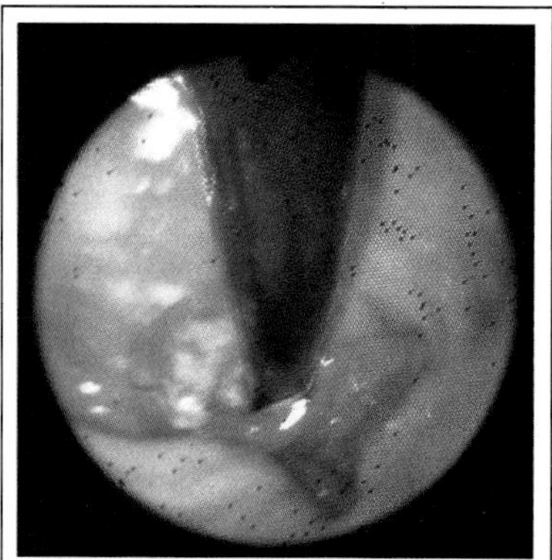

FIG. 1-11.

FIG. 1-10. Cricopharyngeus. This is seen as convergence of folds at the base of the posterior hypopharynx, forming a rosette as they converge on a central point.

FIG. 1-11. Retroflexed ("J") view of the hypopharynx. The tip has been deflected off the posterior cricoid (at 6 o'clock) and views the endoscopy entry from below.

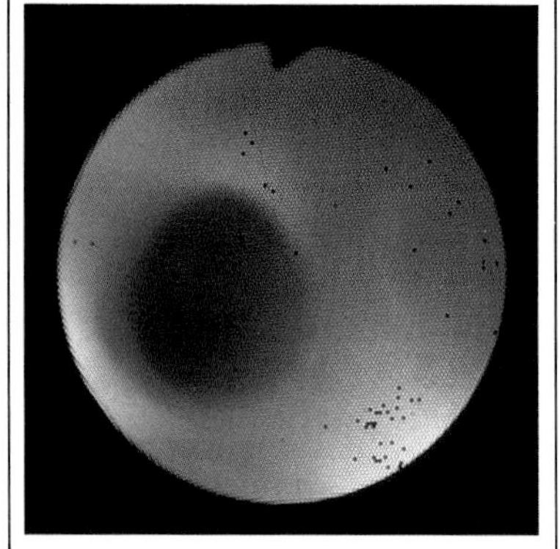

FIG. 1-12.

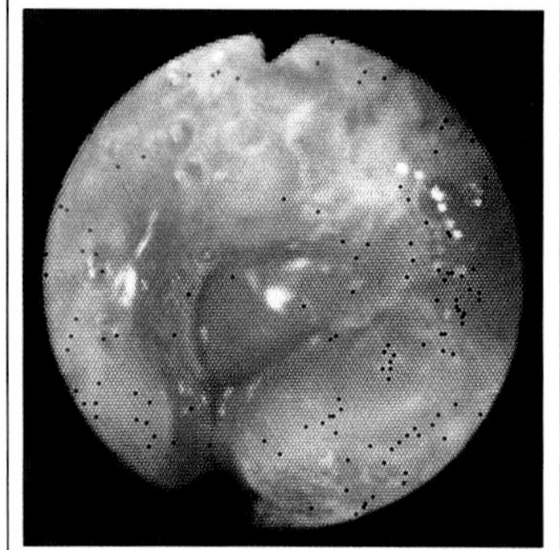

FIG. 1-13.

FIG. 1-12. Benign stricture of the posterior hypopharynx. Note the loss of the rosette (Fig. 1-10).

FIG. 1-13. Carcinoma of the hypopharynx. The smooth rosette has been replaced by irregular friable mucosa.

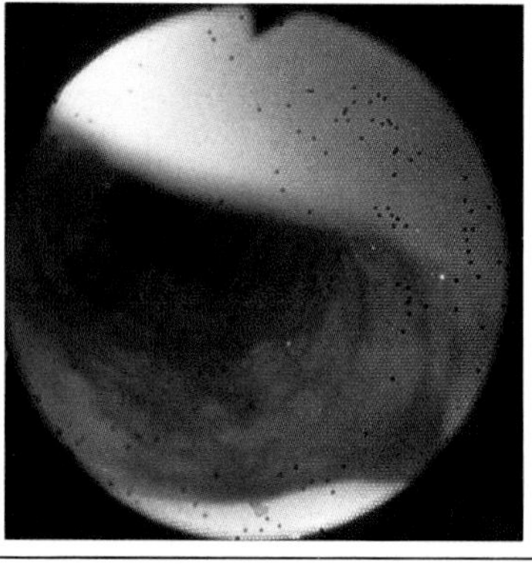

FIG. 1-14.

FIG. 1-14. Cervical esophagus (just distal to the cricopharyngeus). The careful examination in this case was performed on withdrawal.

in the case of a benign stricture (Fig. 1-12), or nodularity and ulceration, in the case of carcinoma (Fig. 1-13).

Examination of the Esophagus

The cricopharyngeus is usually found 15 to 18 cm from the incisor teeth.[9] The cervical and upper thoracic esophagus between this point and 20 cm is not well seen unless special care is taken to examine it, usually as the instrument is being withdrawn (Fig. 1-14).

Beyond 20 cm, the endoscope is advanced slowly enough to allow careful examination of structural features, e.g., the contour of the lumen and mucosal columns. The examination should not be done so quickly that mucosal detail is not observed, especially in the distal esophagus.

Examination of the esophagus ends with inspection of the gastroesophageal (GE) junction, determining its level in relation to the diaphragmatic hiatus (see "Gastroesophageal Junction," this chapter). After examination of the stomach and duodenum, it is wise to re-examine the esophagus as the endoscope is being withdrawn so as to be certain that important structural or mucosal details were not overlooked because the initial intubation was too rapid.

Biopsy and Cytology Techniques

In the course of the examination, the endoscopist may encounter either discrete lesions or simply areas of mucosa that differ from their surroundings, which he will wish to sample. The techniques of endoscopic biopsy and brushing cytology are critically important adjuncts to visual diagnosis, often greatly extending the information provided from the endoscopic appearance alone. In the section which follows we present a brief discussion of the various techniques for obtaining and handling biopsy and cytology specimens.

Biopsy

Forceps.

The adequacy of a biopsy depends on the size of the specimen as well as its depth. Both are greatly influenced by the diameter of the biopsy forceps used, as its "bite" is directly proportional to the diameter; hence the forceps having the greatest diameters provide the largest specimens.[7] In addition, large forceps have a central bayonet which adds to the depth of the bite. The use of a Williams' (hot biopsy) forceps with its large cup is another means of obtaining a large specimen. A large (8 Fr) biopsy forceps with a central bayonet can be used, providing the biopsy channel has a diameter greater than 2.6 mm; the Williams' and other jumbo forceps[7] (diameter 3.6 mm) require a biopsy channel of 3.7 mm.

To make up for the tiny samples provided by small forceps, the endoscopist can perform a greater number of biopsies, but because this is tedious there is a tendency not to do it. Therefore it is important that the largest forceps possible be used for a given lesion, especially if there is a question of its being malignant.

"Large particle" biopsy.

In the case of a discrete polypoid mass or a large fold, one may obtain an even larger sample than that retrieved by forceps biopsy—a "large particle"—by means of an electrosurgical snare. This snare is looped over a portion of the mass or a convenient part of the fold, so that when the snare is closed and current applied a 1-cm specimen is obtained.[10] To use this technique, however, the examiner must be thoroughly familiar with the principles of electrosurgical technique, as discussed elsewhere.[11]

Handling the specimen.

A biopsy specimen must be submitted to the pathologist in a manner which yields maximum diagnostic information. The endoscopist and pathologist must therefore agree about the specifics regarding the handling of histologic samples. In general, pathologists wish the endoscopist to orient a specimen prior to its being placed in fixative by teasing it out of the biopsy forceps with a needle onto a small portion of either Gel-foam or a Millipore filter and then placing it in fixative, generally 10% formalin. The specimen should then be submitted to the pathologist with appropriate identifying information.

Cytology

Two cytologic techniques are currently available: the older targeted brush method and the newer needle aspiration method.

Targeted brushing.

Brushing cytology may increase the diagnostic yield over that seen with biopsy, especially for strictures and other lesions from which the endoscopist cannot obtain an adequate sample with a biopsy forceps.[12] Sheathed brushes are preferred so as to minimize loss of material as the brush is withdrawn from the endoscope. These are now available in sizes which permit their use with even small-caliber instruments. As a lesion must be brushed vigorously using an "up and down" hard rubbing motion, some bleeding is expected even from normal mucosa but especially where the mucosa is inherently friable. Therefore a decision must be made as to whether biopsy or brushing stands the greatest likelihood of success for establishing the tissue diagnosis. In cases where the lesion is polypoid or ulcerated, and histologic sampling is likely to be successful, biopsies would be performed first, whereas in the case of a stricture[12] one would brush before performing a biopsy.

Needle aspiration.

A new technique for obtaining cytologic specimens was recently introduced. In one report it was successfully performed in 54 cases using a 0.5-cm retractable, hollow-bore 23-gauge needle. This was introduced into the mucosa of the lesion or area in question and air suction applied.[13] The aspirated material was then handled in the usual manner (see below). In this series the technique produced a positive result in 31 of 32 cancers (97%) with no false positives.[13] Such a technique may be especially valuable for nonulcerative, infiltrating carcinomas of the gastric cardia where a combined positivity of biopsy and cytology is only 70%.[12]

Handling the specimen.

As in the handling of biopsy material, the method used should be the one best suited to the individual cytopathologist. The standard technique has been to apply the brush directly to a clear or frosted slide and then place it in 95%

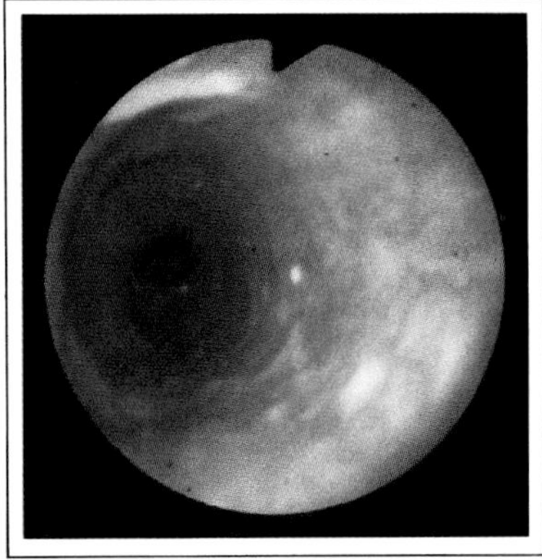

FIG. 1-15.

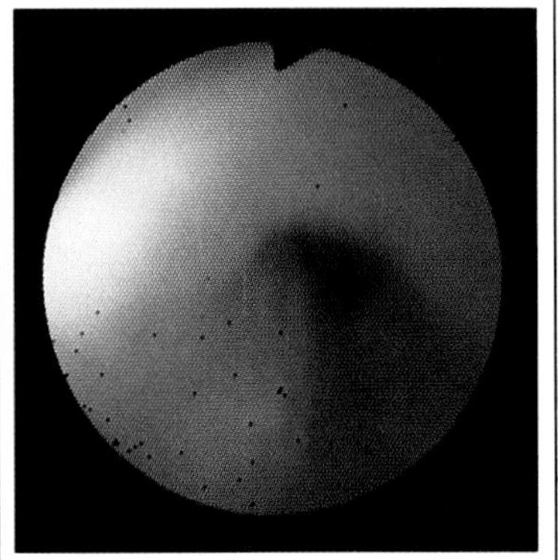

FIG. 1-16.

FIG. 1-15. Lumen of the mid-esophagus, normal diameter.

FIG. 1-16. Lumen of the mid-esophagus with compression by a prominent aortic arch.

alcohol. The slides are then delivered to the cytology service, with appropriate identifying information, where they are stained by the Papanicolaou technique and examined.[14]

NORMAL ENDOSCOPIC APPEARANCE OF THE ESOPHAGUS

Structural Features

Length

The length of the esophagus varies, relating directly to the height of the individual. On the average, when measured from the cricopharyngeus to the GE junction, it is 25 cm.[9] The examiner does not measure this distance, but rather one where esophageal length is reflected as the distance between the GE junction and the incisor teeth, a convenient reference point. The distance includes the 15- to 18-cm distance traversed by the endoscope in the oro- and hypopharynx. Short-statured individuals, particularly women, may have an esophageal length of only 15 cm so that the GE junction is seen 30 to 33 cm from the incisors[9] whereas for some extremely tall men the esophageal length may be up to 35 cm, with the GE junction at 50 cm.[9]

Lumen

Upon entering the esophagus, the single most impressive feature is its tubular lumen. This has a diameter of usually 1.5 to 2.5 cm (Fig. 1-15)[9] with the width increasing to a maximum in the distal portion. The lumen at a level approximately 25 cm from the incisors may show compression from the aortic arch and cardiac structures (see Chapter 2), which because of their placement anterior and just to the left of the esophagus is seen to indent slightly the left anterior wall (between 9 and 1 o'clock) (Figs. 1-16 and 1-17).

One may conveniently divide the esophagus into three

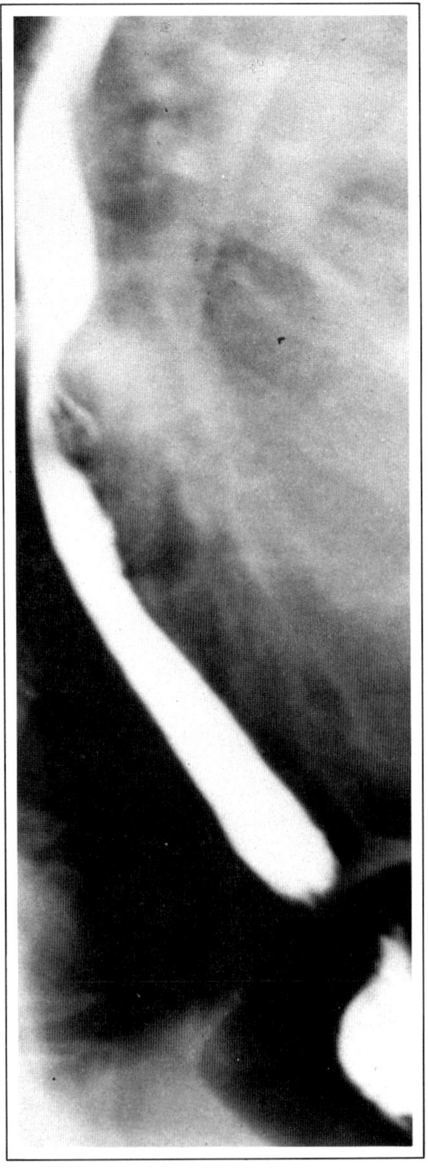

FIG. 1-17. Esophagram of the patient in Fig. 1-16 with an indentation made by a prominent aortic arch.

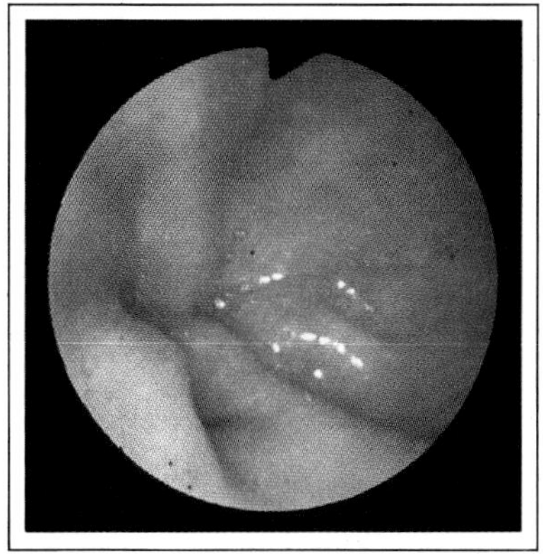

FIG. 1-18.

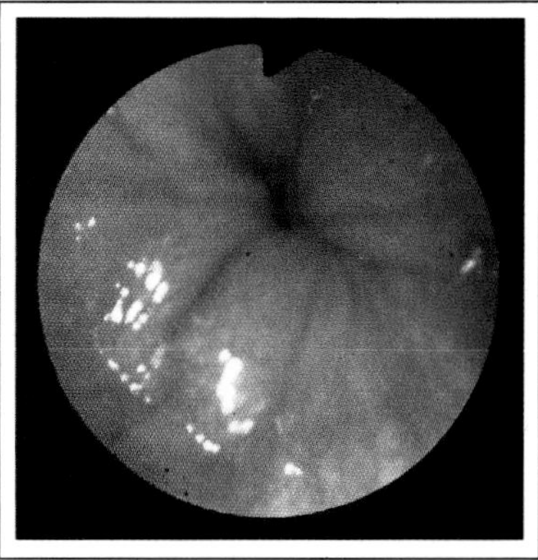

FIG. 1-19.

FIG. 1-18. Esophageal columns.

FIG. 1-19. Cardial folds. Terminating point of the esophageal mucosal columns.

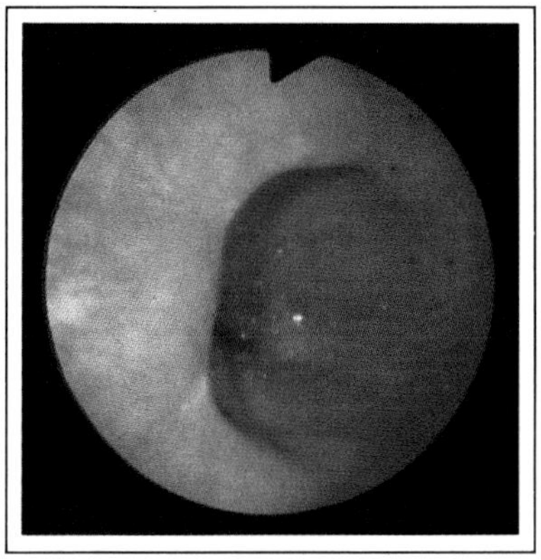

FIG. 1-20.

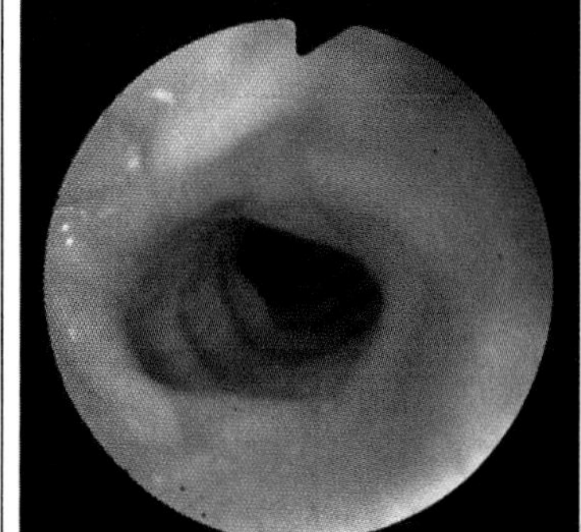

FIG. 1-21.

FIG. 1-20. Gastroesophageal junction, with the "A" ring (lower esophageal sphincter) in the foreground.

FIG. 1-21. Esophageal mucosa with the typical gray-pink coloration.

portions: the upper esophagus (running between the cricopharyngeus and 25 cm), the mid-esophagus (between 25 and 32 cm), and the distal portion (from 32 cm to the GE junction, which generally lies at a level of 39 to 41 cm).

Mucosal Columns

Only when the esophagus is fully insufflated does one see a smooth mucosal surface. With less insufflation, the mucosa is displayed with its characteristic columns (Fig. 1-18). These may be 2 to 4 mm wide and run parallel to each other down to the diaphragm and slightly below, converging at a central point to become the "cardial rosette" (Fig. 1-19).

Lower Esophageal Sphincter

Approximately 2 cm above the GE junction one may observe the physiological "A" ring (Fig. 1-20), which is the proximal extent of the lower esophageal sphincter (LES).[15] This ring-like narrowing can be seen to open and close during the examination as peristaltic waves run through. The 2-cm segment between the "A" ring and the GE junction, the usual location of the LES, has been referred to as the esophageal vestibule.

Mucosal Appearance

Color

The mucosa is typically grayish-blue-pink (Fig. 1-21), being in most cases grayer but in others more pink, or even red (see Chapter 2). However, even with variations in color, the mucosa may be histologically normal.

Character

Esophageal mucosa appears visually to be perfectly smooth (Fig. 1-22). It may actually be bumpy, however, with innumerable tiny irregularities. Some of this irregular character is due to a failure to completely distend the esophagus, but even with adequate distention an irregular character may still be observed, suggesting considerable normal variation in mucosal texture: smooth, slightly coarsened, or bumpy (Fig. 1-23).

Vascular Pattern

The submucosal capillaries of the esophagus tend to be seen as long branching vessels (Fig. 1-24a) running parallel with each other, especially in the distal esophagus (Fig. 1-24b).

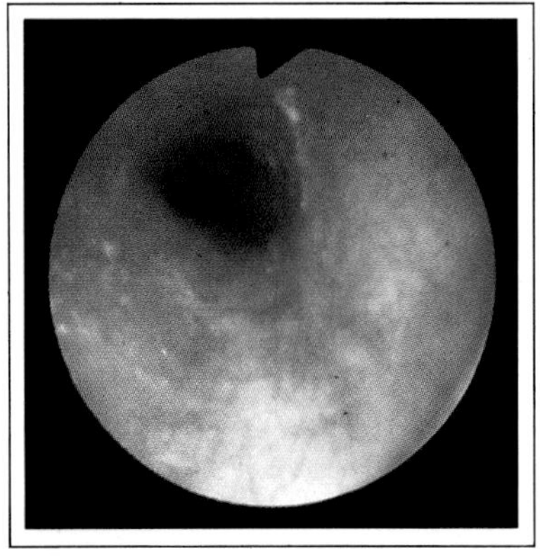

FIG. 1-22.

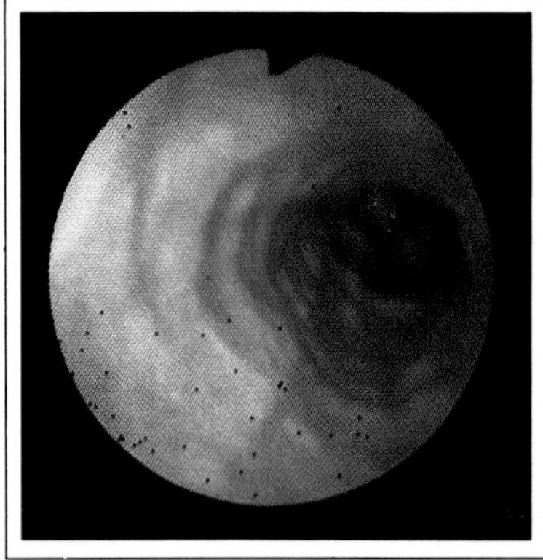

FIG. 1-23.

FIG. 1-22. Esophageal mucosa. Note the smooth texture.

FIG. 1-23. Esophageal mucosa with a bumpy texture; the biopsy was normal.

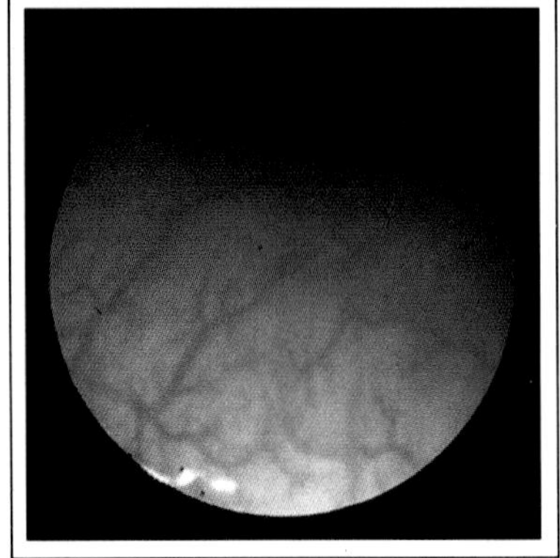

FIG. 1-24a.

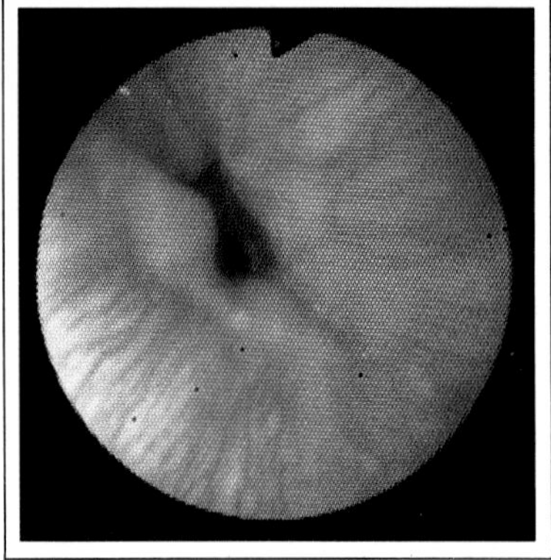

FIG. 1-24b.

FIG. 1-24. Esophageal vascular pattern. **a:** Mid-esophagus. **b:** Distal esophagus.

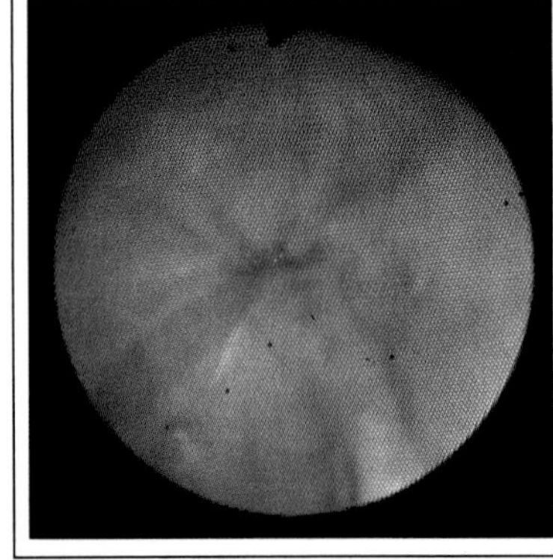

FIG. 1-25.

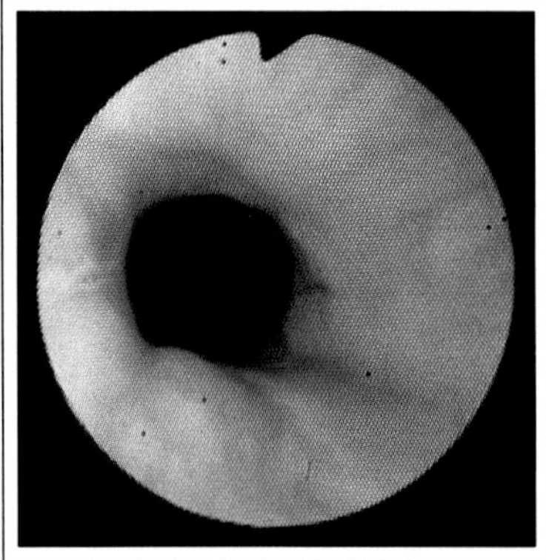

FIG. 1-26.

FIG. 1-25. Gastroesophageal junction, irregular (serrated) type.

FIG. 1-26. Gastroesophageal junction. Normal (<2 cm) interval to hiatal impression below.

GE Junction

As already noted, the distance of the GE junction from the incisors varies with the height of the individual, being generally between 35 cm (in short-statured individuals) and 45 cm (in tall people). It is recognized as an abrupt change from the gray-pink color of esophageal mucosa to the yellow-orange of the cardia (Fig. 1-20) at or just below the diaphragm. The GE junction in an asymptomatic patient can be either uniform (Fig. 1-20) or irregular (Fig. 1-25). This irregular, or serrated, appearance has led to the use of the term "Z" line (short for zig-zag) for the GE junction. Because it is common in asymptomatic patients, one regards a serrated appearance of the GE junction, even though striking, as a normal variant (see Chapter 2), particularly when the gastric mucosal projections are less than 5 mm long and 3 mm wide. Longer (>1 cm) and wider (>5 mm) projections can be abnormal, indicating either the presence of esophagitis (see Chapter 3) or early Barrett's changes (gastric metaplasia; see Chapter 6). In such cases the endoscopist would wish to biopsy this area to determine the nature of the mucosal changes, if any, associated with this appearance.

GE Junction in Relation to the Diaphragmatic Hiatus

Generally the diaphragmatic hiatus is encountered within 1 to 2 cm of the GE junction. The hiatus is identified at the point at which diaphragmatic motion is seen to change the shape of the cardial lumen. This is brought out by the "sniff" test, where the cardia is carefully observed as the patient sniffs in order to move the diaphragm. The point of movement on the cardia is sought and its distance determined in relation to that of the GE junction. Normally, the point of diaphragmatic impression is within 1 to 2 cm of the GE junction (Fig. 1-26). If this exceeds 2 cm, a hiatus hernia is likely.[15] If the endoscopist wishes to confirm the presence of a hiatus hernia suggested on x-ray, this maneuver must be performed before, rather than after, the stomach is entered, as entry tends to draw the intrathoracic portion of the stomach back down below the diaphragm, so as to reduce the hernia.

REFERENCES

1. Epstein, L. I. (1981): Orientation in endoscopy. *Endoscopy,* 13:77–80.
2. McDonald, G. B., O'Leary, R., and Stratton, C. (1978): Preendoscopic use of oral simethicone. *Gastrointest. Endosc.,* 24:283.
3. Gordon, M. J., Mayes, G. R., and Meyer, G. W. (1976): Topical Lidocaine in preendoscopic medication. *Gastroenterology,* 71:564–569.
4. Castiglioni, L. J., Allen, T. S., and Patterson, M. (1973): Intravenous diazepam: an improvement in pre-endoscopic medication. *Gastrointest. Endosc.,* 19:134–136.
5. Gordon, M. J., Mayes, G. R., Landsbaum, C. J., and Meyer, G. W. (1977): Meperidine and topical Lidocaine in pre-endoscopic medication. *Gastrointest. Endosc.,* 24:14–16.
6. Cattan, E. L., Artnak, E. J., Meyer, G. W., and Castell, D. O. (1981): Efficacy of atropine as an endoscopic premedication. *Gastrointest. Endosc.,* 27:120.
7. Siegel, M., Barkin, J., Rogers, A., and Clark, R. (1981): Gastric biopsy: a comparison of biopsy forceps. *Gastrointest. Endosc.,* 27:119.
8. Urakami, Y., Nokihara, M., Kishi, S., and Seifert, E. (1979): The GIF-P2 as a panendoscope. *Gastrointest. Endosc.,* 25:88–92.
9. Hightower, N. C. (1974): Applied anatomy and physiology of the esophagus. In: *Gastroenterology,* Vol. 1, p. 127. Saunders, Philadelphia.
10. Deyhle, P., Sauberli, H., Nuesch, H. J., Huni, R., and Jenny, S. (1974): Endoscopic "jumbo biopsy" in the stomach with a diathermy loop. *Acta Hepatogastroenterol. (Stuttg.),* 21:228–232.
11. Barlow, D. E. (1982): Endoscopic applications of electrosurgery: a review of basic principles. *Gastrointest. Endosc.,* 28:73–76.
12. Kobayashi, S., and Kasugai, T. (1978): Brushing cytology for the diagnosis of gastric cancer involving the cardia or the lower esophagus. *Acta Cytol. (Baltimore),* 22:155–157.
13. Raskin, J. B., Welch, P., Zara, E., Gould, E., and Nadji, M. (1981): Tranendoscopic needle aspiration cytology—a comparison with standard biopsy techniques. *Gastrointest. Endosc.,* 27:128.
14. Prolla, J. C., and Kirsner, J. B. (1972): *Handbook and Atlas of Gastrointestinal Exfoliative Cytology.* University of Chicago Press, Chicago.
15. Morrissey, J. F. (1978): Endoscopic evaluation of gastroesophageal sphincter dysfunction. *South. Med. J. (Suppl. 1),* 71:56–61.

2

THE ESOPHAGUS—VARIATIONS FROM THE NORMAL APPEARANCE

The esophageal appearance encountered by the endoscopist may differ importantly from that of a simple straight tube with gray-pink mucosa down to the gastroesophageal (GE) junction, as described in the previous chapter. Variations in the shape of the lumen, the appearance of the mucosa, and the GE junction give the impression of abnormality. Yet many of these appearances have an uncertain (if any) pathologic significance.

VARIATIONS IN THE SHAPE OF THE LUMEN

Aortic Arch

The aortic arch is noted as an indentation at the junction of the upper and mid-esophagus from the aortic arch as it runs just anterior to the left of the esophagus (see Fig. 1-3a). This indentation of the wall of the esophagus into the lumen is therefore seen in the 9 to 12 o'clock (left anterior) position (Fig. 2-1) if the 12 o'clock lens position is aligned with the anterior wall (see Chapter 1). In some cases the indentation is prominent and suggests a submucosal mass; however, the pulsatile nature of this "mass" and its location indicate that it is simply the aortic arch.

Distal Thoracic Aorta

Tortuosity and dilatation of the thoracic aorta, common in elderly patients, may produce mild compression of the distal esophagus just above the diaphragmatic hiatus.[1,2] Because the aorta lies posterior and to the right of the esophagus (Fig. 1-3c), the resulting indentation of the wall is seen posteriorly (6 o'clock) (Fig. 2-2) and to the right (3 o'clock). Most patients with this appearance are asymptomatic, but some have dysphagia,[2] especially those with associated cardiac enlargement, poor dentition, or significant esophageal motor disturbance (see Chapter 10).

VARIATIONS IN MUCOSAL APPEARANCE

The three appearances of the mucosa to be discussed below—lower esophageal erythema, glycogenic acanthosis, and prominent esophageal veins—are a concern for the endoscopist because of their potential for being confused for true pathologic findings. Yet the endoscopist's awareness of their uncertain significance and the use of this designation in the endoscopic report will hopefully prevent unnecessary additional testing or inappropriate therapy from being instituted.

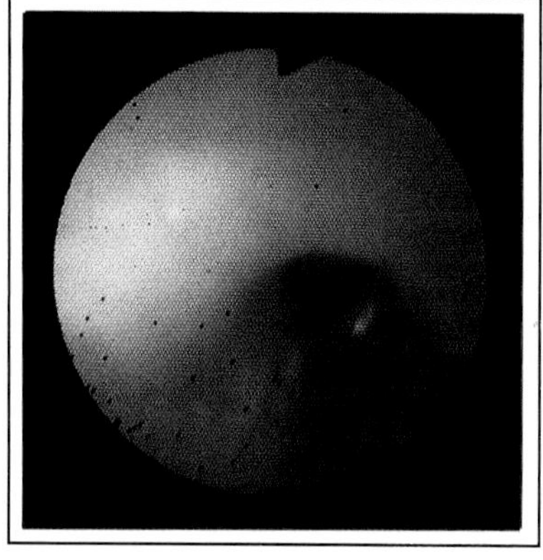

FIG. 2-1.

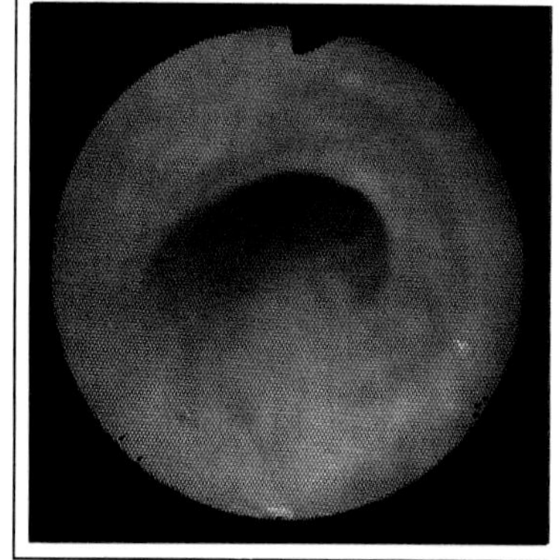

FIG. 2-2.

FIG. 2-1. Aortic arch compression. An indentation is noted on the anterior aspect of the left wall, seen here at 9 o'clock.

FIG. 2-2. Distal thoracic aorta compression, resulting in an indentation on the posterior (6 o'clock) wall.

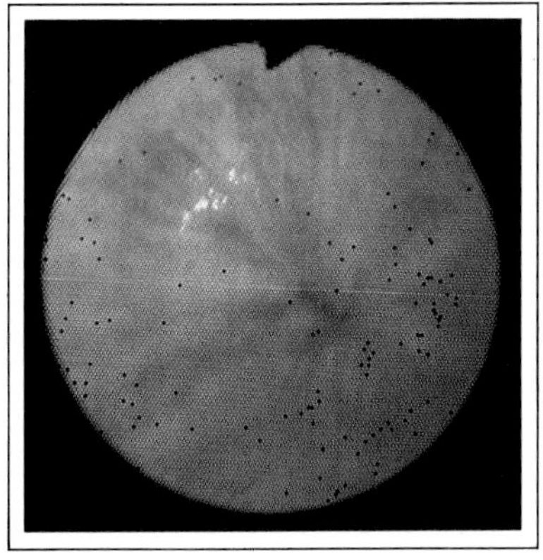

FIG. 2-3.

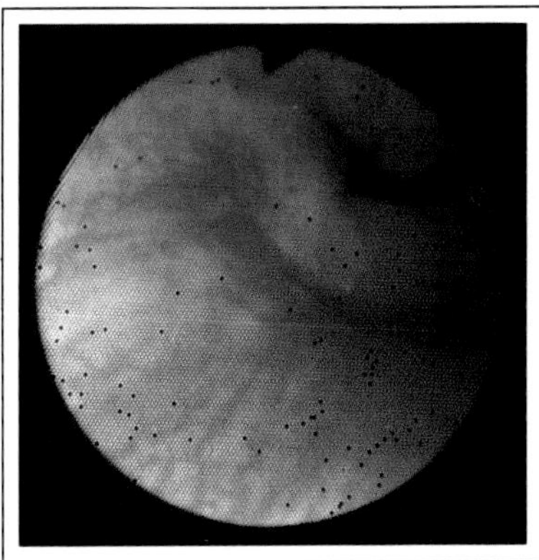

FIG. 2-4.

FIG. 2-3. Lower esophageal erythema with a prominent vascular pattern in a patient with reflux symptoms.

FIG. 2-4. Traumatic lower esophageal erythema after examination of the stomach and duodenum. Patchy erythema is noted along with a prominent and distorted vascular pattern (compare with the normal appearance in Fig. 1-24b). The patient had no reflux symptoms.

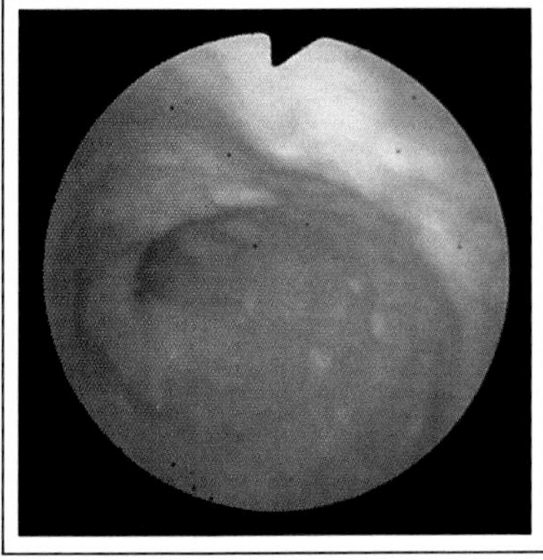

FIG. 2-5.

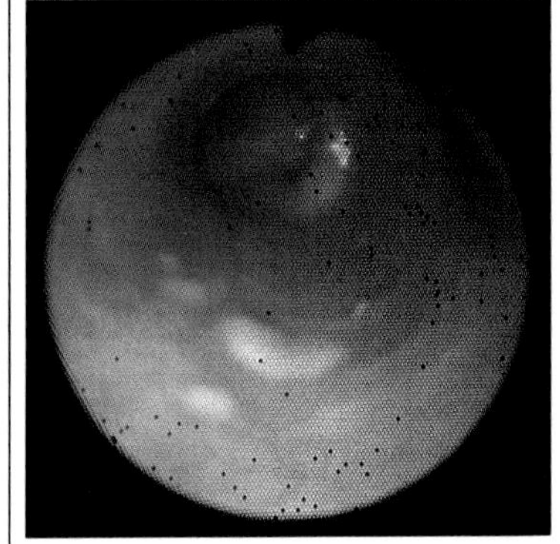

FIG. 2-6.

FIG. 2-5. Glycogenic acanthosis. These 2- to 3-mm pale mucosal excrescences are scattered throughout the esophagus.

FIG. 2-6. Glycogenic acanthosis. In two lesions, the largest of which was 4 mm, biopsy showed increased glycogen content compared with that in the surrounding mucosa.

Lower Esophageal Erythema

We find a distinct reddened appearance (erythema) of the distal esophagus in 5 to 10% of examinations, irrespective of whether reflux symptoms are present. Some authorities regard diffuse or patchy erythema[3,4] as evidence of "mild" esophagitis, especially if accompanied by an accentuation of the vascular pattern[4,5] (Fig. 2-3) over what is considered normal (see Chapter 1). We believe, however, that this is unwise as the false-positive rate for this finding is unknown, i.e., the percent of patients with this finding but lacking either typical reflux symptoms or positive results from other objective tests of reflux, e.g., 24-hr pH monitoring. It is our impression that up to 50% of patients in whom this appearance is found do not have symptomatic reflux. In many of these, lower esophageal erythema is actually related to the endoscopic procedure in that the erythema is noted only on withdrawal. What is probably being observed in these cases is traumatic erythema which occurs with forceful movement of the esophagus around the endoscope that accompanies retching, choking, or coughing (Fig. 2-4). The erythema which occurs with a sudden forceful collapse of the distal esophagus around the endoscope is much like the erythema of the skin which occurs after one's wrists are slapped.

Glycogenic Acanthosis

In up to 2% of examinations we find discrete tiny elevations, generally five or more, scattered about the mucosa (Fig. 2-5). Using double contrast radiography, followed by endoscopy, these have been noted in more than 25% of the cases.[5a] Individually they are 3 mm or less in size and appear whiter than the surrounding gray-pink mucosa (Fig. 2-6). Biopsy of these tiny lesions when appropriately stained with periodic acid Schiff (PAS) reagent reveals an increased glycogen content compared with that in the surrounding mucosa.[6] Occasionally one sees a single focal, perfectly white lesion, called esophageal leukoplakia (Fig. 2-7), in which biopsies reveal the same increased glycogen content as in glycogenic acanthosis, or simply mucosal thickening. The origin of these lesions is unclear. There is no histologic evidence that either appearance is related to esophageal reflux.[6] Even as larger lesions (leukoplakia), they are not generally regarded as premalignant, as is leukoplakia of the mouth,[7] though we have observed one case where a polypoid carcinoma was found in an area where leukoplakia had been noted 5 years before. The importance of glycogenic acanthosis for the most part lies in its potential for being confused with other lesions, especially *Candida* lesions (Fig. 2-8).

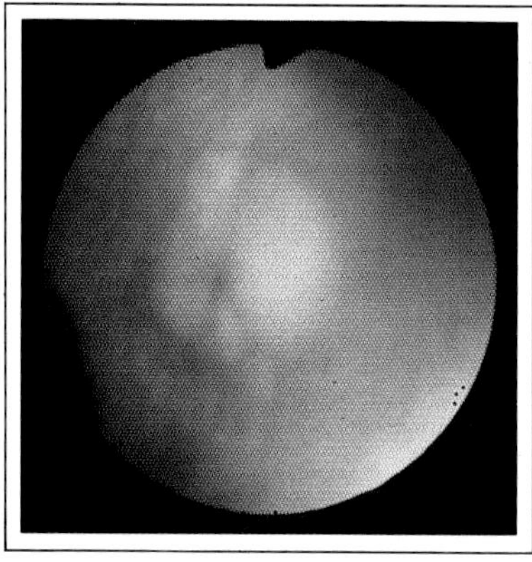

FIG. 2-7.

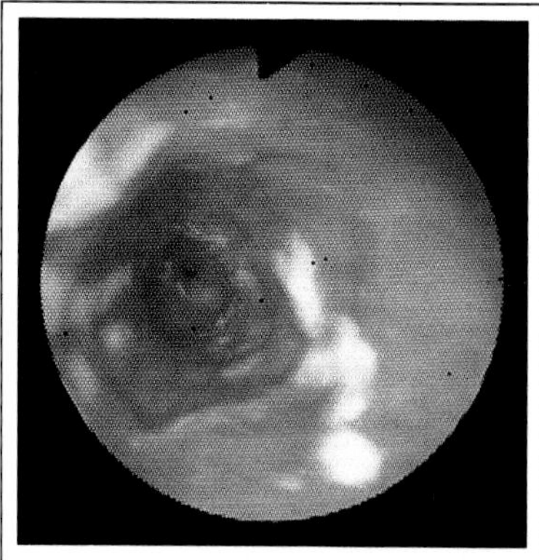

FIG. 2-8.

FIG. 2-7. Leukoplakia. Biopsy of this single lesion showed mucosal thickening without increased glycogen.

FIG. 2-8. *Candida* plaques. These characteristic yellow-white pseudomembranes are readily seen as exudative rather than intermucosal lesions as in the case of glycogenic acanthosis.

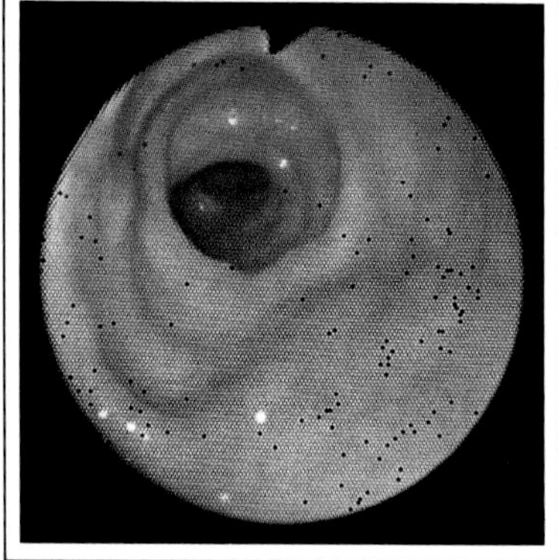

FIG. 2-9.

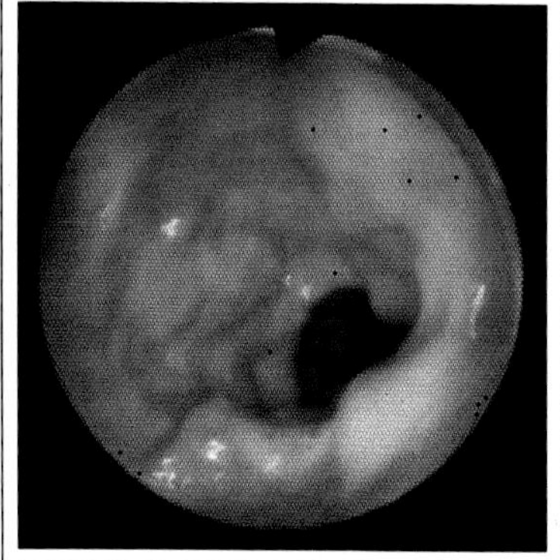

FIG. 2-10.

FIG. 2-9. Prominent esophageal vein. This is seen as a single blue vein in the mid to distal esophagus.

FIG. 2-10. Esophageal varices. Multiple interconnecting venous structures are easily distinguished from the solitary esophageal vein seen in Fig. 2-9.

Prominent Esophageal Veins

Occasionally, especially in elderly patients, one encounters a solitary, often blue structure (Fig. 2-9) in the mid or distal esophagus suggesting a vein and raising the question of esophageal varices (Fig. 2-10) and portal hypertension. In contrast to these veins, however, esophageal varices are never solitary (Fig. 2-10); varices are part of an interconnected system. Moreover, varices, being further from the surface than these veins, appear gray-white rather than blue. Factors which promote the appearance of these veins are unknown.

VARIATIONS IN THE APPEARANCE OF THE GE JUNCTION

As suggested earlier (see Chapter 1), considerable variation exists in the appearance of the GE junction. In this section we present three appearances of the GE junction which are seen without other abnormalities and which we have come to regard as normal variations. These are: (a) angulation; (b) an indistinct transition from esophageal to gastric mucosa; and (c) a GE junction accentuated by the presence of broad interdigitating bands of gastric and esophageal mucosa.

Angulation at the GE Junction

Although the esophageal columns may converge directly onto the cardia to form a "cardial rosette" with no angulation (Fig. 2-11), in most cases there is some angulation because of the turn of the left wall of the esophagus as it becomes the greater curve of the stomach (see Fig. 1-3c). This is seen as an angulus made with the cardial rosette (see Chapter 1) coming off its left (9 o'clock) aspect (Fig. 2-12). In some cases this is marked (Fig. 2-13).

Indistinct GE Junction

In order for the GE junction to be distinct, gastric mucosa must have its expected orange-red (salmon) color. In elderly patients or others with atrophic gastritis (see Chapter 14), or in the presence of profound anemia (hematocrit less than 25), the gastric mucosa becomes so pale its junction with the esophageal mucosa is not easily seen. Furthermore, in atrophic gastritis the gastric mucosal capillary bed, which is otherwise not seen, becomes prominent and merges indistinguishably with that of the distal esophagus (Fig. 2-

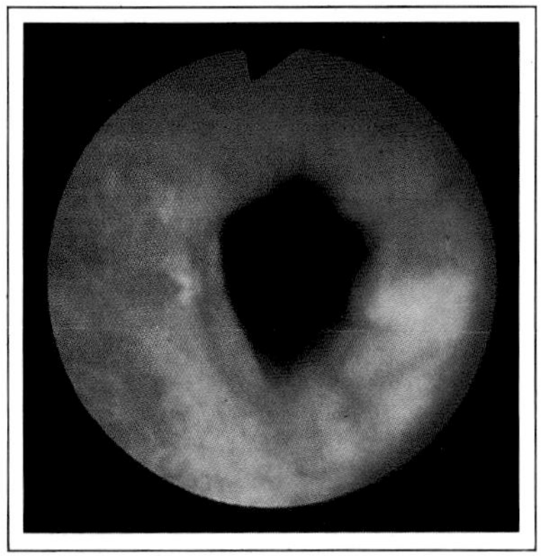

FIG. 2-11.

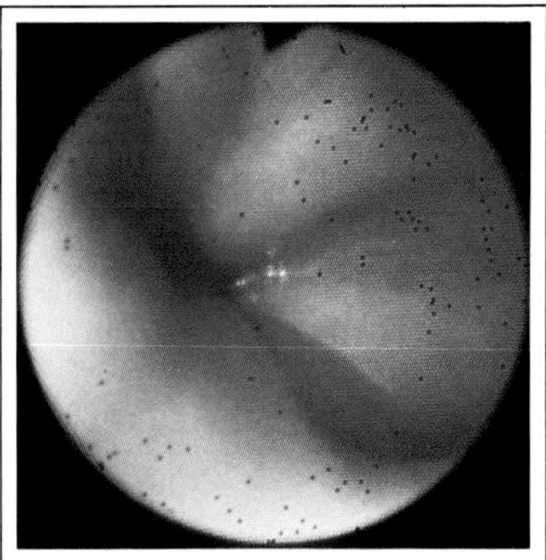

FIG. 2-12.

FIG. 2-11. GE junction, no angulation.

FIG. 2-12. GE junction, slight angulation.

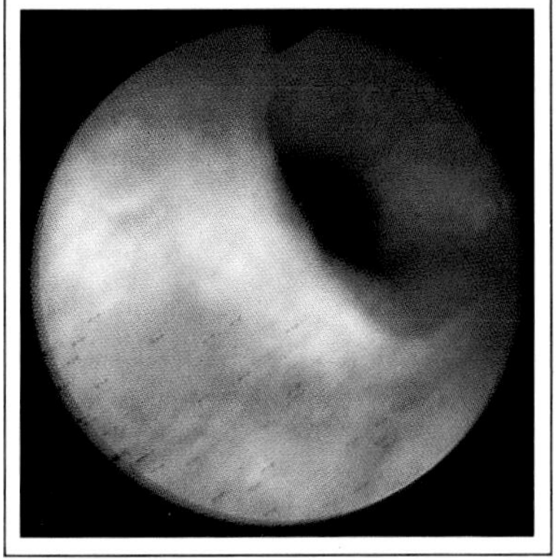

FIG. 2-13.

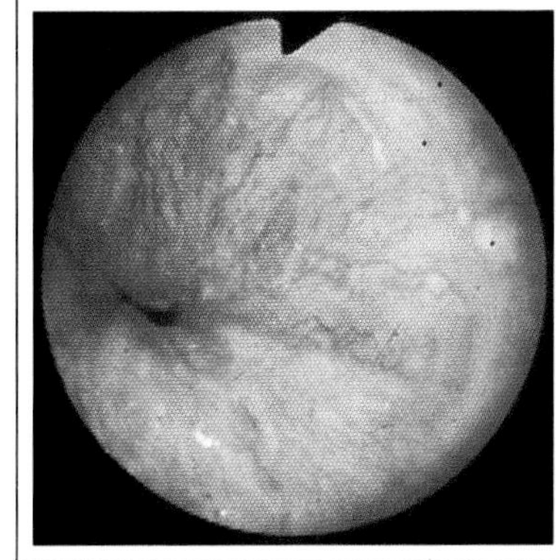

FIG. 2-14.

FIG. 2-13. GE junction, marked angulation; but a sharp angulation is seen at the left (9 o'clock) with respect to the cardia.

FIG. 2-14. Indistinct GE junction in a patient with atrophic gastritis and a prominent capillary pattern.

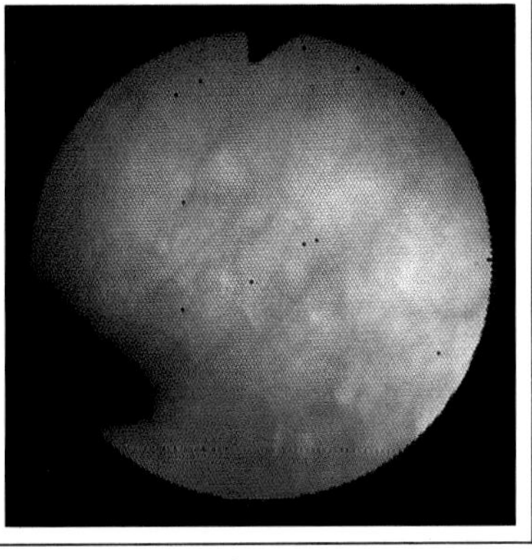

FIG. 2-15.

FIG. 2-15. Accentuated (serrated) GE junction. Bands of orange gastric mucosa of variable width interdigitate with the gray-pink esophageal mucosa in a patient with reflux symptoms.

14). Despite the fact that gastric capillaries tend to be short and tortuous, whereas esophageal vessels tend to be long and parallel, the junction may not be evident.

We are impressed by the proportion of cases (up to 15% in our Unit) where the actual GE junctional point cannot be determined. Although an indistinct junction may cause the examiner to suspect the presence of Barrett's Esophagus (see Chapter 7), we have not encountered a case where the sole endoscopic clue to its presence was an indistinct GE junction.

Accentuated (Serrated) GE Junction

In some cases the GE junction is accentuated by the presence of bands (serrations) of gastric mucosa ascending as much as 1 cm above the most distal point of the squamocolumnar junction (Fig. 2-15). The cause of this ap-

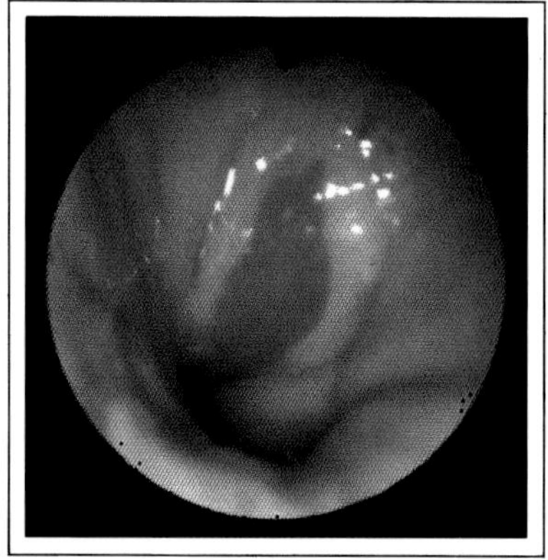

FIG. 2-16.

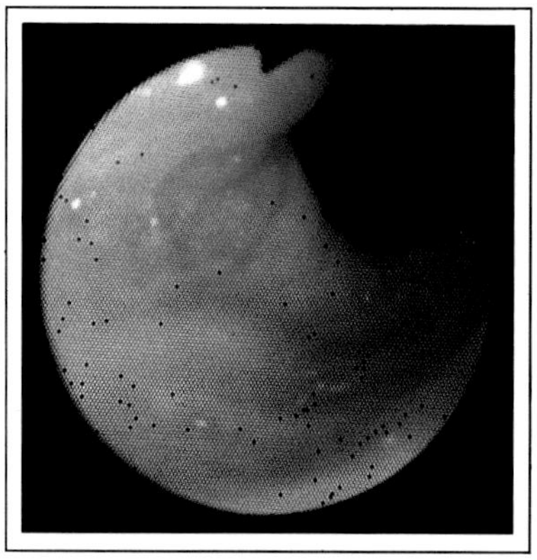

FIG. 2-17a.

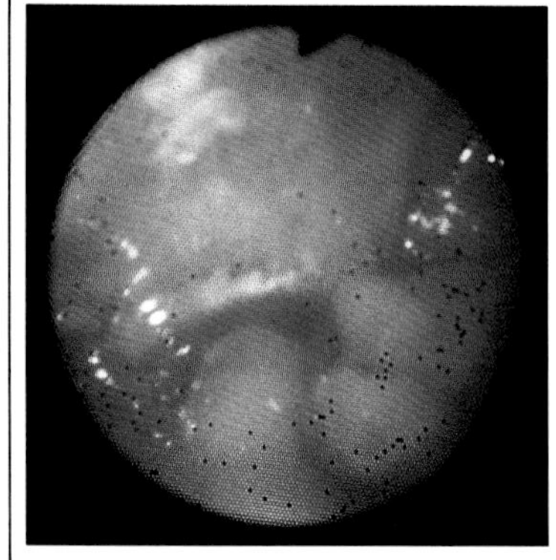

FIG. 2-17b.

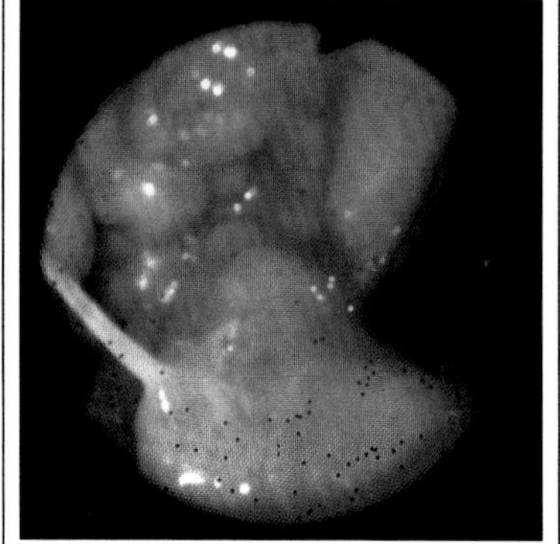

FIG. 2-17c.

FIG. 2-16. Early Barrett's changes. Biopsies of these "tongues" of orange-red cardial mucosa show typical Barrett's changes (see Chapter 6).

FIG. 2-17. a: Accentuated GE junction. A single band of gastric mucosa was noted in the 9 o'clock position, giving the GE junction an asymmetrical appearance. Biopsy of this and the cardia just beyond was negative for malignancy. **b:** Accentuated GE junction in a patient with carcinoma of the gastric cardia [see (c)]. The isolated band of erythematous mucosa running toward the left wall (in the 9 o'clock position) causes the examiner to note the asymmetry of the GE junction (absence of folds in the left anterior quadrant). **c:** Carcinoma of the gastric cardia. The asymmetrical appearance of the GE junction [in (b)] resulted from the erosion of the infiltrating malignancy (enlarged nodular folds) seen on a retroflexed view of the cardia.

pearance is unknown. We have found it in patients with reflux symptoms but more often in those with nonspecific symptoms. If the bands of gastric mucosa are especially broad (>1 cm) and long (>1.5 cm), they may suggest to the examiner the early form of Barrett's esophagus, where one sees "tongues" of Barrett's-type epithelium (Fig. 2-16) rising above the GE junction (see Chapter 6). However, in no case in our experience where the band of gastric epithelium is less than 1 cm has a diagnosis of Barrett's epithelium been proved histologically.

Finally, while an isolated band of gastric mucosa rising above the GE junction may be an innocent finding (Fig. 2-17a) if it is observed in the context of marked asymmetry of the GE junction (Fig. 2-17b), it can also be a sign of cardial carcinoma (Fig. 2-17c).

In all cases in which the accentuated GE junction causes the endoscopist to suspect the presence of a lesion, biopsy is extremely important in determining whether the appearance is simply a normal variation.

REFERENCES

1. McMillan, I. K. R., and Hyde, I. (1969): Compression of the esophagus by the aorta. *Thorax,* 24:32–38.
2. Beachley, M. C., Siconolfi, E. P., Madoff, H. R., and Chaudhry, R. M. (1980): Dysphagia aortica. *Dig. Dis. Sci.,* 25:807–810.
3. Kobayashi, S., and Kasugai, T. (1974): Endoscopic and biopsy criteria for the diagnosis of esophagitis with a fiberoptic esophagoscope. *Am. J. Dig. Dis.,* 19:345–352.
4. Geboes, K., Desmet, V., Vantappen, G., and Mebis, J. (1980): Vascular changes in the esophageal mucosa: an early histologic sign of esophagitis. *Gastrointest. Endosc.,* 26:29–32.
5. Hattori, K., Winans, C. S., Archer, F., and Kirsner, J. B. (1974): Endoscopic diagnosis of esophageal inflammation. *Gastrointest. Endosc.,* 20:101–104.

5a. Glick, S. N., Teplick, S. K., Goldstein, J., Stead, J. A., and Zitomer, N. (1982): Glycogenic acanthosis of the esophagus. *Am J. Roentgenol.,* 139:683–688.

6. Bender, M. D., Allison, J., Cuartas, F., and Montgomery, C. (1973): Glycogenic acanthosis of the esophagus: a form of benign epithelial hyperplasia. *Gastroenterology,* 65:373–380.
7. Silverman, S., and Rozen, R. (1968): Observations on the clinical characteristics and natural history of oral leukoplakia. *J. Am. Dent. Assoc.,* 76:772–777.

3

ESOPHAGITIS

Esophagitis is the commonest pathologic condition of the esophagus. However, the endoscopist finds it a perplexing entity because of: (a) the absence of universally accepted criteria for diagnosis and grading severity; and (b) the difficulty in differentiating the peptic and nonpeptic types because of their similarity in appearance, especially in the presence of severe mucosal injury common to both—pseudomembranous esophagitis.

We present our approach to these difficulties in this chapter. First we look at peptic esophagitis, especially regarding minimal diagnostic criteria and its grading. Following this, we discuss *Candida* and other nonpeptic causes. In a concluding section we consider the appearance of pseudomembranous esophagitis, common to both *Candida* and severe peptic esophagitis.

PEPTIC (REFLUX) ESOPHAGITIS

Peptic (reflux) esophagitis is the commonest type of esophagitis, being diagnosed in 5 to 7% of patients who undergo endoscopy in our Unit. Because reflux of gastric acid, along with pepsin and possibly other noxious agents from the stomach, is a key pathogenetic mechanism, one might expect to find free reflux evident at endoscopy (Fig. 3-1). As this is not observed in most cases, one believes factors other than free reflux are likely to be involved and to be as important, e.g., delayed clearance of reflux material from the esophagus, prolonging its contact with the esophageal mucosa and thereby increasing its potential for injury.[1]

Appearance

For patients even with classic symptoms the examiner does not encounter "typical" findings but, rather, a spectrum, including at one end an appearance which is entirely normal and at the other end severe mucosal injury with ulceration or adherent inflammatory exudate, i.e., pseudomembrane (see below). Between these two extremes are the various grades of endoscopic esophagitis, including that which constitutes for the examiner "minimal changes" or the least altered appearance on which a diagnosis of peptic esophagitis can still be confidently based.

In this section we concentrate first on the minimal requirements for a diagnosis and then follow this by a description system we use to grade severity. The section concludes with a brief consideration of other findings associated

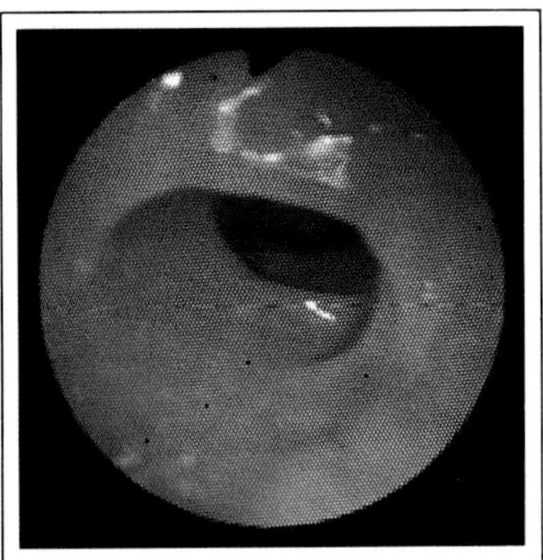

FIG. 3-1.

FIG. 3-1. Free esophageal reflux in a patient with a large hiatus hernia. With the patient lying on the left side, gastric contents with free access to the esophagus would be noted along the left (8 o'clock) wall.

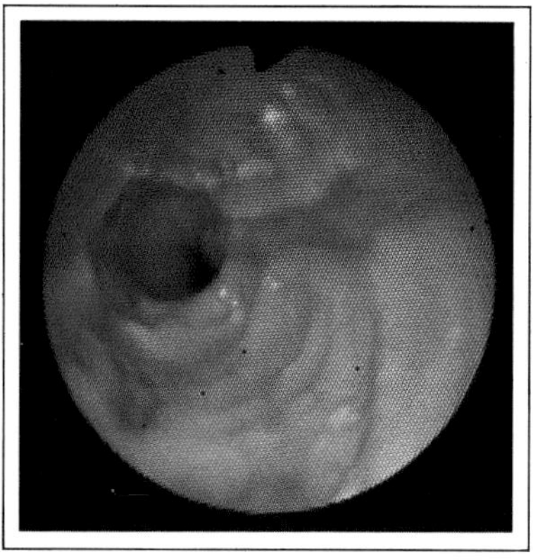

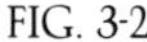

FIG. 3-2.

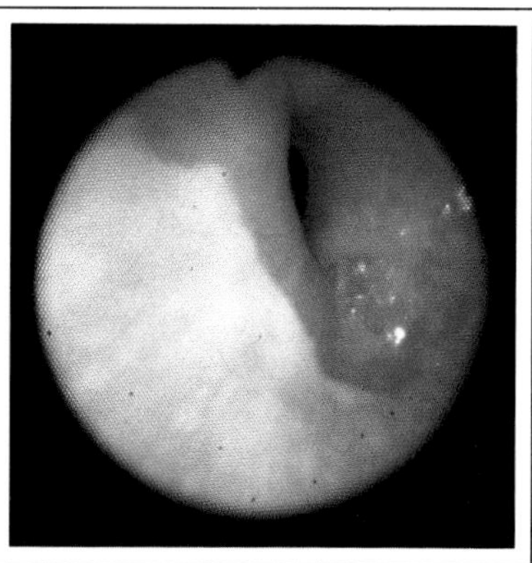

FIG. 3-3.

FIG. 3-2. Esophageal erosions. This is our minimal requirement for a diagnosis of esophagitis. The erosions appear as depressed, reddened, linear areas within a zone of avascular, thickened, gray-white distal mucosa.

FIG. 3-3. Thickened distal esophageal mucosa. This avascular, pearly white appearance was found in an obese patient without reflux symptoms.

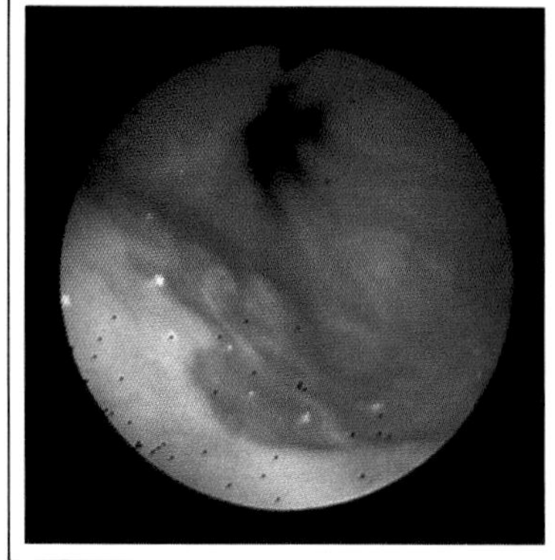

FIG. 3-4.

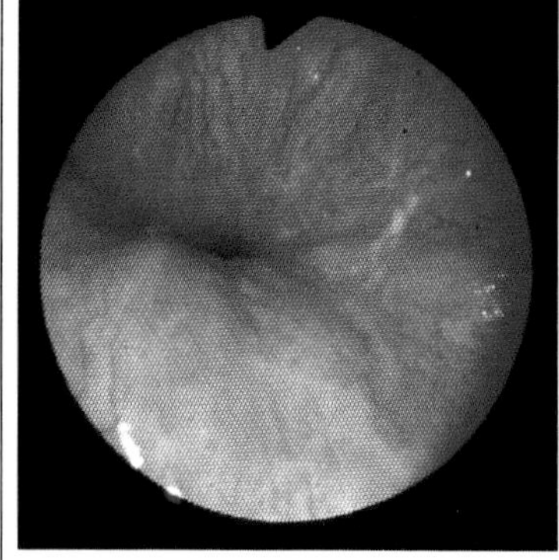

FIG. 3-5.

FIG. 3-4. Esophageal erosions. The depressed nature of the erosion can be best appreciated from its appearance at 6 o'clock. The intervening mucosa is erythematous rather than thickened, as in Fig. 3-2.

FIG. 3-5. Mild esophagitis. There is an indistinct GE junction, along with lower esophageal erythema and a prominent capillary pattern. Alhough this may be the first definite appearance of peptic esophagitis, it does not meet our minimal requirement for a definite diagnosis.

with reflux injury as well as the clinical setting associated with severe peptic esophagitis.

Minimal Changes

Ideally, the minimal finding(s) required for a diagnosis of esophagitis would be so sensitive as to be found in a high percentage of patients with typical symptoms and other evidence of reflux, while specific enough to be absent in most patients who do not have reflux. Furthermore, biopsies taken from the area showing minimal changes would hopefully confirm the presence of esophagitis by fulfilling the standard histologic criteria.

Unfortunately, no minimal requirements for a diagnosis of esophagitis are completely satisfactory. First, many patients, up to 40%, with symptomatic esophageal reflux would fail to meet any criteria because their examinations are entirely normal.[2] A second reason any set of minimal changes are unsatisfactory lies in our inability to confirm these histologically, as these findings would be expected in the distal 2.5 cm of esophagus where histologic changes suggestive of reflux may be found in up to 60% of biopsies taken from normals.[3]

Accepting these limitations, the minimal finding we require for our endoscopic diagnosis of esophagitis is the appearance of discrete zones of erythema called "erosions." This is in contrast to appearances acknowledged by others as indicative of peptic esophagitis (e.g., lower esophageal erythema[4]), accentuated (irregular) gastroesophageal (GE) junction,[5] or "granularity" and friability,[6] all of which we believe are nonspecific. All authorities accept erosions as evidence of definite esophagitis.[4–6]

We believe the term erosion is appropriate for these areas as they are seen, in contrast to surrounding mucosa, as being slightly depressed (Fig. 3-2). This we believe represents "thinning" or "erosion" of the surface epithelium, allowing the basal capillaries to occupy a position closer to the surface, giving it a red appearance (Fig. 3-2). Erosions are typically seen contiguous with or just above the GE junction, giving it an irregular appearance. In many patients the appearance of the mucosa between erosions suggests thickening, as it exhibits a gray or pearly white appearance in association with a loss of submucosa capillaries. This thickening we believe may represent an adaptive response to chronic reflux, as not infrequently it is seen in asymptomatic patients who at endoscopy exhibit free reflux (Fig. 3-1). The appearance of erosions in such areas may be thought of as a sign of the breakdown of an otherwise successful adaptive response to reflux (Fig. 3-3), whereas erosions in a diffusely erythematous mucosa may indicate the absence or disappearance of a prior adaptive response (Fig. 3-4).

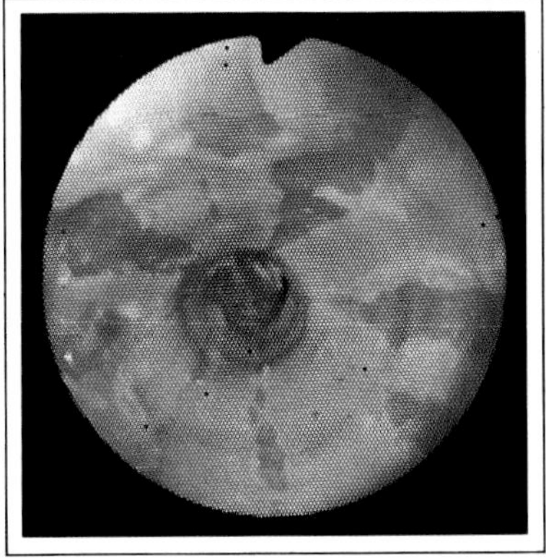

FIG. 3-6.

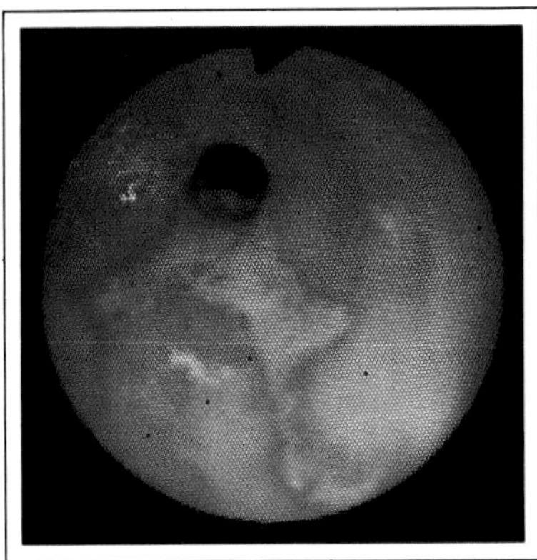

FIG. 3-7.

FIG. 3-6. Moderate esophagitis. Discrete erosions (slightly depressed, erythematous linear areas) are found running within the thickened distal esophageal mucosa.

FIG. 3-7. Severe esophagitis. Acute inflammatory exudate seems to arise focally from the central portion of the erosions. The erosions are now seen only in the periphery of the exudates. The intervening mucosa appears thickened, suggesting longstanding reflux.

Grading of Esophagitis

Like the minimal requirements for diagnosis, there is no general agreement as to the grading of esophagitis. In our system, three grades of esophagitis are recognized: ***mild, moderate,*** and ***severe*** (Table 3-1). This system has evolved out of the need for a simple yet objective means of comparing endoscopic appearances based on the severity of injury indicated histologically. For us, ulceration and an exudate composed of granulation tissue found routinely in biopsies taken from endoscopically severe esophagitis suggests worse injury than the other histologic abnormalities found for the moderate or mild disease.

TABLE 3-1. *Grading of peptic esophagus*

Grade	Endoscopic appearance
Mild	(?) Capillary dilatation; erythema; friability
Moderate	Definite erosions
Severe	Ulceration and/or pseudomembranes

Mild esophagitis.

In cases of "mild" esophagitis, the endoscopist may find a combination of an indistinct GE junction, lower esophageal erythema, and a distorted (tortuous appearing) capillary pattern (Fig. 3-5). Friability (contact bleeding) may also be noted both because reflux-induced thinning of the mucosa causes the capillary bed to come closer to the surface and because the size of these vessels increases.[6a]

Moderate esophagitis.

With "moderate" esophagitis, often in a background of what has been called thickened or pearly white avascular mucosa, the endoscopist notes discrete erosions. These are recognized as slightly depressed, linear or rectangular reddened areas whose blood-red coloration distinguishes them from the more orange gastric mucosa seen contiguously and just below the GE junction (Fig. 3-6). In some cases the erosions themselves are confluent and form broad rectangular areas ascending in a tongue-like fashion into the distal esophagus.

Severe esophagitis.

The presence of granulation tissue, seen either as an acute inflammatory exudate (Fig. 3-7) or the base of an ulcer (Fig. 3-8), marks the esophagitis as being severe. More commonly, the granulation tissue is part of an acute inflammatory exudate which appears to arise from the central portion of the erosions. In some cases much of the mucosal surface is covered by such exudates, often confluent (Fig. 3-9). The term pseudomembranous esophagitis seems appropriate for this appearance (see below). In cases where there has been previous injury with scarring or where the injury penetrates the submucosa, the granulation tissue appears to be the base of an ulceration. In these cases there is often a pronounced tissue reaction around the ulceration, which together with any previous scarring causes these areas to appear nodular (Fig. 3-10). If present at the GE junction, this type of scar deformity may be observed to continue in the cardia as focally enlarged ("sentinel") folds.[5]

It should be recalled that our minimal requirement for esophagitis (see below) was the presence of erosions, which we would grade as moderate esophagitis. What we refer to as mild esophagitis therefore designates an appearance which we do not accept as diagnostic of esophagitis, although some have suggested that a definite association exists between this type of lower esophageal erythema and reflux symptoms (see Chapter 2). Because of the uncertainty concerning this appearance, it is advisable to add the qualifying term "possible" to the mild esophagitis diagnosis to indicate that a definite endoscopic diagnosis cannot be made.

Significantly, in our grading system, in contrast to others, we do not allow the presence or absence of a peptic stricture to influence the grade of esophagitis. A stricture may be present but entirely free of esophagitis both endoscopically and histologically (see Chapter 4).

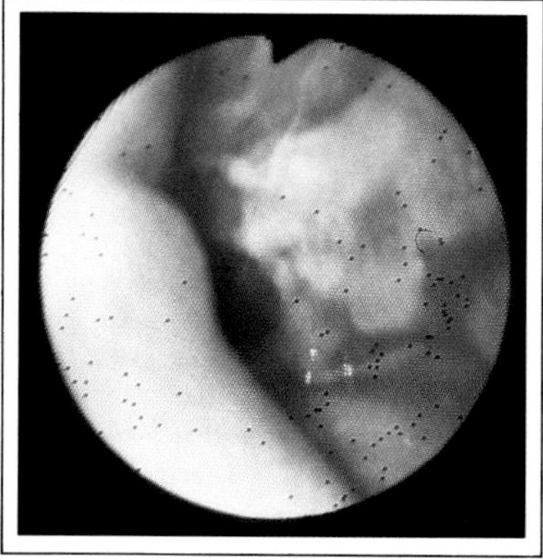

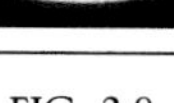

FIG. 3-8.

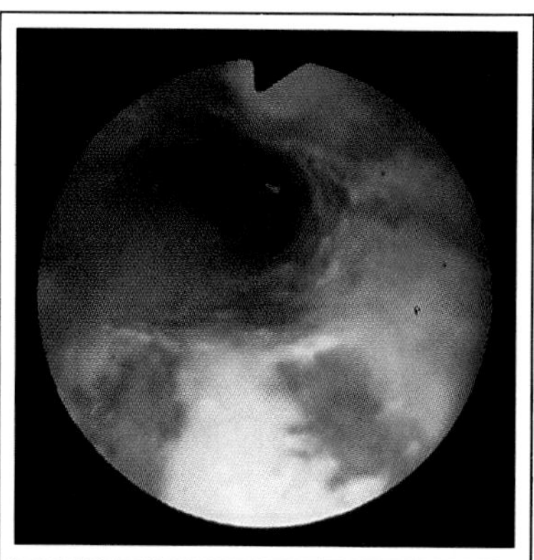

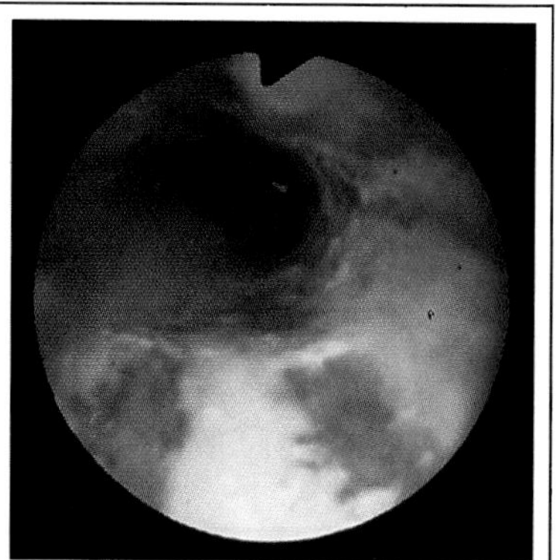

FIG. 3-9.

FIG. 3-8. Severe esophagitis. An ulceration is set in an area of scarred deformity from a previous reflux injury.

FIG. 3-9. Severe esophagitis. A dense confluent (pseudomembranous) acute inflammatory exudate above a hiatus hernia. Brushings were negative for *Candida*.

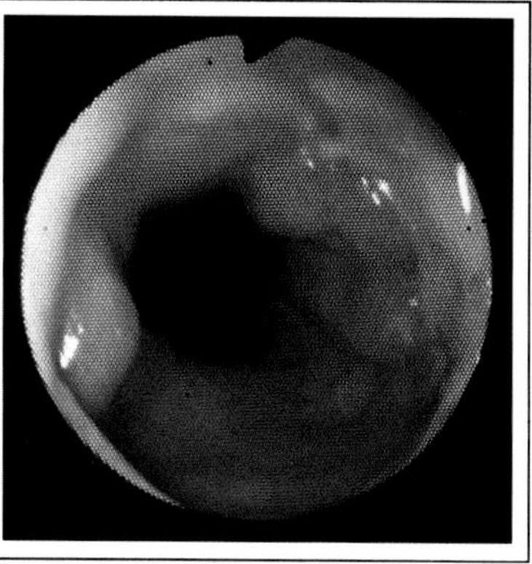

FIG. 3-10.

FIG. 3-10. Inflammatory nodules. Severe esophagitis with inflammatory exudate at the GE junction is associated with nodularity, seen at 3 o'clock.

So that serial comparisons can be made, the endoscopist describes the extent of the changes of esophagitis from the GE junction to the point where definite esophagitis (erosions) is first identified. In addition, the grades of esophagitis seen are noted, i.e., whether moderate or severe, or both, as well as the point at which the transition between them has occurred. Finally, in cases where severe esophagitis is present, a description of the exudate or ulcerations is given, whether focal (confined to the central portions of erosions, e.g., Fig. 3-7), or diffuse (seen as confluent zones, e.g., Fig. 3-9).

Associated Findings

Three additional findings seem to many endoscopists to be linked to esophageal reflux by more than just a chance association. These are: (a) hiatus hernia; (b) the Schatzki ring; and (c) prepyloric gastric erythema and pyloroduodenal ulcers.

Hiatus hernia.

Although it remains controversial as to whether the presence of a hiatus hernia predisposes to reflux, we and others are impressed with the increased frequency of definite esophagitis, moderate or severe (Fig. 3-9), in patients with a hiatus hernia in contrast to others referred for endoscopy.[7] Among our patients, 30 to 40% of those with hiatus hernia have definite esophagitis as opposed to an overall incidence of 10% in patients endoscoped, making it at least three to four times more likely to find esophagitis if a hiatus hernia is present.

Schatzki ring.

The Schatzki ring is widely accepted as a diaphragm-like structure resulting from mucosal hyperplasia of the GE junction. Its relation to esophageal reflux is controversial, although in one study evidence of reflux was found in association with the Schatzki ring in 16 of 18 patients.[8] Two features make us believe it is related to reflux. First, the mucosa above the Schatzki ring, like the ring itself, is often devoid of esophageal submucosa vessels and therefore similar to the thickened esophageal mucosa which is seen in association with chronic reflux. Second, the ring itself may be associated with endoscopic evidence of esophagitis (Fig. 3-11b) as well as early stricture formation. In the latter case the ring is not tissue-thin, as one would expect with pure mucosal hyperplasia, but is thickened ($\geq$4 mm) to suggest the additional component of submucosal fibrosis. This makes us believe that Schatzki's rings may be closer in nature to actual peptic strictures than is generally thought.

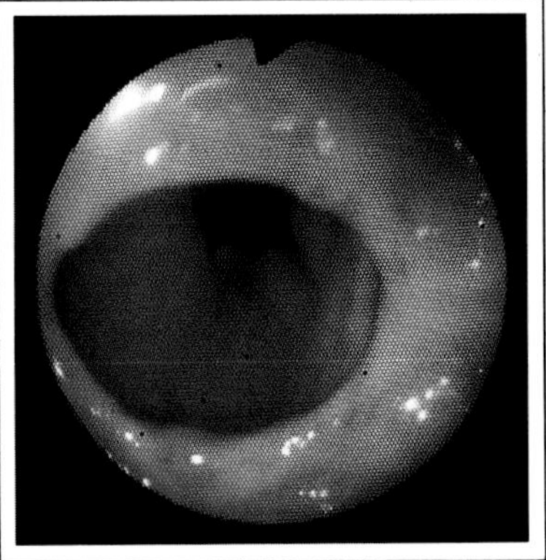

FIG. 3-11a.

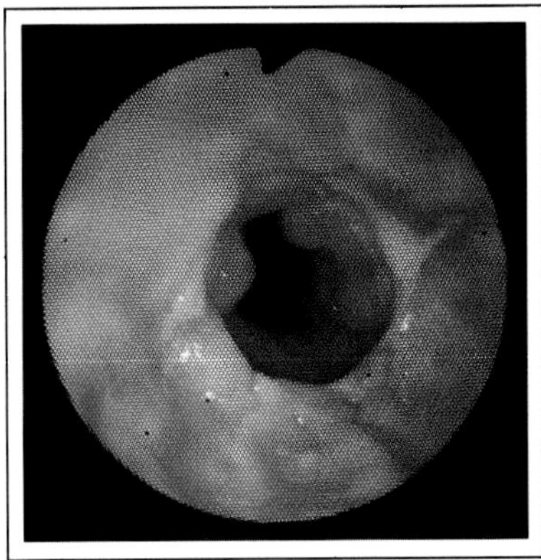

FIG. 3-11b.

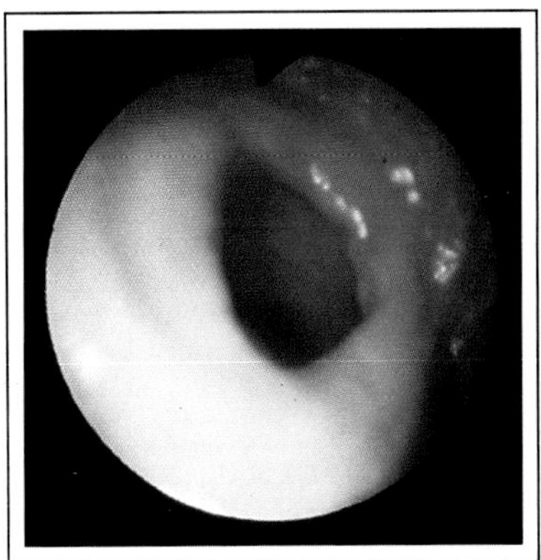

FIG. 3-11c.

FIG. 3-11. a: Schatzki ring. The 2-mm thick ring appears to be composed of avascular esophageal mucosa similar to that found in association with longstanding reflux (Fig. 3-3). **b:** Schatzki ring associated with peptic esophagitis, with the latter indicated by the presence of focal erosions with inflammatory exudates. **c:** Schatzki ring versus early stricture. The 4-mm ring-like deformity of the GE junction may be the earliest indication of a peptic stricture.

Prepyloric gastric erythema and pyloroduodenal ulcerations.

Patients with peptic esophagitis may have peptic ulcer disease of the pyloroduodenal junction which contributes to the severity of the esophagitis if an increased volume of intragastric fluid results.[1] This can be a factor responsible for failure of medical therapy to control reflux symptoms, a result which often prompts endoscopy; therefore examination in such patients always includes careful inspection of the antrum (see Chapter 11) and duodenal bulb (see Chapter 24) for evidence of peptic ulcer disease. Another interesting association has been the finding of antral "gastritis" with areas of linear or confluent erythema (see Chapter 12). Biopsies from the antrum even in patients without erythema may show acute or chronic inflammation, possibly a marker for duodenogastric reflux, a factor which may contribute to the genesis of reflux symptoms.[9]

Clinical Settings Associated with Severe Esophagitis

Vomiting.

Unusually severe and extensive peptic esophagitis is found in patients who have had prolonged vomiting (≤48 to 72 hr), which we refer to as "emetogenic" esophagitis. We have seen severe emetogenic esophagitis, especially in women with vomiting during the third trimester of pregnancy (Fig. 3-12); it may be due to a continued reflux injury after the vomiting, related to the pregnancy itself.[1] Another instance where we have seen emetogenic esophagitis is in patients with protracted vomiting associated with acute pancreatitis. In cases of emetogenic esophagitis, the entire esophagus may be involved with severe esophagitis characterized by ulcerations and pseudomembrane formation (Fig. 3-12).

Nasogastric tube placement.

In rare patients placement of a nasogastric tube may be associated with profound esophagitis even after as short a period as 24 to 36 hr, but usually after periods of more than 1 week. The tube may predispose to reflux by interfering with lower esophageal sphincter function,[10] as well as prolonging the contact time in the esophagus of whatever material is refluxed. As in emetogenic esophagitis (see above), the findings of pseudomembrane and ulcerations often extend to involve the entire esophagus (Fig. 3-13).

Scleroderma involving the esophagus.

See Chapter 7.

Effect of Treatment

The natural history of peptic esophagitis is, in most cases, to improve clinically and endoscopically over an 8-week period even if no specific treatment has been used.[10a] Nevertheless, there can be a marked disparity between clinical improvement following treatment and endoscopic appearance,[10b] with some patients noting a marked decrease in symptoms despite the persistence of endoscopically severe esophagitis. In some cases we have observed, it has taken 3 to 6 months of treatment to achieve a completely normal endoscopic appearance. It is our impression that patients with delayed healing are more prone than others to symptomatic and endoscopic recurrence following discontinuation of treatment.

Biopsy

The endoscopist considers performing a biopsy if: (a) the endoscopic diagnosis is uncertain; (b) the degree of associated

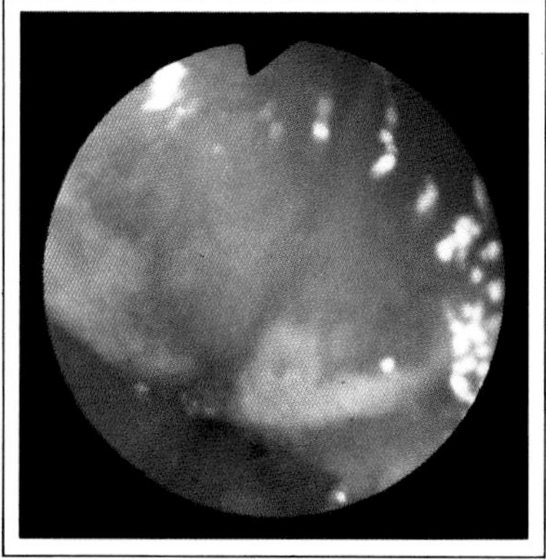

FIG. 3-12.

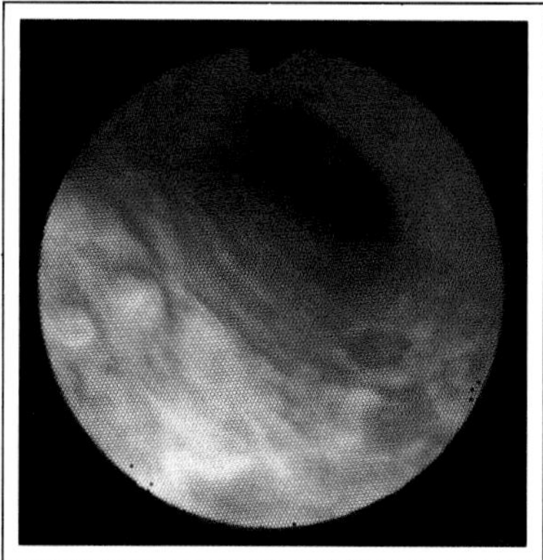

FIG. 3-13.

FIG. 3-12. Emetogenic esophagitis. Discrete inflammatory exudates were present throughout the entire esophagus of this patient with protracted vomiting during the third trimester of pregnancy.

FIG. 3-13. Severe esophagitis (with pseudomembrane formation) in the upper mid-portion after prolonged (1 week) nasogastric tube placement.

nodularity or mass-like deformity raises the question of malignancy; and (c) the location of the esophagitis and appearance of esophageal mucosa below make one suspect Barrett's esophagus (see Chapter 6).

An Uncertain Endoscopic Diagnosis

There are two situations where the endoscopist would perform a biopsy in the case of an uncertain diagnosis: (a) to confirm the presence of histologic esophagitis in cases which endoscopically appear as mild esophagitis; and (b) where there is a questionable exudate or ulceration.

Mild esophagitis.

When the appearance suggests mild esophagitis, the endoscopist may seek histologic confirmation by obtaining biopsies from the area in question. Unfortunately, this is often within a zone 2.5 cm above the GE junction where histologic changes (e.g., basal cell hyperplasia) and elongated dermal papillae may be found in almost 60% of biopsies taken from asymptomatic subjects.[3] Still, such biopsies may show neutrophils in the lamina propria[2] or intraepithelial eosinophils[2a] which would support a diagnosis of esophagitis,[2] although for the most part, with this appearance, biopsy will not establish a diagnosis of symptomatic esophageal reflux.

A questionable exudate.

In some cases, foreign material (e.g., antacids) may adhere to the distal esophagus just above its termination at the cardial rosette and simulate the appearance of pseudomembranous esophagitis. Biopsies taken from such areas can establish unequivocally the presence or absence of an inflammatory exudate; moreover, if the exudate is truly present, its nature, either peptic or from *Candida* or other opportunistic organisms, can be established.

Mass-like Deformity Suggesting Malignancy

The commonest appearance of esophageal malignancy is that of a single ulcerated mass (see Chapter 5). Nevertheless, the finding of nodules or a mass-like deformity in and around an ulcerated area, especially if a stricture is present, raises the question of malignancy. In such cases the endoscopist wisely obtains a series of at least six biopsy specimens from the nodular area(s), as well as brushings (see below).

The Question of Barrett's Esophagus

The location of severe esophagitis above 32 cm (from the incisors), especially where there is some uninvolved-appearing esophageal mucosa below, should always cause one to suspect Barrett's changes (see Chapter 6). To confirm this, multiple biopsy specimens are required, beginning at the level of the cardia and extending above the area of esophagitis.

Brushing

Brushing an area suggestive of esophagitis is useful in two circumstances: (a) where there is considerable irregularity and ulceration at the mouth of a stricture (see Chapter 4); and (b) to determine, in the presence of extensive pseudomembranous esophagitis, if opportunistic infection, i.e., *Candida* or herpes simplex, is present (see "Pseudomembranous Esophagitis," this chapter).

NONPEPTIC ESOPHAGITIS

A specific causative organism, noxious agent, or associated condition other than reflux can be found in 10 to 50% of the cases of esophagitis. We refer to this group of cases as nonpeptic esophagitis, recognizing, however, that reflux may play a yet unidentified role in the initiation or perpetuation of esophageal injury from these other causes. We consider nonpeptic esophagitis in four categories in this section: (a) those associated with specific causative organisms, e.g., *Candida;* (b) those associated with cancer treatment, including irradiation; (c) those associated with other drugs and noxious agents, including lye; and (d) other conditions associated with esophagitis, e.g., eosinophilic gastroenteritis and bullous disorders of the skin.

Esophagitis Associated With a Causative Organism

Candida Esophagitis

Candida esophagitis is the most common type of nonpeptic esophagitis, and *Candida* is the most frequent specific causative organism identified. It accounts for almost all such cases in our Unit, which is approximately 10% of the total cases of esophagitis. The reported incidence of *Candida* esophagitis among the total cases of esophagitis seen at endoscopy has varied from 11%[11] to more than 40%.[12,13] In series that reported a high percentage, *Candida* was intensively sought by means of brushings or biopsies, even in cases where neither a typical appearance of *Candida* (see below) was present nor any of the usual predisposing conditions. It remains to be seen whether others will confirm this high incidence.

In our experience, patients with *Candida* esophagitis usually have some predisposing condition, e.g., diabetes or treatment with antibiotics or immunosuppressive drugs. Others, however, have found predisposing conditions in only a minority (10%) or cases.[12]

Endoscopic appearance.

Typically, *Candida* is recognized by the appearance of discrete 3- to 5-mm raised plaques (pseudomembranes) composed of candidal organisms and adherent granulation tissue (Fig. 3-14). The plaques may appear as discrete lesions (Fig. 3-14) or dense confluent exudates (Fig. 3-15) with the latter seen especially in patients with mucocutaneous candidiasis or who are immunocompromised as a result of cancer treatment. The candidal pseudomembranes are usually firmly adherent, so that any attempt to remove them with a brush or biopsy forceps is accompanied by bleeding. We have seen on occasion, however, especially in patients who have received prior treatment or diabetics without esophageal symptoms, that the *Candida* exudate is loosely adherent and appears as particulate matter, which may be confused with ingested material (Fig. 3-16). The mucosa between the plaques may either be intact or suggest prior involvement, being erythematous and friable (Fig. 3-14).

There is no one typical location for *Candida* esophagitis. In roughly one-third it is present in the upper and midesophagus, being continuous with oral lesions (thrush) and hypopharyngeal lesions. In another one-third it is confined largely to the distal esophagus, with the throat, pharynx, and upper esophagus skipped entirely. In the remaining one-third it involves the entire esophagus with or without the presence of oral thrush. In two-thirds of the cases, therefore, the proximal esophagus is involved. When this occurs, it provides a useful point for differentiation from severe peptic esophagitis in which pseudomembrane formation rarely appears in the proximal esophagus.

Diagnosis.

The diagnosis is readily established by means of brushing the candidal plaque (pseudomembrane) and smearing this material on a clear glass slide, allowing it to dry, then applying 10% potassium hydroxide (KOH). It is then examined for the appearance of typical branched hyphae and budding yeast (Fig. 3-17). This test can be performed directly by the endoscopist if a microscope is available, or the slides may be sent to the pathology laboratory for fungal stains (Fig. 3-17) and examination. Brushing a plaque for the purpose of preparing a KOH smear and examining the smear for the presence of branched hyphae and budding yeast appears to be the best available means of establishing the diagnosis of *Candida* esophagitis, although the number of cases missed with this technique because of inadequate sampling is unknown.

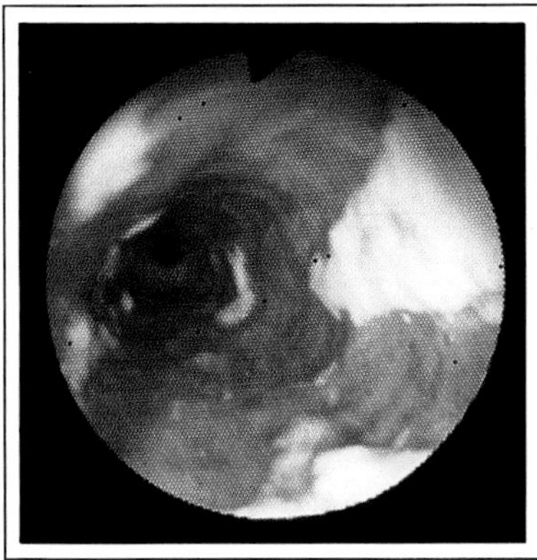

FIG. 3-14a.

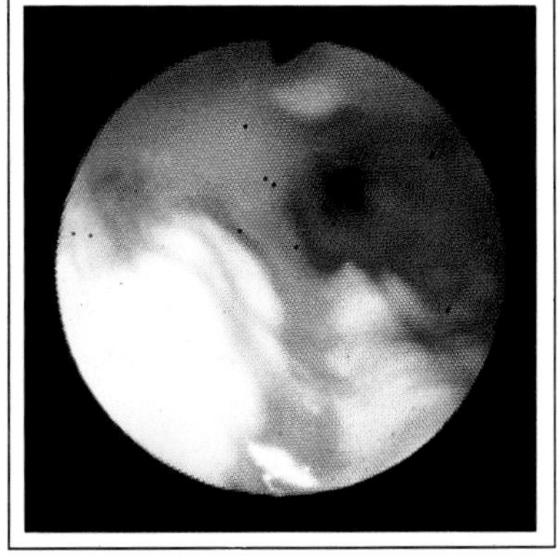

FIG. 3-14b.

FIG. 3-14. *Candida* esophagitis. **a:** Multiple 5- to 10-mm yellow-white adherent plaque-like pseudomembranes are present throughout the esophagus. **b:** Involvement stops short of the GE junction (indicated by the pool at 10 o'clock) because of acid reflux.

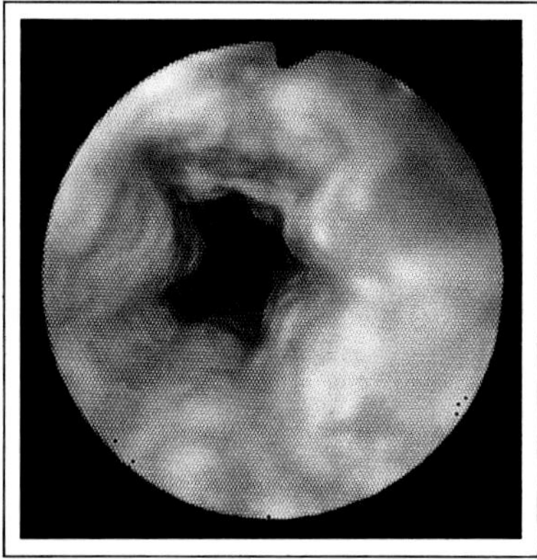

FIG. 3-15.

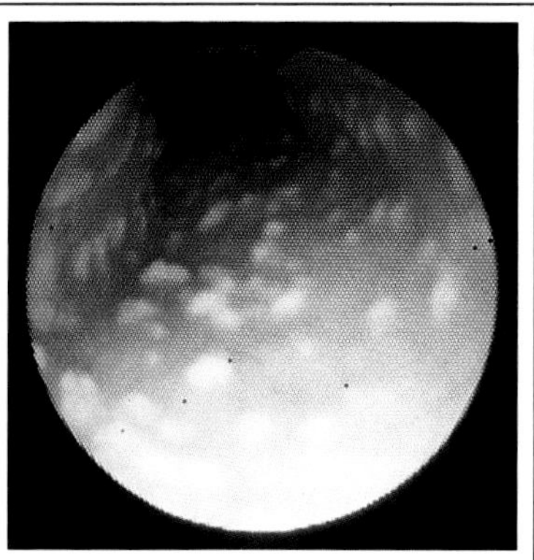

FIG. 3-16

FIG. 3-15. *Candida* esophagitis. Extensive and confluent *Candida* pseudomembranes were found in a patient with mucocutaneous candidiasis.

FIG. 3-16. *Candida* esophagitis. Punctate exudate, loosely adherent, was found in a diabetic without esophageal symptoms. Brushings, however, showed typical candidal organisms, as in Fig. 3-17.

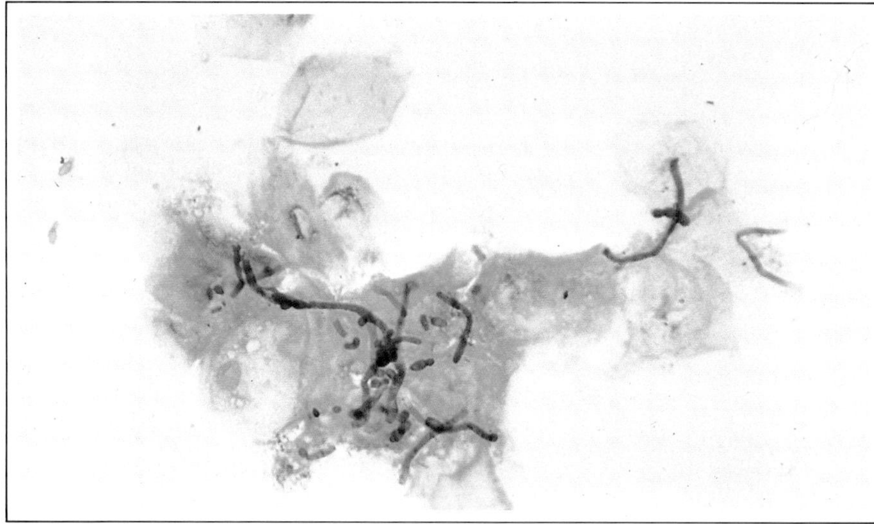

FIG. 3-17.

FIG. 3-17. *Candida,* yeast, and mycelium. This smear was obtained from brushings of a plaque-like pseudomembranous lesion like those of Fig. 3-14. The material was air-dried, but rather than its being examined immediately after the application of a drop of 10% potassium hydroxide it was sent to the pathology department where a fungal (Gomori-methenamine-silver) stain was performed.

Whether a specimen should be sent for fungal culture (if available) is unclear. If hyphae and yeast forms are seen on the KOH preparation, then a fungal culture for typing and determination of the sensitivity of the organism to antifungal agents seems highly desirable, especially for seriously ill, immunocompromised patients undergoing chemotherapy for hematologic malignancies who might require systemic antifungal therapy for *Candida* esophagitis. However, in up to 50% of such patients (Table 3-2), candidal forms are not found on KOH preparations, even from areas of dense pseudomembrane (Fig. 3-23, below). Although there are no data to determine the percentage of false-negative KOH preparations in patients who actually have *Candida* esophagitis, there is information which suggests that the rate of false positivity from fungal cultures is prohibitive. In a study by Kodsi *et al.*[12] positive cultures were found in 6 of 15 patients with classic reflux esophagitis and 12 of 18 patients with normal mucosa (all with negative KOH preparations). These data suggest that it would not be at all unusual to find cultures positive for *Candida* in immunosuppressed patients who do not actually have *Candida* esophagitis, making it unwise, therefore, to culture routinely for *Candida* in patients whose KOH preparations did not show candidal forms.

TABLE 3-2. *Causes of esophagitis determined by endoscopy in 67 patients with hematologic malignancies (1975–1981)*

Cause	No.	%
Candida[a]	34	50
Herpes simplex[b]	9	13
Candida and herpes	1	2
Radiation/Adriamycin	1	2
Esophageal involvement by malignancy	1	2
No explanation	21	31
Total	67	100

[a] By KOH preparation.
[b] By cytology.

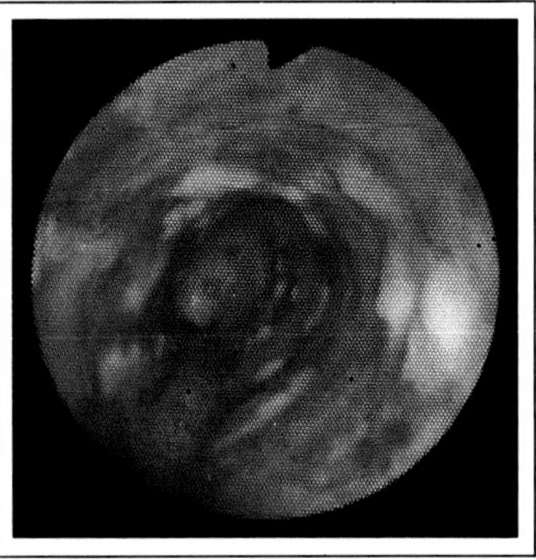

FIG. 3-18.

FIG. 3-18. Herpetic esophagitis. Multiple, small, focal pseudomembranes are observed with the adjacent mucosa intensely erythematous, as if denuded.

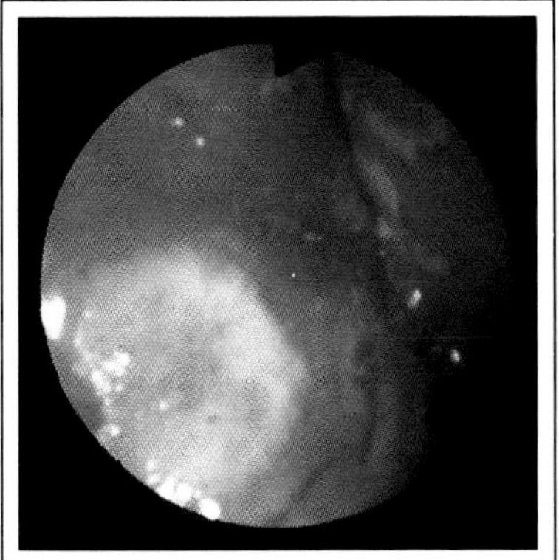

FIG. 3-19a.

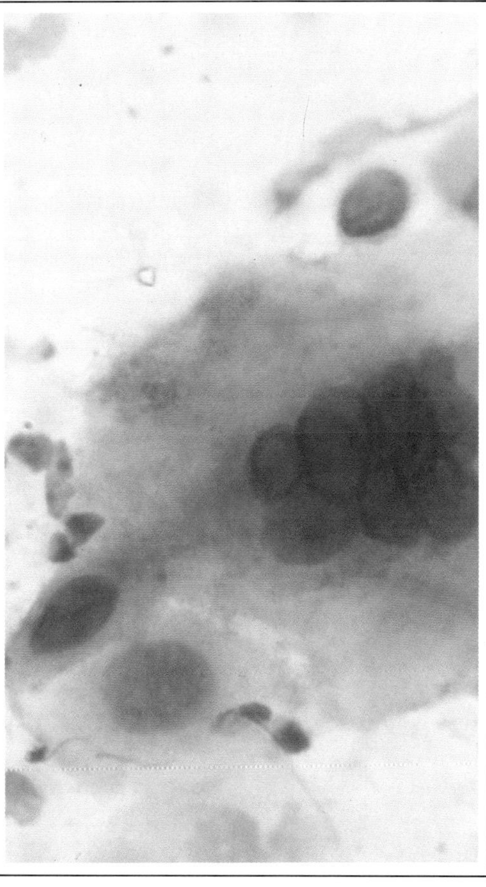

FIG. 3-19b.

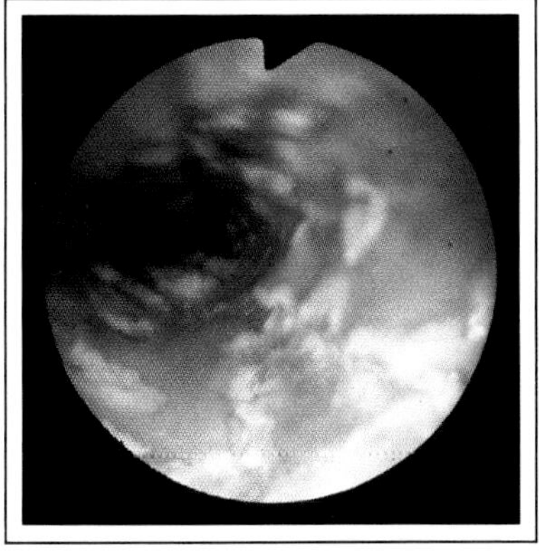

FIG. 3-19c.

FIG. 3-19. a: Herpetic esophagitis. One of many focal pseudomembranes whose central portion appears denuded (causing it to look umbilicated). **b:** Brushing cytology in a patient with herpetic esophagitis. Characteristic multinucleated giant cells are found along with other degenerated epithelial cells with large, irregular, and smudged nuclei. **c:** Concomitant herpetic and *Candida* esophagitis. Dense, plaque-like pseudomembranes (at 6 o'clock) suggestive of *Candida* (similar to Fig. 3-14) were found in a patient with acute myelogenous leukemia recently begun on chemotherapy. In addition, focal exudates with central clearing were observed (at 3 o'clock) similar to those in (a). Brushings from these areas revealed evidence of *Candida* (similar to Fig. 3-16) as well as herpes simplex [similar to that in (b)].

Herpetic Esophagitis

Although an uncommon cause of esophagitis overall, herpetic esophagitis may account for up to 15% of cases in patients with hematologic malignancies undergoing chemotherapy (Table 3-2), the single setting where herpes simplex is most likely to occur.[14] Over a 7-year period in which 5,000 patients were examined, including 600 with endoscopic evidence of esophagitis, 12 (2.0%) had evidence of herpes simplex. Of those, 10 were undergoing chemotherapy. However, it is noteworthy that the remaining two patients were not immunosuppressed, being examined because of longstanding reflux symptoms. One, in fact, had early Barrett's changes (see Chapter 6). Other investigators have noted the occurrence of herpes simplex esophagitis in otherwise healthy individuals.[15]

The appearance of this disorder may be entirely nonspecific with simply discrete pseudomembrane (Fig. 3-18) or ulcerations. In contrast to *Candida* (see above) involvement, the pseudomembranes tend to be smaller and more focal (Fig. 3-18). Their central portions sometimes appear denuded (Fig. 3-19a), as may the mucosa surrounding them (Fig. 3-18). Brushings[16] taken from such areas may show cytologic features suggestive of herpes infection (Fig. 3-19b).

Concomitant Herpetic and Candida Esophagitis

As *Candida* may be cultured from the esophagus in up to two-thirds of individuals with normal-appearing mucosa,[12] it is not surprising that *Candida* is found in immunosuppressed patients with herpetic esophagitis.[14] The precise incidence of these two organisms occurring together is uncertain. In an autopsy study, Nash and Ross [14] found *Candida* in 3 of 14 (22%) cases of herpetic esophagitis, or 6% (3 of 55) of all cases with evidence of esophagitis. At endoscopy the incidence of concomitant ***herpes simplex*** and *Candida* esophagitis appears to be lower. In reviewing our experience with a group of 67 patients with hematologic malignancies undergoing endoscopy to determine the cause of esophagitis (Table 3-2), we found in only 1 of 10 cases where ***herpes simplex*** was the cause of esophagitis was *Candida* present (10%), an incidence of 1.5% (1 of 67) for the group as a whole. In this case the diagnosis was suggested by the appearance (Fig. 3-19c) of both dense *Candida*-type pseudomembranes and focal herpetic type inflammatory exudates and ulcerations.

Cytomegalovirus Esophagitis

Cytomegalovirus (CMV) is a cause of esophagitis in immunosuppressed patients following kidney[16a] and bone marrow transplantation,[16b] as well as in homosexuals with acquired immunodeficiency syndrome (AIDS).[16c] Its highest incidence appears to be following bone marrow transplantation where in one series alone, or in combination with the ***herpes simplex*** virus, it accounted for 10 of 21 cases where an infectious organism was found as a cause of esophagitis.[16b] When present, CMV esophagitis appears as an extensive area of mucosal injury with inflammatory exudate and ulceration.[16c] As in at least one reported case, the ulceration may be deep and progress in size over several weeks.[16c] More often than not CMV will be present elsewhere, especially in gastric or duodenal ulcers.[16a] Biopsies, brushing cytology, or viral cultures may show evidence of CMV.[16b]

Histoplasmosis

Although esophageal involvement from histoplasmosis is occasionally the subject of case reports, the endoscopist rarely, if ever, sees it. When it occurs, it is localized, contiguous involvement from large mediastinal masses (mediastinal granuloma).[17] The esophageal involvement has been uniformly noted as a discrete, mass-like appearance, having an eroded or ulcerated overlying mucosa. This appearance is indistinguishable from that of primary esophageal malignancy, secondary involvement of the esophagus by contiguous lung cancer, mediastinal lymphoma, or esophageal tuberculosis (Fig. 3-20). Biopsies from an esophageal mass associated with mediastinal histoplasmosis may show typical organisms.

Tuberculosis

Like histoplasmosis, mediastinal involvement with tuberculosis may be associated with contiguous involvement of the esophagus.[18] In these occasional cases there is the appearance of a localized mass with eroded, sometimes ulcerated mucosa which may simulate primary esophageal carcinoma (Fig. 3-20). Biopsy may demonstrate typical caseating granulomas.

Esophagitis Associated With Cancer Treatment

Esophageal injury occurs in one of three ways in patients in whom cancer treatment has been instituted: (a) the emergence of *Candida* or ***herpes simplex*** (see above); (b) the effects of irradiation; and (c) the effects of chemotherapy. We have already discussed the *Candida* and herpetic esophagitis, which together constitute the commonest identifiable causes of esophageal injury associated with cancer treatment. In the following section we discuss the two other causes of esophagitis in these patients.

Radiation

Radiation injury to the esophagus mainly occurs during the treatment of carcinoma of the lung and lymphomatous involvement of the mediastinum. In most cases an excess of 6,000 rads will have been administered to patients who subsequently develop esophagitis.[19] However, in one series, one-fourth of the patients who developed significant injury received only 3,000 to 4,000 rads.[19] With the administration of adriamycin, which has a significant "recall" or radiometric effect, esophageal injury may be produced with radiation doses of less than 3,000 rads.[20]

The endoscopic appearance of these lesions is that of severe, acute injury with ulceration and pseudomembranes being observed for the duration of the radiation support (Fig. 3-21). Submucosal injury may also occur, leading to stricture formation (see Chapter 4).

Esophagitis Associated with Cancer Chemotherapy

Although as yet unreported, we find that for almost one-third (30%) of patients who develop esophagitis during the course of treatment neither *Candida* nor ***herpes simplex*** are found when sought by means of brushings or biopsies (Table 3-2). Other investigators, using viral cultures in addition to brushing cytology and histology, found a similar proportion (15 of 46 or 32%) of unexplained cases of esophagitis in immunosuppressed patients after bone marrow transplantation.[16] We see this otherwise unexplained

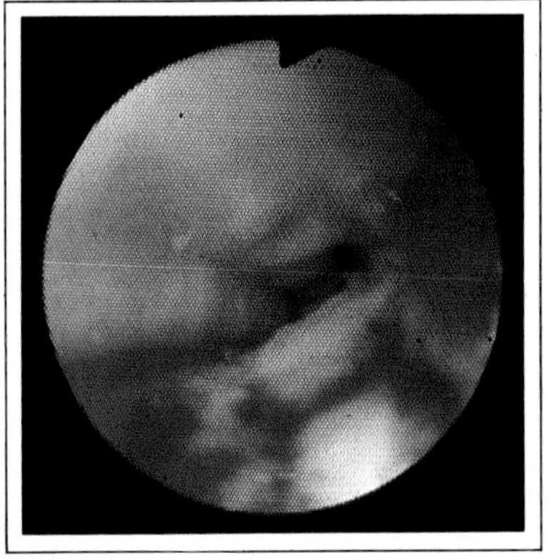

FIG. 3-20.

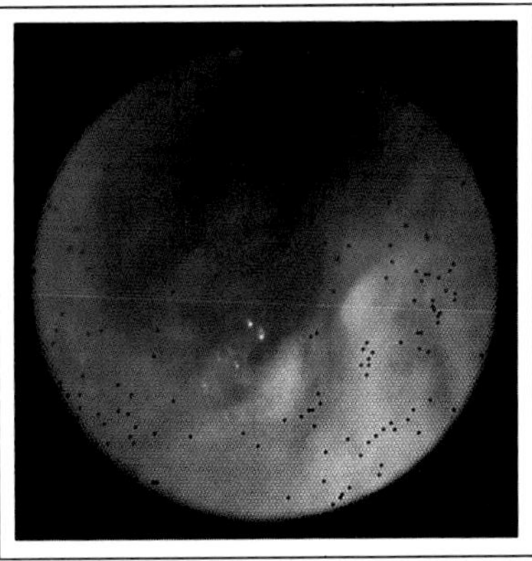

FIG. 3-21.

FIG. 3-20. Esophageal tuberculosis. A large ulcerated mass is seen on the right posterior wall. Although the mass at endoscopy was thought to be malignant, biopsy showed caseating tuberculous granulomas in a patient with a right hilar mass.

FIG. 3-21. Radiation injury. Plaque-like pseudomembranes like this were seen throughout the esophagus 4 weeks after the administration of 6,500 rads to the chest for bronchogenic carcinoma.

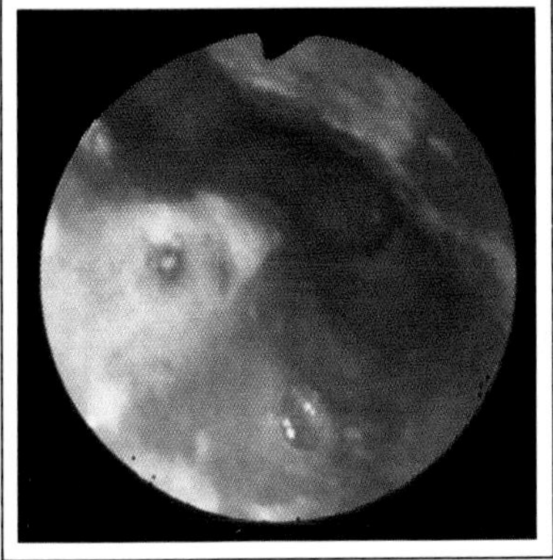

FIG. 3-22.

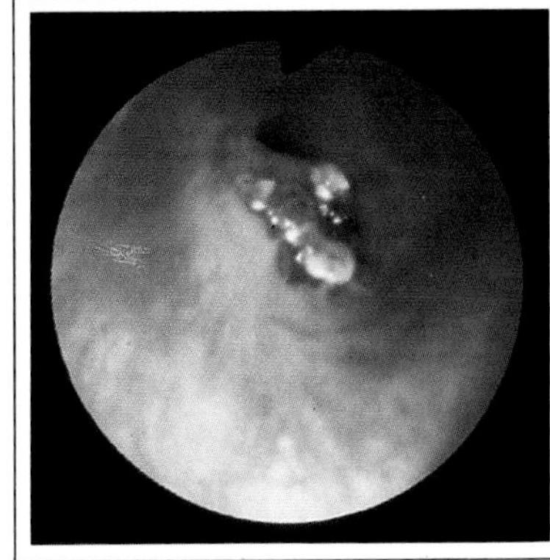

FIG. 3-23.

FIG. 3-22. Esophagitis associated with chemotherapy. Pseudomembranes with erythema and marked friability of the intervening mucosa of the upper midesophagus in a patient who had recently received two cytotoxic agents, methotrexate and cystosine arabinoside.

FIG. 3-23. Esophagitis associated with chemotherapy. An exuberant pseudomembrane lesion in the distal esophagus of a granulocytopenic patient who developed protracted vomiting while on chemotherapy. Florid bacterial colonization was found on smears taken from these lesions.

esophagitis typically in patients receiving combined cytotoxic and immunosuppressive agents, especially for treatment of leukemia or lymphoma. Because the esophagitis seen in such patients is usually found with ulceration and inflammatory exudate (see below) which may be ports of entry for gram negative bacteria that can be cultured from the endoscope and give rise to bacterial sepsis,[20a] we routinely disinfect the endoscope with 2% glutcraldehyde[21] immediately prior to starting the examination.

Appearance.

The esophagitis in these cases is generally severe endoscopically, characterized by the presence of extensive pseudomembranes. The entire esophagus may be involved or the injury be confined to the proximal one-half or two-thirds (Fig. 3-22). In cases where vomiting has occurred, we find a pattern of distal involvement (Fig. 3-23).

Etiology.

As already stated, biopsies and brushings from the areas of involvement provide no clue to the etiology. The cause of this injury is probably multifactorial. Some patients are observed to have had protracted vomiting during the course of chemotherapy making the injury possibly emetogenic. This may apply, however, to only a minority of patients. More likely, two additional factors play an important role in the pathogenesis: (a) the inhibitory effects of the cytotoxic agents on epithelial cell proliferation[22]; and (b) an increased susceptibility to bacterial growth and further tissue injury related to the granulocytopenia (Fig. 3-23) not infrequently present in such patients, especially those undergoing treatment for leukemia.[23] These factors may act separately or in combination. It may be that inapparent reflux injury which is compensated by increased epithelial cell proliferation[24] becomes progressive in these patients in the face of cytotoxic suppression. Moreover, as their response to esophageal mucosal injury often (in up to 60%) involves a granulocyte response,[24a] granulocytopenia could conceivably lead to an even more marked tissue effect than would have occurred if the granulocytic response were intact. Furthermore, the granulocytopenic state may allow bacterial colonization, which is indeed frequently found when these areas are brushed. These bacteria may themselves promote further injury.

We must await further studies to define the mechanisms of this interesting but perplexing phenomenon of severe esophageal injury that occurs in some patients receiving cancer chemotherapy.

Esophagitis Associated With Corrosive Agents and Drugs

Esophagitis and Corrosive Agents

Esophagitis caused by the ingestion of corrosive agents is rarely encountered in adult patients. We have seen only two cases over a 5-year period during which time 3,500 examinations were performed. However, a recent series noted 17 cases endoscoped over a 3-year period.[25] The most common corrosive agent is lye (NaOH) in the form of Drano. It is now generally agreed that endoscopy is safe and indicated in adult patients with a history of recent ingestion to determine the extent of the injury, which may be misjudged from symptoms and physical examination alone.[25,26] The finding of severe, extensive esophageal or gastric injury alerts the physician to the need for intensive observation in a hospital setting, as well as consideration of antibiotics and steroids.

The endoscopic findings are unrelated to the time the examination is performed, reaching maximum severity within 2 hr of ingestion.[27] Severity of mucosal injury in one series[27] was graded as: stage I—simple inflammation (erythema); stage II—ulcerations (focal necrosis) of the esophagus; and stage III—multiple ulcerations (extensive necrosis) throughout the entire esophagus (Fig. 3-24). Each grade had prognostic significance. Delayed healing and stricture formation were found only among stage III patients. This is seen most commonly in patients ingesting strong liquid alkali,[25,26] e.g., Drano. In some patients, gastric erosions and ulcerations are observed along with the esophagitis, although in cases of ammonia or acetic acid ingestion gastric injury may predominate.[25,26]

Drug (Pill)-Induced Esophagitis

A number of drugs in tablet or capsule form have been reported to produce esophagitis; the commonest in the United States are doxycycline, wax-matrix (Slow-K) potassium chloride, and quinidine (especially in the form of quinidine gluconate).[27,28] Injury effects, especially with these agents, are generally marked with the appearance of ulceration and pseudomembranes (Fig. 3-25) and, for potassium chloride, stricture formation. For doxycycline, these effects are especially noted in the upper and mid-esophagus, with the site of injury possibly the result of a "hangup" of this potentially caustic (pH 2.6) medication just above the aortic arch (see Chapter 1). For potassium chloride injury, cardiac (especially left atrial) enlargement has been found in almost all cases,[28] predisposing to injury just above the cardiac (left atrial) impression in the mid-esophagus. In many cases of drug (pill)-induced esophagitis, one can elicit a history of a bedtime dose of the medication, taken with little or no water, and while in a recumbent position, conditions which predispose to the delayed esophageal transit.[27a] This would allow the medication to disintegrate within the esophagus, and cause contact injury.

Although not widely reported,[28,28a] aspirin has been observed to produce injury if taken in large amounts. Like that due to doxycycline, aspirin injury may be in the upper and mid-esophagus, possibly also the result of the "hang-up" of this potentially caustic agent,[29] especially when taken in recumbency, without adequate (>100 cc) liquid. In patients with esophageal motor disorders, especially achalasia, we find the site of injury to be just above the GE junction, possibly resulting from retention of the aspirin in this location.

Severe esophagitis (ulceration and/or pseudomembranes) of the proximal or mid-esophagus with a normal distal appearance should always cause the examiner to inquire about the use of medications in pill form capable of producing esophageal injury. In patients under 30, this would be doxycycline while in older individuals one may find use of either wax-matrix potassium chloride or quinidine gluconate.

Other Conditions Associated With Esophagitis

Eosinophilic Esophagitis

We have noted in two patients, both with peripheral eosinophilia, a form of eosinophilic gastroenteritis involving the esophagus. Unlike other cases where esoinophilic esophagitis has been described either in patients with a normal endoscopic appearance[30] or in those with achalasia with nonspecific "erythema and focal exudate,"[31] in both our cases the esophagitis was severe with ulcerations and pseudomembranes along with stricture formation (Fig. 3-26). In both cases the involvement of the proximal third of the esophagus served to distinguish them endoscopically from peptic esophagitis. In both cases biopsy showed a prominent eosinophilic infiltrate.

Esophagitis Associated with Inflammatory Bowel Disease

In occasional patients with ulcerative colitis or Crohn's disease, esophagitis may be present which neither appears peptic nor is associated with opportunistic organisms (Fig. 3-27). In the case of ulcerative colitis, esophageal involvement has been reported with diffuse ulceration involving the entire esophagus,[32] whereas in Crohn's disease a variety of appearances have been reported,[33] most often stricture formation,[34] or that of multiple ulcerations set in nodular edematous mucosa, creating a "cobblestone" appearance.[33] As with some cases of Crohn's disease that involve the stomach or duodenum (see Chapters 20 and 28), Crohn's disease may not be apparent elsewhere.[34]

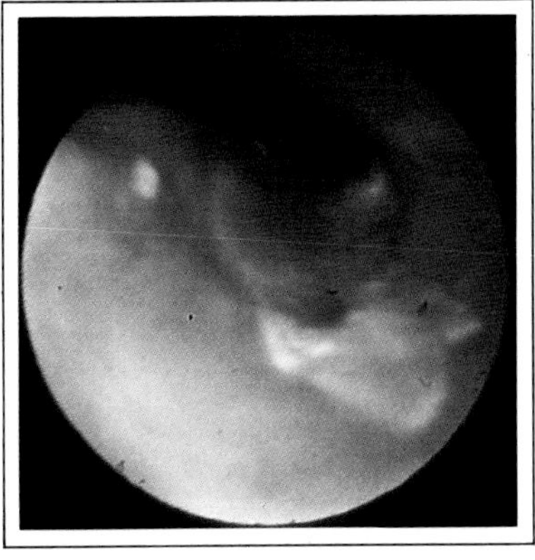

FIG. 3-24.

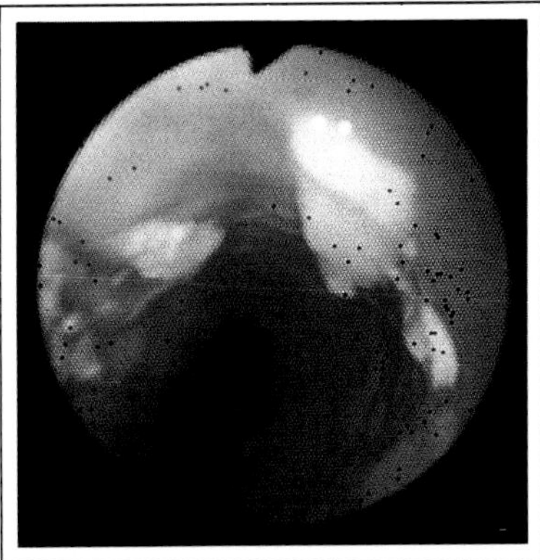

FIG. 3-25.

FIG. 3-24. Lye esophagitis. Severe (stage III)[27] injury is seen with extensive pseudomembrane formation throughout the esophagus.

FIG. 3-25. Drug (wax-matrix potassium chloride) induced esophagitis. Evidence of mid-esophageal severe injury (pseudomembrane) is evident in this patient with congestive heart failure and an enlarged atrium (see text).

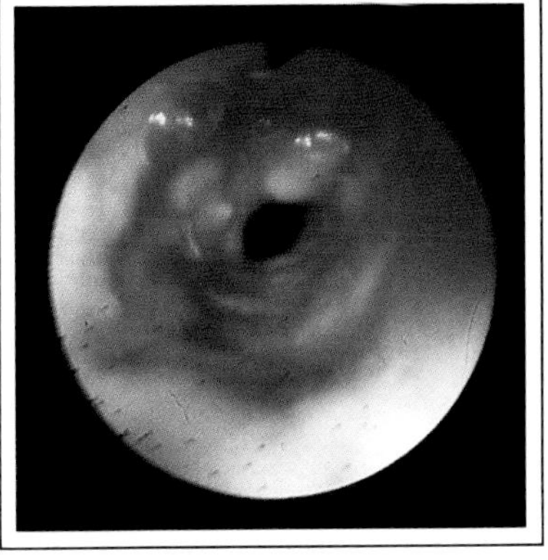

FIG. 3-26.

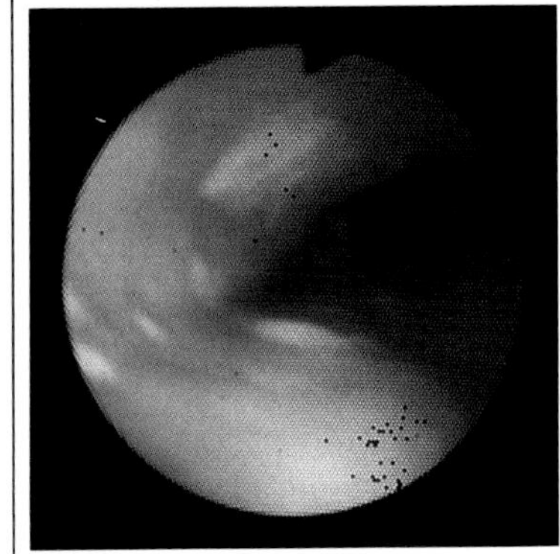

FIG. 3-27.

FIG. 3-26. Eosinophilic esophagitis. Pseudomembrane and marked mucosal friability are seen just above a stricture of the upper third of the esophagus. Biopsies showed a prominent eosinophilic infiltrate.

FIG. 3-27. Crohn's esophagitis. Focal areas of ulcerations and nodularity of the mid-esophagus in a patient with ileocecal Crohn's disease. Biopsy showed focal ulceration thought to be compatible with Crohn's disease.

Esophagitis Associated with Bullous Disorders of the Skin

Patients with epidermolysis bullosa[35] as well as bullous pemphigoid[36] may have involvement of the upper esophagus as a direct extension from the oropharynx. At endoscopy, bullae may be observed along with frank ulcerations and pseudomembranes.[35] In some cases esophageal involvement is followed by stricture formation, especially with epidermolysis bullosa.[35] Extensive necrosis of the entire esophagus has been reported with bullous pemphigoid.[36]

PSEUDOMEMBRANOUS ESOPHAGITIS

Endoscopically, severe mucosal injury may appear as a raised, adherent membrane composed of granulation tissue. The term we use for this is "pseudomembrane," which has in other contexts where it is used the connotation of adherent granulation tissue, the product of mucosal injury. Some authorities prefer to use the term pseudomembrane only in the context of *Candida* esophagitis and employ other terms (e.g., adherent mucus,[5] adherent exudate,[5,6] or superficial ulceration[6]) to describe what we have called the pseudomembranous appearance of severe peptic (reflux) esophagitis (Figs. 3-7 and 3-9). We believe "pseudomembrane" is the proper descriptive term to be applied to an adherent membrane which when stripped off leaves a bleeding undersurface. Biopsy of such tissue invariably shows granulation tissue or marked acute inflammation and is indistinguishable histologically from an ulcer base. For us, the difference between esophageal ulceration (Fig. 3-10) and pseudomembrane (Figs. 3-7 and 3-9) is that in the former the granulation tissue is depressed (Fig. 3-8), whereas in the latter it is slightly raised (Figs. 3-7 and 3-9).

Pseudomembranous esophagitis (severe esophagitis associated with pseudomembrane formation) should not be considered pathognomonic of *Candida* esophagitis. Although it is a usual finding in that condition, it may also be seen in up to one-third of the cases of peptic esophagitis, where it is the most severe manifestation. Because *Candida* esophagitis represents only 10% of our total cases of esophagitis with 30% of our cases of peptic esophagitis being severe, usually with inflammatory exudate, for any given case of pseudomembranous esophagitis there is a three times greater likelihood of a peptic etiology.

Although peptic and *Candida* pseudomembranous esophagitis can closely resemble each other, there are several distinguishing features. First, peptic pseudomembranes are usually found in the distal esophagus, contiguous with the GE junction at the point of presumed maximal exposure to refluxed acid (Fig. 3-7). Only in cases associated with severe peptic injuries, e.g., prolonged nasogastric tube placement, is the proximal esophagus involved with pseudomembranes (Fig. 3-13). Second, in peptic pseudomembranous esophagitis, one expects to see areas above the pseudomembranes of less severe injury characterized by erosions or evidence of chronic reflux as suggested by the presence of mucosal thickening. *Candida* pseudomembranes, unlike those associated with peptic esophagitis, appear throughout the involved portions of the esophagus and do not show lessening of injury for the more proximal esophagus (Fig. 3-14). In many cases there is an abrupt transition between the appearance of pseudomembranes and normal contiguous mucosa. In cases where the distal esophagus is involved, there is usually an abrupt transition just above the GE junction because below this junction the acidic environment is inhospitable to *Candida* (Fig. 3-14b).

The distribution of pseudomembranes is also potentially helpful in distinguishing *Candida* esophagitis from peptic pseudomembranous esophagitis. In two-thirds of the cases we find that *Candida* pseudomembranes are in the proximal esophagus, an unusual location for peptic pseudomembranes. Often these proximal lesions are accompanied by similar plaques in the mouth and throat. However, in up to one-third of the patients with *Candida* esophagitis, the lesion is confined to the distal esophagus, and the throat and proximal esophagus are totally uninvolved.

An uncommon appearance for both *Candida* and peptic pseudomembranous esophagitis is that of a dense confluent exudate where little else is seen (Figs. 3-12 and 3-15). With such an appearance, the diagnosis of *Candida* esophagitis is favored, especially in the absence of a history of other clinical settings for severe esophagitis, i.e., protracted vomiting or nasogastric tube placement.

Diagnosis

Although the clinical setting and endoscopic appearance help differentiate peptic from *Candida* pseudomembranous esophagitis, the most useful means of differentiation are brushings of the pseudomembrane for a KOH preparation, which can be examined microscopically for budding yeast and mycelia (Fig. 3-17).[12] Brushing therefore should be performed in all cases of pseudomembranous esophagitis to determine if *Candida* is present prior to the institution of antifungal therapy. Unfortunately, the accuracy of the test, especially in terms of how often it fails to detect *Candida* actually present with the pseudomembrane, is unknown. In addition, we have occasionally found budding yeast (without mycelial forms) in cases which would, by their clinical setting, be considered peptic pseudomembranous esophagitis. This has been noted especially in patients in whom the peptic pseudomembranous esophagitis was severe and extensive, e.g., in cases associated with vomiting or prolonged placement of a nasogastric tube. In these, because the organisms lack hyphae, which signify the invasive form of *Candida,*[11] we were reluctant to call this *Candida* esophagitis; moreover, the antifungal therapy instituted in some of these cases was not clearly beneficial.

REFERENCES

1. Dodds, W. J., Hogan, W. J., Helm, J. F., and Dent, J. (1981): Pathogenesis of reflux esophagitis. *Gastroenterology,* 81:376–394.
2. Behar, J., Biancani, P., and Sheahan, M. B. (1976): Evaluation of esophageal tests in the diagnosis of reflux esophagitis. *Gastroenterology,* 71:9–15.

2a. Winter, H. S., Madara, J. L., Stafford, R. J., Grand, R. J., Quinlan, J., and Goldman, H. (1982): Intraepithelial eosinophils: a new diagnostic criterion for reflux esophagitis. *Gastroenterology,* 83:818–823.

3. Weinstein, W. M., Bogoch, E. R., and Bowes, K. L. (1975): The normal human esophageal mucosa: a histological reappraisal. *Gastroenterology,* 68:40–44.
4. Kobayoshi, S., and Kasugai, T. (1974): Endoscopic and biopsy criteria for the diagnosis of esophagitis with fiberoptic esophagoscope. *Am. J. Dig. Dis.,* 19:345–352.
5. Morrissey, J. F. (1978): Endoscopic evaluation of gastroesophageal sphincter dysfunction. *South. Med. J. (Suppl. 1),* 71:56–61.
6. Johnson, L. F., DeMeester, T. R., and Haggitt, R. C. (1976): Endoscopic signs for gastroesophageal reflux objectively evaluated. *Gastrointest. Endosc.,* 22:151–155.

6a. Geboes, K., Desmet, V., Vantrappen, G., and Mebis, J. (1980): Vascular changes in esophageal mucosa: An early histological sign of esophagitis. *Gastrointest. Endosc.,* 26:29–32.

7. Wright, R. A., and Hurwitz, A. L. (1979): Relationship of hiatus hernia to endoscopically proved reflux esophagitis. *Dig. Dis. Sci.,* 24:311–313.
8. Scharschmidt, B. F., and Watts, H. D. (1978): The lower esophageal ring and esophageal reflux. *Am. J. Gastroenterol.,* 69:544–549.
9. Volpicelli, N. A., Yardly, J. H., and Hendrix, T. R. (1978): The association of heartburn with gastritis. *Am. J. Dig. Dis.,* 22:333–339.
10. Nagler, K., and Spiro, H. M. (1963): Persistent gastroesophageal reflux induced during prolonged gastric intubation. *N. Engl. J. Med.,* 269:495–500.

10a. Bright-Asare, P., and El-Bassoussi, M. (1980): Cimetidine, metaclopramide, or placebo in the treatment of symptomatic gastroesophageal reflux. *J. Clin. Gastroenterol.,* 2:149–156.

10b. Behar, J., Brand, D. L., Brown, F. C., Castell, D. O., Cohen, S., Crossley, R. J., Pope, C. E., and Winans, C. S. (1978): Cimetidine in the treatment of symptomatic gastroesophageal reflux. A double blind controlled trial. *Gastroenterology,* 74:441–448.

11. Jones, J. M. (1981): The recognition and management of Candida esophagitis. *Hosp. Pract.,* April:64A–64V.
12. Kodsi, B. E., Wickremesinghe, P. C., Kozinn, P. J., Iswara, K., and Goldberg, P. K. (1976): Candida esophagitis: a prospective study of 27 cases. *Gastroenterology,* 71:715–719.
13. Rumfeld, W., Jenkins, D., and Scott, B. B. (1980): Unsuspected gastroesophageal candidiasis: an endoscopic survey. *Gut,* 21:895A.
14. Nash, G., and Ross, J. S. (1974): Herpetic esophagitis. *Hum. Pathol.,* 5:339–345.
15. Osenby, L. C., and Stammer, J. L. (1978): Esophagitis associated with herpes simplex infection in an immunocompetent host. *Gastroenterology,* 74:1305–1306.
16. Lightdale, C. J., Wolf, D. J., Murcucci, R. A., and Salyer, W. R. (1977): Herpetic esophagitis in patients with cancer: ante-mortem diagnosis by brush cytology. *Cancer,* 39:223–225.

16a. Allen, J. I., Silvis, S. E., Sumner, H. W., and McClain, C. J. (1981): Cytomegalic infusion disease diagnosed endoscopically. *Dig. Dis. Sci.,* 26:133–135.

16b. McDonald, G. B., Sharma, P., Sale, G., Shulman, H., Hackman, R., and Meyers, J. (1982): Infectious esophagitis in immunosuppressed patient after marrow transplantation. *Gastroenterology,* 82:1127.

16c. St. Onge, G., and Bezahler, G. H. (1982): Giant esophageal ulcer associated with cytomegalovirus. *Gastroenterology,* 83:127–130.

17. Goodwin, R. A., Loyd, J. E., and DesPrez, R. M. (1981): Histopiasmosis in normal host. *Medicine,* 60:231–266.

18. Dow, C. J. (1981): Oesophageal tuberculosis: four cases. *Gut,* 22:234–236.

19. Nelson, R. S., Hernandez, A. J., Goldstein, H. M., and Saca, A. (1979): Treatment of irradiation esophagitis. *Am. J. Gastroenterol.,* 71:17–23.

20. Boal, D. K. B., Newburger, P. E., and Teele, R. L. (1979): Esophagitis induced by combined radiation and Adriamycin. *Am. J. Roentgenol.,* 132:567–570.

20a. Green, W. H., Moody, M., Hartley, R., Effman, E., Aisner, J., Young, V. M., and Wiernik, P. H. (1974): Esophagoscopy as a source of *Pseudomonas aeruginosa* sepsis in patients with acute leukemia: The need for sterilization of endoscopes. *Gastroenterology,* 67:912–919.

21. Axon, A. T. R., Phillips, I., Cotton, P. B., and Avery, S. A. (1974): Disinfection of gastrointestinal fibre endoscopes. *Lancet,* 1:656–658.

22. Smith, F. P., Kisner, D. L., Widerlite, L., and Schein, P. S. (1979): Chemotherapeutic alteration of small intestinal morphology and function: a progress report. *J. Clin. Gastroenterol.,* 1:203–207.

23. Gilver, R. L. (1970): Esophageal lesions in leukemia and lymphoma. *Am. J. Dig. Dis.,* 15:31–36.

24. Livstone, E. M., Sheahan, D. G., and Behar, J. (1977): Studies of esophageal epithelial cell proliferation in patients with reflux esophagitis. *Gastroenterology,* 73:1313–1319.

24a. Seefeld, U., Krejs, G. J., Siebenmann, R. E., and Blum, A. L. (1977): Esophageal histology in gastroesophageal reflux: morphometric findings in suction biopsies. *Am. J. Dig. Dis.,* 2:956–964.

25. Cello, J. P., Fogel, R. P., and Boland, C. R. (1980): Liquid caustic ingestion: spectrum of injury. *Arch. Intern. Med.,* 140:500–504.

26. DiCostanzo, J., Noirclerc, M., Jouglard, J., Escoffier, J. M., Cano, N., Martin, J., and Gauthier, A. (1980): New therapeutic approach to corrosive burns of the upper gastrointestinal tract. *Gut,* 21:370–375.

27. Mason, S. J., and O'Meara, T. F. (1981): Drug-induced esophagitis. *J. Clin. Gastroenterol.,* 3:155–120.

27a. Hey, H., Jorgensen, F., Sorensen, K., Hasselbalch, H., and Wamberg, T. (1982): Oesophageal transit of six commonly used tablets and capsules. *Brit. Med. J.,* 285:1717–1719.

28. Kikendall, J. W., Friedman, A. C., Oyewole, M. A., Fleischer, D., and Johnson, L. F. (1983): Pill-induced esophageal injury: case reports and review of the medical literature. *Dig. Dis. Sci.,* 28:174–182.

29. Smith, V. M. (1978): Association of aspirin ingestion with symptomatic esophageal hiatus hernia. *South. Med. J. (Suppl. 1),* 71:45–47.

30. Dobbins, J. W., Sheahan, D. G., and Behar, J. (1977): Eosinophilic gastroenteritis with esophageal involvement. *Gastroenterology,* 72:1312–1316.

31. Landres, R. T., Kuster, G. G. R., and Strum, W. B. (1978): Eosinophilic esophagitis in a patient with virus achalasia. *Gastroenterology,* 74:1248–1301.

32. Rosendorff, C., and Grieve, N. W. T. (1967): Ulcerative oesophagitis in association with ulcerative colitis. *Gut,* 8:344–347.

33. Huchzermeyer, H., Paul, F., Seifert, E., Frohlich, H., and Rasmussen, C. W. (1976): Endoscopic results in five patients with Crohn's disease of the esophagus. *Endoscopy,* 8:75–81.

34. LiVolsi, V., and Jeretzske, A. J. (1973): Granulomatous esophagitis: a case of Crohn's disease limited to the esophagus. *Gastroenterology,* 64:313–319.

35. Orlando, R. C., Bozynski, E. M., Briggaman, R. A., and Bream, C. A. (1974): Epidermolysis bullosa: gastrointestinal manifestations. *Ann. Intern. Med.,* 81:203–206.

36. Sharon, P., Greene, M. L., and Rachmilewitz, D. (1978): Esophageal involvement in bullous pemphigoid. *Gastrointest. Endosc.,* 24:122–123.

4

ESOPHAGEAL STRICTURES

Esophageal strictures are not rare. In our Unit they occur on the order of 1 or 2 per 100 cases, which is consistent with the experience of others.[1] As a group, strictures constitute 10 to 20% of all the pathologic appearances of the esophagus.

A stricture is seen in endoscopy as compromise of the lumen by concentric narrowing at which point the esophageal mucosal columns (see Chapter 1) appear to terminate (Fig. 4-1). The concentric narrowing of the lumen caused by a stricture distinguishes its appearance from that of extrinsic compression, which is seen as one-sided, or eccentric, narrowing (Fig. 4-2a). The obliteration of the mucosal columns also allows one to differentiate the appearance of a stricture from that of extrinsic compression (Fig. 4-2a) as well as achalasia (Fig. 4-2b), where in both cases the columns pass through the point of narrowing.

The length of strictures varies considerably.[2] Although most are between 1 and 8 cm, some are very short (≤3 mm) but at the same time have marked luminal narrowing (≤2 mm). An interpretive problem arises for short (<5 mm) strictures which produce only slight luminal compromise (≥11 mm) and are located at the gastroesophageal (GE) junction above a hiatus hernia because they have an appearance similar to that of a Schatzki ring (see Chapter 10). We believe there is actually a spectrum of stricture-like findings at the GE junction ranging from a simple membrane-like Schatzki ring on the one hand (see Chapter 10) to an unequivocal peptic stricture having a width of 1 cm or more on the other. As a true Schatzki ring is mucosal, its diameter should be less than 3 mm (see Chapter 10). We believe that any ring-like deformity with a width of more than 3 mm, whether called a Schatzki ring or not, is likely to have a component of submucosal fibrosis and therefore be the earliest appearance of a peptic stricture that can be identified.

For the various types of esophageal stricture, the endoscopist has three goals: (a) identify the stricture; (b) assess its nature—benign or malignant—and, if malignant, take the appropriate additional steps, i.e., biopsy and brushing, to confirm the diagnosis of cancer; and (c) if benign, determine from its appearance and the clinical context its most likely origin, i.e., whether it is a peptic type or one of the nonpeptic types. In addition to these steps, in some cases the endoscopist may wish to attempt dilatation of the stricture under direct vision.[3]

The plan of this chapter is first to examine the range of appearances of peptic strictures, identify the commonest type, and then discuss other benign strictures. In the final section we present the contrasting features of malignant strictures.

PEPTIC STRICTURES

Stricture formation is a complication of peptic esophagitis in about 10% of the cases,[4] although a history of antecedent reflux symptoms is not invariable.[4] Typically, peptic strictures are located at or just above the GE junction.[4] An accompanying hiatus hernia (Fig. 4-3) is found in 40% of our cases and in over 80% in a reported series,[1] suggesting more than just a chance relationship between hiatus hernia and peptic strictures. The distance of the stricture from the incisor teeth depends on the location of the GE junction, but this is usually between 33 and 45 cm. A stricture located above 32 cm should always raise the question of its being either malignant (see below) or associated with a Barrett's Esophagus (see Chapter 6).

Appearance

Endoscopically a ring-like opening of the stricture is noted that obliterates the converging mucosal columns (Fig. 4-1). Recalling this, one can identify the stricture even if its diameter freely admits the endoscope (Fig. 4-3a).

In the absence of esophagitis, the mucosa around the mouth of the stricture and within it appears smooth (Fig. 4-1). Even when the mouth of the stricture appears distorted

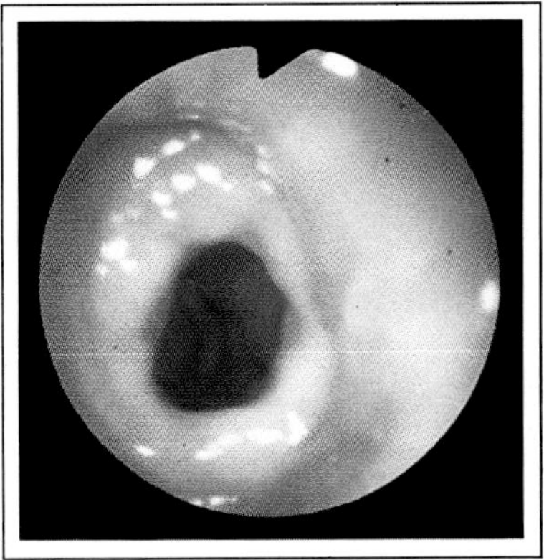

FIG. 4-1.

FIG. 4-1. Peptic stricture. There is a smooth, concentric, ring-like narrowing of the lumen at which point the mucosal column of the right (3 o'clock) wall terminates.

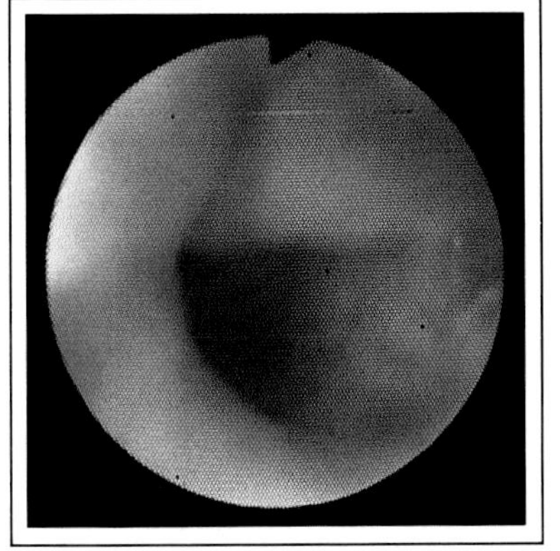

FIG. 4-2a.

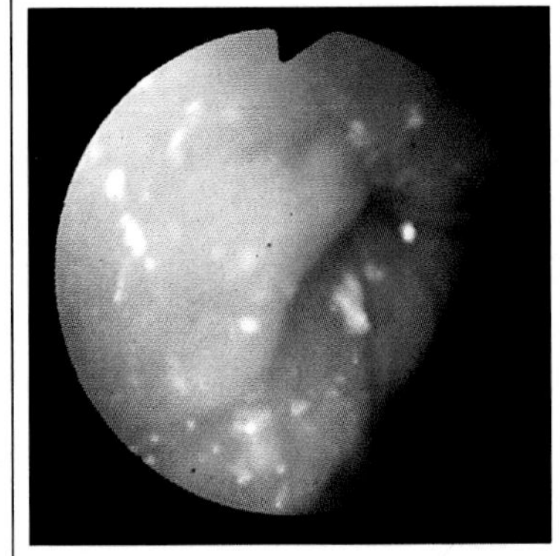

FIG. 4-2b.

FIG. 4-2. a: Extrinsic compression at the GE junction by carcinoma. The lumen is narrowed by a mass denting the right posterior wall (3 to 6 o'clock). The mucosal columns of the opposite wall pass through this point, however. **b:** Achalasia. Mucosal columns forming the rosette run through the point of luminal narrowing, differentiating this appearance from that of a stricture (Fig. 4-11).

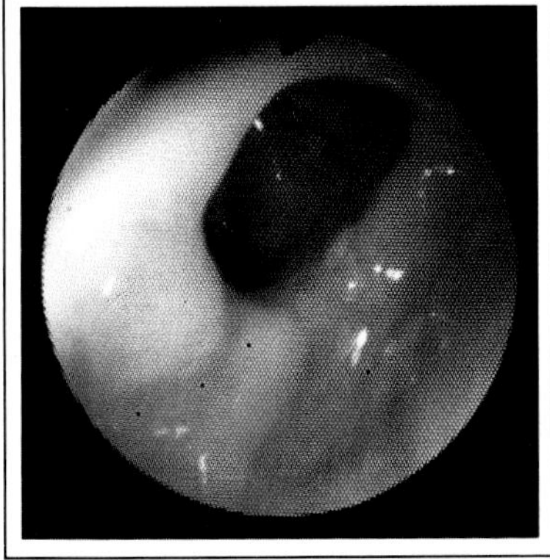

FIG. 4-3a.

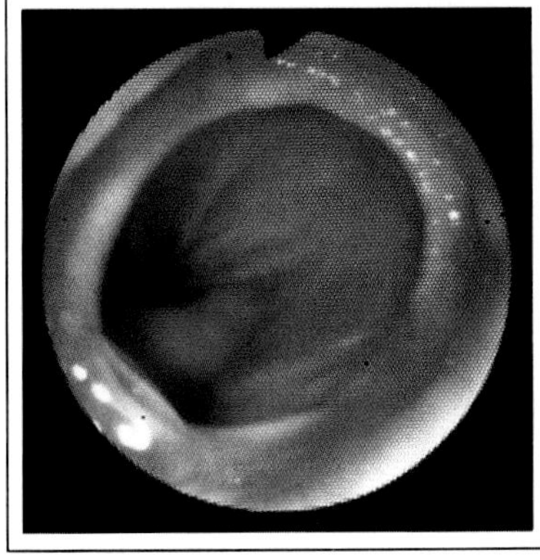

FIG. 4-3b.

FIG. 4-3. a: Mild stricture. An 11-mm stricture above a hiatus hernia to which a 9-mm pediatric-type endoscope passes with ease. **b:** Schatzki ring. The somewhat thickened (3 to 4 mm) ring makes some consider this an early peptic stricture.

(Fig. 4-4) with areas of depression either from previous ulceration or attempts at dilatation, the mucosa is nevertheless smooth and uniform, in sharp contrast to the completely disorganized and irregular appearance of carcinoma with tumor nodules and ulcerations (Fig. 4-5).

Associated Peptic Esophagitis

In approximately half our cases, the stricture has evidence of moderate (Fig. 4-6) or severe esophagitis within the stricture, at its mouth, or just above it (Fig. 4-7), with, in the latter case, ulcerations, pseudomembranes, or both being present. Even though there may be some irregularity associated with the appearance of these features, especially junctional areas between ulcerations which may themselves appear nodular or mass-like (Fig. 4-8), there is still an underlying uniformity to the appearance that suggests esophagitis rather than malignancy. Moreover, the individual nodules are almost invariably less than 4 to 5 mm.[1] Nodules which exceed this size would be considered as suspicious for malignancy. Another suspicious feature is an asymmetrical appearance (Fig. 4-9) around the mouth of a stricture

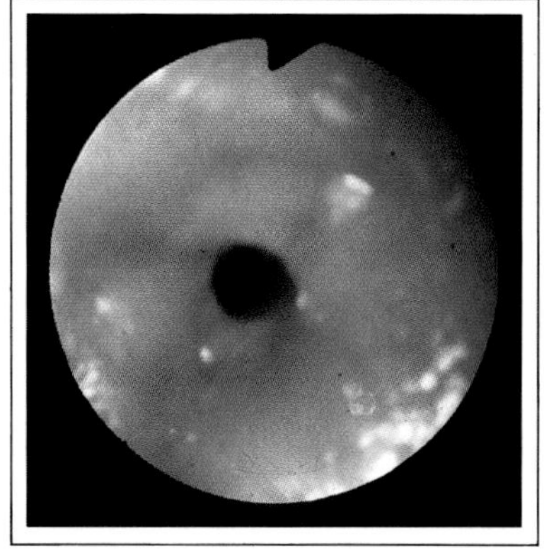

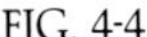

FIG. 4-4.

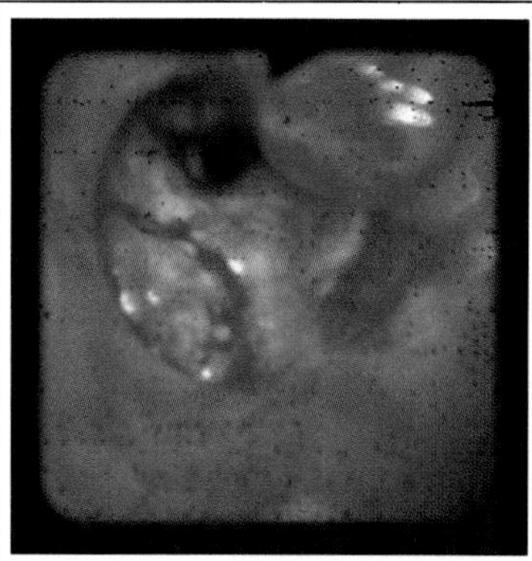

FIG. 4-5.

FIG. 4-4. Peptic stricture, slighly distorted ring. This distortion may be due to repeated prior dilations.

FIG. 4-5. Malignant stricture. Frank tumor nodules can be seen comprising the mouth of the stricture.

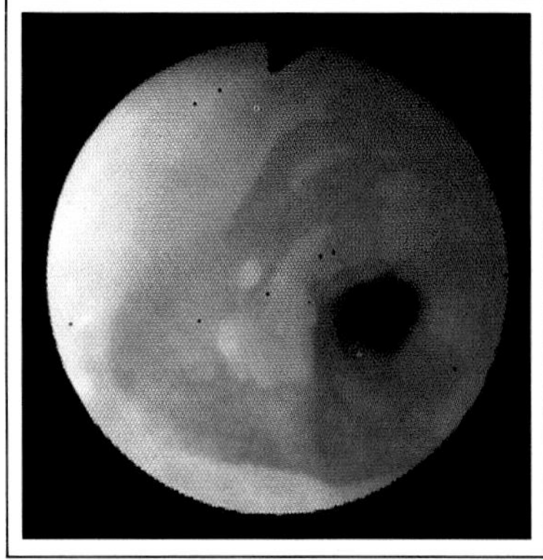

FIG. 4-6.

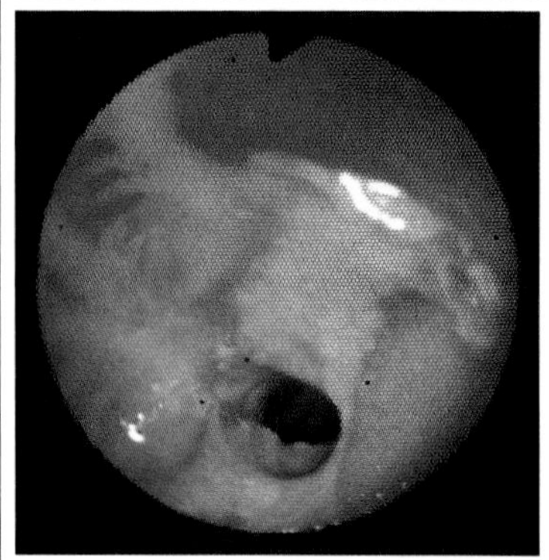

FIG. 4-7.

FIG. 4-6. Peptic stricture with a moderate esophagitis. Confluent areas of erosion are observed just above the mouth of the stricture with intervening islands of intact squamous epithelium.

FIG. 4-7. Peptic stricture with severe esophagitis. The pseudomembrane seen within and just above the stricture indicates severe esophagitis. Although somewhat distorted, possibly from the acute changes, the symmetry of the underlying stricture is preserved.

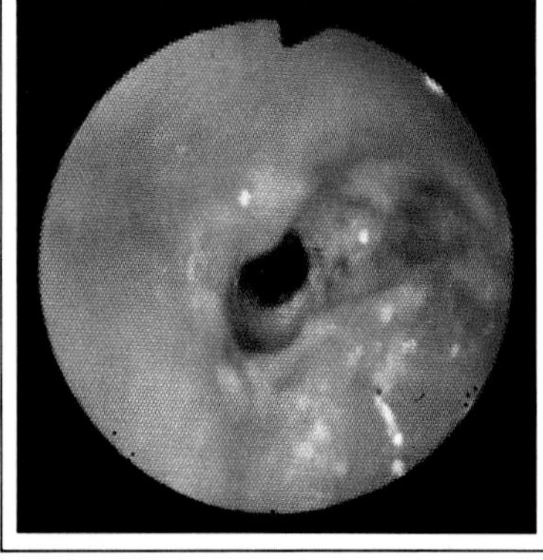

FIG. 4-8.

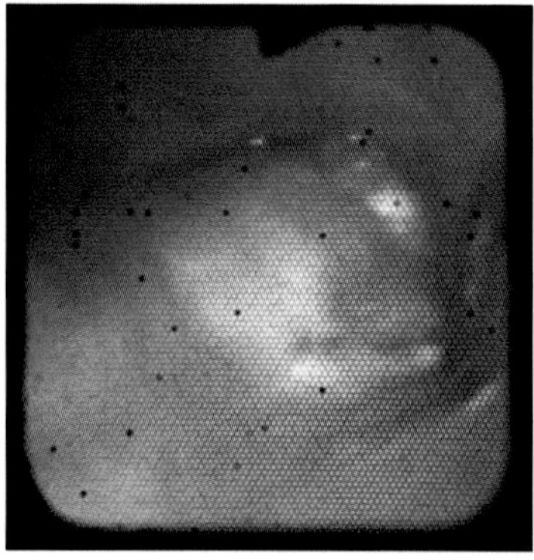

FIG. 4-9.

FIG. 4-8. Peptic stricture with severe esophagitis. The margin of the ulceration on the right posterior (3 to 6 o'clock) wall appears nodular, raising the question of malignancy because of its resemblance to Fig. 4-5. Still, the individual nodules are less than 5 mm, making malignancy unlikely.

FIG. 4-9. Malignant stricture. The asymmetrical appearance of the mouth of the stricture because of a 1-cm nodule is a highly suspicious feature.

in which, for example, an elevated portion is present on only one side (Fig. 4-13, below).

Grading Strictures

Once a stricture is identified, it is graded according to its diameter. This can be estimated by comparing it to the known distance between the "cups" of an open biopsy forceps (called the "open forceps" or "open bite width" method). A less exact "sense" of a diameter of a stricture can be estimated by the "fit" of the endoscope (which has a known diameter).

The grading of strictures (Table 4-1) is done according to the following: Those with diameters between 11 and 13 mm are called minimal (Fig. 4-3), those with diameters between 7 and 11 mm moderate (Fig. 4-1), and those with

TABLE 4-1. *Grading of peptic strictures*

Estimated diameter (mm)	Grade
11–13	Minimal
7–11	Moderate
<7	Marked (high-grade)

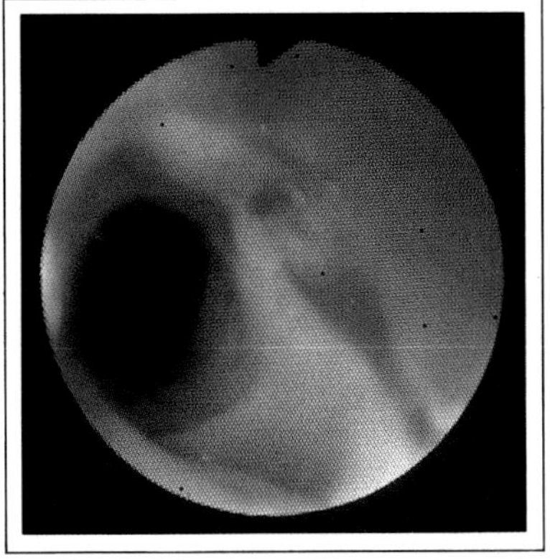
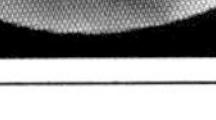

FIG. 4-10.

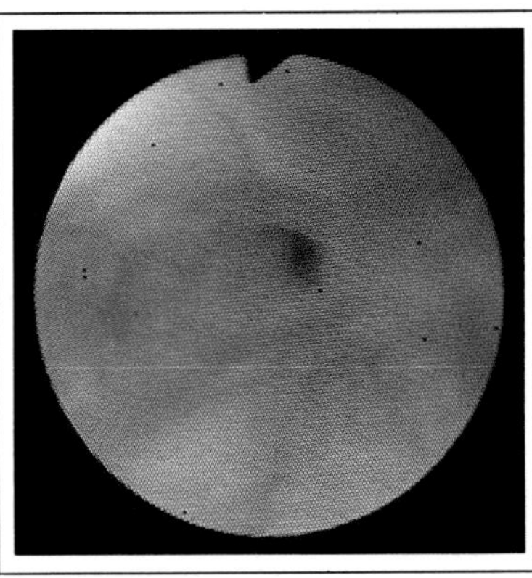

FIG. 4-11.

FIG. 4-10. Moderate stricture. The pediatric endoscope (8.8 mm) enters but does not cross the stricture, estimated by the open forceps method (see text) to have a 7.5 mm diameter.

FIG. 4-11. Marked (high-grade) stricture. The diameter of this short (<5 mm) stricture at the GE junction is only 2 mm. Etiology was thought to be the prolonged (1 year) placement of a feeding tube.

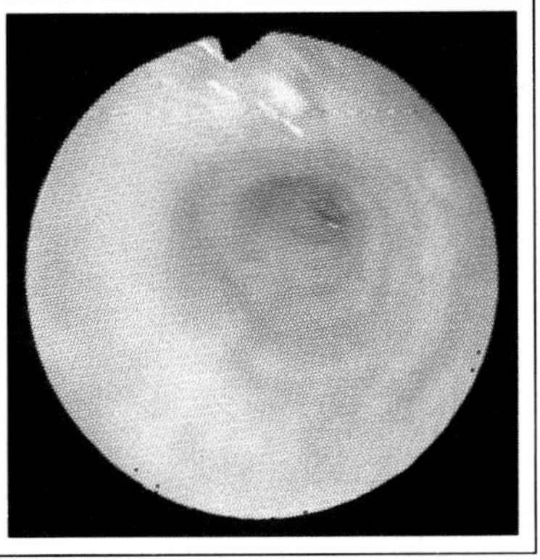

FIG. 4-12.

FIG. 4-12. Marked (high-grade) stricture. The pinpoint lumen and location (30 cm) were suspicious features for malignancy, revealed by brushings taken within the stricture.

diameters less than 7 mm marked or high grade (Fig. 4-6). Generally, a peptic stricture has a diameter of at least 3 mm. If the diameter is less than this (Fig. 4-10), the possibility of another etiology, especially malignancy (Fig. 4-11), is considered.

Indeterminate Peptic Strictures

Because of the deforming appearance of prior severe esophagitis or striking nodularity associated with current severe esophagitis (Fig. 4-12), it may not be possible to state categorically that the stricture is benign. Other suspicious features are an asymmetrical appearance to the mass-like deformity (Fig. 4-13) or a stricture having a diameter of less than 3 mm. In these cases it is proper to refer to the stricture as indeterminate, aggressively pursue biopsy and brushing from the stricture itself, and recommend endoscopic follow-up at 2- to 3-month intervals or sooner if the examiner's index of suspicion is high (Fig. 4-13).

Biopsy and Brushing

One may wish to biopsy all strictures, even those with a typical peptic appearance; certainly those considered indeterminate warrant an aggressive approach. Ideally, biopsy specimens are taken from the mouth of the stricture using the large 2.5-mm forceps. At least four specimens should be taken from every stricture. With any suspicious feature, the number should increase to 8 to 10 in order to decrease the probability of missing a cancer.[5] Because of the inevitable difficulty of biopsy sampling from within a stricture, brushing cytology is the more crucial maneuver, especially from within the stricture.[6]

Even with the aggressive pursuit of biopsies and brushing, it is possible to fail to obtain positive material from malignant strictures. Therefore, for any stricture suspicious enough to call indeterminate one should insist on a follow-up examination within 3 to 4 weeks of the initial endoscopy. In cases where because of the location or appearance of the stricture the index of suspicion is high, one would recommend surgery despite negative biopsies and brushing cytology.

OTHER BENIGN STRICTURES

Benign-appearing strictures located above the GE junction or occurring in other nonreflux clinical settings cause the endoscopist to consider a nonpeptic etiology. In this section we discuss three types of nonpeptic strictures. In the first, the stricture results from a specific, severe esophageal injury,

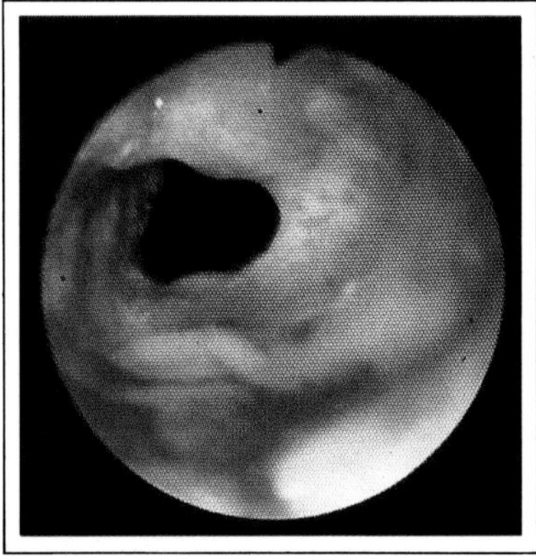

FIG. 4-13a.

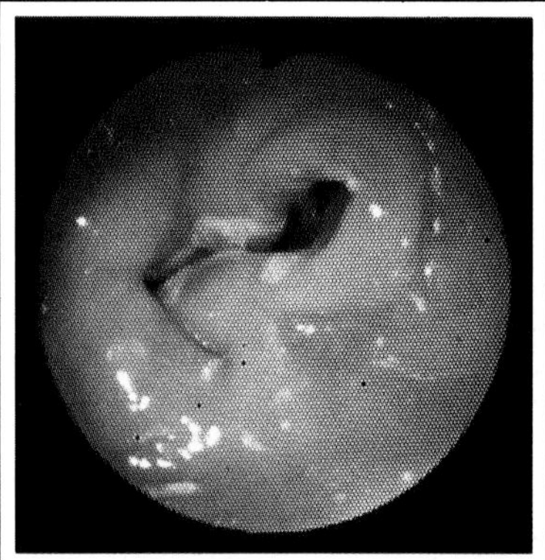

FIG. 4-13b.

FIG. 4-13. a: Indeterminate peptic stricture. The distortion of the lumen by the deep ulceration of the right (3 o'clock) wall caused this stricture to be regarded as indeterminate. Even though biopsies and brushings were negative, close endoscopic follow-up was advised. **b:** Indeterminate stricture, ultimately proved malignant. The mouth of the stricture appears asymmetrical with one side (3 o'clock) heaped up, whereas within the other (9 o'clock) there is a deep ulceration. Biopsy and brushing cytology were positive, but had they not been so repeat endoscopy would have been performed 2 to 4 weeks later for additional histologic and cytologic sampling. In view of the highly suspicious appearance, surgery would have been advised even if the biopsy and brushing cytology were negative.

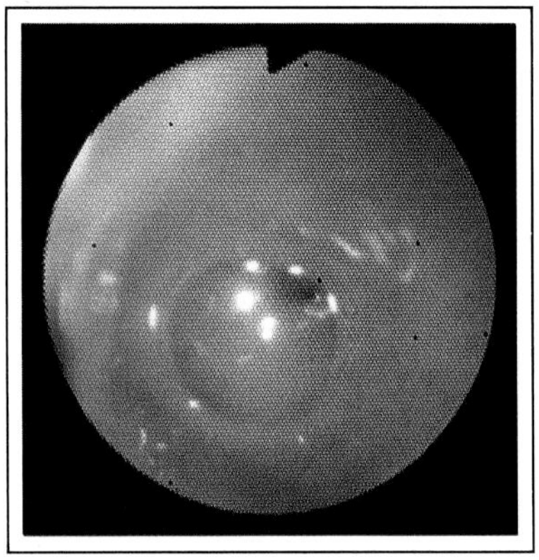

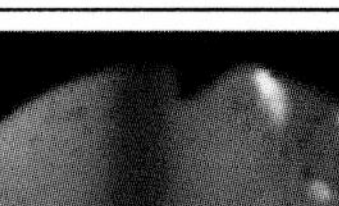

FIG. 4-14a.

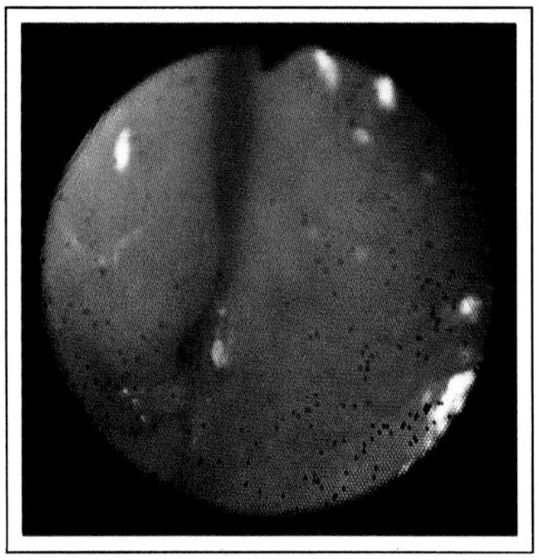

FIG. 4-14b.

FIG. 4-14. a: Radiation stricture. Abrupt transition of the lumen to a pinpoint stricture gives this area a shelf-like appearance, especially from the left posterior (6 to 9 o'clock) wall. The patient had received 4,500 rads for treatment of an esophagogastric lymphoma. **b:** Lye strictures of the cricopharyngeus (in the 7 o'clock position) in a 50-year-old man having suffered lye injury to the esophagus during infancy. The examination was performed because of newly worsening dysphagia, which raised the question of carcinoma (see text) although none was evident.

e.g., irradiation or lye ingestion. In the second, the stricture is associated with esophageal injury which may accompany the placement of a nasogastric tube or previous esophageal surgery. Finally, we discuss a third group of strictures which occurs as part of other diseases, i.e., Crohn's disease, eosinophilic gastroenteritis, and bullous disorders of the skin.

Strictures Associated With Specific Prior Injury

Radiation Strictures

Radiation strictures are found in the mid or upper esophagus after the administration of 3,000 to 6,000 rads for the treatment of carcinoma (breast or lung) or lymphoma.[7,8] In some cases the total dose may have been 3,000 rads or less. These strictures may often be associated with concurrent administration of the radioimetic chemotherapeutic agent, e.g., adriamycin, which can amplify the radiation injury effect, possibly by interfering with the reparative response of the esophageal mucosa to radiation-induced damage.[9]

A radiation stricture is usually seen as an abrupt, marked narrowing of the lumen, often with considerable dilatation of the esophagus above the stricture. Because of the abrupt transition, there is a shelf-like appearance to the mucosa just above the stricture (Fig. 4-14a). The mucosa of the mouth of the stricture is smooth and regular. On close examination, distorted submucosal capillaries or even telangiectasias can be seen as in radiation injury elsewhere in the gastrointestinal (GI) tract.

Not infrequently the radiation stricture is associated with complete obstruction, in which case it is impossible to pass even a 2-mm brush through.[6] In these cases, the differential diagnosis is recurrent carcinoma or lymphoma, and it is not possible to exclude this diagnosis endoscopically, even with multiple biopsies and brushings taken from the stricture.[8]

Lye Strictures

Lye strictures are exceedingly rare; we encountered only one case over a 7-year period in which approximately 5,000 examinations were performed. These are nevertheless a frequent complication of lye ingestion, especially when it occurs during infancy, being found in up to 25% of patients who have ingested lye.[10] The strictures begin to be seen 11 to 16 days after ingestion,[11] at which time one may see only a stricture of the mid or upper esophagus (Fig. 4-14b) and no esophagitis.

Some patients undergo endoscopy as adults because they have had a lye injury and stricture formation as children.

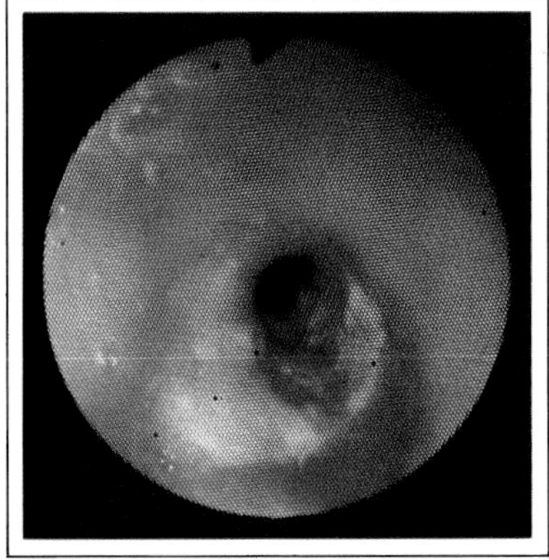

FIG. 4-15.

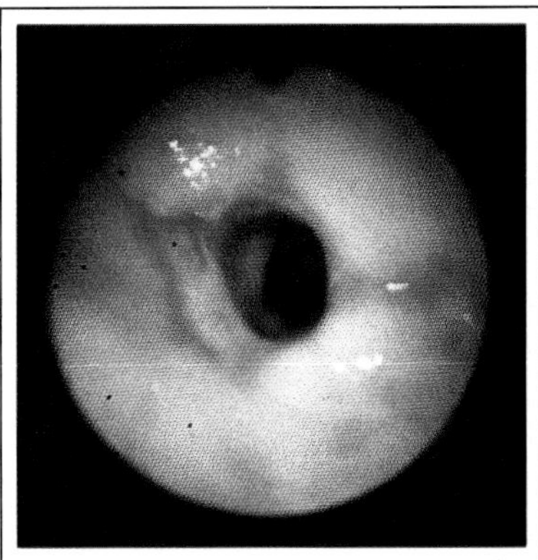

FIG. 4-16.

FIG. 4-15. Postoperative stricture. Marked stricture with ulcerations at the anastomotic point in the mid-esophagus after a distal esophageal and gastric pull-through procedure (see Chapter 9) for carcinoma of the cardia. No evidence of cancer was found at subsequent surgery.

FIG. 4-16. Possible Crohn's stricture. A mid-esophageal ulceration stricture. Biopsy showed acute and chronic inflammation without granuloma. Because of the patient's excellent response to dilatation, no subsequent surgery was performed.

In these patients one looks for asymmetry, nodularity, or any irregular features above the stricture, which would be regarded as suspicious for malignant change, especially because individuals with lye strictures have an increased risk of esophageal malignancy over others in the general population, with cancer occurring in up to 30% of such patients.[12] All patients with lye strictures, especially those sustained during infancy should have periodic endoscopic surveillance probably at yearly intervals. Because of the cancer potential of a lye stricture, the presence of cytologic dysplasia in biopsies taken from nodular, irregular mucosa above lye strictures for us is a strong argument in favor of resection, even in the absence of a definite histologic diagnosis of malignancy.

Nasogastric Tube and Postoperative Strictures

Nasogastric Tube Induced Strictures

Strictures caused by nasogastric tubes are rare complications of tube placement, probably occurring in less than 0.1% of these patients although accounting for up to 10% of benign esophageal strictures.[13] Usually they are associated with nasogastric tube placement of more than 7 days, but occasionally they occur after only 3 to 4 days of placement and rarely after only 24 hr.

Characteristically, the stricture which appears in the mid or mid-distal esophagus is longer than the ordinary peptic stricture, running for as much as 10 to 15 cm down to the GE junction. Luminal narrowing is marked, with a diameter of 3 to 6 mm (Fig. 4-12) and sometimes even less than 3 mm, although it is unusual to find the lumen entirely occluded.

Postoperative Strictures

Like nasogastric tube induced strictures, postoperative strictures are uncommon, accounting for 13% of strictures in one series.[14] These generally occur after a distal esophageal resection for carcinoma (Fig. 4-15), a myotomy for achalasia alone, or with an unsuccessful antireflux operation. The stricture is typically located at the esophagogastric anastomosis or, in the case of achalasia, just above the myotomy site. Typically there is evidence of acute mucosal injury above the stricture, suggesting that reflux is an important factor, although the way the surgery itself was performed (i.e., if it left excessive tension on an esophagogastric anastomosis) may be even more important.

Strictures Occurring as Part of Other Diseases

The conditions we noted in Chapter 3 that give rise to esophagitis may also be associated with stricture formation. The appearances of these strictures are considered in this section.

Crohn's Disease

Esophageal strictures may be found in rare patients with Crohn's disease. They may be the sole focus of the disease, or it may be found elsewhere in the GI tract. In some but not all of the reported cases, the histologic findings were compatible with Crohn's disease after surgical resection.[14]

These strictures are typically located in the mid-esophagus (Fig. 4-16), which is the important feature differentiating them from common peptic strictures. In some cases several foci of Crohn's disease, including the stricture, have been noted within the esophagus with intervening "skip areas." In other cases a "cobblestone" appearance may be seen around the mouth of the stricture as would be true of Crohn's disease in the colon (see Chapter 43). Biopsies of these areas rarely if ever show granulomas.

Strictures Associated With Eosinophilic Gastroenteritis

Eosinophilic gastroenteritis may be associated with esophageal involvement (see Chapter 3). We have seen one

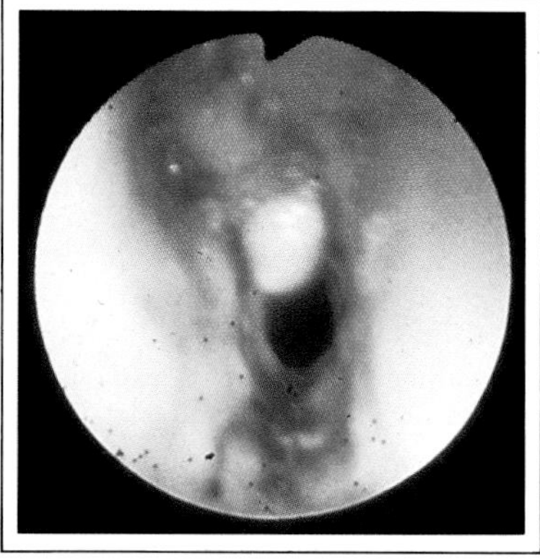

FIG. 4-17

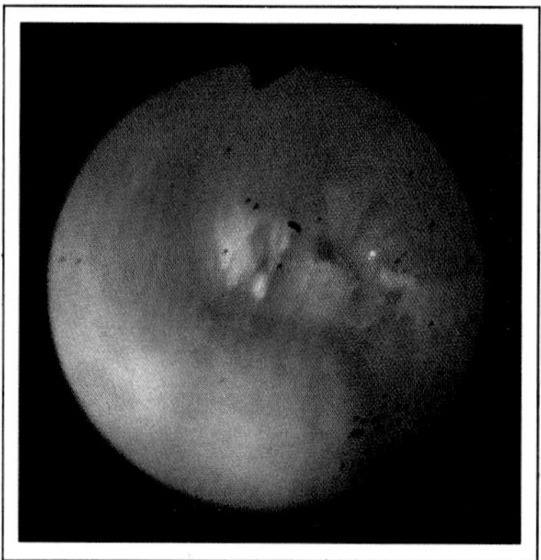

FIG. 4-18.

FIG. 4-17. Eosinophilic esophagitis with stricture. The stricture of the proximal third in this case was found with severe esophagitis (ulceration and pseudomembrane) in a 17-year-old male with peripheral eosinophilia, presenting with dysphagia. Biopsy showed granulation tissue with striking numbers of eosinophils.

FIG. 4-18. Malignant stricture, squamous carcinoma of the distal esophagus. The mouth is asymmetrical and somewhat nodular, and the adjacent left posterior wall (in the 7 o'clock position) had a shelf-like appearance. Biopsies were negative, although brushing cytology within the mouth was diagnostic.

case where peripheral eosinophilia (percent of eosinophils in excess of 20) was associated with stricture formation and severe esophagitis of the upper third of the esophagus (Fig. 4-17). Biopsies showed marked eosinophilic infiltrates of the mucosa. We have seen a similar histologic picture in biopsies taken from an otherwise unexplained stricture of the proximal esophagus in which peripheral eosinophilia was not present. A diagnosis of eosinophilic esophagitis should be considered in any patient with an unexplained stricture of the proximal third of the esophagus, providing malignancy (see below) and Barrett's esophagus (see Chapter 6) can be excluded.

Bullous Disorders of the Skin

Both epidermolysis bullosa and bullous pemphigoid can be associated with esophageal involvement by contiguous extension from the pharynx (see Chapter 3). In these cases the strictures may form at or around the cricopharyngeus or just below it and may be accompanied by high-grade upper esophageal obstruction. In some cases there are no accompanying esophageal lesions that correspond to skin lesions at the time the strictures appear.

MALIGNANT STRICTURES

Malignant strictures are relatively uncommon, occurring with only one-third the frequency of the peptic type. We therefore expect to encounter one malignant stricture per 250 to 300 examinations.

Malignant strictures may originate in one of the following ways: (a) as infiltrating squamous carcinoma; (b) as infiltrating adenocarcinoma arising in the cardiofundic portion of the stomach, extending into the distal esophagus; and (c) as metastatic carcinomas to hilar or cardial lymph nodes with encirclement. Because the origin of a malignant stricture has an important bearing on its endoscopic appearance, we use this division as the basis of the discussion which follows.

Infiltrating Squamous Carcinoma

The infiltrating squamous carcinoma is the most common type of malignant stricture,[15] especially in the proximal or mid-esophagus where it is eight times more common than adenocarcinoma.[16]

Apart from its location, the key feature which suggests the presence of a malignant stricture is the irregularity, asymmetry, and nodularity of the mucosa that forms the mouth of the stricture (Fig. 4-18). This asymmetry is continued just proximal to the stricture, giving it a shelf-like appearance. One carefully examines the mouth of the stricture for the appearance of breaks in the mucosa by frank tumor nodules which have a deep pink-gray appearance and are extremely friable, therefore bleeding when even gently touched. The mucosa proximal to these nodules may appear surprisingly intact. One must remember that a malignant stricture implies that the tumor is infiltrating largely within the submucosa, and that the occasional break of the mucosa may be the only point from which biopsy or brushing will yield a positive result (Fig. 4-5).

Infiltrating Adenocarcinoma

Infiltrating adenocarcinomas may arise from the cardiofundic area and infiltrate the distal esophagus to produce high-grade obstruction within 5 to 6 cm of the GE junction. In our experience and that of others,[15,16] this is the most frequent origin, being up to 25 times more common than primary adenocarcinoma, even for those arising in Barrett's epithelium (see Chapter 6).

In these cases one expects an asymmetrical stricture (Fig. 4-13) with its mouth having a coarse, nodular appearance where the infiltrating tumor is breaking through the squamous mucosa. Here one sees nodules or small masses of tumor which exceed 5 mm; their size, reddish-gray coloration, and friability suggest the presence of carcinoma[17] (Fig. 4-13b).

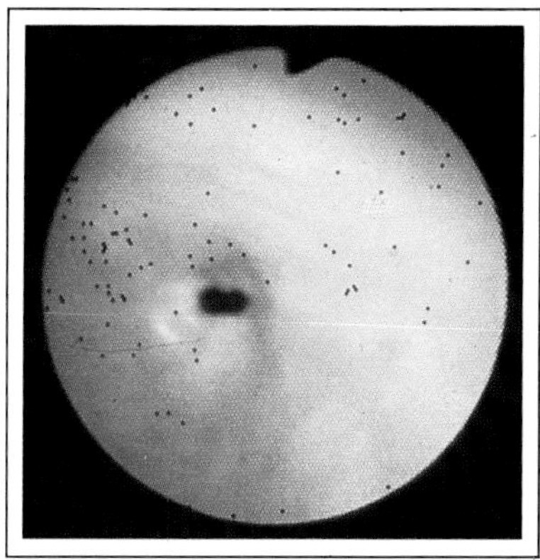

FIG. 4-19. "Benign" stricture from metastatic breast carcinoma. The tumor has metastasized into the mediastinum at the level of the esophagus. The resulting fibrosis produces an annular compression of the lumen with the mucosa completely intact. Not unexpectedly, biopsies and brushings were negative.

FIG. 4-19.

Metastatic Carcinoma

Metastatic carcinoma is the least common of all malignant strictures. The best and most widely quoted example of this is probably the "breast-dysphagia" syndrome, in which there is late metastasis to the mediastinum 5 to 10 years after mastectomy, leading to extrinsic compression of the esophagus by dense fibrous tissue.[18] Typically, the stricture forms in the mid-esophagus, often adjacent to involved hilar lymph nodes.[19]

Often only a tight mid-esophageal stricture is seen, usually with completely intact mucosa; it may therefore be thought to be benign (Fig. 4-19). The history as well as the location of the stricture in the mid-esophagus should cause one to consider this diagnosis.

If the carcinoma is located in the cardial area, breast, lung, or pancreas, it may metastasize to lymph nodes, producing a concentric narrowing at or just below the GE junction. This may give a smooth, short, "rat tail" type stricture with mucosal columns left intact—features which resemble achalasia (see Chapter 8).

Biopsy and Brushing

The decision as to which modality—biopsy or brushing—to pursue vigorously depends on both the visual appearance as well as the likely origin of the lesion.

Malignant Strictures of Squamous Origin

For malignant strictures of squamous origin, evidence of tumor is often found around the mouth of the stricture as either a mass or tumor nodule (Fig. 4-5). If the junction between intact mucosa and the tumor itself can be clearly defined, then directed forceps biopsy is the best choice as it will yield a positive diagnosis. At least six biopsy specimens should be obtained, and preferably 10 or more.[5] They must be taken as forcefully as possible. Some bleeding is to be expected, but it is rarely of any consequence. In cases where the tumor is apparent, cytologic studies are adjunctive. They should not be pursued first, as they may be associated with bleeding, which will obscure the critical junction between the intact squamous epithelium and the cancer, making biopsy less successful. If cytologic study is desired, sheathed brushes should be employed initially; areas within the stricture are brushed, and then as a last step, the mouth of the stricture itself.

Malignant Strictures from Infiltrating Adenocarcinoma

Malignant strictures from an infiltrating adenocarcinoma are commonly located in the distal 5 cm of the esophagus. Whereas the columns around the strictures are enlarged, the overlying mucosa shows only nonspecific erythema or is entirely normal (Fig. 4-20a). For these cases, if a small-caliber endoscope cannot be advanced into the stomach so as to sample the origin of the tumor directly, brushing cytology is the modality which is most likely to give a positive result. The sheathed brush is advanced well within the stricture before the brush itself is extended. After sampling, the brush is returned to the sheath before the sheath is withdrawn from the stricture. In patients in whom the folds at the mouth of the stricture appear both prominent and fixed, multiple biopsies are taken from a single point or the large-particle biopsy technique (see Chapter 1) may be necessary.

Malignant Strictures from Metastatic Carcinomas

In cases of malignant stricture from a metastatic carcinoma, especially strictures of the mid-esophagus from a breast primary, the mucosa of the mouth and the area above it may appear completely intact. Nevertheless, in these cases because the tumor both encircled and invaded the esophagus, repeated forceful biopsies taken from the mouth of the stricture occasionally produce positive results. In these cases cytologic studies of the inside of the stricture should be pursued. Cytologic studies performed after multiple biopsies of the area sometimes produce a positive result

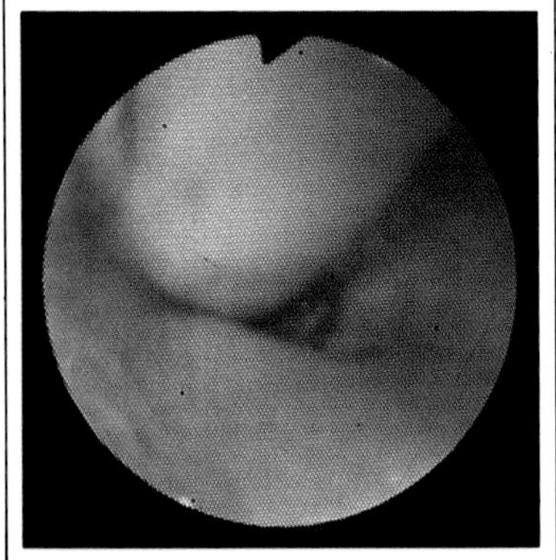

FIG. 4-20a.

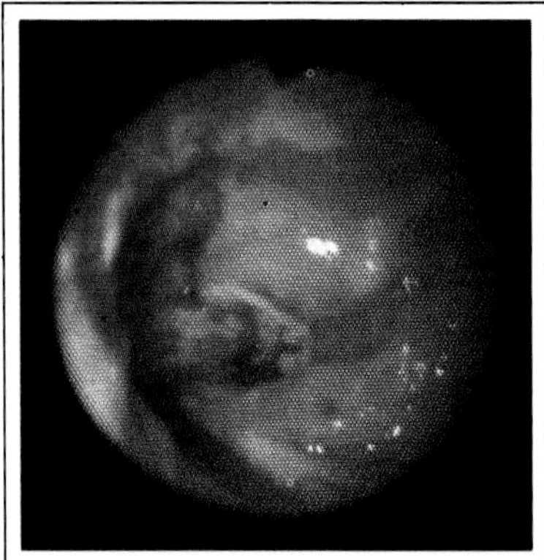

FIG. 4-20b.

FIG. 4-20. Malignant stricture, infiltrating adenocarcinoma arising in the cardia. **a:** The lumen is completely closed and asymmetrical with the mucosal column enlarged. Biopsies were negative, but brushing cytology taken from within the stricture walls were positive. **b:** Tumor nodules were seen at the mouth of the stricture.

when the material obtained prior to biopsy and the biopsies themselves are unrevealing.

Differentiating Benign from Malignant Strictures

The two most important features to consider in the differentiation of benign from malignant strictures are: (a) location of the stricture; and (b) the appearance of its mouth and adjacent mucosa.

Regarding location, a stricture of the upper or mid-esophagus in a patient over age 40 with no history of reflux symptoms to suggest Barrett's esophagus (see Chapter 6) should be considered highly suspicious for cancer. While most strictures of the distal esophagus prove to be peptic, particularly those at the GE junction, it may not be possible to determine a stricture's relation to the GE junction with absolute certainty. Even a stricture with an otherwise benign appearance (see below) should be regarded as suspicious if there is the suggestion radiologically of its being located above the GE junction.

Of primary importance to differentiation is the appearance of the mouth of the stricture. The presence of nodules greater than 5 mm (Figs. 4-5 and 4-9), an asymmetrical appearance (Figs. 4-13b and 4-18), and esophagitis confined to a shelf-like area (Fig. 4-18) should all be viewed as highly suspicious findings for carcinoma. On the other hand, nodules less than 5 mm between ulcerations or pseudomembranes are legitimate appearances for severe peptic esophagitis (Fig. 4-13), even if asymmetrically distributed, so long as the esophagitis itself involves the entire circumference of the esophagus (Fig. 4-8). One may designate such an appearance as "probably benign," though atypical (because of the asymmetric distribution of the nodules), and request follow-up. By contrast, for larger, asymmetric masses (Figs. 4-9 and 4-18) one would use the phrase "highly suspicious for malignancy" and advise surgery, even if biopsies and brushing cytology (see above) were negative.

REFERENCES

1. Hiatt, G. (1977): The roles of esophagoscopy vs. radiography in diagnosing benign peptic esophageal strictures. *Gastrointest. Endosc.*, 23:194–195.
2. Mukhopadhyay, A. K. (1980): Idiopathic lower esophageal sphincter incompetence and esophageal stricture. *Arch. Intern. Med.*, 140:1493–1499
3. Huchzermeyer, H., Freise, J., and Becker, H. (1977): Dilation of benign esophageal strictures by peroral fiberendoscopic bougienage. *Endoscopy*, 9:207–211.
4. Palmer, E. D. (1968): The hiatus hernia-esophagitis-esophageal stricture complex—twenty year prospective study. *Am. J. Med.*, 44:566–579.
5. Witzel, L., Halter, F., Gretillat, P. A., Scheurer, U., and Keller, M. (1976): Evaluation of the specific value of endoscopic biopsies and brush cytology for malignancy of the oesophagus and stomach. *Gut*, 17:375–377.
6. Prolla, J., Reilly, R. W., Kirsner, J. B., and Cockerham, L. (1977): Direct-vision endoscopic cytology and biopsy in the diagnosis of esophageal and gastric tumors: current experience. *Acta Cytol. (Baltimore)*, 21:399–402.
7. Nelson, R. S., Hernandez, A. J., Goldstein, H. M., and Saca, A. (1979): Treatment of irradiation esophagitis. *Am. J. Gastroenterol*, 71:17–23.
8. Blackstone, M. O., Levin, B., Kinzie, J. J., Horneff, J. A., and Skinner, D. B. (1979): Stricture of the esophagogastric junction with adjacent extraluminal cavity following radiation. *Am. J. Gastroenterol.*, 71:290–294.
9. Greco, F. A., Brereton, H. D., Kent, H., Zimbler, H., Merrill, J., and Johnson, R. E. (1976): Adriamycin and enhanced radiation reaction in normal esophagus and skin. *Ann. Intern. Med.*, 85:294–298.
10. Kirsch, M. M., and Ritter, F. (1976): Caustic ingestion and subsequent damage to oropharyngeal and digestive passages. *Ann. Thorac. Surg.*, 21:74–82.
11. Muhletaler, G. A., Gerlock, A. J., de Soto, L., and Halter, S. A. (1980): Acid corrosive esophagitis: radiographic findings. *Am. J. Roentgenol.*, 134:1137–1340.
12. Imre, J., and Kopp, M. (1971): Arguments against long-term conservative treatment of oesophageal strictures due to corrosive burns. *Thorax*, 27:595–598.
13. Buchin, P. J., and Spiro, H. M. (1981): Therapy of esophageal stricture: a review of 84 patients. *J. Clin. Gastroenterol.*, 3:121–128.
14. LiVolsi, V., and Jeretzski, A. J. (1973): Granulomatous esophagitis: a case of Crohn's disease limited to the esophagus. *Gastroenterology*, 64:313–319.
15. Hanson, J. T., Thoreson, C., and Morrissey, J. F. (1980): Brush cytology in the diagnosis of upper gastrointestinal malignancy. *Gastrointest. Endosc.*, 26:33–35.
16. Webb, J. N., and Busuttil, A. (1978): Adenocarcinoma of the oesophagus and the oesophagogastric junction. *Br. J. Surg.*, 65:475–479.
17. Kobayoshi, S., and Watanabe, H. (1976): Endoscopic identification of esophageal involvement by carcinoma of the stomach. *Am. J. Gastroenterol.*, 65:416–421.
18. Polk, H. C., Camp, F. A., and Walker, A. W. (1967): Dysphagia of esophageal stenosis: manifestation of metastatic mammary cancer. *Cancer*, 20:2002–2007.
19. Vansant, J. H., and Davis, R. K. (1971): Esophageal obstruction secondary to mediastinal metastasis from breast carcinoma. *Chest*, 60:93–95.

5

ESOPHAGEAL MALIGNANCIES

Esophageal cancer represents one of the less common gastrointestinal malignancies overall in the United States, with only an expected 8,000 new cases per year, compared with an anticipated 100,000 colorectal or 25,000 gastric cancers.[1] Yet in practice, they are not rare, with one case being found in our Unit for every 70 to 100 patients studied. In some settings cases may be encountered more often than this. This is particularly true for municipal and other hospitals serving an inner city black population for whom there is an increased incidence of esophageal cancer,[2] probably linked to the high incidence of alcoholism among such patients,[3] which together with smoking are major risk factors.[4] The increased risk appears to be especially true for black males, where in one study the esophageal cancer was nearly four times more common than for comparable whites (26.3 versus 7.1 per 100,000), twice as common as gastric cancer (26.3 versus 12.7 per 100,000), and slightly more common than colon cancer (26.3 versus 22.5 per 100,000).[2]

SQUAMOUS CARCINOMA

The majority of esophageal cancers are squamous, but the figure varies among series from 60%[5] to 95%,[6] although when the esophagogastric junction is considered to be part of the esophagus the figure is in the 55 to 60% range.[5] By the time these cancers produce symptoms which prompt endoscopy, there is already evidence of local spread in at least 75%, even in those with only the recent onset of dysphagia.[7] Not surprisingly, even surgical resection provides only a modest improvement in survival.[8]

At the time the patient is referred for endoscopy, the diagnosis is usually suggested on the basis of dysphagia, weight loss, and the radiographic appearance of an irregular mass.[7] At this point the endoscopist wishes to provide both descriptive information about the cancer (i.e., location and extent) as well as histologic or cytologic confirmation, even if this does not in itself greatly affect outcome. It is still necessary to provide a tissue diagnosis of malignancy for patients who are considered inoperable, but where irradiation may still be an option. Furthermore, for such patients, the examiner will wish to determine the feasibility of endoscopic placement of a prosthetic tube across the tumor for palliation.[7a]

Location

Most workers find 60% of squamous carcinomas to originate in the proximal two-thirds (upper third 20%, middle third 40%) of the esophagus, with the remaining 40% found in the distal third,[8] although we find 75% in the upper two-thirds with 60% of these in the mid-esophagus (25 to 32 cm) and the remaining 25% in the distal esophagus.

Appearance

Squamous carcinomas may be considered to have three appearances; they may appear as: (a) a polypoid mass; (b) an ulcerating mass; or (c) a malignant stricture. We have already discussed the appearance of malignant strictures (see Chapter 4), which represent approximately 20% of the squamous cancers we see. In this section we take up the other two, which are more common.

Polypoid Mass

In 60 to 70% of our cases, the appearance is of a polypoid mass (Fig. 5-1). This appears as an irregular, hard, friable lesion projecting into the lumen (Fig. 5-1). It may be superficially ulcerated, with the mass still the principal endoscopic feature (Fig. 5-1). Its color is a mixture of deep pink and gray in contrast to the grayish-white appearance of the uninvolved esophagus. Adjacent to the mass there may be evidence of submucosal infiltration by an abrupt

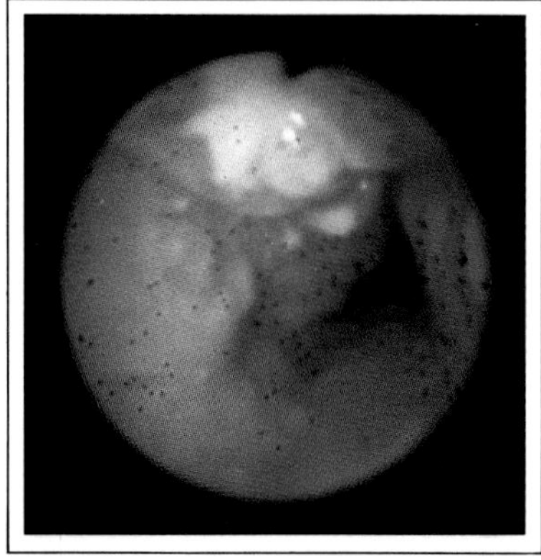

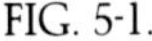

FIG. 5-1.

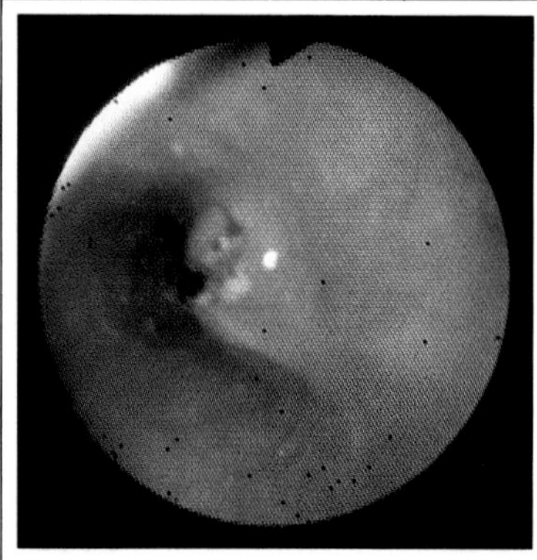

FIG. 5-2.

FIG. 5-1. Esophageal carcinoma, polypoid mass. A large friable mass is seen superficially protruding into the lumen from the left anterior (9 to 12 o'clock) wall.

FIG. 5-2. Esophageal carcinoma, submucosal infiltration. This gives a shelf-like compression of the right (3 o'clock) wall.

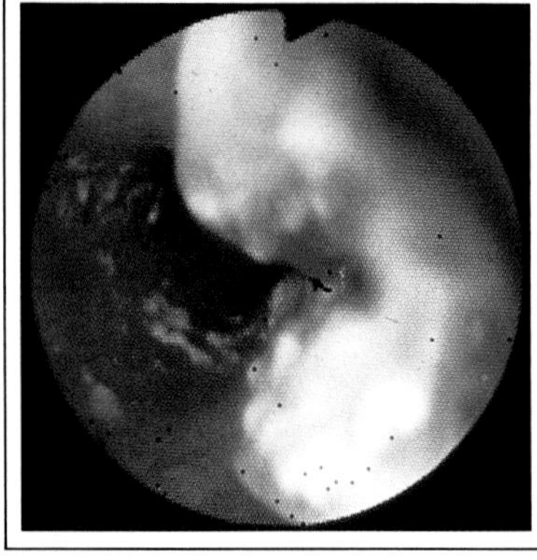

FIG. 5-3.

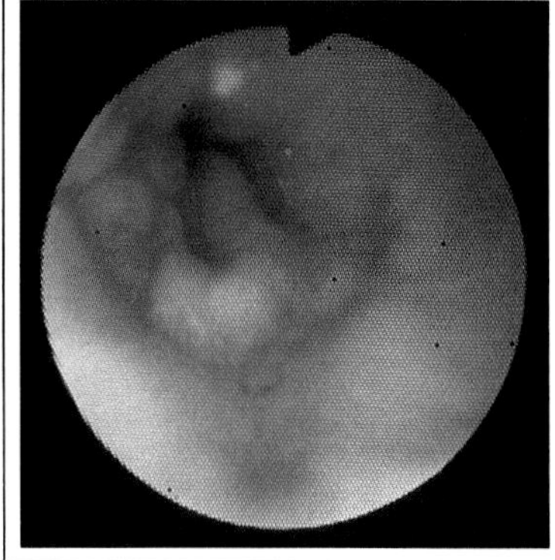

FIG. 5-4.

FIG. 5-3. Esophageal carcinoma, ulcerated mass. The central ulceration is seen at the apex of the mass, which is the most conspicuous endoscopic feature. Carcinoma which has broken through the mucosa is seen adjacent to the central ulceration.

FIG. 5-4. Peptic esophagitis (severe) accompanied by inflammatory polyps. The size of these (<5 mm) suggests that they are inflammatory.

elevation of the wall of the esophagus having essentially normal overlying mucosa, creating the "shelf" appearance (Fig. 5-2).

Ulcerating Mass

In 20% of squamous carcinomas the predominant endoscopic feature is that of an ulceration which is usually large and irregular (Fig. 5-3). The margins of this ulcer are heaped-up and nodular, giving it the appearance of an ulcer set in a mass. The margin is deep pink or red and is set off from the gray-white of the surrounding normal mucosa. The margin of the ulcer is composed of deep pink or reddish-gray tumor nodules (Fig. 5-3). Even without seeing the margin, however, one would suspect carcinoma simply on the basis of the appearance of an ulcerating mass lesion, especially of the proximal or mid-esophagus. Ulcerating cancer of the distal esophagus at the gastroesophageal (GE) junction must be differentiated from severe peptic esophagitis (with ulceration) accompanied by inflammatory polyps (Fig. 5-4).[9] Their size and distribution are the most helpful features in the differentiation. Polyps of less than 5 mm which appear symmetrically are most likely to be related to severe peptic injury of this area, particularly ulceration (Fig. 5-4). Larger polyps with a maximum dimension of greater than 5 mm are more worrisome (Fig. 5-5). Even though some inflammatory polyps may exceed 1 cm[8] (Fig. 5-6), any isolated mass of this size or larger must be aggressively biopsied and brushed to exclude cancer.

Uncommon Appearances of Squamous Carcinoma

Three uncommon appearances for squamous carcinoma are: (a) superficially spreading carcinoma; (b) multifocal carcinoma; and (c) varicoid carcinoma.

Superficially Spreading Carcinoma

Superficially spreading carcinoma represents less than 0.1% of all esophageal cancers.[10] The appearance is that of multiple, tiny plaque-like mucosal nodules running throughout the entire esophagus (Fig. 5-7a). These can be differentiated from other plaque-like appearances (Fig. 5-8), e.g., glycogenic acanthosis (see Chapter 2), by their larger size (greater than 5 mm), their raised appearance, and their rubbery, hard consistency on biopsy. The latter feature distinguishes these lesions from the exudates of *Candida* or severe peptic esophagitis. Biopsy may show only marked dysplasia or *in situ* carcinoma and not reveal occasional foci of invasion which are infrequent even on histologic

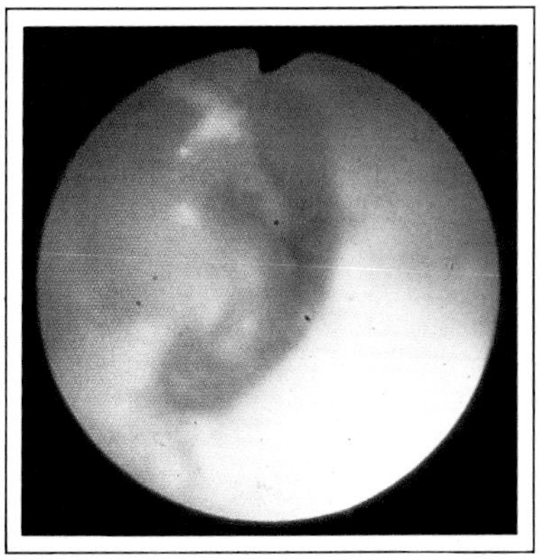

FIG. 5-5.

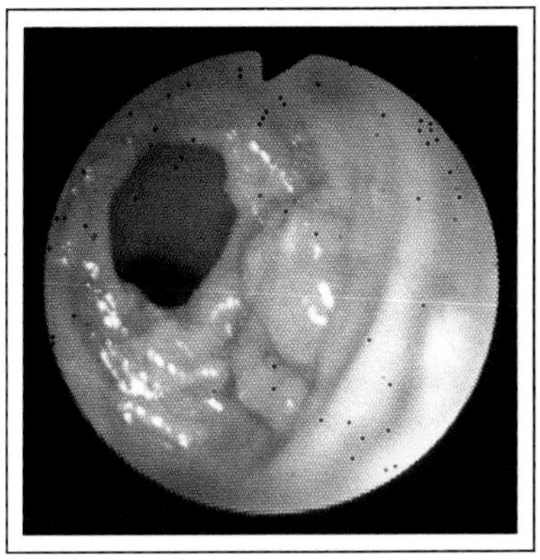

FIG. 5-6.

FIG. 5-5. Esophageal carcinoma, polypoid mass. This was seen endoscopically as an asymmetrical mass (>1 cm) at the GE junction. Note the similarity of its appearance to that in Fig. 5-6.

FIG. 5-6. Large inflammatory (fibroepithelial) polyp. This 1.5-cm polyp with a somewhat irregular appearance was seen adjacent to a peptic stricture and esophagitis, which suggested an inflammatory nature and which was ultimately proved by biopsy and its subsequent course.

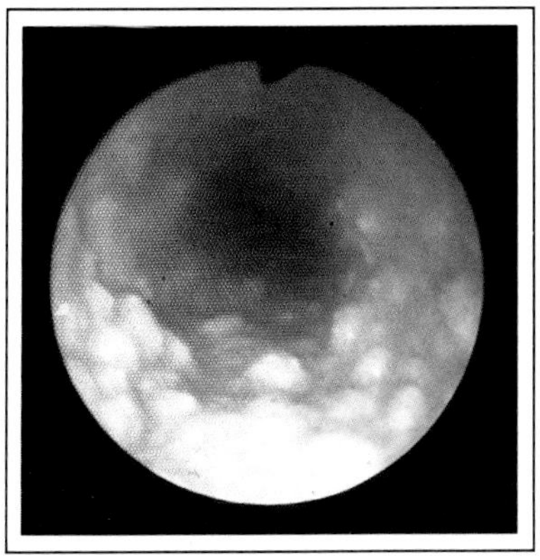

FIG. 5-7a.

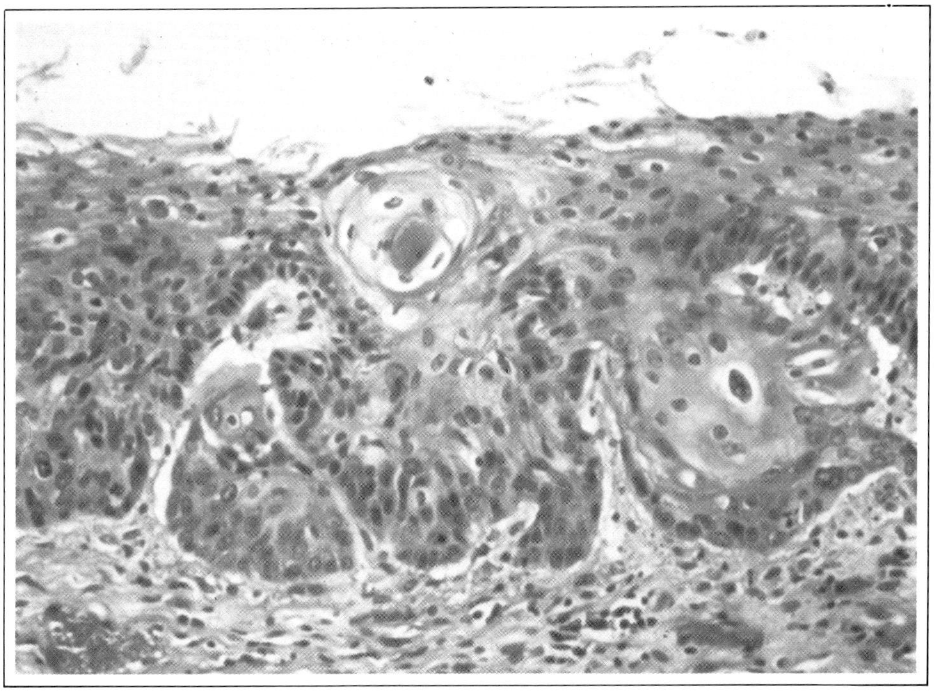

FIG. 5-7b.

FIG. 5-7. a: Esophageal carcinoma, superficially spreading. Endoscopy shows multiple raised, rubbery, hard nodules, ranging in size from several millimeters to 0.7 cm. **b:** Histologic appearance of the superficially spreading esophageal carcinoma [seen in (a), resected specimen]. The cancer is largely intraepithelial.

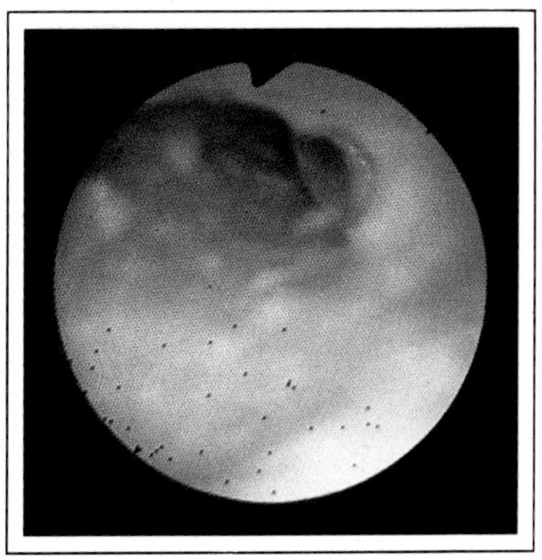

FIG. 5-8.

FIG. 5-8. Glycogenic acanthosis. The typical lesions are small (<5 mm) pale, soft, mucosal excrescences.

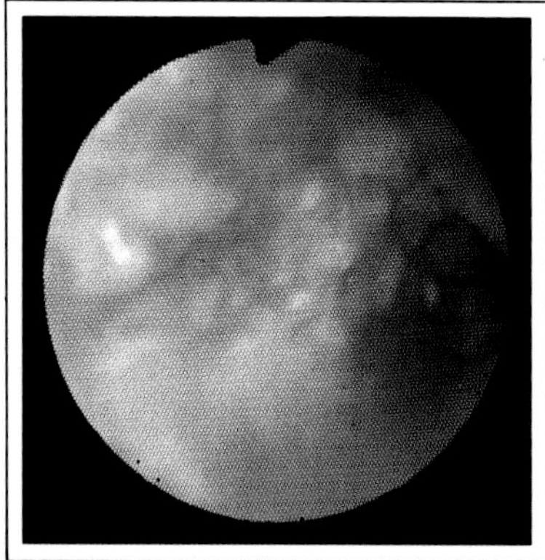

FIG. 5-9a.

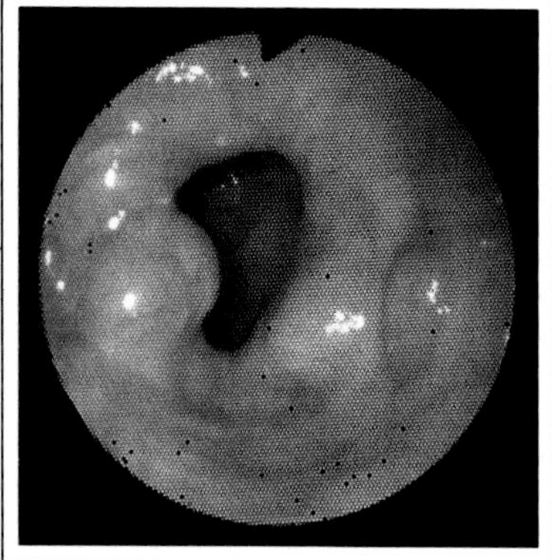

FIG. 5-9b.

FIG. 5-9. Multifocal carcinoma. **a:** The main focus is seen to have a tail-like extension on the left anterior (9 o'clock) wall for approximately 5 cm. This was proved histologically in the resected specimen to represent intraepithelial spread. **b:** A separate 5-mm focus is seen 5 cm from the distal main focus but adjacent to the tail-like (intraepithelial) extension.

examination of the resected specimen (Fig. 5-7b). It is important to attempt to define the proximal and distal extent of the lesion and provide histologic and cytologic confirmation prior to treatment of what may be the most curable form of all esophageal carcinomas.[10]

Multifocal Carcinoma

In most cases esophageal cancer arises from one location. However, in a small percentage of patients a second focus is present.[11] We have observed two types of multifocal carcinoma. In one case, the second focus seen was completely separate (5 cm) from the original carcinoma, whereas in the other there was intraepithelial spread down from the original focus in a tail-like fashion for approximately 5 cm (Fig. 5-9a), which was proven histologically in the resected specimen. In addition, there was a 5-cm satellite tumor in the vicinity of, but separate from, this interepithelial extension (Fig. 5-9b).

Varicoid Carcinoma

In rare cases the carcinoma grows by longitudinal submucosal extension without producing luminal encroachment.[12] This results in the appearance of cylindrical masses which radiographically simulate esophageal varices[13] (Fig. 5-10a), hence the descriptive term varicoid carcinoma. At endoscopy these masses must not be confused with varices (see Chapter 8), which have a grayish-blue or white appearance, are easily compressible, and run up from the GE junction (Fig. 5-10b). By contrast, varicoid carcinomas have a deep pink or reddish-gray appearance and are rubbery, hard masses (Fig. 5-10c) running down from the mid to distal esophagus.

Biopsy and Brushing Cytology

The approach to biopsy and cytology of these lesions to a large extent depends on their appearance.

Polypoid Mass

If one chooses the proper biopsy site, a positive result may be expected in well over 90% of the cases. For the yield to be high, it is often important to carefully observe the mass in its entirety, searching for the point where the intact overlying esophageal mucosa becomes disrupted by the cancer itself, i.e., mucosal "breakthrough." Cancerous mucosa may be recognized by its deep pink or red-gray appearance, which is the predominant mucosa of the mass (Fig. 5-1). Along with this, there is gross nodularity and friability of the surface of the mass. When a mass is present, we believe biopsy should always be attempted first, rather than obscuring the field with blood from brushing. If there is a well-defined mass and point of mucosal breakthrough (Fig. 5-1), little additional yield will result from brushing cytology[14,15] providing the endoscopist can perform at least six, but preferably 10, biopsies of the lesion.[14] If, on the other hand, either the mass (Fig. 5-10) or the point of mucosal breakthrough is not well defined (Fig. 5-5) or for other technical reasons cannot be biopsied adequately, brushing cytology should be aggressively pursued.[14,15]

Ulcerated Mass

As in the case of the polypoid mass, for an ulcerated mass the endoscopist must first carefully observe where the cancer first breaks through to the surface (Fig. 5-3). The yield from biopsy or brushing cytology will be the greatest at this point. If the endoscopist fails to observe the demarcation between intact mucosa and tumor, as well as tumor and ulceration, the opportunity for obtaining a positive histologic or cytologic result is lost.

The number of biopsies taken from an ulcerous lesion is more critical than those taken from a mass because the inflammatory tissue of the ulcer base tends to be sampled, and this is generally not helpful in establishing a diagnosis. It would be well to obtain a minimum of six and generally 10 or more biopsies of any suspicious ulcer,[15] especially

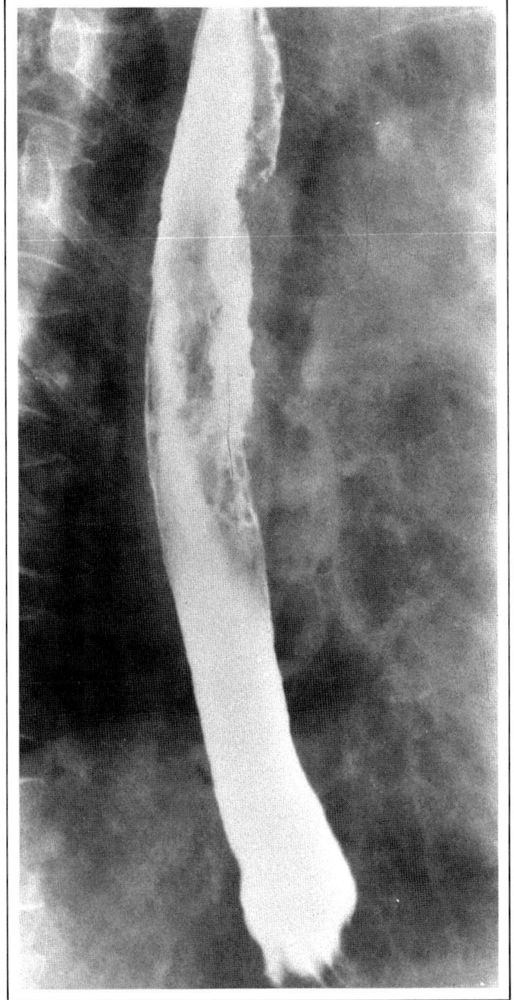

FIG. 5-10a.

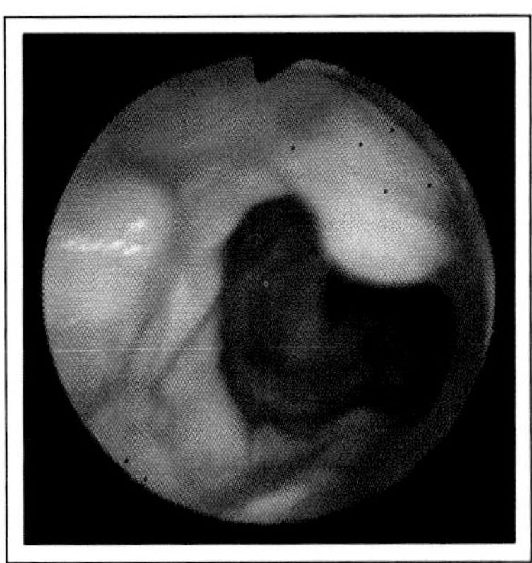

FIG. 5-10b.

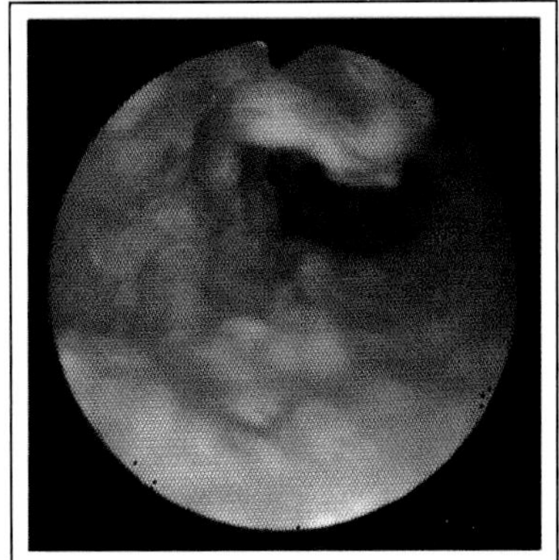

FIG. 5-10c.

FIG. 5-10. a: Varicoid carcinoma. An esophagram shows several irregular polypoid filling defects of the mid-esophagus, resembling esophageal varices. **b:** Esophageal varices. These easily compressible structures must not be confused endoscopically with varicoid carcinoma. **c:** Varicoid carcinoma. Multiple masses of tumor are seen circumferentially projecting into the lumen from 12, 6, and 9 o'clock, largely from the mid-esophagus but sparing the distal portion.

where the boundaries of its margin are not clear-cut. In cases where it is impossible to biopsy the entire margin, brushing cytology would be pursued especially for that part of the lesion.

Stricture

See Chapter 4.

Planned Follow-Up

The endoscopist's concern and suspicion regarding any abnormality, especially an "ulcer," must be communicated as a crucial part of his interpretation. Although his impression may be "severe peptic esophagitis with ulceration" (Fig. 5-4), it would not be wrong for him to communicate his uncertainty using the phrase "but with atypical features" and state precisely what his concern is. Moreover, he should suggest a time, i.e., 3 to 4 weeks after the institution of treatment for peptic esophagitis, for repeat endoscopy for biopsy and cytologic studies.

Cancer Surveillance

Preexisting conditions, e.g., lye stricture (see Chapter 4), achalasia (see Chapter 7), and Barrett's esophagus (see Chapter 6), are all well known to predispose to esophageal carcinoma.[16] Another predisposing condition which is now receiving increasing recognition is that of carcinoma of the oral cavity,[17] hypopharynx, or larynx.[18] For patients presenting with untreated squamous carcinomas of the oropharynx or upper respiratory tract, an overall incidence of 1.6% has been found of esophageal cancer as an unsuspected second primary when screening endoscopy was employed.[18a] This is more than 30 times its expected frequency in the general population.[17] For this reason we recommend endoscopy be routinely performed in all such patients prior to treatment. For male patients with treated cancers of the oral cavity and upper airways, the incidence of a second primary involving the esophagus is also 30 times that of the general population,[17] with that of treated glottic carcinomas, specifically, in one study, 0.5%.[18] Assuming an already increased incidence of esophageal carcinoma for black males, the additional risk for treated oral or glottic carcinomas could approach 1% per year (30 per 100,000 × 30 = 900 per 100,000, i.e., about 1%). This would make this group of patients an important subset for surveillance for squamous carcinoma of the esophagus on a yearly basis. We have ourselves observed two such cases which were examined for surveillance. In both cases the early cancer found proved to be completely amenable to irradiation.

The cancers one finds as a result of surveillance are small, inconspicuous areas of focal nodularity and superficial ulceration (Fig. 5-11). They must be carefully searched for in the mid and distal esophagus. For any such lesion found, biopsy and cytology are pursued aggressively.

ADENOCARCINOMA

In one study where the esophagogastric junction (including the cardia) was considered part of the esophagus, 45% of the esophageal malignancies were adenocarcinoma.[19] This would not be unexpected, as up to two-thirds of cardial adenocarcinomas invade the distal 1 to 2 cm of the esophagus.[19] When present, adenocarcinomas are found principally in the distal esophagus within 5 to 10 cm of the GE junction,[6,19,20] with most, in actuality, being carcinomas of the cardia which have infiltrated across the GE junction into the distal esophagus. Less than 5% of esophageal adenocarcinomas are primary,[6,19] with many if not most of these arising in association with Barrett's esophagus[21] (see Chapter 6).

Appearance

Adenocarcinomas may display both an infiltrative as well as an exophytic growth pattern but most often are infiltrative[20] and appear as fixed, enlarged, asymmetrical nodular folds (Fig. 5-12). Those having an exophytic growth pattern are seen as 5-mm to 1.5-cm, reddish-orange-gray masses at or just below the GE junction (Fig. 5-13). A characteristic feature of these masses is their extreme friability; they bleed copiously even when only gently touched by the endoscope.

Biopsy and Brushing Cytology

The caliber of the endoscope used determines where biopsies and brushings are taken for these lesions. Although

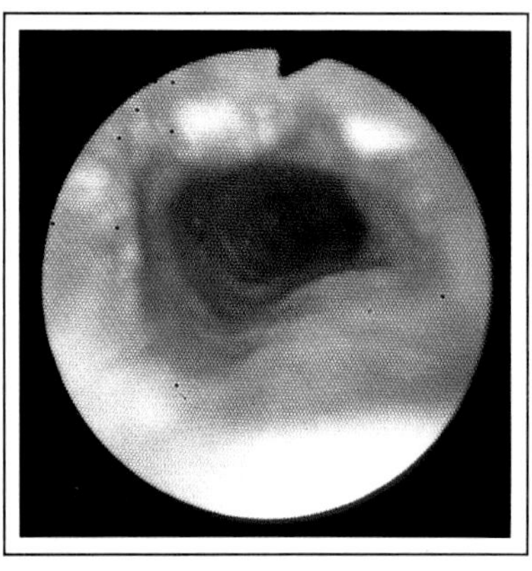

FIG. 5-11.

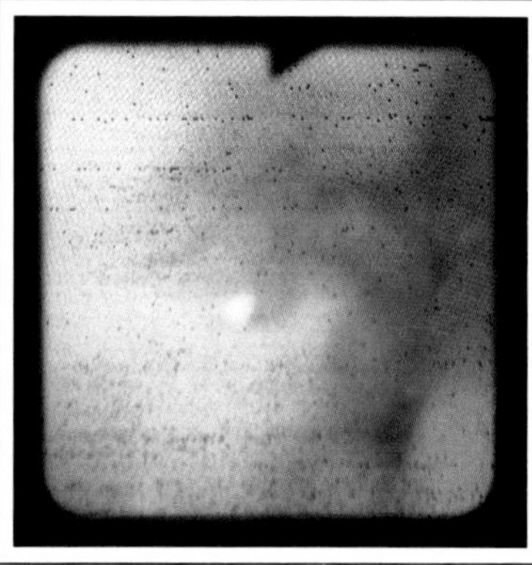

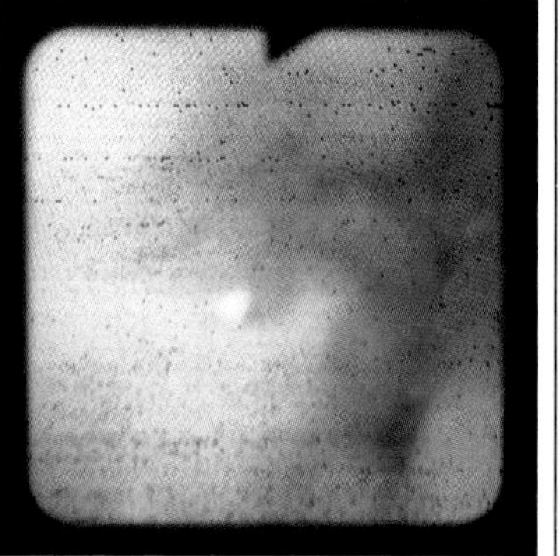

FIG. 5-12.

FIG. 5-11. Esophageal carcinoma as a second primary. This was found as a result of periodic screening in a patient with treated carcinoma of the larynx. The early cancer is seen as several small eroded nodules at 12 o'clock. Biopsies showed squamous carcinoma, and the lesion was satisfactorily treated with irradiation.

FIG. 5-12. Esophageal carcinoma, adenocarcinoma, arising in a cardia. An infiltrated nodular fold with tumor breakthrough is seen with the appearance of orange-red nodules.

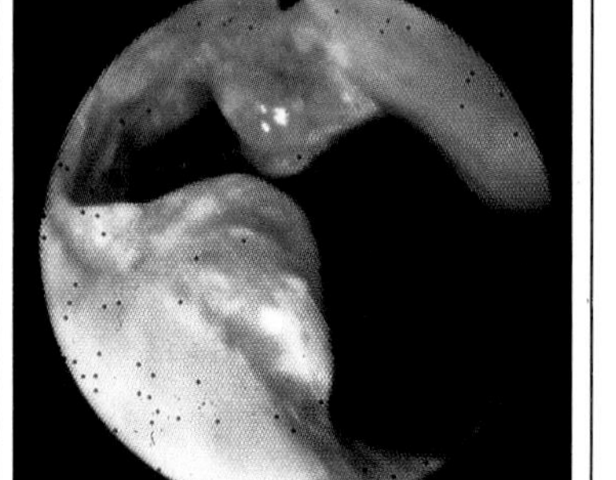

FIG. 5-13.

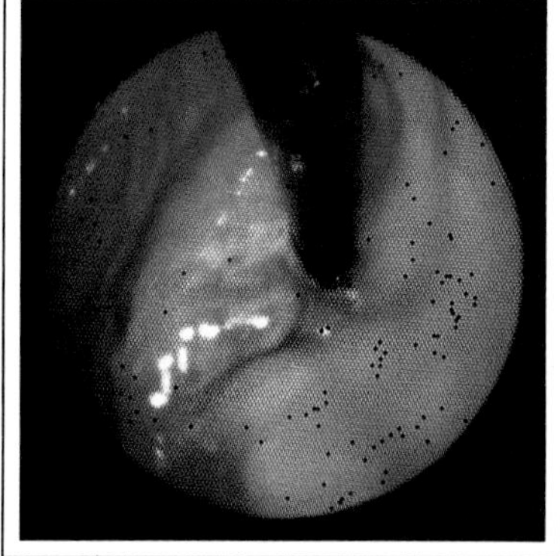

FIG. 5-14.

FIG. 5-13. Esophageal carcinoma, adenocarcinoma, arising from the cardia. In this case eccentric polypoid masses are seen at the GE junction.

FIG. 5-14. Cardial adenocarcinoma. A 9-mm narrow-caliber pediatric-type endoscope views the lesion with its tip in the U-turn (retroflexed) position. The cardia is replaced by tumor.

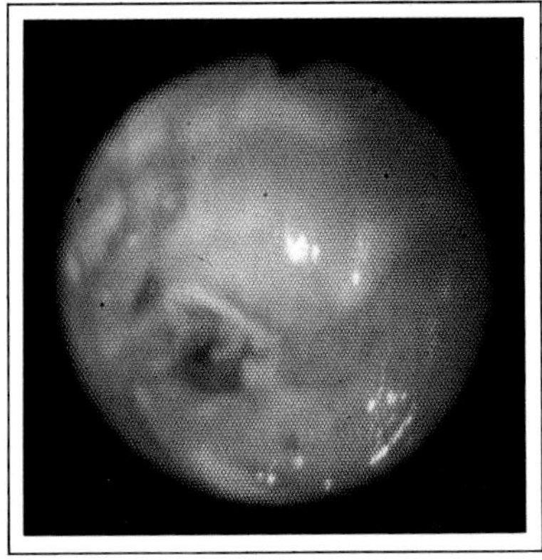

FIG. 5-15.

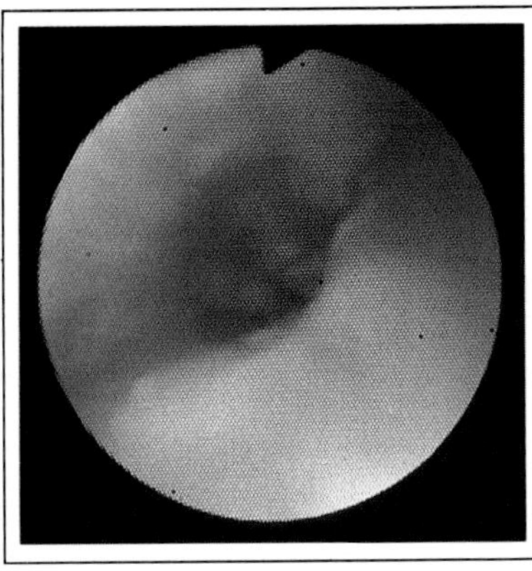

FIG. 5-16.

FIG. 5-15. Esophageal lymphoma, primary. An ulcerated mass at the GE junction was noted from which biopsies showed histiocytic lymphoma.

FIG. 5-16. Esophageal lymphoma, secondary. Mediastinal lymphoma (poorly differentiated lymphoma type) with contiguous esophageal involvement is seen as a large right posterior (3 to 6 o'clock) ulcerated mass.

it is desirable to obtain a tissue diagnosis, it often is not possible to force a larger caliber (11 to 13 mm) endoscope across an area into which the lesion has extended (Fig. 5-13) to obtain biopsies directly from the cardia. If one attempts to pass this instrument across, in many cases bleeding results, which reduces the chance of obtaining tissue from the point of tumor breakthrough. Our approach is to initially examine such patients with the small-caliber (9 mm) endoscope, which affords the best chance of observing the actual site of origin (Fig. 5-14) in the cardia. If this can be accomplished, multiple brushings and biopsies are taken from the cardia with the instrument in a retroflexed U-turn (Fig. 5-14). Care is taken not to apply excessive force when crossing the cardia as this would cause the area to be obscured with blood. As with any esophageal cancer, care is taken first to observe the point at which the mucosa appears disrupted by deep pink or erythematous superficially ulcerated nodules (Fig. 5-14), where six to 10 biopsies[15] would be taken to maximize the changes of a positive result. Brushing cytology has an adjunctive role in these cases, increasing the yield over biopsy, especially in cases in which the lesion appears somewhat stenotic or where the area of mucosal breakthrough cannot be biopsied.[14]

UNCOMMON ESOPHAGEAL MALIGNANCIES

Rarely, the endoscopist encounters a lymphoma, leukemic involvement, sarcoma, or metastatic carcinoma of the esophagus, a group which comprise about 1 to 2% of all malignant lesions at this site. Of these, we have already considered carcinoma metastatic to the esophagus leading to stricture formation (see Chapter 4). In this section, we consider lymphoma, leukemic involvement, and polypoid sarcoma.

Lymphoma

The esophagus is the least common site of gastrointestinal involvement for lymphoma, representing less than 1% of the total. Like lymphomatous involvment elsewhere in the gastrointestinal tract, the histiocytic type predominates, with Hodgkin's disease occurring least often.[22] Lymphoma involving the esophagus may be a primary process or secondary to contiguous spread from mediastinal involvement, each having a distinctive appearance.

Primary Esophageal Lymphoma

Primary esophageal lymphomas are typically located in the GE junction and are indistinguishable from carcinoma arising in this area, having the appearance of a polypoid or ulcerating mass (Fig. 5-15) composed entirely of tumor, which in most cases is histiocytic lymphoma.[23]

Esophageal Involvement by Contiguous Spread

In patients with evidence of mediastinal lymphoma, the esophagus may be involved by contiguous spread (Fig. 5-16). In these cases extrinsic compression of the posterior aspect of the esophagus may be noted, giving rise to a "mass." At the point where there is mucosal infiltration, there may be superficial ulceration or a pseudomembrane. The mucosa overlying most of the "mass," however, is intact or shows only nonspecific changes.

Biopsy and Brushing

In the case of primary esophageal lymphoma, the tumor mass is brushed and biopsied as would be done with any esophageal malignancy. The endoscopist carefully observes the lesion specifically for points of mucosal breakthrough. For secondary involvement, it is the ulcerated portion of the mass which should be sought specifically for biopsy (Fig. 5-16).

Leukemic Involvement

Gross leukemic involvement of the esophagus which could potentially be recognized by the endoscopist is un-

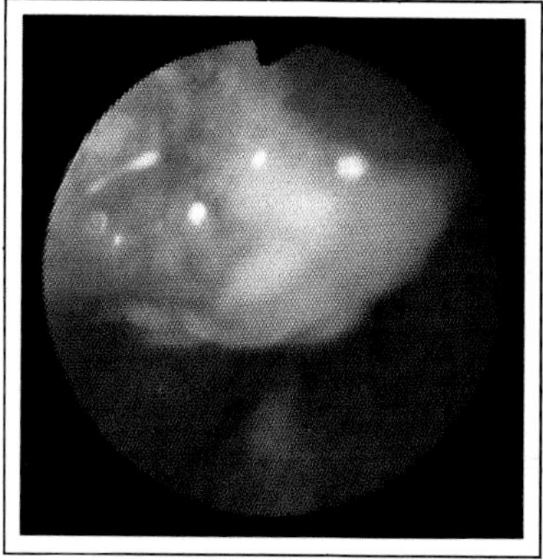

FIG. 5-17.

FIG. 5-17. Liposarcoma of the esophagus. A rare mesenchymal tumor appeared as a bulky, polypoid mass, from which large pieces broke off on biopsy.

usual. Even at autopsy, in one study[23a], it was found in only 2% (4 of 235 cases with leukemia). When present, this appeared as discrete nodules (3 cases) or as a long (7 cm) stricture (1 case). Because of the infrequency of gross leukemic involvement, the endoscopist would regard any abnormal appearance encountered in leukemia as much more likely from opportunistic infection (*candida* or *herpes simplex*) or otherwise associated with treatment (Chapter 3).

Polypoid Sarcoma

A variety of rare mesenchymal tumors, including leiomyosarcoma and carcinosarcoma, are encountered rarely.[24] These tumors grow to enormous proportions and as such should be considered in the differential diagnosis of any extensive malignant lesion of the esophagus, especially where there is marked mucosal friability with large pieces of the tumor breaking off on biopsy (Fig. 5-17).

REFERENCES

1. American Cancer Society (1981): *Cancer Facts and Figures.* ACS, New York.
2. Miller, I. M., and Chapman, T. W. (1981): Reviewing cancer in American Blacks: a Baltimore study. *J. Natl. Med. Assoc.*, 73:127–132.
3. National Institutes of Mental Health (1972): *Alcohol and Health.* First Annual Report to the Congress. The National Institute on Alcohol Abuse and Alcoholism of the National Institutes of Mental Health. U.S. Government Printing Office, Washington, D.C.
4. Wynder, E. L., and Bross, J. J. (1961): A study of etiological factors—cancer of the esophagus. *Cancer,* 14:389–413.
5. Heck, H. A., and Ross, N. P. (1981): Esophageal and gastroesophageal junctional carcinoma. *Cancer,* 46:1873–1878.
6. Turnbull, A. D., and Goodner, J. T. (1968): Primary adenocarcinoma of the esophagus. *Cancer,* 22:915–918.
7. Rubin, P. (1973): Cancer of the gastrointestinal tract. I. Esophagus: detection and diagnosis. *JAMA,* 226:1540–1546.

7a. Peura, D. A., Heit, H. A., Johnson, L. F., and Boyce, H. W. (1978): Esophageal prosthesis in cancer. *Dig. Dis. Sci.*, 23:796–800.

8. Parker, E. F., and Gregorie, H. B. (1976): Carcinoma of the esophagus: long-term results. *JAMA,* 235:1019–1020.
9. Bleshman, M. H., Banner, M. P., Johnson, R. C., and DeFord, J. W. (1978): The inflammatory esophago-gastric polyp and fold. *Radiology,* 128:590–593.
10. Ushigome, S., Spjut, H. J., and Noon, G. P. (1967): Extensive dysplasia and carcinoma in situ of esophageal epithelium. *Cancer,* 70:1022–1029.
11. Suckow, E. E., Yokoo, H., and Brock, D. R. (1962): Intraepithelial carcinoma concomitant with esophageal carcinoma. *Cancer,* 15:733–739.
12. Odes, H. S., Maor, E., Barki, G., Charuzi, I., Krawiec, J., and Bar-Ziv, J. (1980): Varicoid carcinoma of the esophagus: report of a patient with adenocarcinoma and review of the literature. *Am. J. Gastroenterol.*, 73:141–145.
13. Yates, C. W., LeVine, M., and Jensen, K. M. (1978): Varicoid carcinoma of the esophagus. *Radiology,* 122:605–608.
14. Hanson, J. T., Thoreson, C., and Morrissey, J. F. (1980): Brush cytology in the diagnosis of upper gastrointestinal malignancy. *Gastrointest. Endosc.*, 26:33–35.
15. Witzel, L., Halter, F., Gretillat, P. A., Scheurer, U., and Keller, M. (1976): Evaluation of specific value of endoscopic biopsies and brush cytology for malignancies of the oesophagus and stomach. *Gut,* 17:375–377.
16. Wynder, E. L., and Mabuchi, K. (1973): Etiological and environmental factors (cancer of the gastrointestinal tract and esophagus). *JAMA,* 226:1546–1548.
17. Tepperman, B. S., and Fitzpatrick, P. J. (1981): Second respiratory and upper digestive tract cancers after oral cancers. *Lancet,* 2:547–549.
18. Wagenfeld, D. J. H., Hardwood, A. R., Bryce, D. P., VanNostrand, A. W. P., and DeBoer, G. (1981): Second primary respiratory tract malignancies in glottic cancers. *Cancer,* 46:1883–1886.

18a. Gluckman, J. L., Crissmann, J. D., and Donegan, J. O. (1980): Multicentric squamous-cell carcinoma of the upper aerodigestive tract. *Head-Neck Surg.*, 3:90–96.

19. Webb, J. N., and Busuttil, A. (1978): Adenocarcinoma of the oesophagus and oesophago-gastric junction. *Br. J. Surg.*, 65:475–477.
20. Kobayashi, S., and Watanabe, S. (1976): Endoscopic identification of esophageal involvement by carcinoma of the stomach. *Am. J. Gastroenterol.*, 65:416–421.
21. Haggitt, R. C., Tryzelaar, J., Ellis, E., and Colcher, H. (1978): Adenocarcinoma complicating columnar epithelium-lined (Barrett's) esophagus. *Am. J. Clin. Pathol.*, 70:1–5.
22. Carnovale, R. L., Goldstein, H. M., Zornoza, J., and Dodd, G. (1977): Radiologic manifestations of esophageal lymphoma. *Am. J. Roentgenol.*, 128:751–754.
23. Berman, M. D., Falchuk, K. R., Trey, C., and Gramm, H. F. (1979): Primary histocytic lymphoma of the esophagus. *Dis. Dig. Sci.*, 24:883–886.

23a. Gilver, R. L. (1970): Esophageal lesions in leukemia and lymphoma. *Am. J. Dig. Dis.*, 15:31–36.

24. DeMeester, T. R., and Skinner, D. B. (1975): Polypoid sarcomas of the esophagus: a rare, but potentially curable neoplasm. *Ann. Thorac. Surg.*, 20:405–416.

6

BARRETT'S ESOPHAGUS

Between 13%[1] and 20%[2] of patients with endoscopic evidence of peptic esophagitis have visual evidence of gastric metaplasia (Barrett's changes) involving some part of the distal esophagus. As only 60% of patients with symptomatic reflux have endoscopic evidence of esophagitis,[3] one might expect the actual incidence of Barrett's changes in patients with symptomatic reflux to be 5 to 10%, which is our experience. In addition, we find that patients with Barrett's changes generally have had reflux symptoms of longstanding duration. Because of the malignant potential of Barrett's esophagus,[1] it is particularly important to identify patients with this condition for whom periodic endoscopic surveillance will be necessary.

APPEARANCE

In a patient with Barrett's esophagus, the squamocolumnar junction is located above the 32 cm level, generally between 26 and 30 cm from the incisors (Fig. 6-1). It may be relatively uniform, like the gastroesophageal (GE) junction, but often it is strikingly irregular with tongue-like projections (Fig. 6-2) of the deep orange-red Barrett's epithelium extending up into the squamous epithelium; in addition, there may be islands of pearly white squamous epithelium just below the junctional line, entirely surrounded by Barrett's epithelium (Fig. 6-1). At and just above the junction may be reflux changes, which are often those of severe esophagitis (Fig. 6-3).

Barrett's mucosa itself, like gastric mucosa, has an orange coloration but differs from gastric mucosa (see Chapter 11) in being more erythematous, giving it a deep orange-red coloration in contrast to the orange-yellow or pink-yellow of gastric mucosa (Fig. 6-4). Within Barrett's epithelium, tiny filamentous mucosal vessels can sometimes be identified (Fig. 6-4) which lack the usual parallelism of esophageal capillaries (see Chapter 1).

Barrett's mucosa can be followed down to the end of the tubular esophagus (Fig. 6-5), but it is usually not possible to find the junction between Barrett's mucosa and the cardia, even at close range.

HISTOLOGIC CONFIRMATION OF THE DIAGNOSIS

Even though there may be considerable histologic heterogeneity,[4] the commonest appearance found for Barrett's

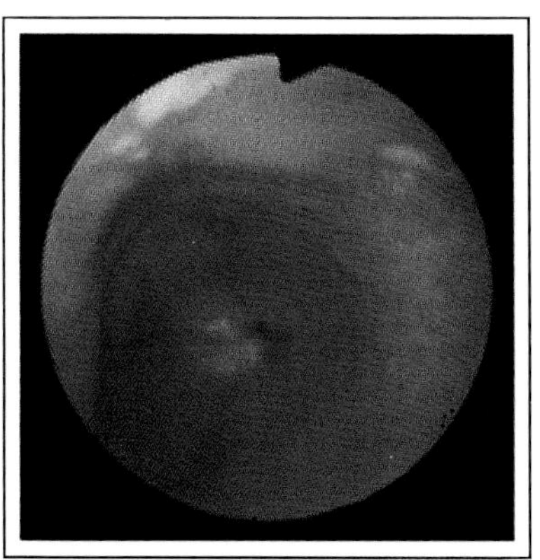

FIG. 6-1.

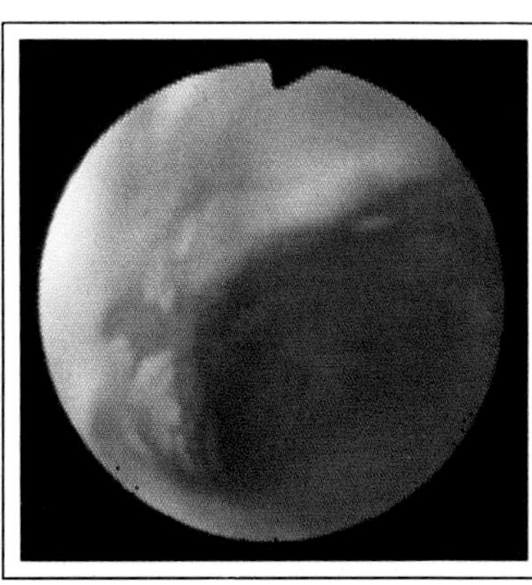

FIG. 6-2.

FIG. 6-1. Barrett's esophagus. The distal third of the esophagus (to the cardia in the distance) is lined with typical (orange-red) Barrett's-type mucosa. Several islands of residual pearly white squamous epithelium are noted at 11 and 1 o'clock.

FIG. 6-2. Barrett's esophagus. Tongue-like projections of Barrett's epithelium are seen at the junction of the Barrett's and squamous epithelium (same case as in Fig. 6-1).

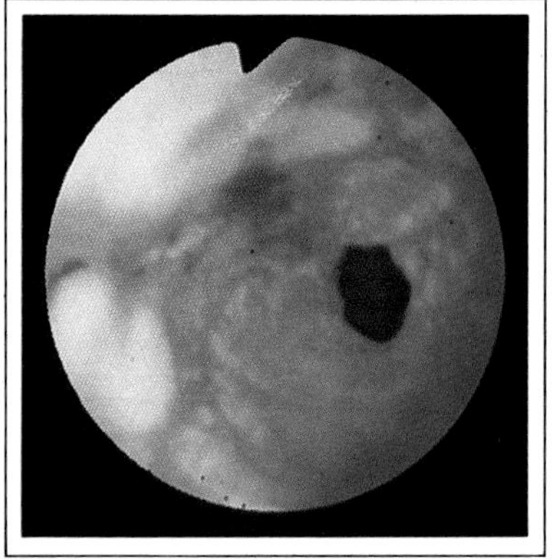

FIG. 6-3.

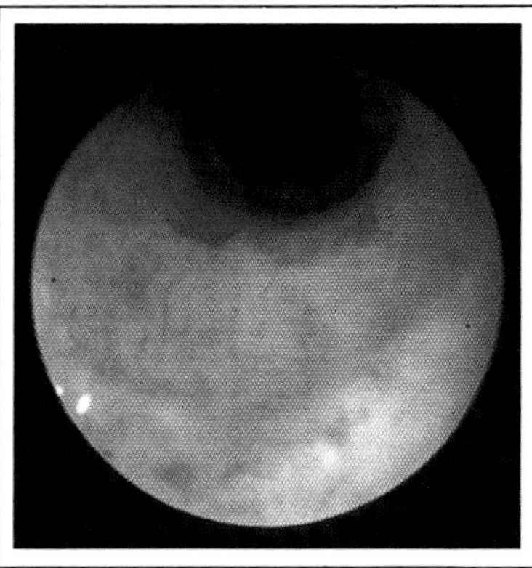

FIG. 6-4.

FIG. 6-3. Barrett's esophagus. This was suggested by the presence of confluent erythema of the distal 2 cm of the esophagus, just distal to a 5-cm zone of focal adherent inflammatory exudate.

FIG. 6-4. Barrett's esophagus. In addition to erythema, there are short, stubby vessels, in contrast to those of normal mucosa, which are longer and run in parallel (see Fig. 1-24b).

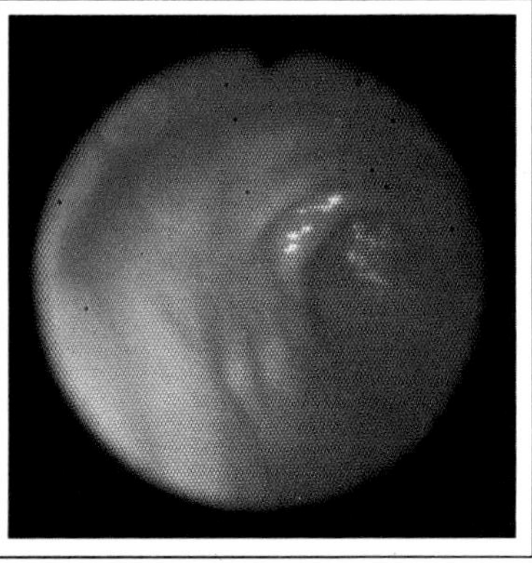

FIG. 6-5.

FIG. 6-5. Barrett's esophagus. In this case Barrett's esophagus and the cardia (in the distance) were indistinguishable.

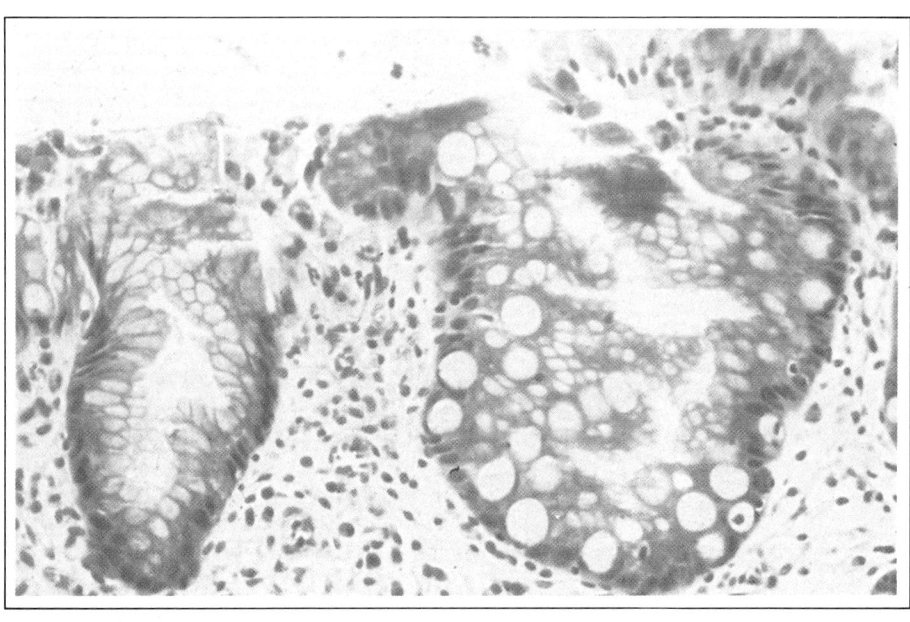

FIG. 6-6.

FIG. 6-6. Biopsy of Barrett's epithelium, distal esophagus. This shows specialized columnar epithelium with intestinal-type goblet cells, in contrast to that of normal cardia (seen on the left-hand side of the field).

epithelium is that of specialized columnar epithelium with intestinal-type goblet cells (Fig. 6-6).[4,4a] To confirm a diagnosis of Barrett's esophagus, one takes advantage of the fact that intestinal-type goblet cells are not found in the cardia, even with atrophic gastritis (see Chapter 14). One therefore takes biopsies beginning from the cardia and continuing into the presumed Barrett's esophagus, anticipating an abrupt transition from cardial glandular mucosa to the specialized columnar type of Barrett's epithelium (Fig. 6-6). We find that, more than any other histologic change, it is the presence of intestinal-type epithelium in biopsies taken from above the hiatal impression which is most

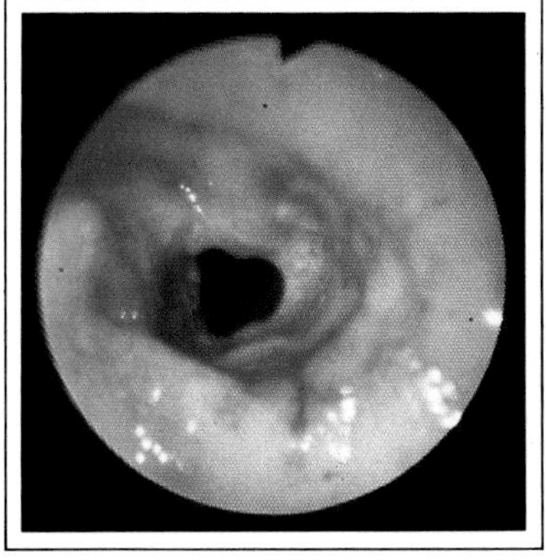
FIG. 6-7.

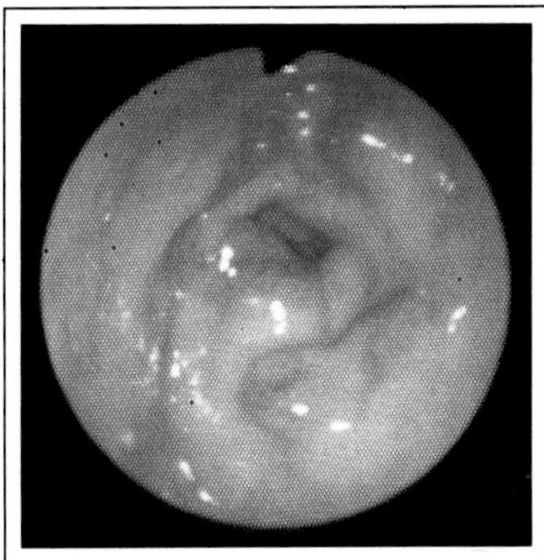
FIG. 6-8.

FIG. 6-7. Mid-esophageal stricture associated with Barrett's esophagus. There is severe esophagitis (ulceration and pseudomembrane) just above this stricture at the squamocolumnar junction.

FIG. 6-8. Mid-esophageal stricture at the squamocolumnar (Barrett's) junction with erosions (moderate esophagitis) only.

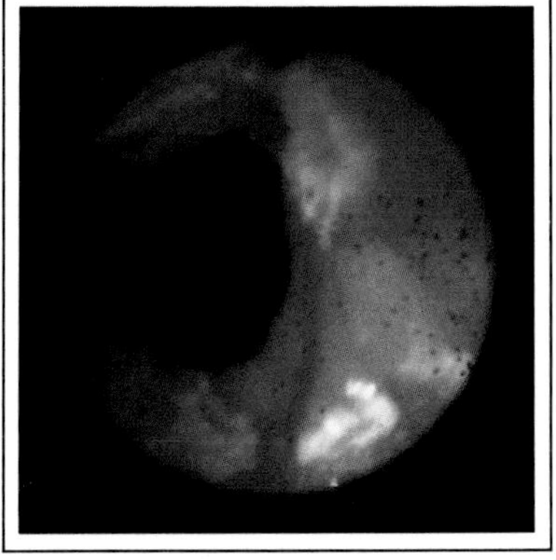
FIG. 6-9.

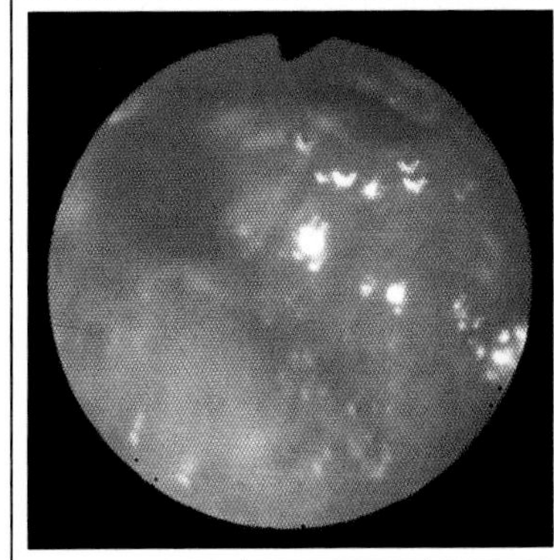
FIG. 6-10.

FIG. 6-9. Mid-esophageal stricture in a 13-year-old boy arising exclusively within Barrett's epithelium in association with extensive (Barrett's type) ulceration. The stricture probably resulted from ulcer scarring. At surgery the ulcer of the anterior wall (12 o'clock) was found to have penetrated into the pericardium.

FIG. 6-10. Malignant stricture arising in Barrett's esophagus. The marked stricture at 12 o'clock would not admit even a 1.7-mm brush. Biopsies around it showed typical Barrett's epithelium. In contrast to Fig. 6-9, this appearance was considered highly suspicious because of the degree of narrowing even though the mucosa above the stricture was intact.

suggestive of the diagnosis of Barrett's esophagus, especially where biopsies from below this show cardia-type mucosa. Additional biopsies are taken through the length of the presumed Barrett's esophagus, especially within 2 cm of the squamocolumnar junction, where at least four biopsies are taken for evidence of dysplasia, i.e., cytologic changes suggestive of neoplastic transformation (see "Endoscopic Surveillance," this chapter).

OTHER APPEARANCES

Benign Mid-Esophageal Strictures

Some patients with Barrett's changes have endoscopy because of dysphagia due to a mid-esophageal stricture (Fig. 6-7) which forms at the junction of squamous and Barrett's epithelium.[5] Apart from their location, these are indistinguishable from a benign peptic stricture (see Chapter 4) at the GE junction. Just as with a peptic stricture of the GE junction, there may be evidence of esophagitis within the mouth of the stricture and just above it (Fig. 6-8); in some cases this is striking (Fig. 6-7), whereas in others it is less apparent (Fig. 6-8). Rarely, a stricture (Fig. 6-9) forms within Barrett's esophagus in association with Barrett's ulcers. These strictures can be differentiated from malignant strictures (see below) arising within Barrett's epithelium (Fig. 6-10) by virtue of the ulcer itself (generally not present in cancer), providing there are no obvious tumor masses or nodules. Nevertheless, any stricture arising within Barrett's epithelium (as opposed to the junction) deserves an especially aggressive effort at biopsy and brushing cytology.

Barrett's Ulcers

Within Barrett's epithelium, frank peptic ulcers are encountered, ranging in size between 1 and 2 cm.[6] These are often but not invariably within 2 cm of the squamocolumnar (Barrett's) junction. Some may be considerably below this point, especially if Barrett's segment is long. The ulcers themselves are for the most part sharply marginated with a punched-out appearance (Fig. 6-11).

Early Barrett's Changes

We have observed several cases of tongue-like extensions of typical Barrett's-appearing orange-red mucosa for 2 to 3 cm above the GE junction in patients with longstanding reflux (Fig. 6-12). They differ from an accentuated GE junction (Fig. 6-13) or from esophageal erosions (Fig. 6-14) in that they are longer ($\geq$1 cm) and wider ($\geq$1 cm). Biopsies taken from these areas have revealed specialized columnar

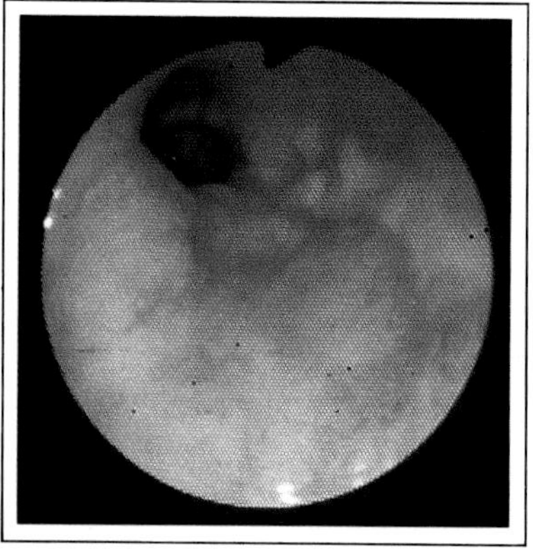

FIG. 6-11.

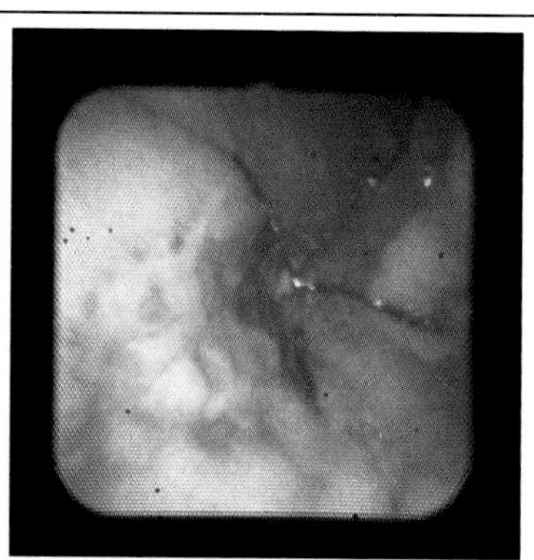

FIG. 6-12.

FIG. 6-11. Barrett's ulcer. A 2-cm ulcer is located 3 cm from the squamocolumnar (Barrett's) junction, 2 cm above the cardia. This was found in the mid-portion of a long Barrett's esophagus.

FIG. 6-12. Early Barrett's changes. Broad bands of intestinalized (biopsy proved) columnar epithelium ascending into the distal esophageal mucosa, which appears thickened in a patient with longstanding reflux symptoms. Whether this evolves into the picture seen in Fig. 6-1 or has the same malignant potential is unknown.

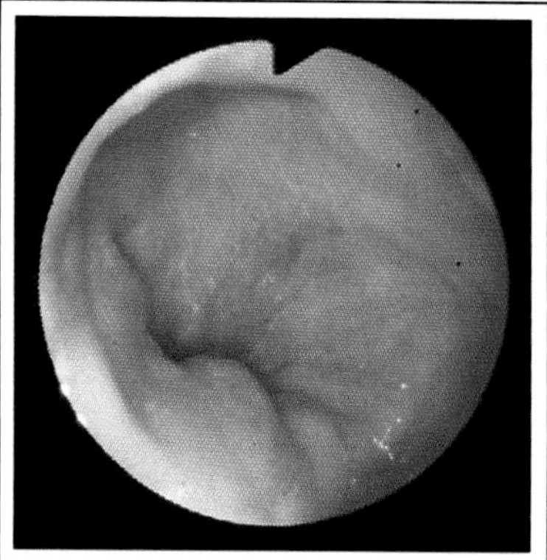

FIG. 6-13.

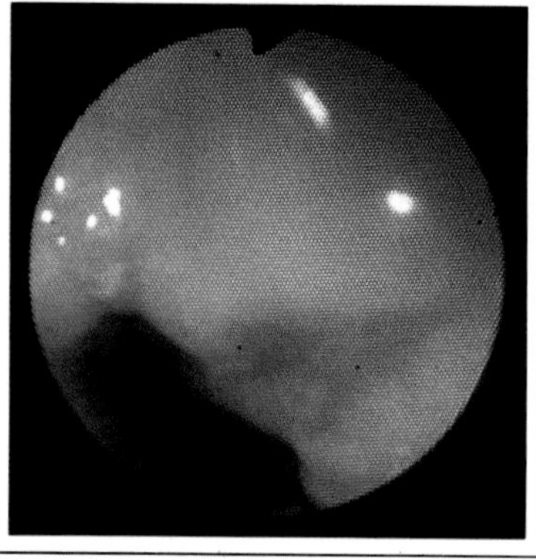

FIG. 6-14.

FIG. 6-13. Accentuated (serrated) GE junction. This appearance is nonspecific. The shorter (<1 cm) and thinner bands were points against a diagnosis of early Barrett's changes. Biopsies failed to reveal evidence of Barrett's esophagus.

FIG. 6-14. Moderate esophagitis. Erosions of the GE junction may also be confused with early Barrett's changes; however, they are generally shorter (<1 cm) and thinner (<5 mm) than tongues indicative of early Barrett's changes (see Fig. 6-12).

epithelium, an abrupt change from that found in biopsies of the cardia. The natural history of these early Barrett's changes is uncertain. Prospective studies are necessary to determine if the changes evolve into the more visual Barrett's appearance and if there is a predisposition to cancer (see below).

CANCER ASSOCIATED WITH BARRETT'S ESOPHAGUS

There seems little doubt that Barrett's epithelium is precancerous.[1,7,8] The cumulative incidence of cancer may be as high as 10%,[1] although in most series it is only 2 to 3%[7]; still, this is more than 100 times that of the general population.

The carcinoma associated with Barrett's esophagus is adenocarcinoma arising in Barrett's epithelium itself. Barrett's changes associated with carcinoma are generally extensive, involving the entire distal esophagus.[1] The extent of these changes plus the long history of reflux symptoms generally obtained in such patients suggest that cancer is a late manifestation which may require the presence of well-established Barrett's changes for at least 5 to 10 years.

Location

Cancers arising in Barrett's epithelium have their proximal margin generally 2 to 3 cm distal to the junction of squamous epithelium with the Barrett's. For a Barrett's esophagus confined to the distal 5 cm of the esophagus, this may mean a carcinoma arising close to the cardia. In most cases the proximal extent of the Barrett's is substantially 2 to 3 cm higher than this, making the mid-esophagus the commonest site.

Appearance

As these cancers tend to infiltrate as well as grow into the lumen, the most frequent endoscopic appearance is that of a malignant stricture of the mid-esophagus, situated 2 to 5 cm below the squamocolumnar junction.[1] The stricture may have an irregular, nodular mouth comprised of deep pink or reddish-gray nodules or frank tumor masses (Fig. 6-15). Occasionally, the mucosa of the mouth appears intact, with only the tightness of the stricture and an irregular shelfed appearance just proximal to it as clues to the presence of cancer (Fig. 6-16). In addition, the location of the stricture

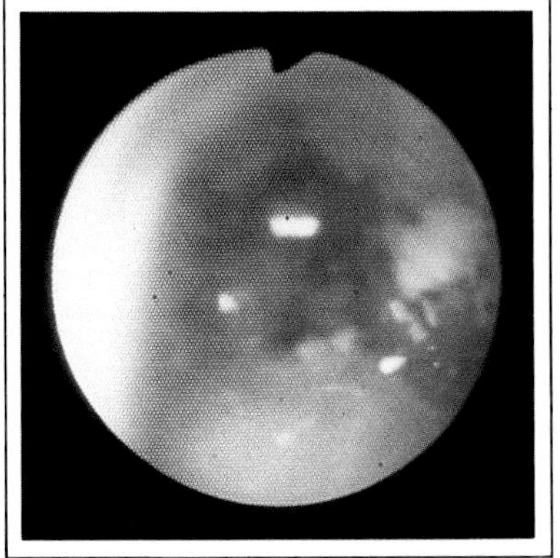

FIG. 6-15.

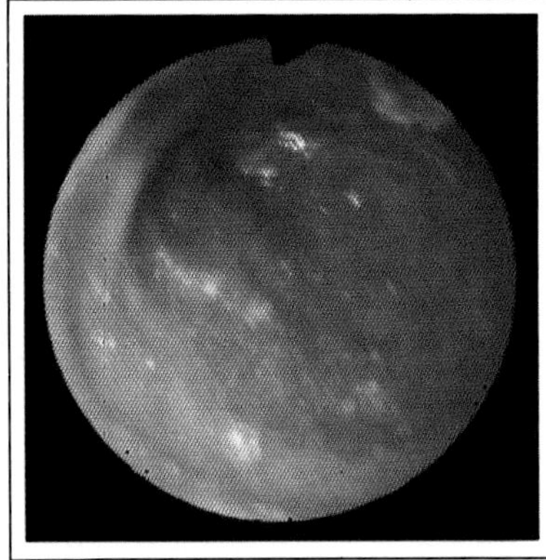

FIG. 6-16.

FIG. 6-15. Adenocarcinoma arising in Barrett's esophagus. A nodular area is seen growing into a stricture at the squamocolumnar (Barrett's) junction.

FIG. 6-16. Adenocarcinoma arising within Barrett's esophagus. This tight but otherwise benign-appearing stricture was found within the Barrett's esophagus 2 cm distal to the squamocolumnar (Barrett's) junction. The location and tightness of the stricture suggest malignancy.

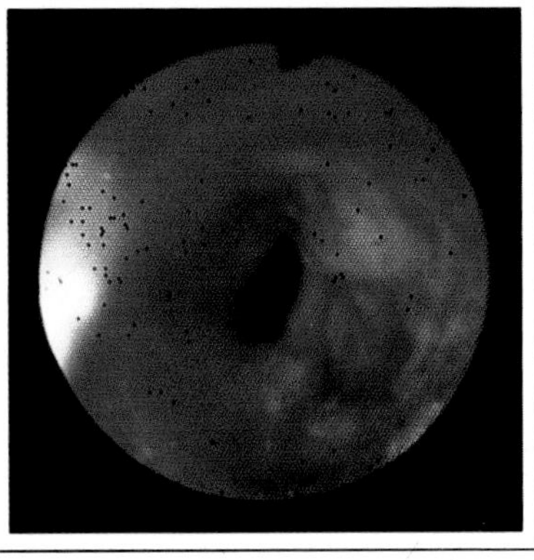

FIG. 6-17.

FIG. 6-17. Adenocarcinoma arising within Barrett's esophagus. A nodular area was noted 3 cm down from the squamocolumnar (Barrett's) junction.

below, rather than at, the squamocolumnar junction is an important sign, indicating a high likelihood of cancer. Another occasional finding is that of nodular polypoid masses within the proximal 2 cm of the Barrett's epithelium (Fig. 6-17).

Biopsy and Brushing Cytology

Biopsy and brushing cytology should be pursued as in the case of any malignant stricture (see Chapter 4) or suspected malignant lesion (see Chapter 5). Biopsy specimens are taken from suspicious areas around the mouth of the stricture as well as any from other irregular areas within Barrett's epithelium (Fig. 6-15 through 6-17). Brushings are taken within the stricture as well as in areas previously biopsied. Because the cancers tend to be infiltrating, the biopsy may not show frank invasive changes but only dysplasia (i.e., the presence of cytologic features suggestive of neoplastic transformation). Because dysplasia is not uncommonly found in association with cancer in Barrett's epithelium,[8] we believe that a biopsy showing definite dysplasia especially in association with a mass or stricture is tantamount to a diagnosis of carcinoma (Fig. 6-18a and b). Rarely, severe dysplasia (cancer *in situ*) is found in resected esophagus without frank invasion. The two cases where this has been reported were unique in that in one the patient had severe dysplasia but no evidence of a mass or other macroscopic abnormalities, whereas in the other there was a diffuse polypoid lesion throughout the esophagus.[9] The absence of frank carcinoma in these cases does not detract from the significance of dysplasia found in association with the typical endoscopic appearance of cancer in Barrett's esophagus, i.e., a stricture (Fig. 6-16) or mass (Fig. 6-17).

CANCER SURVEILLANCE

The cumulative incidence of cancer in Barrett's esophagus has been reported to be between 2%[8] and 8.5%.[1] Unlike squamous cancers, which are almost uniformly fatal within 1 year following diagnosis regardless of treatment, adenocarcinomas seen with Barrett's esophagus may be associated with a prolonged survival (greater than 2 years), even with lymphatic spread, provided a curative resection can be performed.[8] The depth of invasion appears to influence resectability. In one study four cancers confined to the wall of the esophagus all proved uniformly resectable with no recurrence evident from 6 months to 7 years after surgery.[8]

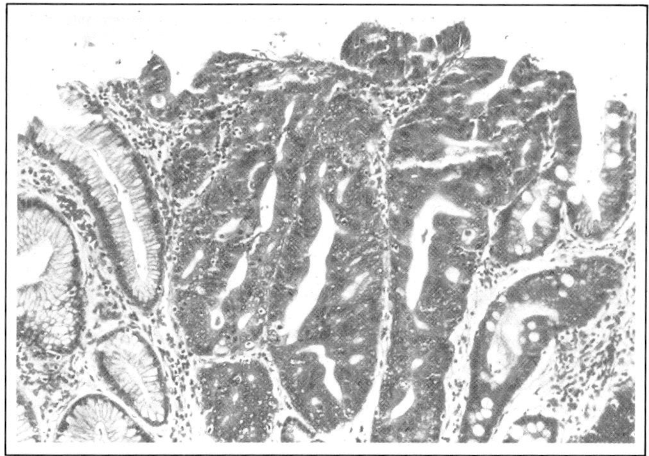

FIG. 6-18a.

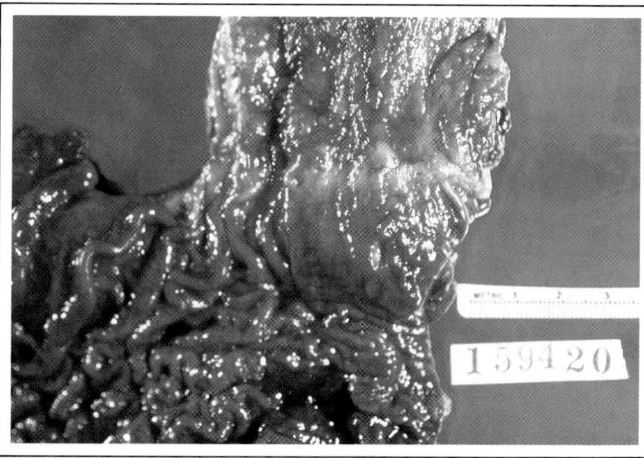

FIG. 6-18b.

FIG. 6-18. a: A biopsy (same patient as in Fig. 6-16) shows focal severe dysplasia without invasion. Nevertheless, surgery was advised and a resection performed. **b:** The surgically resected specimen revealed infiltrating adenocarcinoma.

Among eight patients in whom carcinoma was found to extend through the wall, recurrence was evident within 6 to 8 months of the operation in three of the six who survived the surgery.[8] It is therefore highly desirable from the standpoint of effecting a surgical cure to detect carcinoma in these patients while it is still confined to the wall of the esophagus. More advantageous than this would be to detect neoplastic change before the lesions become frankly invasive. Using endoscopy with biopsy and cytology, cancer *in situ* has been detected in patients with a macroscopic abnormality (nodular masses projecting to the lumen), as well as in those without any such change.[10] Because of the cancer risk in these patients, as well as the endoscopic means to detect premalignant change, we believe that endoscopy should be performed periodically in patients with Barrett's esophagus regardless of whether there has been a change in their symptoms. Endoscopy is, of course, mandatory in those for whom there has been a change in symptoms, especially if associated with weight loss.

There are no precise guidelines at present regarding the frequency of such examinations. We find that examination at 2-year intervals is acceptable for most patients with Barrett's changes. We generally examine patients with strictures or macroscopic changes (e.g., nodularity and irregularity of the squamocolumnar junction) at 6- to 12-month intervals. Biopsies are taken throughout the extent of the Barrett's changes. The finding of definite dysplasia would be an indication for repeat examination within 6 months. We consider the presence of either of the following to be an indication for surgery: (a) severe dysplasia, i.e., cancer *in situ;* and (b) any degree of definite dysplasia associated with a macroscopic lesion. For those who have less than severe dysplasia without a mass, we recommend periodic follow-up every 6 to 12 months and regard progression to severe dysplasia as an indication for esophagectomy.

Recently, regression of Barrett's changes has been reported to occur after reflux surgery.[11] Such regression, however, did not occur in all patients, especially in those who continued to have measurable acid reflux after surgery.[11] In one of the six patients in whom Barrett's changes persisted, carcinoma developed within 4 years of surgery.[11] It therefore appears prudent to closely follow all patients who have had

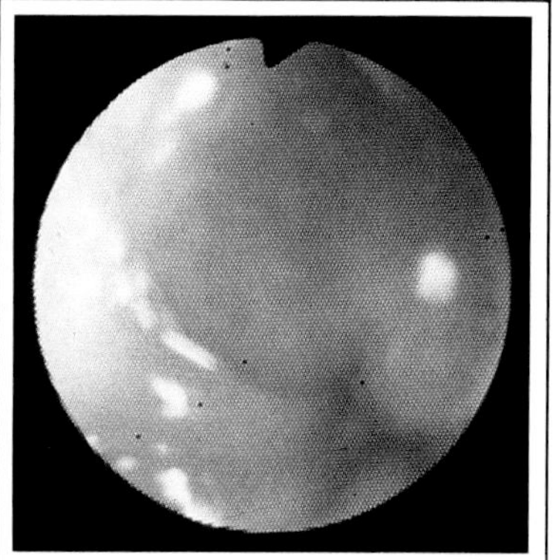

FIG. 6-19.

FIG. 6-19. Heterotopic gastric mucosa at the level of the cricopharyngeus. A 2 × 3 cm discrete, orange-yellow patch was observed at this level, entirely surrounded by gray-white squamous mucosa. Biopsies showed glandular epithelium.

a diagnosis of Barrett's esophagus at any point in time, even those subjected to antireflux operations, especially in whom Barrett's changes persist.

HETEROTOPIC GASTRIC MUCOSA OF THE PROXIMAL ESOPHAGUS

Distinct from the usual appearance and location of Barrett's epithelium, which begins in the mid or distal esophagus and is continuous with gastric mucosa, is heterotopic gastric mucosa of the proximal esophagus which is entirely surrounded by squamous epithelium (Fig. 6-19). The commonest location is within the cricopharyngeus or just distal to it in the cervical esophagus. If this area is examined carefully, one may find this on the order of one case per 400 to 800 examinations.

Heterotopic gastric mucosa is thought to derive from rests of gastric cells left in the esophagus during embryonic life.[12] It is typically an incidental finding, unrelated to esophageal reflux. Although cancers have been found in areas of proximal gastric heterotopia,[13] its malignant potential is not yet defined. Whether periodic endoscopic surveillance should be undertaken for patients with proximal gastric heterotopia is unknown.

REFERENCES

1. Naef, A. P., Savary, M., and Ozzello, L. (1975): Columnar-lined lower esophagus: an acquired lesion with malignant predisposition: report on 140 cases of Barrett's esophagus with 12 adenocarcinomas. *J. Thorac. Cardiovasc. Surg.*, 70:826–835.
2. Burbige, E. J., and Radigan, J. J. (1979): Characteristics of the columnar-cell lined (Barrett's) esophagus. *Gastrointest. Endosc.*, 25:133–136.
3. Behar, J., Biancani, A., and Sheahan, D. G. (1976): Evaluation of esophageal tests in the diagnosis of reflux esophagitis. *Gastroenterology*, 71:9–15.
4. Paull, A., Trier, J. S., Dalton, M. D., Camp, R. C., Loeb, P., and Goyal, R. K. (1976): The histologic spectrum of Barrett's esophagus. *N. Engl. J. Med.*, 295:476–480.

4a. Sjogren, R. W., and Johnson, L. F. (1983): Barrett's esophagus: a review. *Am. J. Med.*, 74:313–321.

5. Musher, D. E. (1978): Mid-esophageal stricture. *Am. J. Gastroenterol.*, 69:331–336.
6. Kothari, T., Mangla, J. C., and Kalra, T. M. S. (1980): Barrett's ulcer and treatment with cimetidine. *Arch. Intern. Med.*, 140:475–477.
7. Hawe, A., Payne, W. S., Weiland, L. H., and Fontana, R. S. (1973): Adenocarcinoma in the columnar lined lower (Barrett) oesophagus. *Thorax*, 28:511–514.
8. Haggitt, R. C., Tryzelaar, J., Ellis, F. H., and Colcher, H. (1978): Adenocarcinoma complicating columnar epithelium-lined (Barrett's) esophagus. *Am. J. Clin. Pathol.*, 70:1–5.
9. McDonald, G. B., Brand, D. L., and Thorning, D. R. (1977): Multiple adenomatous neoplasms arising in columnar-lined (Barrett's) esophagus. *Gastroenterology*, 72:1317–1321.
10. Belladonna, J. A., Hajdu, S. I., Bains, M. S., and Winawer, S. J. (1974): Adenocarcinoma in situ of Barrett's esophagus diagnosed by endoscopic cytology. *N. Engl. J. Med.*, 291:895–896.
11. Brand, D. L., Ylvisaker, J. T., Gelfand, M., and Pope, C. E. (1980): Regression of columnar esophageal (Barrett's) epithelium after antireflux surgery. *N. Engl. J. Med.*, 302:844–848.
12. De la Pava, S., Pickren, J. W., and Adler, R. H. (1964): Ectopic gastric mucosa of the esophagus: a study of histogenesis. *N.Y. State J. Med.*, 64:1831–1835.
13. Carrie, A. (1950): Adenocarcinoma of the upper end of the esophagus arising from gastric epithelium. *Brit. J. Surg.*, 37:474–477.

7

ESOPHAGEAL MOTOR DISORDERS

In this chapter we consider endoscopic aspects of: (a) achalasia; (b) scleroderma; and (c) other motor disturbances resulting from diabetes, chronic alcoholism, diffuse esophageal spasm, and aging (presbyesophagus). These conditions present a challenge to endoscopists for different reasons. In the case of achalasia, the examination itself, particularly entry into the stomach, is difficult because of esophageal dilatation and retention. In the case of scleroderma, the endoscopic appearance may be confusing because of the severity and extensiveness of the esophagitis present. In these cases, as well as with esophagitis occurring with diabetes and chronic alcoholism, there is the need to determine if *Candida* or other opportunistic organisms are present. Finally, in all of these cases, but especially in achalasia, there is the inevitable obligation to exclude an underlying carcinoma.

ACHALASIA

Patients with achalasia are generally referred for endoscopy having had at least radiologic study of the esophagus, if not manometry as well. Even in these cases—where the esophagram shows the classic appearance of a dilated, aperistaltic esophagus with a short and "beak-like" appearance of the cardia, and manometry shows a loss of peristaltic activity in the body of the esophagus and incomplete relaxation of an otherwise hypertensive sphincter[1]—the physician will wisely request an endoscopic examination in every patient over the age of 40. This is because no radiologic appearance, regardless of how typical, effectively excludes carcinoma because the latter can produce a similar if not identical radiographic appearance.[2]

In other patients it may be unclear from the radiographic appearance whether the abnormality is achalasia or a peptic stricture; hence endoscopy is done to determine the nature of the cardial obstruction, mechanical or motor. Finally, in patients with known achalasia for whom pneumatic dilatation is being considered, the physician may wish to be aware of mechanical factors, e.g., the presence of associated diverticula of the cardia or distal esophagus, which may place the patient at increased risk.

Our consideration of achalasia focuses on these concerns. First, we examine the classic endoscopic findings in achalasia, especially those of the cardia. Next we consider the alterations in this classic appearance produced by prior treatment, or others such as associated diverticula. In the final section we are concerned with the endoscopic findings which suggest the presence of carcinoma in patients thought to have achalasia.

Appearance

Untreated Achalasia

The striking feature in patients with untreated achalasia is often the degree of esophageal dilatation (Fig. 7-1). This is difficult to quantify objectively, but one can easily imagine placing four, and in some cases five or six (9 mm), open biopsy forceps end to end at the widest point of the esophagus. Within the body of the esophagus there is generally retained foreign material (Fig. 7-2), in some cases appearing formed like gastric bezoars. Occasionally, the foreign material is so dense that the examination must be abandoned until it is removed with an Ewald tube. A wise policy is to place an Ewald tube prior to endoscopy in any patient with presumed achalasia and lavage until clear.

If on entry into the esophagus the 12 o'clock lens position is aligned with the anterior wall as the endoscope is advanced into the distal esophagus (between 32 and 40 cm), the lumen may be seen to go off in the 3 o'clock (right-sided) direction (see Chapter 1). This is true in cases where the esophagus is markedly dilated and assumes a "sigmoid" shape (Fig. 7-1). In the most distal portion, the esophagus veers toward the left-hand (9 o'clock) side where the "cardial rosette" actually arises (Fig. 7-3).

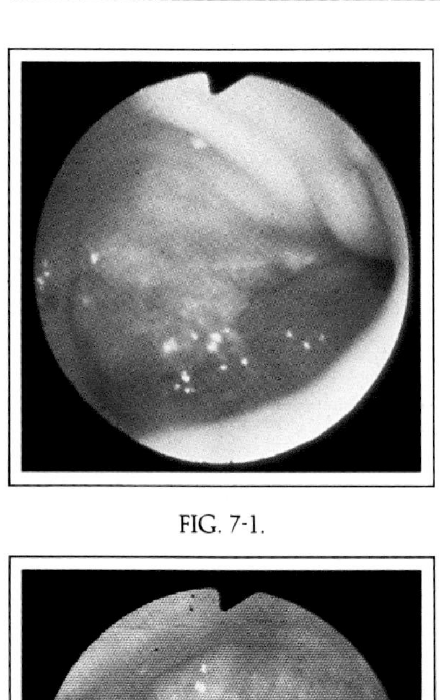

FIG. 7-1.

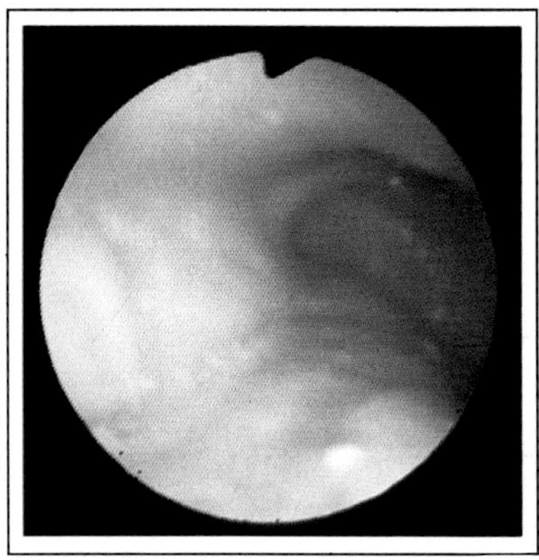

FIG. 7-2.

FIG. 7-1. Achalasia. There is marked dilatation of the body of the esophagus, as well as deviation of the lumen to the right (3 o'clock) wall just above the cardia.

FIG. 7-2. Achalasia. Note the dilatation of the body of the esophagus with fluid retention along the left (9 o'clock) wall (with the patient lying on his left side).

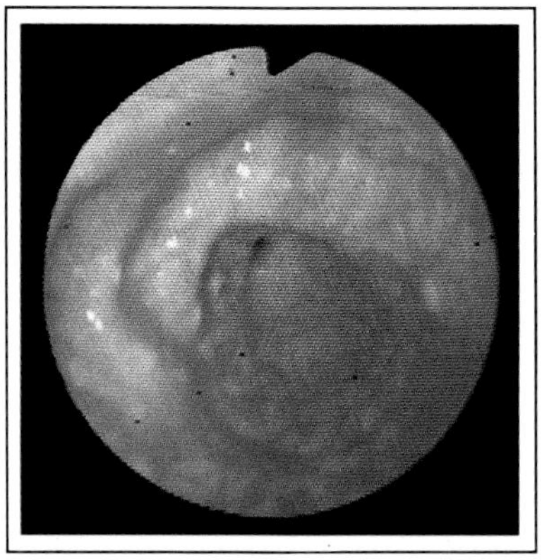

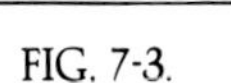

FIG. 7-3.

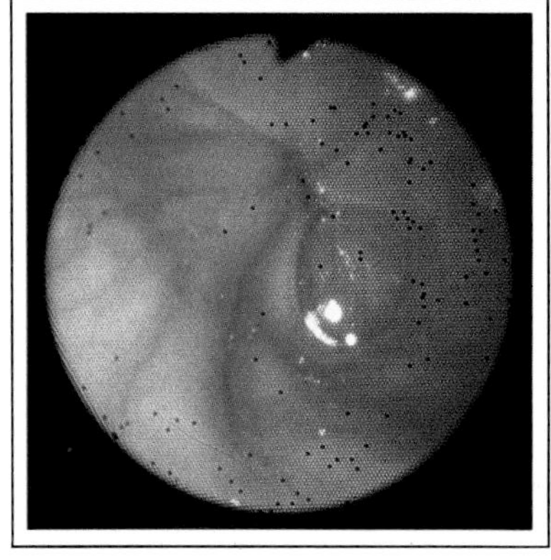

FIG. 7-4a.

FIG. 7-3. Achalasia. Deviation of the lumen to the left (9 o'clock) just above its junction with the cardial high-pressure zone. Some irregularity of the mucosa in the distal esophagus is noted, probably as a stasis change.

FIG. 7-4. Achalasia. **a:** The high-pressure zone is closed, although mucosal columns are seen to run through. **b:** The gentle pressure applied to the instrument tip succeeds in opening the cardia. **c:** The cardia is now wide open, permitting the instrument to pass through. Ordinarily in untreated achalasia the GE junction is not seen.

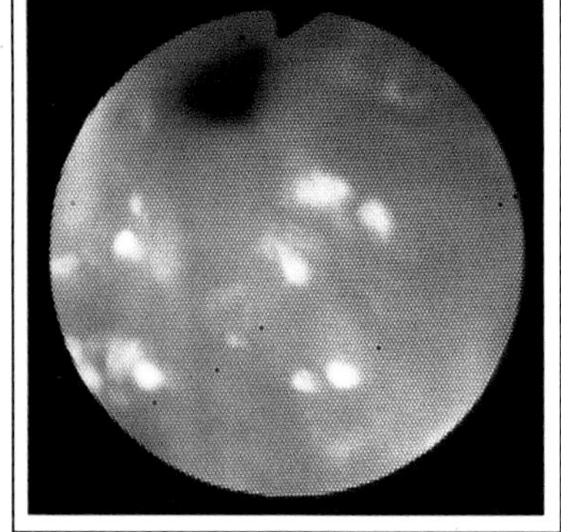

FIG. 7-4b.

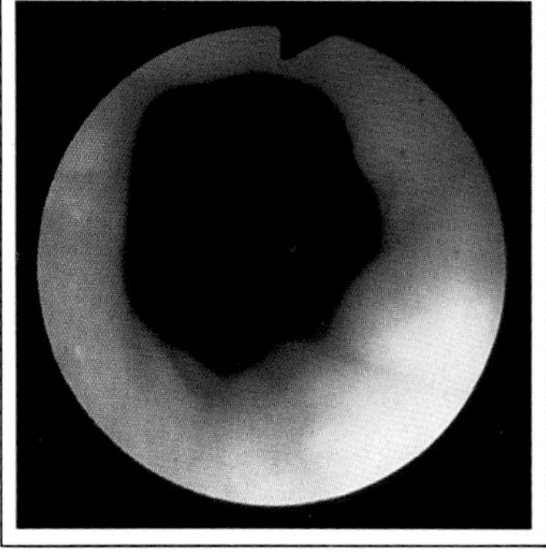

FIG. 7-4c.

The cardial rosette (high-pressure zone) actually begins 1 to 2 cm above the gastroesophageal (GE) junction, so that the GE junction lying within the high-pressure zone is usually not seen in patients with untreated achalasia. The esophageal columns can be seen to radiate into the rosette and beyond, forming the mucosal folds of the cardia. The mucosa is intact throughout the rosette. If the endoscope is placed within the center of the rosette, it is usually able to dilate the rosette such that even an endoscope of 11 to 13 mm will have no difficulty being advanced into the stomach, though initially the rosette may be tightly closed (Fig. 7-4a). Advancing the endoscope into the stomach is facilitated if it is recalled that the direction of the fundus and body where the endoscope is to be advanced is to the left and anterior to the distal esophagus (see Chapter 11). Counterclockwise torquing of the instrument shaft and upward deflection (toward the 10 o'clock position) will direct the tip toward the anterior wall of the body of the stomach, thereby facilitating passage across the cardia entry into the stomach.

Prior to entering the stomach, the endoscopist carefully observes the mucosa of the distal esophagus. This can be

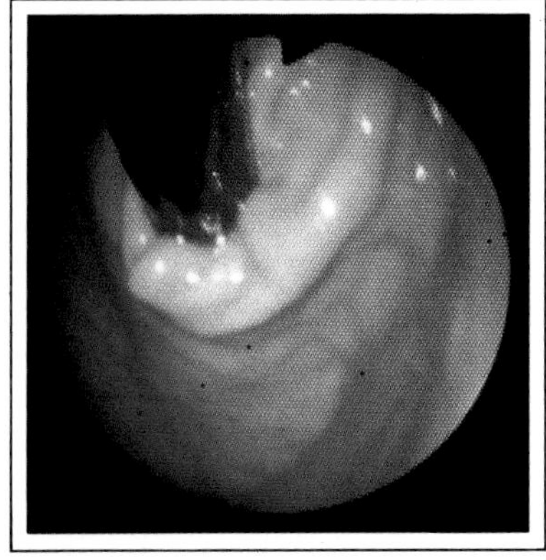

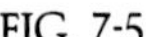

FIG. 7-5.

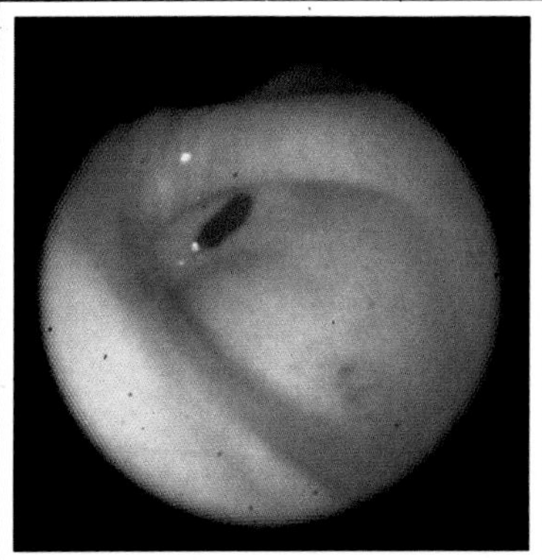

FIG. 7-6.

FIG. 7-5. Achalasia. Normal cardia is seen with the U-turn maneuver (see Chapter 11). The cardia must be visualized completely to exclude malignancy.

FIG. 7-6. Achalasia, prior treatment with a Heller myotomy. There is marked deformity of the distal esophagus just above the cardia with a V-shaped scar deformity.

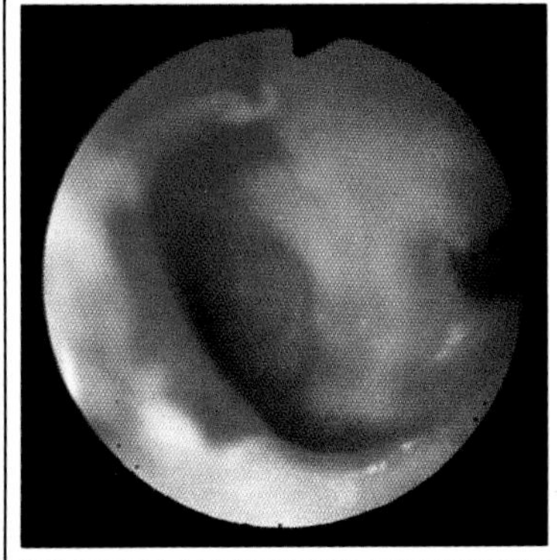

FIG. 7-7.

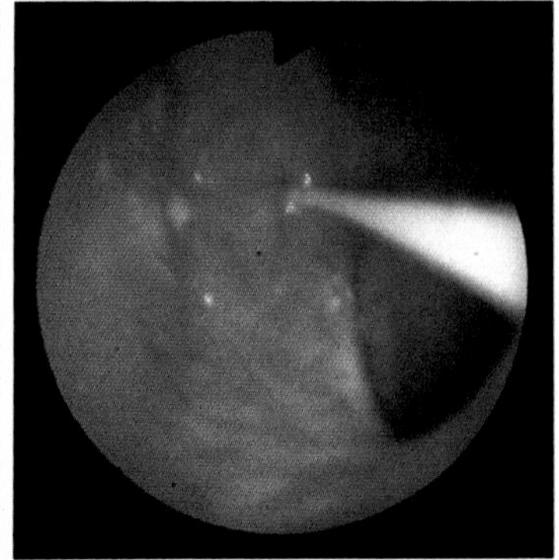

FIG. 7-8.

FIG. 7-7. Achalasia, prior treatment with a Heller myotomy. There is ulceration (3 o'clock) and pseudomembrane formation suggestive of severe peptic injury and reflux.

FIG. 7-8. Achalasia with a large (4 to 5 cm) diverticulum. The mouth of the diverticulum was noted at the right of a cardial rosette through which a polyethylene cannula has been passed.

entirely normal or show mucosal irregularity (Fig. 7-3), nonspecific erythema, or mucosal thickening suggested by the loss of the normal vascular pattern (see Chapter 3). Frank erosions between nodules of hyperplastic epithelium can be seen in some patients, especially those with marked esophageal dilatation and the sigmoid appearance suggesting long standing achalasia. The origin of this esophagitis is uncertain but is possibly an effect of stasis.

Once in the stomach, it is necessary to complete the examination of the cardia with a U-turn retroflexion maneuver (see Chapter 11). The cardia appears perfectly smooth and symmetrical, with the cardial folds being entirely distinct and separate from the fundus, hugging the endoscope as it passes through (Fig. 7-5).

Previously Treated Achalasia

The goal of treatment in achalasia, whether surgery or pneumatic dilatation, is destruction of the integrity of the lower esophageal motor unit. The injury itself may be associated with scarring. Moreover, if in the case of surgery an antireflux operation is not performed coincidentally, or if the pneumatic dilatation is completely effective, esophageal reflux may be significant and cause further distortion from peptic injury. One can therefore see a variety of appearances of the cardial rosette after treatment, ranging from that of untreated achalasia (Fig. 7-1) to one of either stricture formation alone (Fig. 7-6) or with esophagitis. In some cases the reflux esophagitis following myotomy is severe, with ulceration and pseudomembrane formation (Fig. 7-7).

Diverticula Associated With Achalasia

Esophageal motor disorders, especially achalasia and diffuse esophageal spasm, are a setting for esophageal diverticula.[4] When diverticula occur in achalasia, they are most often small, 2 cm or less. Less commonly, they are larger (Fig. 7-8) or even of the giant type (Fig. 7-9) where they exceed 5 cm. They are generally found just above the high-pressure zone (Fig. 7-10), but on occasion they are seen to originate from within the cardia. In either case, their presence in and around the cardial high-pressure zone (Fig. 7-8) is a potential risk factor for pneumatic dilatation, especially the presence of large diverticula which may compromise placement of the pneumatic bag. The finding of a diverticula in achalasia, therefore, should always be communicated directly to the physician planning pneumatic dilatation.

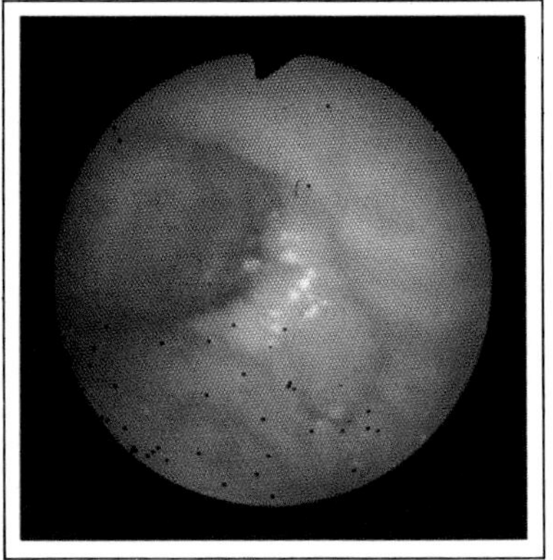

FIG. 7-9.

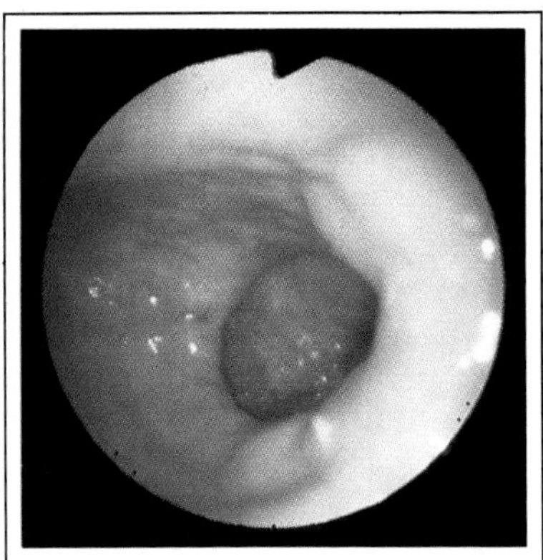

FIG. 7-10.

FIG. 7-9. Achalasia with a giant diverticulum. The endoscope has entered a 10-cm diverticulum on the right side (3 o'clock) with the lumen seen at the left (9 o'clock).

FIG. 7-10. Achalasia with two diverticula of the body of the esophagus. A wide-mouth diverticulum is noted to the left at 9 o'clock and a second smaller diverticulum just below.

Achalasia and Cancer

Achalasia as a Precancerous Lesion

The incidence of cancer in patients with well-established achalasia from a large series was 41 cases per 100,000 per year, about seven times the incidence of esophageal cancer in the general population.[5] The achalasia had been present in these patients with cancers for at least 10 years.[5,6] The cancers arise in the mid or distal esophagus, several centimeters above the cardial high-pressure zone and in all other ways are indistinguishable from ordinary squamous carcinomas.[5,6]

Achalasia Secondary to Carcinoma

Gastric carcinoma,[2,7] lymphoma[8] originating in the cardiofundic area, or cancer metastasizing[2] from the lung, breast, or pancreas to pericardial lymph nodes can produce radiographic and manometric features which are identical with those of idiopathic primary achalasia. We find the incidence of achalasia secondary to malignancy approaches 2 to 3% of patients referred for endoscopy because of achalasia; hence the exclusion of cancer in a patient over the age of 40 with symptoms of achalasia for less than 1 year is an important concern for the endoscopist. Although there are no published data, we believe, based on our own experience (four cases of achalasia secondary to carcinoma during a 5-year period and none of cancer arising in well-established achalasia) that cancer producing an achalasia-like picture is by far more common than cancer arising in patients with well-established achalasia.

The best defense against missing a diagnosis of cancer is a high index of suspicion for patients in the cancer age range, especially for those presenting with achalasia over the age of 60 in whom the onset of dysphagia within 1 year has been associated with marked weight loss.[2]

Appearance

Examination of the distal esophagus may reveal evidence of mucosal involvement as in other infiltrating malignancies of this area (see Chapter 5). Asymmetrical, enlarged, erythematous or friable folds would be regarded as very suspicious in such patients (Fig. 7-11). Occasionally, a distinct ulcerative mass lesion is found, but in half the cases the mucosa of the distal esophagus is entirely intact[2] (Fig. 7-12). In these cases there may be two additional findings: (a) failure to pass the endoscope into the stomach; and (b) appearance of a cardial mass.

Failure to enter the stomach.

The endoscopist expects to enter the stomach with an endoscope 11 to 13 mm in diameter in most cases of primary achalasia (Fig. 7-4c) and certainly with an endoscope of pediatric size (9 mm). Failure to enter the stomach should raise the suspicion of cancer especially in an elderly patient. However, the endoscopist must remember that if the distal esophagus is markedly dilated and tortuous (Fig. 7-1), one may not enter the stomach because of marked bowing of the instrument within the dilated esophagus, which dissipates the force applied to advance it. Therefore in the face of marked esophageal dilatation, failure to enter the stomach is not by itself a worrisome finding, as it would be with minimal or no esophageal dilatation. Unfortunately, the passage of a standard (11 to 13 mm) adult endoscope into the stomach does not exclude cancer. In one series, an endoscope could be passed into the stomach of six of seven patients with cancer-associated achalasia[2]; in four it was an adult (12 to 13 mm) sized instrument, and in two it was the pediatric (8 to 9 mm) type. One expects that if an intermediate (11 mm) or small (8 to 9 mm) caliber instrument is used, the stomach can be entered in a large percentage of patients with cancer-associated achalasia.

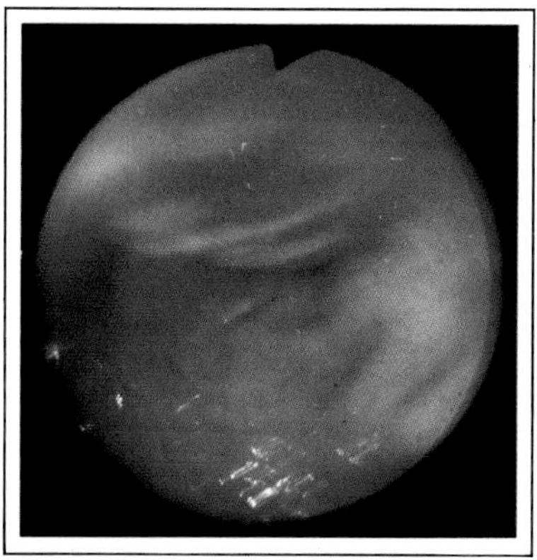

FIG. 7-11.

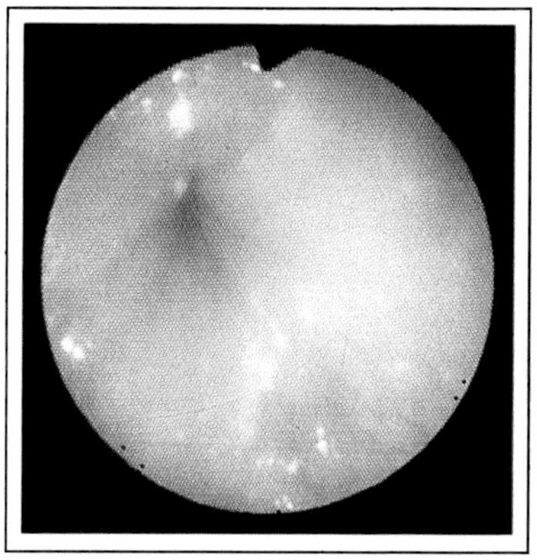

FIG. 7-12a.

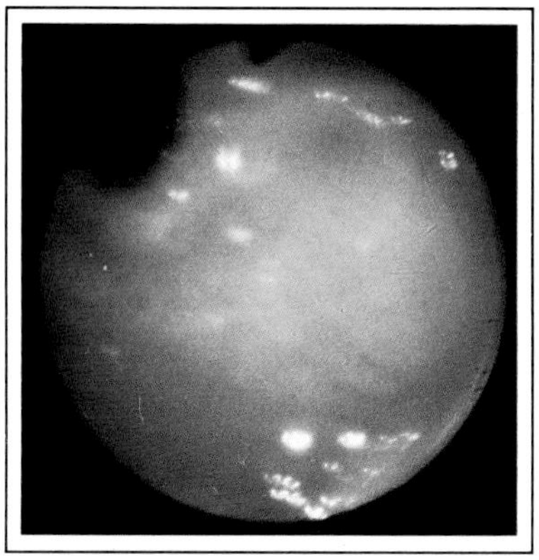

FIG. 7-12b.

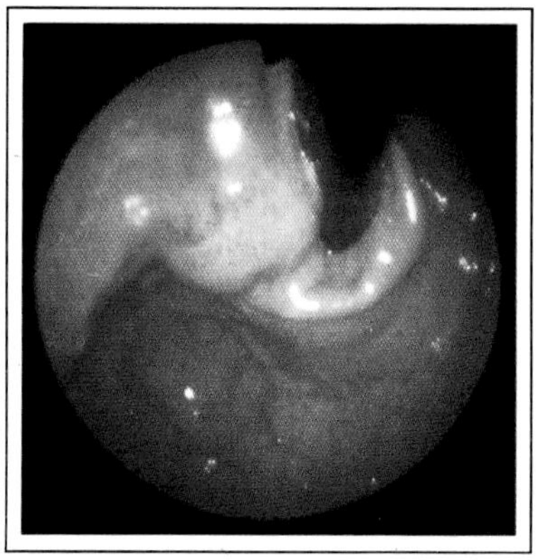

FIG. 7-12c.

FIG. 7-11. Achalasia secondary to cancer. The large, indurated, friable folds at the GE junction in a patient with achalasia suggest malignancy as a cause of the motor disturbance.

FIG. 7-12. a: Achalasia secondary to cancer. The mucosa of the distal esophagus running through the high-pressure zone appears completely intact. **b:** An incomplete, retroflexed (U-turn) view of the cardia (same patient). The passage of an 11-mm endoscope and this view (although incomplete) was taken as evidence of uncomplicated achalasia. **c:** Two months later, repeat endoscopy with a complete retroflexed view of the cardia now shows an asymmetrically distorted fold. Surgical exploration 2 weeks later revealed carcinoma of the tail of the pancreas invading the cardia.

Appearance of the cardia.

For patients suspected of achalasia secondary to carcinoma involving the cardia, it is essential to examine the cardia from the retroflexed "U" appearance (see Chapter 11) and to see it in its entirety (Fig. 7-12b). Normally the cardial folds are perfectly smooth and symmetrical (Fig. 7-5). The appearance of an asymmetrical cardial mass, even if it is entirely submucosal (Fig. 7-12c), is a highly suspicious finding for carcinoma, especially one metastatic to the pericardial lymph nodes. Other carcinomas of the cardiofundic area produce a nodular, indurated appearance to the folds of this area (Fig. 7-13). Biopsies taken from these areas may well show carcinoma. However, it should be appreciated that biopsies taken from areas with only nonspecific changes or having a normal appearance are not likely to be positive. Nevertheless, the endoscopist must make his suspicions concerning cancer known to the referring physican. Although the examiner may believe endoscopic follow-up is a viable alternative to nonsurgical intervention, the efficacy of such an approach is questionable as the cancer may continue to reside outside the cardia or in the wall and still not be amenable to a tissue diagnosis even months later. The best policy may well be to encourage surgery so that at least a definite diagnosis is established. In some cases a curative resection or other palliative surgical procedure is then feasible.

SCLERODERMA

Scleroderma esophagus occurs as part of a multisystem disorder in a patient with skin changes and pulmonary and renal findings.[9] Rarely, it is found in a patient having only Raynaud's phenomenon.[10] The esophageal motor disorder is characterized by decreased to absent peristaltic activity in the body of the esophagus, with a diminished or absent lower esophageal high-pressure zone.[9] These abnormalities are thought to result from atrophy and replacement of the smooth muscle of the distal esophagus by fibrous tissue.[11] The result of these motor disturbances is to increase the frequency of esophageal reflux as well as to diminish the rate of acid clearance and prolong its contact time with the mucosa.[12] As a result of these disturbances, the peptic esophagitis seen in such patients may be unusually extensive and severe, leading to stricture formation.[13] Contributing to the severity of the esophagitis may be the presence of *Candida,* which in one series[12] was found in almost one-third of the patients with scleroderma who had erosive esophagitis at endoscopy.

Appearance

One may observe severe esophagitis in these patients, with evidence of ulceration and pseudomembrane along with free reflux (Fig. 7-14). Often the GE junction and

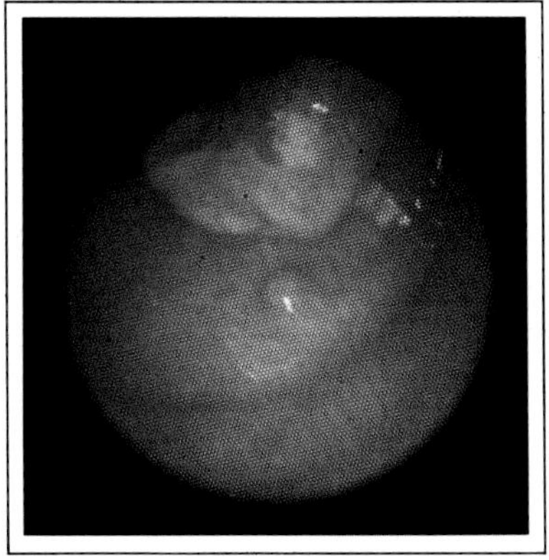

FIG. 7-13.

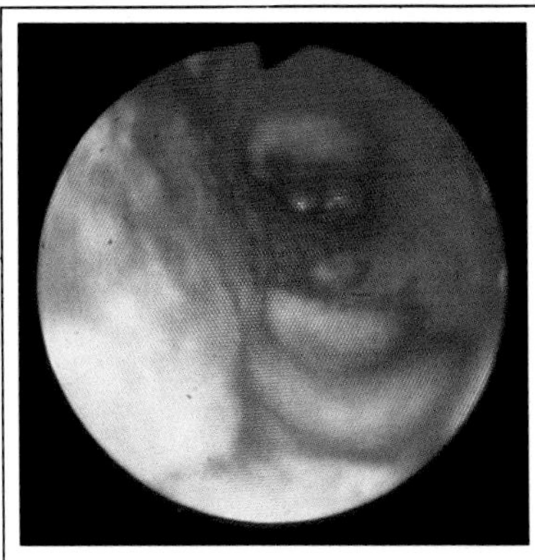

FIG. 7-14.

FIG. 7-13. Achalasia secondary to gastric cancer. This is a cardial tumor mass with mucosal nodules. Biopsies were positive for carcinoma.

Fig. 7-14. Scleroderma of the esophagus with severe free reflux and mucosal injury. Free reflux from the cardia (bile-stained material) is apparent at 12 o'clock with erythema and pseudomembrane formation from the GE junction to the mid-esophagus (28 cm).

cardial area remain remarkably patulous as evidence of the absent lower esophageal high-pressure zone (Fig. 7-14).

The esophagitis is unusual in the extent of severe changes, which may be found as high as the upper mid-esophagus, as in patients with prolonged vomiting prior to nasogastric tube placement or diabetes mellitus (see below). In some patients there is evidence of esophagitis, although less severe, extending up to the cricopharyngeus.

Peptic Stricture

Stricture formation occurs in about 3% of patients with scleroderma[13] (Fig. 7-15). These strictures may be unusually tight, with frequent recurrences after dilatation, ultimately requiring surgery.[9]

Barrett's Esophagus

We have observed one case of Barrett's esophagus in a patient with a 10-year history of scleroderma and occasional reflux symptoms. In this case, the distal esophagus showed the typical orange-red appearance of Barrett's epithelium.

OTHER MOTOR DISORDERS

Diabetes Mellitus

Patients with diabetes mellitus may have evidence of severe, extensive reflux injury at endoscopy. The cause of this injury appears to be multifocal, derived from increased numbers of nonperistaltic contraction,[14] as well as a decreased incidence of peristalsis after swallowing, especially in patients with peripheral neuropathy.[14] In addition, there appears to be in some a weakening of the lower esophageal sphincter,[15] and delay in esophageal emptying in the supine position.[16] As in scleroderma, the presence of *Candida* esophagitis,[17] which can be especially severe in uncontrolled diabetes, may be a contributing factor to the severity of peptic changes. Added to this can be diabetic gastroparesis[18] in which an increased gastric volume may lead to an increased number of reflux episodes.[19]

Patients with diabetes mellitus may show evidence of injury in the mid or proximal esophagus (Fig. 7-16), at sites above those seen in patients with ordinary peptic esophagitis. Furthermore, the injury at these proximal sites is severe, i.e., with ulcerations and pseudomembranes (Fig. 7-16), in contrast to the usual case of peptic esophagitis where generally if there is any definite involvement in this location only erosions are present (see Chapter 3).

Chronic Alcoholism

Chronic alcoholics are generally referred for endoscopy as part of a workup for gastrointestinal (GI) bleeding or because of the question of varices associated with alcoholic liver disease. Evidence of peptic esophagitis may be present at endoscopy which in some cases may be severe. The basis for this injury may lie in the acute and chronic effects of alcoholism,[20] especially in the weakening of the lower esophageal sphincter, which appears to be a concomitant of large (greater than 200 cc) daily alcohol consumption.[21] This, combined with a decrease in the amplitude of peristaltic waves,[21] may promote reflux injury because of both an increased number of reflux episodes and diminished clearance.

Diffuse Esophageal Spasm

Diffuse esophageal spasm is being increasingly recognized as a cause of chest pain and dysphagia.[1] Such patients are referred for endoscopy so as to exclude mechanical obstruction from carcinoma as a cause of this motor disturbance. At endoscopy the appearance is that of ring-like contractions (Fig. 7-17c), corresponding to the x-ray appearance of the corkscrew esophagus (Fig. 7-17a). Despite the striking appearance of these ring-like contractions, the endoscopist

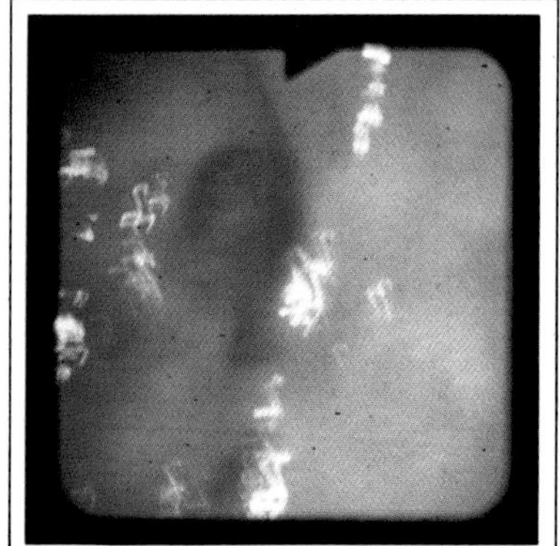

FIG. 7-15.

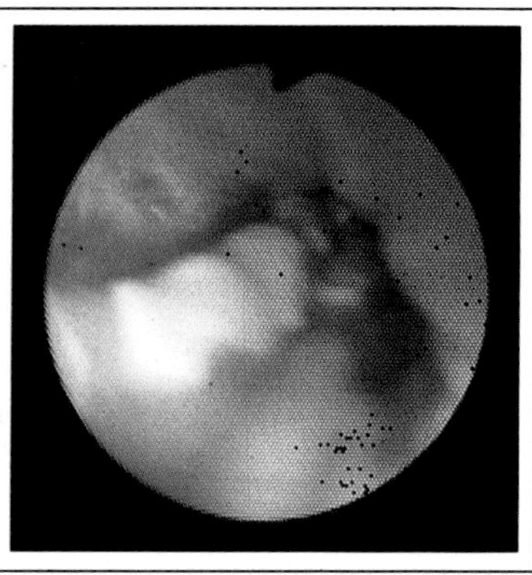

FIG. 7-16.

FIG. 7-15. Scleroderma of the esophagus with peptic stricture. A marked (4 mm) stricture is seen in the distal esophagus, with the esophagus somewhat dilated above.

FIG. 7-16. Diabetes mellitus with severe esophagitis. There are extensive linear erosions and pseudomembranes throughout the entire esophagus. Probably contributing to the extent and severity of the injury was the coexisting gastroparesis (see Chapter 20). Although the pseudomembrane suggests *Candida* esophagitis, multiple smears for *Candida* were negative.

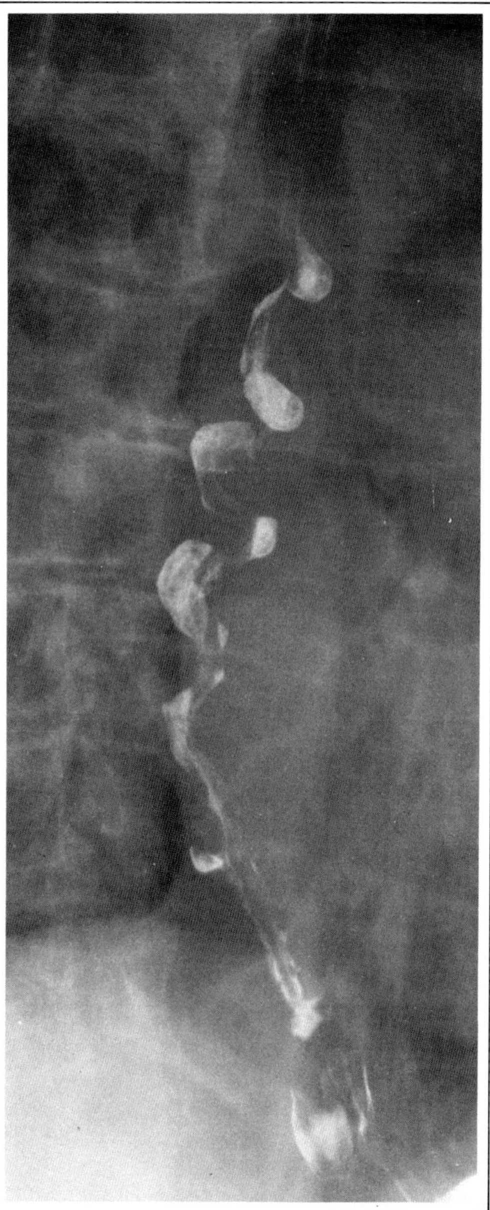

FIG. 7-17a.

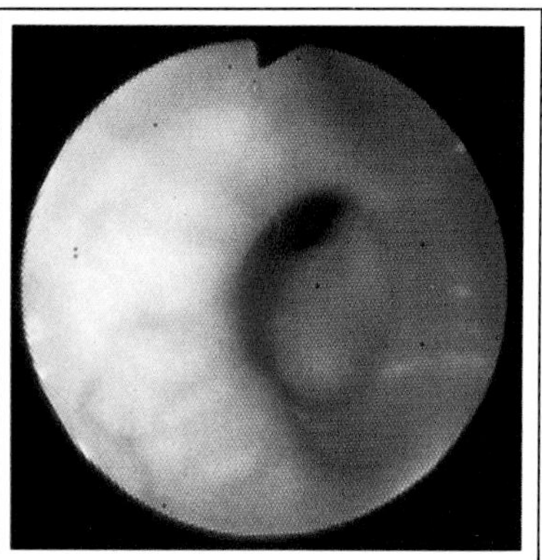

FIG. 7-17b.

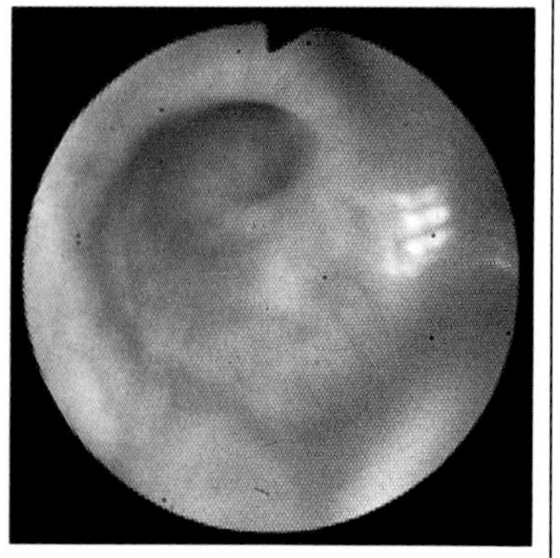

FIG. 7-17c.

FIG. 7-17. Diffuse esophageal spasm. **a:** This patient has a history of intermittent dysphasia and chest pain brought on by eating, with an esophagram showing a corkscrew esophagus suggestive of diffuse esophageal spasm. **b:** An endoscopic view of the mid-esophagus shows a nonperistaltic high-pressure wave at 9 o'clock. **c:** The same view as in (b), except that now the waves have disappeared.

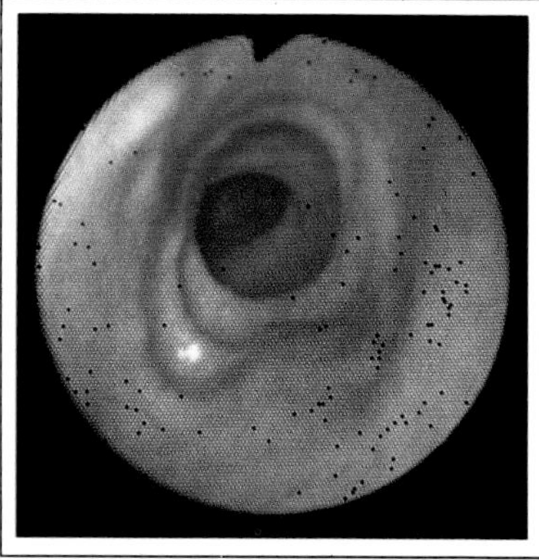

FIG. 7-18.

FIG. 7-18. Motor disturbance of aging (presbyesophagus). Multiple concentric rings are seen in the mid and distal esophagus; these are expected in up to 25% of patients over the age of 60 and are indicative of a nonspecific motor disturbance.

generally has no difficulty negotiating through the esophagus and into the stomach for a retroflexed view of the cardia (see Chapter 11).

Motor Disturbances of Aging (Presbyesophagus)

With aging there is the appearance of disordered contractions of the esophagus in up to 25% of subjects studied.[22] At endoscopy, one often sees in patients over age 60 concentric ring-like waves which appear and disappear as the endoscope is advanced distally. These correspond to the increased number of nonperistaltic contractions (tertiary waves) in manometric studies and the pattern of "curling" of presbyesophagus seen radiographically.

The endoscopic appearance of multiple concentric rings (Fig. 7-18) is generally of no consequence, although in patients with ill-fitting dentures who chew poorly or with extrinsic compression in the aortic arch or distal thoracic aorta (see Chapter 10) intermittent dysphagia may result.

REFERENCES

1. Castell, D. O. (1976): Achalasia and diffuse esophageal spasm. *Arch. Intern. Med.*, 136:571–579.
2. Tucker, H. J., Snape, W. J., and Cohen, S. (1978): Achalasia secondary to carcinoma: manometric and clinical features. *Ann. Intern. Med.*, 89:315–318.
3. Vantrappen, G., and Hellemans, J. (1980): Treatment of achalasia and related motor disorders. *Gastroenterology*, 79:144–154.
4. Debas, H., Payne, W. S., Cameron, A. J., and Carlson, H. C. (1980): Pathophysiology of lower esophageal diverticulum and its implications for treatment. *Surg. Gynecol. Obstet.*, 151:593–600.
5. Wychulis, A. R., Woolam, G. L., Anderson, H. A., and Ellis, F. H. (1971): Achalasia and carcinoma of the esophagus. *JAMA*, 215:163–164.
6. Lortat-Jacob, J. L., Richard, C. A., Fekete, F., and Tcstart, J. (1969): Cardiospasm and esophageal carcinoma: report of 24 cases. *Surgery*, 66:969–975.
7. McCallum, R. W. (1979): Esophageal achalasia secondary to gastric carcinoma: report of a case and a review of the literature. *Am. J. Gastroenterol.*, 71:24–29.
8. Davis, J. A., Kantrowitz, P. A., Chandler, H. L., and Schatzki, S. (1975): Reversible achalasia due to reticulum-cell sarcoma. *N. Engl. J. Med.*, 293:130–132.
9. Mukhopadhyay, A. K., and Graham, D. Y. (1976): Esophageal motor dysfunction in systemic diseases. *Arch. Intern. Med.*, 136:583–588.
10. Stevens, M. B., Hookeman, P., Siegel, C. I., Esterly, J. R., Schulman, L. E., and Hendrix, T. R. (1964): Aperistalsis of the esophagus in patients with connective tissue disorders and Raynaud's phenomenon. *N. Engl. J. Med.*, 270:1218–1222.
11. Treacy, W. L., Baggenstoss, A. H., Slocomb, D. H., and Codè, C. E. (1963): Scleroderma of the esophagus: a correlation of histological and physiologic findings. *Ann. Intern. Med.*, 59:351–356.
12. Zamost, B. J., Hirschberg, J. M., Ippoliti, A. F., Clements, P. J., Furst, D. E., and Weinstein, W. M. (1981): Pathogenesis of erosive esophagitis in scleroderma. *Gastroenterology*, 80:1322.
13. Poirier, T. J., and Rankin, G. B. (1972): Gastrointestinal manifestation of progressive systematic scleroderma based on a review of 364 cases. *Am. J. Gastroenterol.*, 58:30–44.
14. Hollis, J. B., Castell, D. O., and Bradon, R. L. (1977): Esophageal function in diabetes mellitus and its relation to peripheral neuropathy. *Gastroenterology*, 73:1098–1101.
15. Mandelstam, P., Siegel, C. I., Lieber, A., and Siegel, M. (1969): The swallowing disorder in patients with diabetic neuropathy-gastroenteropathy. *Gastroenterology*, 56:1–12.
16. Stewart, I. M., Hasking, D. J., Preston, B. J., and Atkinson, M. (1976): Oesophageal motor changes in diabetes mellitus. *Thorax*, 31:278–283.
17. Eras, P., Goldstein, M. J., and Sherlock, P. (1972): Candida infection of the gastrointestinal tract. *Medicine*, 51:367–379.
18. Goyal, R. K., and Spiro, H. M. (1971): Gastrointestinal manifestations of diabetes mellitus. *Med. Clin. North Am.*, 55:1031–1034.
19. Dodds, W. J., Hogan, W. J., Helm, J. F., and Dent, J. (1981): Pathogenesis of reflux esophagitis. *Gastroenterology*, 81:376–394.
20. Winship, D. H., Catlisch, C. R., Zboralske, F. E., and Hogan, W. J. (1968): Deterioration of esophageal peristalsis in patients with alcoholic neuropathy. *Gastroenterology*, 55:173–178.
21. Mayer, E. M., Grabowski, C. J., and Fisher, R. S. (1978): Effects of gradual doses of alcohol upon esophageal motor function. *Gastroenterology*, 75:1133–1136.
22. Khan, T. A., Shragge, B. W., Crispin, J. S., and Lind, J. F. (1977): Esophageal motility in the elderly. *Am. J. Dig. Dis.*, 22:1049–1054.

8

ESOPHAGEAL VARICES

One generally thinks of esophageal varices in the context of upper gastrointestinal bleeding. Yet they are often encountered in cirrhotic patients who are not bleeding[1] in whom endoscopy may be performed for other reasons, e.g., the evaluation of anemia or gastrointestinal symptoms. In our Unit, on a yearly basis, we encounter nonbleeding varices one and a half to two times more often then bleeding varices (see Chapter 34). In this chapter, we consider the following aspects of varices in the nonbleeding state: (a) the usual appearances; (b) the estimation and grading of variceal size; (c) appearances which may be confused with varices; (d) appearances following endoscopic treatment (sclerosis); and (e) the uncommon "downhill" type of varices.

Esophageal varices are submucosal veins which form as a result of portal hypertension, allowing decompression of the portal venous system into the systemic circulation through the azygos vein. The endoscopist expects, therefore, to first encounter varices in the mid-esophagus at the level of the azygos vein (Fig. 8-1a), at 25 to 30 cm. In probably no more than 10% the varices will extend into the proximal (cervical) esophagus, indicating inadequate decompression by the azygos vein. In the distal esophagus, the varices progressively enlarge (Fig. 8-1b) finally crossing the gastroesophageal (GE) junction into the cardia (Fig. 8-1c) to become the short gastric veins of the fundus. Once the cardia is entered, however, the endoscopist finds it difficult, if not impossible, to follow the course of the varices, because of their now deep submucosal location in contrast to their position in the esophagus, just slightly below the mucosal surface.[1] The superficial location in the esophagus, in contrast to the stomach, probably best accounts for why, for varices of equal size (distal esophagus compared with cardia), the commonest location of variceal rupture is within a 2 cm zone above, rather than below, the GE junction[1] (see Chapter 34).

APPEARANCE

Esophageal varices may appear as a single blue-gray column with other less apparent elevations (Fig. 8-2), as multiple elevated columns, or as multiple elevated blue-gray or multiple interconnecting raised areas (Fig. 8-3) with no columns. The columns themselves have a distinct, undulating quality giving them a serpiginous appearance (Fig. 8-4), which is their most distinctive visual characteristic. The undulating course of the varices may also cause their surfaces to seem uneven, almost nodular. The combination of these features provides for their distinctive appearance (Fig. 8-5).

Basic Coloration

Their coloration varies from blue-gray to gray-white. Large varices tend to be blue-gray, but often we observe them to be gray-white or even yellow-white (with intense illumination). Small varices frequently have a gray-white coloration, but this is not invariably so, with some having a striking gray-blue appearance (Fig. 8-6).

Associated Erythema

Within the distal esophagus, both diffuse and linear erythema may be found in the mucosa overlying the varices (Fig. 8-7). The origin of this erythema is uncertain. Some have suggested that the linear-appearing erythema is vascular (i.e., telangiectasis of the *vasa vasorum* or "varices overlying varices"),[2] but this is unproved. As the linear erythema resembles erosions, it is tempting to view this appearance as esophagitis of uncertain cause. Contrary to what might be expected, esophageal reflux has not been consistently

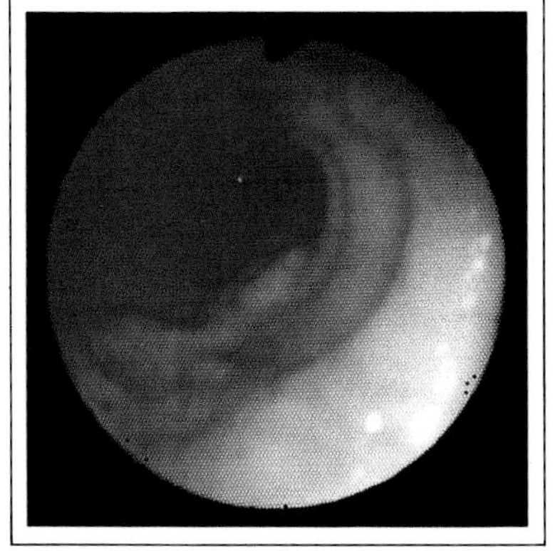

FIG. 8-1a.

FIG. 8-1b.

FIG. 8-1. a: Esophageal varices. These are relatively inconspicuous at the point of maximum decompression, the level of the azygos vein, but are nevertheless recognized as serpiginous, blue elevations. **b:** Esophageal varices. At the point of least decompression (at the cardia), the varices are most conspicuous. **c:** Cardial varices. These are seen with the retroflexed view of the cardia in direct continuity with the distal esophageal varices seen in (b).

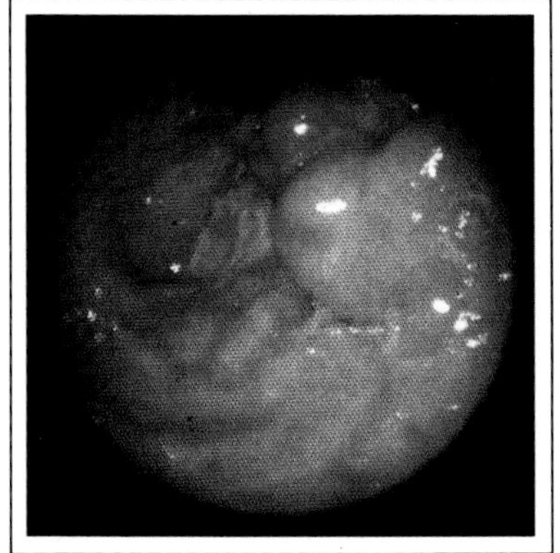

FIG. 8-1c.

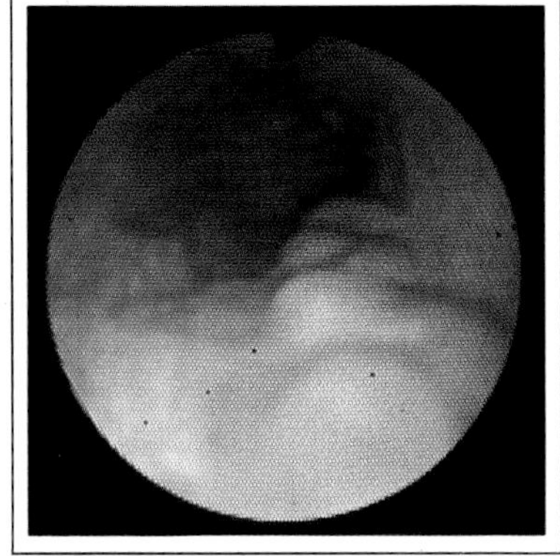

FIG. 8-2.

FIG. 8-2. Esophageal varices. One prominent varix is seen at 6 o'clock, with the others less apparent.

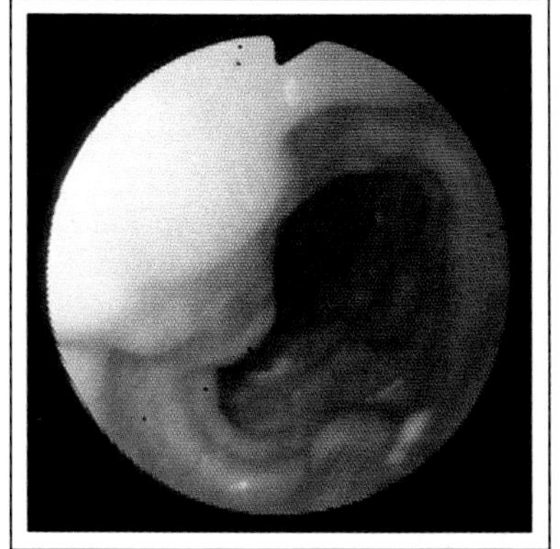

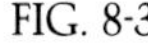

FIG. 8-3.

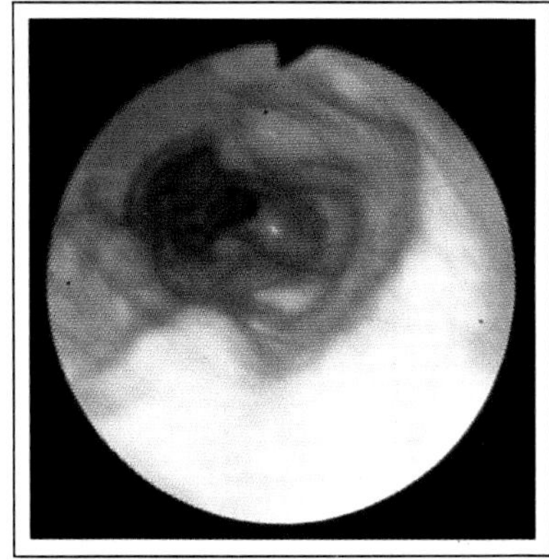

FIG. 8-4.

FIG. 8-3. Esophageal varices. Note the multiple, interconnecting blue-gray raised areas.

FIG. 8-4. Esophageal varix, as an undulating mucosal column.

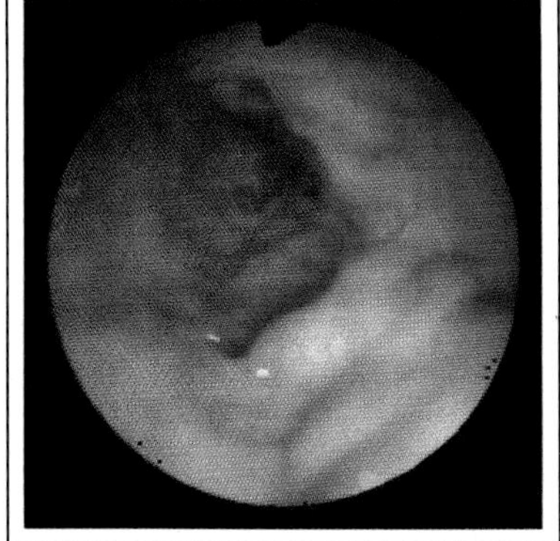

FIG. 8-5.

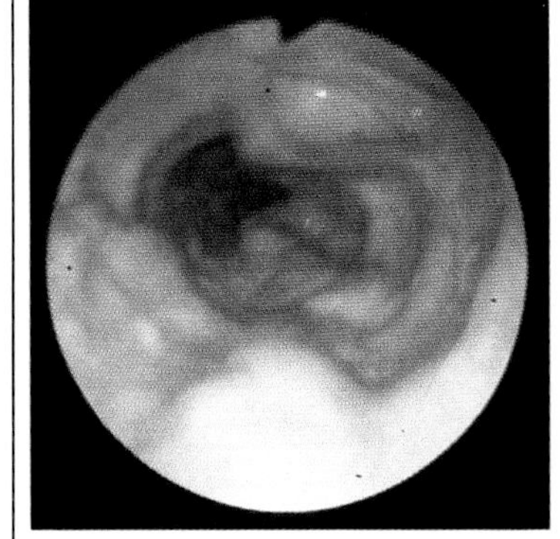

FIG. 8-6.

FIG. 8-5. Esophageal varices. This is the most characteristic appearance with undulating interconnecting mucosal columns.

FIG. 8-6. Esophageal varices. The large varix at 12 o'clock appears gray-white, being most intensely illuminated, whereas the smaller ones at 6 o'clock reflect less light and appear gray-blue.

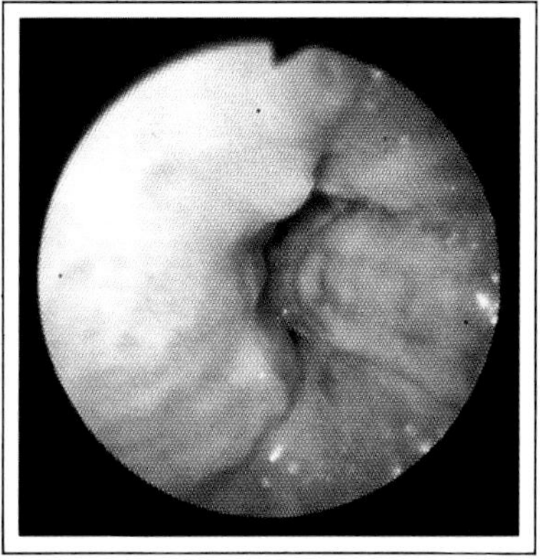

FIG. 8-7.

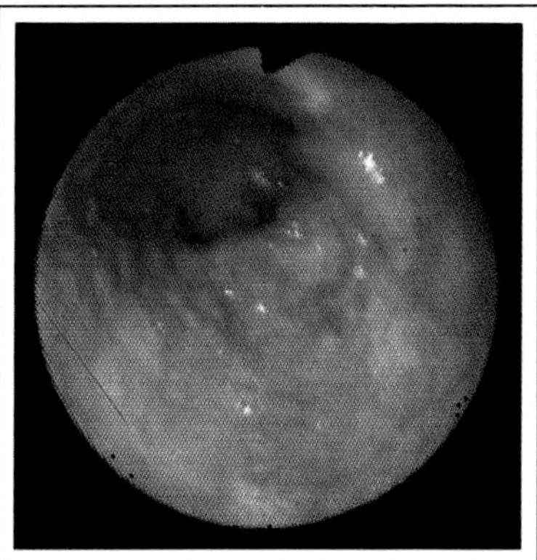

FIG. 8-8.

FIG. 8-7. Esophageal varices with erosions. Large varices project into the lumen at 3 o'clock and show surface erosions. The origin and significance of these erosions remain uncertain.

FIG. 8-8. Esophageal varices 1+. These can just barely be identified, having a height equal to one-fourth the bite width of an open pediatric biopsy forceps (see text), or between 1 and 2 mm.

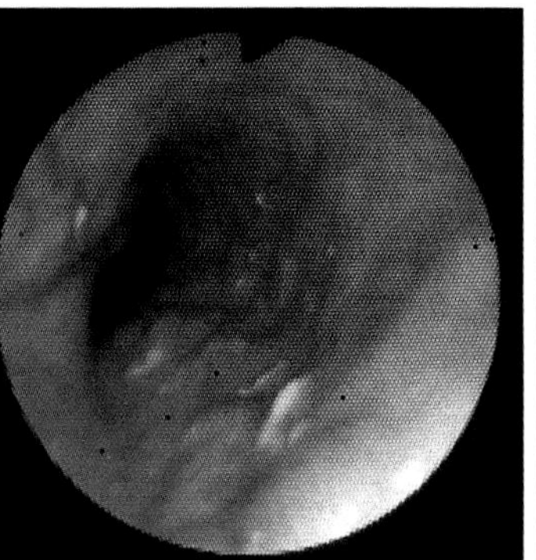

FIG. 8-9.

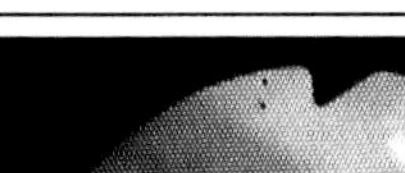

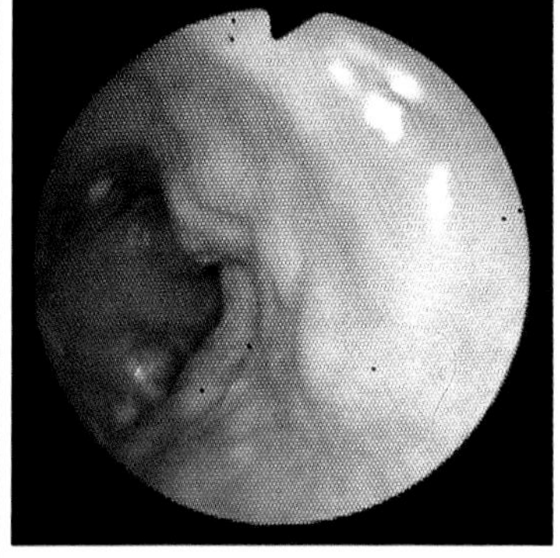

FIG. 8-10.

FIG. 8-9. Esophageal varices 2+. These are better recognized with a height equal to one-half the open bite width, or between 2 and 3 mm.

FIG. 8-10. Esophageal varices 3+. These are clearly recognized with a height of three-fourths the bite width, or between 3 and 4 mm.

demonstrated in patients with esophageal varices, even those with tense ascites.[3] It may be that because the varices project out into the lumen, erosions occur as a wear-and-tear phenomenon.

The significance of the color changes associated with varices is unclear. Although the tendency of esophageal varices to bleed has been related to size,[1] it is unsettled whether color changes (i.e., the so-called "red color sign")[2] independent of variceal size (Fig. 8-7), increase the likelihood of bleeding as was suggested in one report.[2]

GRADING OF VARICEAL SIZE

There is no universally accepted system for grading the size of varices. Some use the system of small-size or large-size varices according to the subjective impression of the degree of protrusion into the lumen.[1] Many use a 1+ to 4+ system based on the same idea, where the numbers are entirely subjective. Our approach, derived from the method of Conn and Brodoff,[4a] is an attempt at objectivity. First, we choose a standard point for estimating maximum height, which we take to be 2 cm above the GE junction, a location where varix height would be maximum and easily determined. In addition, we assign grades on the basis of estimating the variceal height (Table 8-1), which compares the height of the varix to a known standard, which for us is the distance (5 mm) between the "cups" of an open Olympus FA (1.7 mm) biopsy forceps (Olympus Corporation of America, New Hyde Park, New York). This distance we refer to as the "open bite." The varix height of one-fourth of this is considered to be 1+ (Fig. 8-8), one-half of this 2+ (Fig. 8-9), three-fourths of this 3+ (Fig. 8-10), and equal to or greater than this length 4+ (Fig. 8-11). Each number corresponds roughly to the millimeters of varix height. Using this system, one can compare the size of varices over time, which bears importantly on the likelihood of variceal bleeding.[1]

TABLE 8-1. *Grading of esophageal variation used on varix height at 2 cm for gastrointestinal junction*

Grade	Standard employed to estimate varix height (where the bite width of 1.7 mm forceps = 5 mm)
1+	One-fourth bite width
2+	One-half bite width
3+	Three-fourths bite width
4+	One or more bite width(s)

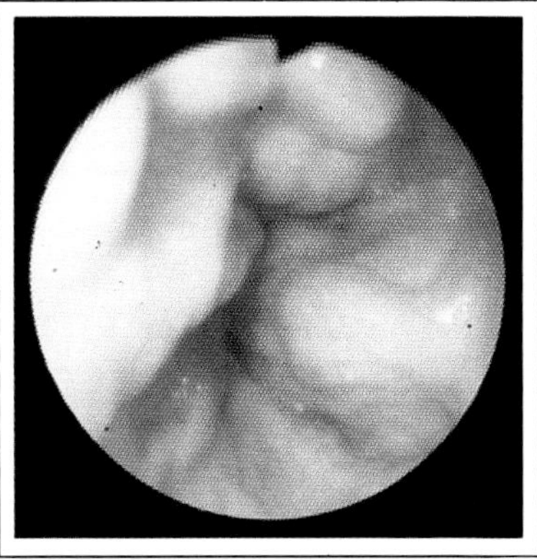

FIG. 8-11.

FIG. 8-11. Esophageal varices 4+. The height of these is equal to a full bite width, 4 mm or more.

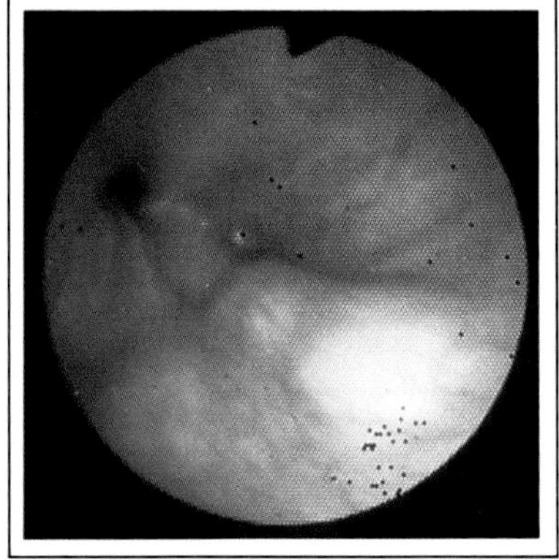

FIG. 8-12a.

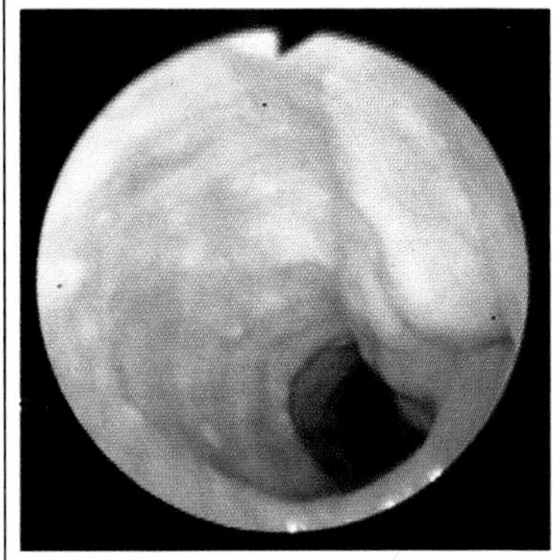

FIG. 8-12b.

FIG. 8-12. a: Prominent esophageal mucosal columns. The parallel mucosal columns may be prominent and if slightly tortuous may suggest varices. However, unlike varices, mucosal columns generally disappear with continued insufflation. **b:** Esophageal varix, isolated. The large (4+) varix at 3 o'clock is actually part of a system, with others at 7 o'clock.

APPEARANCES CONFUSED WITH VARICES

Two appearances may be confused with esophageal varices and require special consideration. These are: (a) prominent esophageal columns; and (b) dilated esophageal veins.

Prominent Esophageal Mucosal Columns

Prominent esophageal mucosal columns constitute a common appearance, especially if an insufficient amount of air has been administered (Fig. 8-12). To avoid confusing this appearance with that of varices, the endoscopist attempts better insufflation of the esophagus with more air, which effaces mucosal columns but not varices. Those esophageal columns which are not effaced may be distinguished from varices by their course, which is perfectly straight, rather than undulating (Fig. 8-5).

Dilated Esophageal Veins

In some patients, especially the elderly, one may see short, dilated, gray-blue veins (Fig. 8-13) which may be confused with varices. Usually these dilated veins are single, straight, and short (<2 cm), stopping proximal to the distal esophagus (Fig. 8-13), unlike the common varices, which can be seen to extend into the cardia (Fig. 8-3). Occasionally, these veins are particularly long and appear to extend into the mid-esophagus to the level of the azygos vein; these may represent a kind of "downhill" varix from elevated superior vena cava pressure secondary to congestive heart failure.

APPEARANCES FOLLOWING ENDOSCOPIC TREATMENT (SCLEROSIS) OF VARICES

The endoscopic injection of varices with a sclerosing agent (in the United States either sodium morrhuate or sodium tetradecyl sulfate) is an increasingly performed procedure for control of acute bleeding and for prevention of its recurrence.[4b] As tissue necrosis both within and around a successfully treated varix is a frequent sequella,[4c] it is not surprising that small (5 mm–1 cm) ulcerations or inflammatory exudates (pseudomembranes) are found as frequently as they are[4d]—in our experience, in all cases. In these cases one may see evidence of injury of the distal esophagus for as long as one month following treatment. Deeper ulcerations may be associated with stricture for-

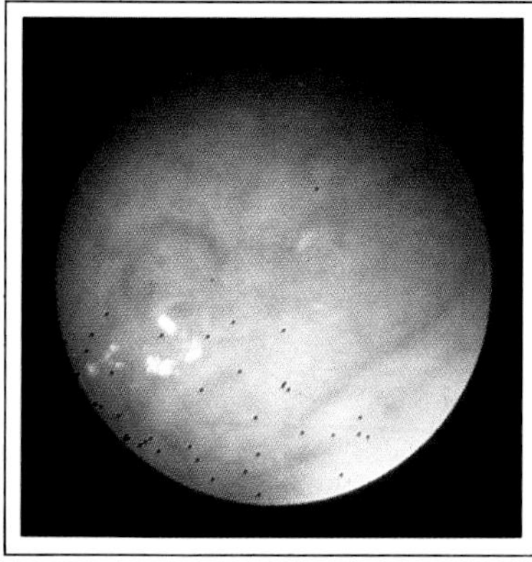

FIG. 8-13.

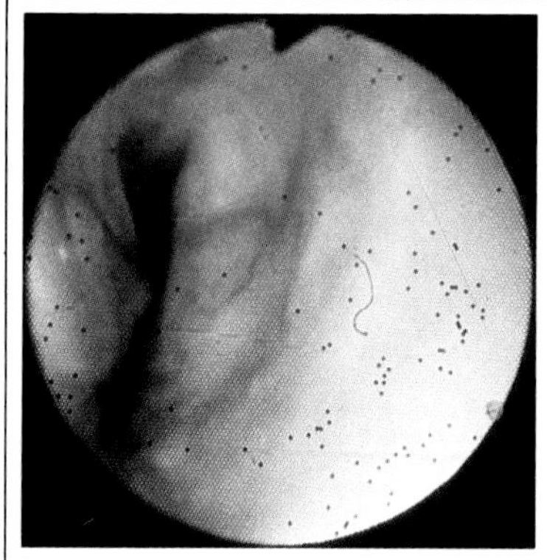

FIG. 8-14.

FIG. 8-13. Dilated esophageal vein. The isolated gray-blue vascular structure on the left (9 o'clock) wall is a part of a system. It does not extend proximally or distally and therefore is unlikely to be a varix.

FIG. 8-14. Downhill varices. These grade 1+ to 3+ varices were seen immediately upon entering the esophagus and extended down to 30 cm in a patient with a mediastinal mass. In this case the superior vena cava obstruction was ultimately proved. The fact that the varices stopped at 30 cm suggests that the obstruction did not occlude the azygos vein, allowing it to serve for decompression.

mation. The endoscopist who encounters a patient with varices and extensive ulceration of the distal esophagus should now suspect prior recent endoscopic sclerosis and should not perform additional injections at that time for fear of serious bleeding,[4e] unless mandated by a desperate clinical situation.

DOWNHILL VARICES

Esophageal varices most frequently form as a result of portal hypertension in which the submucosal veins of the esophagus which drain into the azygos system "above" are used to decompress the portal system "below." In these cases the flow is termed "uphill." In rare cases, with obstruction of the superior vena cava and azygos vein, blood from the upper extremities, head, and thorax may flow through inferior thyroid vein and mediastinal collaterals into the esophageal veins and then into the portal vein via the left gastric (coronary) vein. These are called "downhill" varices, with the best known cause for these being bronchiogenic carcinoma,[5] which produces obstruction of the superior vena cava. Mediastinal fibrosis, a substernal thyroid gland,[5] and achalasia[6] have also been reported as causes. In some, the level of obstruction determines the extent of the varices. Obstruction of the superior vena cava of the azygos vein (Fig. 8-14) still allows for compression via the azygos vein so that the varices terminate 30 cm from the incisors. With obstruction of the azygos vein itself, the varices continue into the distal esophagus, crossing the cardia to decompress by way of the left gastric vein.

REFERENCES

1. Liebowitz, H. R. (1961): Pathogenesis of esophageal varix rupture. *J.A.M.A.*, 175:874–879.
2. Beppu, K., Inokuchi, K., Koyanagi, N., Nakayama, S., Sakata, H., Kitano, S., and Kobayaski, M. (1981): Prediction of variceal hemorrhage by esophageal endoscopy. *Gastrointest. Endosc.*, 27:213–218.
3. Eckhardt, V. F. G., and Grace, N. D. (1979): Gastroesophageal reflux and bleeding esophageal varices. *Gastroenterology*, 76:39–42.
4. LeBrec, D., Defleury, P., Rueff, B., Nahum, H., and Benhamou, J.-P. (1980): Portal hypertension, size of esophageal varices, and risk of gastrointestinal bleeding in alcoholic cirrhosis. *Gastroenterology*, 79:1139–1144.

4a. Conn, H. D., and Brodoff, M. (1964): Emergency esophagoscopy in the diagnosis of upper gastrointestinal hemorrhage: a critical evaluation of its diagnostic accuracy. *Gastroenterology*, 47:505–512.

4b. Allison, J. G. (1983): The role of injection sclerotherapy in the emergency and definitive management of bleeding esophageal varices. *J.A.M.A.*, 249:1484–1487.

4c. Evans, D. M. D., Jones, D. B., Cleary, B. K., and Smith, P. M. (1982): Oesophageal varices treated by sclerotherapy: a histopathological study. *Gut*, 23:615–620.

4d. Sanowski, R. A., Brayko, C. M., Kozarek, R. A., and Howells, T. (1983): Endoscopic injection sclerotherapy of esophageal varices. *Gastrointest. Endosc.*, 29:242–243.

4e. Ayres, S. J., Goff, J. S., Warren, G. H., and Schaefer, J. W. (1982): Esophageal ulcerations and bleeding after flexible fiberoptic esophageal vein sclerosis. *Gastroenterology*, 83:131–136.

5. Sorokin, J. J., Levine, S. M., Moss, E. G., and Biddle, C. M. (1977): Downhill varices: report of a case 29 years after resection of a substernal thyroid gland. *Gastroenterology*, 73:345–348.
6. Kraft, A. R., Frank, H. A., and Glotzer, D. J. (1973): Achalasia of the esophagus complicated by varices and massive hemorrhage. *N. Engl. J. Med.*, 288:405–406.

9

POSTSURGICAL APPEARANCES OF THE ESOPHAGUS

The endoscopist may be asked to examine symptomatic patients after surgery involving the esophagus. The commonest operations he encounters are: (a) antireflux surgery; (b) vagotomy; (c) esophagectomy with gastric pull-through; and (d) colon interposition. When examining such patients, the endoscopist should have fixed in mind the expected appearances for these operations so as not to confuse them with others which suggest a pathologic condition.

ANTIREFLUX SURGERY

Patients are symptomatic after antireflux surgery for one of three reasons: (a) an ineffective operation; (b) an effective operation with new symptoms related to the surgery; and (c) an effective antireflux operation for symptoms unrelated to reflux. To best assist the referring physician, the endoscopist must establish in his examination, first, if there is evidence of esophagitis (see Chapter 3) and, second, if the appearance of the esophagogastric junction is the expected one for the operation which has been performed. In this section we present the appearances the endoscopist is most likely to encounter for the particular esophageal operations performed.

Nissen Fundoplication

In the Nissen fundoplication the gastric fundus is sewn around the lower esophageal high-pressure zone, augmenting it.[1] This has several results that concern the endoscopist. In the first place, it lowers the position of the gastroesophageal (GE) junction to a point clearly below the diaphragm. In addition, as the wrap is sewn on the right-hand side, there will be extrinsic compression from this side as well as leftward deviation of the esophagus position below the diaphragm.

Appearance

The anatomic changes of the surgery have important consequences as far as the endoscopic appearance is concerned. In contrast to the unoperated patient, the examiner now observes the diaphragmatic hiatal impression, established by the "sniff" test (see Chapter 1), well above the GE junction (Fig. 9-1). Just below the diaphragmatic hiatal impression, there is a new high-pressure zone for the portion of the cardia and upper body which has been "wrapped." The entrance to this has what has been described as a "hooded"[3] or "nipple-like" appearance (Fig. 9-1). Because of the fundoplication itself, the segment which runs through is usually tightly constricted, although not invariably, as some surgeons create a "floppy" fundoplication, which is said to allow for normal but not pathologic reflux.[3]

The examination should always include a "U" retroflexed view of the cardia (see Chapter 11), where one expects to see a mass-like deformity of the cardia with prominent though pliant symmetrical folds (see Chapter 19).

Disrupted Fundoplication ("Slipped Wrap")

Symptomatic patients may be referred for endoscopy following Nissen fundoplication to determine whether the surgical "wrap" is intact or disrupted.[2] In contrast to the intact case (see above), the GE junction is located at or above the diaphragmatic hiatus, rather than below it. The nipple-like or hooded deformity is not seen just below the hiatal impression as it would be for the intact case. Rather a band-like constriction of the upper body is found 3 to 4 cm distal to the hiatus (Fig. 9-2), representing the malpositioned fundoplication. This band creates a separate chamber of proximal stomach and continues for about 3 to 4 cm, with its lumen finally opening into the remainder of the body.

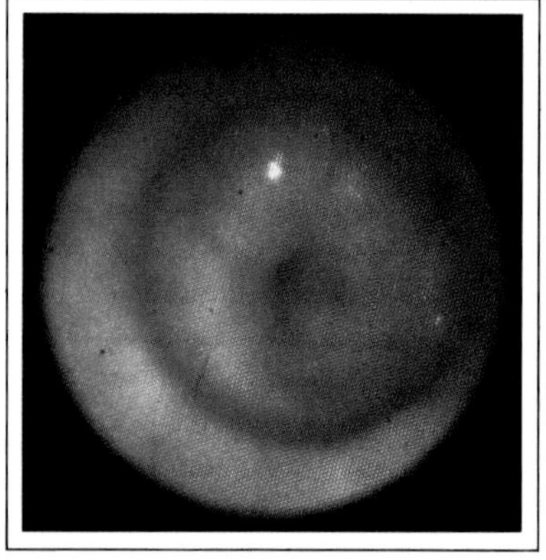

FIG. 9-1.

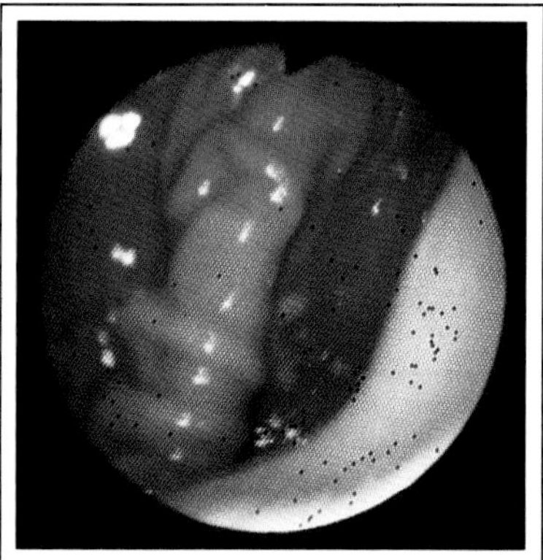

FIG. 9-2.

FIG. 9-1. Nissen fundoplication. Note the nipple-like opening at the GE junction into a 3-cm narrowed area just below. Above is the ring-like diaphragmatic hiatal impression.

FIG. 9-2. Disrupted Nissen fundoplication. The endoscope tip is just above a 3- to 4-cm band-like constriction 7 cm below the GE junction. This creates above it (at 9 o'clock) a gastric pouch, separate from the rest of the stomach (entered at 6 o'clock).

FIG. 9-3a.

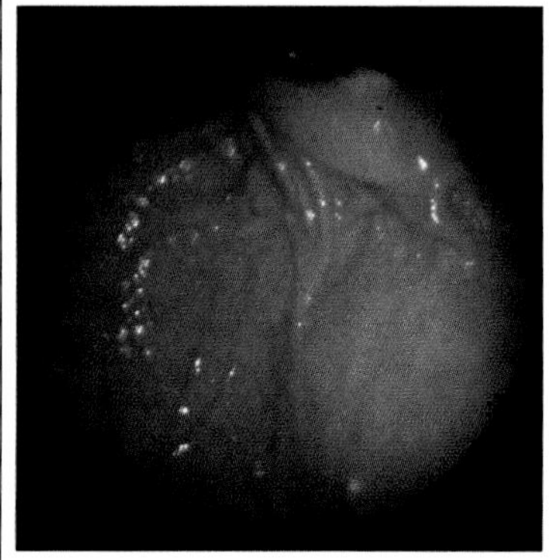

FIG. 9-3b.

FIG. 9-3. a: Belsey (Mark IV) procedure. The diaphragmatic hiatal impression is seen at 12 o'clock, and the GE junction is 2 cm distal to this point. The indentation at 12 o'clock results from the anterior gastropexy. **b:** Retroflexed view of the cardia. The converging folds leading to the cardia are the result of the posterior closure of the anterior gastropexy.

Belsey (Mark IV) Procedure

The Belsey (Mark IV) procedure, which utilizes an intrathoracic approach, is an anterior gastropexy (causing a short segment of distal esophagus to become intraabdominal by attaching it to the diaphragm) and posterior closure of the diaphragmatic hiatus.[4]

In patients having had this operation, the examiner can expect to encounter the GE junction slightly below the diaphragmatic hiatus as determined by the sniff test. The point at which the esophagus is attached to the diaphragm is observed as 2 to 3 cm of anterior (12 o'clock) compression (Fig. 9-3a) beginning at the hiatal impression. Evidence of anterior deformity is also noted on examination of the cardia (Fig. 9-3b) when viewed by means of U-type retroflexion (see Chapter 11).

Hill Gastropexy Repair

In the Hill gastropexy repair, which is performed less often in recent years, the surgeon essentially sews the distal 3 to 5 cm of the esophagus into the diaphragm as he closes the diaphragmatic hiatus. This firmly secures the intraabdominal portion of the esophagus and cardia below the diaphragm.[4]

As in the fundoplication, the endoscopist expects to find the diaphragmatic hiatal impression above, rather than below, the GE junction. There may be some narrowing of the distal portion of the esophagus and cardia resulting from the plicating sutures placed on the anterior and posterior walls. As such, the endoscopic appearance for the Hill procedure does not differ markedly from that for the Belsey operation (Fig. 9-3).

OTHER SURGICAL PROCEDURES

Vagotomy

Vagotomy is the most commonly performed operation which can potentially distort the appearance of the cardioesophageal junction. Yet this occurs rarely, probably in no more than 1 to 2% of truncovagotomy procedures,[5] although it may be more common after selective (proximal) vagotomy.[6] Such patients are referred for endoscopy because of dysphagia,[5,6] which has been attributed to narrowing of the distal esophagus because of periesophageal fibrosis, edema, or hematoma formation. In addition, an achalasia-like picture has been described,[7] possibly from vagal denervation of the lower esophageal sphincter, i.e., "neurogenic dysphagia." Whatever the cause, the condition tends

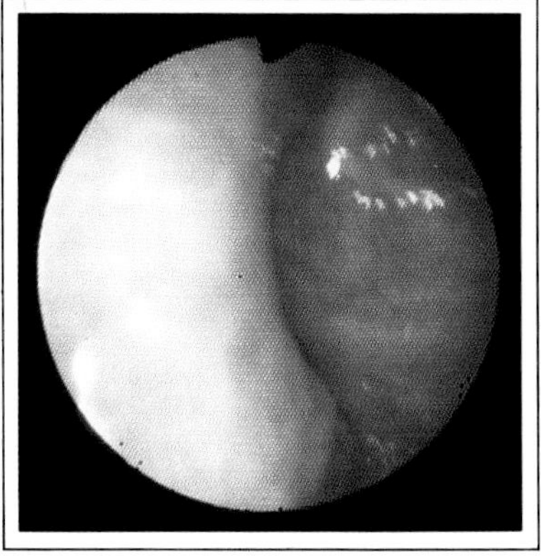
FIG. 9-4.

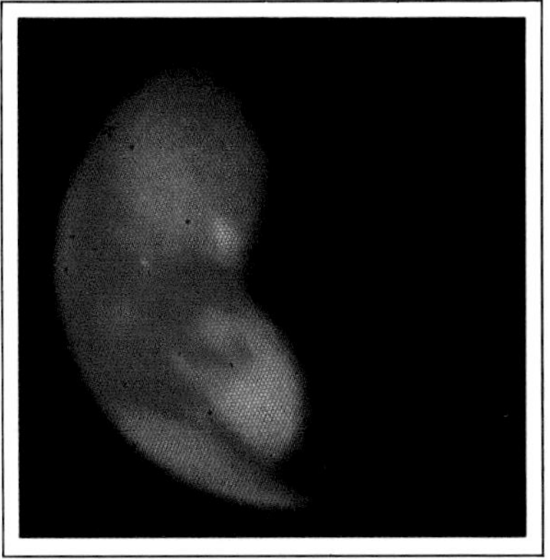
FIG. 9-5.

FIG. 9-4. Postvagotomy dysphagia. The expected left-sided (9 o'clock) compression from periesophageal fibrosis is noted. The mucosal columns pass across the GE junction from the right (3 o'clock) wall as evidence against a stricture.

FIG. 9-5. Esophagogastric anastomosis. The nodularity seen results from the interrupted sutures used in the surgery, and some friability (ease of bleeding) at the anastomosis is also an expected finding.

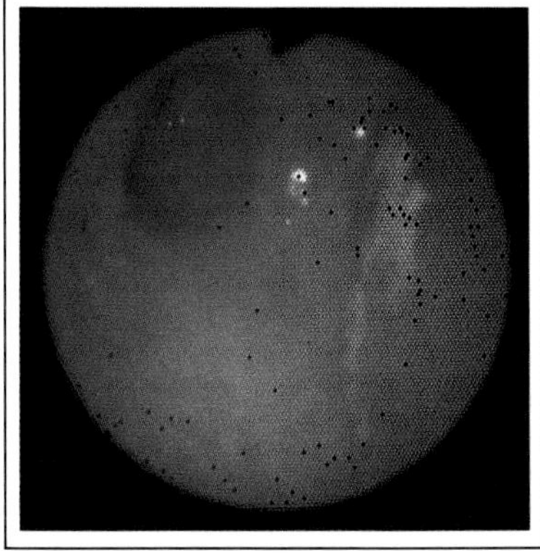
FIG. 9-6.

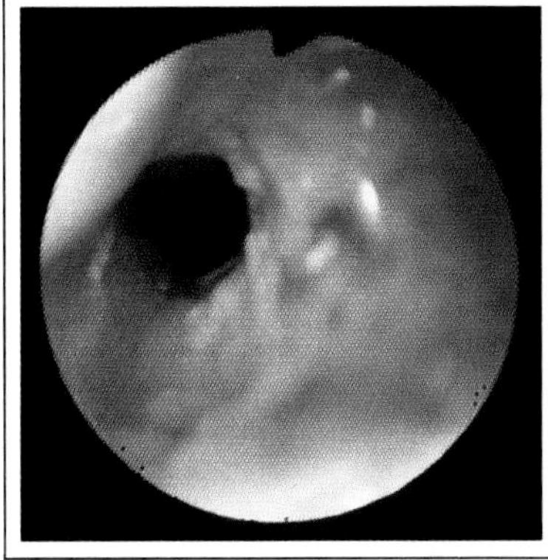
FIG. 9-7.

FIG. 9-6. Distal esophagectomy with gastric pull-through. The intrathoracic stomach has been entered. As a result of the pull-through, the orientation is the reverse of normal (see Chapter 11), with the lesser curve observed toward 9 o'clock and the greater curve and gastric lake at 3 o'clock.

FIG. 9-7. Esophagogastric anastomosis. A stricture has resulted from severe reflux injury, now seen with obvious ulceration at its mouth.

to subside over a 3- to 6-month period during which time it is often amenable to esophageal dilatation.[5,6] In patients in whom the dysphagia persists beyond this period, surgical exploration may become necessary.

In patients with postvagotomy dysphagia, the endoscopist may simply find the esophageal column intact and radiating into the esophagogastric junction (Fig. 9-4). Resistance is encountered within the area at or just below the diaphragmatic hiatal impression; however, in most cases the resistance gives way, especially if a small-caliber (9 mm) endoscope is employed. As the columns are intact, the appearance will be indistinguishable from that of achalasia regardless of whether esophageal motility studies demonstrate typical features. Endoscopy therefore does not differentiate between cases of postvagotomy dysphagia from periesophageal fibrosis and those of the "neurogenic" type with manometric and radiologic features of classic achalasia.[7]

Esophagectomy (Subtotal) With Gastric Pull-Through

Subtotal esophagectomy with gastric pull-through is often performed for resectable carcinoma of the mid or distal esophagus.[8] The esophagogastric anastomosis is found between 22 and 32 cm with approximately 10 to 15 cm of intrathoracic stomach.

The esophagogastric anastomosis has a somewhat nodular appearance (Fig. 9-5) because of the use of interrupted sutures in its construction; however, the mucosal appearance is either normal or shows such nonspecific features as erythema and friability. As a result of the surgery the stomach is rotated on its long axis, resulting in an orientation with the esophagus just opposite of the expected (see Chapter 11); therefore as the pull-through portion of the stomach is entered, one finds the lesser curve coming off the left wall at 9 o'clock and the greater curve toward 3 o'clock (Fig. 9-6). On the esophagus side of the stoma, there may be evidence of moderate or severe esophagitis (Fig. 9-7) because of free reflux. In some cases, changes are severe and lead to stricture formation (Fig. 9-7). Contributing to this tendency would be technical problems in the creation of the anastomosis, e.g., excessive tension or the use of irradiation postoperatively in patients having cancer operations.

Appearance of Recurrent Cancer

The appearance of recurrent carcinoma depends largely on whether the initial resection was curative or palliative. If the resection of the original carcinoma was believed surgically and histologically to be complete (curative), recurrence will be largely limited to lymph nodes and serosal

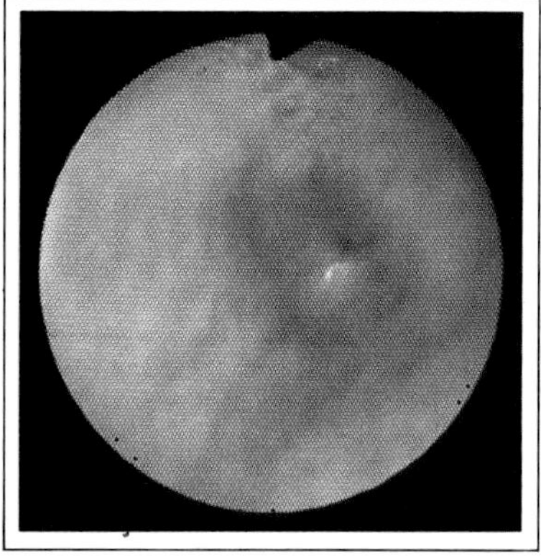

FIG. 9-8.

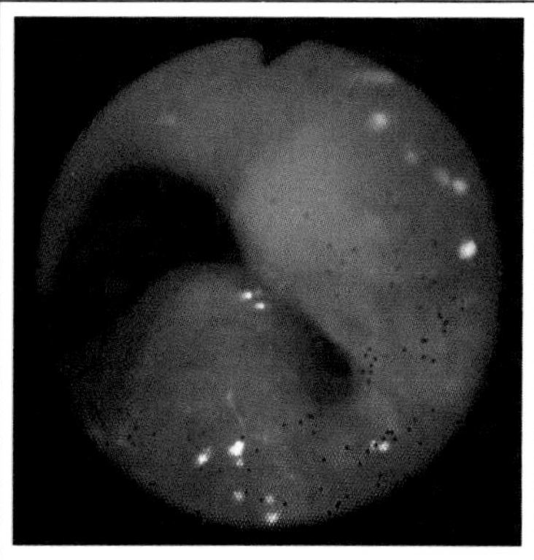

FIG. 9-9.

FIG. 9-8. Recurrence of a cardial carcinoma as a benign stricture. One year after a curative resection, a smooth, pinpoint stricture appeared just above the anastomosis. Because of the intact mucosa, this was thought benign, although recurrence was proved at subsequent surgery.

FIG. 9-9. Recurrent cardial carcinoma after palliative resection. At the time of the original surgery, there was cancer in the resected margins. Six months later there is a rigid, indurated cardial fold—evidence of recurrent carcinoma at the anastomosis.

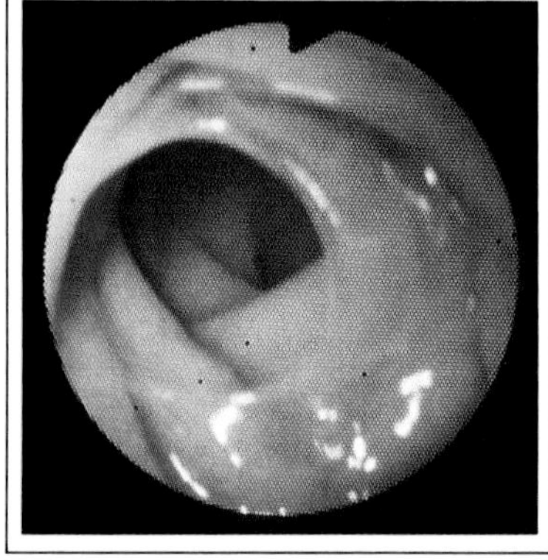

FIG. 9-10.

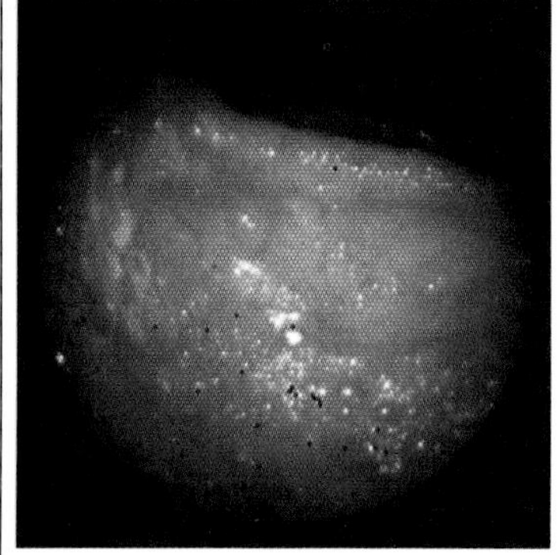

FIG. 9-11.

FIG. 9-10. Colon interposition. An interhaustral colonic type fold denotes this segment as interposed between esophagus and stomach.

FIG. 9-11. Colon interposition. The colonic section has been entered and a prominent vascular pattern typical of colonic mucosa is observed.

invasion, without involvement of the mucosa. In these cases evidence of recurrence would be that of a stricture with a marked degree of narrowing but an intact mucosa (Fig. 9-8).

In cases where there was evidence surgically or histologically of an incomplete resection, recurrence may occur within the mucosa of the anastomosis. In such cases any irregular appearance of the stoma is important and suggests the need for multiple (six to 10) biopsies and brushings. In particular, one looks for the presence of nodular masses having a rock-hard consistency and being larger than 5 mm (Fig. 9-9). Such findings strongly suggest recurrence.

Colon Interposition

Placement of a length of transverse colon, usually from the left side, in isoperistaltic fashion between the resected margin of the esophagus and stomach is being increasingly performed for both malignancy and benign esophageal disease; this includes patients having strictures with failed medical management[9] and those having achalasia with failed prior surgical myotomy.[9 10]

Although excellent results have been reported, some patients do have recurrent obstructive-type symptoms after this surgery. The endoscopist's task is to determine the cause—whether it is "functional," having to do with the length of the isoperistaltic segment used, or mechanical, the result of stricture formation either at the proximal (esophagocolic) or distal (cologastric) anastomosis.

Upon entry into the colonic segment, one views the characteristic interhastral folds (Fig. 9-10), and vascular pattern (Fig. 9-11) (see Chapter 39). The esophagus is just above this, with mucosa which is either normal or showing nonspecific erythema (Fig. 9-12). At approximately 40 cm from the incisors, the diaphragmatic hiatus can be appreciated. In some cases the colon is redundant below the diaphragm prior to the cologastric anastomosis such that the stomach is not entered. More often, however, the cologastric anastomosis is found within 5 cm of the diaphragmatic hiatal impression. At this point, one notes the abrupt transition between the pale yellow-white colonic epithelium and the orange-yellow gastric mucosa.

Total Gastrectomy

Esophagitis may complicate the postoperative course after total gastrectomy for nearly 30%[11] of patients or more.[12,13]

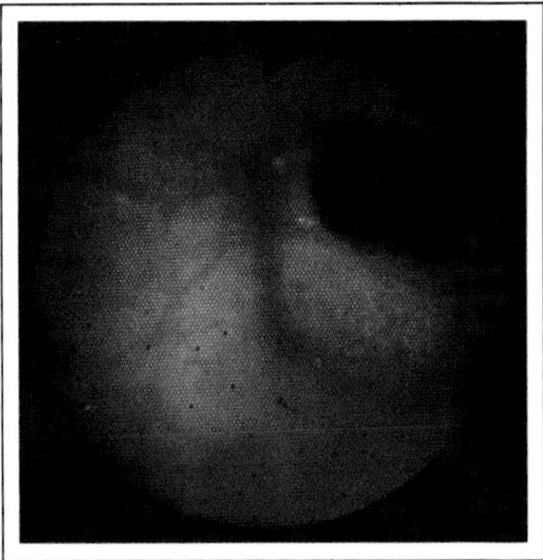

FIG. 9-12.

FIG. 9-12. Colon interposition. The esophagus shows nonspecific erythema just above the anastomosis.

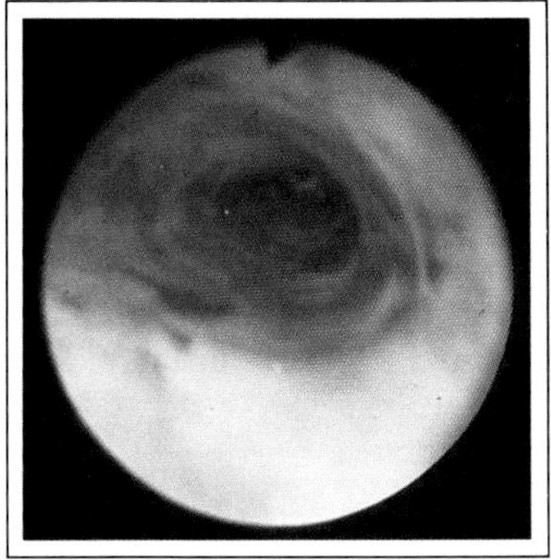

FIG. 9-13a.

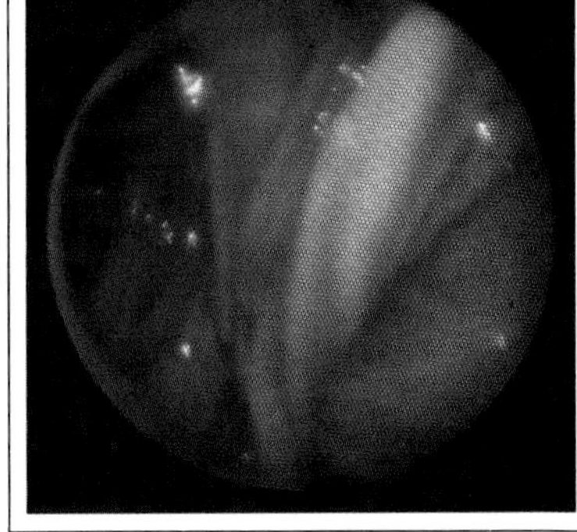

FIG. 9-13b.

FIG. 9-13. a: Alkaline reflux esophagitis after total gastrectomy. In this patient with an end-to-side esophagojejunostomy with distal enteroenterostomy (b) extensive areas of adherent inflammatory exudate were present along with marked friability indicative of severe esophagitis (see Chapter 3). One expects this appearance to completely resolve after a Roux-en-Y loop 50 cm distal to the esophagojejunal anastomosis. **b:** The jejunal aspects of an end-to-side esophagojejunostomy in a patient after total gastrectomy for a leiomyosarcoma. Bile delivered from the afferent loop freely refluxes into the esophagus to produce in one-third of the cases moderate to severe esophageal injury (a).

It is seen no less often after surgery for the Zollinger-Ellison syndrome, where unlike after resections for cancer adjuvant irradiation and chemotherapy are not administered.[12] In all cases where esophagitis occurs, the injury is generally believed to be the result of the effects on esophageal mucosa of bile and pancreatic secretion,[13] and has been termed alkaline reflux esophagitis.[12] This is readily reversed after the operation with the creation of Roux-en-Y diversion at 50 cm from the esophagojejunal anastomosis.

Patients with this condition are examined because of symptoms of retrosternal pain, sour brash, bilious vomiting, and dumping after total gastrectomy. Dysphagia may also occur, especially in the minority (10%+) who develop an anastomotic stricture in association with the esophagitis.[13]

Although the esophagitis generally involves the distal esophagus, it may be more extensive, especially if the distal esophagus including the lower esophageal sphincter has been resected. In these cases the proximal esophagus is involved. Ulcerations and inflammatory exudate may be expected in half the cases (Fig. 9-13a) in the area within 5 cm of the esophagojejunal anastomosis (Fig. 9-13b). In 10% an anastomotic stricture is associated with the esophagitis.[13]

REFERENCES

1. Fisher, R. S., Malmud, L. S., Lobis, I. F., and Maier, W. P. (1978): Antireflux surgery for symptomatic gastroesophageal reflux: mechanism of action. *Am. J. Dig. Dis.*, 13:152–160.
2. Donahue, P. E., de Tarnowski, G. O., and Bombeck, C. T. (1981): Endoscopic assessment of a floppy Nissen fundoplication. *Gastrointest. Endosc.*, 27:121.
3. Saik, R. P., Greenberg, A. G., and Peskin, G. W. (1977): A study of fundoplication disruption and deformity. *Am. J. Surg.*, 134:19–26.
4. Brindley, C. V., and Hightower, N. C. (1979): Surgical treatment of gastroesophageal reflux. *Surg. Clin. North Am.*, 59:841–851.
5. Spencer, J. D. (1975): Postvagotomy dysphagia. *Br. J. Surg.*, 62:354–355.
6. Skjennald, A., Stadaas, J. D., Syversen, S. M., and Aune, S. (1979): Dysphagia after proximal gastric vagotomy. *Scand. J. Gastroenterol.*, 14:609–613.
7. Sharp, J. R. (1979): Mechanical and neurogenic factors in postvagotomy dysphagia. *J. Clin. Gastroenterol.*, 1:321–324.
8. Chassin, J. L. (1978): Esophagogastrectomy. *Ann. Surg.*, 188:22–27.
9. Wilkins, E. W. (1980): Long-segment colon substitution for the esophagus. *Ann. Surg.*, 192:722–725.
10. Glasgow, J. C., Cannon, J. P., and Elkins, R. C. (1979): Colon interposition for benign esophageal disease. *Am. J. Surg.*, 137:175–179.
11. Schrock, T. R., and Way, L. W. (1978): Total gastrectomy. *Am. J. Surg.*, 135:348–355.
12. Morrow, D., and Passaro, E. R. (1976): Alkaline reflux esophagitis after total gastrectomy. *Am. J. Surg.*, 132:287–290.
13. Matikainen, M., Laatikainen, T., Kalima, T., and Kivilaakso, E. (1982): Bile acid composition and esophagitis after total gastrectomy. *Am. J. Surg.*, 143:196–198.

10

UNCOMMON ESOPHAGEAL APPEARANCES

In this chapter we present a variety of uncommon appearances which fall into two categories: (a) structural abnormalities, encompassing vascular compression, esophageal rings, webs, and diverticula; and (b) other abnormalities, including esophageal polyps and foreign bodies.

STRUCTURAL ABNORMALITIES

Extrinsic Compression from Vascular Structures

Ordinarily, the crossing of the esophagus by the aortic arch proximally and the thoracic aorta itself distally usually produces only a barely noticeable indentation of the wall, proximally at 10 o'clock (left anterior) and distally at 5 o'clock (right posterior). These crossings may slightly affect the shape of the lumen (see Chapter 2). In rare patients, however, the crossing of the esophagus by the aorta or anomalous branches may compress the lumen and produce intermittent or even persistent dysphagia. In this section, we consider extrinsic compression produced by: (a) anomalies of the aortic arch; (b) cardiac enlargement; and (c) a thoracic aorta.

Anomalies of the Aortic Arch

Two cases of dysphagia from aortic arch anomalies have been described recently.[1,2] Both involved the subclavian artery. In one case, the right subclavian artery took off directly from the aortic arch and ran posteriorly to the esophagus, causing a band-like compression of the lumen on the posterior (6 o'clock) side.[1] In this report the condition was called "dysphagia lusoria" (derived from arteria lusoria, the term for anomalous origin for the right subclavian artery). Surgery was required in this case. We have encountered what we believe to be a similar, though less severe, case having a comparable radiographic (Fig. 10-1a) and endoscopic (Fig. 10-1b) appearance. In our case the dysphagia was relieved with mild sedation so that arteriography to prove the diagnosis was never performed.

A corresponding anomaly of the left subclavian artery[2] has also been described, although the endoscopic details were not given. In this case there was posterior, ring-like compression of the esophagus by the ligamentum arteriosum as it coursed over to the left subclavian artery. This occurred in association with an anomalous right aortic arch and required surgical intervention.

Cardiac Enlargement

The left atrium lies in close proximity to the anterior wall of the middle and distal esophagus. In some patients this is reflected in a modest compromise of the lumen, with cardiac pulsations being apparent on the anterior (12 o'clock) aspect of the distal esophagus. With cardiac enlargement, especially the left atrium, there may be significant compression of the lumen (Fig. 10-2). In an occasional elderly patient, this is associated with intermittent dysphagia, especially after the ingestion of poorly chewed meat.[3]

Compression from the Distal Thoracic Aorta (Dysphagia Aortica)

Tortuosity, dilatation, and true aneurysms of the thoracic aorta are capable of producing significant right posterior (3 to 6 o'clock) compression (Fig. 10-3). The anatomic basis for this is that the aorta is fixed within its diaphragmatic hiatus by a sling originating from the two crura of the diaphragm posteriorly which encircles the esophagus anteriorly preventing additional anterior movement.[14] The dysphagia associated with compression by the descending thoracic aorta has been called dysphagia aortica.[3,4] It may be a particular problem in elderly patients, who have increased numbers of nonperistaltic motor waves,[5] chew poorly because of missing teeth or ill-fitting dentures, and

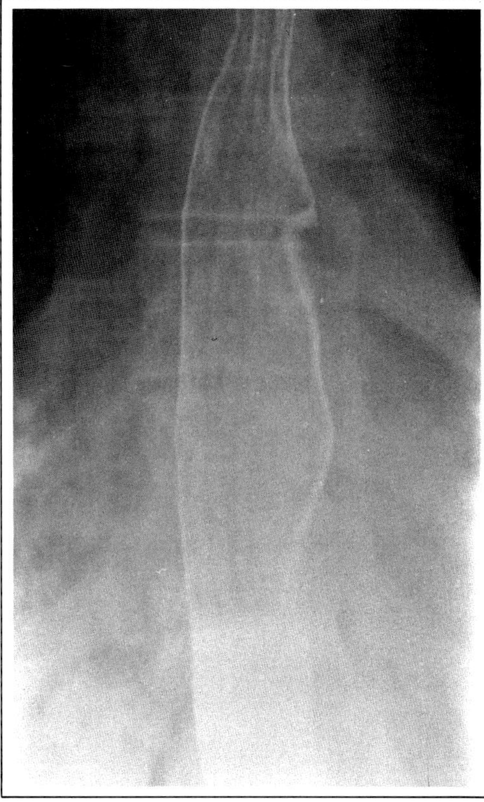

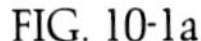

FIG. 10-1a.

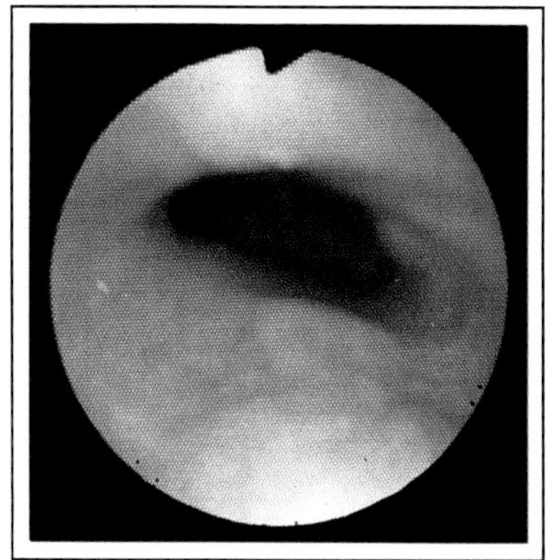

FIG. 10-1b.

FIG. 10-1. Possible dysphagia lusoria (anomalous origin of the right subclavian artery from the aortic arch). **a:** The esophagram shown here suggests an impression from the aortic arch which is seen obliquely from left to right. Other views (not shown) suggest this to be posterior to the esophagus and would be compatible with an anomalous right subclavian artery. **b:** A band-like posterior compression of the esophagus at the level of the aortic arch (25 cm) would be compatible with vascular compression from an anomalous right subclavian artery.

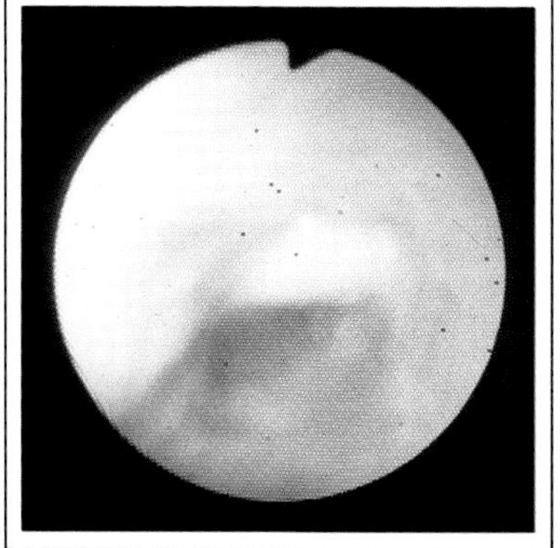

FIG. 10-2.

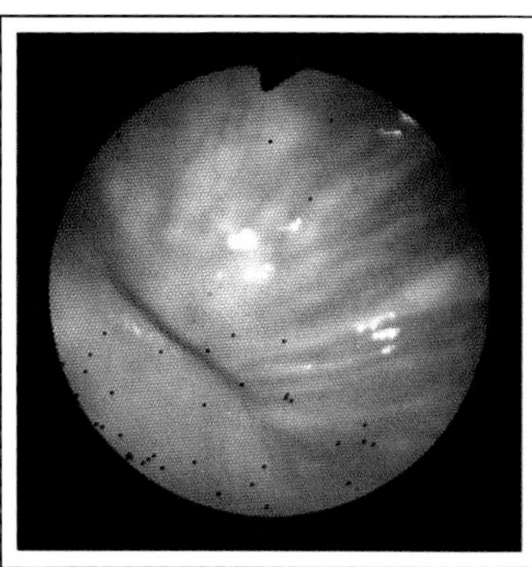

FIG. 10-3.

FIG. 10-2. Left atrial compression of the mid-esophagus. A pulsating indentation of the anterior wall with sharp angulation at 30 cm caused intermittent dysphagia in a patient with congestive heart failure and an enlarged left atrium.

FIG. 10-3. Dysphagia aortica. Marked extrinsic compression of the right wall of the distal esophagus just above the diaphragm in a patient with a proven aneurysm of the thoracic aorta.

periodically trap large food particles in the distal esophagus causing intermittent dysphagia. Some actually present with food impaction and complete obstruction.[4]

Rings and Webs

Projections into the lumen called rings and webs typically prompt the performance of endoscopy because of intermittent dysphagia which results from swallowing large food boluses. These become temporarily trapped by the ring.

Mucosal (Schatzki) Rings

Most mucosal rings encountered by the endoscopist are of the Schatzki type, located at the gastroesophageal (GE) junction in association with a hiatus hernia (Fig. 10-4). Endoscopically, this is a thin membrane or diaphragm-like ring 2 to 3 mm thick. In the classic study by Schatzki and Gary,[6] the thickness of the ring measured radiographically did not exceed 4 mm. Similarly, we find at endoscopy that the typical Schatzki ring has a thickness of about 3 mm, estimated using the "open bite width" method (see Chapter 4).

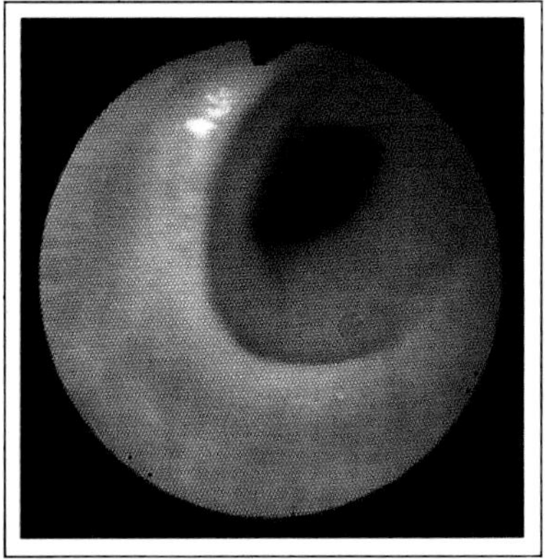

FIG. 10-4.

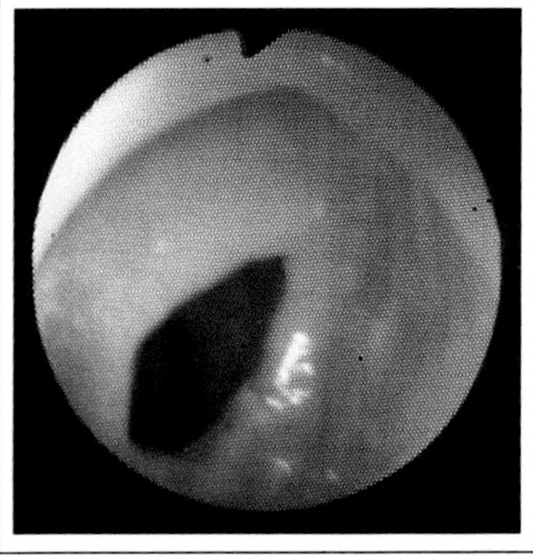

FIG. 10-5.

FIG. 10-4. Schatzki ring. A diaphragm-like, membranous ring is seen at the GE junction above a hiatus hernia. The thickness of the ring is estimated to be about 2 mm, distinguishing it from a thicker, though ring-like, peptic stricture (Fig. 10-5).

FIG. 10-5. Schatzki ring versus a peptic stricture. The width of this ring-like deformity was estimated to be 4 mm, more than would be expected even from a double ply of mucosa. Although it has the appearance of a Schatzki ring, its width suggests at least the presence of submucosal fibrosis, if not an early stricture. Whether this appearance progresses to that of a typical stricture (width ≥1 cm) is uncertain.

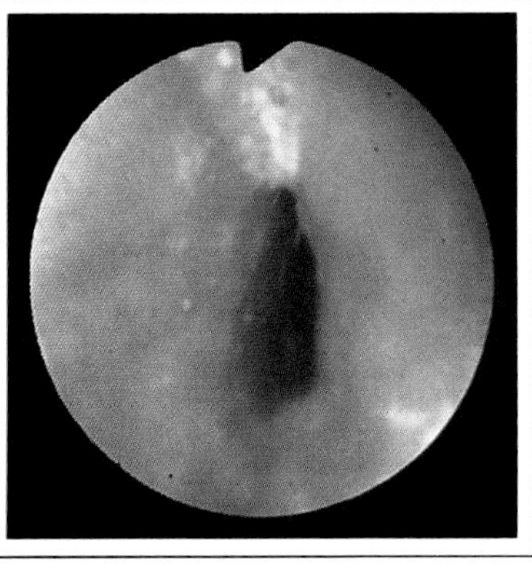

FIG. 10-6.

FIG. 10-6. Muscular ring. A stricture-like opening of 6 mm is seen in the mid-esophagus through which an 11-mm endoscope was passed with minimal resistance, suggestive of a muscular ring.

In most cases (74% in one series[7]) the lumen is compromised negligibly by the ring (Fig. 10-4), with a diameter ranging between 15 and 23 mm, resulting in no dysphagia.[7] In about 25%, the diameter of the ring is smaller, between 7 and 18 mm. In these patients there is intermittent dysphagia, with large boluses becoming trapped periodically above the ring.

The relationship of a Schatzki ring to esophageal reflux and peptic stricture is unsettled. As already mentioned (see Chapter 3), we generally observe the mucosa above the Schatzki ring to be thickened (Fig. 10-4), a finding we associate with chronic reflux. Others have reported reflux symptoms and evidence of peptic esophagitis in association with Schatzki rings.[7,8] Our belief is that the Schatzki ring appearance, along with mucosal thickening above it, is the result of squamous hyperplasia which has occurred within the distal esophagus as a response to chronic reflux. The presence of a hiatus hernia generally in evidence with a Schatzki ring may predispose to such reflux (see Chapter 3) and because of the spherical shape of its lumen (in contrast to the tubular esophagus), cause the termination of the thickened mucosa of the GE junction to appear ring-like (Fig. 10-4). Additional squamous hyperplasia may cause further narrowing of the lumen, but a Schatzki ring ought to remain thin if it consisted only of a mucosal layer, even one of double thickness, with a width of only 3 mm or less. Yet many Schatzki rings appear thicker. A ring with a greater width (3 to 4 mm or more) suggests to us the presence of submucosal fibrosis, which has been observed in autopsy studies.[9] These Schatzki rings with a component of submucosal fibrosis we regard as early peptic strictures (Fig. 10-5), although to what extent this appearance progresses to that of a typical peptic stricture (a width of 1 cm or more) is unknown.

Muscular Rings

Muscular rings can be distinguished from the Schatzki ring by their location above the GE junction.[10] They may have the appearance of a tight stricture radiographically and even at endoscopy. Esophageal columns may appear obliterated by a muscular ring (Fig. 10-6), but in contrast to a stricture, the larger, adult type (11 to 13 mm) endoscope can generally be passed through a muscular ring with ease.

Esophageal Webs

Esophageal webs are essentially semilunar mucosal projections confined to one wall of the esophagus (Fig. 10-7). They are best known as part of the Plummer-Vinson syndrome, in which the web occurs at the level of the cri-

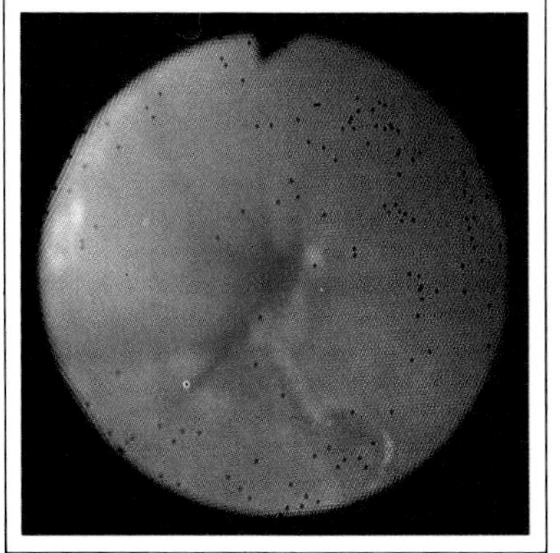

FIG. 10-7a.

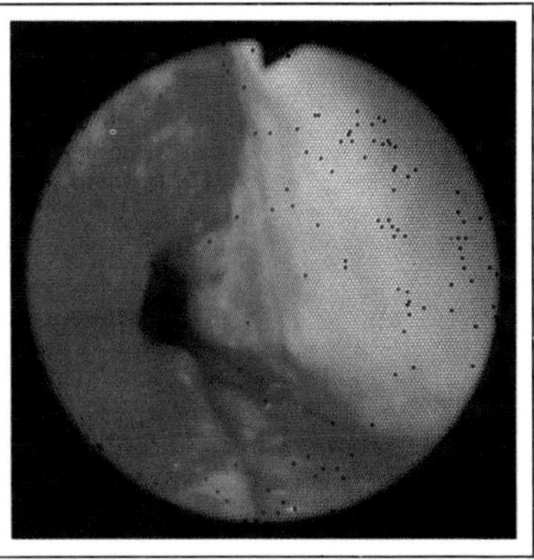

FIG. 10-7b.

FIG. 10-7. Upper esophageal web. **a:** A semilunar, whitish mucosal projection can be seen off the 3 o'clock wall at 20 cm from the incisors in a patient with intermittent dysphagia to large pills. **b:** Bleeding has occurred after passage of the endoscope.

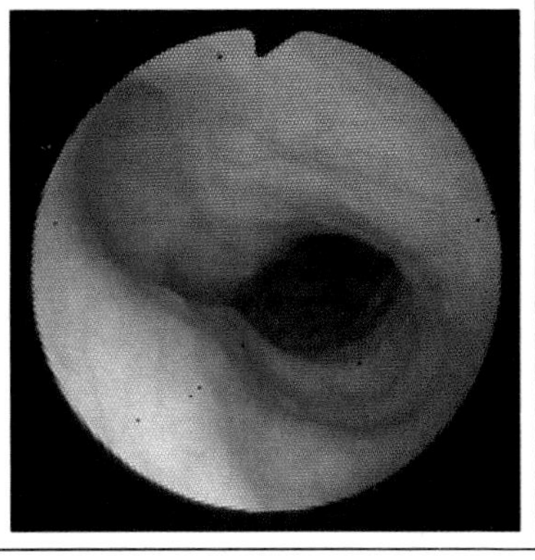

FIG. 10-8.

FIG. 10-8. Mid-esophageal (traction type) diverticulum. This blind passage at 9 o'clock (the lumen goes off to 3 o'clock) located in the mid-esophagus was seen radiographically to be just above several calcified hilar lymph nodes.

copharyngeus in association with iron deficiency anemia. Webs, however, may occur in the absence of anemia, being noted in one series in 5.5% of all patients referred for gastrointestinal radiographic studies, and occurring with the same frequency in patients with anemia as in those without it.[11] Endoscopy may be requested to confirm the presence of a suspected web, based on an esophagram; however, webs, especially of the cricopharyngeus, are difficult to demonstrate by endoscopy, being broken by the endoscope as it passes into the esophagus (Fig. 10-7, a and b).

In addition to single, cricopharyngeal webs, they have been found both singly[12] and multiply[13] in the mid and distal portions.

Esophageal Diverticula

There are three types of diverticula which are recognized at endoscopy: (a) mid-esophageal (traction type); (b) epiphrenic and others (pulsion type) associated with esophageal motor disorders; and (c) diffuse esophageal diverticulosis.

Mid-Esophageal (Traction Type) Diverticula

The mid-esophageal diverticula are the most common type recognized in our Unit. They appear as small (<1.5 cm) projections off the main course of the lumen. They are found within the mid-esophagus at the level of the hilum (25 cm) (Fig. 10-8). Radiographic studies of the esophagus show the diverticulum to be situated just above a calcific density representing old granulomatous disease.[11] It is thought that the diverticulum results from the motor wave front continuously meeting resistance at the point of adherence of the esophagus to the adjacent lymph nodes, causing the wall of the esophagus to project out at just above this point, creating the diverticulum.[14,15]

Epiphrenic and Other (Pulsion Type) Diverticula (Including Zenker's) Associated with Motor Disorders

Epiphrenic diverticula form within or just proximal to a persistent high-pressure zone[15] associated with achalasia (Fig. 10-9a) or diffuse spasm.[15] In achalasia we have seen diverticula elsewhere in the esophagus, including a giant diverticulum of the upper esophagus (Fig. 10-9b).

Zenker's diverticula form just above the cricopharyngeus, off the posterior wall of the hypopharynx (Fig. 10-10a). These may be found in association with a motor disorder of the cricopharyngeus resembling achalasia,[16] although this need not always be the case.[17] As one would predict

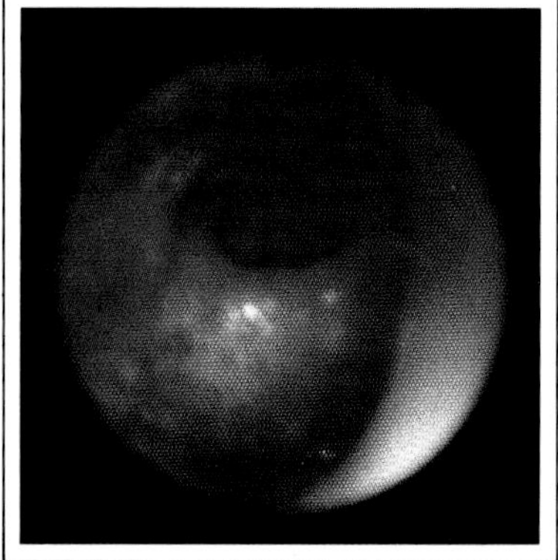

FIG. 10-9a.

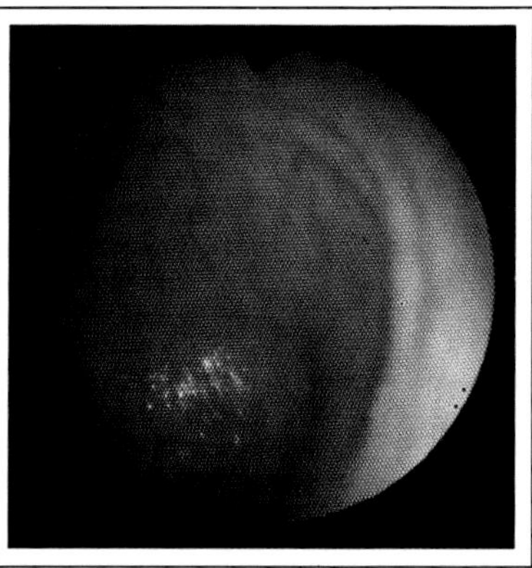

FIG. 10-9b.

FIG. 10-9. a: Epiphrenic (pulsion type) diverticulum in achalasia. This is seen at 6 o'clock just above the high-pressure zone at 12 o'clock. **b:** Large upper esophageal diverticulum and achalasia. The opening to the body of the esophagus from this huge (5 × 10 cm) saccular diverticulum is seen in the distance at 6 o'clock.

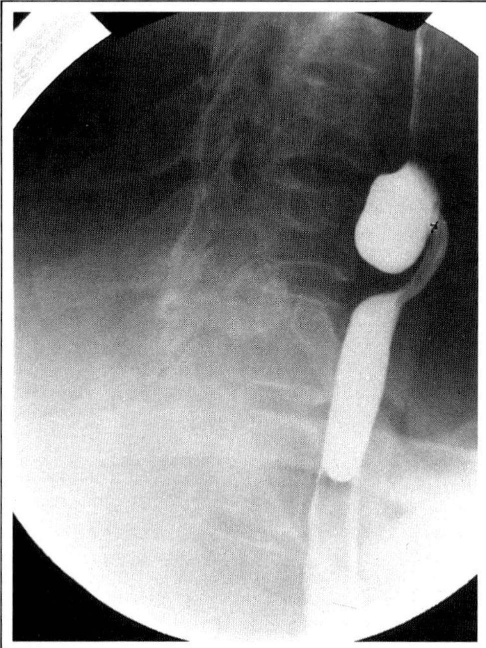

FIG. 10-10a.

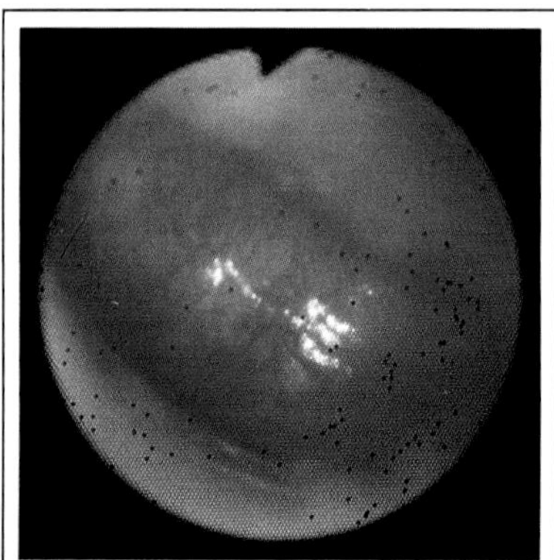

FIG. 10-10b.

FIG. 10-10. Zenker's diverticulum. **a:** A radiographic demonstration of the classic pulsion diverticulum which forms just above the cricopharyngeus. **b:** The endoscope tip is in the mouth of the diverticulum, a direct extension of the lumen of the posterior hypopharynx.

from the radiographic appearance, at endoscopy Zenker's diverticulum appears as a pouch-like extension of the posterior hypopharynx (Fig. 10-10b). In these cases it is difficult to intubate the cricopharyngeus because of the tendency of the tip, even when properly aligned, to either reenter the diverticulum or assume a completely retroflexed position within the hypopharynx. We find that if the cricopharyngeus can be identified, a biopsy forceps can be passed across into the esophagus to serve as a "guide wire" to facilitate entry.

Diffuse Intramural Diverticulosis

Diffuse intramural diverticula are actually tiny invaginations of the esophageal mucosa in the wall of the esophagus. As such, the disorder is sometimes referred to as diffuse intramural pseudodiverticulosis because the diverticula consist only of the mucosal layer.[18] Radiographically, these appear as multiple small projections found in association with strictures, especially of the upper esophagus (Fig. 10-11a). Because the diverticula tend to fill up with debris and bacteria, they may appear endoscopically as pinpoint exudates (Fig. 10-11b). *Candida* may be found in up to half the cases and when present may be associated with a severe motility disturbance.[19] In other cases the pseudodiverticulosis is thought to be due to irritation from an unknown source, leading to dilatation and squamous metaplasia of the esophageal mucous glands which become the diverticula. Esophageal reflux is not considered part of the pathogenesis.

OTHER UNCOMMON APPEARANCES

Esophageal Polyps

Esophageal polyps are not rare if one includes glycogenic acanthosis (see Chapter 2), which may be found in up to 25% of examinations as multiple 1- to 4-mm, whitish mu-

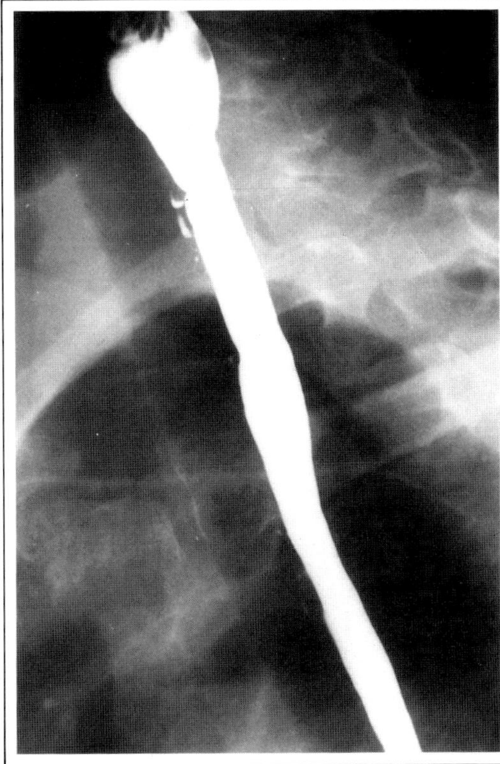

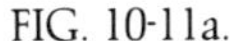

FIG. 10-11a.

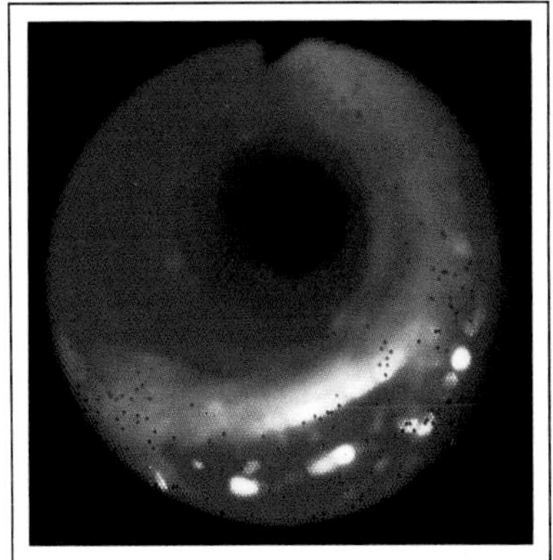

FIG. 10-11b.

FIG. 10-11. Esophageal intramural pseudodiverticulosis. **a:** Radiologically, multiple intramural collections of contrast material were observed just distal to a cricopharyngeal stricture [same as in (b)]. **b:** With cricopharyngeal stricture. Tiny exudates are observed distal to the stricture (KOH preparation negative for *Candida*) representing the mouths of diverticula filled with bacteria and cellular debris.

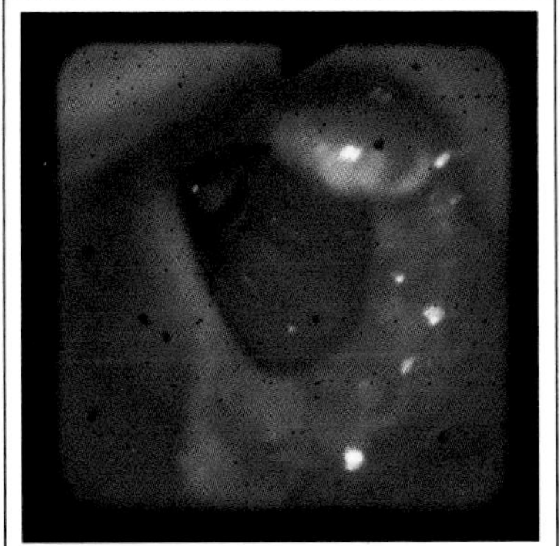

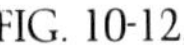

FIG. 10-12.

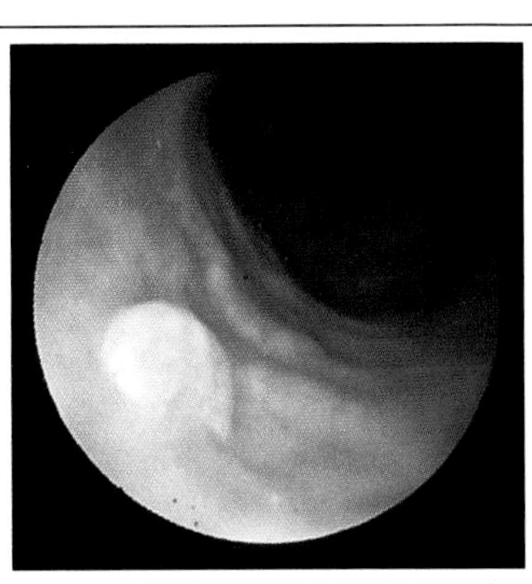

FIG. 10-13.

FIG. 10-12. Inflammatory polyp. A 6-mm polyp is seen just above a stricture along with erosions indicative of peptic esophagitis.

FIG. 10-13. Squamous papilloma. Multiple biopsies showed this isolated, whitish 4-mm mid-esophageal polyp to be a squamous papilloma.

cosal excrescences.[19a] Apart from glycogenic acanthosis, simple hyperplastic polyps are the chief diagnostic consideration for polyps of this size. Esophageal polyps larger than 4 mm are found much less commonly. There are a variety of diagnostic possibilities for these entities depending on whether the polyp is epithelial or submucosal.

Epithelial Polyps

Epithelial polyps generally appear singly, having an altered mucosal color or texture to denote them as epithelial polyps; they are mostly inflammatory and are commonly associated with esophageal reflux (Fig. 10-12) (see Chapter 3). Other single epithelial polyps, less often observed, are hyperplastic squamous papillomas[20] (Fig. 10-13), areas of leukoplakia (Fig. 10-14) (see Chapter 2), ecotopic sebaceous glands,[20a] and small (<3 cm) squamous carcinomas.[21] The endoscopist considers any given epithelial polyp benign (Fig. 10-12), especially if it is less than 5 mm (Fig. 10-13) and associated with peptic eophagitis (Fig. 10-12). In the absence of frank peptic changes (Fig. 10-15), one should consider any polypoid appearance as suspicious, especially if it is larger than 1 cm (Fig. 10-16), and proceed with vigorous biopsy and brushing cytology (see Chapters 1 and 5). Even though benign polyps,

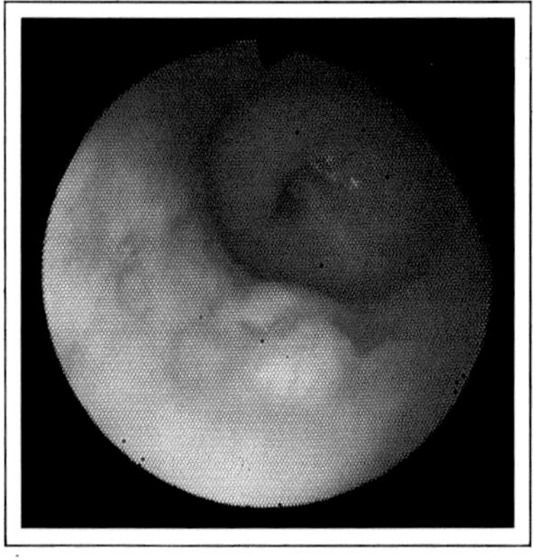

FIG. 10-14.

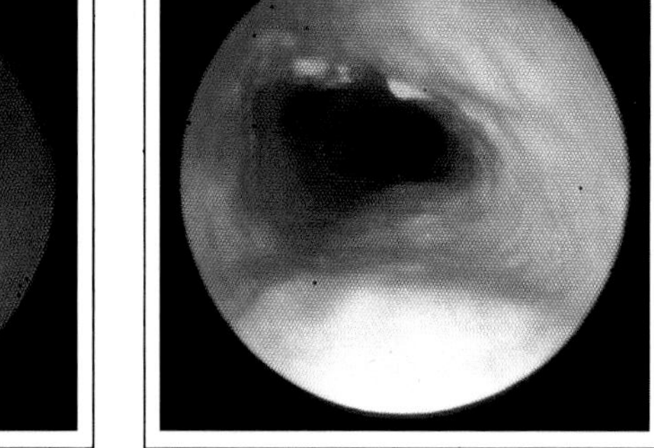

FIG. 10-15.

FIG. 10-14. Leukoplakia. One of many areas of leukoplakia is seen as a gray-white, 3 × 8 mm elevated lesion. Biopsy showed thickening of the squamous layer, compatible with leukoplakia. Although the lesion is similar in appearance to glycogenic acanthosis (see Chapter 2), the glycogen content histologically was not increased.

FIG. 10-15. Small squamous carcinoma. A 2.5-cm eroded elevated area is seen on the anterior (12 o'clock) wall of the mid-esophagus which, in view of its location and the absence of other reflux changes, was viewed as highly suspicious. Biopsy showed squamous carcinoma.

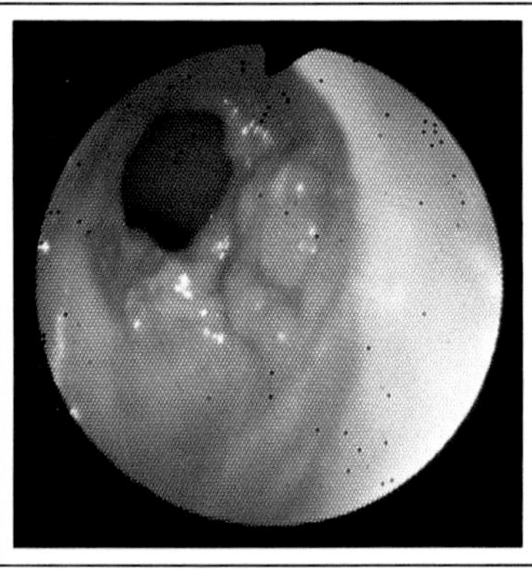

FIG. 10-16.

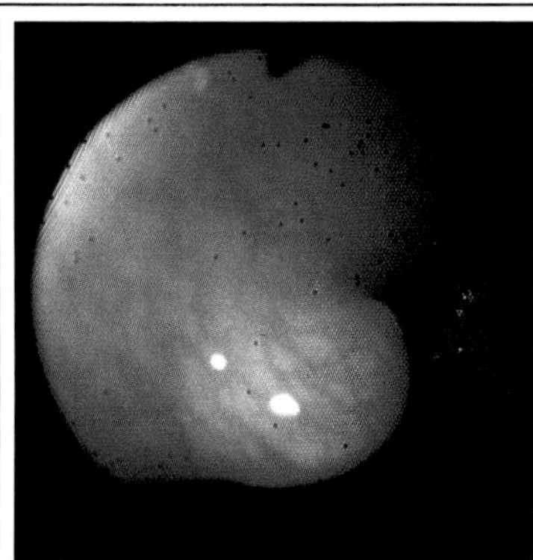

FIG. 10-17.

FIG. 10-16. Inflammatory polyp. The appearance of this 1.5-cm polypoid mass of the right (3 o'clock) wall just above a peptic stricture has a corrugated surface similar to that of the cancer shown in Fig. 10-15. The presence of a peptic stricture as well as moderate esophagitis (with erosions) were reassuring, although its size still warranted an aggressive approach to biopsy (6 to 10 samples). These showed the lesion to be inflammatory.

FIG. 10-17. Submucosal polyp, possibly leiomyoma. The smooth overlying mucosa suggests this to be a submucosal mass. Biopsy showed squamous mucosa compatible with a submucosal polyp.

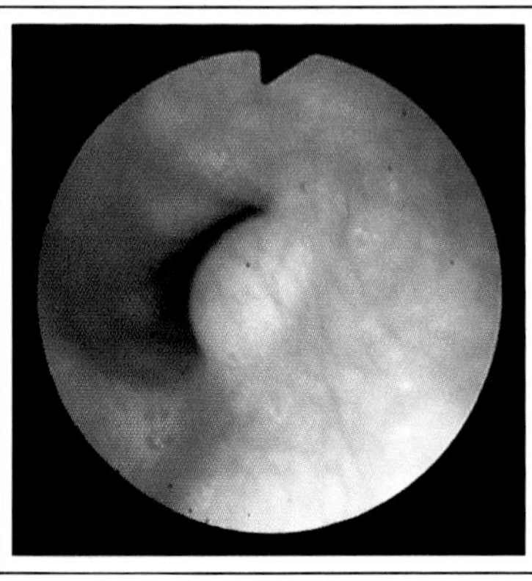

FIG. 10-18.

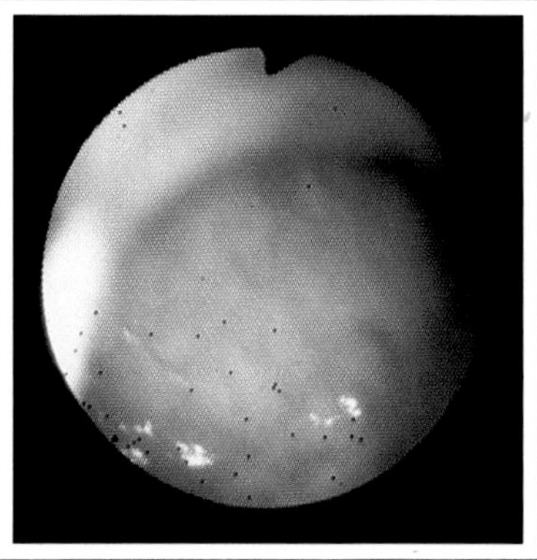

FIG. 10-19.

FIG. 10-18. Submucosal polyp, esophageal cyst. This pale, 7.5-mm polyp was unusually compressible when biopsied. Despite its endoscopic appearance and a biopsy which showed only squamous epithelium, the referring physician elected to have it removed surgically. Histologic sections through it showed it to be a submucosal cyst.

FIG. 10-19. Esophageal vein. A focal submucosal elevation was seen which proved quite compressible. Its bluish discoloration, however, suggested that it was a vein.

e.g., squamous papillomas,[20,22] or inflammatory polyps (Fig. 10-16) can achieve a size of up to 1.5 cm, one is aggressive in these cases so as not to miss the rare opportunity to diagnose esophageal cancer while it is still at a treatable stage,[21] appearing as a small (1 to 2 cm) sessile, polypoid mass.

Submucosal Polyps

Submucosal polyps are recognized by the intactness of the overlying mucosa (Fig. 10-17) which is for the most part smooth and regular. For large polyps, though, the mucosa may appear eroded, erythematous, or irregular. Even so, biopsy will show for the most part intact squamous epithelium to suggest a submucosal origin.

In the main, submucosal polyps of the esophagus are single leiomyomas[23] and are located in the distal esophagus. Rarely, multiple leiomyomas have been observed.[24] Other submucosal polyps observed include carcinoids, fibromas, granular cell tumors,[24a] and fibrovascular polyps.[25] Removal either surgically or endoscopically is indicated for larger polyps (>1.5 cm) associated with intermittent dysphagia.

An interesting though rare submucosal polyp that we

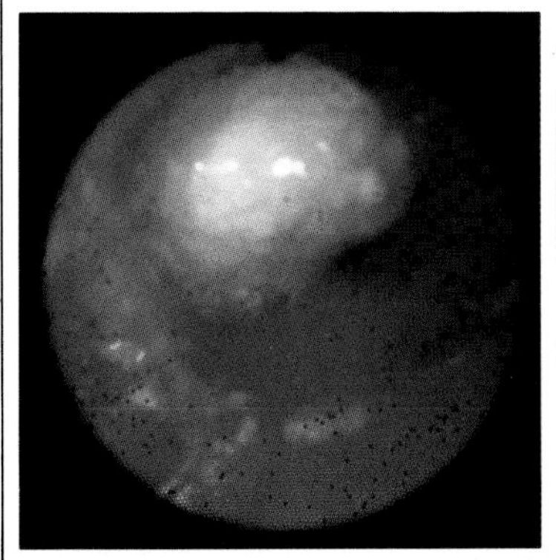

FIG. 10-20a.

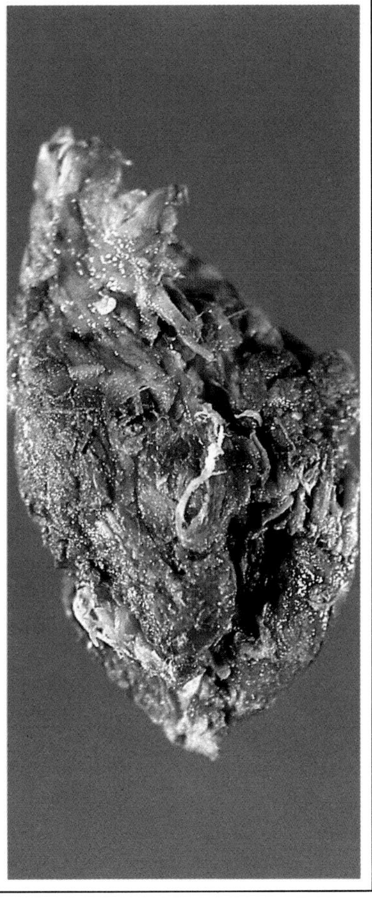

FIG. 10-20b.

FIG. 10-20. Foreign body (chicken wing). **a:** The yellow-gray irregular appearance of a distal esophageal luminal mass suggests it to be a large piece of impacted meat, possibly chicken. The patient is known to have achalasia. **b:** This was extracted by means of an electrosurgical snare.[28]

have seen is the submucosal inclusion cyst arising from the submucosal glands of the distal esophagus.[26] This appears as a soft, grayish-white, smooth mass which is remarkably compressible with biopsy forceps (Fig. 10-18). The white or gray color of the submucosal cyst helps distinguish it from dilated esophageal veins, which tend to be blue (Fig. 10-19).

Foreign Bodies of the Esophagus

In adults, foreign bodies in the esophagus are most often large pieces of solid meat or bones which are ingested rapidly and become lodged at the GE junction. Coins, pieces of dentures, and other objects are also encountered from time to time.[27]

In the more common ingested-food impactions, endoscopically one most often sees either the yellow-brown (chicken) mass (Fig. 10-20, a and b) or a similar dark red (beef) mass. These may be smooth but more often have surface irregularities from their having been partially chewed. When the foreign body is a bolus of meat, one expects to find in association some kind of mechanical obstruction (usually a Schatzki ring or peptic stricture), motor disorder such as achalasia (Fig. 10-20), or diffuse esophageal spasm. The possibility of one or the other should always be evaluated after the impaction is removed. Depending on the size and nature of the foreign body, endoscopy is used to either remove the object[29] or push it into the stomach.[30]

REFERENCES

1. Berenzweig, H., Baue, A. E., and McCallum, R. W. (1980): Dysphagia lusoria: Report of a case and review of the diagnostic and surgical approach. *Dig. Dis. Sci.*, 25:630–636.
2. Leonardi, H. K., Naggar, C. Z., and Ellis, F. H. (1980): Dysphagia due to aortic arch anomaly: diagnostic and therapeutic considerations. *Arch. Surg.*, 115:1229–1232.
3. Birnholtz, J. C., Ferrucci, J. T., and Wyman, S. M. (1974): Roentgen features of dysphagia aortica. *Radiology*, 111:93–96.
4. Beachley, M. C., Siconolfi, E. P., Madoff, H. R., and Chudhry, R. M. (1980): Dysphagia aortica. *Dig. Dis. Sci.*, 25:807–810.
5. Khan, T. A., Shragge, B. W., Crispin, J. S., and Lind, J. F. (1977): Esophageal motility in the elderly. *Dig. Dis. Sci.*, 22:1049–1054.
6. Schatzki, R., and Gary, J. E. (1953): Dysphagia due to a diaphragm-like localized narrowing in the lower esophagus ("lower esophageal ring"). *Am. J. Roentgenol.*, 70:911–922.
7. Arvanitakis, C. (1977): Lower esophageal ring: endoscopic and therapeutic aspects. *Gastrointest. Endosc.*, 24:17–18.
8. Scharschmidt, B. F., and Watts, H. D. (1978): The lower esophageal ring and esophageal reflux. *Am. J. Gastroenterol.*, 69:544–549.
9. Ottinger, L. W., and Wilkins, E. W. (1980): Late results in patients with Schatzki rings undergoing destruction of the ring and hiatus herniorrhaphy. *Am. J. Surg.*, 139:591–594.
10. Snape, W. J. (1979): Diagnosis and management of esophageal rings and webs. *Pract. Gastroenterol.*, 3:34–42.

11. Nosher, J. L., Campbell, W. L., and Seaman, W. B. (1975): The clinical significance of cervical esophageal and hypopharyngeal webs. *Radiology*, 117:45–47.
12. Tedesco, F. J., and Morton, W. J. (1975): Lower-esophageal and hypopharyngeal webs. *Radiology*, 117:45–47.
13. Shiflet, D. W., Gilliam, J. H., Wallace, C. W., Austin, W. E., and Ott, D. J. (1979): Multiple esophageal webs. *Gastroenterology*, 77:556–559.
14. Kaye, M. D. (1974): Oesophageal motor dysfunction in patients with diverticula of the mid-thoracic esophagus. *Thorax*, 29:666–672.
15. Hurwitz, A. L., Way, L. W., and Haddad, J. K. (1975): Epiphrenic diverticulum in association with an unusual motility disturbance: report of surgical correction. *Gastroenterology*, 68:795–798.
16. Palmer, E. D. (1976): Disorders of the cricopharyngeus muscle: a review. *Gastroenterology*, 71:510–519.
17. Knuff, T. E., Benjamin, S. B., and Castell, D. O. (1980): Zenker's diverticulum: a reappraisal. *Gastroenterology*, 78:1196.
18. Castillo, S., Aburashed, A., Kimmelman, J., and Alexander, L. C. (1977): Diffuse intramural esophageal pseudodiverticulosis: new cases and review. *Gastroenterology*, 72:541–545.
19. Lewicki, A. M., and Moore, J. P. (1975): Esophageal moniliasis: a review of common and less frequent characteristics. *Am. J. Roentgenol.*, 125:218–225.
19a. Glick, S. N., Teplick, S. K., Goldstein, J., Stead, J. A., and Zitomer, N. (1982): Glycogenic acanthosis of the esophagus. *Am. J. Roentgenol.*, 139:683–688.
20. Zeabart, L. E., Fabian, J., and Nord, H. J. (1979): Squamous papilloma of the esophagus: a report of 3 cases. *Gastroenterol. Endosc.*, 25:18–20.
20a. Ramakrishnan, T., and Brinker, J. E. (1978): Ecotopic sebaceous glands in the esophagus. *Gastrointest. Endosc.*, 24:293–294.
21. Koehler, R. E., Moss, A. A., and Margulis, A. R. (1976): Early radiographic manifestations of carcinoma of the esophagus. *Radiology*, 119:1–5.
22. Ravry, M. J. R. (1979): Endoscopic resection of squamous papilloma of the esophagus. *Am. J. Gastroenterol.*, 71:398–400.
23. Plachta, A. (1962): Benign tumors of the esophagus—review of the literature and report of 99 cases. *Am. J. Gastroenterol.*, 38:639–652.
24. Fernandes, J. P., Mascarenhas, M. J., daCosta, J. C., and Correia, J. P. (1975): Diffuse leiomyomatosis of the esophagus: a case report and review of the literature. *Am. J. Dig. Dis.*, 20:684–690.
24a. Reyes, C. F., Kathuria, S., and Molnar, Z. (1981): Granular cell tumor of the esophagus: a case report. *J. Clin. Gastroenterol.*, 2:365–368.
25. Jang, G. C., Clouse, M. E., and Fleischner, F. (1969): Fibrovascular polyp—a benign intraluminal tumor of the esophagus. *Radiology*, 92:1196–1200.
26. Kahle, M., and Weber, E. G. (1980): Cysts of the esophagus. *Hepatogastroenterol.*, 27:372–376.
27. Nandi, P., and Ong, G. B. (1978): Foreign body in the esophagus: a review of 2394 cases. *Br. J. Surg.*, 65:5–9.
28. DeLuca, R. F., Ferrer, J. P., and Wortzel, E. L. (1976): Polypectomy snare extraction of foreign bodies from the esophagus. *Am. J. Gastroenterol.*, 66:374–376.
29. Rogers, B. H. G. (1979): A new method for extraction of impacted meat from the esophagus utilizing a flexible fiberoptic endoscope and an overtube. *Gastrointest. Endosc.*, 25:47.
30. Jackson, F. W. (1981): Push-through technique for rapid removal of esophageal foreign bodies. *Gastrointest. Endosc.*, 27:123.

Section 2

THE STOMACH AND PYLORIC CHANNEL

11

THE STOMACH—ENDOSCOPIC ORIENTATION, TECHNIQUE OF EXAMINATION, AND NORMAL APPEARANCE

ENDOSCOPIC ORIENTATION

Entry into the Stomach

Anatomically, the esophagus is related to the stomach at the esophagogastric junction so that its anterior and posterior walls are continuous with those of the stomach, its left wall becomes the greater curve of the stomach, and its right wall becomes the lesser curve (Fig. 11-1a). As the esophagus is, for the most part, a straight, relatively short (20 to 25 cm) tube, the alignment of the anterior wall with the 12 o'clock lens position (see Chapter 1), which can be established on entry, is easily maintained down to the gastroesophageal (GE) junction (Fig. 11-1a). Thus the anterior wall of the esophagus is still seen in this position of the eyepiece (Fig. 11-1b), the left wall in the 9 o'clock position, the right wall in the 3 o'clock, and the posterior wall in the 6 o'clock position.

Based on the above considerations, upon entering the stomach one expects to see the anterior and posterior walls in the 12 and 6 o'clock positions, with the greater curve (the extension of the left wall of the esophagus) observed in the 9 o'clock position and the lesser curve (the extension of the right wall) in the 3 o'clock position (Fig. 11-2).

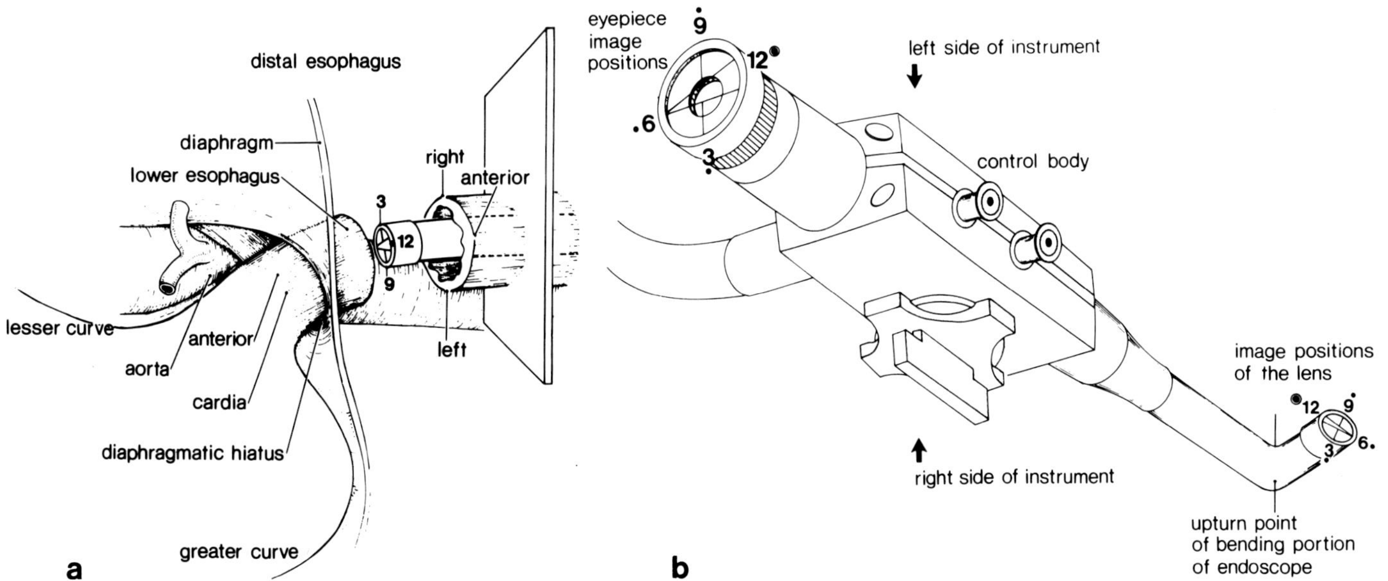

FIG. 11-1. a: Lens image positions in the distal esophagus with the 12 o'clock position still aligned with the anterior wall. **b:** Eyepiece image positions in relation to those of the lens (see Chapter 1).

Alignment Along the Longitudinal Axis of the Stomach

Because the longitudinal axis of the esophagus lies perpendicular to that of the stomach (Fig. 11-2), continued advancement in this direction, once the stomach is entered, would cause the tip to become wedged against the anterior wall or to achieve a retroflexed view of the cardia and fundus (see below). What is desired at this point, however, is advancement of the tip distally, along the longitudinal axis of the stomach toward the posteriorly lying lower body and antrum. This change in alignment is readily accomplished by means of clockwise rotation (torquing) of the insertion tube (endoscope shaft) of 60° to 90°, causing the tip to align itself with the longitudinal axis of the stomach toward the posterior antrum (Fig. 11-3).

The visual clue to the alignment being correct is the appearance of rugal folds running in the same direction (Fig. 11-4b) in which the endoscope is being advanced rather than obliquely to it (Fig. 11-4a) as was the case on entry. In this orientation where the tip is aligned with the longitudinal axis of the stomach, one expects to find the lesser curve in the 12 o'clock position (Fig. 11-3) with the greater curve at 6 o'clock, the anterior wall at 9 o'clock, and the posterior wall at 3 o'clock (Fig. 11-4b).

Gastric Angle

The gastric angle is a landmark denoting both the junction of the body and the antrum, as well as the lesser curve. It is seen with the commonly used forward-viewing endoscope as a crescent-shaped fold coming off the lesser curve (Fig. 11-5), separating the gastric body from the antrum. As a result of the 60° to 90° clockwise rotation, the midline of the angle is aligned in the 6 o'clock to 12 o'clock axis of the visual field. As in the case of the gastric body, following alignment of the tip to the longitudinal axis of the stomach, the anterior and posterior walls are seen in the 9 and 3 o'clock positions of the visual field, respectively, with the greater curve in the 6 o'clock position.

Antrum

As the antrum is the direct continuation of the lower body (Fig. 11-6), the orientation is the same, with the lesser curve seen in the 12 o'clock position, the anterior and posterior walls in the 9 and 3 o'clock positions, respectively, and the greater curve in the 6 o'clock position. The prepyloric antrum and pyloric channel are then seen as a convergence of the walls of the antrum, generally at a central point. With the use of currently available small-caliber (9 to 11 mm) endoscopes capable of wide tip deflection, the pyloric channel is visualized in most cases with the tip in the mid or distal antrum. If the pyloric ring is not seen because it occupies an unusually high position just off the lesser curve, tip alignment with the midline of the antrum nevertheless allows the endoscope to be advanced blindly with sufficient retroflexion in the distal antrum to locate a high pyloric channel (Fig. 11-7).

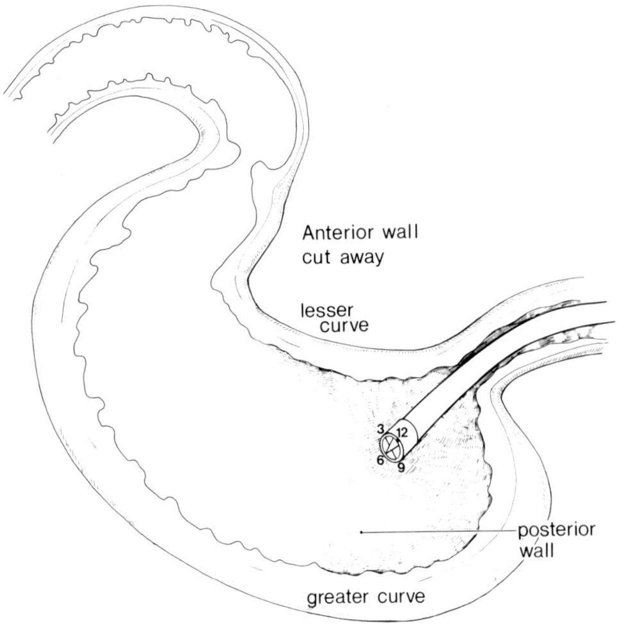

FIG. 11-2. Lens image positions on entry into the stomach.

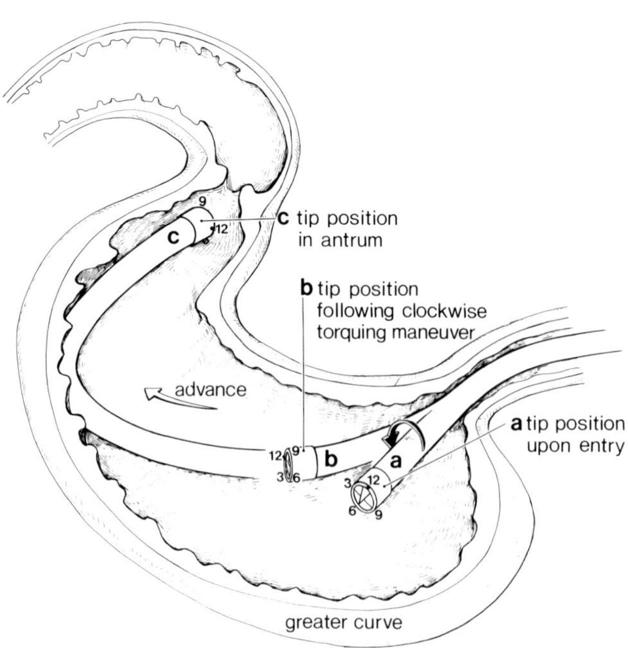

FIG. 11-3. Lens image positions after a 60° to 90° clockwise torquing maneuver.

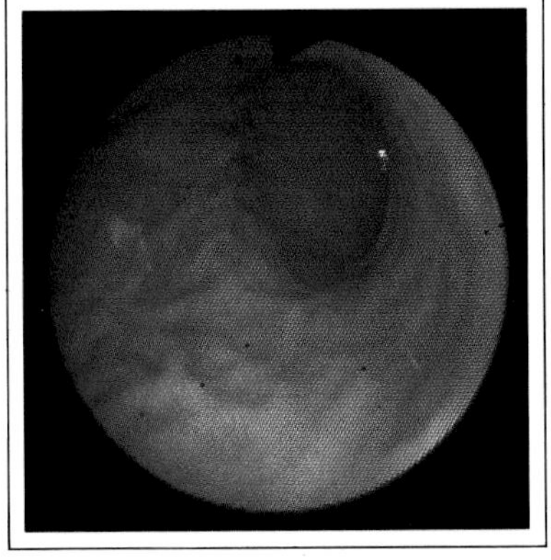

FIG. 11-4a.

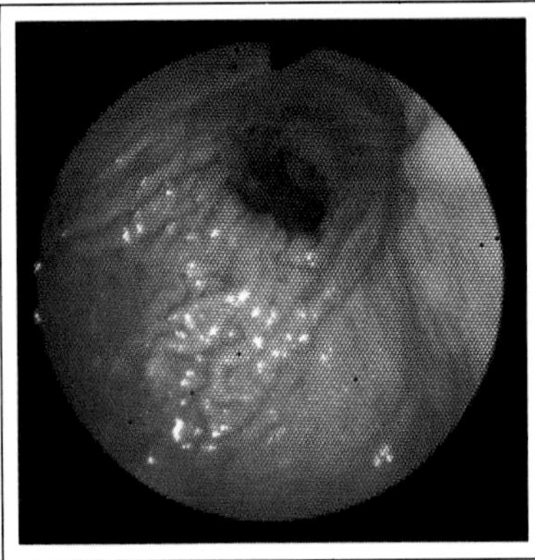

FIG. 11-4b.

FIG. 11-4. a: Rugal folds on entry prior to the clockwise torquing maneuver. These run obliquely toward the forward direction of the tip. **b:** Rugal folds after a 60° to 90° clockwise torquing maneuver. These are observed to run parallel to the forward direction of the tip. The gastric lake, as a marker of the anterior aspect of the greater curve, has shifted from the 9 o'clock (a) to the 7 o'clock position, with the lesser and greater curves in the 12 and 6 o'clock positions, respectively.

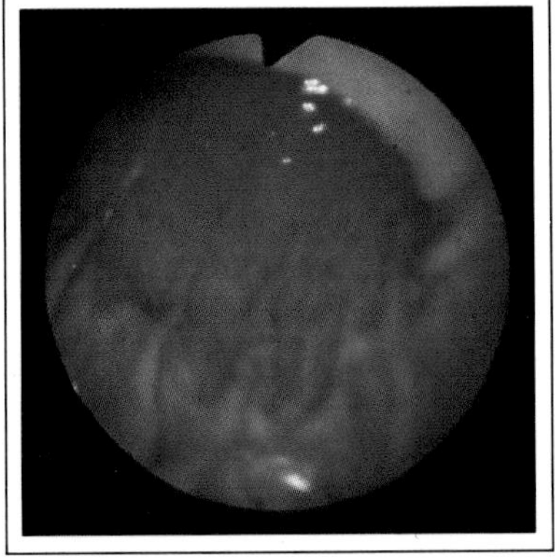

FIG. 11-5.

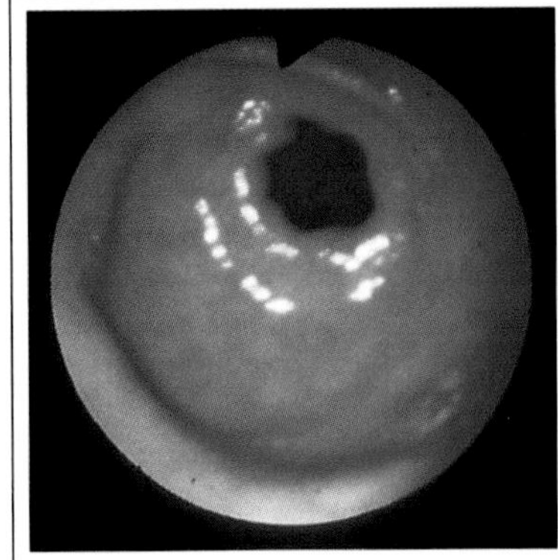

FIG. 11-6.

FIG. 11-5. Gastric angle. The lesser curve landmark is seen as a crescent-shaped fold at 12 o'clock after a clockwise torquing maneuver (Fig. 11-2). In this orientation, the midline of the angle is in the 12 o'clock position.

FIG. 11-6. Prepyloric antrum and pyloric channel. The lesser curve is observed in the 12 o'clock position, and the anterior and posterior walls are in the 9 and 3 o'clock positions, respectively. Note that the greater curve is in the 6 o'clock position. The pyloric channel is seen as a ring-like opening just off the lesser curve.

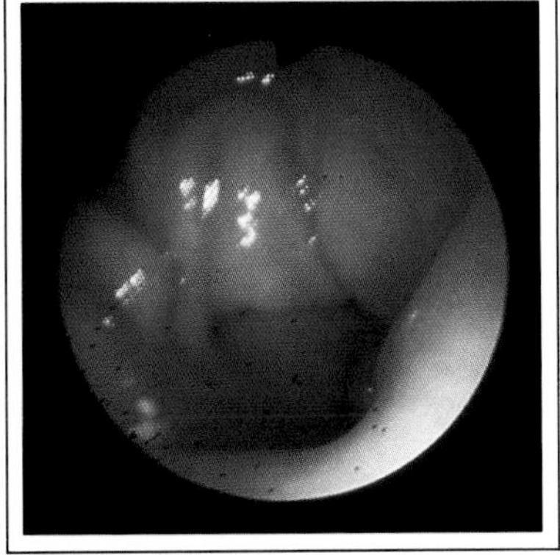

FIG. 11-7.

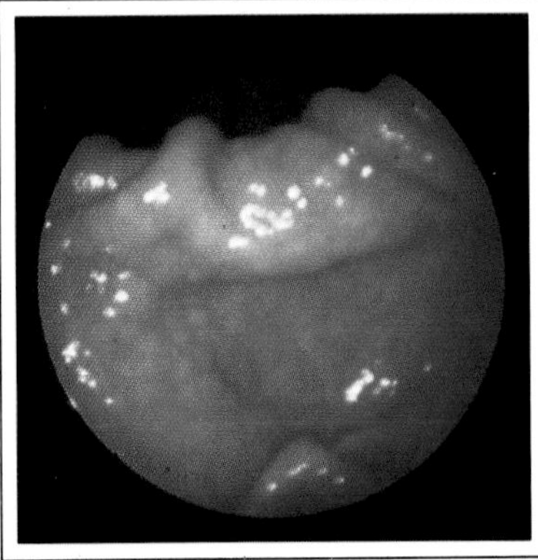

FIG. 11-8.

FIG. 11-7. Locating the pylorus. After maximum upward deflection of the tip and further insertion with the tip in the midline, the additional retroflexion brings the pylorus into view.

FIG. 11-8. Angle and lesser curve of the antrum, J-type retroflexed view. The lesser curve aspect of the antrum which is not well seen immediately on entry (Fig. 11-6) is observed to better advantage. The pyloric channel is now just barely seen at 6 o'clock, and the body is off at 12 o'clock just above the angle

Retroflexion in the Antrum and Body

With forward-viewing instruments, because the lesser curve is seen obliquely or not at all, it is often necessary to establish a retroflexed (J-type) position in the antrum (Fig. 11-8) or lower body (Fig. 11-9). In the antrum (Fig. 11-8) the anterior and posterior walls are still seen in the 9 and 3 o'clock positions. Because of the tip deflection, which may approach 180°, the greater curve, which prior to retroflexion had been seen in the 6 o'clock position (Fig. 11-4a), is now observed at 12 o'clock following the maneuver (Fig. 11-10), with the lesser curve now observed at 6 o'clock (Fig. 11-10).

Retroflexion in the Fundus

Once the gastric angle and body have been examined, the endoscopist turns attention toward the cardia and fundus which can be satisfactorily observed only by means of retroflexion. This is accomplished either by J-type or, as we prefer, U-type retroflexion.

J-Type Retroflexion

For some endoscopists, simple upward deflection and withdrawal of the endoscope tip is sufficient for an examination of the cardia and fundus (Fig. 10-10). With currently available narrow-caliber (9 to 11 mm) endoscopes, it is possible to achieve close to 180° tip deflection so that the cardia and fundus can be observed in this fashion (Fig. 11-10). As with retroflexion in the antrum and lower body (Fig. 11-9), the 12 o'clock position views the endoscope itself lying along the greater curve, in this case of the fundus, with the anterior and posterior walls viewed in the 9 and 3 o'clock positions, respectively, and the lesser curve seen at 6 o'clock (Fig. 11-10). The posterior cardia coming off the lesser curve would be expected to be found somewhere in the 3 to 6 o'clock quadrant.

The problems of J-type retroflexion are apparent from a consideration of its orientation. First, it may not be possible in all cases to withdraw the tip into the fundus because of anatomic considerations, causing the tip to abut against the lesser curve. In the second place, part of the fundus is obscured by the endoscope, and finally the cardia itself may be seen only tangentially or not at all.

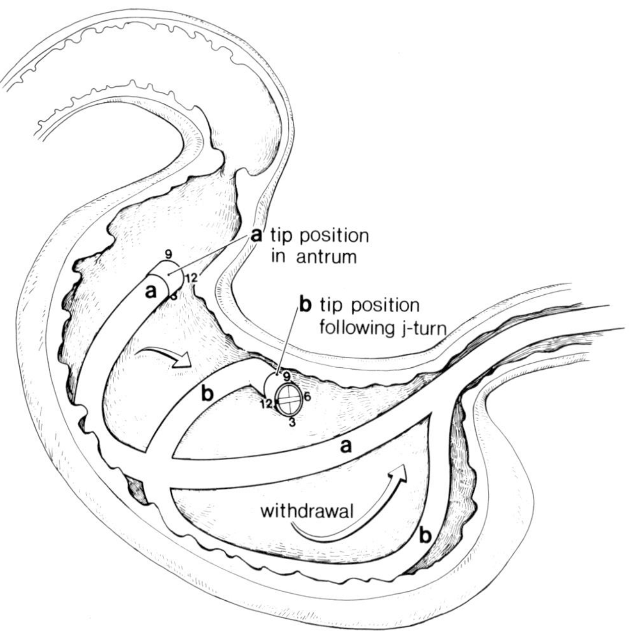

FIG. 11-9. Lens image positions after J-type retroflexion.

U-Type Retroflexion

Because of the limitations of J-type retroflexion for examining the cardiofundic area, we perform a U-type procedure in all cases. The basis of this maneuver is deflection of the endoscope tip of the anterior wall of the fundus, resulting in a completely unobscured view of the cardia and fundus.

To understand the orientation of this maneuver (Fig. 11-11), we must reconsider that which was encountered upon entry into the stomach (Fig. 11-2). It is this orientation which must be re-established, first by a 60° to 90° counterclockwise rotation (torquing maneuver) when the gastric lake (denoting the junction of the body and fundus) is seen (Fig. 11-12). The success of the counterclockwise rotation is judged by noting the rugal folds of the anterior wall that run toward the bile lake, now seen at 12 o'clock, and denoting the anterior wall. With the tip fully in the "up" position, with continued insertion, it is deflected off the anterior wall toward the cardia. With perfect alignment (the midline of the endoscope in the same plane as the midline of the cardia), the cardia as the most posterior structure comes into view at 12 o'clock with the anterior wall at 6 o'clock and the greater curve at 9 o'clock (Fig. 11-13).

In most cases, however, because the patient lies on his left side, with continued insertion of the endoscope, the tip may be expected to slip toward the most proximal anterior and greater curve aspect of the fundus ("leftward slippage") and provide an obscured view (Fig. 11-14a). The cardia and some of the fundus are seen in the 3 o'clock position, but the remainder is seen poorly or not at all.

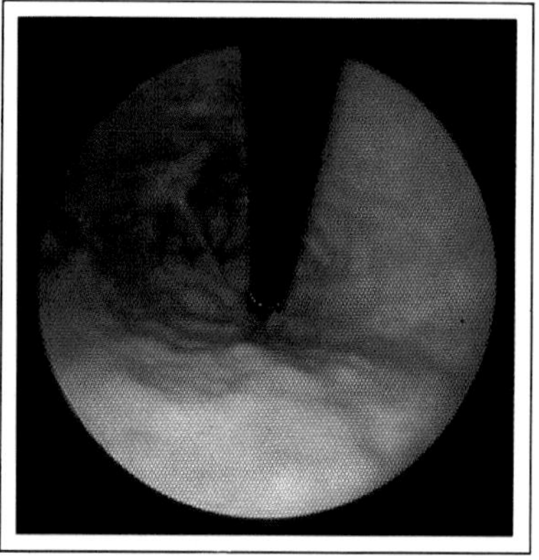

FIG. 11-10.

FIG. 11-10. Upper body, fundus, and cardia; J-type retroflexion. The cardia is observed toward the 5 o'clock position, and the endoscope runs along the greater curve toward 12 o'clock with the lake at 9 o'clock marking the anterior wall and with the posterior wall in the 3 o'clock position.

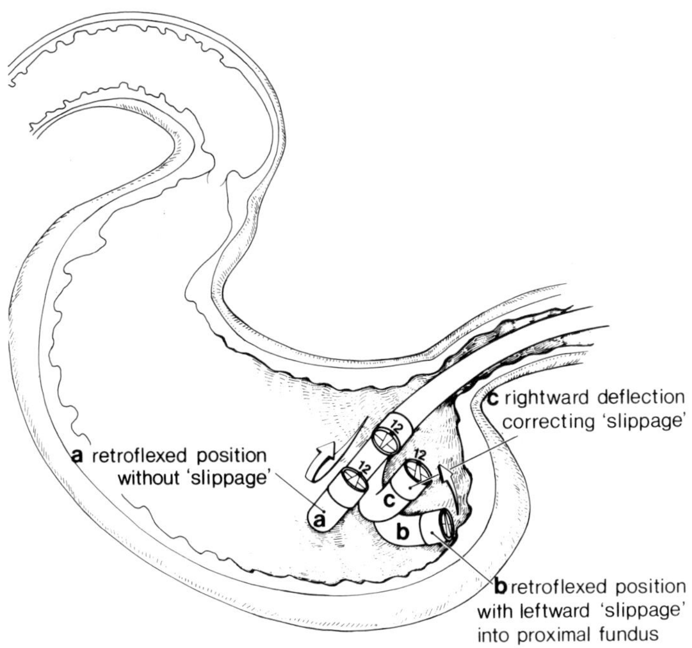

FIG. 11-11. Lens image position after U-type retroflexion.

However, rightward deflection of the tip corrects this (Fig. 11-11), with the entire fundus coming into view, its anterior wall being in the 6 to 9 o'clock position and its greater curve aspect between 9 and 12 o'clock (Fig. 11-14b).

TECHNIQUE OF EXAMINATION

Intubation

Body

Once the stomach has been entered (Fig. 11-1) and the tip position is determined to be in the upper body adjacent to the anterior wall aspect of the greater curve (see "Endoscopic Orientation, Entry into the Stomach," this chapter), the endoscopist aligns the tip along the longitudinal axis of the stomach by means of a 60° to 90° clockwise torquing maneuver (Fig. 11-4a). The adequacy of this maneuver can be checked from the position of the gastric lake which marks the anterior aspect of the greater curve with the patient in the usual endoscopy position (lying on his left side toward the anterior abdominal wall). This will have shifted from its original 9 to 11 o'clock position in the visual field on entry to a 6 to 9 o'clock position (Fig. 11-4b). The rugal folds are also seen to run in the direction of the 12 o'clock position, now aligned to the posteriorly running lesser curve midline, rather than perpendicular or obliquely to it as was true on entry. With proper alignment of the tip in the longitudinal axis of the stomach, advancement proceeds with gentle insertion of the instrument, the tip being deflected downward to offset its inclination toward retroflexion.

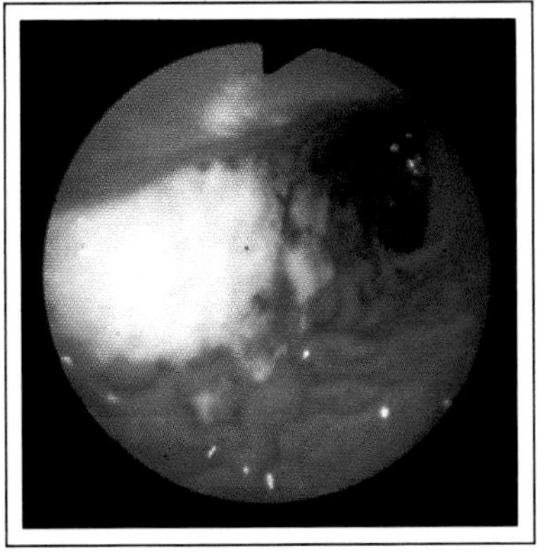

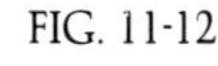

FIG. 11-12.

FIG. 11-13.

FIG. 11-12. Gastric lake during counterclockwise rotation to align in the horizontal axis. Ideally, this continues until the gastric lake is seen in the 12 o'clock position at which point the tip is deflected upward.

FIG. 11-13. U-type retroflexion, ideal alignment with the cardia. In this case no slippage into the fundus has occurred so the cardia is seen directly at 12 o'clock with a greater curve at 9, the anterior wall at 6, and the lesser curve at 3 o'clock.

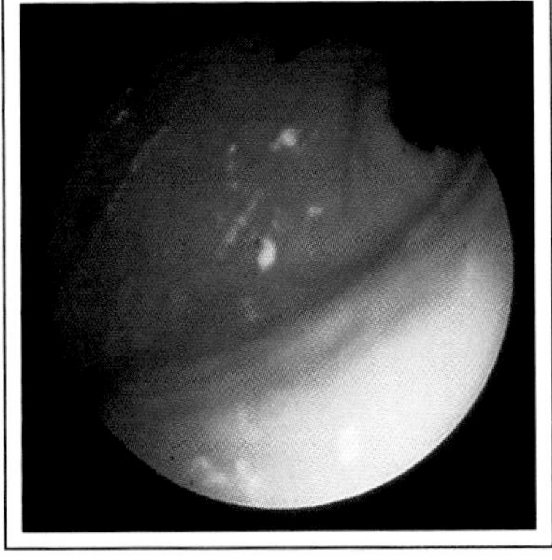

FIG. 11-14a.

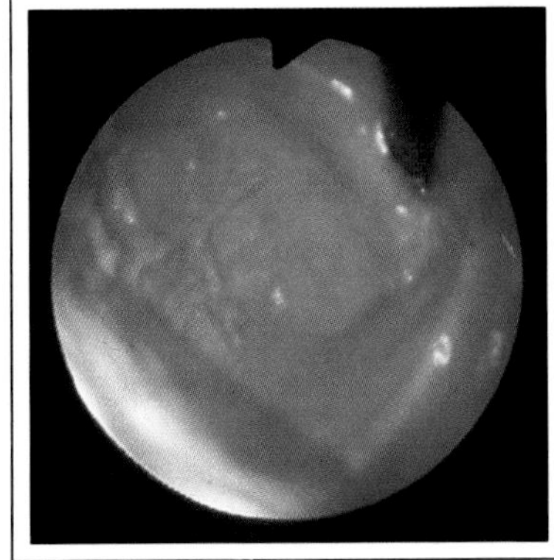

FIG. 11-14b.

FIG. 11-14. a: U-turn maneuver with leftward slippage (anteriorly) into the proximal fundus. The cardia is seen at 3 o'clock, but the remainder of the fundus is incompletely visualized because the tip has slipped proximally (Fig. 11-11). **b:** U-turn maneuver with slippage corrected with rightward deflection. The tip is moved off the anterior wall, allowing the proximal fundus to be viewed (Fig. 11-11). The cardia is still seen at 3 o'clock, and the gastric lake is between 6 and 9 o'clock, with the greater curve between 9 and 12 o'clock.

Antrum

The junction of the body and antrum is recognized by the appearance of the angulus, seen as a crescentic or half-moon-shaped fold projecting off the lesser curve (Fig. 11-5), running from 9 to 3 o'clock. Once the antrum is entered, continued intubation with downward deflection in the same manner as is used in the body allows for intubation to the prepyloric region (Fig. 11-6).

The pyloric channel is often seen in this position and is intubated directly (see Chapter 21). Should the pylorus not be seen, upward deflection with continued insertion allows the tip to rise up in the distal antrum and bring a high-set pylorus (just off the lesser curve) (Fig. 11-7).

Detailed Examination of the Stomach

There are many ways to examine the stomach. The important point is to be both systematic and deliberate so as to minimize the amount of unexamined surface area. To this end, our approach in general is to observe the stomach in detail after, rather than before, the duodenum has been examined (see Chapter 24). Once having returned to the stomach, the antrum is examined first, followed by careful inspection of the angle and body, and finally a retroflexed examination of the cardiofundic area.

Antrum

Examination of the antrum begins with careful inspection of its entire distal portion, using arc-like torquing movements (antral arcs). These begin on the anterior (9 o'clock) wall side with upward deflection along the lesser curve and then swinging over to the posterior (3 o'clock) wall (Fig. 11-15). The endoscope is withdrawn approximately 3 cm between each arc, at which time the greater curve, being in a direct line of view (at 6 o'clock), is examined. The arc should be made within the antrum until the angle is reached. At this point, J-type retroflexion is performed so that the angle is observed *en face* as a strut-like fold projecting off the lesser curve of the antrum (Fig. 11-16). Just below the angle, the tip is deflected up, with insertion pressure applied so that in a J-type retroflexed position the antral side of the gastric angle is observed as well as the antral aspect of its anterior and posterior walls (Fig. 11-8).

Angle

As it is a common location of gastric pathology, especially ulcer disease, special care is taken to inspect completely the angle from below (Fig. 11-8), *en face* (Fig. 11-20, below), and from above (Fig. 11-17). It should be kept in mind that the commonly used forward-viewing endoscopes tend to cause one to observe the angle tangentially and therefore incompletely unless special efforts are made to view it in its entirety.

Body

Within the body, arc-like movements are continued, being made at 5-cm intervals until the junctional area between the body and fundus is reached. This is denoted by a change in the direction of the rugal folds from 6 o'clock to 9 o'clock (Fig. 11-18). A further indication of this location is the appearance of the gastric lake, which because of the elevation of the patient's head (often between 30° and 60°) is seen in the distal fundus, just above its junction with the body (Fig. 11-12). At this point, preparation is made for the examination of the cardia and fundic area by means of retroflexion.

Retroflexed View of the Fundus and Cardia: J-Type Retroflexion

Once the upper body is reached, some endoscopists prefer simply to deflect the tip maximally in the "up" position and withdraw the instrument until the cardia and fundus come into view. In many cases this provides an adequate although somewhat obscured view of the fundus and cardia (Fig. 11-10). If the view obtained is not ideal, it is often possible, even with the tip fully deflected up, to rotate the instrument in the counterclockwise direction so as to move the shaft off the greater curve of the fundus, where it is obscuring the view, onto the posterior wall curve. This in effect converts the J-type retroflexed position (Fig. 11-19a) into a U-type position (Fig. 11-19b).

U-Type Retroflexion

As mentioned above, we believe the cardia and fundus are best examined in virtually all cases if a formal U-type retroflexion is performed. As will be recalled (see above), to perform this the orientation on entry into the stomach (Fig. 11-2) must be re-established by means of a 60° to 90° counterclockwise rotation which corrects for the initial clockwise torquing necessary to align the tip along the longitudinal axis. This clockwise rotation is performed at a point at or just below the level of the gastric lake (Fig. 11-12) where the direction of the rugal folds of the greater curve is seen to go off in an anterior (9 o'clock) direction. The effect of the counterclockwise rotation now causes the tip to become aligned with the transverse axis of the stomach at the junction of the fundus and body, which must occur if U-type retroflexion is to be successful. Upward deflection and forceful, blind insertion of the instrument are continued

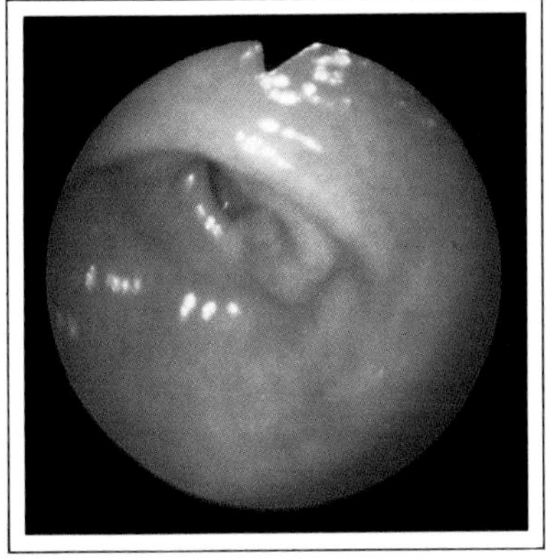

FIG. 11-15.

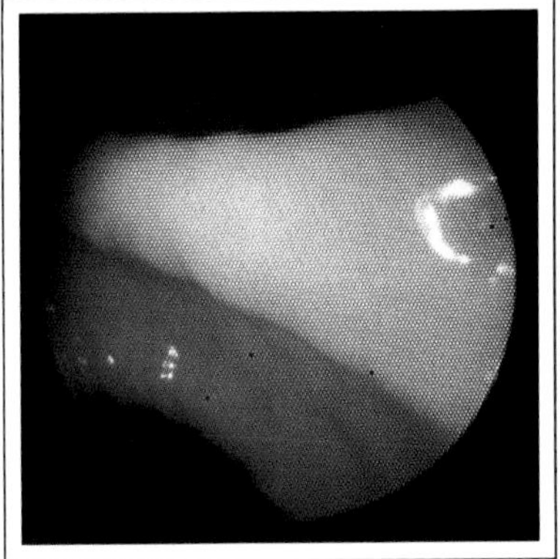

FIG. 11-16.

FIG. 11-15. Antrum, posterior wall, and lesser curve observed as part of an antral arc.

FIG. 11-16. Gastric angle, *en face* view, by J-type retroflexion within the antrum, with the lesser curve now running toward 6 o'clock.

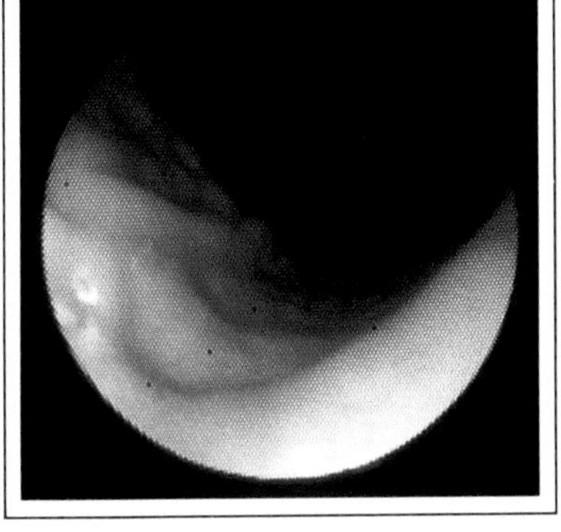

FIG. 11-17.

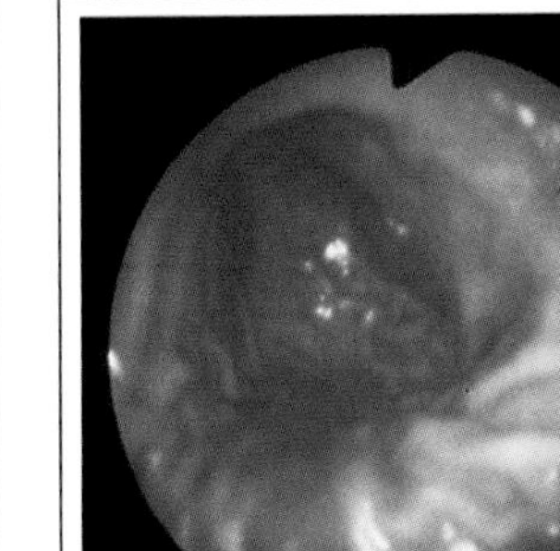

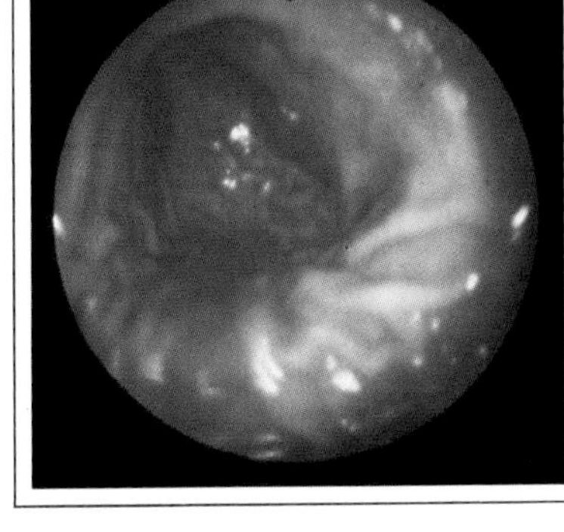

FIG. 11-18.

FIG. 11-17. Lesser curve, just proximal to the gastric angle (at 6 o'clock) viewed from above by J-type retroflexion.

FIG. 11-18. Gastric body (proximal) on completion of multiple arcs at its junction with the fundus (off toward 6 o'clock).

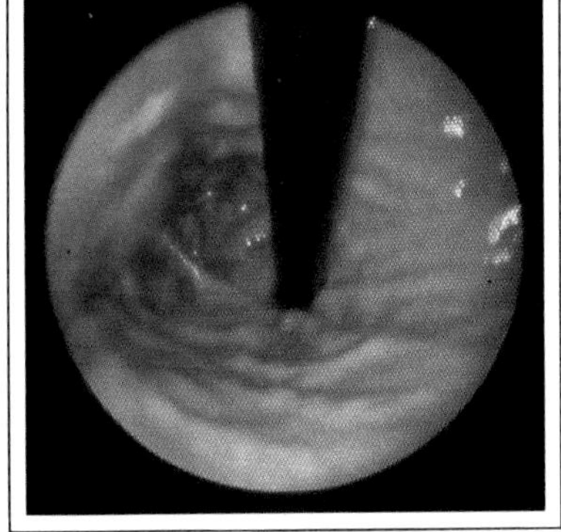

FIG. 11-19a.

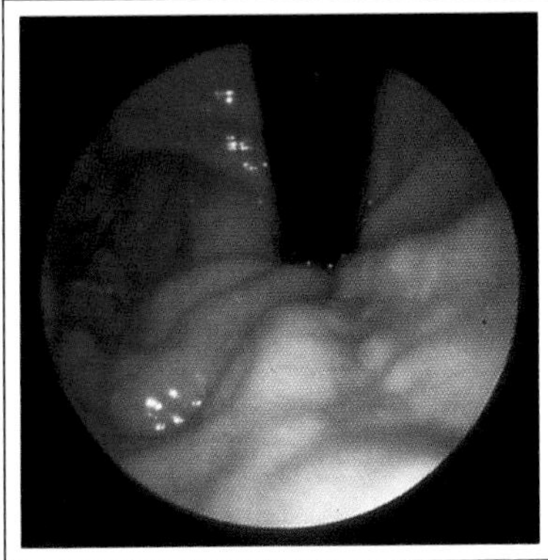

FIG. 11-19b.

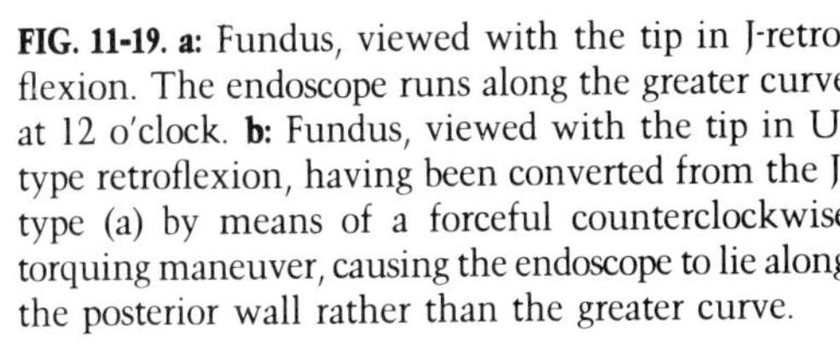

FIG. 11-19. a: Fundus, viewed with the tip in J-retroflexion. The endoscope runs along the greater curve at 12 o'clock. **b:** Fundus, viewed with the tip in U-type retroflexion, having been converted from the J-type (a) by means of a forceful counterclockwise torquing maneuver, causing the endoscope to lie along the posterior wall rather than the greater curve.

until the cardia is seen either in the 12 o'clock position or, as is more often the case because of leftward slippage (see above), in the 3 o'clock position. To correct for this leftward slippage, rightward tip deflection generally brings the entire fundus into view (Figs. 11-13 and 11-14). In addition, forceful insertion often causes slippage at the point of retroflexion in the upper body, causing it and, most importantly, the tip to lie further from the cardia and fundus. This is corrected by withdrawing the instrument in the retroflexed position for short distances, while maintaining continuous air injection, until the fundus comes into view. At this point, reinsertion is again attempted for a definitive view of the cardia.

Upper Body, Cardia, and Diaphragmatic Impression

After examination of the cardia and fundus by retroflexion, the endoscope tip is returned to the original position in the upper body. The endoscope is withdrawn with arc-like movements made at 3-cm intervals to examine the upper body and cardia. As a final determination, we note

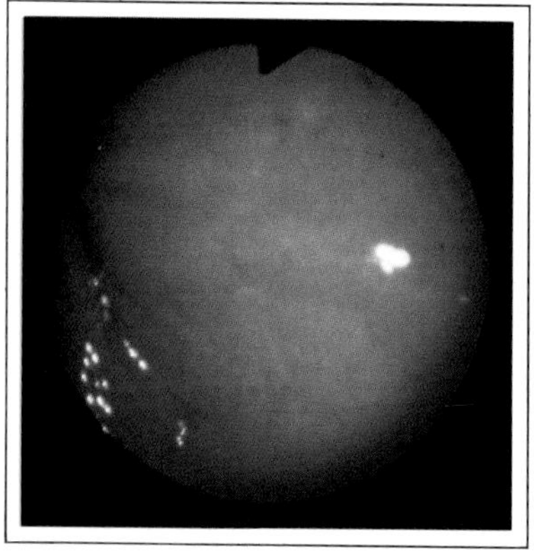

FIG. 11-20.

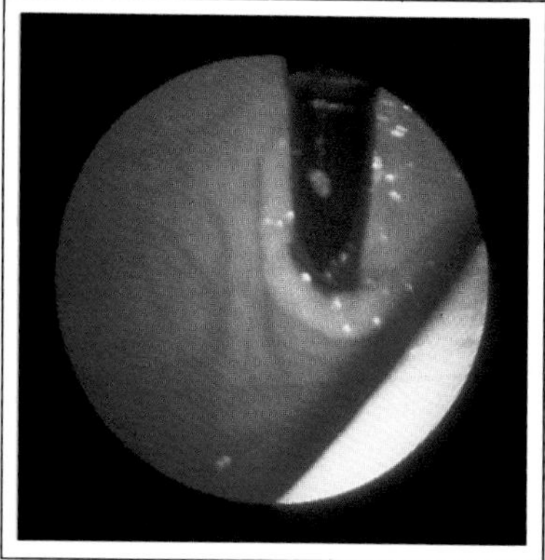

FIG. 11-21a.

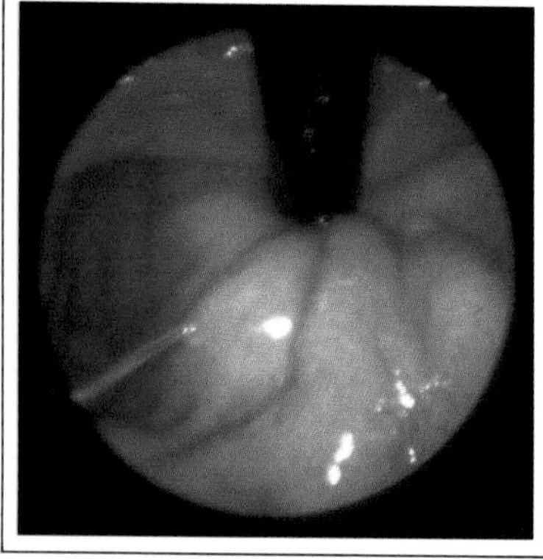

FIG. 11-21b.

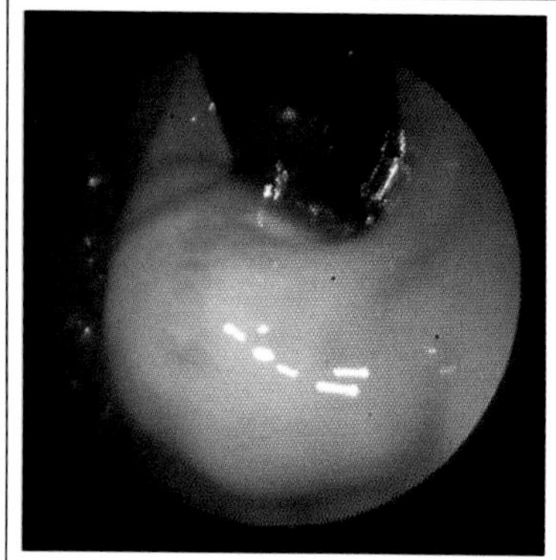

FIG. 11-21c.

FIG. 11-20. Cardia, direct entry, just beyond the GE junction. Folds within the cardia can be seen to run toward the diaphragmatic hiatal impression at 9 o'clock.

FIG. 11-21. a: Normal cardia (retroflexed view). A smooth ring-like fold is seen surrounding the endoscope. **b:** Redundant cardial folds (retroflexed view). Multiple redundant mucosal folds in the cardia cause it to appear nodular. **c:** Cardial mass. A single persistent area of deformity appearing as a small nodule is a suspicious finding for carcinoma.

the location of the GE junction in relation to the diaphragmatic hiatus. Some prefer to do this on entering the stomach because the examination itself can force the position of the GE junction toward the level of the diaphragm and thus eliminate the chance of determining if a hiatus hernia is present. Either way, the patient is asked to sniff in order to determine the level of the diaphragm. This causes a movement in the diaphragm which is seen as an indentation against the right posterior (3 o'clock) aspect of the cardia. The level at which this occurs is compared to the level of the GE junction. A separation of up to 2 cm may be considered normal; one which is greater than 2 cm is taken to be indicative of the presence of a hiatus hernia (see Chapter 13).[1]

NORMAL ENDOSCOPIC APPEARANCE OF THE STOMACH

Regions of the Stomach

Cardia

The cardia is tubular, like the esophagus, with parallel running mucosal folds (the cardial rosette) which are seen as an extension of the esophageal mucosal columns. However, the mucosa of the cardia stands in sharp contrast with the gray-white of the esophagus (see Chapter 1), having an orange-pink (Fig. 11-20) or yellow-white coloration. Also, in contrast to distal esophageal mucosa, in most (but not all) cases a mucosal vascular pattern is absent.

When the cardia is viewed in a retroflexed position, the mucosal folds which were seen on entry become effaced, so that the cardia may appear as a perfectly smooth ring-like fold (Fig. 11-21a). In cases where the cardial folds are prominent, complete effacement may not occur and a certain degree of irregularity or nodularity is observed because of redundancy (Fig. 11-21b). These nodules are, in fact, simply redundant mucosa, being extremely pliant and easily tented (see below), unlike the case when a cardial mass (Fig. 11-21c) is present.

Fundus

As seen in the U-type retroflexed position, the fundus appears as a hollow, rounded area anterior and proximal to the cardia. Usually the mucosa is flat, and whatever folds are initially present disappear with continued insufflation. Prominent mucosal capillaries are typical (Fig. 11-22a); their presence by itself does not imply mucosal atrophy as it would if they were found in the body as well (see Chapter 14). In addition to capillaries, veins may be seen which may be sizeable, up to 5 mm in diameter. Fundic veins, because of their smaller size and straight appearance (Fig. 11-22b), are usually not confused with gas-

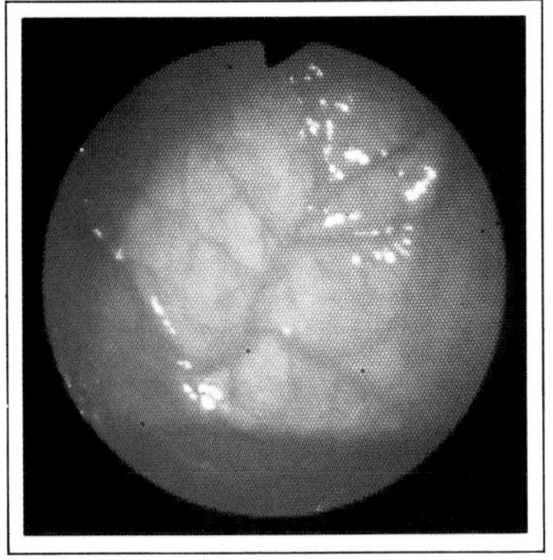

FIG. 11-22a.

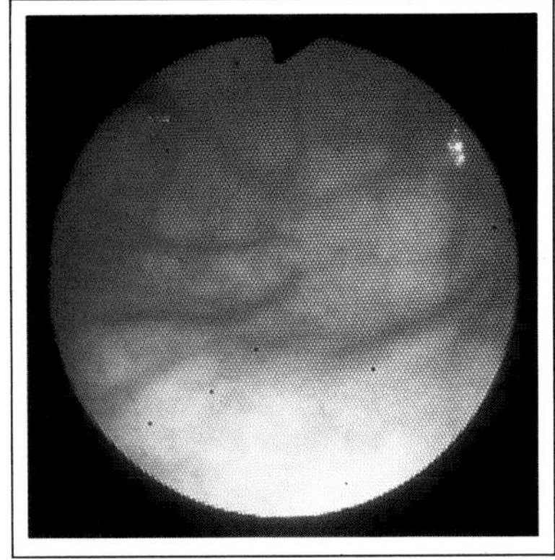

FIG. 11-22b.

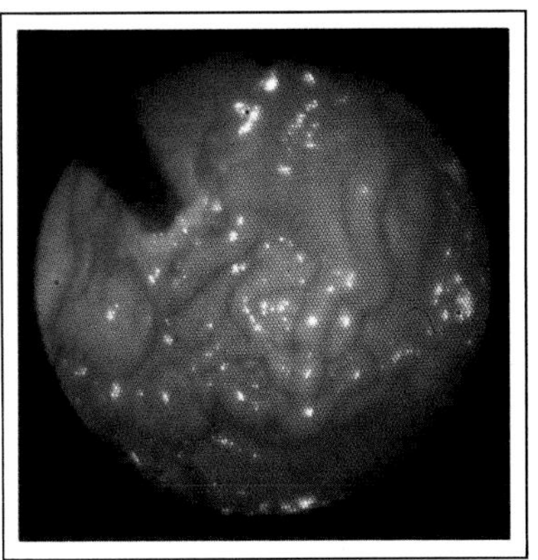

FIG. 11-22c.

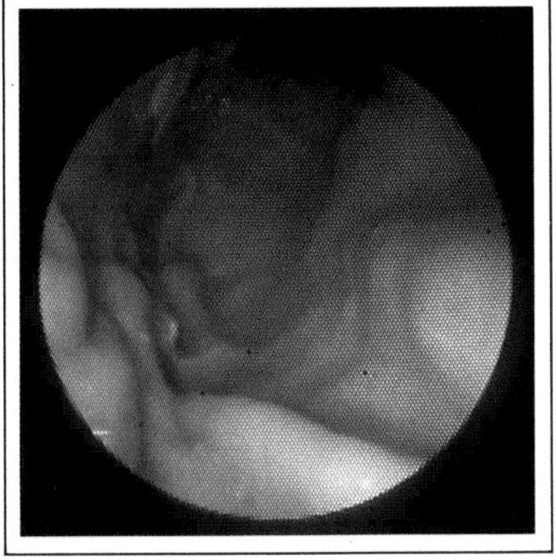

FIG. 11-23a.

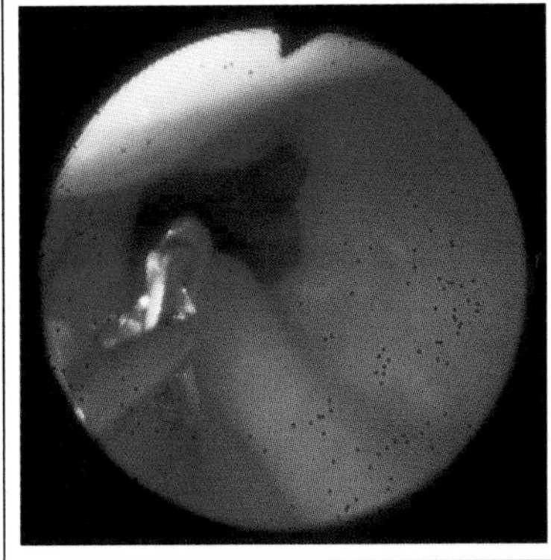

FIG. 11-23b.

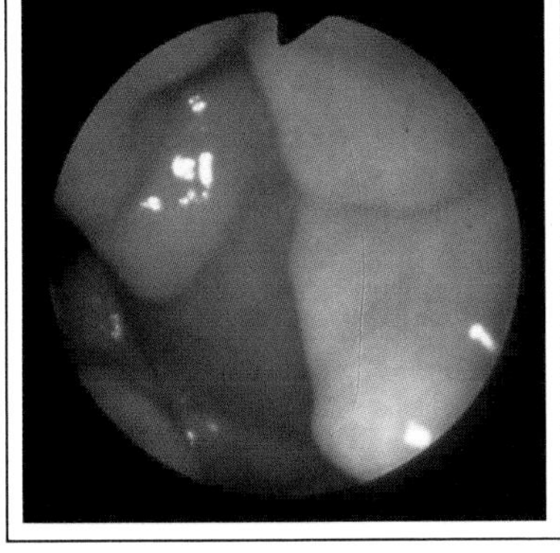

FIG. 11-23c.

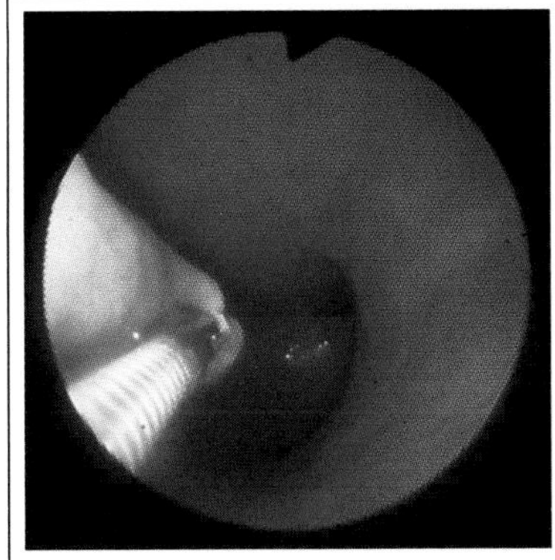

FIG. 11-23d.

FIG. 11-22. a: Fundus (retroflexed view), with a prominent submucosal capillary pattern. This is frequently seen in the fundus and by itself does not warrant a diagnosis of mucosal atrophy. **b:** Fundus (retroflexed view) with 2- to 3-mm veins, a normal finding. **c:** Fundic (gastric) varices. Multiple 5-mm serpiginous varices run in the direction of 9 to 3 o'clock, perpendicular to a rugal fold going toward 12 o'clock (see Chapter 37).

FIG. 11-23. a: Rugal folds, body normal, 3 to 5 mm. **b:** Measurement of rugal fold height using the open bite width method. The open bite width (from edge to edge) has a measured length of 5 mm. In this case the estimated height of the rugal fold is 4 mm. **c:** Large rugal folds, body. Using the open forceps method, these were estimated to have a height of 1.0 to 1.5 cm. **d:** Tenting sign. A small portion of mucosa is seen to tent up, i.e., be picked up and drawn out into the lumen. This indicates that although the fold may be prominent the mucosa is not bound to the submucosa in a way to suggest an infiltrative process.

tric varices (see Chapter 37), which are wider than 5 mm and appear serpiginous or even ridge-like (Fig. 11-22c).

Gastric Lake

With the patient lying on his left side toward the anterior abdominal wall, with his head elevated 30° to 45°, fluid will collect along the most dependent portion of the greater curve, which is the distal fundus (Fig. 11-4b). This collection of fluid is known as the gastric lake. The fluid is generally grayish-white in the absence of bile; the presence of bile imparts a greenish-yellow coloration to it (Fig. 11-25, below). The presence of bile in the gastric lake is of uncertain clinical significance (see Chapter 12).

Body

The rugal folds (Fig. 11-4a) are the dominating feature within the body of the stomach. These are principally located on the greater curve and adjacent portions of the anterior and posterior walls, becoming less prominent on the lesser curve, where with air insufflation they can be effaced. Generally, the mucosa of these folds has the same yellow-gray-orange appearance as that of the cardia, although variations toward increasing redness must be expected (see Chapter 12). The most variable feature within the body is probably the height and thickness of the rugal folds. Generally, after sufficient insufflation the folds are 4 to 5 mm high, as estimated using the open forceps method (Fig. 11-23b). Folds with a height between 5 mm and 1 cm we arbitrarily designate as "prominent," whereas those with a height exceeding 1 cm are called "large" (Fig. 11-23c). The appearance of large folds is designated "gastric hyperrugosity" (see Chapter 12). Some of this variability in size has to do with the ability or the lack thereof to produce adequate air insufflation. Prominent or large rugal folds are found even in those cases where air is retained.

In cases where prominent or large folds are encountered, there is often a concern about the possibility of infiltrating malignancy. In this regard, more important than height or width in predicting the absence of an infiltrating malignancy is the pliancy of the folds, especially its mucosa. This should tent up easily when grasped with a biopsy forceps (Fig. 11-23d), so that only a small portion of the fold at its mucosal surface is actually raised. The absence of tenting suggests the possibility of an infiltrative process (see Chapter 16).

Gastric Angle

The major landmark for the lesser curve and separation of the body and antrum is the gastric angle. If no particular effort is made to view the angle, it is seen with forward-viewing instruments only tangentially as a crescent-shaped structure descending from the lesser curve (Fig. 11-1). If seen *en face* by means of J-retroflexion, it appears as a strut-like fold, separating the body above from the antrum below (Fig. 11-16). Viewed in this way, it is seen to have a thickness between 5 and 10 mm and to be perfectly symmetrical and smooth.

Antrum

There is actually no one typical antral appearance. The antrum may be short (<3 cm) or long (>10 cm). It may have an upward or downward deviation, and may run off in either an anterior or posterior direction rather than staying in the midline. In addition to variations in the course of the antrum, a multitude of mucosal fold patterns ranges from single folds (i.e., ***incisurae***) running vertically or horizontally for short distances, to folds which are entirely circumferential (see Chapter 12).

Prepyloric Antral Region

The prepyloric antral region, within 2 cm of the pyloric channel, is one of enormous variation, especially regarding mucosal folds (see Chapter 12). Although one might expect to find a prominent central pyloric channel with only a slight mucosal prominence, this appearance (Fig. 11-6) is actually less common than one where the pyloric channel

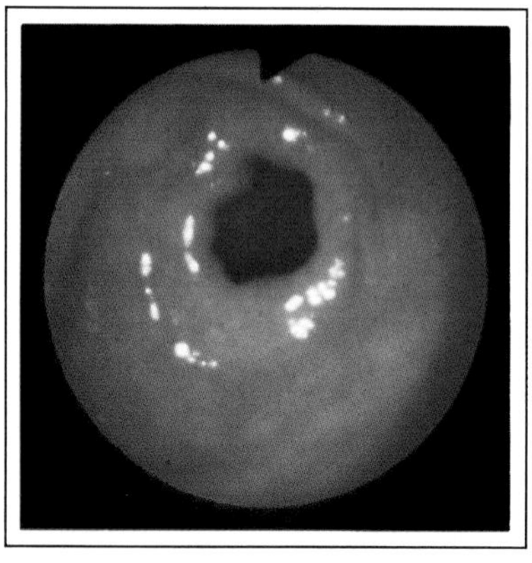

FIG. 11-24a.

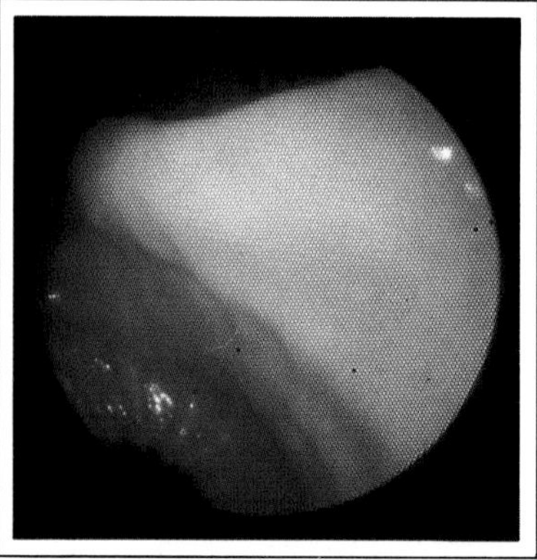

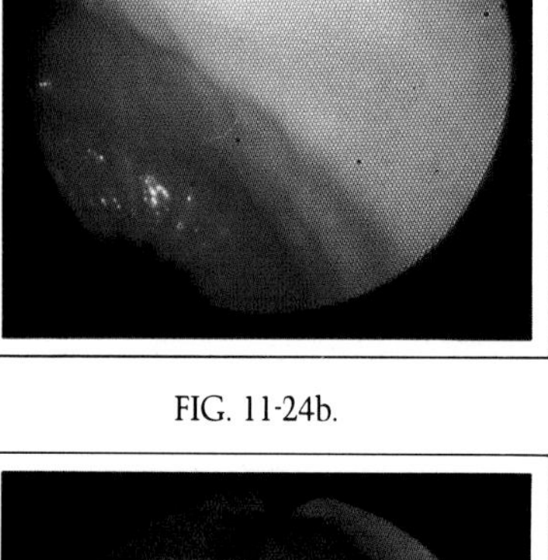

FIG. 11-24b.

FIG. 11-24. a: Normal gastric mucosa, yellow-orange color. **b:** Normal gastric mucosa, gray-white color in a close-up view of a relatively foldless antrum with intense illumination. **c:** Normal gastric (body) mucosa, reddish-orange color, associated with bile in the gastric lake. **d:** Normal gastric (body) mucosa, deep pink to red because of poor illumination. **e:** Normal gastric mucosa [same as in (d)], gray-white because of more intense illumination.

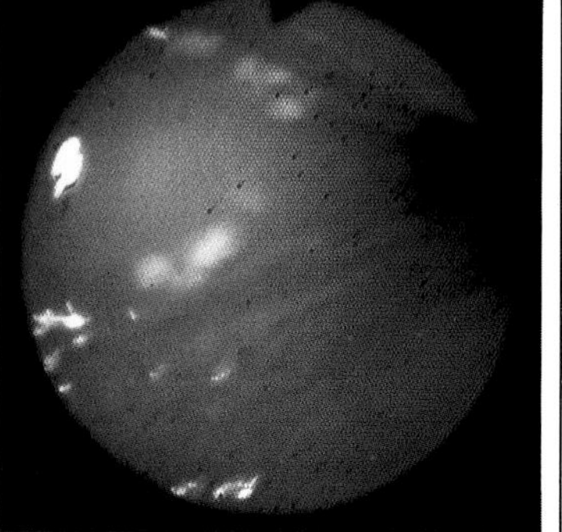

FIG. 11-24c.

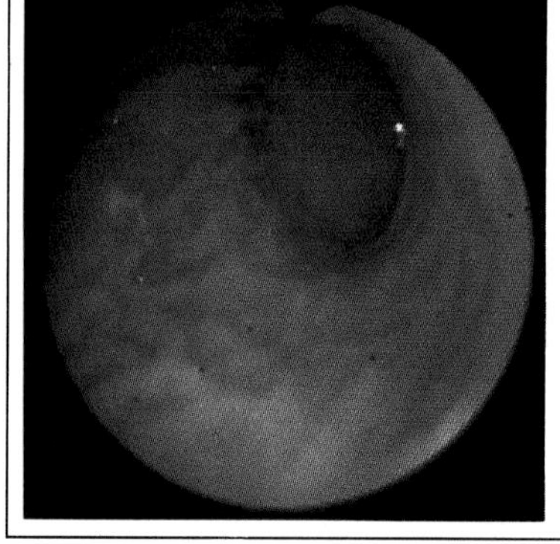

FIG. 11-24d.

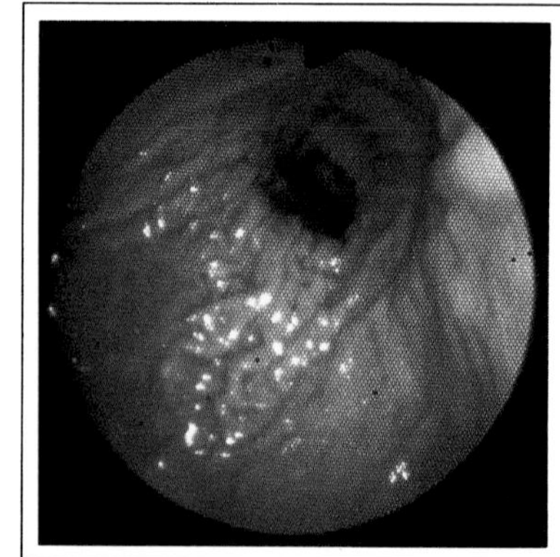

FIG. 11-24e.

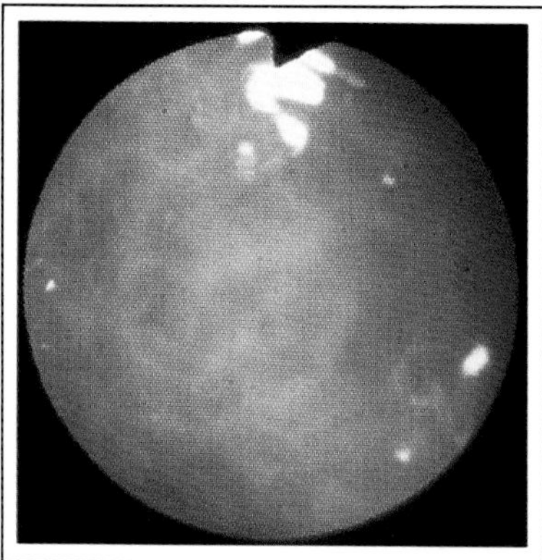

FIG. 11-25.

FIG. 11-25. Normal gastric (body) mucosa, close-up view. The mucosal character is geographic with the erythematous areas corresponding to the areae gastricae (see text), around which run white linear depressions, the lineae gastricae. Although the appearance may be designated "patchy erythema," biopsies are generally normal.

is obscured by prominent prepyloric antral folds (see Chapter 12).

Normal Mucosal Appearance

Orange-yellow is the single most common mucosal color (Fig. 11-24a). However, rather than a single typical color, one expects to find a range of colors, from yellow-gray-white to orange red. Mucosal color depends on the intensity of the illumination provided by the endoscope, as well as the light reflected by the structure(s) illuminated. For example, a short antrum (Fig. 11-24a) may appear yellow-gray because as a relatively closed, tubular space it reflects light more intensely. The lack of mucosal folds also allows greater reflection of light and hence a yellow-white appearance (Fig. 11-24b). Another factor that affects coloration (in the absence of histologic change) is the presence of bile in the gastric lake (Fig. 11-24c), which gives mucosa a reddened appearance because of altered reflection of light (with greater absorption of the white end of the light spectrum) as well as a possible direct mucosal effect of bile leading to capillary dilatation but no other histologic change. Probably more than any structural factor, mucosal color depends on the adequacy of the illumination. Less intense lighting causes the mucosa to appear deep pink, even reddened (Fig. 11-24d), whereas the same mucosa would appear orange-pink or gray-white (Fig. 11-24e) if properly illuminated.

Character

One expects gastric mucosa to be perfectly smooth and glistening, yet close-up views, especially with currently available instruments with a magnification factor of 10×, tend to bring out the underlying mucosal architecture of zones of slightly erythematous elevations (areae gastricae) and intervening mucosal linear depressions (lineae gastricae).[2] This pattern (Fig. 11-25) is common on close-up views without the histologic abnormality which may accompany the same appearance when seen at a distance of 2 to 3 cm from the mucosal surface (see Chapter 12).

Vessels

Capillaries.

Submucosal vessels may be regularly observed in isolated regions, e.g., the cardia, fundus (Fig. 11-22a), or antrum, and still not be associated with an altered histology (i.e., atrophic gastritis). Only when capillaries are found in the body as well as the adjacent region is the likelihood high that a biopsy will show atrophic gastritis.[3]

Veins.

Veins (<5 mm) are commonly found in the fundus (Fig. 11-22b) or body, especially when the mucosal folds can be completely effaced with insufflation. They are completely normal findings for the fundus. Even when found in the body in the absence of submucosal capillaries[3] to suggest atrophic gastritis, biopsies usually show normal mucosa.

Normal Appearance in Relation to Histology

A normal endoscopic appearance does not exclude the possibility of chronic gastritis. Taor et al.[4] found atrophic gastritis on biopsy in the face of a normal endoscopic appearance in 10% of patients examined, and other histologic changes were seen in an additional 30%. Even though the histologic appearance can be at variance with a normal endoscopic appearance, we do not routinely perform biopsies in these cases because no study has yet been reported which provides the necessary guidelines for dealing with such discrepancies.

REFERENCES

1. Morrissey, J. F. (1978): Endoscopic evaluation of gastroesophageal sphincter dysfunction. *South. Med. J. (Suppl. 1)*, 71:56–61.
2. Mackintosh, C. E., and Kreel, L. (1977): Anatomy and radiology of the areae gastricae. *Gut*, 18:855–864.
3. Meshkinpour, H., Orlando, R. A., Arguello, J. F., and DeMicco, M. P. (1979): Significance of endoscopically visible blood vessels as an index of atrophic gastritis. *Am. J. Gastroenterol.*, 71:376–379.
4. Taor, R. E., Fox, B., Ware, J., and Johnson, A. G. (1975): Gastritis—gastroscopic and microscopic. *Endoscopy*, 7:209–215.

12

THE STOMACH—VARIATIONS FROM THE NORMAL APPEARANCE

Five gastric appearances can be singled out as being different from normal (see Chapter 11) yet having uncertain clinical significance. These appearances are: (a) nonspecific gastric erythema; (b) bile in the gastric lake; (c) a large rugal fold (hyperrugosity) pattern; (d) (nodular) cardial folds; and (e) prominent (prepyloric) antral folds. These are not infrequent occurrences. At least one (most often bile in the gastric lake) may be expected in 30 to 40% of gastric examinations. Unfortunately, even experienced endoscopists disagree about significance of these appearances.

NONSPECIFIC ERYTHEMA

As previously noted (see Chapter 11), the color of gastric mucosa is orange-pink, becoming yellow-orange (Fig. 12-1) or gray-white with more intense illumination. We find, however, in approximately 5 to 10% of gastric examinations, even without previous gastric surgery[1] (see Chapter 19), that the mucosa has a distinctly red coloration (Fig. 12-2) either diffusely or linearly along rugal folds. Views of the mucosa from 2 to 3 cm, especially that with a diffuse pattern, show the erythema to be discontinuous, actually composed of innumerable tiny (1 to 3 mm) raised dots of erythema (Fig. 12-3). These, we believe, individually are the areae gastricae, the innumerable surface elevations which careful anatomic studies[2] have suggested comprise the characteristic topographic arrangement of gastric mucosa. Separating these slightly raised dots of erythema are yellow-white lines which are observed anatomically to be the lineae gastricae, or mucosal depressions between the elevations.

A variety of terms have been used to designate this appearance. Many of these include the word gastritis, e.g., acute gastritis, chronic gastritis, or superficial gastritis. Because superficial gastritis has been histologically associated with this appearance in 40% or more of cases, some believe it to be the appropriate designation for this appearance[2,3]. Because we find no histologic abnormality in up to 60% of these cases, we prefer the simple descriptive term "nonspecific gastric erythema."

The erythema may be diffuse, involving both body and antrum (Fig. 12-2), or it may be confined to either the body (Fig. 12-4) or the antrum (Fig. 12-5). When the antrum alone is involved (Fig. 12-5), the term "antral gastritis" has been used. The significance of localized erythema as opposed to the more generalized variety is unknown.

We find that in approximately 25% of our cases of nonspecific gastric erythema, bile in the gastric lake occurs (Fig. 12-6), although the relationship between the two findings is unclear. As we have already suggested (see Chapter 11), the bile present in the gastric lake may alter the illumination of the mucosa as well as the state of the mucosal capillaries, leading to dilatation and thereby creating a reddened mucosa (Fig. 12-6).

A variety of histologic appearances may be seen in biopsies taken from areas shown in nonspecific gastric erythema, including superficial gastritis, diffuse gastritis, and mucosal atrophy. We note that in almost 60% of biopsies taken the histologic appearance is normal or shows only capillary dilatation. Others[1,3] also find normal histology with this appearance, although in less than 20%. We find the most consistent histologic abnormality is capillary dilatation in combination with glandular epithelium showing mucin depletion (Fig. 12-7a). We believe it is the combination of capillary dilatation and mucin depletion which alters light transmission from the mucosal surface, giving it its reddened appearance. In addition to capillary dilatation and mucin depletion, a pleomorphic infiltrate of lymphocytes, eosinophils, and plasma cells may be present. This infiltrate may appear in the upper third of the mucosa, for which the term superficial gastritis is used, or it may occur diffusely throughout the mucosa. In approximately 5 to 10% of the cases polymorphonuclear leukocytes cause the histologic appearance to receive the designation "acute gastritis."[4] In

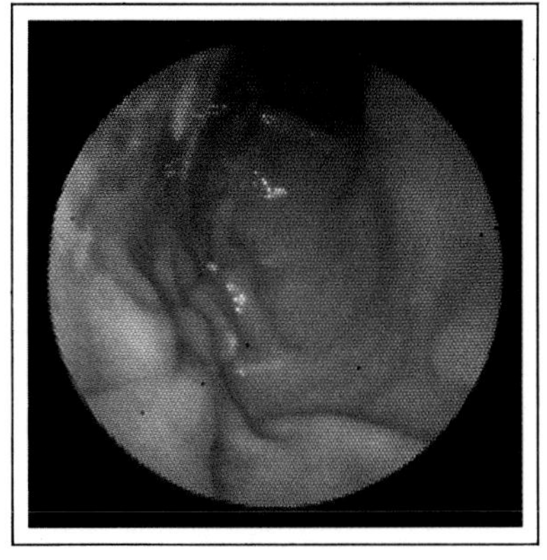

FIG. 12-1.

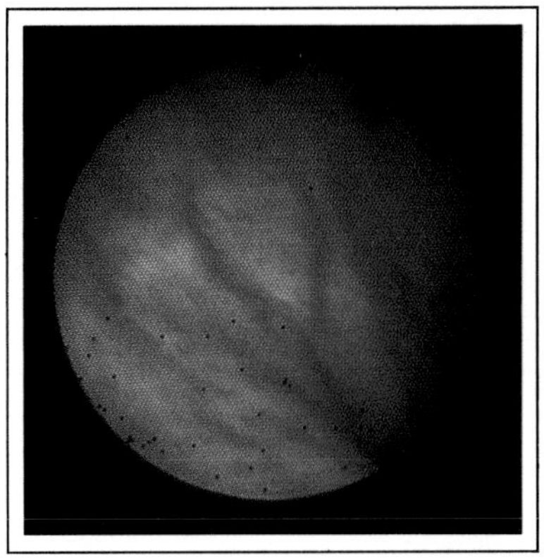

FIG. 12-2.

FIG. 12-1. Gastric mucosa with an orange-gray color.

FIG. 12-2. Nonspecific gastric erythema. The mucosal color is a reddish-orange.

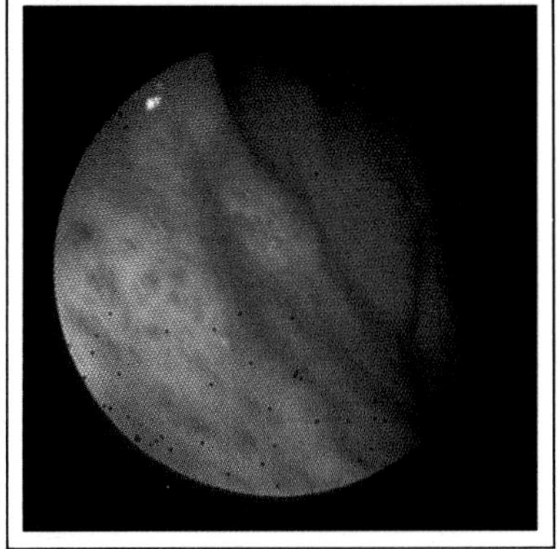

FIG. 12-3.

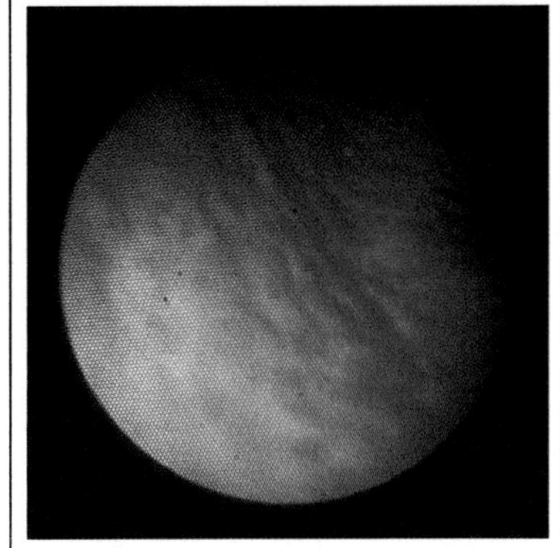

FIG. 12-4.

FIG. 12-3. Nonspecific gastric erythema, mucosal detail. The erythema seen in Fig. 12-2 actually consists of innumerable raised dots of erythema (scarletina, morbiliform pattern) which may represent the areae gastricae with linear pale areas between as the lineae gastricae (see text).

FIG. 12-4. Nonspecific gastric erythema in the body. The erythema in this case ended abruptly at the level of the gastric angle.

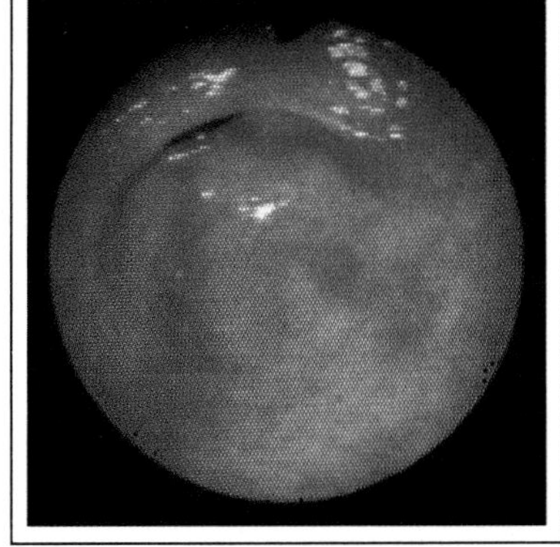

FIG. 12-5.

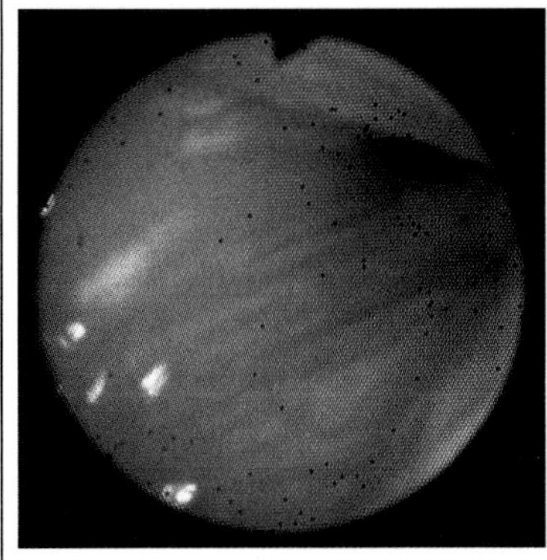

FIG. 12-6.

FIG. 12-5. Antral erythema. Erythematous streaks are seen to radiate to the pyloric channel.

FIG. 12-6. Bile in the gastric lake in association with nonspecific gastric erythema.

upward of 20% of our cases, where the endoscopic appearance is identical to that associated with mucin depletion and inflammation, only capillary dilatation is found histologically (Fig. 12-7b).

The clinical significance of nonspecific gastric erythema continues to be a subject of controversy. In a study of symptomatic patients having endoscopy performed in our Unit, those with diffuse, nonspecific erythema were contrasted with other symptomatic patients having no final diagnosis for symptoms except "irritable digestive tract syndrome." Thirty patients with erythema were contrasted with 40 patients without erythema. Among those with erythema, we found a higher percentage (60% versus 30%) of cases having a short duration (<1 year) of symptoms prior to endoscopy, as well as a higher percentage of cases with vomiting (30% versus 15%) and epigastric "burning" (40% versus 15%). This clustering is interesting as it may indicate in symptomatic patients with gastric erythema an alteration in the state of the gastric mucosa, conceivably from an as yet unidentified infectious agent,[5] an alteration in gallbladder function enhancing mucosal injury from bile reflux,[6] or the sudden onset of delayed gastric emptying.[7]

Although in our study the histology was not examined in every patient, an important subgroup of symptomatic

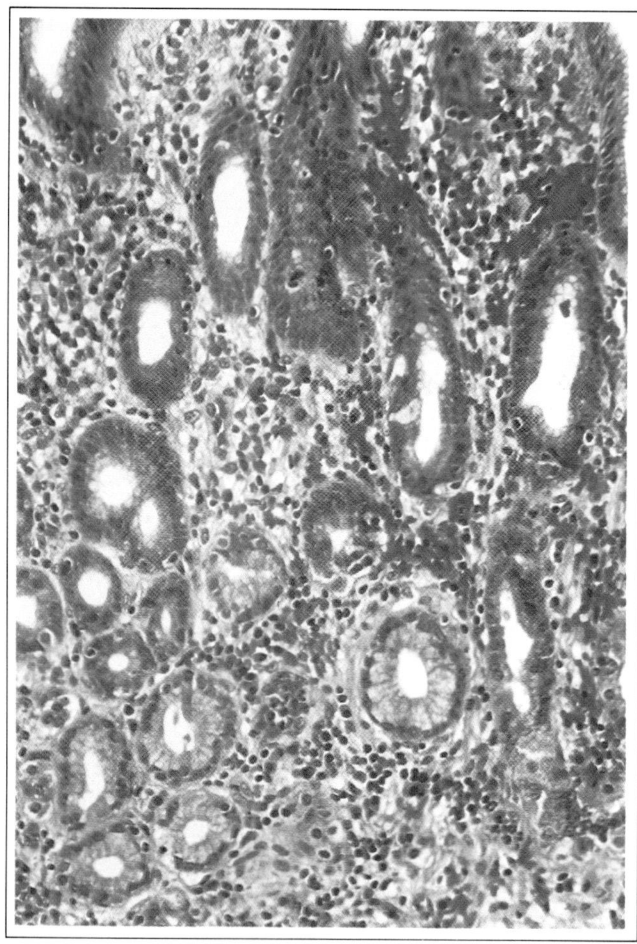

FIG. 12-7a.

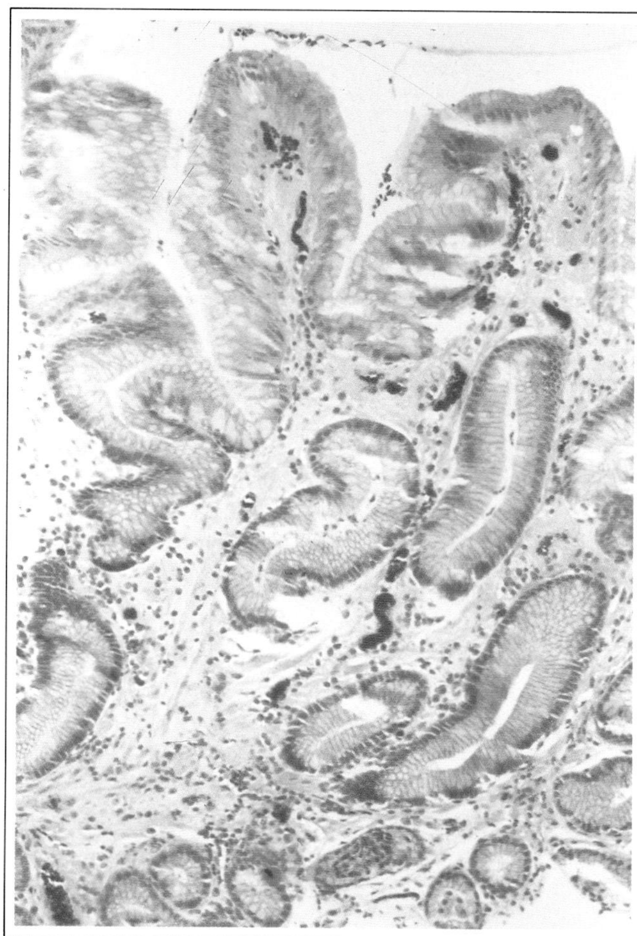

FIG. 12-7b.

FIG. 12-7. a: Superficial gastritis. Biopsy of mucosa pictured in Fig. 12-2 shows capillary dilatation, mucin depletion of glandular epithelium, and an inflammatory infiltrate confined to the outer third of the mucosa. **b:** Biopsy of an erythematous streak (Fig. 12-5) shows only capillary dilatation.

patients with nonspecific erythema may be those whose biopsies show polymorphonuclear leukocytes, i.e., those with acute gastritis.[4] Such changes are indistinguishable from those in biopsies taken from the margins of peptic ulcers. In one study, two-thirds of patients with these acute changes had symptoms which were indistinguishable from those of peptic ulcers, even though macroscopic ulcers were not found. The natural history of these acute changes in relation to the development of frank ulceration is not known, however; nor is it known if treatment influences the natural history of this appearance.

At present, for patients who are found at endoscopy to have nonspecific gastric erythema, we believe it is wise to resist the temptation to attribute symptoms to this endoscopic appearance or any associated histologic changes.

BILE IN THE GASTRIC LAKE

Bile in the gastric lake may be encountered in as many as 30% of unoperated stomachs. Like erythema, with which it is associated in 20 to 30% of the cases, it is an entirely nonspecific finding (Fig. 12-6). It is an almost invariable finding in patients with previous gastric surgery (see Chapter 19) and is often found in those with prior cholecystectomy who may have continuous secretion of bile into the duodenum which periodically is refluxed back into the stomach.[6] It may also be found in occasional patients with gallbladder disease in whom there is diminished gallbladder filling,[8] presumably because of fibrous scarring of the gallbladder or cystic duct. In addition, it may be seen with vomiting, especially if the patient reports the vomiting as bilious. We find the range of histologic findings to be identical in those patients with vomiting as in asymptomatic patients in whom bile is found at endoscopy performed for other reasons. In more than 60 to 70% of either group, there is a completely normal histologic appearance. Therefore, like nonspecific erythema, we view the finding of bile as being of uncertain clinical significance.

HYPERRUGOSITY PATTERN (LARGE RUGAL FOLDS)

We find large rugal folds with a height in excess of 1 cm (Fig. 12-8a) in approximately 1% of examinations. These correspond to large gastric folds (>8 mm in width) dem-

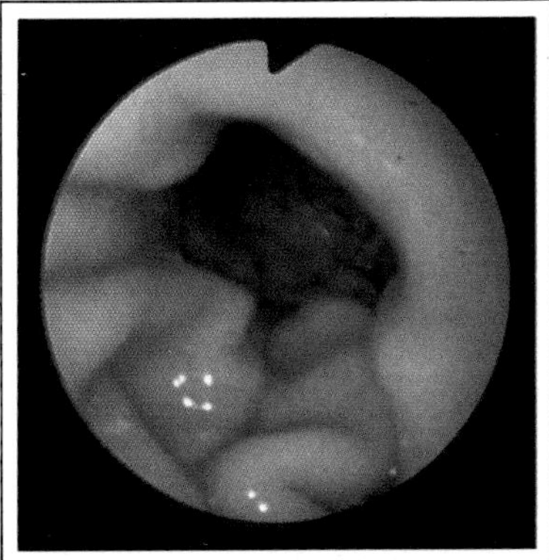

FIG. 12-8a.

FIG. 12-8. a: Large gastric folds (1 cm) corresponding to those seen radiographically in (**b**).

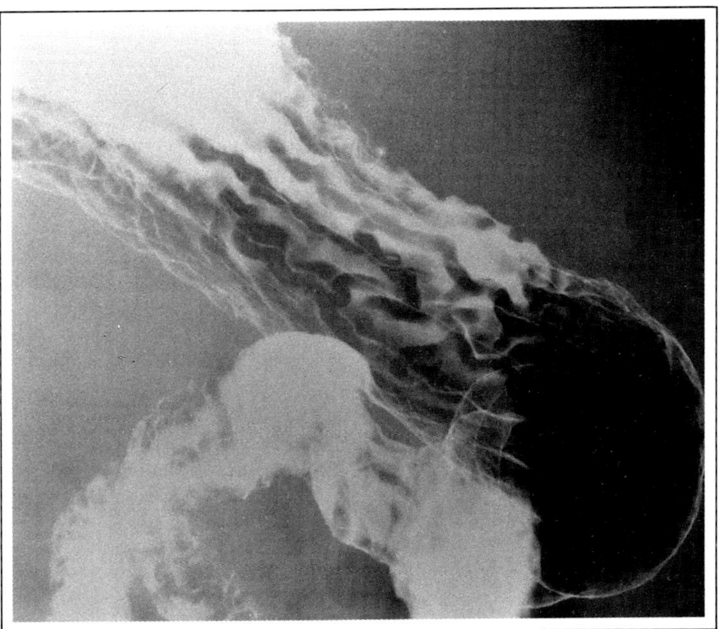

FIG. 12-8b.

onstrated radiographically (Fig. 12-8b). Like gastric erythema, which may be seen on the ridges of these folds (Fig. 12-9), or bile in the gastric lake, which is sometimes also found (Fig. 12-9), the folds themselves are a nonspecific finding, with forceps or large-particle snare biopsies[9] showing variable amounts of gastritis. It is unclear as to whether this gastritis is responsible for the folds or simply a response to the wear-and-tear effects on the superficial mucosa residing on the ridges. The important question, however, is not what is responsible for the fold, but whether the fold is simply large or is indicative of an infiltrating malignancy. It is our impression that an assessment of pliancy by means of the mucosal tenting sign (see Chapter 11) is often helpful in this regard. Finding the mucosa to be pliant (Fig. 12-10a), although reassuring, does not allow the endoscopist categorically to conclude that infiltrating malignancy is not present (Fig. 12-10c), as the accuracy of this test (particularly the false-negativity rate) has never been systematically evaluated. On the other hand, the absence of mucosal tenting (Fig. 12-10b) strongly points to malignancy, especially if symptoms such as pain and weight loss are present. If forceps biopsies in such a case were unrevealing, one would then perform a full-thickness mucosal (large particle) snare biopsy[9] (see Chapter 1). Laparotomy might still be necessary in cases where even with a negative large-particle biopsy the clinical index of suspicion remains high because of weight loss and suggestive computed tomography of the stomach.[10] In other cases (Fig. 12-11), where mucosal pliancy estimated by the tenting sign was present, large-particle biopsy, if negative, might alone serve as a definitive measure in that the likelihood of an infiltrating process seems to be low. However, like the tenting sign itself, the miss (false-negativity) rate of this type of biopsy in cases of infiltrating malignancy is unknown.

NODULAR CARDIAL FOLDS

As already noted (see Chapter 11), redundant cardial mucosa causes the cardial ring seen in the retroflexed position

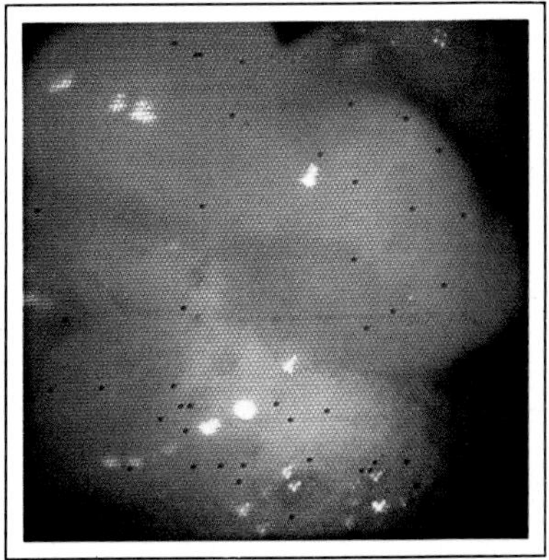

FIG. 12-9.

FIG. 12-9. "Giant" rugal folds (>1.5 cm). Bile and nonspecific erythema are also noted.

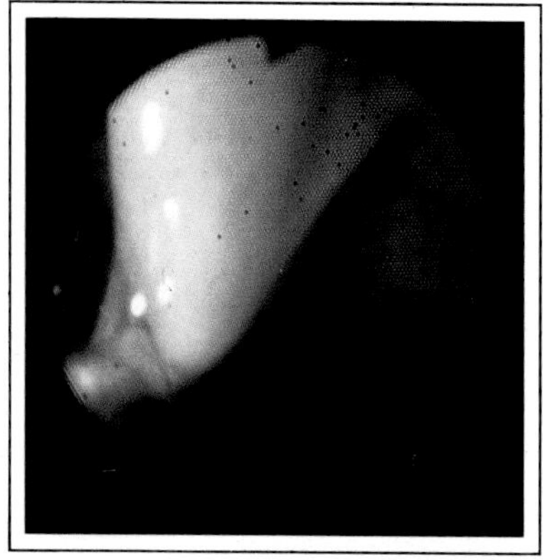

FIG. 12-10a.

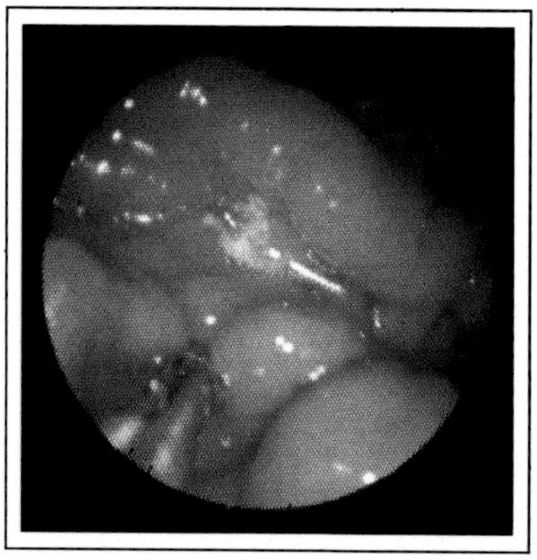

FIG. 12-10b.

FIG. 12-10. **a:** Tenting of large (1 cm) rugal folds. To establish its pliancy, a small zone of mucosa is being lifted up into the lumen by the biopsy forceps. **b:** Infiltrating gastric malignancy. In this case the prominent mucosal folds are rigid and do not tent. **c:** Infiltrating gastric (cardial) malignancy. In this case there was tenting of these folds; nevertheless, the patient had surgery because of a 60-pound weight loss and suspicious computed tomography of the stomach. The infiltrating carcinoma of the cardia with widespread metastasis underscores the fallibility of the tenting sign.

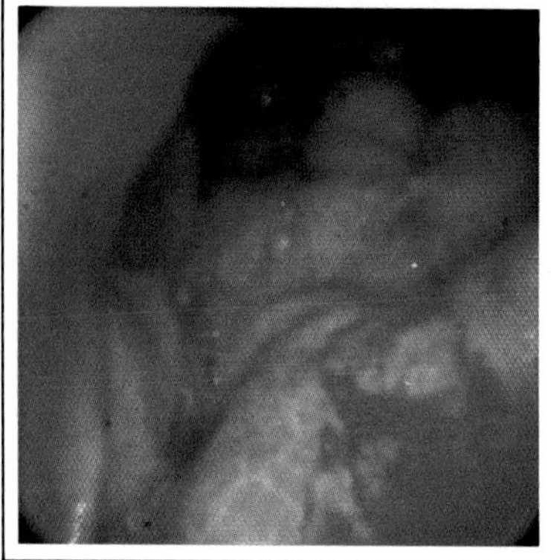

FIG. 12-10c.

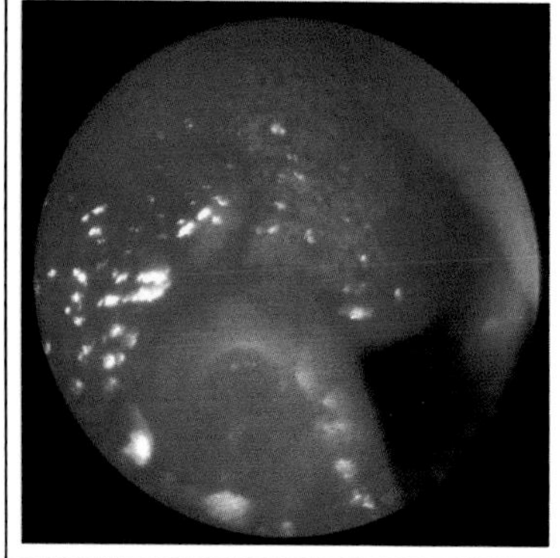

FIG. 12-11.

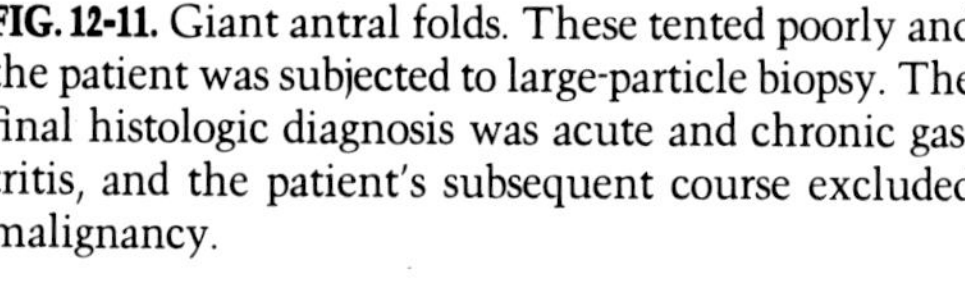

FIG. 12-11. Giant antral folds. These tented poorly and the patient was subjected to large-particle biopsy. The final histologic diagnosis was acute and chronic gastritis, and the patient's subsequent course excluded malignancy.

to appear nodular (Fig. 12-12). We find this appearance in approximately 0.5% of the cases. The symmetrical folds which make up this appearance suggest its true nature (Fig. 12-12). This must be differentiated from the asymmetrical firm nodular mass of carcinoma (Fig. 12-13) and cardial varices, which, although pliant, are asymmetrical and part of a system of fundic varices (Fig. 12-14).

ANTRAL FOLDS

One expects that with adequate insufflation the antrum will appear perfectly flat or with only slightly elevated prepyloric folds (Fig. 12-15). Prominent antral folds (>5 mm height and 1 cm width) are present in 10%. There are two patterns of antral folds: (a) a single (sometimes two) roofing fold which forms and arches over the pyloric channel (Fig. 12-16); and (b) a system of large pyloric antral folds (Fig. 12-17).

Patients with prominent antral folds are likely to be referred for endoscopy because of a question on a radiologic study of the stomach of either a mass (produced by a filling defect from the folds) or an ulcer (resulting from barium collecting between the folds).[11] For endoscopists there are two interpretive questions: (a) Are the folds to be taken as evidence of prior peptic disease? (b) Are the folds infiltrated?

With regard to the question of prior peptic ulcer disease,

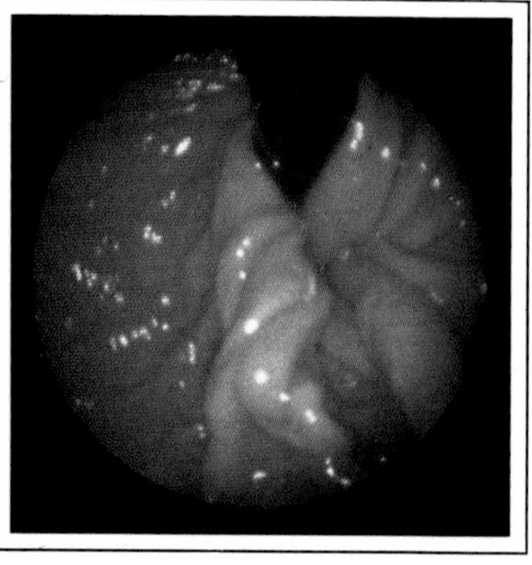

FIG. 12-12.

FIG. 12-12. Prominent cardial folds (retroflexed view). These result from redundant mucosa of the cardia. Some nodularity is suggested, but the folds are symmetrical and pliant.

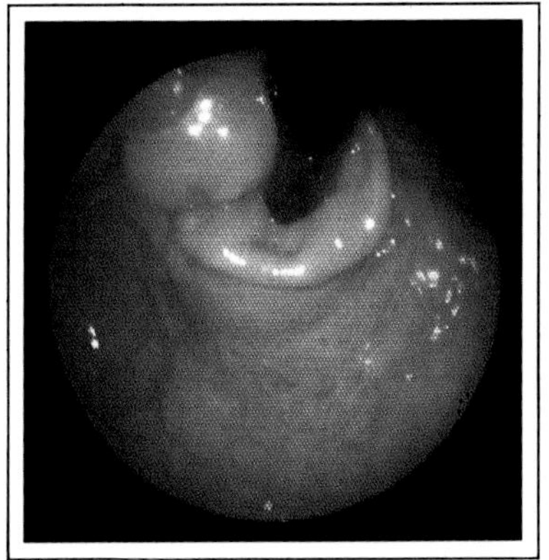

FIG. 12-13a.

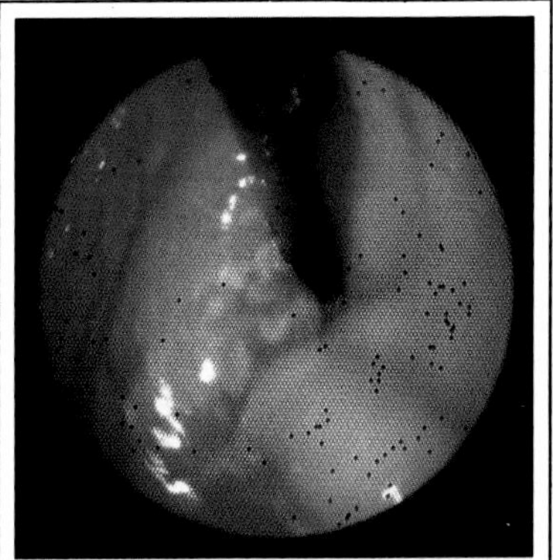

FIG. 12-13b.

FIG. 12-13. a: Metastatic carcinoma to the cardia. An asymmetrical cardial, nodular fold is observed. This 1-cm nodule proved to be relatively fixed. At surgery it was found to represent a serosal implant from a neighboring carcinoma of the tail of the pancreas. **b:** Primary cardial carcinoma. In this case, unlike that in (a), there is a tumor mass on the anterior (9 o'clock) aspect of the cardia.

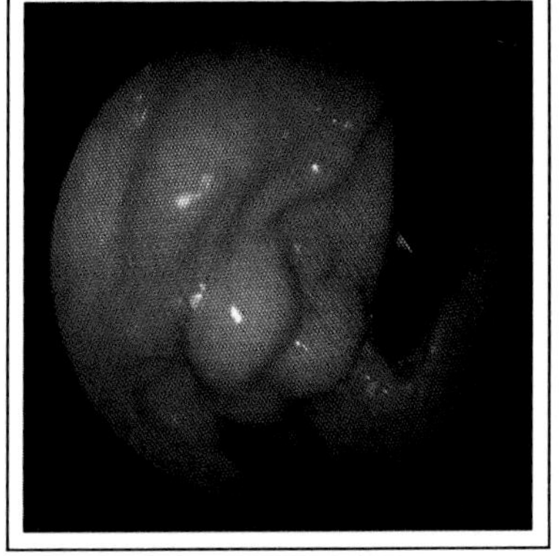

FIG. 12-14.

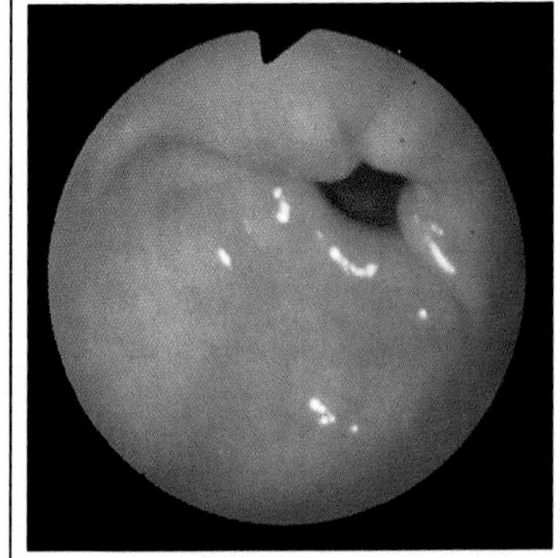

FIG. 12-15.

FIG. 12-14. Cardial varices. The asymmetrical folds are part of a system of nodular folds extending into the fundus and are suggestive of gastric varices. The diagnosis was confirmed arteriographically.

FIG. 12-15. Antrum prepyloric region. There are slightly elevated prepyloric folds, a common appearance.

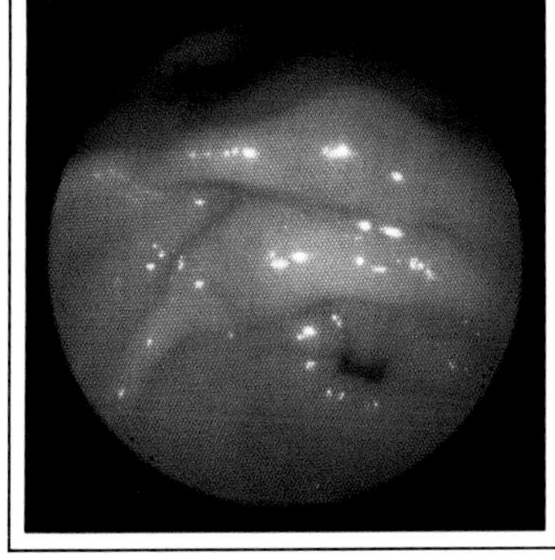

FIG. 12-16.

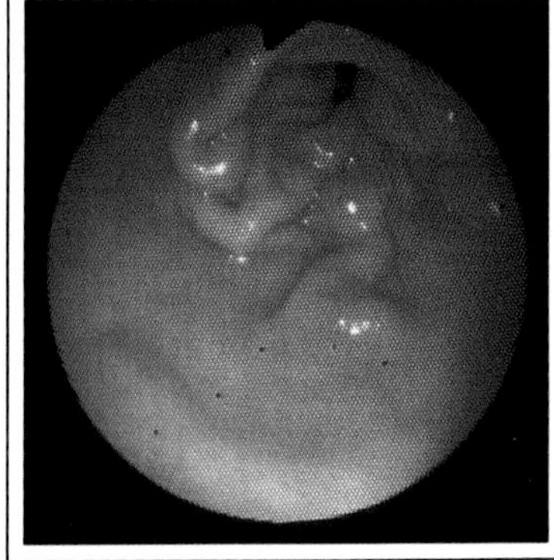

FIG. 12-17.

FIG. 12-16. Antrum prepyloric region. Prominent roofing folds form an archway over the pyloric channel, a common variation.

FIG. 12-17. Large antral folds. Folds such as these or larger may be expected in 10% or more of examinations and are especially common among black patients (30% of the cases).

antral folds are a common finding in patients both with and without a suggestive history. We find this particularly true for black patients, in whom prominent prepyloric folds are noted in up to 30% of the cases studied for any reason. We do not, therefore, use the finding of folds themselves as evidence of peptic disease. This is similar to the case of the congenital antral mucosal diaphragm (Fig. 12-18)—which may closely resemble the scar deformity associated with peptic ulcer disease (Fig. 12-19) and yet can be found in patients with no ulcer history whatsoever.[12]

The question of infiltration in the antrum can be more difficult to resolve than in the body because antral folds, especially prepyloric ones, tend to be less pliant and therefore tent poorly (Fig. 12-20a). If individual folds themselves can be defined (Fig. 12-20a), one may still, in the absence of symptoms suggestive of malignancy (e.g., weight loss), regard them simply as antral folds. Snare biopsy, however, must be considered if there is a question about their nature because of symptoms or the appearance of a mass (Fig. 12-20b). In patients with liver disease (Fig. 12-21) in whom prominent antral folds are seen, especially those with a serpiginous character, arteriography should be considered prior to biopsy to determine if the folds are in fact large gastric varices (see Chapter 37).

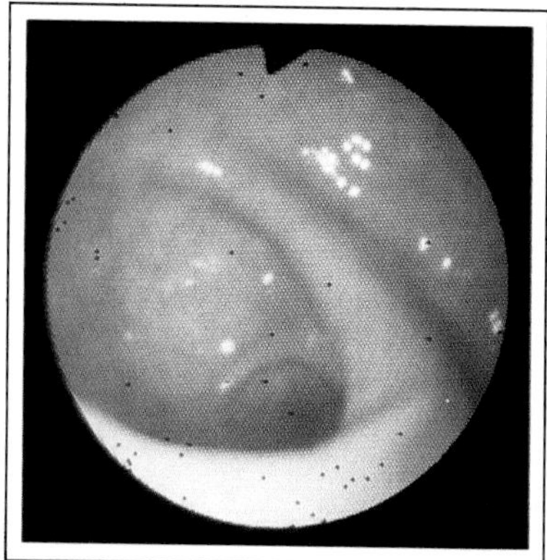

FIG. 12-18.

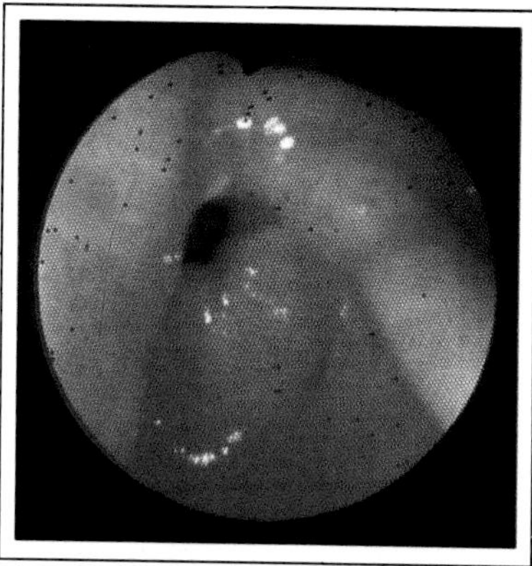
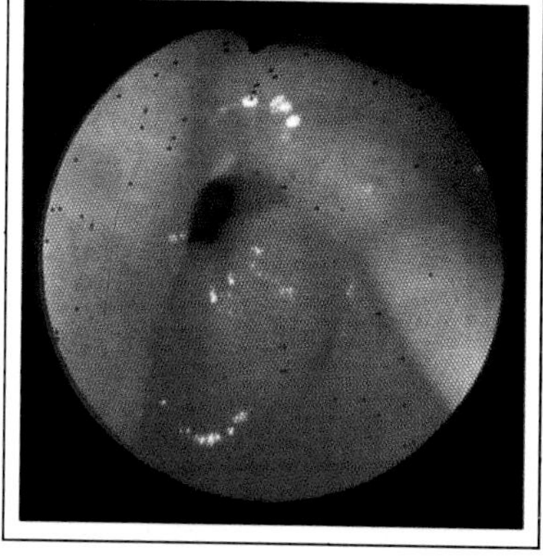

FIG. 12-19.

FIG. 12-18. Antral deformity, possibly a congenital mucosal diaphragm (see Chapter 13).

FIG. 12-19. Antral deformity, which is probably converging folds from previous ulcer disease but is similar in appearance to that in Fig. 12-18. Note the small ulcer depression at the point of convergence.

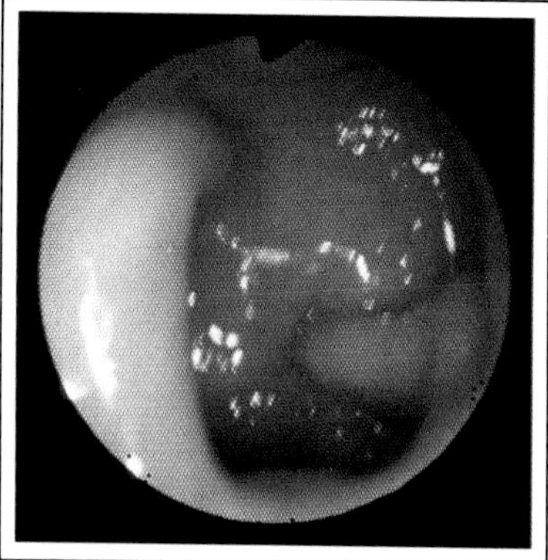

FIG. 12-20a.

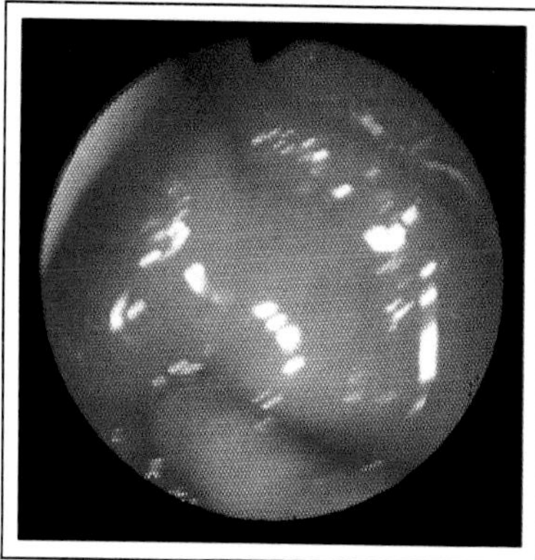

FIG. 12-20b.

FIG. 12-20. a: Prominent prepyloric antral folds. These appeared relatively fixed and tented poorly. Individual folds, however, were easily identified. Because the appearance was symmetrical and the patient asymptomatic, no further work-up was advised. **b:** Antral folds with a mass. An asymmetrical, slightly umbilicated mass was observed in a patient with nonspecific abdominal complaints. Because of recent weight loss, the patient was subjected to surgery, which proved the mass to be a small carcinoid with metastatic implants found elsewhere in the abdomen.

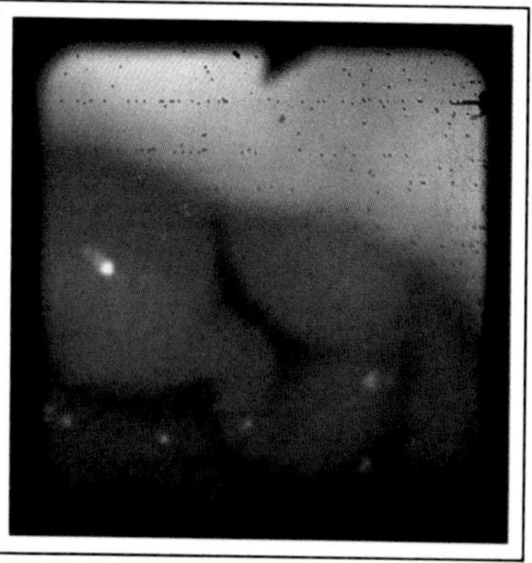

FIG. 12-21.

FIG. 12-21. Antral varices in a patient with liver disease. Arteriography confirmed the diagnosis and allowed large-particle biopsy to be avoided, which would have been catastrophic.

REFERENCES

1. Myren, J., and Serck-Hanssen, A. (1974): The gastroscopic diagnosis of gastritis. *Scand. J. Gastroenterol.*, 9:437–462.
2. Mackintosh, C. E., and Kreel, L. (1977): Anatomy and radiology of the areae gastricae. *Gut*, 18:855–864.
3. Taor, R. E., Fox, B., Ware, J., and Johnson, A. G. (1975): Gastritis—gastroscopic and microscopic. *Endoscopy*, 7:209–215.
4. Greenlaw, R., Sheahan, D. G., DeLuca, V., Miller, D., Myerson, D., and Myerson, P. (1980): Gastroduodenitis: broader concept of peptic ulcer disease. *Dig. Dis. Sci.*, 25:650–672.
5. Ramsey, E. J., Carey, K. V., Peterson, W. L., Jackson, J. J., Murphy, F. K., Read, N. W., Taylor, K. B., Trier, J. S., and Fordtran, J. S. (1979): Epidemic gastritis with hypochlorhydria. *Gastroenterology*, 76:1449–1457.
6. Warshaw, A. L. (1979): Bile gastritis without prior gastric surgery: contributing role of cholecystectomy. *Am. J. Surg.*, 137:527–531.
7. Rhodes, J. B., Robinson, R. G., and McBride, N. (1979): Sudden onset of slow gastric emptying of food. *Gastroenteroscopy*, 77:569–571.
8. Shaffer, F. A., McOrmond, P., and Duggan, H. (1980): Quantitative cholescintigraphy assessment of gallbladder filling and emptying and duodenogastric reflux. *Gastroenterology*, 79:899–906.
9. Bjork, J. T., Geenen, J. E., Soergel, K., Parker, H. W., Leinicke, J. A., and Komorowski, R. A. (1977): Endoscopic evaluation of large gastric folds: a comparison of biopsy techniques. *Gastrointest. Endosc.*, 24:22–23.
10. Balfe, D. M., Koehler, R. E., Karstaedt, N., Stanley, R. J., and Sagel, S. S. (1981): Computed tomography of gastric neoplasms. *Radiology*, 140:431–436.
11. Tawile, N., and Schuman, B. M. (1974): A gastroscopic analysis of antral deformity. *Gastrointest. Endosc.*, 20:160–161.
12. Clements, J. L., Jinkins, J. R., Torres, W. E., Thomas, B. M., Thomas, J., Elmer, R. A., and Weens, H. S. (1974): Antral mucosal diaphragm in adults. *Am. J. Roentgenol.*, 133:1105–1111.

13

STRUCTURAL ABNORMALITIES OF THE STOMACH

Not infrequently, the endoscopist finds himself performing an examination without prior radiologic studies. Some clinicians now refer patients for endoscopy directly because of its recognized superiority over still widely used single-contrast radiographic studies, especially for the detection of peptic ulcers.[1] In other cases, where endoscopy is performed as an emergency measure for upper gastrointestinal bleeding, radiographic studies are again omitted because of their generally low accuracy. In still other cases, a radiographic study may have been performed but neither the study nor even a report of its radiologic interpretation is available. In each of these instances, the endoscopist must be prepared to interpret the findings associated with structural abnormalities of the stomach without other information. For an extremely common abnormality, e.g., a hiatus hernia, this is routine. For other less frequently encountered appearances, e.g., those associated with organoaxial rotation, gastric webs, or diverticula, the examiner must know and understand their anatomy so that whenever the situation arises he can correctly interpret their potentially confusing appearances.

HIATUS HERNIA

Hiatus hernia is commonly found at endoscopy. We observe it in about 10% of examinations and as the sole diagnosis in 3 to 5%, an experience which accords with that of others.[3] The presence of a hiatus hernia is suspected when, on crossing the gastroesophageal (GE) junction, one encounters a pouch-like appearance of the cardia with the proximal end of the pouch being bound by the GE junction and the distal end formed by the diaphragmatic impression on the posterior aspect of the lesser curve (Fig. 13-1). A distance of up to 2 cm between the GE junction and the diaphragmatic impression may be considered normal, whereas a distance in excess of 2 cm and certainly 3 cm suggests a hiatus hernia (see Chapter 11). In cases where the examiner wishes to make a valid determination of whether a hiatus hernia is present, he will measure the distance between the GE junction and the diaphragmatic hiatus prior to entering the stomach proper, rather than on withdrawal, as in the course of the gastroduodenal examination it is possible to slide the herniated portion of

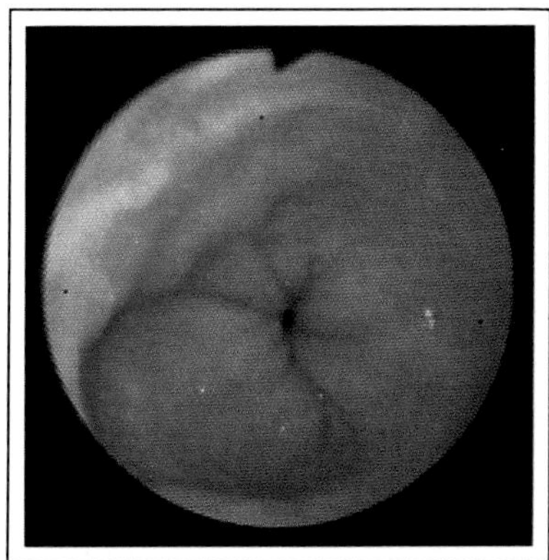

FIG. 13-1.

FIG. 13-1. Hiatus hernia. A ring-like GE junction is noted 3 cm above the diaphragmatic impression observed in the distance, giving the cardia a pouch-like appearance which should always suggest hiatus hernia.

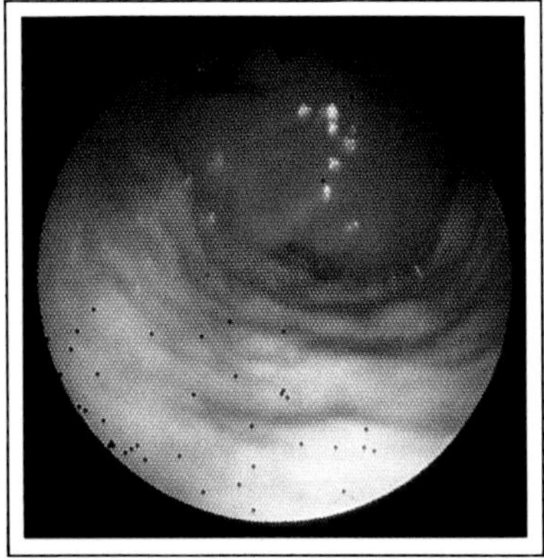

FIG. 13-2a.

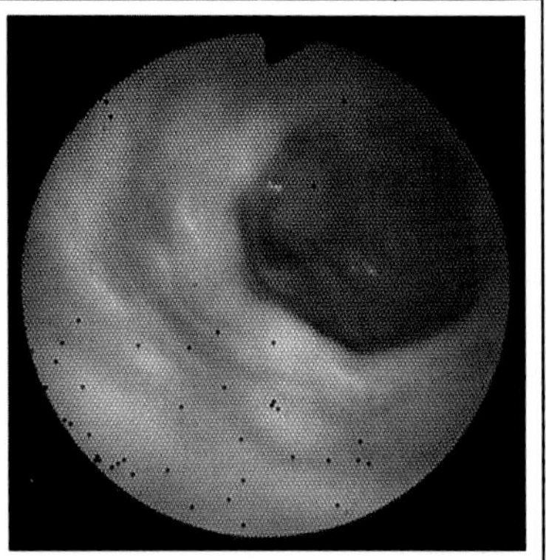

FIG. 13-2b.

FIG. 13-2. a: Prolapsing cardial mucosa. Another appearance which suggests the presence of a hiatus hernia is prolapse of cardial mucosa into the distal esophagus. **b:** Hiatus hernia. After return of the prolapsed cardial mucosa, the typical pouch-like appearance of a hiatus hernia is recognized.

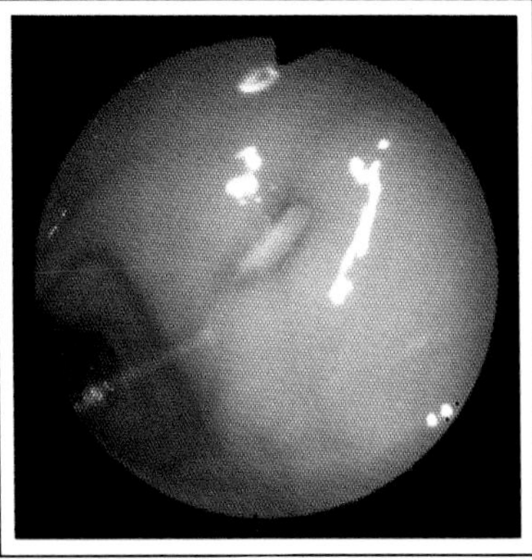

FIG. 13-3.

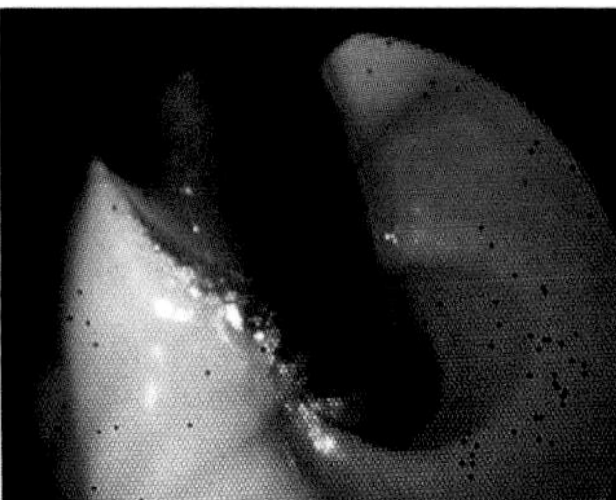

FIG. 13-4.

FIG. 13-3. Hiatus hernia with an ulcer. On the posterior wall, just above the diaphragmatic impression, a 3-mm linear ulcer was observed.

FIG. 13-4. Open cardia sign observed in the U-type retroflexed position. The force necessary to establish the retroflexed position brings out the diaphragmatic hiatus, with a ridge-like impression from the diaphragmatic crus seen just above the open cardia. In addition to this, the fundus is seen in the 12 o'clock direction against the left leaf of the diaphragm.

the stomach back into a position below the diaphragm causing the distance between the GE junction and diaphragmatic impression to appear normal even in the presence of a significant (3 to 5 cm) hiatus hernia.

Another finding which would cause one to suspect the presence of a hiatus hernia is that of prolapsing gastric mucosa into the esophagus (Fig. 13-2a).

The clinical significance of a hiatus hernia is unsettled. While it is common in the general adult population and does not in itself define a group more likely to have symptoms of esophageal reflux,[2a] it does define a group who at endoscopy are more likely to display definite esophagitis (see Chapter 3).[3] This may occur not so much because a hiatus hernia predisposes to reflux, as its presence results in delayed clearance of any acid which has been refluxed.[3a]

The presence therefore of a hiatus hernia, especially in a symptomatic patient, should make the examiner wish to examine carefully the distal 2 cm of the esophagus for endoscopic signs of esophagitis: erosion, ulcerations (Fig. 13-3), or inflammatory exudate. Once within the hernia, a careful search is undertaken for ulcerations (especially at the level of the diaphragm, which seems to be particularly vulnerable).[4]

When the cardia is viewed in the retroflexed position in the presence of a hiatus hernia, it appears "open" (Fig. 13-4); that is, the widened diameter of the diaphragmatic hiatus is appreciated as the intrathoracic cardia is forced across the diaphragm. The retroflexed view is important for examining the hernia for proximal ulcerations, which cannot be seen in any other way, as well as for a cardial carcinoma for which there is said to be an increased incidence in association with hiatus hernia.[5]

Large Hiatus Hernia

Hiatus hernias larger than 5 cm are occasionally encountered (Fig. 13-5). In these, both cardia and fundus are often herniated above the diaphragm and therefore constitute a mixed type of hernia (sliding plus paraesophageal), with the cardia being the sliding component and the fundus constituting the paraesophageal part. The mixed nature of the large hiatus hernia is best appreciated when viewed in the retroflexed position (Fig. 13-6), the hernia being entered through the open cardia (Fig. 13-6). In addition to iron deficiency anemia from occult blood loss,[6] large hiatus hernias are associated with the appearance of organoaxial rotation[7] (Fig. 13-7) and obstruction[8] (see below).

ORGANOAXIAL ROTATION (GASTRIC VOLVULUS)

Uncommonly, but especially in elderly patients, the stomach turns on its longitudinal axis (producing a "flip-flop"), placing the greater curve in the cephalad position

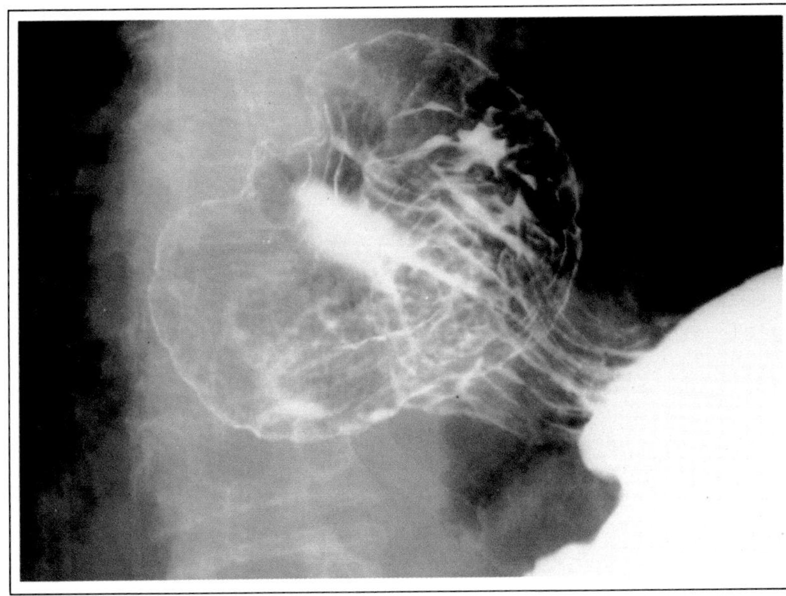

FIG. 13-5.

FIG. 13-5. Large (6 cm) hiatal hernia, radiographic appearance.

and the lesser curve in the caudad position. Although organoaxial rotation may be congenital or a consequence of gastric surgery, in most cases it is found in association with a large paraesophageal hernia (Fig. 13-7). Organoaxial rotation may be of the intermittent or the nonobstructive type, as well as obstructive.[9]

We observed one case which was nonobstructive and associated with a large paraesophageal hiatus hernia. In this instance the body of the stomach, which had undergone organoaxial rotation as it had been herniated above the diaphragm, could be observed and entered only in the retroflexed position (Fig. 13-7b). In this case the body was entered and the endoscope advanced for a short distance, at which time the procedure itself caused the herniated, rotated portion of the stomach to become intra-abdominal again and "flip" back into its normal anatomic position.

It is important to be aware of the fact that with this anatomic appearance there is a potential for the nonobstructive type to become obstructive because of enlargement of the proximal intrathoracic portion, leading to compression of the distal portion at the level of the diaphragm, a complication which occurs in 10 to 30% of the cases.[7]

GASTRIC INCISURAE AND ANTRAL MUCOSAL DIAPHRAGMS (WEBS)

Gastric incisurae and antral mucosal diaphragms are transverse mucosal folds of the body or antrum, being either noncircumferential incisurae or circumferential mucosal diaphragms (also called webs). Incisurae may be in the body or antrum, but mucosal diaphragms occur almost exclusively in the antrum and are therefore called antral mucosal diaphragms.

Incisurae

Single, transverse folds are found in either the body (Fig. 13-8) or the antrum (Fig. 13-9). They are rarely seen in the body, encountered on the order of one per 1,000 exami-

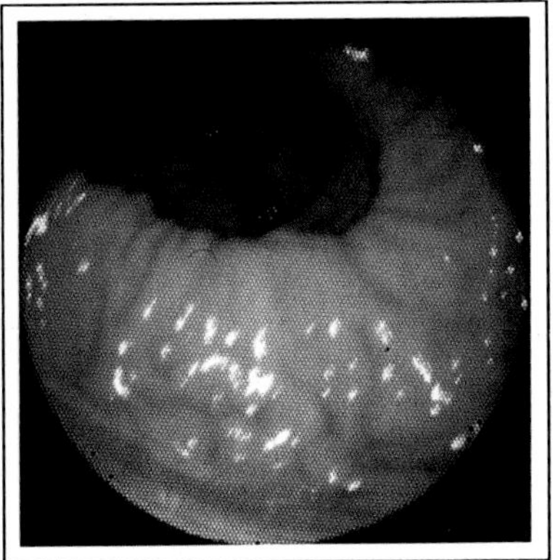

FIG. 13-6a.

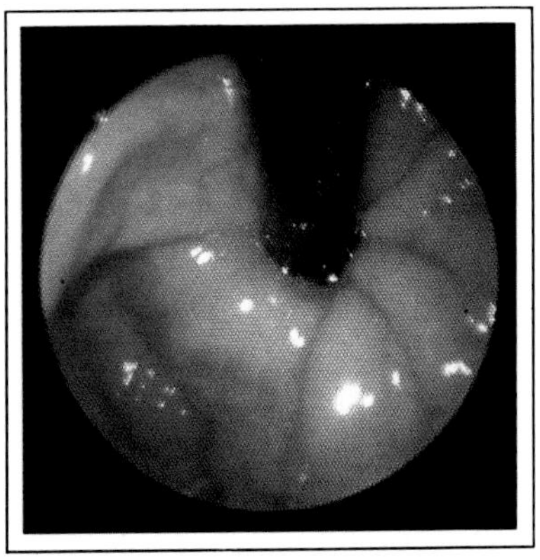

FIG. 13-6b.

FIG. 13-6. a: Large (6 cm) hiatal hernia (the same as in Fig. 13-5), retroflexed view. The junction of the gastric body and hernia are seen within the open cardia. **b:** Large (6 cm) hiatus hernia. The endoscope has been successfully maneuvered into the hernia and inspects the proximal portion.

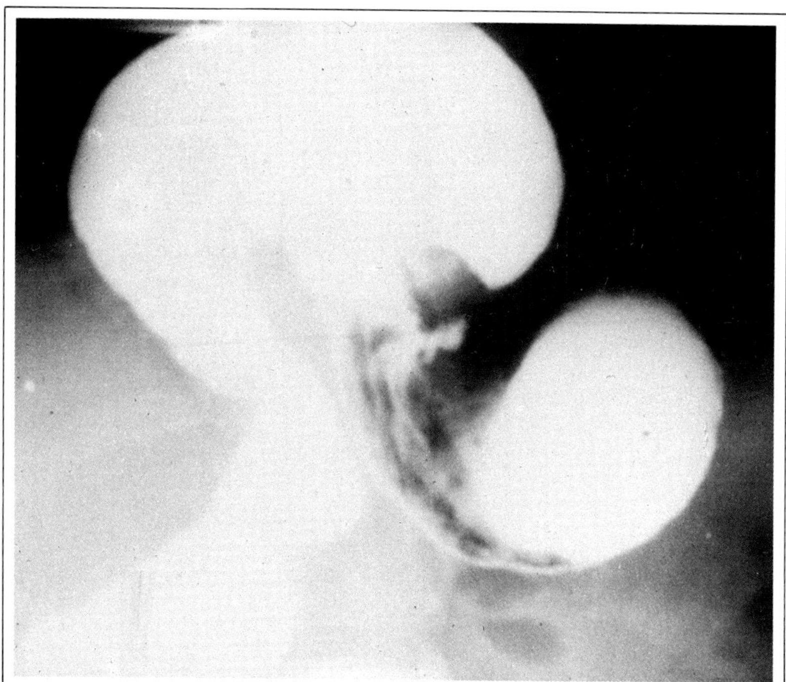

FIG. 13-7a.

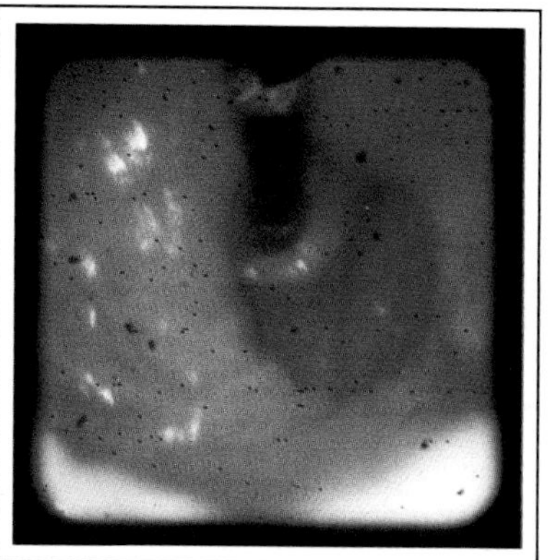

FIG. 13-7b.

FIG. 13-7. a: Large paraesophageal hiatus hernia with organoaxial rotation ("upside-down stomach"), radiographic appearance. The esophagus enters the cardiofundic area below the diaphragm, which is continuous with the body above. **b:** Endoscopic view of the entry point into the paraesophageal hernia seen in (a). The level of the diaphragm is indicated by the ring-like border of the open cardia, which is barely seen running from 7 o'clock to 5 o'clock. The ridge running from 6 o'clock to 11 o'clock is the greater curve, with the gastric body running off toward 9 o'clock. Within the true cardia (the ring-like opening through which the endoscope emerges), the junction point with the esophagus is also seen.

nations but in 1 to 2% of examinations of the antrum. The patients are asymptomatic or have nonspecific complaints that in no way suggest peptic ulcer disease. We regard the incisurae as congenital abnormalities rather than evidence of peptic ulcer disease.

Antral Mucosal Diaphragms (Webs)

Circumferential antral mucosal folds (Fig. 13-10) are found in 0.5%[10] of radiographic studies of the stomach in adults and, in our own experience, in the same percent of endoscopic examinations. Fifty percent are asymptomatic (Fig. 13-10) when the diameter of the mucosal diaphragm exceeds 13 mm. When the narrowing is less than 10 mm, and especially less than 5 mm, symptoms of gastric outlet obstruction are found.[10] In these cases, the antral web may simulate the pyloric channel (as a "pseudopylorus"), causing the endoscopist to mistake the antral portion distal to the web for the duodenal bulb, resulting in a failure to identify the web.[10a]

Most webs are probably congenital[10,12] although some are undoubtedly acquired as a scar deformity from peptic ulcer disease.[10a] In still others, the web may be congenital but predispose to peptic ulcer disease.[11] Ultimately it may be impossible to tell with certainty if the web is congenital or acquired.[12] Furthermore, differentiation of a web from true ulcer scar deformity can be elusive, although, in general, an ulcer scar deformity (see Chapter 17) tends to be thicker (Fig. 13-11) with folds in excess of 3 mm which converge at acute angles with a central depression (often containing an ulcer) while an antral web appears as a continuous, thin (<3 mm) fold or parallel series of such folds running circumferentially (Fig. 13-10).[12] Only in cases where the endoscopist felt secure in the diagnosis of a congenital web, would he attempt endoscopic electrosurgical incision[12a] in symptomatic cases as an alternative to surgery.

GASTRIC DIVERTICULA

Gastric diverticula are rarely encountered in endoscopic practice, occurring on the order of one per 1,000 examinations in our experience. Others have reported an even lower incidence in radiographic and autopsy studies.[13] Although diverticula may be acquired, most are thought to

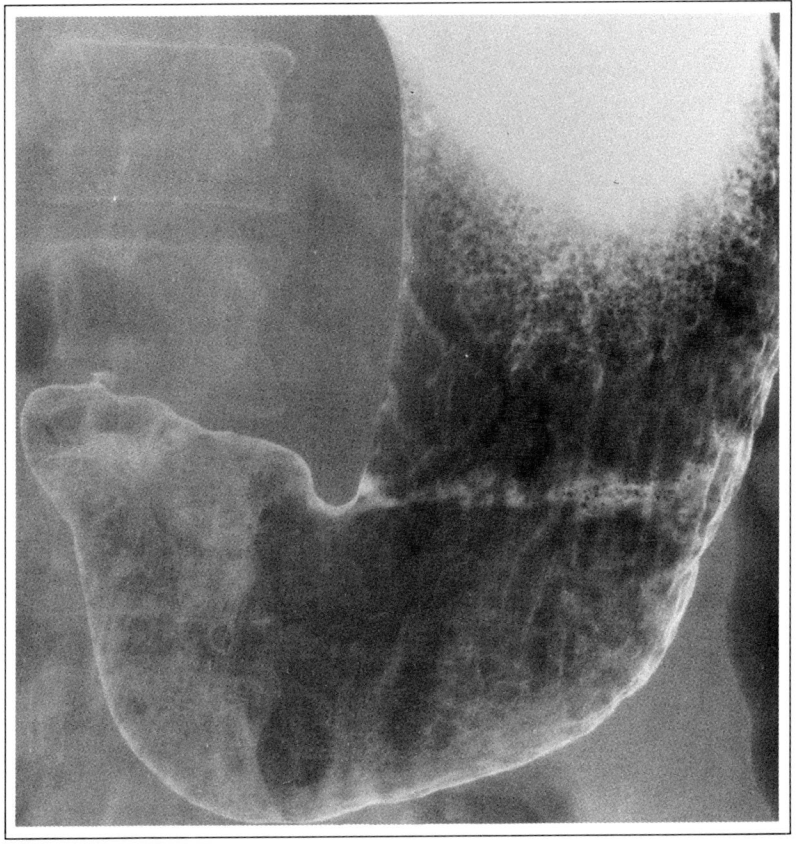

FIG. 13-8a.

FIG. 13-8b.

FIG. 13-8. a: Incisura of the body. A transverse mucosal fold is seen radiographically cutting across the lower body. **b:** At endoscopy, a fixed transverse fold of the greater curve was observed to correspond to that noted radiographically in (a).

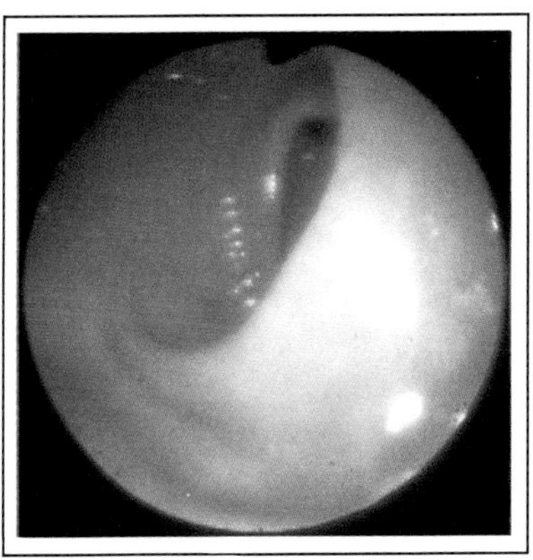

FIG. 13-9.

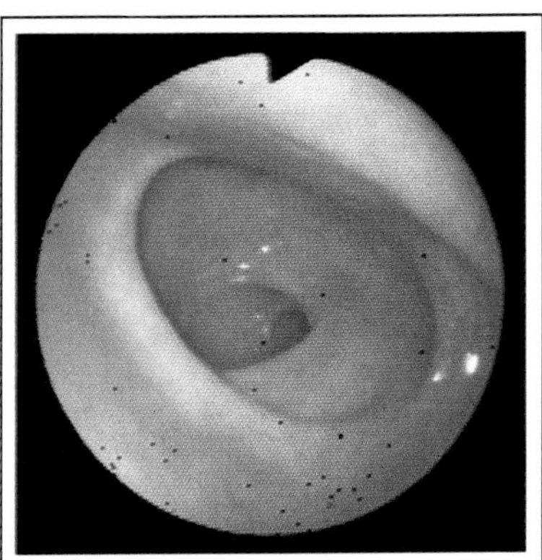

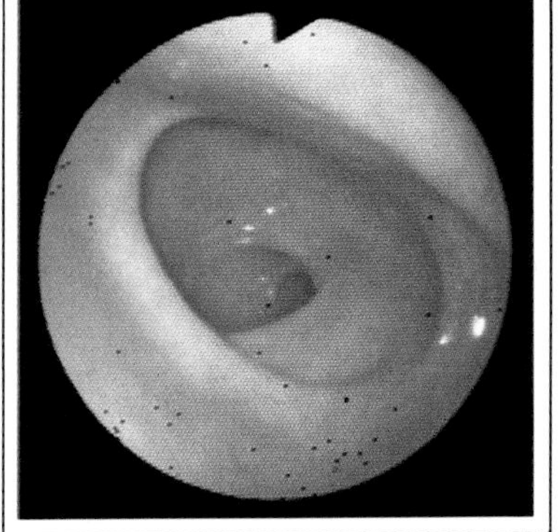

FIG. 13-10.

FIG. 13-9. Antral incisura. A single fixed mucosal fold of the posterior wall of the mid-antrum.

FIG. 13-10. Antral mucosal diaphragm (web). A circumferential mucosal (3 mm) fold is seen in the prepyloric antrum in an asymptomatic patient examined because of anemia.

FIG. 13-11.

FIG. 13-12.

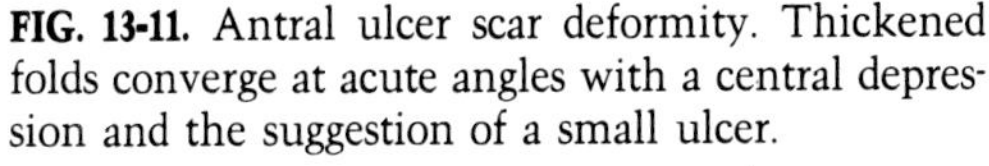

FIG. 13-11. Antral ulcer scar deformity. Thickened folds converge at acute angles with a central depression and the suggestion of a small ulcer.

FIG. 13-12. Gastric diverticulum. This 2-cm opening was noted on the posterior wall of the body just below the cardia.

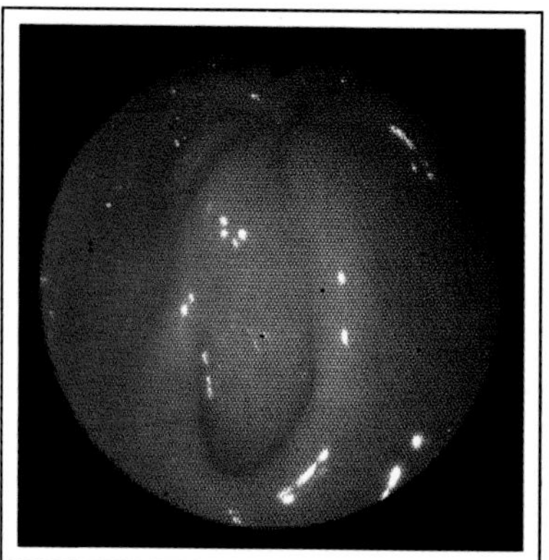

FIG. 13-13.

FIG. 13-13. Gastric diverticulum, incomplete. Two prepyloric folds are joined by a transverse fold (at 6 o'clock), creating a pouch-like deformity, possibly representing an incomplete diverticulum.

be congenital. They contain all the usual layers of the gastric wall and are almost always observed within 5 cm of the GE junction on the posterior wall of the upper body or fundus (Fig. 13-12). The mouth of the diverticulum is often observed as a 1-cm or smaller opening to which rugal folds may radiate (Fig. 13-12). The folds are generally absent within the diverticulum. Usually, one does not wish to enter the diverticulum because of the possibility of endoscopic perforation.

In addition to large diverticula of all layers of the gastric wall, small intramucosal ("incomplete") diverticula may be noted (Fig. 13-13).

Most often, gastric diverticula are incidental findings in patients who are examined because of nonspecific complaints or anemia. Infrequently, as in one reported case, they may be associated with symptoms which can be reproduced by probing in diverticulum with a biopsy forceps and which disappear following its resection.[13a] Another rare manifestation is that of hemorrhage from the diverticulum.[14]

REFERENCES

1. Martin, T. R., Vennes, J. A., Silvis, S. E., and Ansel, H. J. (1980): A comparison of upper gastrointestinal endoscopy and radiography. *J. Clin. Gastroenterol.*, 2:21–25.
2. McGinn, F. P., Guyer, P. B., Wilken, B. J., and Steer, H. W. (1975): A prospective comparative trial between early endoscopy and radiology in acute upper gastrointestinal hemorrhage. *Gut*, 16:707–713.

2a. Palmer, E. D. (1968): The hiatus hernia–esophagitis-esophageal stricture complex. Twenty-year prospective study. *Am. J. Med.*, 44:566–579.

3. Wright, R. A., and Hurwitz, A. L. (1979): Relation of hiatus hernia to endoscopically proven reflux esophagitis. *Dig. Dis. Sci.*, 24:311–313.

3a. Johnson, L. F., DeMeester, T. R., and Haggitt, R. C. (1978): Esophageal epithelial response to gastroesophageal reflux, a quantitative study. *Am. J. Dig. Dis.*, 23:498–509.

4. Smith, V. M. (1978): Association of aspirin ingestion with symptomatic esophageal hiatus hernia. *South. Med. J. (Suppl. 1)*, 71:45–47.
5. Mayer, D. A., Gray, G. F., Teixidor, H. S., and Thorbjarnarson, B. (1976): Carcinoma of the gastric cardia and hiatal hernia. *J. Thorac. Cardiovasc. Surg.*, 71:592–598.
6. Cameron, A. J. (1976): Incidence of iron deficiency anemia in patients with large diaphragmatic hernia: a controlled study. *Mayo Clin. Proc.*, 51:767–769.
7. Groarke, J. F., and Hirschowitz, B. I. (1977): An upside-down view of an upside-down organ. *Gastrointest. Endosc.*, 24:30–31.
8. Culver, B. T., Pirson, H. S., and Bean, B. C. (1962): Mechanics of obstruction in paraesophageal diaphragmatic hernias. *JAMA*, 181:933–938.
9. Carter, R., Brewer, L. A., and Hinshaw, D. B. (1980): Acute gastric volvulus: a study of 25 cases. *Am. J. Surg.*, 140:99–105.
10. Clements, J. L., Jinkins, J. R., Torres, W. E., Thomas, B. M., Thomas, J., Elmber, R. A., and Weens, H. S. (1979): Antral mucosal diaphragms in adults. *Am. J. Roentgenol.*, 133:1105–1111.

10a. Higgins, M. J., Friedman, A. C., Lichtenstein, J. E., and Bova, J. G. (1982): Adult acquired antral web. *Dig. Dis. Sci.*, 27:80–83.

11. Ghahremani, G. G. (1974): Non-obstructive diaphragms or rings of the gastric antrum in adults. *Am. J. Roentgenol.*, 121:236–247.
12. Feliciano, D. V., and van Heerdon, J. A. (1977): Pyloric antral mucosal webs. *Mayo Clin. Proc.*, 52:650–653.

12a. Brandt, L. J., Boley, S. J., Daum, F., and Kleinhaus, S. (1978): Endoscopic resection of an obstructing antral web in an infant. *Am. J. Dig. Dis.*, 23(May Suppl.):6S–8S.

13. Meeroff, M., Gallan, J. R., and Mecroff, J. C. (1967): Gastric diverticulum. *Am. J. Gastroenterol.*, 47:189–203.

13a. Anaise, D., Brand, D. C., Smith, N. L., and Soroff, H. S. (1983): Pitfalls in the diagnosis and treatment of a symptomatic gastric diverticulum. *Gastrointest. Endosc.*, 29:(*in press*).

14. Graham, D. Y., Kimbrough, R. C., and Fagan, T. (1974): Congenital gastric diverticulum as a cause of massive hemorrhage. *Am. J. Dig. Dis.*, 19:174–178.

14

GENERALIZED GASTRIC MUCOSAL ABNORMALITIES

A generalized gastric abnormality such as hemorrhagic gastritis is well known to the endoscopist from his experience with patients examined because of upper gastrointestinal bleeding where this type of lesion may account for up to 30% of the cases (see Chapter 36). Less well appreciated is the frequency with which the endoscopist finds generalized mucosal abnormalities in examinations of the stomach for reasons apart from bleeding where this type of appearance may be found in 10 to 15%, making this group of conditions one of the most frequently encountered. Yet all of the conditions making up this group are different, each with its own particular appearance and clinical relevance. Three types are discussed in this chapter: (a) nonspecific (chronic) gastritis; (b) drug-related chronic mucosal abnormalities; and (c) mucosal abnormalities in several frequently encountered disease states.

NONSPECIFIC (CHRONIC) GASTRITIS

At endoscopy the examiner can recognize one of four types of chronic gastritis: (a) superficial; (b) atrophic; (c) hypertrophic (including Menétrièr's disease); and (d) a newly recognized type, chronic erosive (varioliform) gastritis.

Superficial Gastritis

Superficial gastritis is the commonest type of chronic gastritis, recognized by us in 4 to 5% of gastric examinations and in up to 16% by others.[1] In cases where superficial gastritis is confirmed histologically, the endoscopist often notes diffuse gastric erythema of the body and antrum as the principal finding. When observed exclusively in the antrum, this is referred to as "antral gastritis." In either case, the erythema, when viewed at close range, is seen to consist of tiny, raised dots of reddened mucosa (Fig. 14-1). Even in cases where there is a superficial gastritis histologically (as with mucin depletion, capillary dilatation, and an inflammatory infiltrate), we regard this finding as having an uncertain clinical significance and caution against attributing to it any symptoms or other clinical findings, e.g., anemia or occult blood in the stool (see Chapter 12).

Atrophic Gastritis

In 1 to 2% of our examinations we make an endoscopic diagnosis of atrophic gastritis, based on the appearance of submucosal vessels (giving rise to a mucosal vascular pattern similar to that found in the colon—see Chapter 39). When this is noted diffusely in the fundus and body (Fig. 14-2), the examiner may expect biopsies to show atrophic gastritis (or gastric atrophy) in upward of 75% of cases; however, when this appearance is confined to either the fundus, body, or antrum, normal histology is most often observed.[2] Endoscopically, one cannot differentiate between cases which on biopsy show atrophy (with a decrease in the number of glands, absent parietal and chief cells, and intestinal metaplasia) and those which indicate atrophic gastritis (an inflammatory component in addition to minimal atrophy). However, this is of less importance than the detection of atrophy itself, which seems to place the patient at increased risk for gastric cancer (see below).[3]

The 1 to 2% of patients having atrophic gastritis suggested by the appearance of submucosal vessels is low in comparison to its true prevalence, which for patients coming to endoscopy probably approaches 10%.[3a] Unfortunately, the detection of atrophic gastritis is not enhanced by the use of other features, e.g., mucosal discoloration, smoothness, or flattened rugal folds, which although they may be seen in patients with atrophic gastritis, are entirely nonspecific.

In patients with atrophic gastritis one often finds multiple

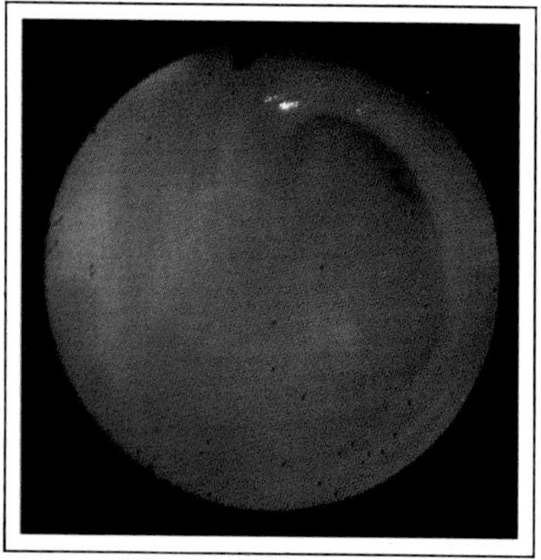

FIG. 14-1a.

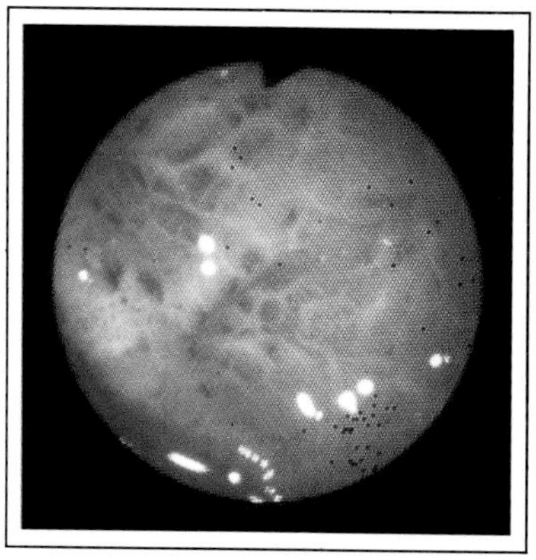

FIG. 14-1b.

FIG. 14-1. Nonspecific gastric erythema (superficial gastritis). The diffuse mucosal erythema (**a**) when viewed at close range (**b**) is actually seen to consist of tiny raised dots of erythema which we believe are the areae gastricae with intervening pale linear zones, the lineae gastricae. Biopsies were interpreted as showing superficial gastritis; nevertheless, the appearance was regarded as having an uncertain relationship to the patient's history of epigastric pain, nausea, and vomiting.

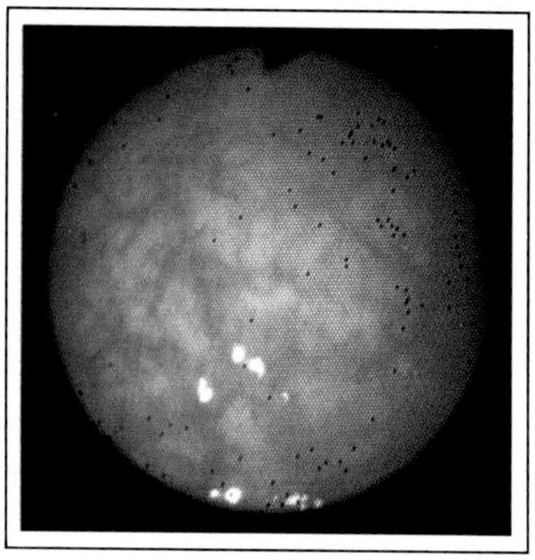

FIG. 14-2a.

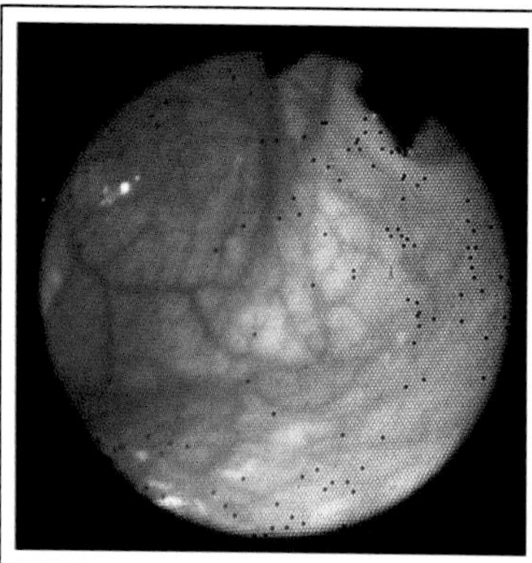

FIG. 14-2b.

FIG. 14-2. Atrophic gastritis. Prominent submucosal capillaries are present in the body (**a**) as well as in the fundus (**b**). The diagnosis of atrophic gastritis was confirmed histologically in this patient with a diffuse submucosal vascular pattern.

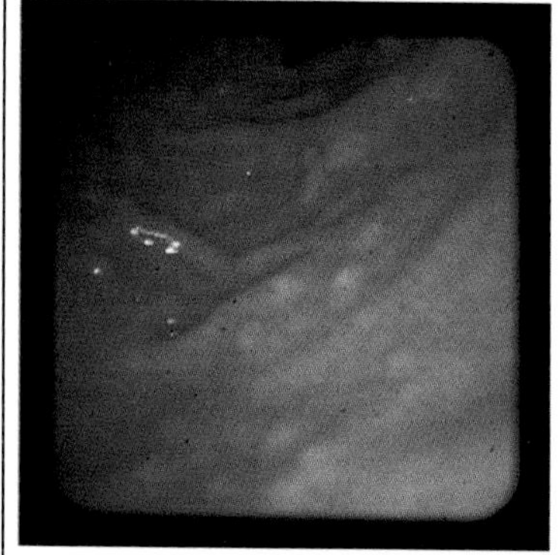

FIG. 14-3a.

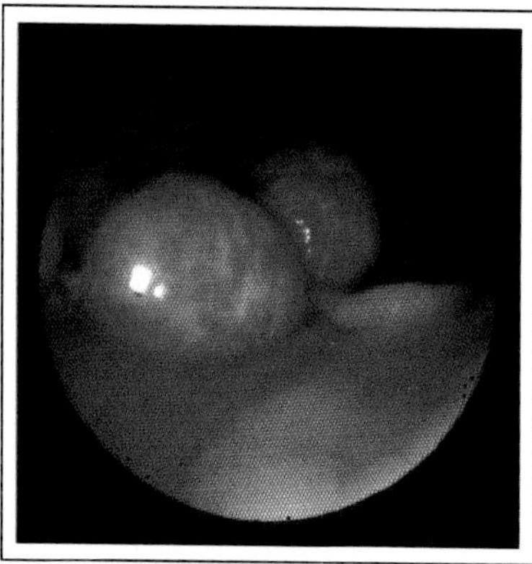

FIG. 14-3b.

FIG. 14-3. a: Atrophic gastritis with tiny (regenerative) hyperplastic polyps. **b:** Atrophic gastritis with large hyperplastic polyps in a patient with known pernicious anemia.

1- to 3-mm mucosal excrescences which are tiny hyperplastic polyps (Fig. 14-3a) (see Chapter 17). Occasionally, larger solitary or multiple polyps are encountered which are usually hyperplastic[3] (Fig. 14-3b).[4]

The symptoms prompting endoscopy in patients with atrophic gastritis are for the most part nonspecific, and one would think that they would be entirely unrelated to the finding of atrophic gastritis. Recently, however, delayed gastric emptying, especially of solids, was found in patients with either atrophic gastritis alone or in association with pernicious anemia; this is in contrast to normal controls and suggests an interrelationship between the mucosal state and antral motor function which could be clinically significant.[5] The importance of atrophic gastritis (gastric atrophy), however, lies not in its relation to symptoms but in its relation to the risk of gastric cancer, which has been found to be about 10% for patients followed for more than 10 years after a histologic diagnosis has been made of atrophic gastritis with intestinal metaplasia.[3] As the yearly rate of cancer appears to be less than 0.5%,[6] it is not surprising that no general consensus has emerged regarding follow-up for these patients. We nonetheless are impressed with a 2% rate of carcinoma (early) and 6% rate of severe dysplasia (cytologic changes suggesting neoplastic transformation of glandular epithelium to, or just short of, cancer *in situ*) found in a British series when endoscopy was performed in 50 asymptomatic patients with atrophic gastritis and pernicious anemia.[7] This is potentially as high a rate of cancer detection as in patients having had gastric resection performed 15 to 20 years previously who are now routinely screened in many parts of the world because of the cancer risk of this condition (see Chapter 19). Our policy, therefore, has been to recommend endoscopic surveillance for patients with atrophic gastritis, particularly those with pernicious anemia or a strong family history of cancer. If multiple (5 to 10) biopsies show no dysplasia, endoscopy would be repeated in 2 years. If mild or moderate dysplasia (epithelial cell changes suggestive only of neoplastic transformation but far short of cancer *in situ*) is present without any suspicious macroscopic appearance, we would examine the patient within a year. For severe dysplasia, particularly if found with a macroscopic lesion suggestive of early gastric cancer (see Chapter 16), we advise surgery.

Hypertrophic Gastritis, Hypertrophic Gastropathy, and Menétrièr's Disease

Hypertrophic Gastritis

Some continue to apply the older term[8] "hypertrophic gastritis" to large rugal folds exceeding 1 cm height, although, as recognized by Palmer[9] more than 25 years ago, biopsies show either a completely normal histology or nonspecific acute and chronic inflammation. Even the deeper large-particle snare biopsy technique in these patients only occasionally shows a histologic picture other than nonspecific inflammation.[10] Because of the absence of specific histology for this appearance, we do not use a histologic term but simply refer to rugal folds greater than 1 cm in height as "large rugal folds" (see Chapter 12).

Hypertrophic Gastropathy

The term "hypertrophic gastropathy" has been used to designate both large rugal folds[11] and another appearance—that of a diffuse, nodular texture of the antrum. Another term used for this is "état mamelonné." We believe that the individual 1- to 3-mm nodules represent prominent areae gastricae. Although at one time this appearance was thought to be highly suggestive of hypertrophic gastritis, biopsies are most often found to be entirely normal.[9,12]

Menétrièr's Disease

Menétrièr's disease is an extremely rare condition. We encountered only one case among 5,000 examinations performed over a 7-year period, although Davis et al. reported six cases encountered over a 10-year period.[13] The histologic hallmark for Menétrièr's disease is mucosal hyperplasia (rather than hypertrophy), especially of mucus-producing cells, leading to cystic dilatation of the gastric glands.[14] The resulting endoscopic appearance is that of highly convoluted, intensely erythematous beefy red folds of the body, fundus, and occasionally the antrum (Fig. 14-4b).

The patient with Menétrièr's disease commonly presents with upper abdominal pain and discomfort, coupled with profound hypoproteinemia and gastric hyposecretion,[13] where the diagnosis is strongly suspected once radiologic examination and/or endoscopy shows giant polypoid folds of the body. While forceps biopsies performed at endoscopy often fail to show the characteristic cystic dilatation of the glands sufficient to establish a histologic diagnosis,[14] the clinical picture may be otherwise so suggestive as to make histologic confirmation seem superfluous. However, infiltrating gastric malignancy may have a similar endoscopic appearance (see Chapter 16), so in cases where the diagnosis is clinically uncertain, especially where weight loss is profound, large-particle snare biopsy is indicated.[10] In some cases, surgery may be necessary for full-thickness biopsy to exclude cancer, especially in the presence of weight loss.

Chronic Erosive (Varioliform) Gastritis

Recent reports from several centers[15–18] in both Europe[15–17] and the United States[18] have identified a distinctive endoscopic appearance of discrete 5- to 10-mm nodules with central erosions (Fig. 14-5b). There are no specific symptoms. Patients with this finding undergo endoscopy because of upper abdominal pain, anorexia, nausea, and weight loss lasting 1 to 3 months[15] and recurring at 3-month to 3-year intervals[15] or being persistent.[16] In some cases the patient is entirely asymptomatic, with endoscopy being performed because of anemia or occult blood in the stool.

The etiology of the condition is unknown. The finding of increased numbers of immunoglobulin E (IgE) cells in biopsies taken from these lesions, the presence of significant allergy histories and elevated serum IgE levels in half of one group studied by Lambert et al.,[15] and the response to sodium cromoglycate[17] suggest an allergic basis. Because of the similarity in symptoms and the response to antacid treatment, some investigators have suggested that this condition may be part of the clinical spectrum of peptic ulcer disease.[18]

The endoscopic appearance is that of prominent gastric folds (5 to 10 mm), most commonly in the fundus, body, and antrum together[15] but also involving the antrum alone.[15,16,18] Characteristically, there is a discrete nodular bulge to the fold, with an erosion in the center. These erosions have been called "aphthoid" if covered by a thin whitish exudate, "active" if this appears as a white or brown crater surrounded by a red halo, or "healed" if only a depression is seen.[15] Biopsies taken from these lesions show a mixed type of inflammatory infiltrate with a relative preponderance of plasma cells, along with lymphocytes, eosinophils, and polymorphonuclear leukocytes.[18]

Both symptoms and endoscopic appearance improve over time.[15,17,18] Whether treatment with prednisolone,[16] cromoglycate,[17] or antacids[18] measurably affects the course remains to be determined.

DRUG-INDUCED MUCOSAL ABNORMALITIES

Patients ingesting drugs capable of producing mucosal injury may be referred to endoscopy for reasons other than acute gastrointestinal hemorrhage. It may be for unexplained anemia, occult blood in the stools, or ulcer-type symptoms. Other patients may be referred for nonspecific complaints. In this section we consider the chronic effects that can be found in patients without acute gastrointestinal hemorrhage. The reader is referred elsewhere in the book (see Chapter 36) for a discussion of the appearances found in association with drug-induced gastric bleeding.

Aspirin

Aspirin is the most common cause of drug-induced chronic mucosal injury. Injury may begin within hours of ingesting the first dose[19] and continues even after the aspirin is stopped. Even small amounts of aspirin in a susceptible individual are capable of producing injury, the pathogenesis of which is considered elsewhere (see Chapter 36). Studies by Baskin et al.[19] indicate that 600 mg given alone produces histologic evidence of gastric injury within 2 hr in approximately 20% of patients. In the presence of 10 mEq HCl, this increases to 50%. Endoscopic evidence of mucosal injury as erosions (see below) may be present after ingestion of only 2.6 g aspirin over 24 hr.[20] Furthermore, we have seen significant aspirin injury, including deep ulcerations, in patients who ingest relatively small amounts—even only two or three aspirin tablets (325 mg) per day. In most cases, however, six to eight tablets or more are being consumed.

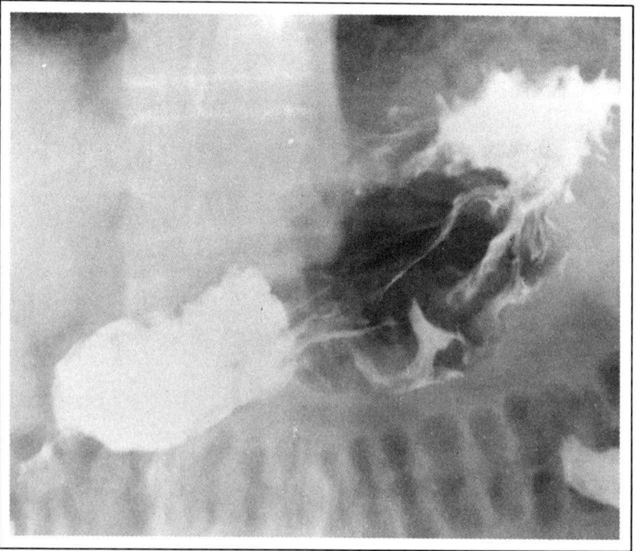

FIG. 14-4a.

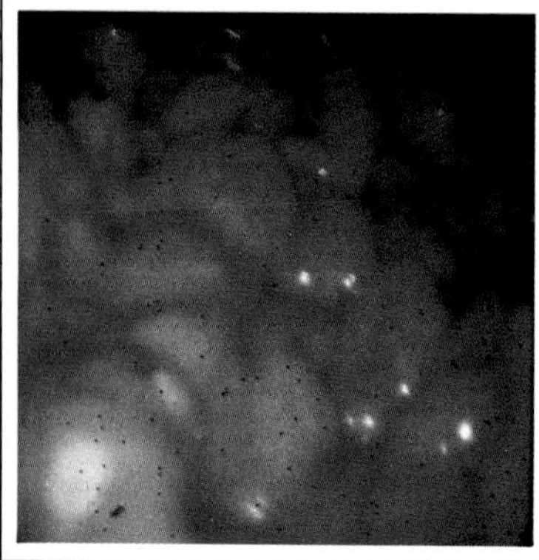

FIG. 14-4b.

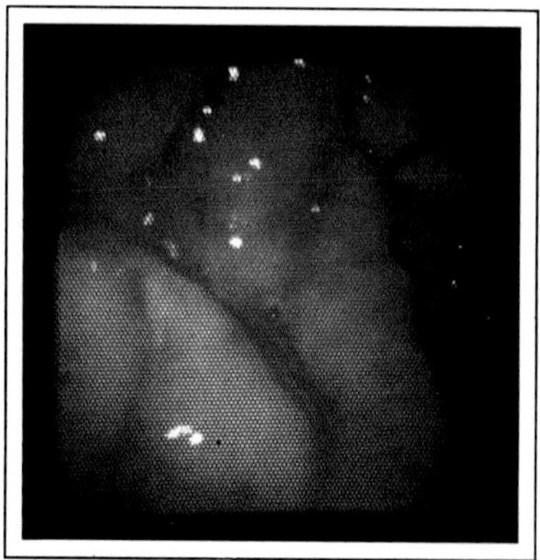

FIG. 14-4c.

FIG. 14-4. a: Hypertrophic gastritis. Giant rugal folds (width >1.5 cm) were noted on a radiographic examination of the stomach. **b:** Hypertrophic gastritis. Large folds (>1.0 cm) were observed in the upper body and were thought to represent hypertrophic gastritis, but forceps biopsies showed only acute gastritis. A large-particle biopsy was refused. **c:** Menétrièr's disease. The giant rugal folds (≥1.5 cm) were indistinguishable from those of hypertrophic gastritis (a). Forceps biopsy in this patient presenting with anemia, hypoproteinemia, and gastrointestinal bleeding showed diffuse hyperplasia of the surface foveolar mucous cells, highly suggestive of Menétrièr's disease.

Location

At endoscopy, aspirin-induced mucosal injury is most often seen in the lower body, gastric angle, and antrum, especially in the prepyloric antral region (Fig. 14-6).

This contrasts with acute aspirin mucosal injury, which commonly involves both proximal (body and fundus) and antral areas.[21] The explanation for the distal predominance in chronic aspirin injury is unknown, especially if the more frequent exposure of antral mucosa to higher concentrations of bile salts known to potentiate aspirin injury plays a role. Of interest in this regard was a study of rats in which aspirin ulceration produced by 250 mg/kg (equivalent to 60 aspirin tablets ingested by a 70-kg man) could be entirely prevented by bile duct pyloric channel ligation.[22]

Appearance

Aspirin-induced mucosal injury characteristically consists of multiple small (≤5 mm), white (fibrin)-based, ulcer-like lesions[23] (Fig. 14-6). They are called erosions when the lesion lacks depth[23] (Fig. 14-7a), i.e., appears two-dimensional, and are called ulcerations when the lesion is depressed, sharply circumscribed, and three-dimensional[18] (Fig. 14-7b). A third type of erosion occurs in the form of a white, fibrinous exudate (Fig. 14-7c). In addition to the white-based erosions or ulcerations, there is focal erythema, either as a rim around the white-based lesion (Fig. 14-7) or, as the commonest injury phenomenon of all, small circumscribed zones of hyperemia (Fig. 14-8). Between these lesions, the mucosa appears normal.

The finding of white-based erosions within the distal stomach, especially in the face of ulcer symptoms, might cause the endoscopist to view them as an ulcer equivalent[22a] and recommend standard ulcer treatment. We believe the finding of multiple antral erosions should first raise in the examiner's mind the possibility of aspirin or other nonsteroidal analgesic usage (see below). Following an examination in which an appearance suggestive of aspirin injury was observed, the patient should be questioned closely about specific aspirin-containing products. As patients frequently do not know the aspirin content of many products sold over the counter, we routinely run through a list of 15 commonly used aspirin-containing products (Table 14-1).

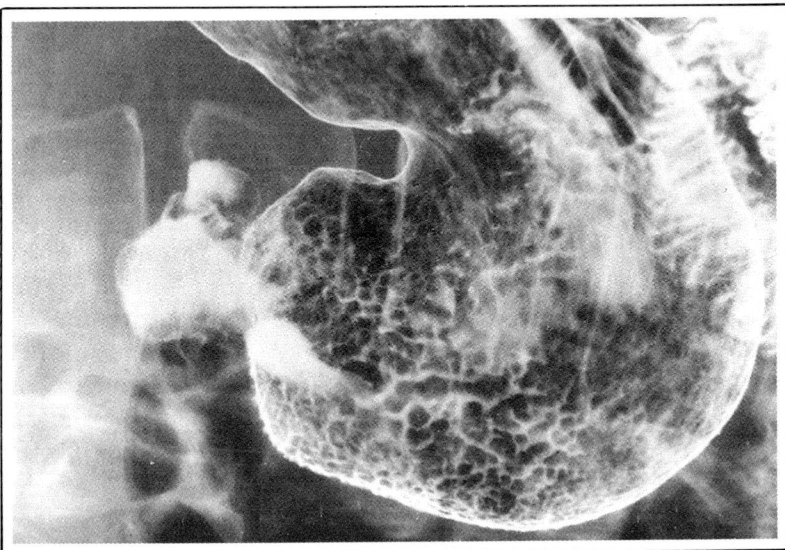

FIG. 14-5a.

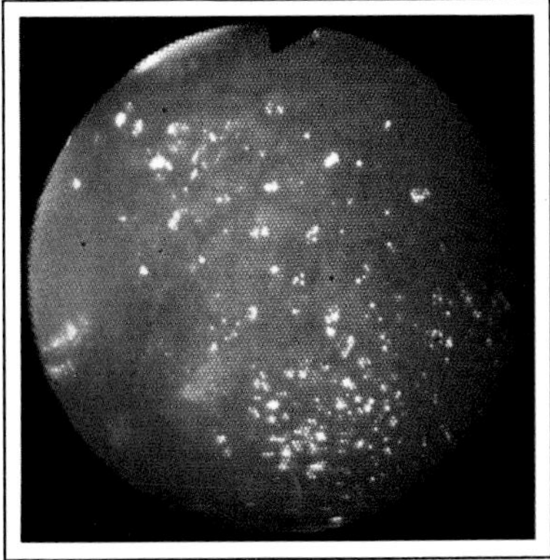

FIG. 14-5b.

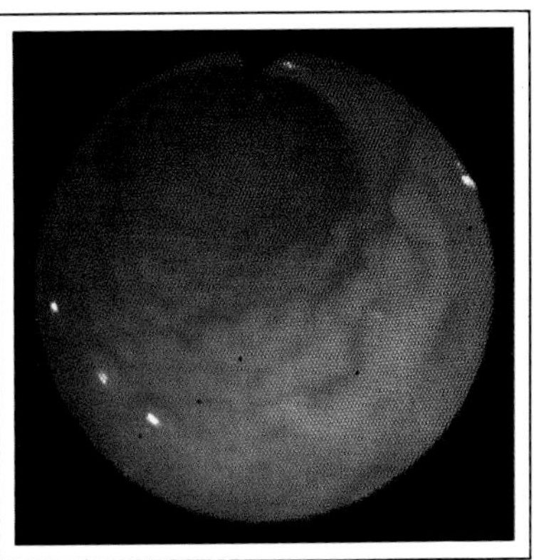

FIG. 14-5c.

FIG. 14-5. a: Hypertrophic gastropathy (état mamelonné). A double-contrast radiographic study of the antrum shows a finely nodular pattern, corresponding to the areae gastricae. **b:** Hypertrophic gastropathy (état mamelonné). Endoscopic view of the antrum shows the granular appearance resulting from the highlighting of prominent, raised areae gastricae. Forceps biopsy showed completely normal antral mucosa. **c:** Chronic erosive (varioliform) gastritis. Multiple 5- to 10-mm nodules were found throughout the lower body and antrum on the greater curve in an asymptomatic patient examined because of anemia. Biopsies showed evidence of acute and chronic inflammation with plasma cells, lymphocytes, eosinophils, and polymorphonuclear leukocytes. Despite the persistence of these nodules over a 2-year period, the patient remains asymptomatic.

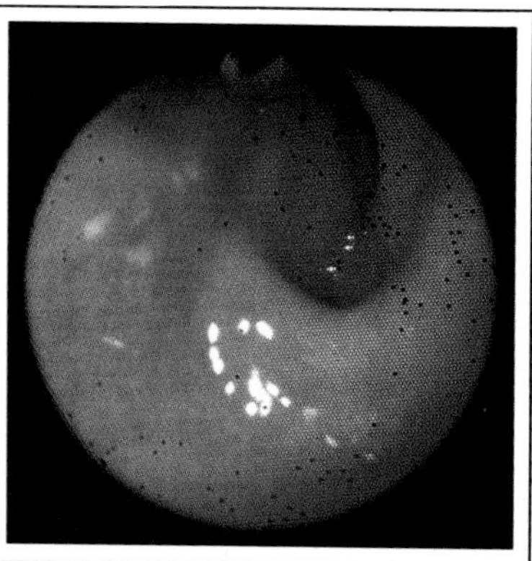

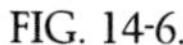

FIG. 14-6.

FIG. 14-6. Aspirin erosions. Several white (fibrin)-based 2- to 3-mm lesions are seen within an erythematous area on the anterior wall of the prepyloric antrum.

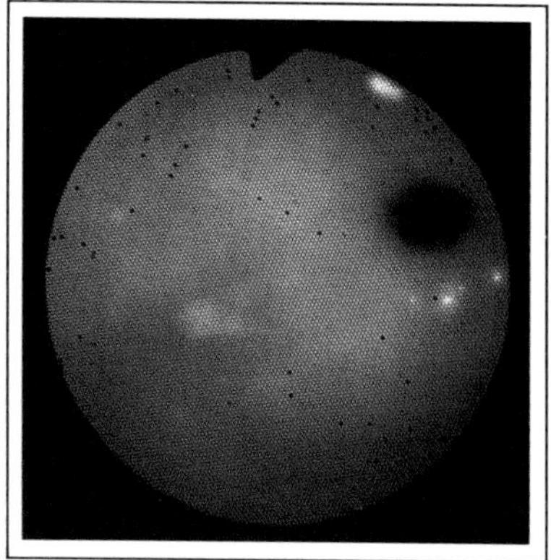

FIG. 14-7a.

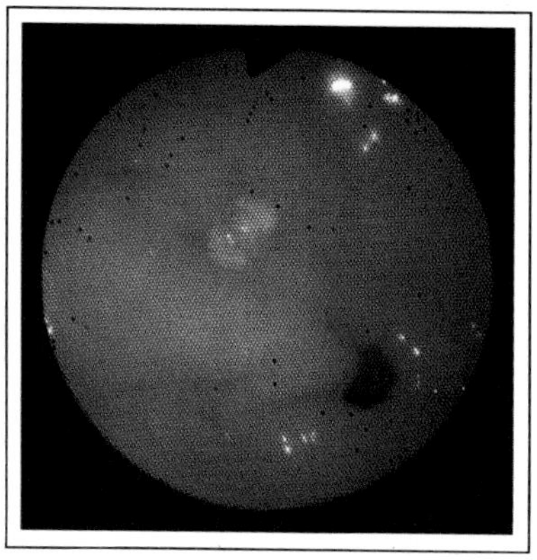

FIG. 14-7b.

FIG. 14-7. a: Aspirin erosions. The 2-mm white (fibrin)-based lesion has no apparent depth (two-dimensional), suggesting it to be mucosal–hence the term erosion. **b:** Aspirin ulceration. The 3-mm white (fibrin)-based lesion is circumscribed with apparent depth (three-dimensional), indicating submucosal penetration—hence the term ulceration. **c:** Aspirin exudate. The 3-mm white (fibrin)-based lesion is situated slightly higher than the surrounding mucosa, suggesting an (acute) inflammatory exudate.

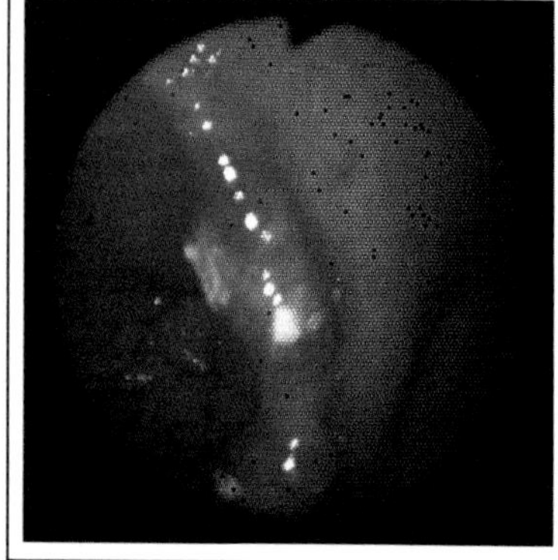

FIG. 14-7c.

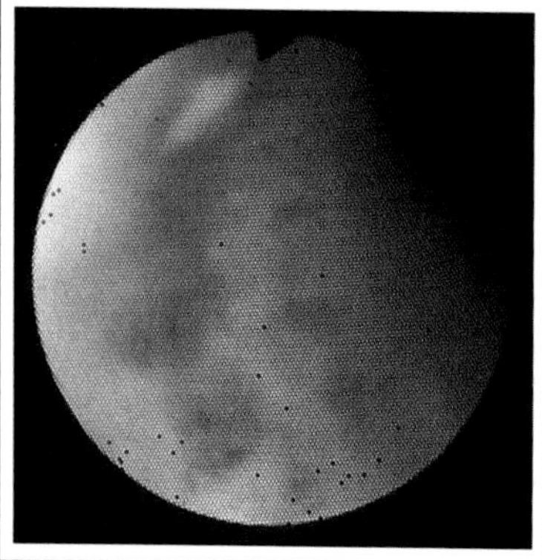

FIG. 14-8.

FIG. 14-8. Aspirin mucosal injury, erythema. No white-based lesions are present, only focal erythema of the prepyloric antrum in an asymptomatic patient on 3.6 g of aspirin endoscoped because of anemia.

The endoscopist thus has a rare opportunity to provide lasting clinical benefit to the patient by informing him of the aspirin content and toxic effect of a product which he may not even suspect is responsible for his symptoms. Discontinuing its use may be all the treatment the patient will need.

Other Nonsteroidal Anti-inflammatory Agents

Drugs such as Indocin (indomethacin),[24] Motrin (ibuprofen),[24] and other newer nonsteroidal agents[24] (Table 14-2) produce toxic effects on gastric mucosa which at endoscopy are indistinguishable from those of aspirin.[24,25] Characteristically, these are multiple, white-based erosions (Fig. 14-9) with focal hyperemia (Fig. 14-10) of the distal stomach.

The nonsteroidal agents vary in terms of their potential for producing injury. Indocin (indomethacin 150 mg/day)[26] and Naprosyn (naproxen 750 mg/day)[26] have the greatest injury potential, and Motrin (ibuprofen 1,600 mg/day),[25] Clinoril (sulindac 350 mg/day),[24] and Dolobid (diflunisal 750 mg/day)[24] the least.

Like aspirin, any of the nonsteroidal anti-inflammatory agents are occasionally associated with large gastric ulcers (see Chapter 15), especially, we find, in patients who continue to take these drugs even with ulcer symptoms because

TABLE 14-1. *Commonly used aspirin-containing products*

Product	Manufacturer
Alka-Seltzer	Miles
Anacin	Whitehall
Ascriptin	Rorer
Aspirin (USP)	Various manufacturers
Bayer Aspirin	Glenbrook
Bufferin	Bristol-Myers
Coricidin	Schering
Darvon Compound	Lilly
Dristan	Whitehall
Ecotrin	Smith Kline & French
Empirin	Burroughs Wellcome
Excedrin	Bristol-Myers
Fiorinal	Sandoz
Percodan	Endo
Sine-Off	Menley & James

From Leist and Banwell (1974): *N. Engl. J. Med.*, 291:710–712.

TABLE 14-2. *Commonly prescribed nonsteroidal anti-inflammatory agents listed in order of their gastrotoxicity*

Trade name	Generic name	Manufacturer
Indocin	Indomethacin	Merck Sharp & Dohme
Naprosyn	Naproxen	Syntex
Motrin	Ibuprofen	Upjohn
Tolectin	Tometin	McNeil
Clinoril	Sulindac	Merck Sharp & Dohme
Dolobid	Diflusinal	Merck Sharp & Dohme

Data from refs. 19, 24, and 26.

neither they nor their physicans are aware of the drug's ulcerogenic potential. As in the case of aspirin, we closely question patients with a suggestive endoscopic appearance as to whether they are using one of the commonly prescribed nonsteroidal agents (Table 14-2).

Corticosteroids

Data are currently lacking as to whether corticosteroids produce mucosal injury similar to that found with aspirin and nonsteroidal agents. Very often patients on steroids in whom ulceration occurs have a condition such as rheumatoid arthritis for which an increased predisposition to peptic ulcer disease may exist, in addition to their taking the aspirin or nonsteroidal agents concurrently with steroid[27]; hence the ulceration, if present, may actually result from any or all of these. That the ulcerogenic potential of corticosteroids alone is low was suggested in a recent study of 21 patients in whom corticosteroids were administered because of rheumatoid arthritis in which prior endoscopy showed no mucosal injury. In only three of the 21 patients did any mucosal injury phenomenon (erosion or ulcerations) develop, contrasted with 13 of 26 patients who developed lesions while taking aspirin.[24] Because of this, it seems prudent to closely question any patient on steroids with an appearance of generalized antral mucosal injury about the use of aspirin-containing products or other nonsteroidal agents which may have been prescribed in addition, rather than to assume the injury was due entirely to the steroids.

Although steroids may have a low potential for initiating injury, we believe they may affect an underlying peptic ulcer diathesis by causing a delay in the healing of a given ulcer. They would thereby increase the predisposition toward complications, e.g., bleeding or perforation.[28]

Potassium Chloride Supplements

Recently, the wax-matrix potassium chloride (KCl) preparation Slow-K has been shown capable of producing mucosal lesions (erosions and ulcerations) in normal volunteers similar to those caused by aspirin and other nonsteroidal analgesic agents.[29] Potentiating the injury effect was delayed gastric emptying brought about by the concurrent administration of a potent anticholinergic agent (glycopyrrolate). A similar injury effect was not observed when a microencapsulated KCl preparation, in which the potassium is widely dispersed in the stomach, was employed. The clinical significance of the observation is uncertain, but it seems prudent to question any patient with an aspirin-type mucosal injury appearance (see above) about the use of Slow-

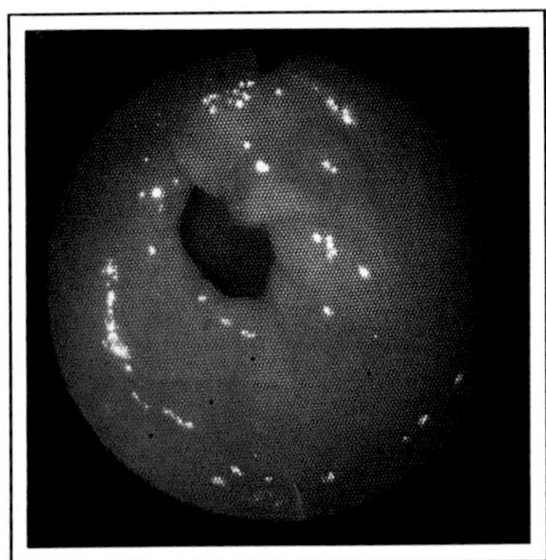

FIG. 14-9.

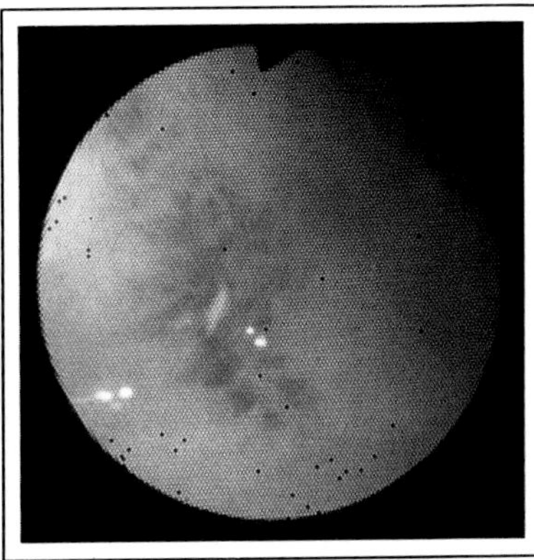

FIG. 14-10.

FIG. 14-9. Indocin (indomethacin) mucosal injury. Focal erosions are present that are similar to those in Fig. 14-6 produced by aspirin.

FIG. 14-10. Motrin (ibuprofen) mucosal injury. Focal erythema with an erosion similar to an aspirin injury (Fig. 14-7a).

K, especially in the face of antral scarring (see Chapter 18) or evidence of gastric retention.

Cancer Chemotherapeutic Agents

There is little evidence that most currently employed cancer chemotherapeutic agents administered either orally or intravenously cause gastric mucosal injury. Although some are capable of producing depressive effects on intestinal mucosal cell proliferation,[30] they cause little or no consistent injury to gastric mucosa. We have seen examples of focal hyperemia (Fig. 14-11) in critically ill patients receiving multiple cytotoxic agents but the potential effects of these agents and that of the "stress" of the underlying illness are difficult if not impossible to separate.

One definite injury which has been observed to be associated with chemotherapy is the extensive ulceration which has occurred with intra-arterial administration of 5-fluorouracil into the liver. In these cases ulceration has occurred when a percutaneously placed arterial catheter became displaced and was positioned in the left gastric or gastroduodenal artery, leading to extensive ulcerations within the distal stomach.[31] We have observed similar injuries in patients with a surgically implanted catheter still within the hepatic artery (Fig. 14-12). The cause of the ulceration in such cases is unknown.

MUCOSAL APPEARANCES ASSOCIATED WITH CIRRHOSIS, UREMIA, AND THROMBOCYTOPENIA

Endoscopy is often requested in hospitalized patients with significant underlying disorders, the commonest being cirrhosis, uremia, and thrombocytopenia. Most often this will be for acute gastrointestinal hemorrhage (see Chapter 37). Many patients, however, will have endoscopy performed because of chronic anemia, or other nonspecific complaints.

Cirrhosis

In patients with cirrhosis, especially accompanied by portal hypertension and thrombocytopenia (platelet count 60,000 to 100,000 cu mm), one may observe in the antrum linear zones of dot-like petechiae, along with 2 to 4 mm areas of focal erythema (Fig. 14-13), particularly on the ridges of mucosal folds. Spontaneous, as well as contact bleeding (mucosal friability), is frequently noted. This appearance should not be confused with that found on close inspection of nonspecific gastric erythema (Fig. 14-1b) where the slightly raised, reddened areas (areae gastricae) are separated by only thin, pale linear zones (lineae gastricae). By contrast, the linear zones of petechiae and focal erythema associated with cirrhosis may be widely separated from each other (Fig. 14-13), 5 mm or more, by larger spaces in between antral folds. In addition, careful inspection of the petechiae will show some to have a brownish discoloration, suggestive of old blood from prior, recent bleeding.

Although studies are unavailable, one imagines daily bleeding would occur from the lesions in amounts comparable to that reported for gastric angiodysplasia of the antral type (see Chapter 37) having a similar appearance which may present as a chronic iron deficiency anemia, requiring repeated transfusions.[31a]

The pathogenesis of the antral petechiae and focal erythema in these cases is almost certainly multifactorial. Thrombocytopenia itself may be associated with a similar appearance (see below), but only at lower levels (platelet counts ≤30,000). It may be, however, that any thrombocytopenia present promotes bleeding from a mucosal vascular abnormality associated with portal hypertension. In this regard, discrete zones of focally raised erythema have been observed in patients with cirrhosis with portal hypertension and chronic gastrointestinal blood loss. An intriguing suggestion for the origin of this focal erythema is that it is the result of capillary dilatation from the presence of intramucosal vascular shunts as a response to portal hypertension.[32,33] Finally, because of the forceful grinding action of the antrum, repeated trauma to the dilated capillaries would occur causing petechiae to form as well as blood loss from the mucosal surface, especially from the ridges of folds which would be most subject to abrasion from luminal contents as well as neighboring folds.

Another pattern for petechiae and focal erythema in cirrhosis is that of a distribution in the body at fundus, similar to that of acute gastric erosion found in patients with upper gastrointestinal bleeding (see Chapter 36). In either proximal or distal location, the appearance of petechiae and erythema is amazingly constant from one examination to another and not influenced by the administration of antacids or antisecretory agents. The presence of proximal lesions appears to predispose a patient to recurrent acute bleeding,[33] especially if one bleeding episode has already occurred. This likelihood of bleeding from the lesions in one study was reduced by the administration of the beta-blocking agent propranolol in an amount known to lower portal pressure.[33]

Uremia

The uremic stage of renal disease is associated with an altered gastric mucosal appearance,[34] particularly in the antrum (Fig. 14-14). The origin of these changes is unknown. In cases where such changes occur, diffuse or focal erythema of the antrum is seen in association with prominent or large gastric folds.

The focal hyperemia seen in nonbleeding uremic patients differs from the hemorrhagic uremic gastritis in patients with a blood urea nitrogen (BUN) level in excess of 100

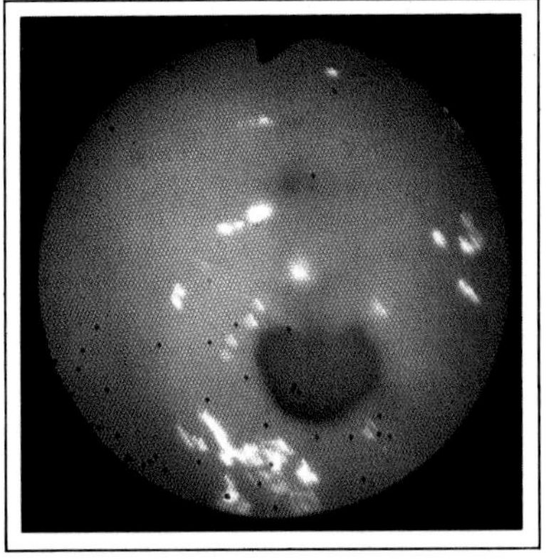

FIG. 14-11.

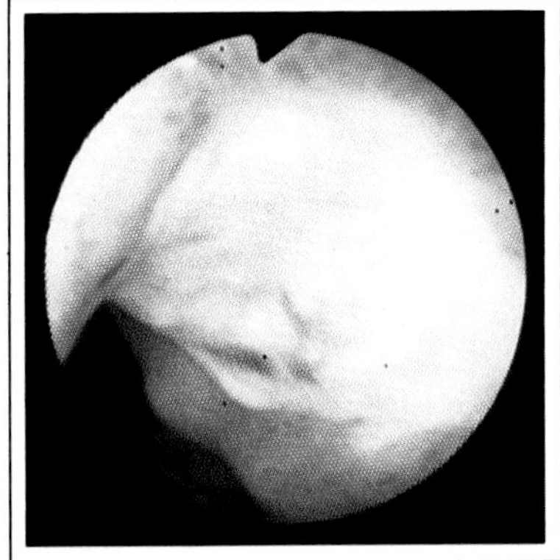

FIG. 14-12.

FIG. 14-11. Gastric mucosal injury effect possibly due to chemotherapy. Focal hyperemia in the prepyloric antrum in a patient treated with cytosine arabinoside and adriamycin who was endoscoped because of dysphagia.

FIG. 14-12. Gastric mucosal injury associated with intra-arterial (hepatic artery) chemotherapy (Floxuridine—FUDR) by means of a surgically implanted (Infusaid) pump. An extensive ulceration of the greater curvature of the antrum is present.

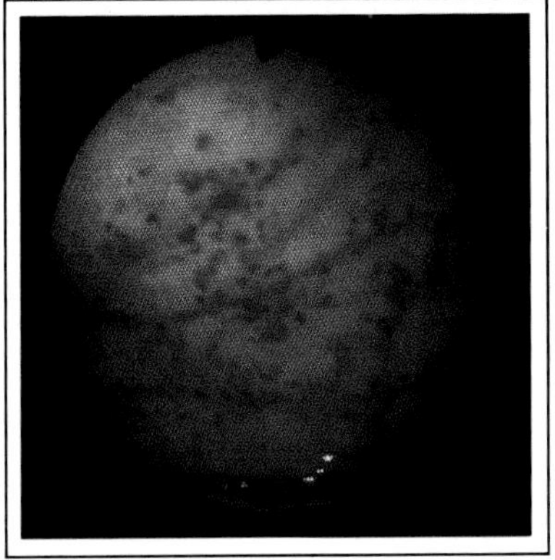

FIG. 14-13.

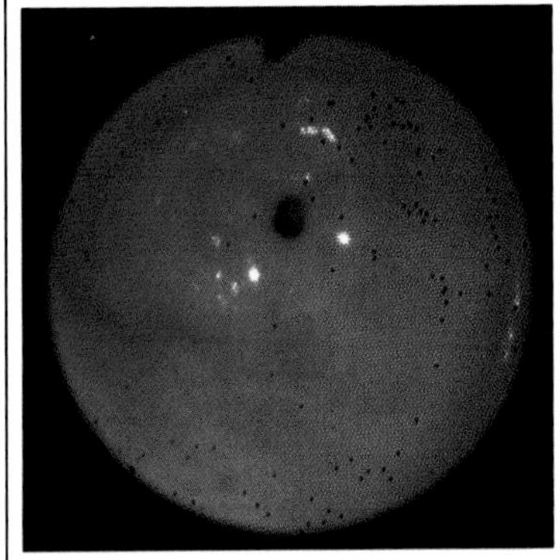

FIG. 14-14.

FIG. 14-13. Gastric mucosal appearance associated with cirrhosis and portal hypertension. Focal pinpoint hyperemia appears in a patient with cirrhosis and a history of bleeding or ingestion of gastrotoxic agent. These lesions may in some way result from intramucosal vascular shunts associated with portal hypertension.

FIG. 14-14. Antral hyperemia associated with uremia. The patient, examined because of vague complaints, had a BUN of 75 mg/dl with no history of bleeding.

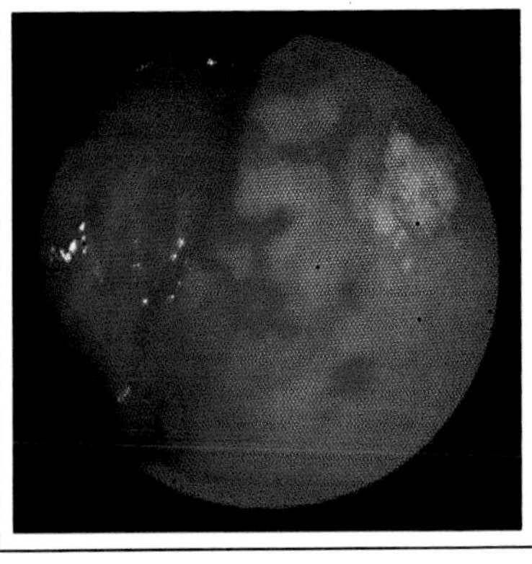

FIG. 14-15.

FIG. 14-15. Thrombocytopenia associated with intramucosal hemorrhage. Focal areas of intramucosal hemorrhage are suggested by the appearance of discrete, intensely erythematous zones seen prior to entering the antrum in a patient with a platelet count of 25,000/cu mm. There was no history of ingestion of any known gastrotoxic agent.

mg/dl in whom frank bleeding erosions (focal red spots with adherent clot or blood oozing from the surface—see Chapter 37) are seen throughout the stomach.

Thrombocytopenia

We find the gastric mucosal appearance to be affected by an altered platelet count only when the count falls below 30,000/cu mm, where resulting capillary fragility[35] leads to the formation of petechiae (1 to 3 mm) and ecchymoses (up to several centimeters) within gastric mucosa, especially of the antrum, similar to the appearance of petechiae in patients with cirrhosis and portal hypertension, but with less marked thrombocytopenia (see above). We believe these lesions to be the result of intramucosal hemorrhage, with the petechiae and ecchymoses occurring at points of increased mucosal trauma, e.g., on the crests of rugal folds, and especially in the antrum along the path of the motor wave front (Fig. 14-15). With restoration of the platelet count to above 30,000/cu mm, these lesions resolve.

REFERENCES

1. Myren, J., and Serck-Hanssen, A. (1974): The gastroscopic diagnosis of gastritis: with particular reference to mucosal reddening and mucous covering. *Scand. J. Gastroenterol.*, 9:457–462.

2. Meshkinpour, H., Orlando, R. A., Arguello, J. F., and DeMicco, M. P. (1979): Significance of endoscopically visible blood vessels as an index of atrophic gastritis. *Am. J. Gastroenterol.*, 71:376–379.
3. Cheli, R., Santi, L., Ciancamerla, G., and Canciani, G. (1973): A clinical and statistical follow-up study of atrophic gastritis. *Am. J. Dig. Dis.*, 18:1061–1066.
3a. Taor, R. E., Fox, B., Ware, J., and Johnson, A. G. (1975): Gastritis—gastroscopic and microscopic. *Endoscopy*, 7:209–215.
4. Deyle, P. (1980): Results of endoscopic polypectomy in the gastrointestinal tract. *Endoscopy* (Suppl.), 35–46.
5. Frank, E. B., Lange, R., and McCallum, R. W. (1981): Abnormal gastric emptying in patients with atrophic gastritis with or without pernicious anemia. *Gastroenterology*, 80:1151.
6. Elsborg, L., and Mosbech, J. (1979): Pernicious anaemia as a risk factor in gastric cancer. *Acta Med. Scand.*, 206:315–318.
7. Stockbrugger, R. W., Menon, G. G., Mason, R. R., Beilby, J. O. W., Bourne, R., and Cotton, P. B. (1978): Gastroscopic survey in pernicious anemia. *Gut*, 19:444a.
8. Schindler, R., and Ortmayer, M. (1942): Histopathology of chronic gastritis. *Am. J. Dig. Dis.*, 9:411–414.
9. Palmer, E. D. (1954); Gastritis: a reevaluation. *Medicine*, 33:199–290.
10. Bjork, J. T., Geenen, J. E., Soergel, K. H., Parker, H. W., Leinicke, J. A., and Komorowski, R. A. (1977): Endoscopic evaluation of large gastric folds: a comparison of biopsy techniques. *Gastrointest. Endosc.*, 24:22–24.
11. Chusid, E. L., Hirsch, R. L., and Colcher, H. (1964): Spectrum of hypertrophic gastropathy. *Arch. Intern. Med.*, 14:621–628.
12. Ona, F. W., and Damevski, K. (1977): Gastroscopic diagnosis of état mamelonné. *Gastrointest. Endosc.*, 23:209–210.
13. Davis, J. M., Gray, G. F., and Thorbjarnarson, B. (1977): Menétrièr's disease: a clinicopathologic study of six cases. *Ann. Surg.*, 185:456–461.
14. Scharschmidt, B. F. (1977): The natural history of hypertrophic gastropathy (Menétrièr's disease): report of a case with 16 year follow-up and review of 120 cases from the literature. *Am. J. Med.*, 63:644–652.
15. Lambert, R., Andre, C., Moulinier, B., and Bugnon, B. (1978): Diffuse varioliform gastritis. *Digestion*, 17:159–167.
16. Farthing, M. J. G., Fairclough, P. D., Hegarty, J. E., Swarbrick, E. T., and Dawson, A. M. (1981): Treatment of chronic erosive gastritis with prednisolone. *Gut*, 22:759–762.
17. Andre, C., Gillon, J., Moulinier, B., Martin, A., and Fargier, M. C. (1981): Randomised placebo-controlled double-blind trial of two dosages of sodium cromoglycate in treatment of varioliform gastritis: comparison with cimetidine. *Gut*, 23:343–352.
18. Elta, G. H., Fawax, K. A., Dayal, Y. L., McClean, A. M., Bloom, S. M., Paul, R. E., and Kaplan, M. M. (1983): Chronic erosive gastritis—a recently recognized disorder. *Dig. Dis. Sci.*, 28:7–12.
19. Baskin, W. N., Ivey, K. J., Krause, W. J., Jeffrey, G. E., and Gemmell, R. T. (1976): Aspirin-induced ultrastructural changes in human gastric mucosa: correlation with potential difference. *Ann. Intern. Med.*, 85:299–303.
20. Hoftiezer, J. W., O'Laughlin, J. C., and Ivey, K. J. (1982): Effects of 24 hours of aspirin, Bufferin, paracetamol and placebo on normal human gastroduodenal mucosa. *Gut*, 23:692–697.
21. Sugawa, C., Lucas, C. E., Rosenberg, B. F., Riddle, J. M., and Walt, A. J. (1973): Differential topography of acute erosive gastritis due to trauma or sepsis, ethanol, and aspirin. *Gastrointest. Endosc.*, 19:127–130.
22. Djahanguiri, B., Abtahi, F. S., and Hemmati, M. (1973): Prevention of aspirin-induced gastric ulceration by bile duct or pylorus ligation in the rat. *Gastroenterology*, 65:630–633.
22a. Greenlaw, R., Sheahan, D. G., DeLuca, V., Miller, D., Myerson, D., and Myerson, P. (1980): Gastroduodenitis. A broader concept of peptic ulcer disease. *Dig. Dis. Sci.*, 25:600–672.
23. Silvoso, G. R., Ivey, K. J., Butt, J. H., Lockard, O. O., Holt, S. D., Sisk, C., Baskin, W. N., Mackercher, P. A., and Hewett, J. (1979): Incidence of gastric lesions in patients with rheumatic disease on chronic aspirin therapy. *Ann. Intern. Med.*, 91:517–520.
24. Caruso, I., and Bianchi Porro, G. (1980): Gastroscopic evaluation of anti-inflammatory agents. *Br. Med. J.*, 1:75–78.
25. Pemberton, R. E., and Strand, L. J. (1979): A review of upper gastrointestinal effects of the newer nonsteroidal anti-inflammatory agents. *Dig. Dis. Sci.*, 24:53–54.
26. Lanza, F. L., Royer, G. L., Nelson, R. S., Chen, T. T., Seckman, C. E., and Rack, M. F. (1979): The effects of ibuprofen, indomethacin, aspirin, naproxen, and placebo on the gastric mucosa of normal volunteers: a gastroscopic and photographic study. *Dig. Dis. Sci.*, 24:823–828.
27. Sun, D. C. H., Roth, S. H., Mitchell, C. S., and Englund, D. W. (1974): Upper gastrointestinal disease in rheumatoid arthritis. *Am. J. Dig. Dis.*, 19:405–410.
28. Spiro, H. S., and Mellis, S. S. (1960): Clinical physiologic implications of the steroid-induced peptic ulcer. *N. Engl. J. Med.*, 263:286–295.
29. McMahon, F. G., Akadamar, K., Ryan, J. R., and Ertan, A. (1982): Upper gastrointestinal lesions after potassium chloride supplements: a controlled clinical trial. *Lancet*, 2:1059–1061.
30. Smith, F. P., Kisner, D. L., Widerlite, L., and Schein, P. S. (1979): Chemotherapeutic alteration of small intestinal morphology and function: a progress report. *J. Clin. Gastroenterol.*, 1:203–207.
31. Narsete, T., Ansfield, F., Wirtanen, G., Ramirez, G., Wolberg, W., and Jarrett, F. (1977): Gastric ulceration in patients receiving intrahepatic infusion of 5-fluorouracil. *Ann. Surg.*, 186:734–736.
31a. Wheeler, M. H., Smith, P. B., Evans, D. M. D., and Laurie, B. W. (1979): Abnormal blood vessels of the gastric antrum: a cause of upper-gastrointestinal bleeding. *Dig. Dis. Sci.*, 24:155–158.
32. Van Vliet, A. C. M., ten Kate, F. J. W., Dees, J., and van Blankenstein, M. (1978): Abnormal blood vessels of the prepyloric antrum in cirrhosis of the liver as a cause of chronic gastrointestinal bleeding. *Endoscopy*, 10:89–94.
33. Lebrec, D., DeFleury, P., Rueff, B., Nahum, H., and Benhamou, J.-P. (1980): Portal hypertension, size of esophageal varices and risk of gastrointestinal bleeding in alcoholic cirrhosis. *Gastroenterology*, 79:1139–1144.
34. Margolis, D. M., Saylor, J. L., Geisse, G., DeSchryver-Kecskemeti, K., Harter, H. R., and Zuckerman, G. R. (1978): Upper gastrointestinal disease in chronic renal failure: a prospective evaluation. *Arch. Intern. Med.*, 138:1214–1217.
35. Freirich, E. (1966): Effectiveness of platelet transfusions in leukemia and aplastic anemia. *Transfusion*, 6:50–59.

15

BENIGN GASTRIC ULCERS

Benign ulcers, the commonest endoscopic abnormality seen in the stomach, are found in about 10% of examinations performed in our Unit. Nevertheless, identification and accurate interpretation of gasric ulcers remain a challenge to all endoscopists, even the most experienced. Mistakes have serious consequences. Overlooking an ulcer could result in a patient's symptoms being attributed to functional causes; and mistaking foreign material (mucus, saliva, or antacid residue) lodged between rugal folds (Fig. 15-1) for an ulcer may cost the patient an unnecessary course of treatment. Finding an ulcer but neglecting to elicit a history of aspirin ingestion means a missed opportunity for identifying a correctable cause of the ulcer which could hasten its resolution and prevent its recurrence. More serious are mistaken diagnoses resulting from a failure to correctly differentiate benign from malignant ulcers. To diagnose cancer in the case of a benign ulcer may cause an unnecessary operation, whereas not to appreciate the appearance of a small malignant ulcer may mean a missed opportunity for diagnosing gastric cancer at a curable stage.

In this chapter we discuss the three types of interpretive challenges that gastric ulcers present: (a) the endoscopic observation of benign gastric ulcers; (b) the endoscopic features of ulcers associated with anti-inflammatory agents; and (c) the differentiation of benign from malignant ulcers, with particular attention to the "indeterminate" ulcer. After our treatment of the interpretive aspects of gastric ulcers, we turn our attention briefly to a consideration of the approach to biopsy and brushing cytology of benign and indeterminate gastric ulcers.

ENDOSCOPIC OBSERVATION OF BENIGN GASTRIC ULCERS

Location

Benign ulcers may be found anywhere in the stomach; however, most (80%+) are found in the distal body on or close to the gastric angle (Fig. 15-2a) or proximal body, or within the antrum (Fig. 15-2b) exclusive of its distal 2 cm. The remainder (20%) occur in the prepyloric antrum[1] (Fig. 15-2c). The location of the gastric ulcer to a large extent depends on whether it is primary (unassociated with duodenal bulb ulcers, duodenal deformity, or gastric hypersecretion) or secondary (associated with duodenal bulb de-

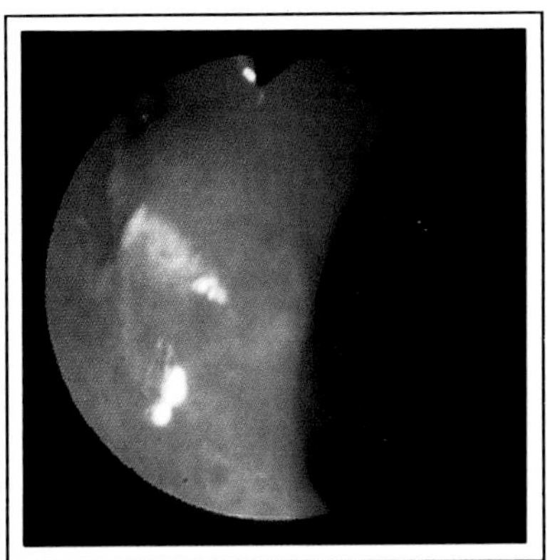

FIG. 15-1a.

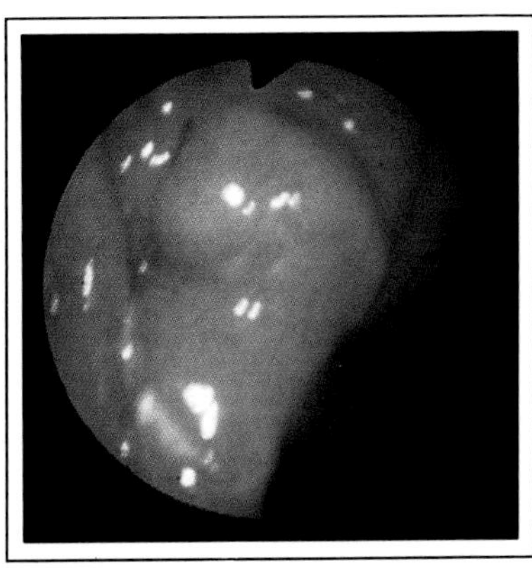

FIG. 15-1b.

FIG. 15-1. a: Foreign material lodged between rugal folds (at 10 o'clock), simulating an ulcer base. **b:** After vigorous washing using a polyethylene cannula, the foreign material appears to have moved onto the folds.

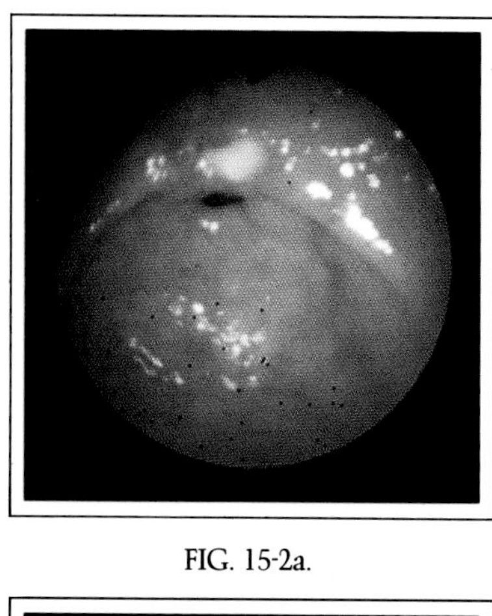

FIG. 15-2a.

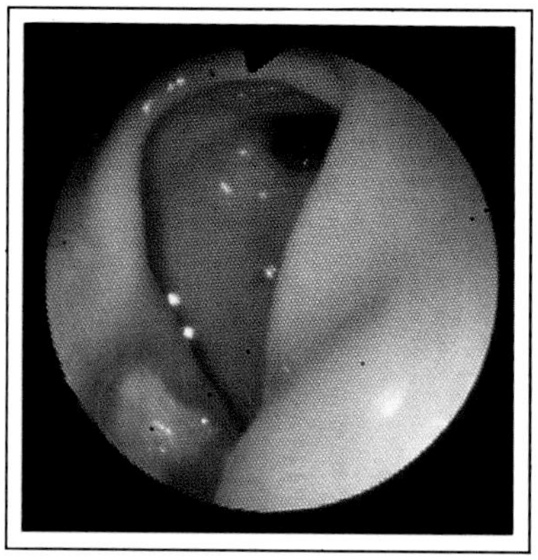

FIG. 15-2b.

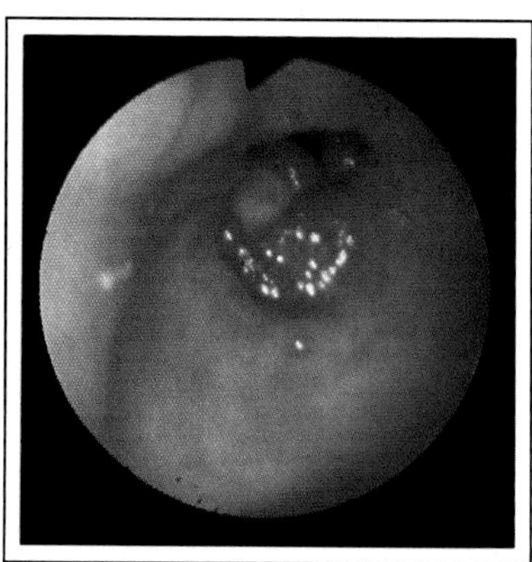

FIG. 15-2c.

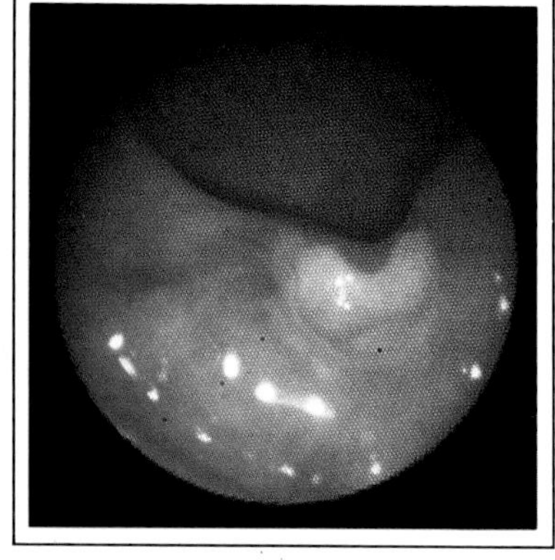

FIG. 15-3a.

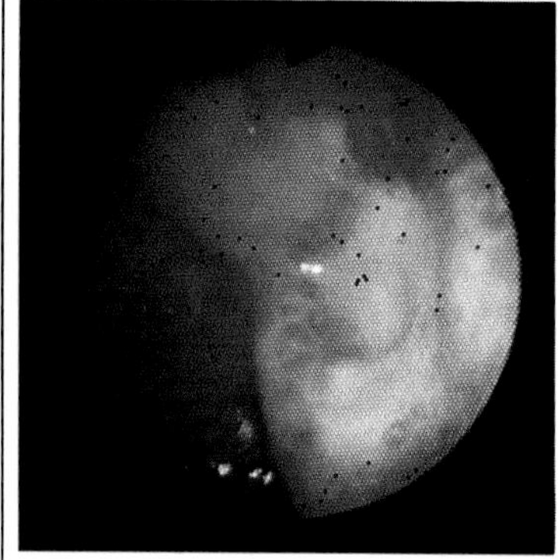

FIG. 15-3b.

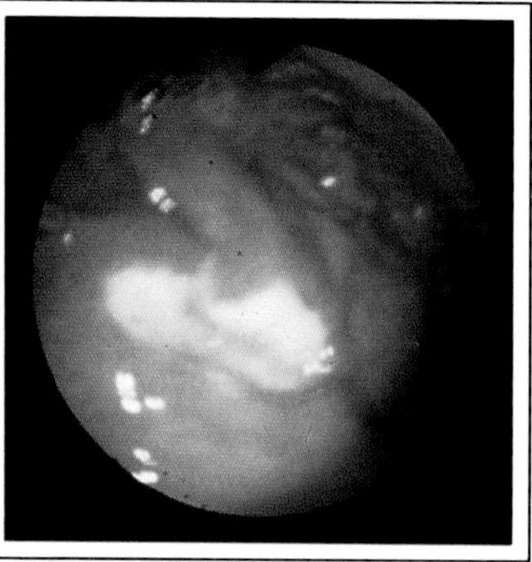

FIG. 15-3c.

FIG. 15-2. a: Benign ulcer in the angle. **b:** Benign ulcer in the antrum. **c:** Benign ulcer in the prepyloric antrum.

FIG. 15-3. a: Benign ulcer in the upper mid-body, posterior wall. **b:** Benign ulcer in the cardia. **c:** Benign ulcer in the fundus, just above its junction with the body.

formity, inactive duodenal ulcer, or gastric hypersecretion). Most primary ulcers are located on the gastric angle or in the immediate vicinity, whereas secondary ulcers tend to be located in the prepyloric antrum as well as on the gastric angle.

Proximal benign gastric ulcers of the body (Fig. 15-3a), especially the upper portion, cardia (Fig. 15-3b), or fundus (Fig. 15-3c), tend to be found in elderly patients. Of 52 patients over the age of 60 with gastric ulcers, Sheppard et al. found 30 to be in the upper body, 16 in the mid-body, and only six on the angle or in the antrum.[1] The reason for this "ascent" of gastric ulcers in elderly patients to the proximal stomach is unknown. One theory holds that the proximal location of these ulcers has to do with the upward migration of the junction of parietal and pyloric mucosa on the lesser curve, with this junctional area a predisposing focus for ulceration.[2]

Appearance

Endoscopically there are three components to any ulcer, all of which require careful observation: (a) the base; (b) the margin; and (c) the relation of the margin to the surrounding folds (Table 15-1). Correct interpretation of an ulcer requires a thorough examination of these features.

TABLE 15-1. *Features which differentiate benign from malignant ulcers*

Feature	Benign	Malignant
Base	Variable; generally smooth and homogeneous	Variable; generally irregular
Margin	Regular; intact mucosal pattern	Irregular mucosal pattern; may be disrupted by the presence of tumor nodules
Margin in relation to surrounding folds	Margin and folds merge uniformly	Folds cut off or disrupted by tumor within the margin
Size	Small ulcer (≤1 cm) (95% benign)	Large ulcer (>2 cm) (20% malignant)

The Base

The white (fibrin) base is the most prominent feature of an ulcer; in untreated patients it is typically round, regular, and punched-out with a smooth, uniform appearance (Fig. 15-4). Generally, the earlier the patient is studied in relation to the onset of symptoms, the more likely it is that his ulcer will be in the active stage and the more typical the ulcer base will be. However, once the ulcer enters the healing stage (see below), the base becomes irregular in both shape and consistency (Fig. 15-5a).

In addition to the stage of the ulcer (active or healing), its size creates interpretive problems as well. The base of large ulcers is often irregular in regard to consistency (Fig. 15-5b) and is especially so if it is deeply penetrating (Fig. 15-5c). In some cases this results from the presence of vascular structures within the base, whereas in other posteriorly penetrating ulcers actual pancreatic tissue may be seen (Fig. 15-5c).

The Margin

The margin of a typical benign gastric ulcer is slightly raised in relation to the ulcer base, but smooth and regular (Fig. 15-6). Often the margin is erythematous (Fig. 15-7), with a closeup appearance similar to that of superficial gastritis (see Chapter 14) with the distinctive lineae and areae gastricae. In the context of an ulcer, this appearance is indicative of the presence of regenerative-type mucosa.[3] Such ulcers may be said to have entered the healing stage (see below), whereas a regular margin (in the absence of mucosal erythema) is characteristic of the active stage of a benign gastric ulcer (Fig. 15-5). As the ulcer enters the

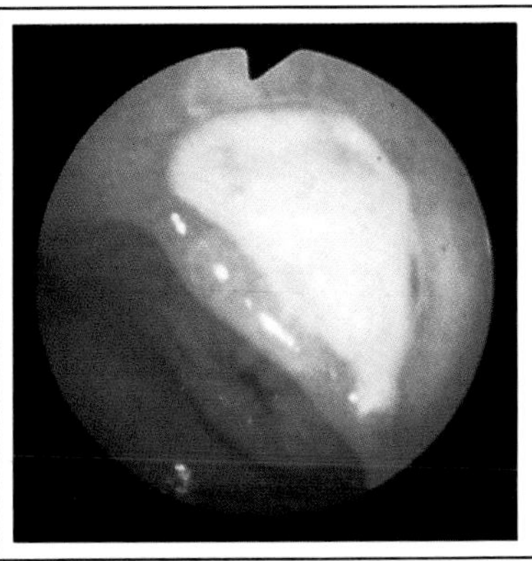

FIG. 15-4.

FIG. 15-4. Benign ulcer base. This has a punched-out, smooth, regular appearance of an active ulcer. The absence of any erythema of the margin suggests that little healing has occurred.

FIG. 15-5. a: Healing ulcer base. The regular base of the ulcer in Fig. 15-4 has become distorted as the ulcer heals. The base is now seen as an irregular erythematous area within which the residual ulcer base is broken up during healing. **b:** Large ulcer base. This is part of a large (>3 cm) ulcer. With an ulcer of this size, the base often appears distorted. **c:** Penetrating ulcer base. Seen within the base and distorting its appearance are raised areas which were found at surgery to be portions of pancreas.

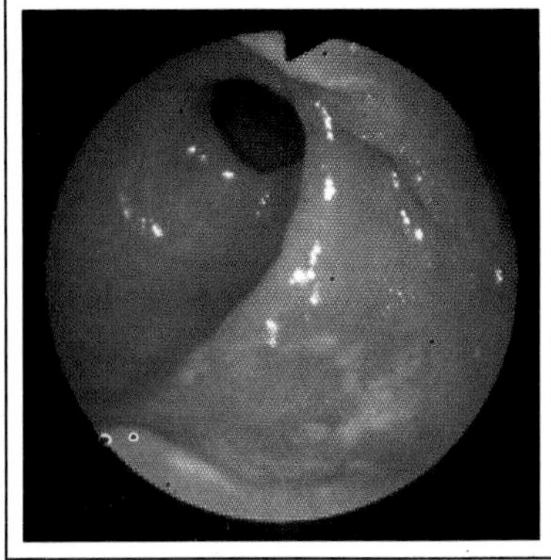

FIG. 15-5a.

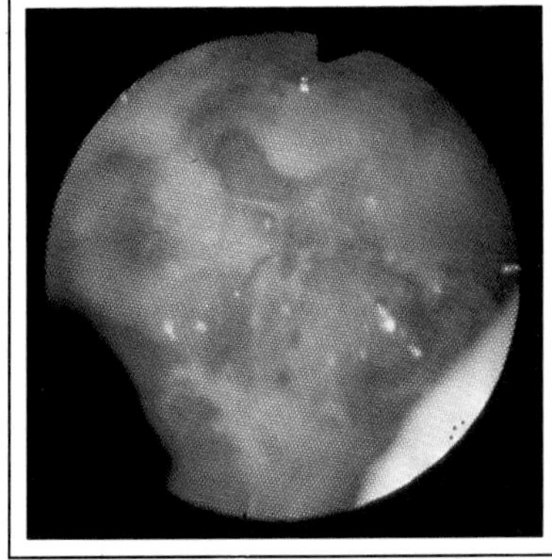

FIG. 15-5b.

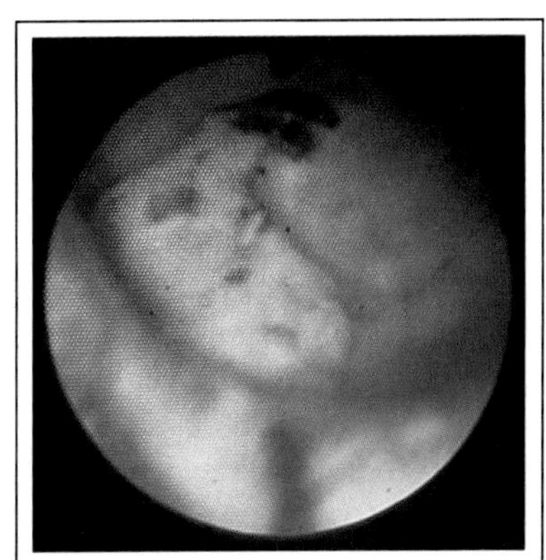

FIG. 15-5c.

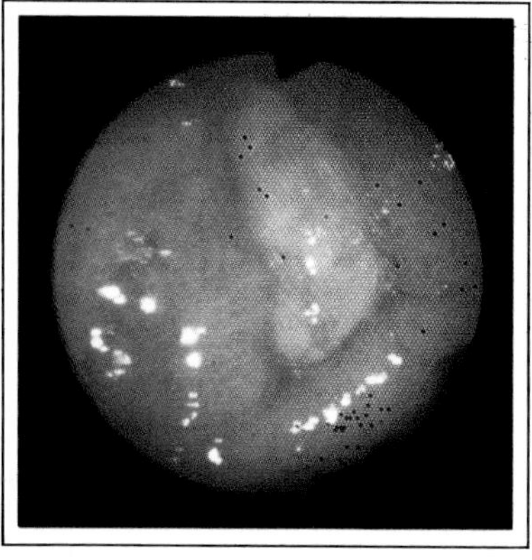

FIG. 15-6.

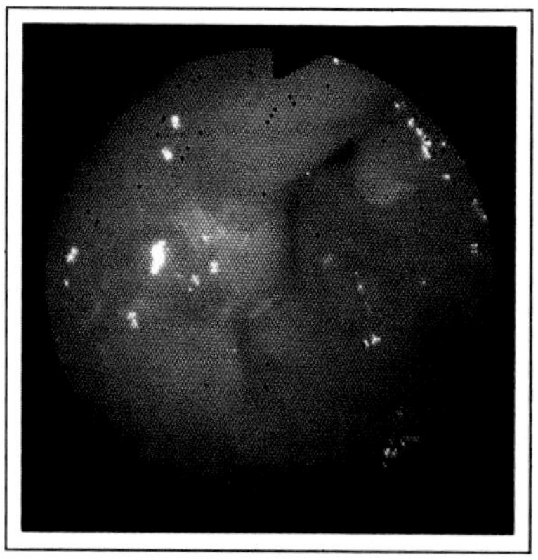

FIG. 15-7.

FIG. 15-6. Benign ulcer margin. A smooth, rounded, regular margin adjacent to the base.

FIG. 15-7. Healing ulcer margin. The margin shows a punctate erythema from which biopsies typically show regenerative-type mucosal changes.[3] The individual reddened points, we believe, represent discrete areae gastricae with regenerative-type mucosa (see text), making this appearance a reliable marker for an ulcer in the healing stage.

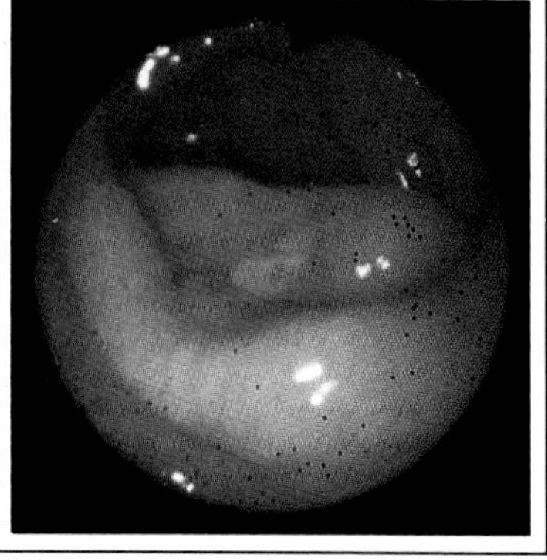

FIG. 15-8a.

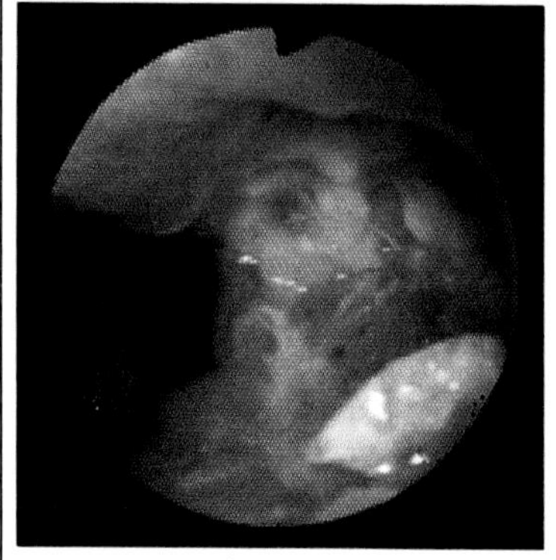

FIG. 15-8b.

FIG. 15-8. a: Deformed (scarred) ulcer margin. Prominent converging folds which distort the margin represent scarring from previous ulceration. **b:** Distorted margin of a large (>3 cm) ulcer margin. The margin of this ulcer is irregular and even nodular, warranting careful follow-up.

healing stage, the margin takes on an irregular, erythematous, often nodular character, as a reflection of the inflammatory and reactive mucosal changes which are associated with healing (Fig. 15-7). Another feature that determines the shape of the margin is scarring from previous ulcerations, which may give the margin a distorted appearance (Fig. 15-8a).

As in the case of the base itself, the size of an ulcer is often a factor in determining the appearance of the margin, with large ulcers often associated with an extremely irregular margin. This is especially the case for ulcers which are over 2 cm maximum dimension (Fig. 15-8b).

Relation of Margin to Surrounding Mucosal Folds

In theory, there should be no separation between an ulcer base and any mucosal folds which surround it. One expects, therefore, that it should be possible in most cases to follow these folds right up to the ulcer base (Fig. 15-9b). However, this may not be possible for several reasons. First, the surrounding folds (Fig. 15-9a) may not be seen unless a special effort is made, as conventional forward-viewing endoscopes view many ulcers (especially those of the lesser curve) at best only tangentially. In many cases a retroflexed position does allow better visualization of the ulcer margin in relation to the surrounding folds (Fig. 15-9b); nevertheless, the location of some ulcers (Fig. 15-11a) altogether precludes visualization of this important relationship with the forward-viewing endoscope. In these cases, only a side-viewing instrument will suffice (Fig. 15-11b).

The size of the ulcer may also be a factor in distorting the expected relation between the surrounding folds and the margin. With larger ulcers (>1.5 cm), the surrounding folds do not run up to the base of the margin but appear to "blend" in with the margin because of the edema and other reactive changes within the margin itself (Fig. 15-10a). In some cases where the ulcers exceed 2 cm, folds running up to the margin may appear to be "cut off" (Fig. 15–10b).

Ulcer Size

An attempt should be made to measure the size of ulcers. With experience, one can estimate the size surprisingly well from the endoscopic appearance alone. However, it is best to employ a more reliable measure. We find that the open bite method (see Chapter 4) provides a reasonably good estimate of ulcer size (Fig. 15-12). In this method the premeasured distance between the cups of an open biopsy forceps (6 to 9 mm) is used to estimate ulcer size by placing the open forceps across the ulcer. The number of open bite widths is estimated for the length and width of the ulcer, which is then converted into centimeters.

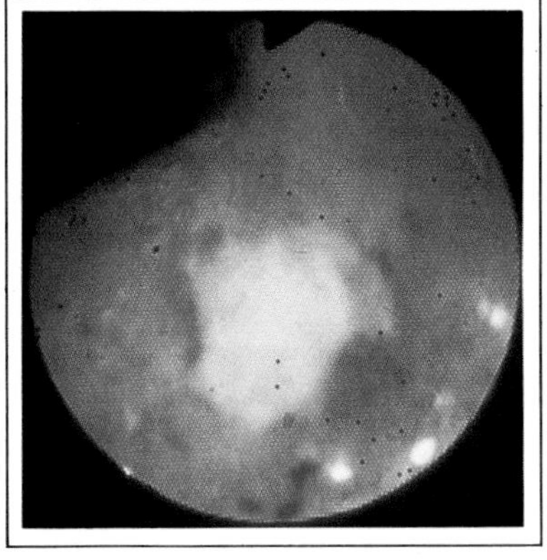

FIG. 15-9a.

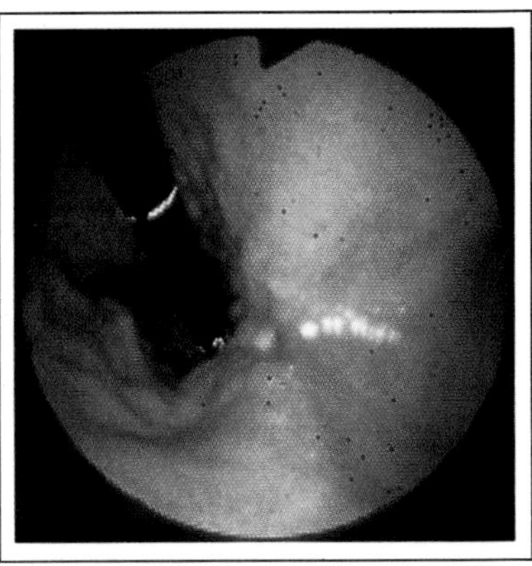

FIG. 15-9b.

FIG. 15-9. a: Benign ulcer. The base and margin are well visualized, but the margin is not seen in relation to the surrounding folds. **b:** Benign ulcer base and margin in relation to surrounding folds. With retroflexion, the surrounding folds are now seen to radiate into the ulcer margin.

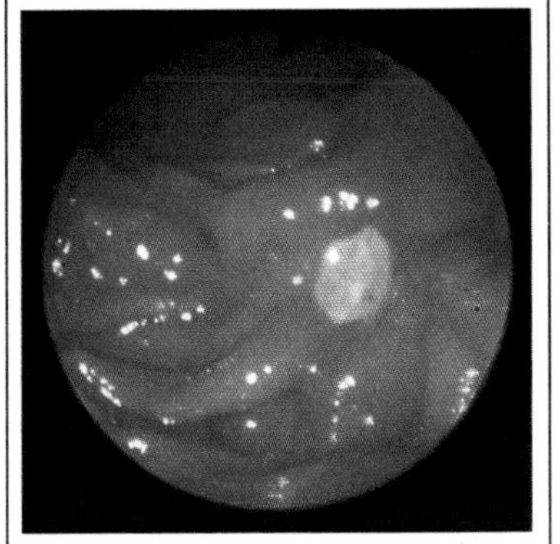

FIG. 15-10a.

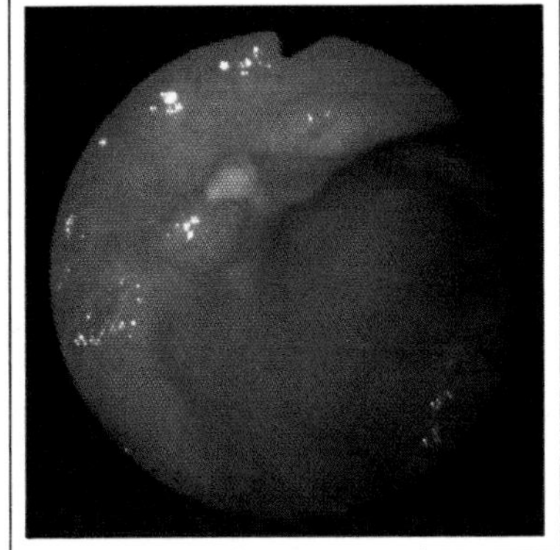

FIG. 15-10b.

FIG. 15-10. a: Benign ulcer. A common pattern is pictured here where a surrounding fold (at 9 o'clock) blends into the margin but does not continue up to the base (as is true at 6 o'clock). **b:** Benign ulcer, atypical relation of folds to margin. The margin, being prominent, appeared to cut off the fold radiating toward it.

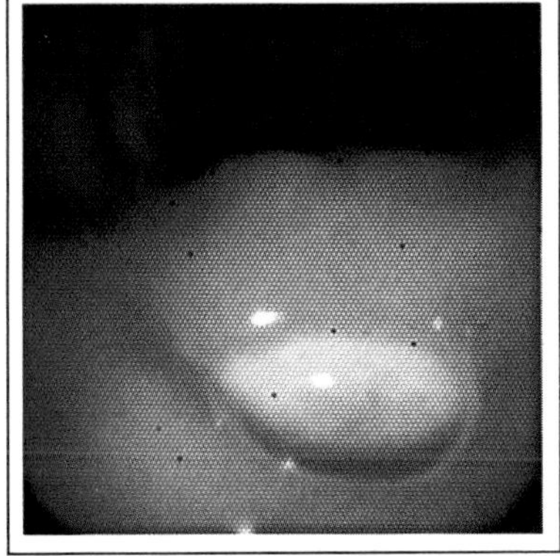

FIG. 15-11a.

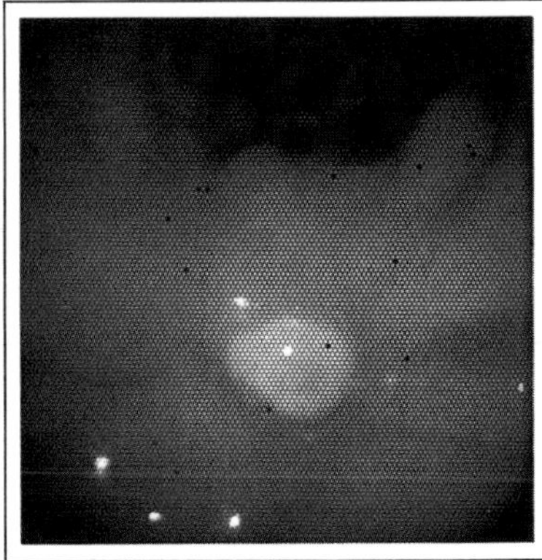

FIG. 15-11b.

FIG. 15-11. a: Benign ulcer, angle observed with a forward-viewing endoscope. The relationship of the margin to the surrounding folds is not seen because a retroflexed view could not be obtained. Biopsy of the proximal (12 o'clock) aspect of the margin was also impossible. **b:** Benign ulcer, observed with a side-viewing endoscope. The relation of the ulcer margin and surrounding fold is now clearly seen, with folds radiating to the base. Biopsy of the proximal margin was also feasible.

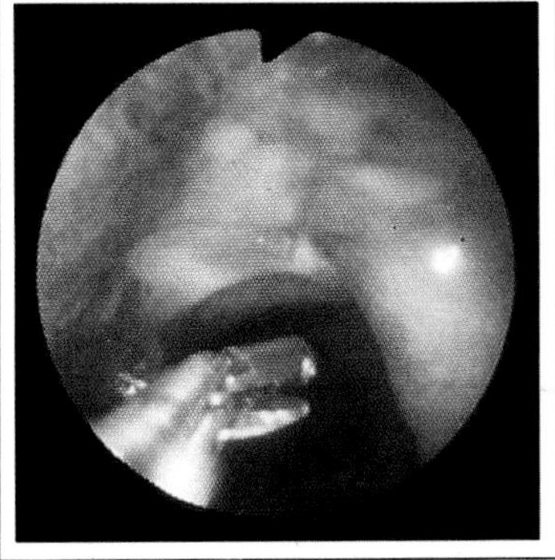

FIG. 15-12.

FIG. 15-12. Measuring a gastric ulcer using the open bite width method. In this case the open bite width measured a segment of 9 mm. Using this standard, the ulcer was found to be 1.3 cm (1.5 segments) in one dimension (9 to 3 o'clock) and 1 cm (just over one segment) in the other dimension (12 to 6 o'clock).

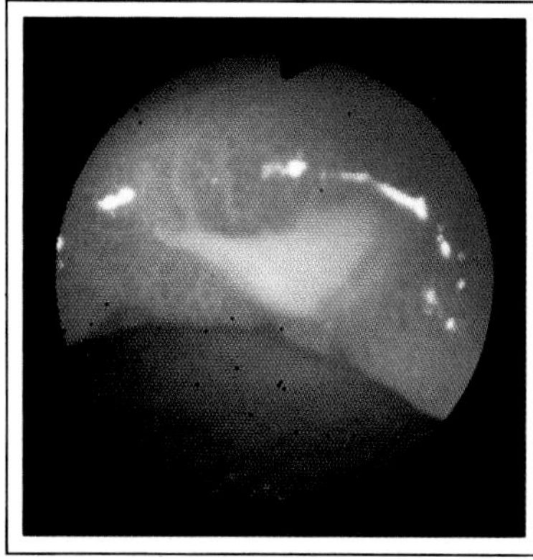

FIG. 15-13a.

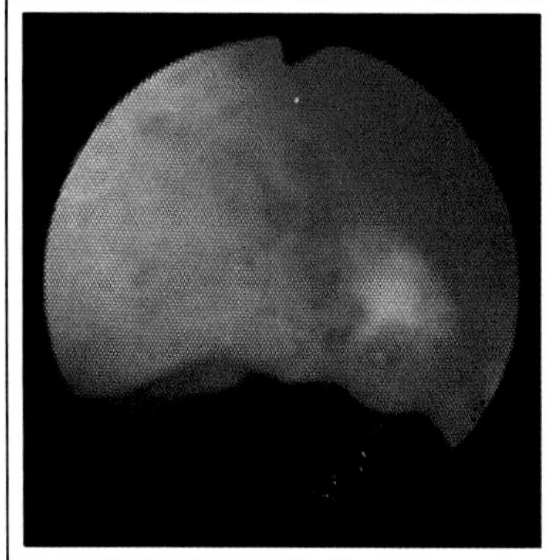

FIG. 15-13c.

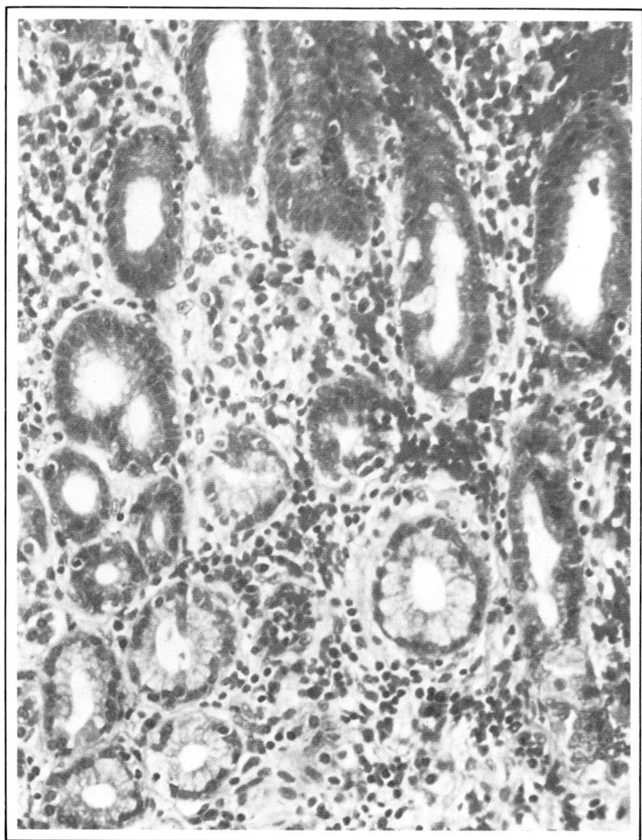

FIG. 15-13b.

FIG. 15-13. a: Ulcer healing, early or initial stage.[3] The margin of the base is sharp. An erythematous rim confined to a 1-cm zone around the ulcer base is noted with apparent areae and lineae gastricae, suggesting the presence of regenerative-type epithelium.[3] This was confirmed histologically. **b:** Biopsy taken from the margin of a healing ulcer. Mucin depletion of the foveal epithelial cells with acute and chronic inflammation and capillary dilatation are the expected histologic features seen in ulcer healing. **c:** Ulcer healing, proliferative stage.[3] The margin of the ulcer base has become irregular—evidence of a later stage of healing—with some re-epithelialization of the base having already occurred.

We, as do others,[1] find that gastric ulcers tend to be equally divided between those less than 1 cm (45%) and those between 1 and 3 cm (45%) (Table 15-2); about 10% are greater than 3 cm (giant gastric ulcers).

Ulcer Healing

The endoscopist must be able to recognize signs of healing both during the initial examination and on subsequent encounters with the ulcer. Healing is evidenced by the substitution of regenerative erythematous mucosa for the white ulcer base itself. Early healing is seen as an erythematous rim around the ulcer base[3] (Fig. 15-13a) consisting of regenerative mucosa (Fig. 15-13b). Later, as the ulcer continues to heal, it loses its symmetry and its perfect, regular, punched-out appearance, with its base especially becoming irregular and less well defined (Fig. 15-13c). This appearance has been referred to as the proliferative stage.[3] With continued healing, the margin predominates and the white base shrinks, ultimately becoming linear and then disappearing altogether. As the base is replaced by regenerative epithelium, one notes what has been called the "red scar," or palisade, stage (Fig. 15-14a). This has the appearance of a focal zone of erythema in the area formerly occupied by the white ulcer base. The endoscopist carefully inspects for atypical features within such areas, e.g., an unusual, pale coloration (Fig. 15-14b) or extremely intense erythema (lacking areae or lineae gastricae-type markings). Such appearances would cause one to pursue biopsy aggressively to exclude early gastric cancer (see Chapter 16).

TABLE 15-2. *Relation of size to type of ulcer for 219 gastric ulcers examined over a 5-year period*

Size (cm)	Benign (No.)	Malignant (No.)	% Malignant
<1	80	5	6
1–2	75	14	15
2–3	22	5	18
>3	15	3	20
Overall	192	27	14

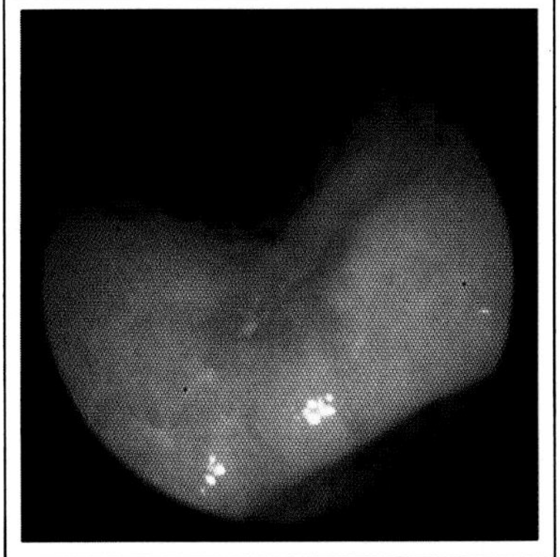

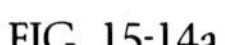

FIG. 15-14a.

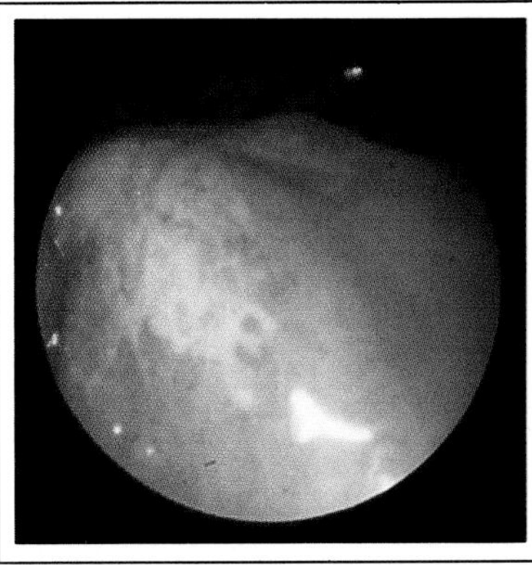

FIG. 15-14b.

FIG. 15-14. a: Ulcer healing, "red scar" (palisade) stage.[3] The ulcer base is indistinct, having been almost completely replaced by regenerative-type epithelium. **b:** Atypical healing, early gastric cancer. Note the zone of atypical healing adjacent to the ulcer base (at 10 o'clock). The extensive gray-white area, an appearance unlike that of typical ulcer healing, was a clue to the presence of cancer (see Chapter 16).

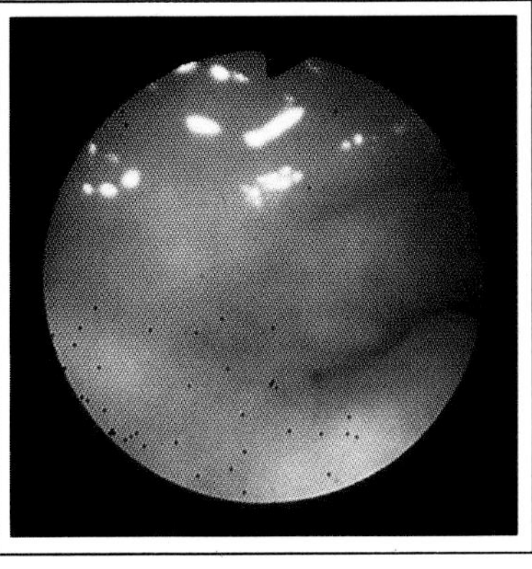

FIG. 15-15.

FIG. 15-15. Ulcer healing, healed, "white scar," cobblestone scar[3] stage. A depression (scar deformity) is seen in the prepyloric antrum at 9 o'clock where previously an ulcer had been described. The appearance of its mucosa is indistinguishable from that of its surroundings and would be expected on biopsy to show mature epithelium having completely replaced the regenerative type associated with the healing stages.

Ultimately, the regenerative epithelium of the red scar is replaced by mature epithelium that is undistinguishable from the surrounding mucosa and at this point is termed a "white scar" or simply "ulcer scar deformity" (Fig. 15-15). All that remains to suggest the former ulcer may be gastric folds which converge on each other toward the point where the ulcer had been rather than running in parallel. Sometimes all that remains is a dimple in the mucosa (Fig. 15-15).

The question of whether to follow every patient with a benign gastric ulcer to the white scar stage must be answered on an individual basis. Overall, if the visual impression of benignity is borne out on biopsy (see below), one's confidence level might be as high as 97% of the cases overall[4] and an even higher percentage for ulcers less than 1 cm, a size found with only a small number of malignant ulcers.[5]

Further follow-up seems unnecessary for an uncomplicated ulcer with typically benign features. However, if any atypical features are observed, especially the mucosal coloration around the margin, it would be extremely important to follow the patient to complete healing, even if in some cases it takes more than a year, so as not to miss the opportunity to diagnose curable gastric cancer (see Chapter 16). For patients who present with a gastric ulcer complication, e.g., bleeding or obstruction, it may be prudent to continue therapy until the white scar stage has been reached thus indicating complete healing. Several Japanese studies have suggested that ulcers which are treated to the point of complete healing may remain in remission longer than those in which treatment is stopped at an arbitrary point or when the patient becomes asymptomatic.[6]

Rates of Ulcer Healing

The healing rate of benign gastric ulcers is variable, but one generally finds it to be on the order of 1 to 4 mm per week, when thought of as a decrease in the maximum dimension of the ulcer. The actual rate is somewhat influenced by treatment, with, as in one study, 86% healed after 8 weeks for patients on cimetidine contrasted with 58% for those on placebo.[6a] Some, nevertheless, will require extended periods of time (>12 weeks) to heal completely. In particular, we find these to be large ulcers (>2 cm), unassociated with anti-inflammatory agent usage (see below), and those where the surrounding mucosa shows histologically atrophic gastritis.[6b]

ULCERS ASSOCIATED WITH ANTI-INFLAMMATORY AGENTS

Aspirin is both widely used and the commonest potentially ulcerogenic drug found in association with gastric ulcers. In one study, 52% of 61 patients with gastric ulcers consumed 15 or more aspirin per week compared with only 10% of the controls.[7] The finding of an ulcer at endoscopy should therefore cause the examiner to suspect regular aspirin usage as a cause or a contributing factor, especially if a suggestive appearance (see below) is present. Because patients are often not aware of the aspirin content of commonly used over-the-counter analgesics, we find it necessary to question each patient from a list of commonly used aspirin-containing products (see Table 14-1).

Like aspirin, commonly prescribed nonsteroidal anti-inflammatory agents are potentially ulcerogenic in a susceptible individual. Some, when used in high dosage, are as ulcerogenic as aspirin (see Chapter 14). As these medications have unfamiliar names, patients may not be able to recall specific medications until the name itself is mentioned. We therefore find it useful to review with a patient a list of commonly prescribed nonsteroidal agents (see Table 14-2), along with the list of products containing aspirin.

Corticosteroids, though having a relatively low potential for initiating gastric mucosa injury,[8] in comparison to aspirin and some other nonsteroidal agents,[8] do appear to double the risk of peptic ulcer disease,[8a] although not specifically that of gastric ulcers. Moreover, the proportion of individuals taking corticosteroids who develop peptic ulcers is low (1.8%).[8a] One would, therefore, think that the patient on corticosteroids at greatest risk for a gastric ulcer would be one either with a prior history of having one or be concomitantly taking aspirin or other nonsteroidal agents.

Some may feel that it is not the endoscopist's place to attempt to find, in the history of a patient with a gastric ulcer, an ulcerogenic agent which the patient may not even be aware he is consuming. However, we believe this should be done because discovery of such ingestion may be as important as finding the ulcer itself. This is true for two reasons. First, with regard to interpretation, an ulcer associated with aspirin or a nonsteroidal agent is often large with atypical features (see below), which may prompt the endoscopist to suspect malignancy. We have ourselves been responsible for advising surgery in several cases where a malignant appearance was present when in retrospect a different interpretation would have been placed on the ulcer had the history of significant aspirin consumption been obtained. In these cases the patients did not know that the analgesic product, used in excess (more than eight tablets per day), contained aspirin (in one case it was Anacin and in the other Excedrin).

A second reason to obtain the history of using an ulcerogenic agent relates to ulcer healing. Even though it is possible to achieve complete healing while a patient continues to use aspirin or nonsteroidal agent,[9] such ingestion may prolong both symptoms and the time required for healing, and it may also place a patient at risk for complication of his ulcer, e.g., bleeding or perforation.

Appearance

Multiple small ulcerations.

Multiple small (<5 mm) shallow ulcers of the prepyloric antrum (Figs. 15-5a and b) is the commonest appearance for ulcerations caused by aspirin[10] and other nonsteroidal anti-inflammatory agents.[8] White-based erosions and focal erythema are often seen in conjunction (Fig. 15-16). This appearance corresponds to the pattern of injury observed in normal volunteers following even 24 hr of aspirin (8 tablets, total 2.6 g)[10a] or one week of nonsteroidal analgesic usage.[10b] The endoscopic finding of multiple scattered superficial white-based lesions, therefore, should always raise in the examiner's mind the possibility that anti-inflammatory agents are responsible and cause him to question the patient, following the procedure about their usage, even, as in the case of aspirin, in amounts taken for only 24 hr.[10a]

Large ulcers.

A less common appearance for ulcers associated with anti-inflammatory agents is that of one or more large, deep ulcers (Fig. 15-17a). Although large ulcers may be present in less than 10% of patients with injury from ulcerogenic medications, they probably account for a large proportion of patients who actually require hospitalization, either for acute bleeding (Fig. 15-17a) or obstructive symptoms (Fig. 15-18a), in some cases suggesting malignancy (Fig. 15-19).

Since the predominant injury pattern for aspirin and other nonsteroidal analgesic agents in studies of volunteers with prior normal endoscopy[10a,10b] and in patients on long term aspirin[10] is that of small ulcers, along with scattered red- and white-based erosions (see above), the finding of one or more (generally two) large ulcers (>1.5 cm), often in the absence of erosions, is curious. The explanation for this may be a selective lack of the expected mucosal adaptation[10c] in areas which subsequently ulcerate deeply because of initial low levels of musocal prostaglandins[10d] that are lowered even further by aspirin or other nonsteroidal agents.[10e]

Despite their size, the large ulcers associated with anti-inflammatory agents will completely heal (Fig. 15-18c) once the offending drug is stopped. However, because of their initial size, with a maximum dimension often in excess of 4 cm, healing may not be complete even after 5 months (Fig. 15-18b). Still, we have observed surprising rates of healing, sometimes exceeding 6 mm per week (as reduction in maximum dimension of the ulcer) once the agent is withdrawn. Even though complete healing of ulcers associated with anti-inflammatory agents can occur with cimetidine,[10f] this is unpredictable especially for large ulcers (>1 cm) which may remain unhealed despite treatment.[10f] Eliciting a history of anti-inflammatory agent usage (see

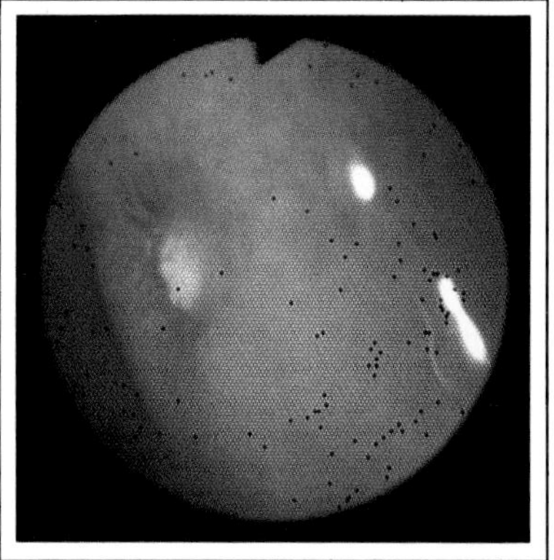

FIG. 15-16.

FIG. 15-16. Small aspirin ulcer. One of several small (<5 mm) ulcers in the prepyloric antrum and focal hyperemia.

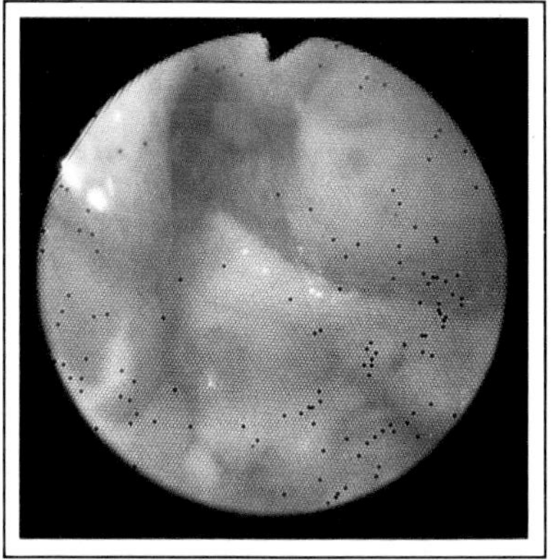

FIG. 15-17a.

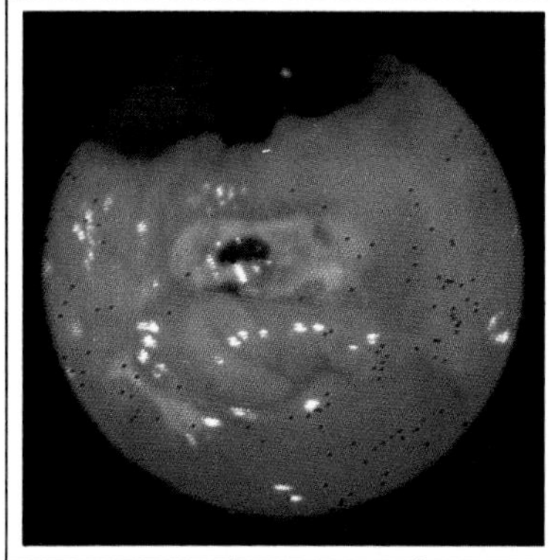

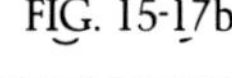

FIG. 15-17b.

FIG. 15-17. a: Large aspirin ulcer. Unlike small aspirin ulcers (such as that in Fig. 15-16), larger ones are often found in the absence of surrounding mucosal erythema endoscopically or of chronic gastritis histologically.[11,12] **b:** Gastric ulcer in the prepyloric antrum, with typical surrounding erythema and a small satellite ulcer (off toward 8 o'clock).

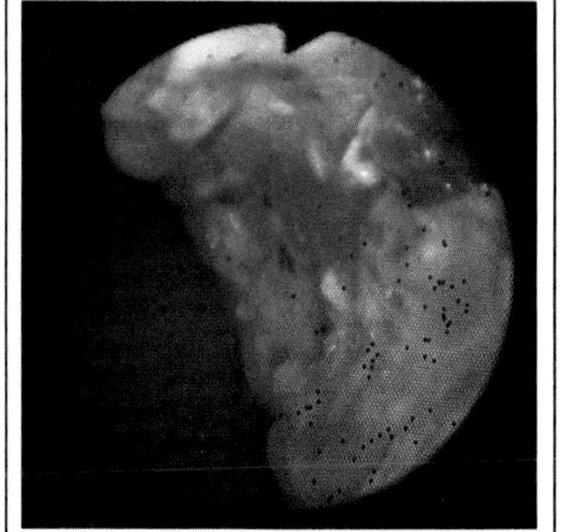

FIG. 15-18a.

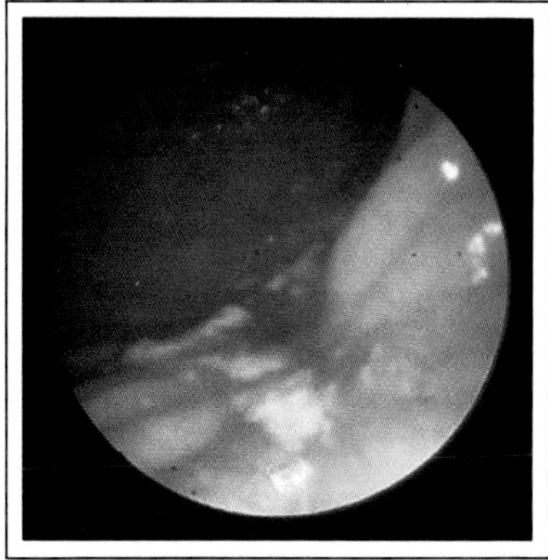

FIG. 15-18b.

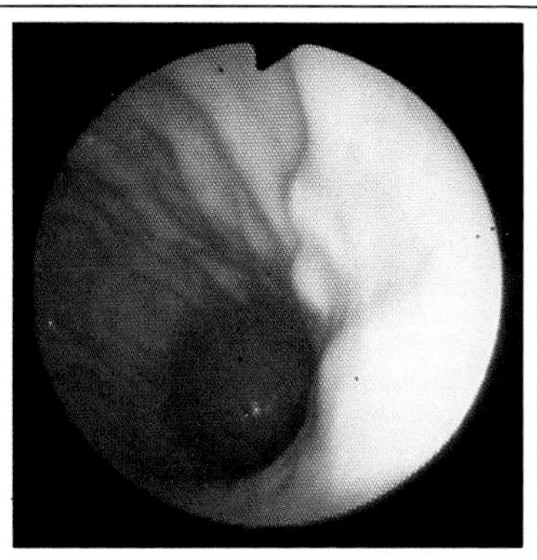

FIG. 15-18c.

FIG. 15-18. a: Large aspirin ulcer. A 6-cm lesser curve ulcer is seen with an irregular base. **b:** Large aspirin ulcer that is healing. At a second examination 5 months later (after the patient had completely stopped taking aspirin), the ulcer was observed to have markedly decreased in size (to 1 to 5 cm). **c:** Large aspirin ulcer, completely healed, 8 months after the initial diagnosis.

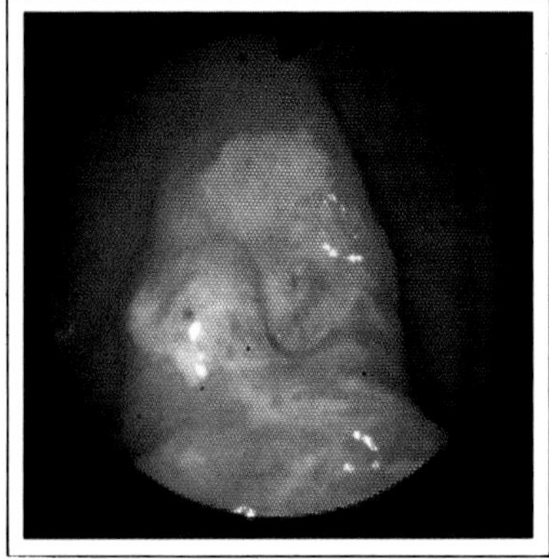

FIG. 15-19.

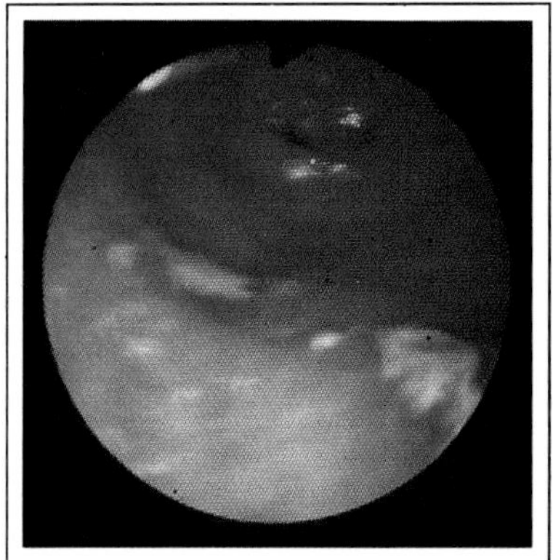

FIG. 15-20.

FIG. 15-19. Large aspirin ulcer, with an irregular margin—an indeterminate ulcer (similar to that in Fig. 15-18c). Complete healing was observed after discontinuation of aspirin.

FIG. 15-20. Multiple gastric ulcers. These small superficial lesions have been called erosions or aphthous ulcers.[13]

Chapter 14) so that they may be stopped can be a critical step to ensure healing, especially of large ulcers.

A potential clue to both the increased vulnerability of the mucosa in which these ulcers are set[11] and their association with aspirin or other nonsteroidal analgesic usage lies in the examination of biopsies taken from surrounding mucosa. Unlike other gastric ulcers (Fig. 15-17b), which usually show marked inflammation of surrounding mucosa, as well as regenerative changes indicative of healing there (see above), these ulcers often appear to be grossly and histologically set in normal mucosa.[11] In one study of large gastric ulcers, ranging in size from 1.2 to 5.5 cm, in which endoscopically obtained biopsies taken from the mucosa surrounding the ulcer failed to reveal chronic gastritis, all were found to be in patients with a history of habitual aspirin use, the daily dose ranging up to 12,000 mg![12]

Other appearances.

Ulcers, especially if large (>2 cm), may be complicated by bleeding (see Chapter 36), penetration, or perforation. We have previously reported the simultaneous penetration of two large aspirin ulcers with the formation of a gastrogastric fistula.[13] Because of the size and the predisposition of these ulcers to penetrate endoscopically, they often appear indeterminate (see below) as to whether malignancy is present (Fig. 15-19) or even frankly cancerous. For this reason the history obtained by the endoscopist of significant aspirin or nonsteroidal agent ingestion may be crucial for correct interpretation.

Multiple Gastric Ulcers

As we have already stated, the finding of multiple—generally three or more—small gastric ulcers constitutes an appearance highly suspicious that aspirin or another nonsteroidal anti-inflammatory agent is the cause. Nevertheless, we find this appearance even in patients who are thoroughly questioned and deny the use of these agents. Of such patients in our Unit up to 30% have two or more ulcers.[14] Generally, the number of ulcers is three with the commonest location the prepyloric region. Others have described multiple, small (<5 mm) superficial lesions (Fig. 15-20) which respond poorly to medical management and occur repeatedly. These have been termed "aphthous" ulcers.[15]

DIFFERENTIATION OF BENIGN FROM MALIGNANT ULCERS

The differentiation of benign from malignant ulcers remains a great challenge. Even though some studies have suggested an accuracy of visual diagnosis in excess of 90%,[4,16] this is misleading from the standpoint of the confidence with which the endoscopist can attach the designation benign or malignant to any given ulcer.

In a recent study[5] where the endoscopist's level of confidence was specifically assessed, the endoscopist called 81% of what in fact were benign ulcers something other than benign. More than half (56%) were called equivocal and 18% malignant. For ulcers which were in fact malignant, the endoscopist did better, calling 78% malignant; however, 22% were still called something else, either equivocal (19%) or benign (3%). These authors found that they needed to use the term equivocal to describe 50% of their cases.[4] Of interest was the outcome of those ulcers in the equivocal group. For 5% the ulcer was ultimately proved to be malignant, contrasted with a 1% incidence of malignancy found in patients whose ulcers were called benign. This higher incidence of cancer among ulcers with equivocal features contrasted with those appearing benign corresponds with our own experience, although we use the term indeterminate (see below) rather than equivocal to describe such ulcers. We employ this term in only 20% of cases but find a fivefold incidence of malignancy when these ulcers are contrasted with those considered benign (15% versus 3%).

Rather than expecting to find a clear differentiation between benign and malignant ulcers, we believe the endoscopist should expect that in 20 to 50% of the cases he will

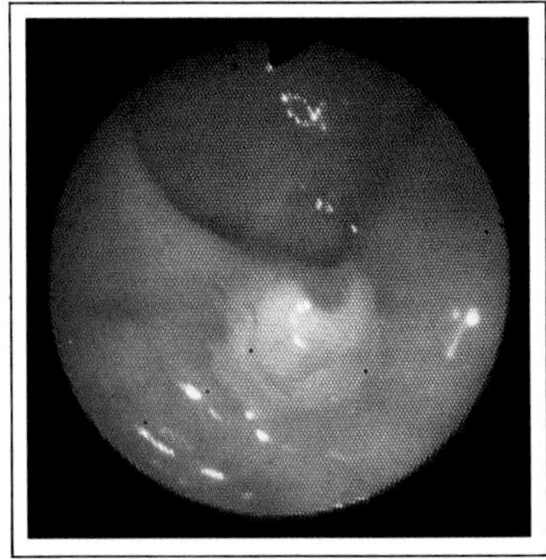

FIG. 15-21a.

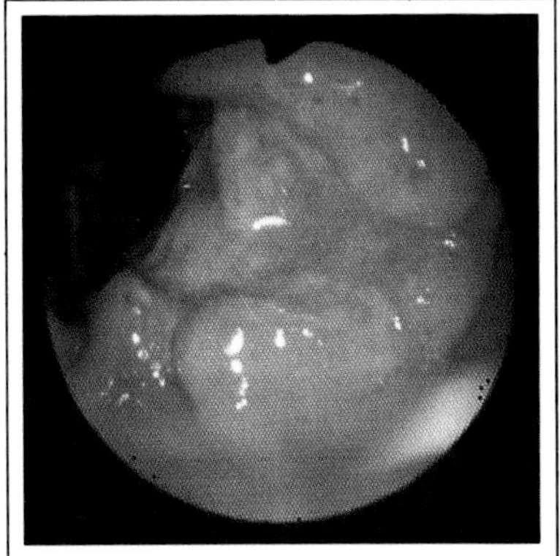

FIG. 15-21b.

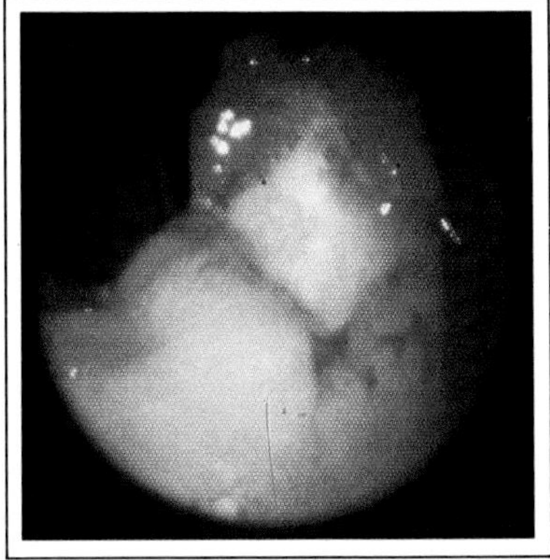

FIG. 15-21c.

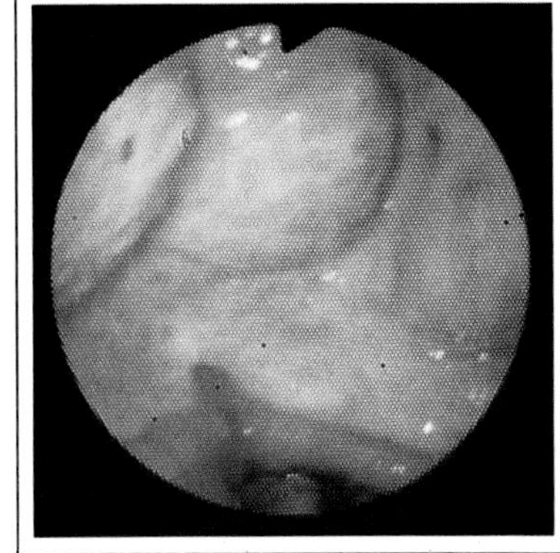

FIG. 15-21d.

FIG. 15-21. a: Benign ulcer base with a smooth, regular appearance. **b:** Malignant ulcer base with its characteristic distorted nodular appearance. This nodularity is also present in the margin. **c:** Malignant ulcer base, early gastric cancer. The ulcer base appears benign, with the cancer confined to its margin, especially at 12 o'clock. **d:** Benign ulcer base in a large (6 cm) ulcer. The base of an ulcer this size often has an irregular, distorted appearance.

not be able to designate the ulcer as either benign or malignant but will need to use some other term, e.g., indeterminate or equivocal, to express his legitimate uncertainty about the nature of the ulcer and to indicate to the referring physician the need for close endoscopic follow-up should biopsy and brushing cytology fail to reveal malignancy.

Differentiating Features

The differentiating features of benign and malignant ulcers are summarized in Table 15-1. Correct interpretation of any ulcer ultimately depends on a complete viewing of its base, margin, and the margin in relation to surrounding folds.

The Base

The base tends to be smooth and regular in benign ulcers (Fig. 15-21a) and irregular in malignant ulcers (Fig. 15-21b). However, the appearance of the ulcer base is actually so variable as to make it the least useful feature of all in differentiation. Contrary to the expectation of a smooth base in all benign ulcers and an irregular one in malignant ulcers, the reverse is often the case. In early gastric cancer appearing as an ulcer (see Chapter 16), the base of the ulcer may be perfectly smooth and regular with the cancer being confined almost entirely to its margin (Fig. 15-21c). Conversely, there is the case of a large benign gastric ulcer (>3 cm) where the base appears irregular, even nodular (Fig. 15-21d). The appearance of the base of the ulcer alone therefore should never be the deciding factor as to how the endoscopist ultimately comes to view an ulcer.

The Margin

More useful, we find, than the appearance of the base is that of the margin. The margin of a typical benign ulcer is discrete and sharply demarcated in relation to its base. In addition, the margin is regular and smooth (Fig. 15-22a). Any deviation from this should call an ulcer into question. Obviously, most disturbing is the finding of a margin which has distinct nodules within it (Fig. 15-21b). Also unsettling is an irregular margin of an ulcer (Fig. 15-22b), particularly where the mucosal coloration is either inhomogenous, lacking the discrete areae and lineae gastricae (Fig. 15-22c) expected of a healing ulcer (see above), or appears uniformly erythematous.[15a]

Margin in Relation to Surrounding Folds

The expected relationship of the margin of a benign ulcer to its surrounding folds is that these would terminate at the base or, if the ulcer is large, merge with the margin

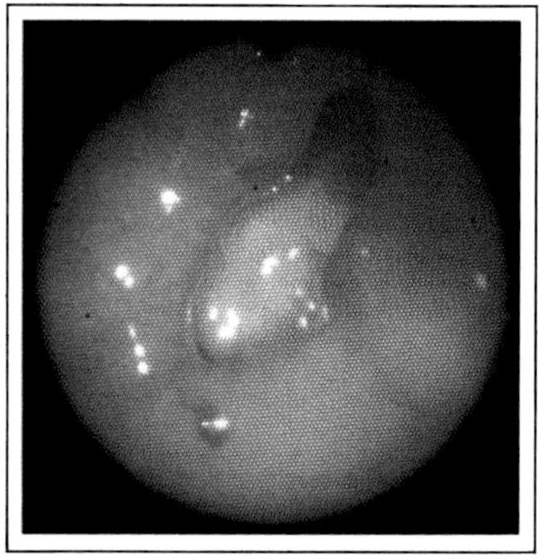

FIG. 15-22a.

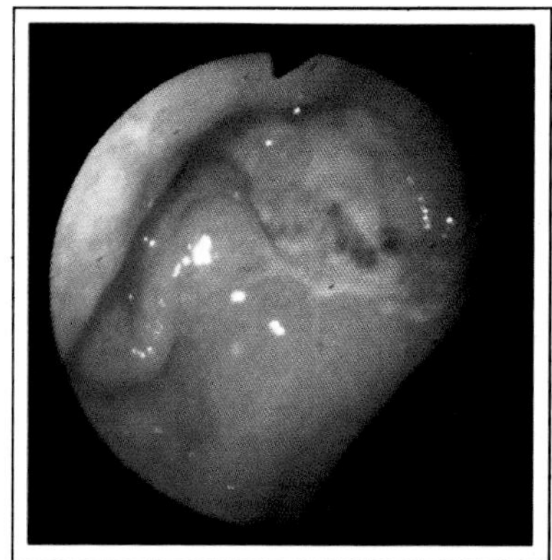

FIG. 15-22b.

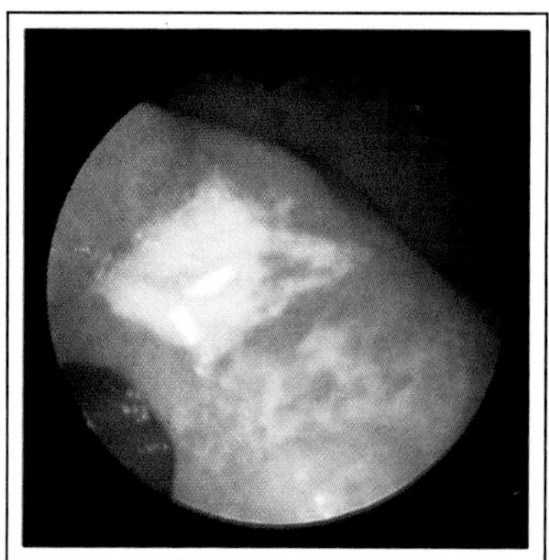

FIG. 15-22c.

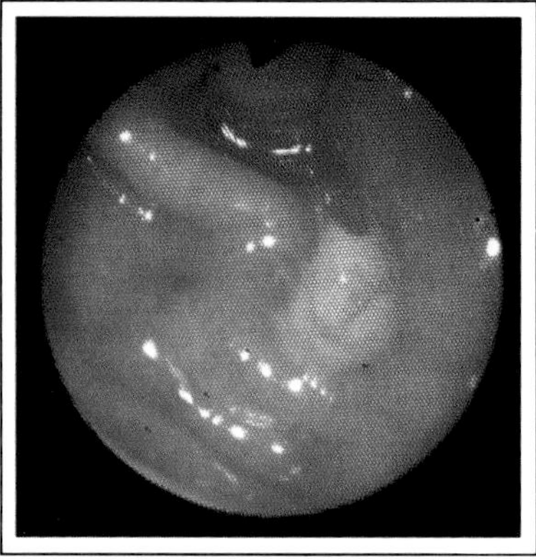

FIG. 15-23a.

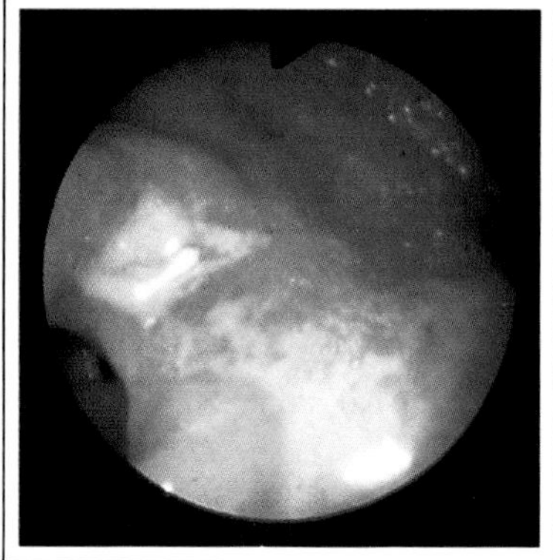

FIG. 15-23b.

FIG. 15-22. a: Benign ulcer margin, which is smooth and regular with intact, glistening mucosa. **b:** Malignant ulcer margin. The indistinct border of the margin (in the absence of erythema due to healing) was the clue to the underlying malignant nature of this ulcer. **c:** Malignant ulcer margin. The inhomogeneous nature of the mucosal coloration of the margin correctly indicated to the endoscopist the possibility of early gastric cancer (see Chapter 16).

FIG. 15-23. a: Benign ulcer, surrounding folds. These come up directly to merge with the ulcer margin. **b:** Malignant ulcer (early gastric cancer), surrounding folds. These terminate at 4 o'clock, short of the ulcer base, and are separated by a margin having atypical mucosa.

(Fig. 15-23a). When differentiating benign from malignant ulcers, one carefully inspects the surrounding folds in search of an atypical relationship to the ulcer margin. The appearance of folds which are cut off at a distance from the ulcer base, or where their termination appears clubbed or palisaded (Fig. 15-23b) would cause the endoscopist to suspect malignancy, as would an ulcer margin which extended out over the surrounding folds in a plateau-like manner, obliterating the folds (Fig. 15-21b). More subtle is the presence of a slight depression of the ulcer margin in relation to the surrounding folds, causing them to appear clubbed, and where the intervening mucosa has an atypical appearance, being neither normal nor regenerative (Fig. 15-23b).[16a]

Indeterminate Ulcers

In practice, 10 to 15% or more of gastric ulcers lack features which clearly designate them either benign or malignant. These we consider indeterminate. Although most are benign either by virtue of complete endoscopic healing or in some cases surgical resection, we find as many as 15% to be cancerous—roughly five times the incidence of malignancy in ulcers which are called benign (approximately 3%).[4] Because of the incidence of malignancy, the endoscopist must pursue biopsy and brushing cytology even more aggressively than he might for typically benign ulcers (see below). Moreover, he advises close endoscopic follow-up for all indeterminate ulcers because of his uncertainty about the nature of the ulcer, and the increased prevalence of gastric cancer for this group of ulcers.

We find three types of ulcer appearance that are more likely to be considered indeterminate than others. These are: (a) large ulcers (≥2 cm); (b) ulcers with distorted margins; and (c) ulcers associated with a mass-like deformity.

Large (>2 cm) Ulcers

Although the majority of ulcers 2 to 3 cm or larger are benign, we find a two- to threefold increased likelihood of cancer in these ulcers (Table 15-2) when compared with ulcers less than 1 cm, with the highest incidence of cancer (20%) being found in ulcers greater than 3 cm. Because of this, we have come to regard any ulcer greater than 2 cm as "indeterminate" (Fig. 15-24a). By doing so, we single out these ulcers in particular for aggressive biopsy and close follow-up (Fig. 15-24b). Another reason related to size is the distortion of the margin, which is often found in association with large ulcers. The heaped-up, enlarged edematous folds which surround such ulcers often suggest malignancy (see below). Finally, we regard large ulcers as indeterminate for one simply technical reason. It may be difficult or impossible to completely examine the margin

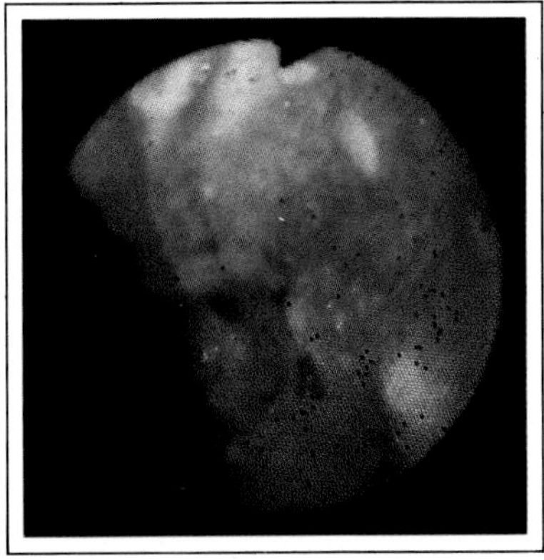

FIG. 15-24a.

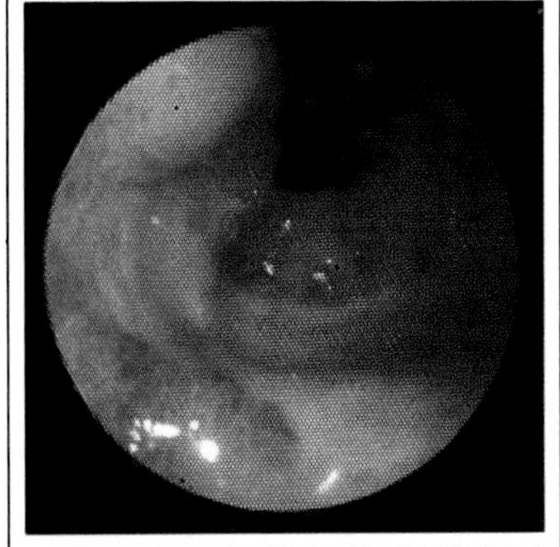

FIG. 15-24b.

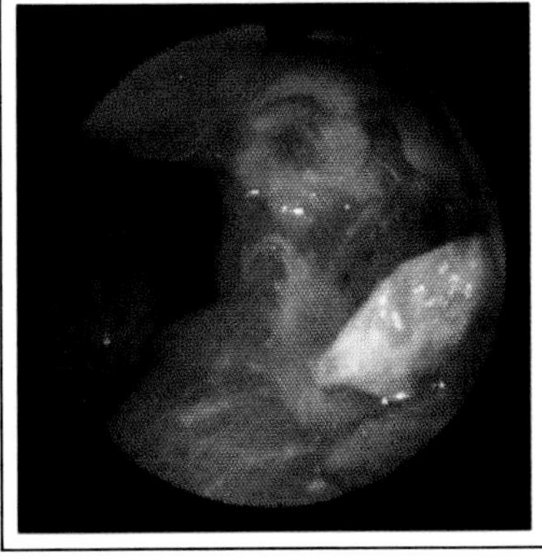

FIG. 15-24c.

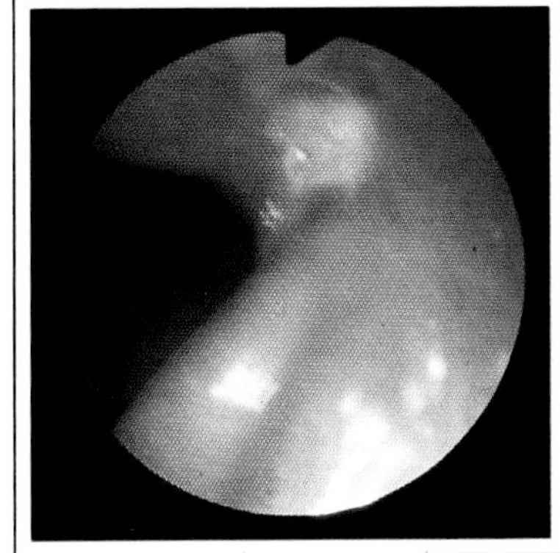

FIG. 15-24d.

FIG. 15-24. a: Indeterminate ulcer, because of size (3 × 5 cm) and the irregular appearance of its base. This was followed endoscopically to the point of complete ulcer healing (see Fig. 15-18). **b:** Indeterminate ulcer, because of size (>6 cm) alone. Initial biopsies and cytology were negative; a subsequent biopsy (9 weeks later) strongly suggested lymphoma, ultimately proved at surgery. **c:** Indeterminate ulcer, because of size (3 cm) and the distorted appearance of the ulcer base and margin. This was impossible to completely examine. Because of the negative brushings and biopsies, as well as a strong aspirin history, it was elected to follow this ulcer. **d:** Indeterminate ulcer seen in (c) after a 10-week period. The margin is distinct and the folds radiate to the ulcer base, signs of the ulcer's being benign.

of a large ulcer (Fig. 15-24c), especially one situated high on the lesser curve of the body or just distal to the angle. For this reason, the endoscopist will wish to see the ulcer again, hopefully at a reduced size for better visual assessment (Fig. 15-24d) as well as for another round of biopsies and, if necessary, brushing cytology.

Ulcers with Distorted Margins

As previously stated, the margin of a benign ulcer may appear distorted if the ulcer is large (Fig. 15-24c), deep (Fig. 15-25a), or observed during the healing stage (Fig. 15-8b). It is not common to find an ulcer with distorted margins for all three reasons. Of these, the changes which result from ulcer healing are the most difficult to be confident about. One finds erratic re-epithelialization around and within the ulcer base accompanied by inflammatory and reactive changes within the mucosa of the margin and surrounding folds to give them a swollen appearance (Fig. 15-25a), especially the folds which merge with the margin of the ulcer. The re-epithelialization around the periphery of the ulcer base may create the impression of a depressed margin (Fig. 15-25c), suggesting the appearance of early gastric cancer (Fig. 15-25a). In some cases the marginal erythema is so intense it obscures the lineae and areae gastricae (Fig. 15-25c), so that the appearance suggests early gastric cancer (Fig. 15-21c). The distorted appearance of the margin during the early healing phases (Fig. 15-24c) may well give way to a more orderly appearance at a later point in healing (Fig. 15-24d). If the endoscopist calls the initial appearance indeterminate and requires a subsequent examination, the appearance he finds at that time better allows the benign nature of the ulcer to be appreciated (Fig. 15-24d).

Ulcers Associated with a Mass-like Deformity

Benign ulcers are often set in areas of scarred deformity from previously existing ulceration. These cases present an interpretive problem, first because the "mass effect" of the deforming folds (Fig. 15-25a) causes them to resemble a malignant ulcer (Fig. 15-21b). Secondly, the mass effect may prevent a close look at the margins, either to establish its completely benign nature (Fig. 15-25a) or to spot a disturbing feature, e.g., an irregular junction between the ulcer base and margin (Fig. 15-25d). Most importantly, the endoscopist may find it difficult to regard an ulcer situated within a mass as benign even though the overlying mucosa appears perfectly intact (Fig. 15-26) because any such mass may be cancer (Fig. 15-27), even though an exceedingly uncommon experience. In all cases where an ulcer is present in association with a mass, we believe the endoscopist's concern about the nature of the lesion is best communicated by

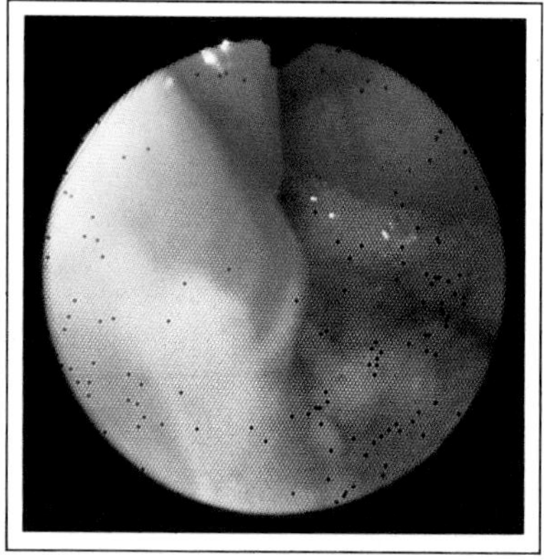

FIG. 15-25a.

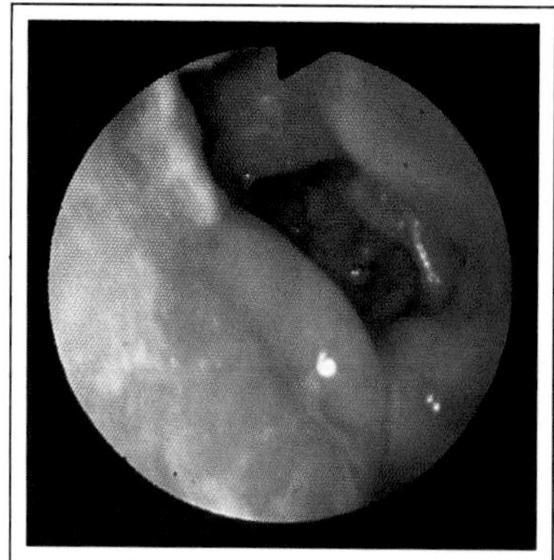

FIG. 15-25b.

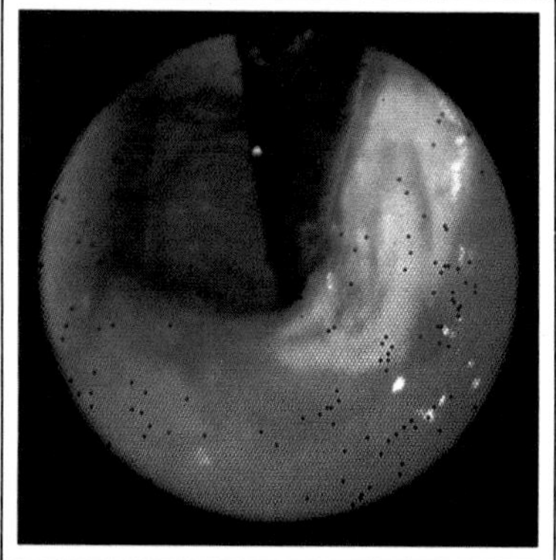

FIG. 15-25c.

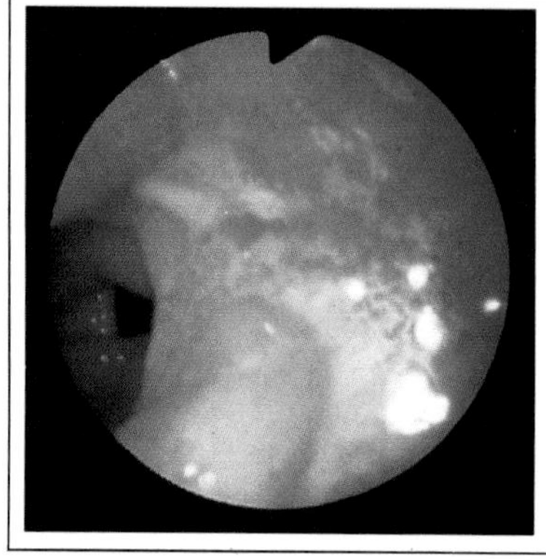

FIG. 15-25d.

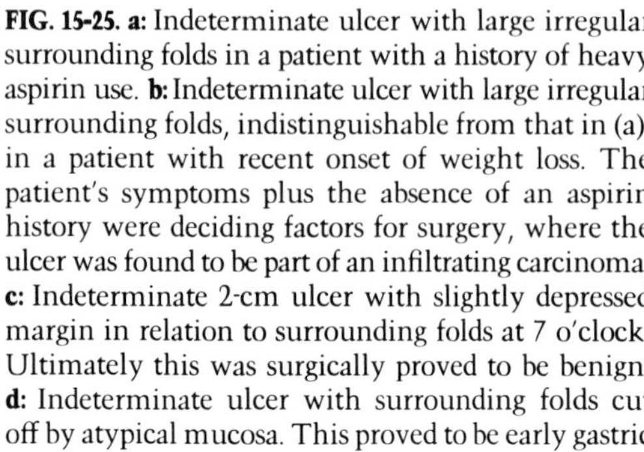

FIG. 15-25. a: Indeterminate ulcer with large irregular surrounding folds in a patient with a history of heavy aspirin use. **b:** Indeterminate ulcer with large irregular surrounding folds, indistinguishable from that in (a), in a patient with recent onset of weight loss. The patient's symptoms plus the absence of an aspirin history were deciding factors for surgery, where the ulcer was found to be part of an infiltrating carcinoma. **c:** Indeterminate 2-cm ulcer with slightly depressed margin in relation to surrounding folds at 7 o'clock. Ultimately this was surgically proved to be benign. **d:** Indeterminate ulcer with surrounding folds cut off by atypical mucosa. This proved to be early gastric cancer.

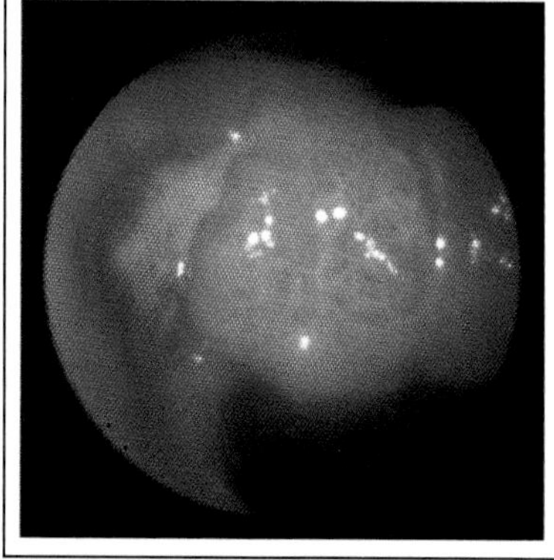

FIG. 15-26.

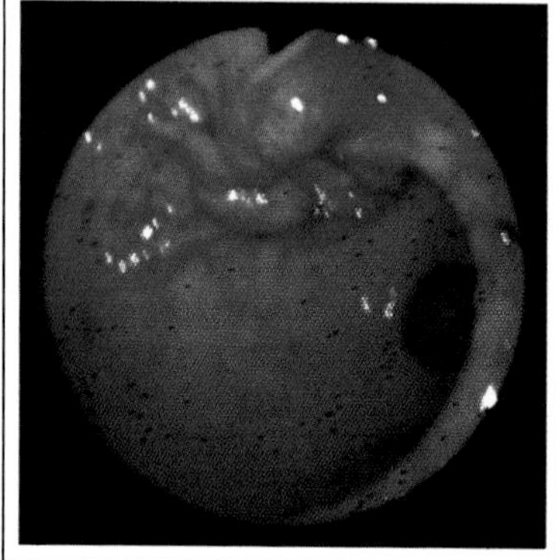

FIG. 15-27.

FIG. 15-26. Indeterminate ulcer in a mass-like deformity with intact overlying mucosa. At surgery this was found to be a deeply penetrating gastric ulcer associated with lymphoid proliferation (called pseudolymphoma—see Chapter 20).

FIG. 15-27. Indeterminate ulcer, submucosal mass-like deformity with central ulceration presenting with gastric bleeding. The ulcer itself was incompletely viewed. At surgery, infiltrating carcinoma was found with the overlying mucosa completely intact.

using the term indeterminate rather than another in which the word malignancy appears—which could be interpreted by the clinician to mean no option except surgery.

BIOPSY AND BRUSHING CYTOLOGY FOR BENIGN AND INDETERMINATE GASTRIC ULCERS

Although biopsy and brushing cytology (see Chapter 1) increase the accuracy of endoscopy for determining the nature of gastric ulcers beyond that which can be achieved from visual assessment alone,[4,17–19] these modalities do not replace the need for careful endoscopic examination of any ulcer because endoscopy to a large extent determines how vigorously one will pursue biopsy and brushing cytology. Naturally, all endoscopists develop their own policy as to the number of biopsies to be taken and when to employ cytologic studies. In this section we present our policy in terms of benign and indeterminate ulcers, where the endoscopic assessment of both the size as well as the nature of the ulcer determines how aggressively biopsy and brushing cytology are pursued. (Our policy concerning malignant ulcers is discussed in Chapter 16.)

Benign Ulcers (<1 cm)

The incidence of cancer in benign-appearing ulcers of less than 1 cm is low enough (<3%)[5] to make biopsy and brushing cytology seem superfluous. For ulcers less than 5 mm, especially if multiple (Fig. 15-20) and if aspirin or another nonsteroidal anti-inflammatory agent can be incriminated, biopsy and brushings may be entirely dispensed with. For ulcers between 5 mm and 1 cm (Fig. 15-23a), we generally prefer to take a set of four-quadrant biopsies and perform at least one brushing of the margin rather than attempt eight or more biopsies, which is often not feasible in these small ulcers. Although the policy of taking only four biopsies could miss up to 10% of cancers present,[17] because the incidence of cancer in this group is so low (only 6% of malignant ulcers are this size) (Table 15-2) the actual miss rate with this policy would probably be less than 1%. Because of the low likelihood of failing to detect cancer for ulcers of this size, unless there were a technical problem in performing biopsies, brushing cytology is not routinely performed.

Benign Ulcer (1 to 2 cm)

For ulcers having a maximum dimension of 1 to 2 cm, we find an incidence of malignancy of 15% contrasted with 6% for ulcers of less than 1 cm (Table 15-2). Because of the incidence of cancer for these ulcers, a more aggressive biopsy policy is necessary. In these cases eight[17] and preferably 10 biopsies[18] (two sets of four quadrants, with two additional biopsies) of the margin should be obtained especially at the junction of the margin with the base. Such a policy would miss fewer than 1% of the cancers actually present. In these cases the role of brushing cytology is adjunctive,[19] being sought particularly where biopsy sampling of the entire margin has not been successful because of poor technical control of the margin, especially for ulcers high on the lesser curve. In these cases the tip of the standard forward-viewing instruments, even those with the capability of 180° retroflexion, still only view the lesser curve tangentially (or obliquely), so that biopsy sampling is achieved from only one (generally the distal) side of the margin (Fig. 15-11a). An alternative approach for ulcers in this location is to employ a large-channel (2.8 mm) side-viewing endoscope (e.g., Olympus JF-1T, Olympus Corporation of America, New Hyde Park, New York) to obtain biopsy as well as cytology samples from all surfaces of the margin (Fig. 15-11b).

Benign Ulcers (>2 cm) and Indeterminate Ulcers

As 20% of ulcers 2 cm or larger are malignant, we consider any ulcer of this size, which is not obviously malignant, as indeteminate, irrespective of other features. While the incidence of malignancy for smaller indeterminate ulcers, including those with either distorted margins or an associated mass-like deformity, is lower, on the order of 5 to 10%, we regard the overall increased likelihood of cancer for the group as a whole as an indication for aggressive tissue sampling with at least 8 to 10 biopsies. Cancer, which appears as a ≥2 cm indeterminate ulcer, may be largely infiltrating except for the ulcer itself (see Chapter 16). Because of this, one needs to take biopsies at the interface of the margin and base (Fig. 15-25b), as well as of nodular areas of the base itself.[20] Nine or more biopsies ensure a low likelihood overall (≤5%) of missing cancer.[17,18] With this many biopsies taken, brushing cytology[19] may be superfluous if sampling from the margin and base is thought to be technically successful. However, if the position or size of the ulcer prevents adequate histologic sampling, brushing cytology is indicated.

REFERENCES

1. Sheppard, M. C., Holmes, G. K. T., and Cockel, R. (1977): Clinical picture of peptic ulceration diagnosed endoscopically. *Gut,* 18:524–530.
2. Oi, M., Ito, S., Kumagai, F., Yoshida, K., Tanaka, Y., Miho, O., and Kijima, M. (1969): A possible dual control mechanism in the origin of peptic ulcer: a study on ulcer location as affected by mucosa and musculature. *Gastroenterology,* 57:280–293.
3. Miyake, T., Suzaki, T., and Oishi, M. (1980): Correlation of gastric ulcer healing features by endoscopy, stereoscopic microscopy, and histology, and a reclassification of the epithelial regenerative process. *Dig. Dis. Sci.,* 25:8–14.
4. Nelson, R. S., Urrea, L. H., and Lanza, F. L. (1976): Evaluation of gastric ulcerations. *Am. J. Dig. Dis.,* 21:389–392.
5. Mountford, R. A., Brown, P., Salmon, P. R., Alvarenga, C., Neumann, C. S., and Read, A. E. (1980): Gastric cancer detection in gastric ulcer disease. *Gut,* 21:9–17.
6. Miyake, T., Ariyoshi, J., Suzaki, T., Oishi, M., Sakai, M., and Ueda, S. (1980): Endoscopic evaluation of the effect of sucralfate therapy and other clinical parameters on the recurrence rate of gastric ulcers. *Dig. Dis. Sci.,* 25:1–7.

6a. Isenberg, J. I., Peterson, W. L., Elashoff, J. D., Sandersfeld, M. A., Reedy, T. J., Ippoliti, A. F., Van Deventer, G. M., Frankl, H., Longstreth, G. F., and Anderson, D. S. (1983): Healing of benign gastric ulcer with low-dose antacid or cimetidine. *N. Engl. J. Med.,* 308:1319–1324.

6b. Wright, J. P., Young, G. O., Klaff, L. J., Weers, L. A., Price, S. K., and Marks, I. N. (1982): Gastric mucosal prostaglandin E levels in patients with gastric ulcer disease and carcinoma. *Gastroenterology,* 82:263–267.

7. Cameron, A. J. (1975): Aspirin and gastric ulcer. *Mayo Clin. Proc.,* 50:565–570.
8. Caruso, I., and Bianchi-Porro, G. (1980): Gastroscopic evaluation of anti-inflammatory agents. *Br. Med. J.,* 1:75–78.

8a. Messer, J., Reitman, D., Sacks, H. S., Smith, H., and Chalmers, T. C. (1983): Association of adrenocorticosteroid therapy and peptic-ulcer disease. *N. Engl. J. Med.,* 309:21–24.

9. Gerber, L. H., Rooney, P. J., and McCarthy, D. M. (1980): Healing of peptic ulcers during continuing anti-inflammatory drug therapy in rheumatoid arthritis. *J. Clin. Gastroenterol.,* 3:7–11.
10. Silvoso, G. R., Ivey, K. J., Butt, J. H., Lockard, O. O., Holt, S. D., Sisk, C., Baskin, W. N., Mackercher, P. A., and Hewett, J. (1979): Incidence of gastric lesions in patients with rheumatic disease on chronic aspirin therapy. *Ann. Intern. Med.,* 91:517–570.

10a. Hoftiezer, J. W., O'Laughlin, J. C., and Ivey, K. J. (1982): Effects of 24 hours of aspirin, bufferin, paracetamol, and placebo on normal gastroduodenal mucosa. *Gut,* 23:692–697.

10b. Lanza, F. L., Royer, G. L., Nelson, R. S., Chen, T. T., Seckman,

C. E., and Rack, M. F. (1979): The effects of ibuprofen, indomethacin, aspirin, naproxen, and placebo on gastric mucosa of normal volunteers. *Dig. Dis. Sci.*, 24:823–828.

10c. Graham, D. Y., Smith, J. L., and Dobbs, S. M. (1983): Gastric adaptation occurs with aspirin administration in man. *Dig. Dis. Sci.*, 28:1–6.

10d. Wright, J. P., Young, G. O., Klaff, L. J., Weers, L. A., Price, S. K., and Marks, I. N. (1982): Gastric mucosal prostaglandin E levels in patients with gastric ulcer disease and carcinoma. *Gastroenterology*, 82:263–267.

10e. Konturek, S. J., Piastucki, I., Brzozowski, T., Kadecki, T., Dembinska-Kiec, A., Zmuda, A., and Gryglewski, R. (1981): Role of prostaglandins in the formation of aspirin-induced gastric ulcers. *Gastroenterology*, 80:4–9.

10f. O'Laughlin, J. D., Silvoso, G. R., and Ivey, K. J. (1981): Healing of aspirin-associated peptic ulcer disease despite continued salicylate ingestion. *Arch. Intern. Med.*, 141:781–783.

11. MacDonald, W. C. (1973): Correlation of mucosal histology and aspirin intake in chronic gastric ulcer. *Gastroenterology*, 65:381–389.

12. Hamilton, S. R., and Yardley, J. H. (1980): Endoscopic biopsy diagnosis of aspirin-associated chronic gastric ulcers. *Gastroenterology*, 78:1176.

13. Ito, Y., Blackstone, M. O., and Hatfield, G. E. (1978): Gastrogastric fistula linking two penetrating ulcers: report of a case. *Gastrointest. Endosc.*, 24:247–248.

14. Winans, C. S., Yoshii, Y., and Kobayashi, S. (1972): Endoscopic diagnosis of multiple benign gastric ulcers. *Gastrointest. Endosc.*, 19:63–66.

15. Morgan, A. G., McAdam, A. F., Pyrah, R. D., and Tinsley, G. F. (1976): Multiple recurring gastric erosions (aphthous ulcers). *Gut*, 17:633–639.

16. Segal, A. W., Healy, M. J. R., Cox, A. B., Williams, I., Slavin, G., Smithies, A., and Levi, A. J. (1975): Diagnosis of gastric cancer. *Br. Med. J.*, 2:669–672.

16a. Kobayaski, S., Kasugai, T., and Yamazaki, H. (1979): Endoscopic differentiation of early gastric cancer from benign peptic ulcer. *Gastrointest. Endosc.*, 25:55–57.

17. Sancho-Poch, F. J., Balanzo, J., Ocana, J., Presa, E., Sala-Cladera E., Cusso, X., and Vilardell, F. (1978): An evaluation of gastric biopsy in the diagnosis of gastric cancer. *Gastrointest. Endosc.*, 24:281–282.

18. Dekker, N., and Tytgat, G. N. (1977): Diagnostic accuracy of fiber-endoscopy in the detection of upper intestinal malignancy: a follow-up analysis. *Gastroenterology*, 73:710–714.

19. Witzel, L., Halter, F., Gretillat, P. A., Scheurer, U., and Keller, M. (1976): Evaluation of specific value of endoscopic biopsies and brush cytology for malignancies of the oesophagus and stomach. *Gut*, 17:375–377.

20. Hatfield, A. R. W., Slavin, G., Segal, A. W., and Levi, A. J. (1975): Importance of the site of endoscopic gastric biopsy in ulcerating lesions of the stomach. *Gut*, 16:884–886.

16

GASTRIC MALIGNANCIES

In keeping with the well-known decline in the incidence of gastric cancer in the United States over the past 40 years,[1] gastric malignancies are seen relatively infrequently at endoscopy. Over a 7-year period (1974–1980) they accounted for only 2 to 3% of 5,000 patients examined. Still, these are the commonest malignancies found at upper gastrointestinal (GI) endoscopy. Therefore, the endoscopist must by familiar with their varied appearances as well as the features which allow their differentiation from benign lesions. Moreover, he must be knowledgeable concerning biopsy and brushing cytology of malignant lesions so that a definitive diagnosis is provided, even if, as is so often the case, this changes neither management nor outcome.

ADENOCARCINOMA

The commonest gastric malignancy is adenocarcinoma, which in our experience (Table 16-1) accounts for 85% of gastric malignancies. Among our patients, adenocarcinoma was 10 times more common than lymphoma, the latter accounting for 8.4% of the cases. Others have found even a greater predominance of adenocarcinoma, with lymphomas representing only 3 to 4% of the cases or less.[2]

Endoscopically, we may recognize adenocarcinoma as advanced or early, in which cases the macroscopic appearance predicts well whether the cancer is extended into or beyond the muscularis propria (advanced gastric cancer) or falls short of it (early gastric cancer).

TABLE 16-1. *Types of gastric malignancy seen over a 7-year period (1974–1980)*

Type	No.	%
Adenocarcinoma	102	85.7
Lymphoma	10	8.4
Carcinoma metastatic to the stomach	5	4.2
Leiomyosarcoma	2	1.7
Total	119	100

ADVANCED GASTRIC CANCER

In the United States most (90%+) gastric cancers are advanced,[3] where the cancer in the resected specimen extends into the muscularis propria, often through the serosa. Unfortunately, the resection rate for cancers of the advanced type is, at best, 50%,[3] with a 5-year survival of only 10 to 20%, especially if the cancer has already penetrated the serosa.[3] Few if any of the patients whose cancers are unresectable survive 5 years.

The impact of endoscopy in these patients is not profound. One study[4] compared the outcome of gastric cancer at a medical center where endoscopy was freely available to that in another where it was available by direct referral to that in a third where there was no regular endoscopy service. The duration of symptoms for diagnosis and the survival rate after surgery were identical for all three centers. Furthermore, radiology proved almost as reliable as endoscopy as a first-line measure for diagnosis in this study.[4]

Although the endoscopist does not affect outcome in patients with advanced gastric cancer, he nevertheless tries to provide the following information: (a) a description of the appearance of the lesion; (b) an estimation of the extent of the lesion, i.e., how much of the stomach is involved and whether the lesion extends into the cardia or across the pyloric channel; and (c) histologic and/or cytologic confirmation of the endoscopic diagnosis.

Location

We and others[5,6] have found that at endoscopy most gastric cancers have a predominantly proximal location, most being located in the body (Fig. 16-1a) and the remainder

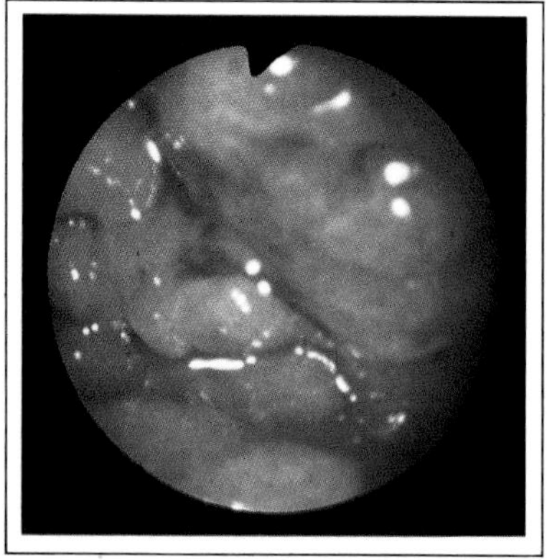

FIG. 16-1a.

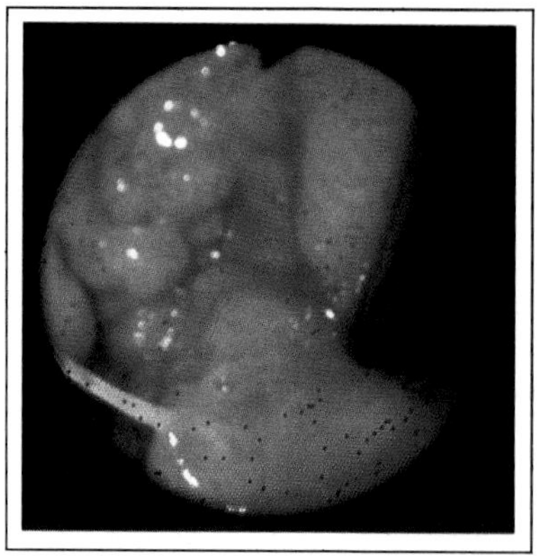

FIG. 16-1b.

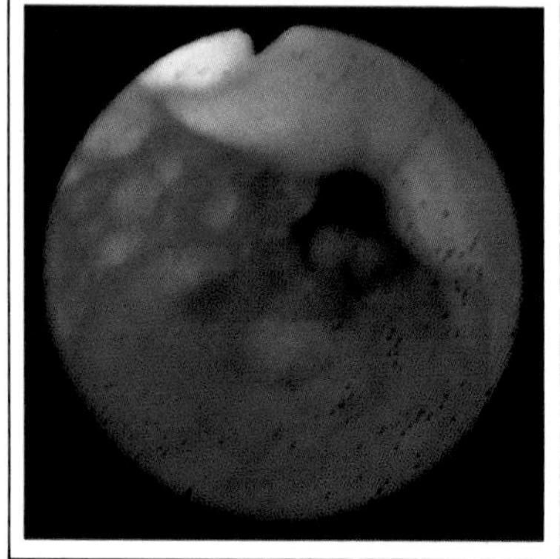

FIG. 16-1c.

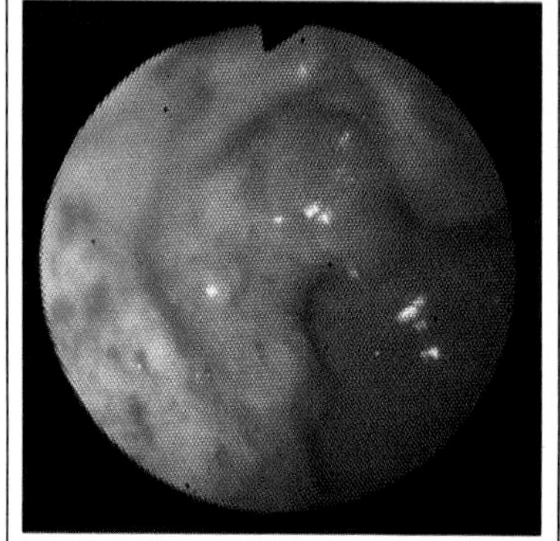

FIG. 16-1d.

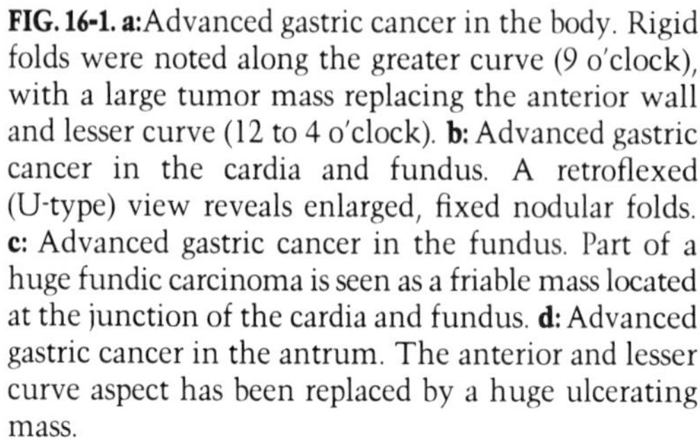

FIG. 16-1. a: Advanced gastric cancer in the body. Rigid folds were noted along the greater curve (9 o'clock), with a large tumor mass replacing the anterior wall and lesser curve (12 to 4 o'clock). **b:** Advanced gastric cancer in the cardia and fundus. A retroflexed (U-type) view reveals enlarged, fixed nodular folds. **c:** Advanced gastric cancer in the fundus. Part of a huge fundic carcinoma is seen as a friable mass located at the junction of the cardia and fundus. **d:** Advanced gastric cancer in the antrum. The anterior and lesser curve aspect has been replaced by a huge ulcerating mass.

in either the cardia (Fig. 16-1b) or the fundus (Fig. 16-1c). Over a 7-year period 56% of 94 advanced gastric cancers were proximal, 39% in the body and 17% in the cardiofundic area (Table 16-2). Others have noted an even greater preponderance of proximal locations. Winawer et al.[5] reported 74%, and Landres and Strum[6] noted 76%, of their cancers to be proximal. This contrasts with distal predominance noted in surgical series, where an antral location has been noted in 50%[7] to 75%[8] of the cases. Among our cases, the antrum (Fig. 16-1d) was the location in only 35%. Least common of all was the appearance of a diffuse carcinoma (Fig. 16-2) involving all or part of both body and antrum.

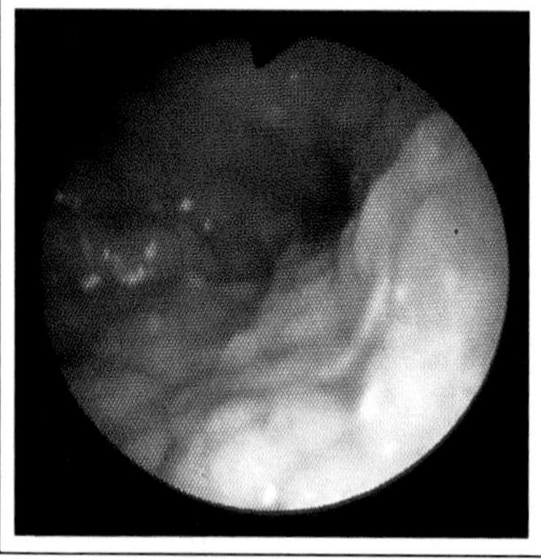

FIG. 16-2. Advanced gastric cancer, diffuse. Nodular, rigid folds extend from the upper body into the antrum, distal to the gastric angle (seen at 12 o'clock).

Appearance

The primary determinant of appearance is the basic growth pattern, i.e., whether it is exophytic (growing out into the lumen) or infiltrating (spreading within the wall). A secondary determinant of appearance for either of these growth patterns is whether the lesion is ulcerated.

Some choose to refer to the appearance of advanced cancers by their basic growth pattern—exophytic or infiltrating[5]—or use a third category, ulcerative, in addition.[6] We, however, favor the four categories of the Borrmann classification (Table 16-3) because these descriptions characterize appearance in the way we have found most useful—first

TABLE 16-2. *Location of 94 advanced gastric carcinomas seen over a 7-year period (1974–1980)*

Location	No.	%
Cardiofundic area	16	17
Body	37	39
Antrum	32	35
Diffuse	9	9
Total	94	100

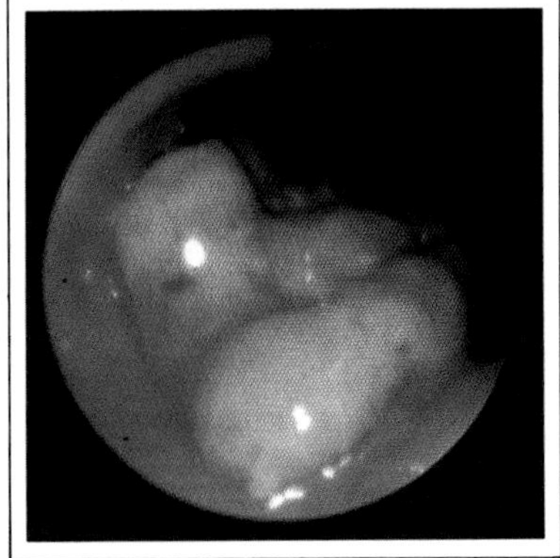

FIG. 16-3a.

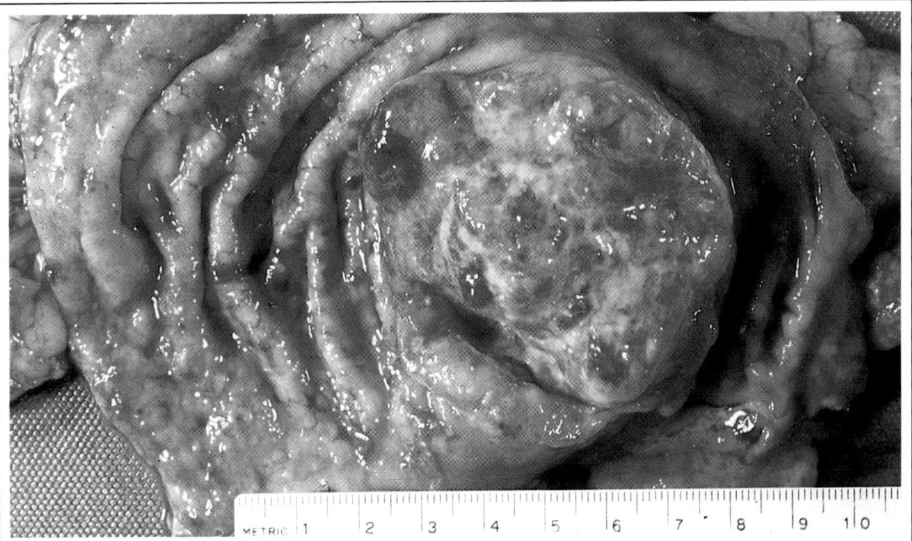

FIG. 16-3b.

FIG. 16-3. Advanced gastric cancer, polypoid (Borrmann I). **a:** The antrum is filled entirely with a huge polypoid carcinoma seen best in the resected specimen. **b:** The size of the polypoid carcinoma in this case can be best appreciated in the resected specimen.

by the growth pattern and then by the presence or absence of ulceration.

Polypoid Mass (Borrmann I)

We find that 20% of advanced cancers (Table 16-4) have the appearance of a polypoid mass (Fig. 16-3). About two-thirds of these are located in the body, one-fourth in the antrum, and the remainder in the cardiofundic area (Table 16-5). The cancer has a strikingly irregular, nodular, gray-pink appearance which stands in contrast to the smooth-textured, orange-pink mucosa surrounding it (Fig. 16-3a). In these cases the surface of the mass consists of frank tumor nodules (Fig. 16-3b).

TABLE 16-3. *Borrmann classification of advanced gastric cancer*

Type	Appearance
I	Polypoid mass
II	Polypoid mass with central ulceration
III	Infiltrating lesion with central ulceration
IV	Diffusely infiltrating lesion

TABLE 16-4. *Appearance of 94 gastric carcinomas seen over a 7-year period*

Endoscopic appearance	Borrmann classification	No.	%	
Exophytic growth pattern				
Mass	I	19	20.2	62.8
Mass with central ulcer	II	40	42.6	
Infiltrating growth pattern				
Infiltration with central ulcer	III	6	6.4	37.2
Infiltration	IV	29	30.8	
Total		94	100.0	

Polypoid Mass with Central Ulceration (Borrmann II)

A polypoid mass with a central ulceration is the commonest appearance of advanced gastric cancer, accounting for more than 40% of our cases. The mass (Fig. 16-4a) or central ulceration may be the dominating feature of the lesion. Rugal folds are seen to terminate at the edge of the mass (Fig. 16-4b). The mass effect of the tumor itself gives the margin in relation to the surrounding mucosa a characteristic palisaded appearance (Fig. 16-4b). The base of the central ulceration is composed largely of granulation tissue, but tumor nodules may be seen within the base. Because of its nodularity and obvious demarcation from the surrounding mucosa, the Borrmann II type, which is an ulcerating cancerous mass, is rarely confused with the appearance of a benign gastric ulcer (see Chapter 15).

TABLE 16-5. *Location in relation to appearance for 94 advanced gastric carcinomas*

Location	Exophytic	Ulcerative	Infiltrative
Cardiofundic area	2	7	7
Body	12	16	9
Antrum	5	23	4
Diffuse	—	—	9
Total	19	46	29

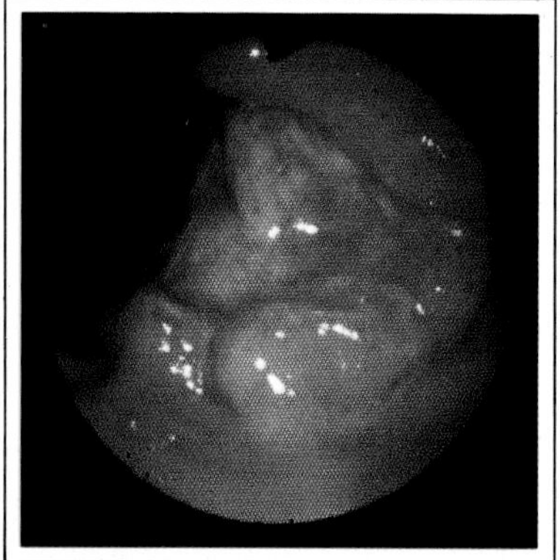

FIG. 16-4a.

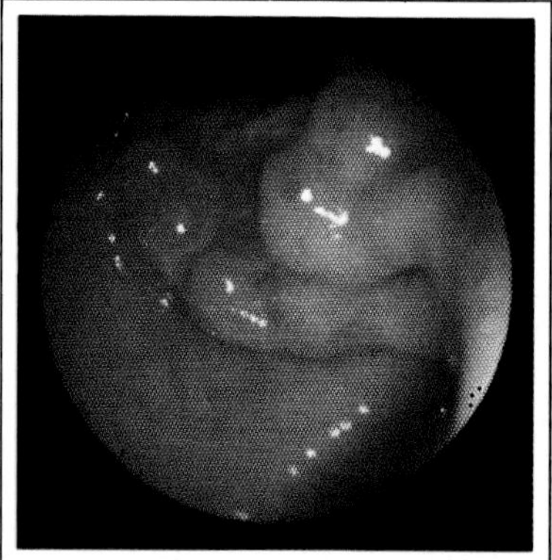

FIG. 16-4b.

FIG. 16-4. a: Advanced gastric cancer, ulcerated mass (Bormann II). In this case the mass itself is the predominant feature, with the central ulceration less apparent. **b:** Retroflexed view of the same lesion as in (a) shows the mass cutting off adjacent rugal folds (seen at 3 o'clock).

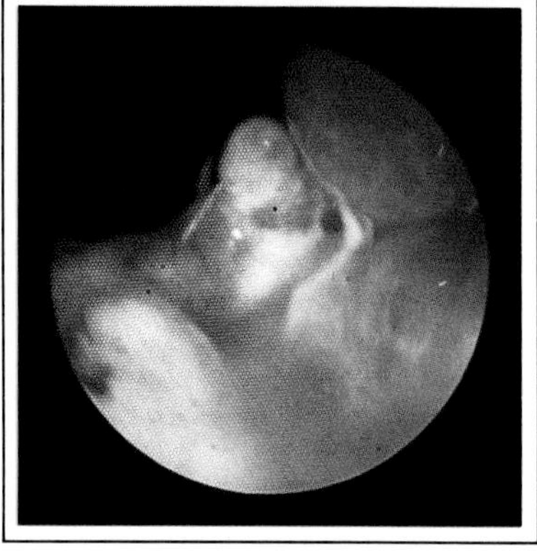

FIG. 16-5a.

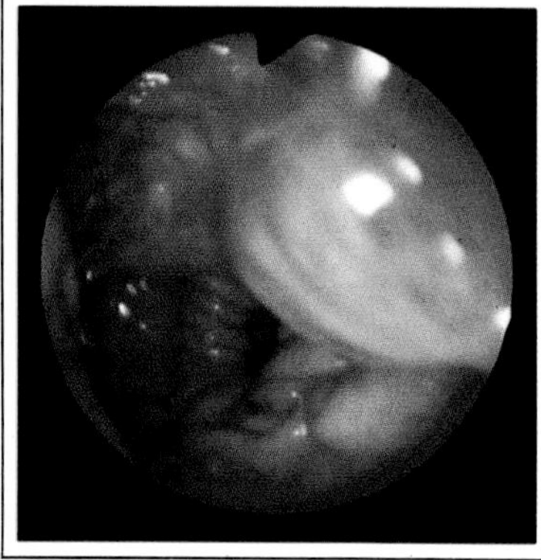

FIG. 16-5b.

FIG. 16-5. Advanced gastric cancer, infiltrating with central ulceration (Borrmann III). **a:** Large, rigid folds surround a deep central ulceration. A tumor nodule is noted at one point on its distal margin (between 12 and 1 o'clock). **b:** The predominant feature of this lesion was a giant (>5 cm) gastric ulcer (a small part of which is seen at 12 o'clock). The margin, while prominent, was nonetheless regular. Biopsies would be sought from the periphery of the base just at its interface at the margin (e.g., at 10 o'clock), rather than the margin itself (at 3 o'clock) where the mucosa appears intact.

Infiltrating Lesion With Central Ulceration (Borrmann III)

The Borrmann III appearance is least common of all, seen by us in less than 10% of the cases. It may be difficult to recognize as cancer when it appears simply as a large (>3 cm) gastric ulcer (Fig. 16-5b). Even cases where tumor nodules have erupted through the mucosa surrounding the ulcer, the examiner may fail to appreciate them as malignant (Fig. 16-5a). In cases where only the ulcer is seen, which can have a surprisingly regular appearance (Fig. 16-5a), the appearance can easily be mistaken for a benign ulcer simply set among large gastric folds.

The really important characteristic of the Borrmann III type lesion is its infiltrative growth pattern. This explains why the margin of the ulcer may consist of large folds (Fig. 16-5b) with intact underlying mucosa. The infiltrating nature of the Borrmann type III lesion is immediately contrasted with the exophytic Borrmann II ulcer whose margin is actually carcinoma (Fig. 16-4b).

Infiltrating Carcinoma (Borrmann IV)

We find the infiltrating carcinoma to be the second most commonly encountered appearance, comprising 30% of cases. Others[5,6] find it even more commonly—in 50% or more of their cases.

We find most of the cancers with this appearance either in the body (Fig. 16-6a) or cardiofundic region (Table 16-5). The smallest number of these lesions occur in the antrum (Fig. 16-6b), whereas in one-third of cases it occurs diffusely (Fig. 16-6, c and d) and warrants the term "linitis plastica."

The extent of an infiltrating gastric carcinoma depends on the principal area involved. In cases involving the body, the carcinoma is usually confined to the stomach. Lesions involving the cardia or antrum may involve contiguous areas of the esophagus or duodenal bulb, though in most cases where there is spread to a contiguous structure it is the esophagus (Fig. 16-7a). In one surgical series,[9] 80% of carcinomas of the cardiofundic region did involve the distal esophagus. Much less common is transpyloric spread from infiltrating carcinomas involving the antrum. Although this has been reported in 10%[10] to 20%[11] of cases, we have observed only one such case (Fig. 16-7b) out of 94 advanced cancers (2%).

For infiltrating cancer, we find that in about two-thirds of the cases there is mucosal breakthrough by the cancer itself (Fig. 16-6c) which facilitates both its recognition and histologic or cytologic confirmation. The difficulty occurs in the one-third of cases where breakthrough does not occur

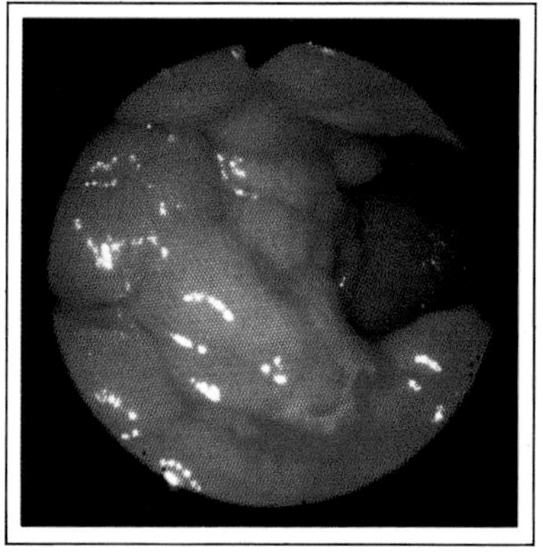

FIG. 16-6a.

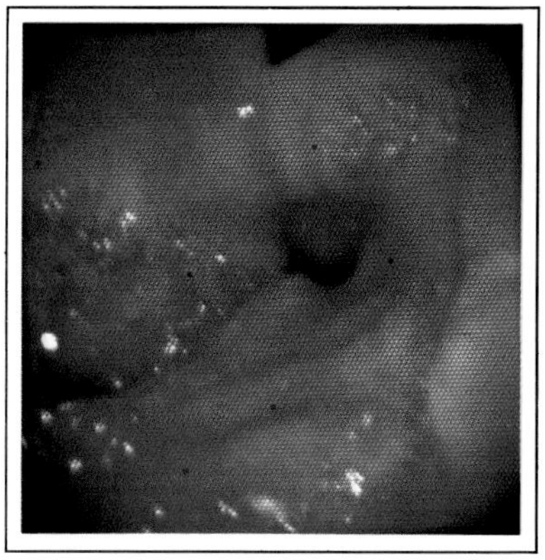

FIG. 16-6b.

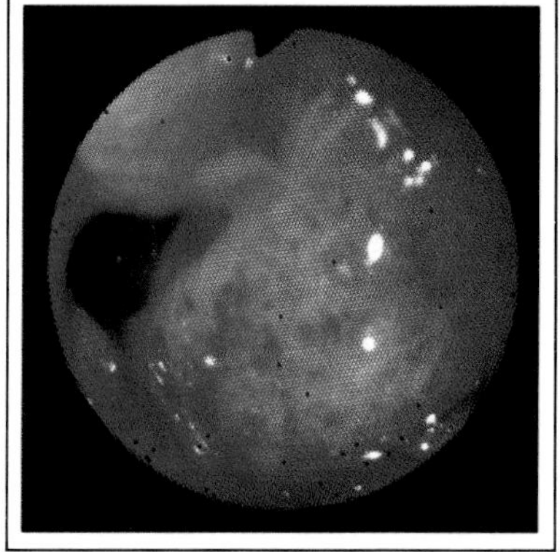

FIG. 16-6c.

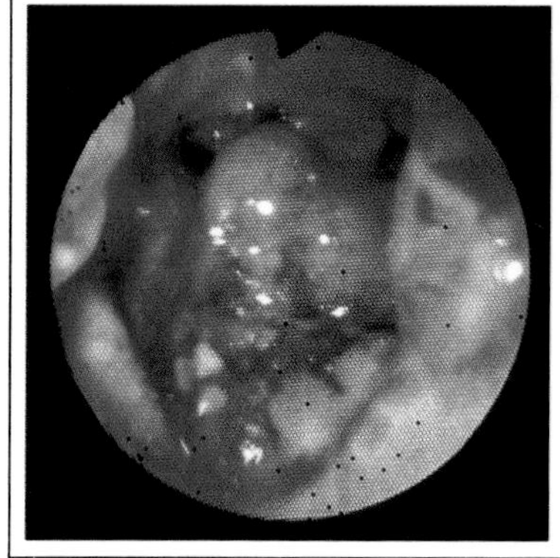

FIG. 16-6d.

FIG. 16-6. a: Advanced gastric cancer, diffusely infiltrating (Borrmann IV). Large, rigid folds are seen in the lower body. **b:** Advanced gastric cancer, diffusely infiltrating (Borrmann IV). Enlarged folds and tumor masses are seen in the antrum. **c:** Linitis plastica type of advanced gastric cancer (Borrmann IV). Infiltrating carcinoma involving the body (in this view) and antrum (d). A large tumor mass replaces the expected rugal folds pattern of the body. **d:** Linitis plastica type of infiltrating gastric cancer (Borrmann IV). Just beyond a large tumor mass in the lower body (c), a similar appearance is found in the antrum, indicating extensive gastric involvement.

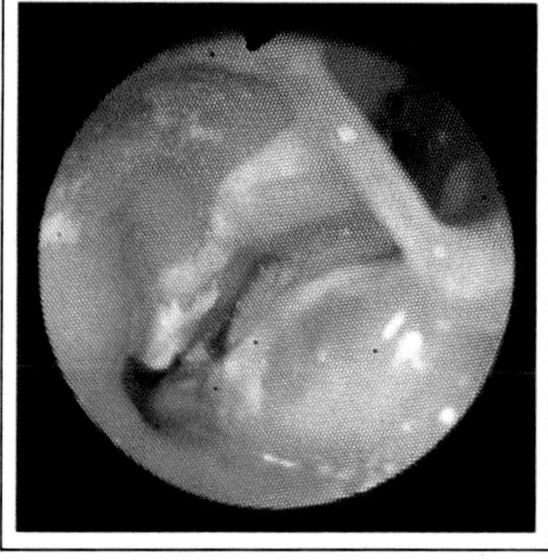

FIG. 16-7a.

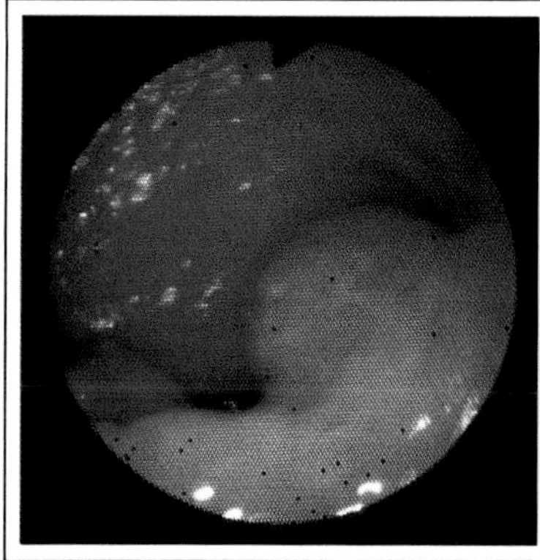

FIG. 16-7b.

FIG. 16-7. a: Esophageal involvement from extension of a cardial carcinoma, appearing as an ulcerated, asymmetrical stricture. **b:** Transpyloric extension. This occurred in a case where the antrum was diffusely involved (Fig. 16-6b). Biopsy of the polypoid mass at 5 o'clock was positive for adenocarcinoma.

(Fig. 16-8a) or is not appreciated (Fig. 16-8b). In these cases the problem is to find the demarcation between normal stomach and that involved by infiltrating malignancy (Fig. 16-8a). To do this, the endoscopist looks for two signs: (a) the shelf effect of infiltrating carcinomas; and (b) the loss of mucosal tenting.

Shelf effect.

Surprisingly, there is often a sharp demarcation between the area of the stomach in which infiltrating carcinoma is present and the adjacent wall of the stomach free of carcinoma. As the infiltrated wall of the stomach is raised in relation to the uninvolved contiguous wall, a shelf-like effect is created (Fig. 16-9a). Because a common location of infiltrating carcinoma is the body, one looks for this shelf effect in the lower body at or just above the gastric angle. When infiltrating carcinoma of the antrum is present, it is seen to produce a shelf effect with the uninvolved contiguous wall of the body (Fig. 16-9b).

Absence of mucosal tenting.

As already noted (see Chapter 12), the presence of infiltrating cancer causes the mucosa of the rugal folds to be bound down to the submucosa. As a result, the mucosa

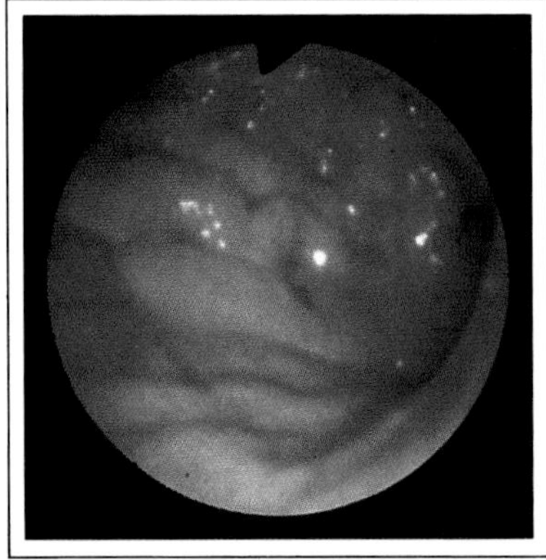

FIG. 16-8a.

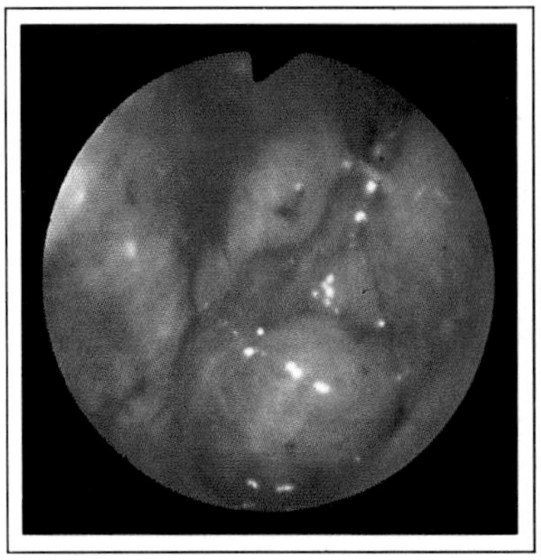

FIG. 16-8b.

FIG. 16-8. a: Advanced gastric cancer, diffusely infiltrating (Borrmann IV). The folds of the anterior wall (12 o'clock) and greater curve (9 o'clock) are of normal size but fixed (i.e., there is an absence of tenting, similar to that seen in Fig. 16-10). There is no obvious mucosal breakthrough of the tumor to biopsy or brush for cytology. **b:** Diffusely infiltrating carcinoma (Borrmann IV) with tumor replacing the anterior (9 o'clock) surface of the mid-body. Note the contrast of the area of mucosal breakthrough at 9 o'clock (erythematous, roughened, and dull) with the smooth, glistening mucosa at 6 o'clock where no breakthrough has occurred.

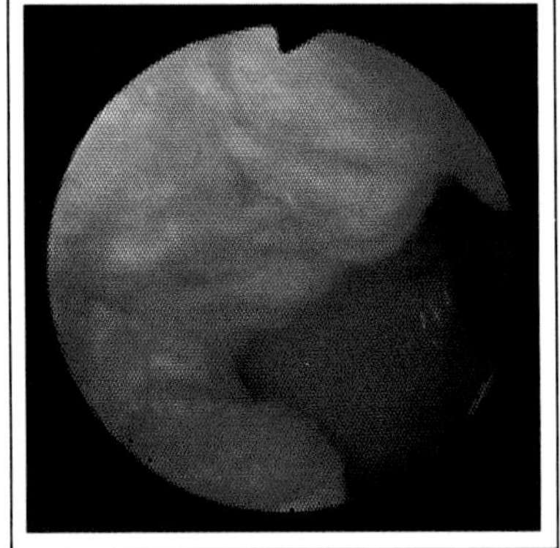

FIG. 16-9a.

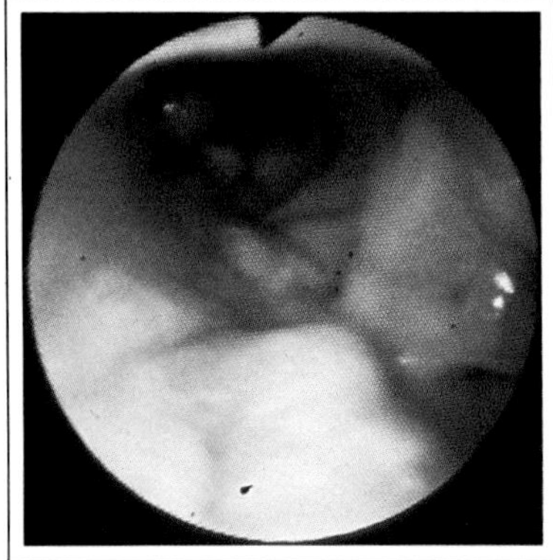

FIG. 16-9b.

FIG. 16-9. Infiltrating carcinoma (Borrmann IV). **a:** The body with a distal shelf effect. The distal extent of the carcinoma is sharply demarcated by the shelf effect where the tumor abruptly stops and normal mucosa begins. **b:** The antrum with a proximal shelf effect.

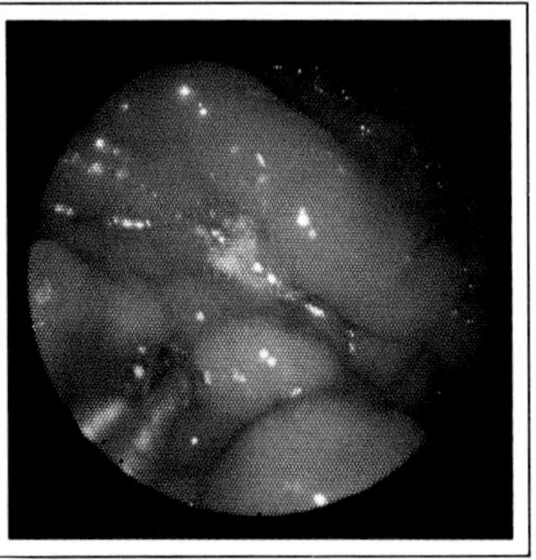

FIG. 16-10.

FIG. 16-10. Infiltrating carcinoma (Borrmann IV). There is an absence of mucosal tenting as evidence of fixation of the mucosa to the submucosa.

cannot be pulled out (tented) into the lumen but it adheres rigidly to the submucosa (Fig. 16-10), which itself is fixed due to the presence of cancer. The lack of mucosal tenting is an important clue to the presence of infiltrating malignancy within a rugal fold; folds with normal pliancy, however, do not exclude malignancy (see Chapter 12).

Biopsy and Brushing Cytology for Advanced Gastric Cancer

Biopsy is successful in most cases if multiple samples are submitted and if these are taken from points where the cancer is actually exposed. For an exophytic lesion (Borrmann I or II), finding such areas (Fig. 16-11) is a relatively simple matter. For infiltrating lesions, it is more difficult to find points of mucosal breakthrough. However, if an area of infiltration is carefully examined, it is often possible to find points where the cancer is actually exposed to the surface, such as in the base of a Borrmann III type ulcerative lesion.[12] In this case, one searches out both the periphery and center of the lesion for breakthrough, evidenced by nodularity, especially at the interface of the base margin (Fig. 16-12, a and b). For the diffusely infiltrating Borrmann IV lesion, one looks for areas where the smooth, glistening,

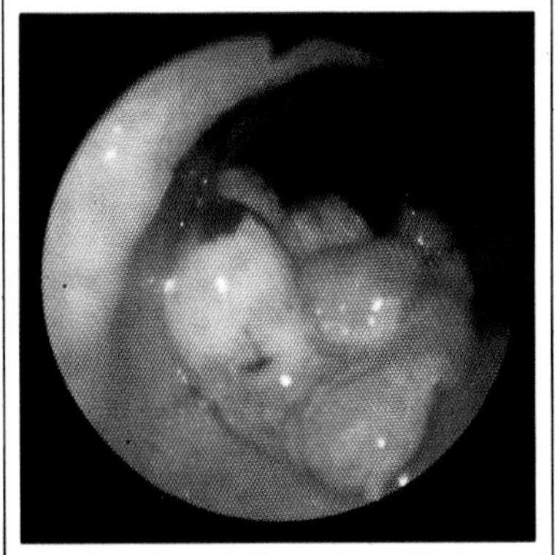

FIG. 16-11a.

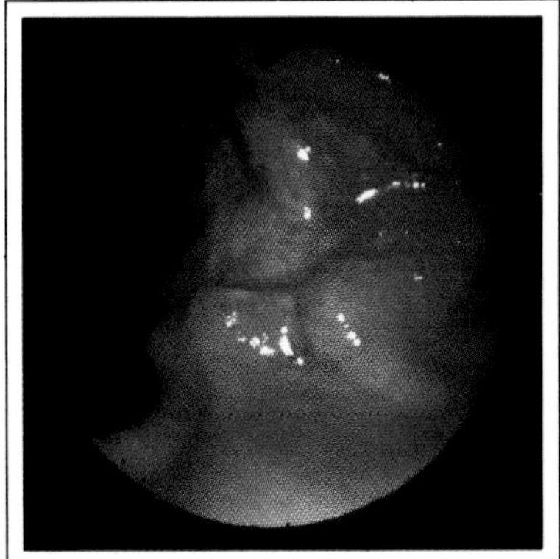

FIG. 16-11b.

FIG. 16-11. a: Biopsy site for polypoid (Borrmann I) type cancer. A high yield may be expected from biopsy from any nodule. **b:** Biopsy site for ulcerating mass (Borrmann II). Biopsies of the nodular margin as well as distorted areas of the base would have a high yield.

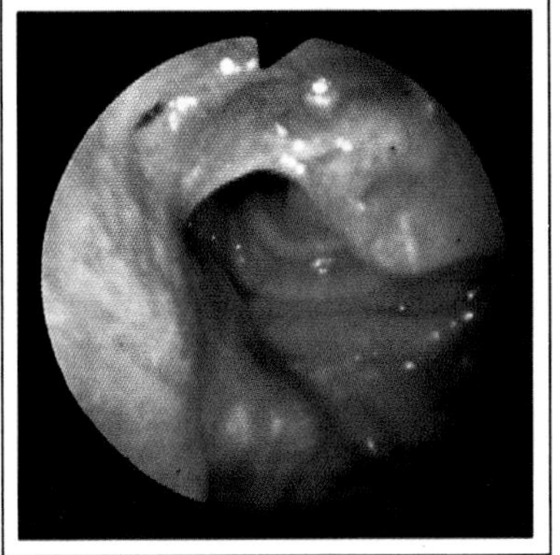

FIG. 16-12a.

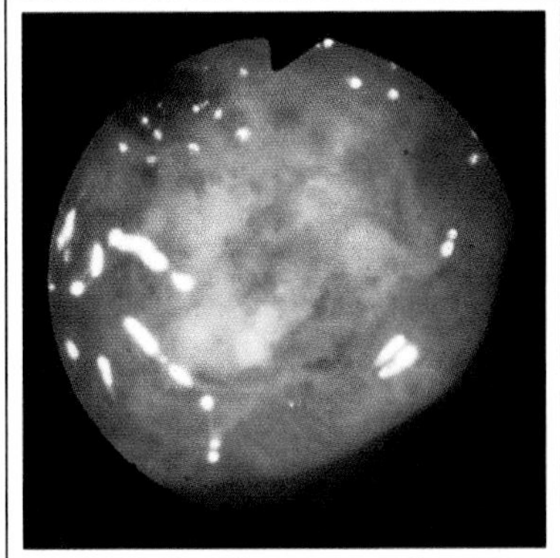

FIG. 16-12b.

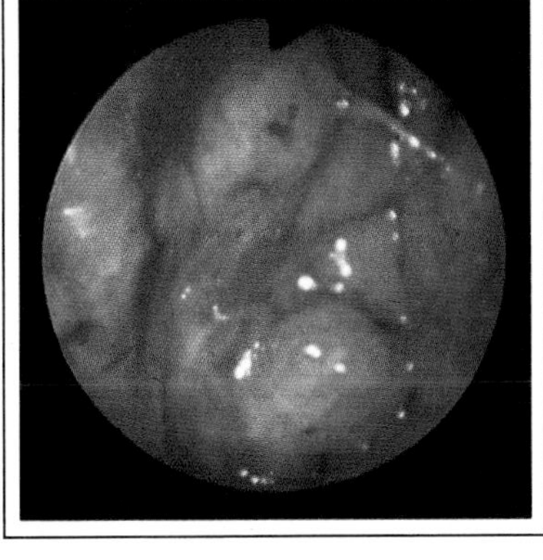

FIG. 16-12c.

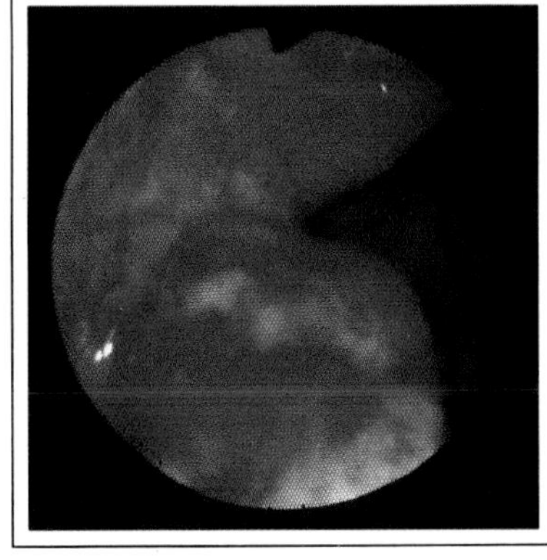

FIG. 16-12d.

FIG. 16-12. a: Biopsy site for infiltrating cancer with central ulceration (Borrmann III). The infiltrating cancer producing this giant ulcer is best sampled at the interface of its deep ulcer base and margin. Several biopsies would be obtained from distorted areas of the base itself (b). **b:** The slightly raised areas, e.g., those at 10 o'clock, as well as its interface with the margin would be expected to have the highest yield. **c:** Biopsy site for diffusely infiltrating carcinoma (Borrmann IV). Biopsies taken from the raised, irregular area at 9 o'clock suggesting tumor breakthrough would be expected to have a higher yield than the glistening, though somewhat nodular, folds at 6 o'clock. **d:** An obvious tumor mass such as that at 6 o'clock would always be a preferred biopsy site.

discrete folds give way to dull, irregular zones (Fig. 16-12c) as well as frank tumor masses (Fig. 16-12d).

Winawer et al.[5] examined the overall effectiveness of endoscopic biopsies in patients with advanced gastric cancer in which four biopsy specimens were obtained from each patient. As would be expected, the yield was highest for exophytic lesions, with or without ulceration: 80 to 90%. However, for infiltrating lesions alone, the yield dropped to 50 to 60%, and for infiltration with ulceration (what we call the Borrmann III lesions) the yield was somewhat higher at 70%. Although cytologic study did not improve the yield for exophytic lesions, it did improve that for the infiltrating type, especially when ulceration was present, bringing the yield up to 80%.

We and others[13] have found that cytology complements biopsy, especially with infiltrative lesions,[5] but that the contribution of cytology overall does not support its routine use; rather, it is useful in cases where for technical reasons (e.g., carcinoma of the cardia) an adequate sampling of the tumor is not obtained by biopsy. Moreover, as gastric cytology is not universally available, one may be forced to rely on aggressive and shrewd biopsy of areas of the lesion where one is likely to have the highest yield, i.e., where the mucosa has given way to frank carcinoma (Fig. 16-12).

In addition to biopsying selected areas of the lesion, the yield from biopsy itself seems to increase with the number of biopsies taken. Sancho-Poch et al.[14] found that the probability of a positive biopsy, regardless of the appearance of the lesion, increases dramatically when the number of biopsies is increased from three to six (from 63% to 97%, respectively). This should make one regard six biopsies as an absolute minimum number, with eight or more (with a probable yield of 99%) highly desirable. Similarly, Dekker and Tytgat[15] found that a high rate of accuracy (99.8%) could be obtained if 10 biopsies were taken from the lesion. Although in our experience the infiltrating carcinoma, as either a Borrmann III or IV type appearance, may elude biopsy, high positivity rates for biopsy are undoubtedly found when a greater number of biopsy specimens are taken.

EARLY GASTRIC CANCER

In cases of early gastric cancer, the lesion is confined to the mucosa or submucosa, stopping short of the muscularis propria. Originally described in Japan, it is being increasingly recognized throughout the world, with many centers, including some in the United States,[16] finding 10 to 20% of gastric cancers to be "early." The legitimacy of the designation of "early" derives from the following. First, as would be expected for any cancer detected in an early stage, there is a high percentage of curative resections (90%) and 5-year survivals (80% to 90%).[17] This contrasts to a much lower percentage of resectability (50%) and 5-year survival (10% to 20%) for gastric cancers which are advanced. Second, as is appropriate for the early stage of a cancer, a substantially higher proportion of gastric cancers of the early type will be found in asymptomatic patients whose cancer is found as a result of mass screening than in symptomatic patients (40% contrasted to 20% or less).[17a] Still one might prefer the purely descriptive term "superficially spreading" gastric cancer because it may be that it is this pattern of spread, one which may be inherently more indolent with a prolonged doubling time,[17b] that accounts for the high rate of curative resection and high 5-year survival (see above). Nevertheless, the term early gastric cancer is now uniformly accepted throughout the world to designate this type of gastric malignancy.

Although the endoscopic diagnosis of early gastric cancer is sometimes delayed because of the similarity in its appearance to that of a peptic ulcer (see below), there is a fortunate tendency of the lesions to remain early for a surprising length of time. In a prospective Japanese study[18] that used the endoscopic appearance to indicate whether the cancer was early or advanced (which is highly accurate in the differentiation of these lesions once familiarity with them is achieved)[19], early appearances were found to have remained unchanged, on average, for 33 months (range 15 to 64 months).[18] We have also seen a patient with an early lesion that appeared as a suspicious ulcer endoscopically. The initial set of biopsies were misread as "benign" (cancer was actually present). When the patient finally came to surgery 3 years later, the cancer was still early.[20] The fact that an early gastric cancer remained in this stage for many months or even years is of little help to the patient whose lesion is misinterpreted as being a benign gastric ulcer and does not receive endoscopic follow-up because he experiences symptomatic improvement with antacids or H_2-receptor blocking agents, e.g., cimetidine.[21] Indeed, a cycle of healing and reulceration is described for early gastric cancer which simulates that of benign ulcers.[22] Rather than rely on the uncertainty of follow-up as a means of detecting these lesions, the endoscopist must recognize their appearances from the outset so that the opportunity for surgical cure is not missed.

Appearance

Early gastric cancer may appear endoscopically in one of three ways: (a) a polypoid lesion (either as a gastric polyp

TABLE 16-6. *Japanese classification of early gastric cancer*

Type		Appearance[a]
I Protruded	Gastric polyp	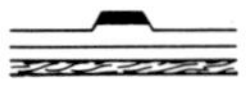
II Superficial		
IIa Elevated	Focal mucosal elevation	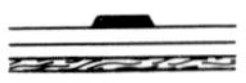
IIb Flat	Focal mucosal discoloration	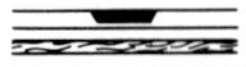
IIc Depressed	Focal mucosal discoloration/depression	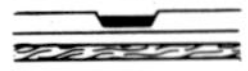
III Excavated	Ulcer	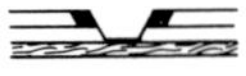
Combined types IIc and III	Ulcer with discoloration/depressed margins	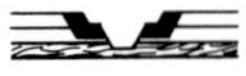

[a] Black areas indicate cancer; shaded areas indicate muscularis propria.

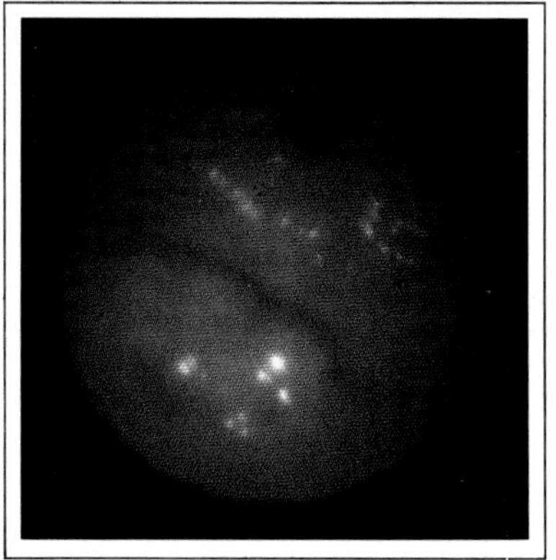

FIG. 16-13a.

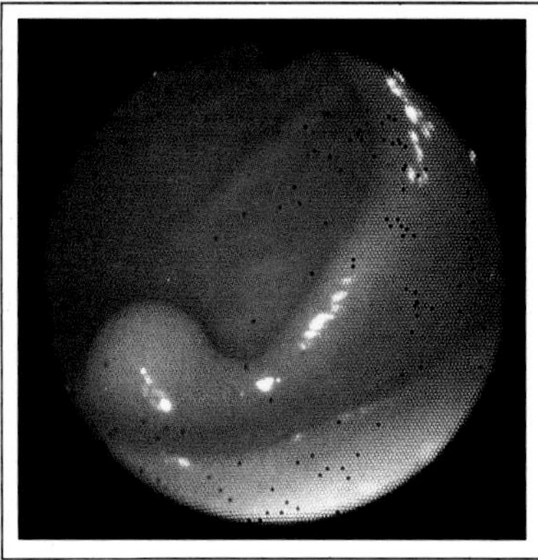

FIG. 16-13b.

FIG. 16-13. a: Early gastric cancer, superficial elevated type (IIa). A 1-cm polypoid lesion stands apart from the surrounding mucosa. The nodular appearance of its surface stands in sharp contrast to that of a common benign gastric polyp (b). **b:** Hyperplastic polyp in the antrum. The uniform, smooth surface distinguishes this polyp from the superficial elevated-type (IIa) early gastric cancer.

or focal mucosal elevation); (b) a focal area of mucosal depression and/or discoloration; or (c) an ulceration, commonly associated with depression or discoloration of its margin. A classification of early gastric cancer (Table 16-6) based on these appearances, originally introduced in Japan in 1962, has become standard throughout the world.[17] For the purposes of our discussion, we present the appearances of early gastric cancer as we actually recognize them in practice: either a small polypoid mass (type I or IIa), a discrete area of focal mucosal discoloration and/or depression (type IIb or IIc), or the combination of a gastric ulcer (type III) associated with focal mucosal discoloration and/or depression (type III + IIc; or type IIc + III, where the first term denotes whether the appearance is largely that of an ulcer or mucosal alteration[20]).

Small Polypoid Mass (Type I or IIa)

The small polypoid mass is a relatively uncommon appearance, accounting for less than 15% of our cases of early gastric cancer.[20] Because they occur infrequently and are not widely known, their significance may not be appreciated, although once aware the endoscopist finds that these are the easiest of the early gastric cancer appearances to identify because these lesions stand apart so clearly from the surrounding mucosa (Fig. 16-13a). Because of the bumpy, irregular, even nodular character of the surface epithelium, these lesions (Fig. 16-13a) are usually not mistaken for common hyperplastic polyps (Fig. 16-13b), which are smooth rather than nodular.

Focal Mucosal Discoloration and/or Depression (Type IIb or IIc)

Focal mucosal changes of discoloration and/or depression that occur as an isolated finding are the most difficult of all the early gastric cancers to recognize. Fortunately, they represent less than 30% of the total.[16,17,20] The problem in recognition arises from the fact that these areas (Fig. 16-14a) can be confused with peptic ulcers in the healing stage (Fig. 16-14b). It may be impossible to differentiate these two appearances in up to 20% of these cases, even when the diagnosis of early gastric cancer is considered,[23] making aggressive biopsy and follow-up examination mandatory whenever early gastric cancer with this appearance is considered. There are, nevertheless, two features which do help to differentiate the healing stage of peptic ulcer disease from early gastric cancer. First, the erythema associated with ulcer healing can be seen on close-up views to consist of raised red dots (areae gastricae) with intervening fine white lines (lineae gastricae). We find this to be a good visual indicator (Fig. 16-14b) of the presence of regenerative epithelium which is expected with healing. By contrast, the erythema associated with early gastric cancer (especially that of the type IIc lesion), is either uniformly intense (Fig. 16-15b) or completely irregular, consisting of some pale, erythematous areas (Fig. 16-14a), possibly representing intact mucosa interspersed between gray-white islands (Fig. 16-14c) of the superficial spreading cancer. In this appearance the cancer itself is broken up by patches of regenerative mucosa ("sanctuary" areas).[24]

In these lesions, aside from mucosal coloration one needs to examine the margin closely (Fig. 16-14a). Here one detects rugal folds which appear to be "cut off" with "clubbed" terminations (Fig. 16-14a). This may be contrasted with the chronic ulcer scar (Fig. 16-14b) in which the rugal folds have a more gentle termination, giving the appearance of converging folds. A uniformly erythematous area (Fig. 16-15b) or a totally irregular one (Fig. 16-14a) especially appearing as a depressed area, sharply demarcated from the surrounding folds, should always make one suspect early gastric cancer of the type IIc appearance. Once suspected, even if biopsies and brushing cytology (see below) are unrevealing, it is essential that the patient have follow-up examinations to provide the maximum opportunity for making the diagnosis of early gastric cancer.

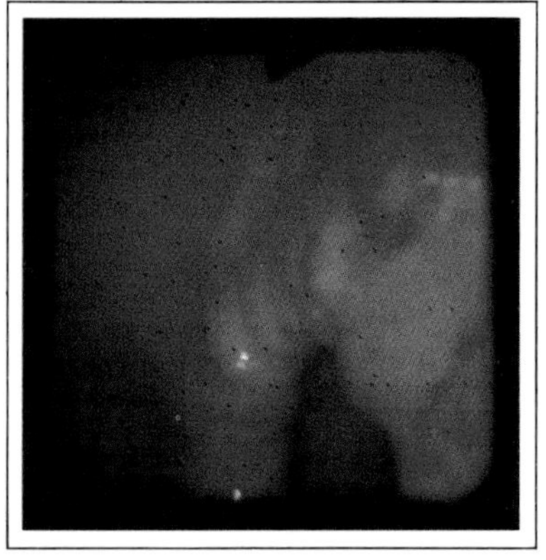
FIG. 16-14a.

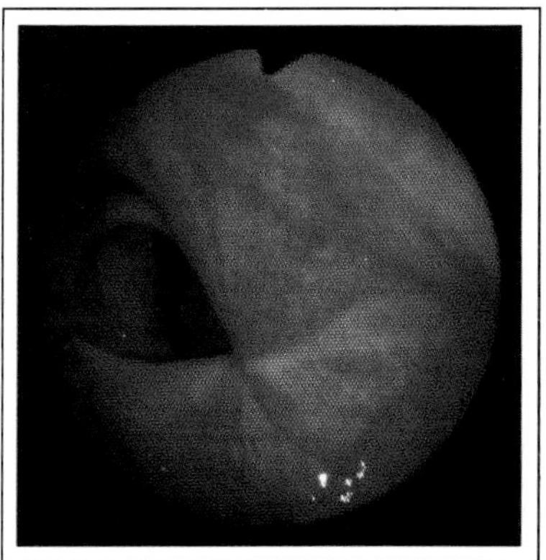
FIG. 16-14b.

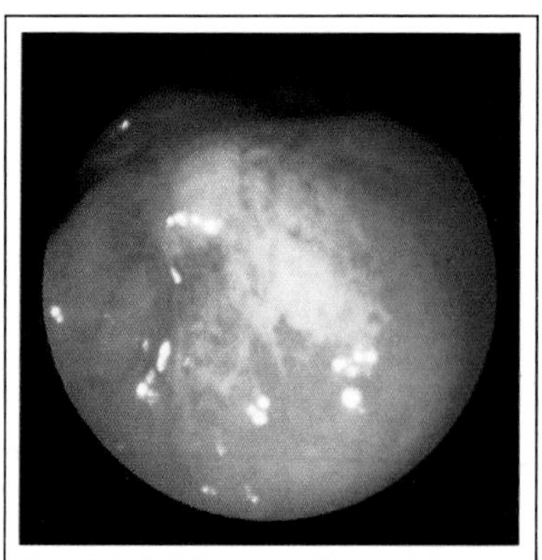
FIG. 16-14c.

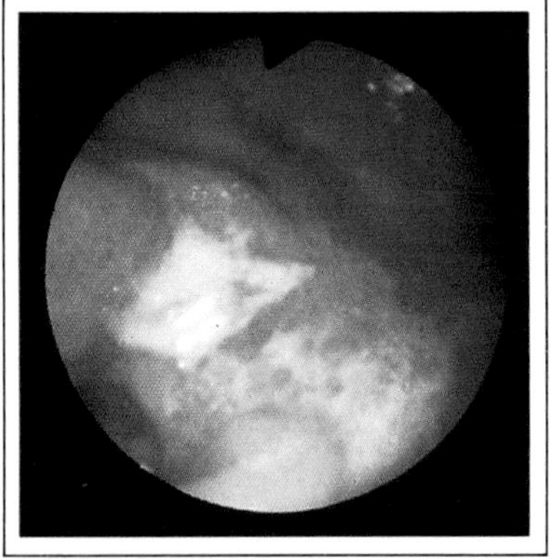
FIG. 16-15a.

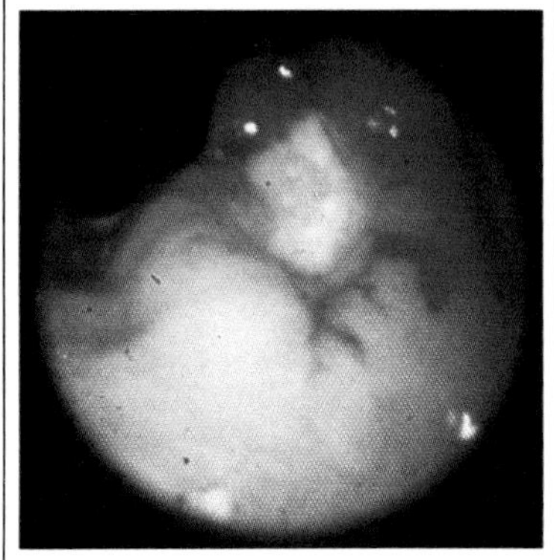
FIG. 16-15b.

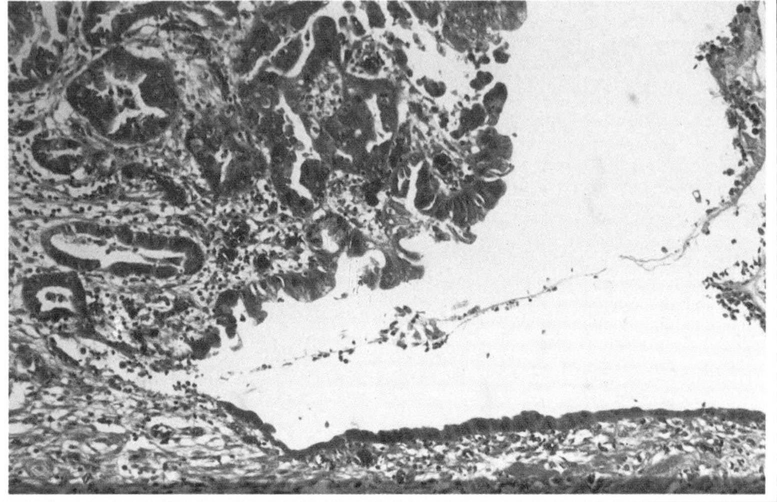
FIG. 16-15c.

FIG. 16-14. a: Early gastric cancer, superficial depressed type (IIc). A zone of yellow-gray mucosa is seen where the expected mucosal folds running to the gastric angle (from 2 o'clock) have been effaced. **b:** Healing gastric ulcer, red scar stage. The erythematous mucosa resembles a IIc area, but unlike the cancer appearance this is broken up by the erythematous areae gastricae, indicative of regenerative epithelium (see Chapter 15). **c:** Early gastric cancer, superficial depressed (IIc) type. The gray-white zone in this case represents the mucosal cancer with the orange-gray areas corresponding to intact gastric mucosa, so-called sanctuary areas.[24]

FIG. 16-15. a: Early gastric cancer, combined type; with features of both the excavated and superficial depressed types (III + IIc). The ulcer appears benign, with the cancer found exclusively in the adjacent IIc zones (same as in Fig. 16-14c). **b:** Early gastric cancer, combined type (III + IIc). The cancer is in the intensely erythematous margin at 12 o'clock and the adjacent depressed zone at 9 o'clock. The ulcer base had a benign appearance both endoscopically and histologically (c). **c:** Section through the margin of a III + IIc lesion (b). The base (middle right) was entirely free of cancer, which was confined to the margin.

Gastric Ulcer Associated With Focal Mucosal Discoloration and/or Depression (Type III + IIc; Type IIc + III)

In our experience[20] and in others' in the United States[16] and elsewhere,[17] the commonest appearance of early gastric cancer is that of an ulcer whose margin shows focal mucosal discoloration and depression[16] (Fig. 16-15a). This accounts for more than half the cases and in some series for over 70%. Although the gastric ulcer makes it easy to identify, in practice it makes recognition of this lesion as a cancer difficult because of the ulcer itself, which is so easily mis-

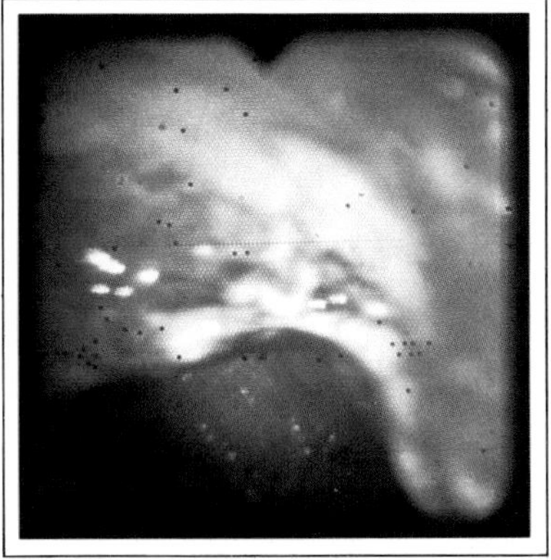

FIG. 16-16a.

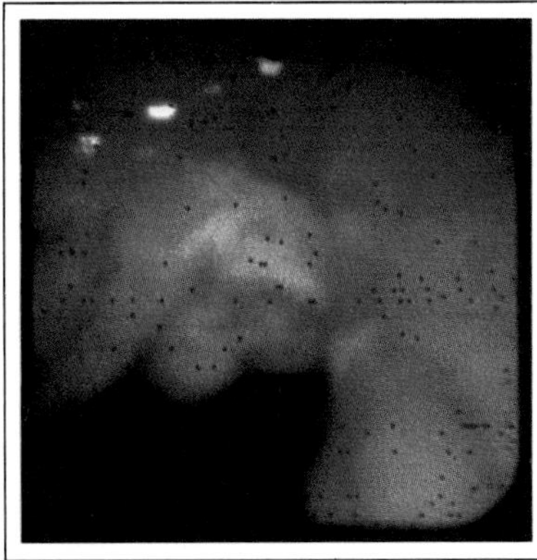

FIG. 16-16b.

FIG. 16-16. a: Early gastric cancer, combined type (III + IIc). The irregular margin with its intensely erythematous appearance raised the question of malignancy. Biopsies were negative. **b:** Partial healing of early gastric cancer, combined type (III + IIc). The lesion appears to have begun to heal with a reduction in the size of the ulcer base, although biopsies of its margin revealed carcinoma.

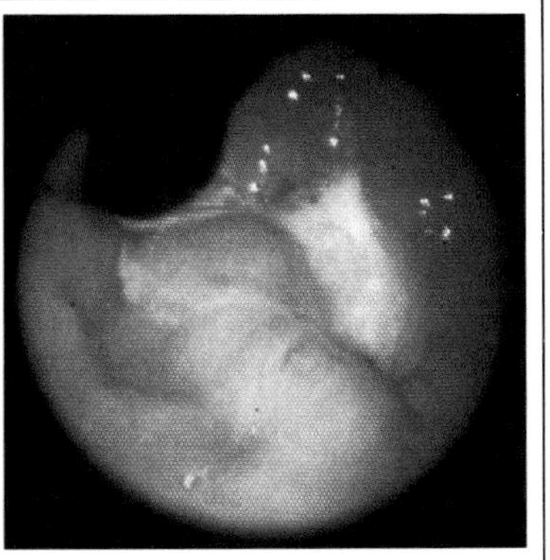

FIG. 16-17a.

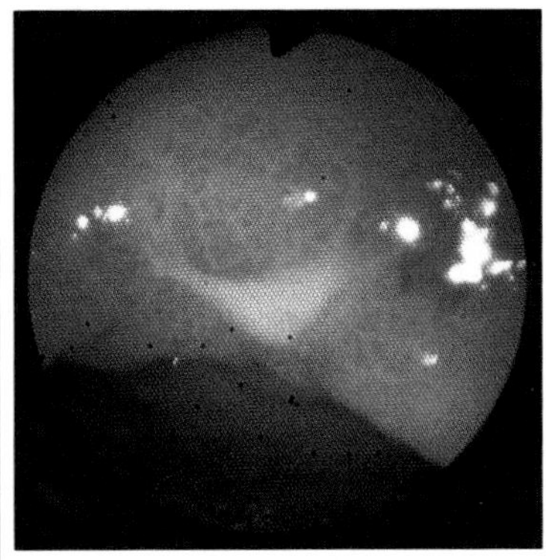

FIG. 16-17b.

FIG. 16-17. a: Early gastric cancer, combined type (III + IIc). The intensely erythematous margin (between 12 and 3 o'clock) as well as the depressed portion at 9 o'clock suggested the possibility of early gastric cancer. Thorough inspection of the margin was required to differentiate this appearance from that of a benign gastric ulcer (b). **b:** Benign gastric ulcer healing. The ulcer base is surrounded by a zone of erythematous mucosa, which on close inspection shows a pattern of tiny red dots (areae gastricae) with intervening white lines (lineae gastricae), the expected appearance of ulcer healing (see Chapter 15).

taken for a simple benign gastric ulcer (Fig. 16-15b), especially when the ulcer base is the predominant visual feature.[21] That these lesions look alike is accounted for by the fact that the base of the ulcer, except at its interface with the margin,[17] is generally free of cancer (Fig. 16-15c). Further adding to the confusion is the fact that the benign ulcer portion (Fig. 16-16a) may actually undergo partial healing (Fig. 16-16b).[22]

As far as the interpretation of these ulcers is concerned, everything rests on the endoscopist's ability to inspect the margins of the ulcer as carefully as possible and to regard any deviation (Fig. 16-17a) from the expected appearance (Fig. 16-17b)—either its coloration or its relation to the base or surrounding folds—as highly suspicious findings worthy of aggressive biopsy (see below) and close endoscopic follow-up. Generally such inspection, if performed with a forward-viewing endoscope, requires viewing the ulcer in several positions, including at least one retroflexed view (see Chapter 15) so that the margin is completely viewed, especially in its relation to the surrounding folds. In many cases such inspection challenges the endoscopist's technical ability to its maximum; nevertheless, the endoscopist must persevere so that he does not miss the opportunity of making the diagnosis of gastric cancer at a stage with such a favorable outcome.[17]

Biopsy and Cytology for Early Gastric Cancer

Because early gastric cancers are often complex lesions, with a cancerous as well as noncancerous portion, for biopsy to be effective the lesion must be carefully studied. Once, however, the suspicious portion is found, because the cancer is mucosal it is quite amenable to forceps biopsy. Still, because the noncancerous portion may be interspersed with that which is cancerous, the key is to obtain enough biopsies of an area to be certain that any cancer present will be sampled. Generally this means taking 6 to 10 biopsies of a lesion suspected of being early gastric cancer, with eight or more biopsies assuring, as in advanced cancer, a low probability of missing any cancer present.[15] For ulcers, this means taking at least two biopsies from each quadrant of its margin (Fig. 16-15a) whereas for a polypoid lesion (Fig. 16-13a) or focally depressed area (Fig. 16-14c), one would obtain biopsies from the central portion of the lesion itself.

The role of cytology in the diagnosis of early gastric cancer appears to be a secondary one. In our experience, cytology by itself had a low (54%) yield and combining it with biopsy did not help.[20] However, because early gastric cancer may be focal, the biopsy must be precisely targeted to what may be a relatively small zone of cancerous epithelium. If the endoscopic control of the lesion necessary

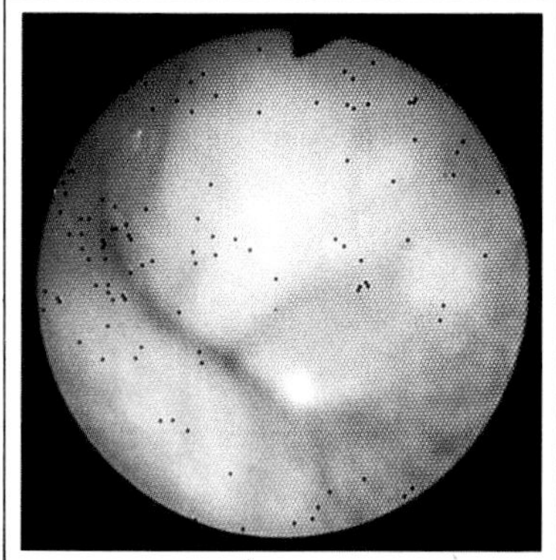

FIG. 16-18a.

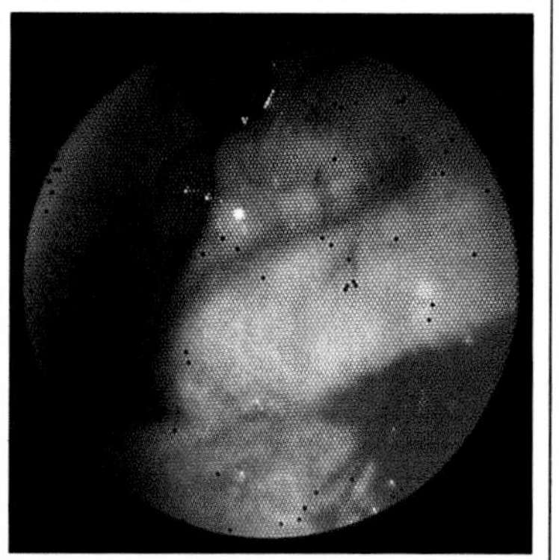

FIG. 16-18b.

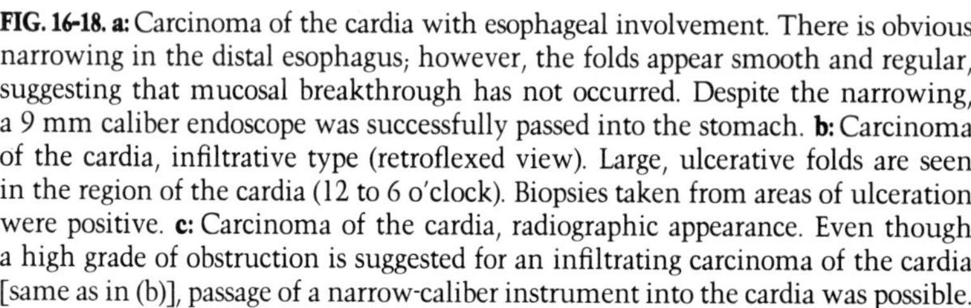

FIG. 16-18. a: Carcinoma of the cardia with esophageal involvement. There is obvious narrowing in the distal esophagus; however, the folds appear smooth and regular, suggesting that mucosal breakthrough has not occurred. Despite the narrowing, a 9 mm caliber endoscope was successfully passed into the stomach. **b:** Carcinoma of the cardia, infiltrative type (retroflexed view). Large, ulcerative folds are seen in the region of the cardia (12 to 6 o'clock). Biopsies taken from areas of ulceration were positive. **c:** Carcinoma of the cardia, radiographic appearance. Even though a high grade of obstruction is suggested for an infiltrating carcinoma of the cardia [same as in (b)], passage of a narrow-caliber instrument into the cardia was possible.

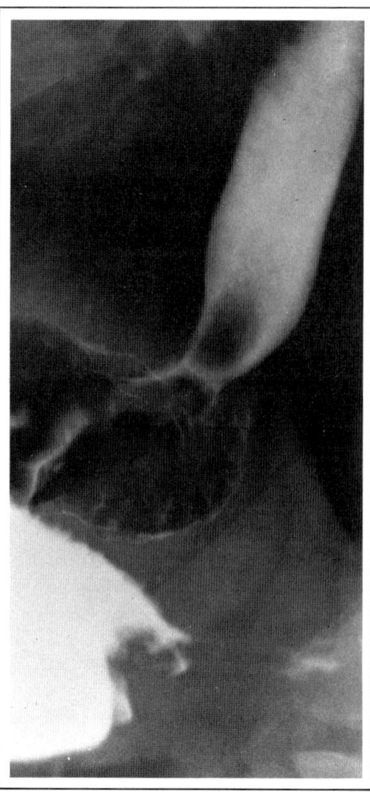

FIG. 16-18c.

to do this is lacking, brushing cytology, if available, offers a better chance of diagnosis than a poorly controlled biopsy. If cytology is to be employed, sampling would be from the central portion of polypoid and focally depressed lesions. In the case of ulcers, brushing would be from the margin, the commonest location of cancerous epithelium for this type of early gastric cancer which may masquerade as a benign ulcer.

SPECIAL PROBLEMS IN RECOGNIZING GASTRIC CANCERS

In this section we present our approach to the three most difficult endoscopic presentations of gastric cancer. These are: (a) cancer of the cardia; (b) linitis plastica (diffusely infiltrating carcinoma); and (c) recurrent gastric cancer.

Cancer of the Cardia

Cancer in this location and the adjacent fundus accounts for 17% of our cases (Table 16-2). With extensive submucosal spread proximally, all that may be seen is a stricture of the distal esophagus with enlarged mucosal folds but without obvious tumor breakthrough (Fig. 16-18a). In most cases, however, especially if a narrow-caliber (9 mm) pediatric-type endoscope is used, one can successfully visualize the cardia. In two-thirds of the cases a polypoid mass (Fig. 16-18b) or ulcerating lesion is seen in the cardia even when radiographic studies suggested that passage into the stomach will not occur (Fig. 16-18c). In all cases, therefore, one should attempt to negotiate such "strictures," which are often extrinsic impressions, i.e., a tumor outside the wall (Fig. 16-18a). It should be the goal in each case to pass a narrow-caliber endoscope across such strictures so that the tumor is viewed directly (Fig. 16-19a) especially at the point of the mucosal breakthrough, e.g., an ulceration within the cardia (Fig. 16-19a); multiple biopsies and, if available, cytology brushings[13] are then obtained from the lesion directly.

In a case where even the narrow-caliber endoscope does not pass through, one needs to use an instrument which is capable of passing the large (7 Fr) sheathed brushes to obtain a cytology specimen directly from within the stricture, thereby affording the greatest opportunity for a positive diagnosis when the stomach cannot be entered.

In cases where the stomach is entered, the finding one expects is that of large nodular asymmetrical folds (Fig. 16-19b) in that more than half of the cancers are predominantly infiltrative in appearance. Large folds therefore constitute a suspicious appearance, especially if asymmetrical

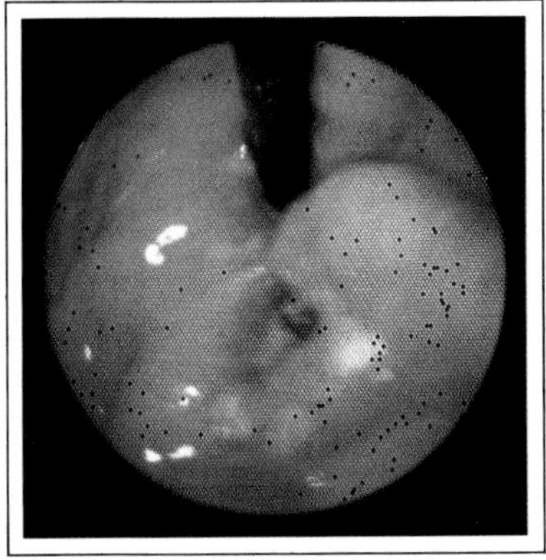

FIG. 16-19a.

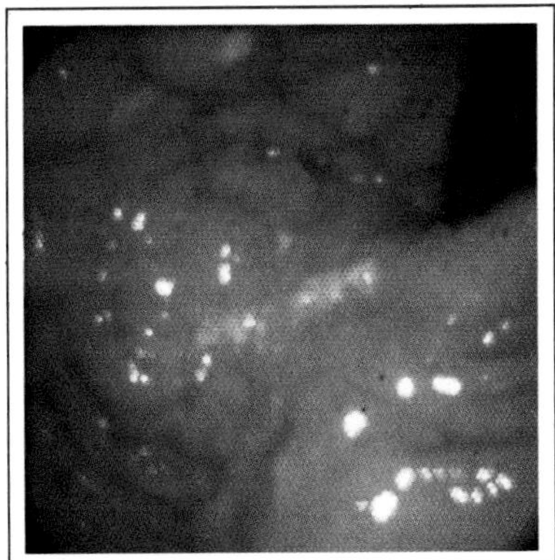

FIG. 16-19b.

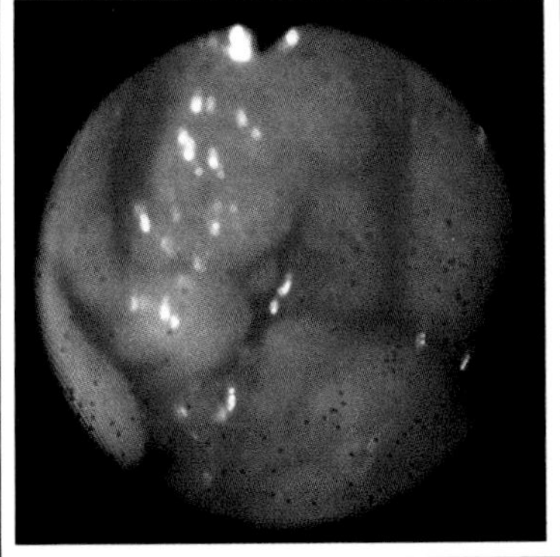

FIG. 16-19c.

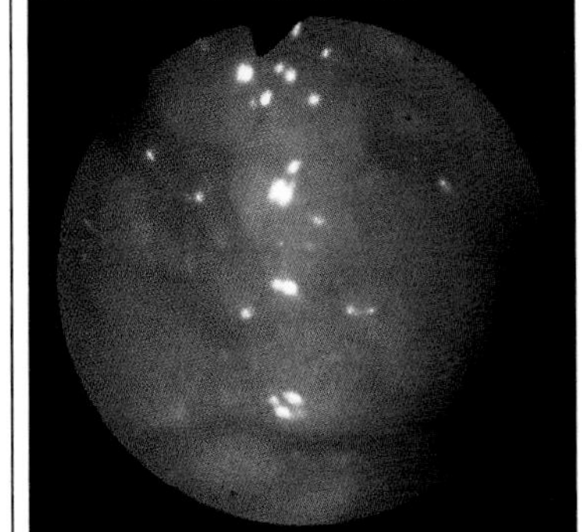

FIG. 16-20.

FIG. 16-19. Carcinoma of the cardia. **a:** The folds are enlarged and rigid. Within the cardia is a large ulceration. The favored site for biopsy and brushing cytology is the ulceration itself. **b:** The finding of asymmetrically enlarged folds (off toward the fundus at 9 o'clock) was the only clue to the presence of an infiltrating malignancy of this area. As the mucosa appears intact, it is not surprising that biopsies and brushing cytology were negative. **c:** Enlarged nodular folds appear as evidence of infiltrating malignancy. Despite their size, the overlying mucosa appeared intact, even glistening (as at 9 o'clock). As is often the case with this appearance, multiple biopsies (>10) and brushing cytology were negative.

FIG. 16-20. A mass-like fold associated with diffuse infiltrating malignancy. Despite the size of this fold, the intact (glistening) overlying mucosa suggests a lower likelihood of a positive result from forceps biopsy. In such a case one could consider large-particle biopsy (see Chapter 1).

(Fig. 16-19b), ulcerated (Fig. 16-19a), or nodular (Fig. 16-19c). Rather than attempting to direct the biopsies and cytology at the folds themselves, these should be specifically directed at the nodular and/or ulcerated areas which indicate a high (Fig. 16-19a) likelihood of tumor breakthrough (Fig. 16-18b), and therefore most likely to yield a positive result.

Linitis Plastica

In 10% of our cases we find diffuse infiltrating carcinoma involving the body and antrum. The term linitis plastica may be applied for this type of diffusely infiltrating carcinoma. It is this appearance which poses the greatest challenge to the endoscopist: First, it is important to recognize the involved folds, which may not appear strikingly different from normal. Second and even more crucial, it is necessary to recognize areas of possible tumor breakthrough where histologic and cytologic sampling would have their highest yield in the type of malignancy where these modalities are least effective.

As mentioned previously (see above) for infiltrating carcinoma (Borrmann IV), careful observation of these folds will reveal them to be indurated, rubbery, and fixed, lacking the normal pliancy of the mucosa which allows it to be tented up (Fig. 16-10). However, one must do more than recognize rugal folds as being abnormal to determine where biopsies and brushing cytology specimens should be taken. For example, if one were to biopsy only large folds, the chance for a positive diagnosis would be low (50 to 60%)[5] especially if the mucosa appeared intact (Fig. 16-20). Therefore the endoscopist examines areas within folds for evidence of mucosal breakthrough by the tumor. This appears as discrete areas where the mucosa becomes nodular, dull (Fig. 16-12c), and often extremely friable.

Biopsies and brushings may fail to reveal malignancy even though the clinical suspicion and appearance at endoscopy make it a strong possibility. In these cases one needs to consider large-particle snare biopsy or needle aspiration cytology (see Chapter 1), especially in the presence of large rugal folds in areas where their appearance is mass-like (Fig. 16-20).[25] Should this measure not be available or fail, if there is a high clinical index of suspicion, especially because of significant weight loss, laparotomy is recommended.

Recurrent Gastric Cancer

Recurrences after surgery for advanced gastric cancer are not uncommon, even when resection was considered cu-

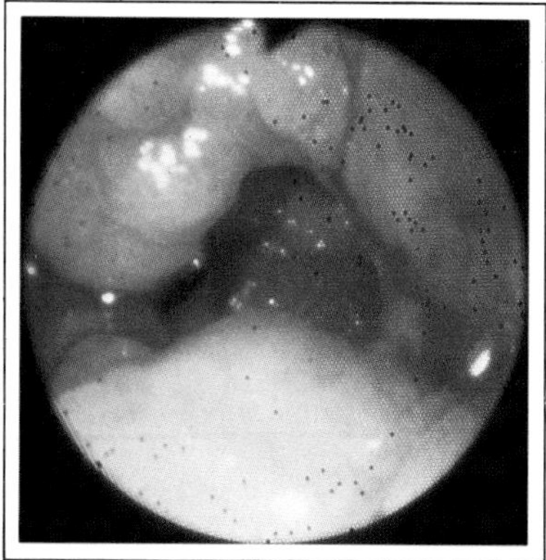

FIG. 16-21a.

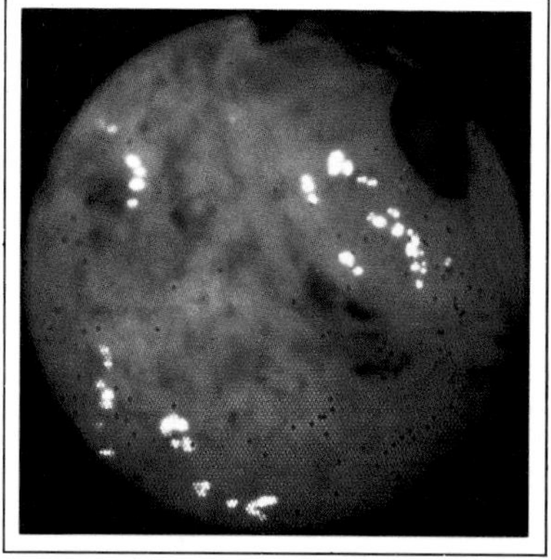

FIG. 16-21b.

FIG. 16-21. a: Prominent gastric folds associated with previous surgery (antrectomy and Billroth I anastomosis). In the context of previous surgery for gastric carcinoma, such folds may be erroneously interpreted as suggesting a recurrence. **b:** Radiation associated with gastric mucosal changes. Friability, edema, and narrowing of the stoma could raise the suspicion of recurrent gastric cancer.

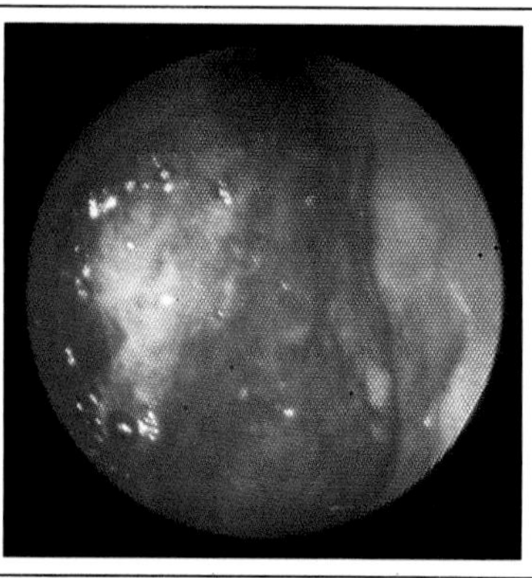

FIG. 16-22.

FIG. 16-22. Recurrent gastric cancer, nonmucosal type, at the gastroenterostomy stoma. The mucosa appeared both indurated and friable, but multiple biopsies were unrevealing. At surgery, recurrent cancer was present in the lymphatics and invading the serosa and submucosa (but not the mucosa).

rative and the patient has survived for 5 years. Between 17%[26] and 30%[27] of such patients have evidence of recurrence at that time or subsequently. For those having resections considered palliative, recurrence is invariable.[27] Determining endoscopically whether recurrence is present may be difficult. Surgery (see Chapter 19) alone (Fig. 16-21a) or in combination with irradiation (see Chapter 20) administered after surgery (Fig. 16-21b) can result in the appearance of prominent gastric folds with diminished pliancy, along with varying degrees of gastric erythema. These changes closely simulate those which would be found in a recurrence. The endoscopist therefore cannot simply regard any abnormal finding as evidence of recurrence. In this section we discuss the specific appearances which we believe to be highly suggestive of recurrence, with and without mucosal involvement.

Recurrence Without Mucosal Involvement

The commonest anatomic site of recurrence is the lymphatic system which drained the original tumor.[26] From these lymphatics the recurrent tumor spreads to involve the wall of the stomach from the serosal side, then the submucosa, and finally the mucosa (if at all). The most common endoscopic appearance in these cases therefore is that of stenosis, which generally occurs at the anastomosis of the residual stomach with the small bowel. The mucosa overlying stenotic areas may show nonspecific stomatitis (Fig. 16-22) or even a normal appearance. The lack of pliancy of the mucosa as evidenced by its failure to tent is suggestive of recurrence, especially in a patient with the stenosis occurring within 1 year of resection. Unfortunately, because of the submucosal location of the tumor, mucosal biopsies and brushing cytology are generally negative. There is as yet no reported experience using needle aspiration cytology or large-particle biopsy in this setting, although it is anticipated that in the case of the latter, its performance would be extremely difficult and possibly associated with a higher complication rate than under other circumstances, and it would still be of low yield. Unfortunately, only a "second-look" surgical procedure may suffice to prove the diagnosis of recurrence.

Recurrence With Mucosal Involvement

Recurrence with mucosal involvement occurs for the most part where the anastomotic margin was not free of tumor and less commonly in cases where 5 years or more

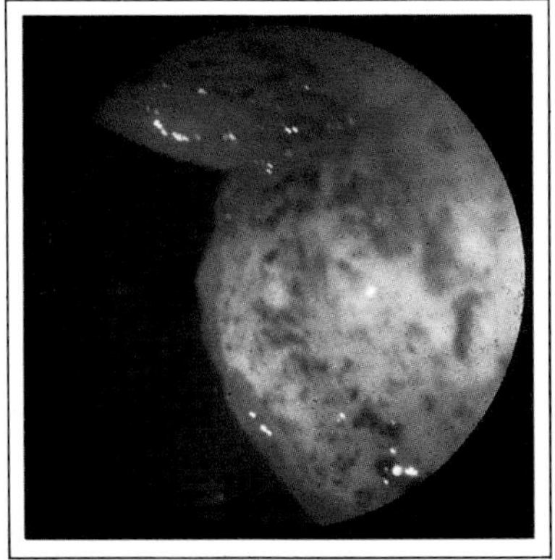

FIG. 16-23a.

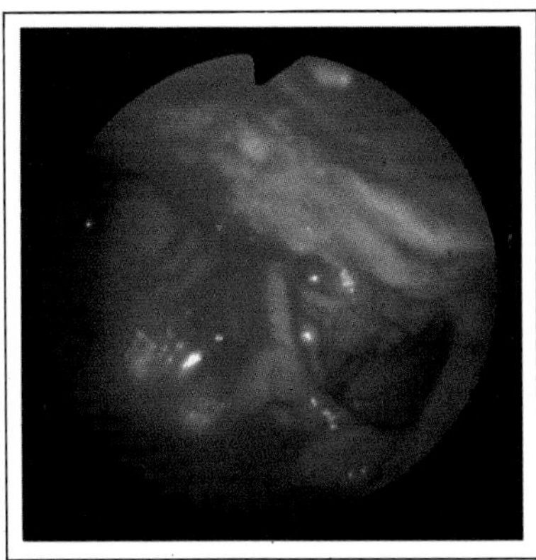

FIG. 16-23b.

FIG. 16-23. Recurrent gastric cancer. **a:** Early mucosal type. This obvious tumor mass was in a patient whose resection and anastomosis were known to be only palliative. **b:** Late mucosal type. A stomal tumor mass appeared 7 years after the initial resection with histology identical to that of the original cancer.

have passed since the surgery.[26] Some of these late recurrences may be a second primary which histologically resembles that of the carcinoma originally resected. The absence of widespread evidence of metastasis at the time of a second-look operation favors a second primary, whereas extensive metastasis with gastric mucosal involvement (noted in 25% in one study[26]) would be more in keeping with the late recurrence.

Common to both early and late mucosal recurrence is the finding of a tumor mass at the anastomosis (Fig. 16-23, a and b). In the case of a late recurrence, we have seen a diffuse infiltrating component as well.

In cases where the recurrence is associated with mucosal involvement, biopsies—if enough are taken (8 to 10)—should have their expected high yield.[14,15] Brushing cytology is reserved for those cases where, for technical reasons, adequate sampling of the tumor cannot be achieved.

GASTRIC LYMPHOMA

Although the incidence of gastric lymphoma is rising, in most series it still comprises less than 5% of gastric malignancies, as was true 20 years ago.[2] As a referral center for lymphoma, we at the University of Chicago find it to comprise 8.4% of our cases of gastric malignancy (Table 16-1); still this is only one lymphoma for every 10 carcinomas. Despite the infrequency with which it is seen, because lymphoma carries substantially better prospects for treatment its recognition deserves particular emphasis.

Of the various types of lymphoma, most which involve the stomach are of the non-Hodgkin's type, either histiocytic lymphoma (also called reticulum cell sarcoma) or lymphocytic lymphoma (either well differentiated or poorly differentiated),[28] with the Hodgkin's type being least common.[28] In addition, regarding the setting of gastric lymphoma, we see it slightly more often in the stomach as part of generalized abdominal lymphoma than as a primary tumor. The endoscopic appearance, however, does not depend on whether the gastric involvement is primary or secondary.[28]

Appearance

Some have suggested that a distinctive endoscopic appearance for gastric lymphoma exists[28]—as a volcano-like ulcer in which a deep ulcer base appears within a prominent raised margin (Fig. 16-24a). However, we noted this finding in only 1 of 10 patients with gastric lymphoma. Even Nelson and Lanza, who proposed it as a "distinctive characteristic," found it in only 9 of 40 cases.[28]

The most commonly reported appearance and that which best accords with our experience is the presence of large, diffusely ulcerated folds that involve either the entire body or the antrum.[29] As in the case of infiltrating adenocarcinoma of the antrum, the thickened folds compromise the lumen, causing a stenotic appearance (Fig. 16-24b). The infiltrative appearance of lymphoma is often indistinguishable from an advanced gastric cancer of the Bormann IV type, although we find that in cases of lymphoma the folds tend to be more diffusely ulcerated (Fig. 16-24b) than in carcinoma (Figs. 16-8 and 16-9). We observed one case of lymphocytic lymphoma that was a poorly differentiated type. The appearance was that of an infiltrating malignancy with a large central ulceration (Fig. 16-24c) similar to that found with advanced gastric cancer of the Borrmann III appearance (Fig. 16-5a).

Even though appearances may be identical, because adenocarcinoma is so much more probable on a statistical basis than lymphoma, it always deserves to be considered as the first diagnosis for any malignant appearance of the stomach in a patient without known lymphoma elsewhere. By the same token, lymphoma always deserves mention as a diagnostic possibility given the appearance of an infiltrating malignancy.

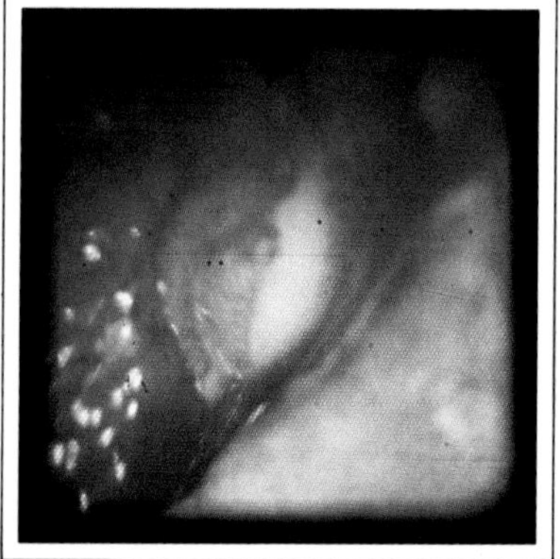

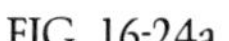

FIG. 16-24a.

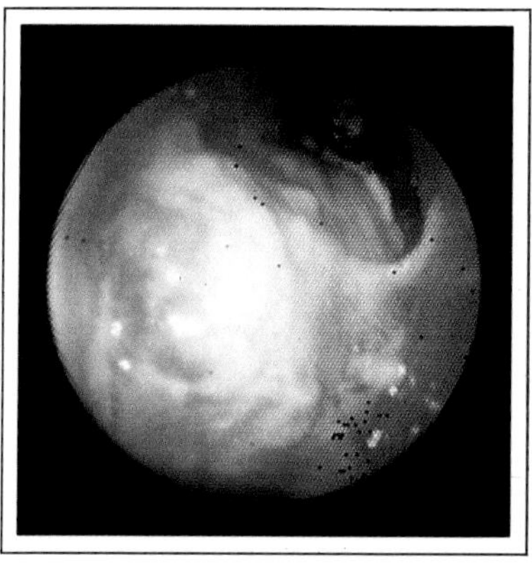

FIG. 16-24b.

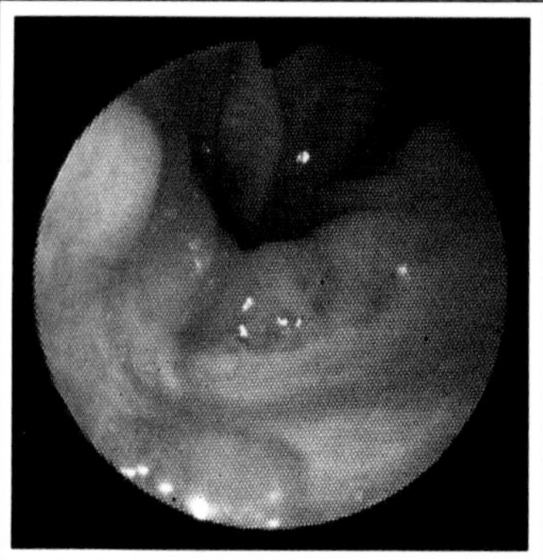

FIG. 16-24c.

FIG. 16-24. a: Gastric lymphoma, volcano-type ulceration. The ulcer appears as part of a mass which is largely submucosal. **b:** Gastric lymphoma, infiltrating appearance, with diffusely ulcerated folds. **c:** Gastric lymphoma, infiltrating, with a large central ulceration simulating the Borrmann III appearance of adenocarcinoma.

A less common appearance for lymphoma is the presence of single (Fig. 16-25a) or multiple (Fig. 16-25b) discrete polypoid masses. When these occur multiply, they are referred to as "lymphoma polyps." Ranging in size from 5 mm to 1.5 cm, they have a firm, rubbery consistency with a somewhat pale mucosal coloration (Fig. 16-25a). This contrasts with the soft consistency and eroded mucosal appearance of common benign hyperplastic polyps (see Chapter 17).

In most cases lymphoma involving the stomach does not extend into the duodenum. At best, involvement of the duodenal bulb occurs only in 25%[10]; among our patients it was only 10% (1 of 10 cases). In this case it had occurred as a separate focus of involvement (Fig. 16-26) in a patient with gastric involvement of the body.

Biopsy and Brushing Cytology

Endoscopic biopsy[29,30] in recent reports has been surprisingly successful for providing tissue diagnosis in lymphoma despite the fact that the predominant appearance is that of an infiltrating malignancy. Biopsy has its lowest yield for advanced gastric cancers with this appearance, being on the order of 60 to 70%.[5] By contrast, in gastric lymphoma the yield from biopsy in one series was 87%[28], whereas in another the figure was somewhat lower (70%)[29] though comparable to the best yield reported for advanced gastric cancer with a similar infiltrating appearance.[5] The explanation for the higher yield in lymphoma may lie in the seemingly higher incidence of diffuse ulceration of the infiltrated fold, possibly exposing deeper areas of mucosa where the yield from biopsy would be expected to be greater. Associated with, and possibly leading to, the diffuse mucosal ulceration seen with lymphoma may be a greater tendency of the lymphoma cells to be close to or at the surface, well within reach of a superficial forceps biopsy or even a cytology brush.

The role of cytology in gastric lymphoma is a complementary one to biopsy. The yield of positive results from combined cytology and biopsy has been reported to be greater than that for biopsy alone.[29] Another virtue of cytology is that it may provide a clue to the presence of a lymphoproliferative disorder by virtue of the finding of lymphocytes when biopsy reveals only granulation tissue or nonspecific changes. The finding of lymphocytes on cytologic study always indicates that deeper biopsies should be pursued, either by means of the large-particle technique (see Chapter 1) or laparotomy, especially in cases where malignancy is strongly suspected.

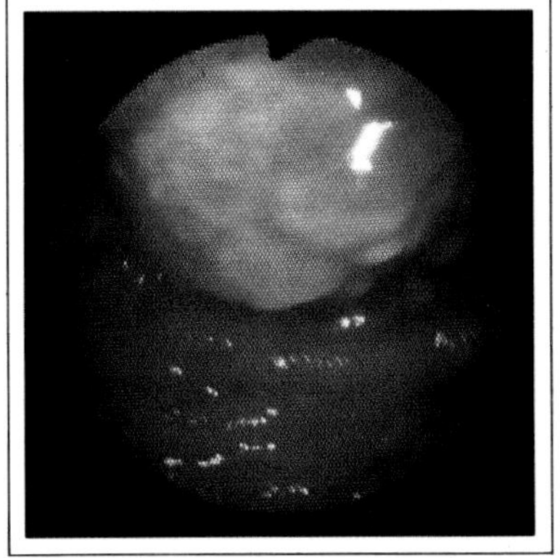

FIG. 16-25a.

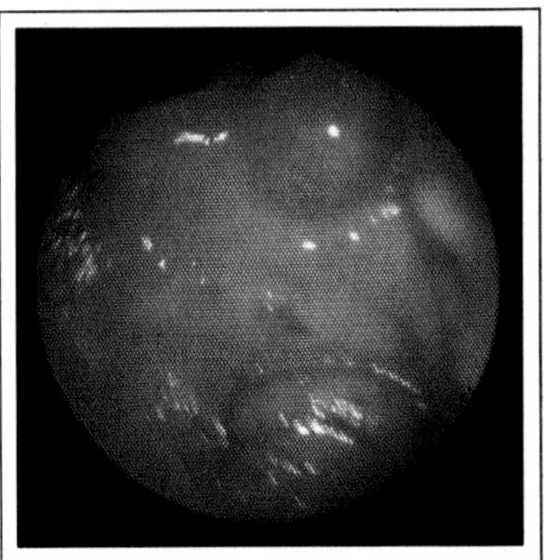

FIG. 16-25b.

FIG. 16-25. a: Gastric lymphoma, large polypoid mass in the upper body. **b:** Gastric lymphoma—multiple lymphoma polyps—were noted in the fundus along with a single large polypoid mass of the upper body (a).

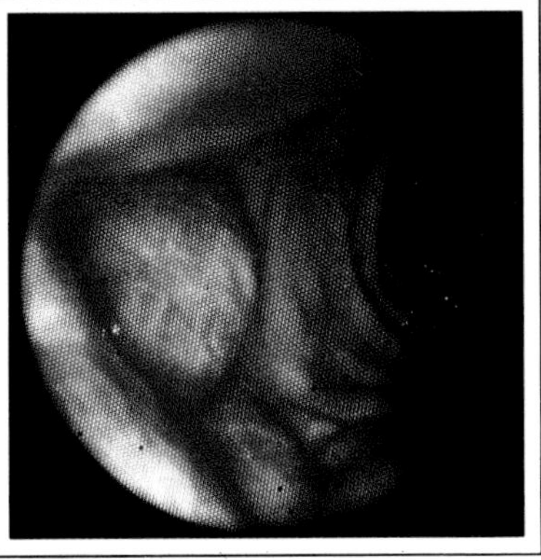

FIG. 16-26.

FIG. 16-26. Lymphoma polyps of the duodenal bulb. A second focus of lymphoma in a patient with an infiltrative lesion of the body of the stomach but without an obvious antral focus.

GASTRIC APPEARANCES IN LEUKEMIA

Leukemic involvement of the stomach is not a rare finding at autopsy. In a study from our institution, it was found in 23% (35 of 148 cases),[29a] with the highest prevalence (33%) in lymphocytic leukemia. For most (27 cases), the lesions appeared as plaque-like thickenings and elevated nodular areas. In two cases, the rugal folds were massive and convoluted to give a brain-like appearance. In the final six cases, part of the lesion was necrotic.

Despite the frequency with which leukemic infiltrates may be found at autopsy, they are rarely encountered by the endoscopist. Even at our institution which is a referral center for the treatment of leukemia, during a 10-year period in which over 300 leukemic patients were examined, none had endoscopic evidence of gastric involvement. Reported instances of gastric involvement are also rare, with only one case since 1970.[29b] In a patient with lymphocytic leukemia, multiple deep ulcers were found in the setting of enlarged, indurated rugal folds similar to the appearance of gastric lymphoma (see above).

A more frequent gastric appearance in leukemic patients is that of nonleukemic lesions which at autopsy are three times commoner than leukemic lesions.[29a] These are generally of the acute mucosal injury type, as focal mucosal hemorrhages or hemorrhagic necroses, often found in association with gastric bleeding, and are similar to those in patients with other malignancies (see Chapter 37). Less often encountered nonleukemic appearances include focally ulcerated nodules associated with opportunistic organisms (*Candida* and *herpes simplex*—see Chapter 20) and frank ulcers occurring in granulocytopenic patients following chemotherapy, which are heavily colonized with bacteria, similar to those found under these circumstances in the esophagus (see Chapter 3).

METASTATIC CARCINOMA TO THE STOMACH

Rarely, a malignant-appearing lesion proves to be a metastatic implant in the wall of the stomach from nongastrointestinal primary cancer. We have observed five such cases over a 7-year period. Among these were examples of the most common carcinomas which metastasize to the stomach: lung, breast, and skin (melanoma).[30] Clinically, the patient with gastric metastases may not have widespread evidence of metastatic disease, with endoscopy being performed for nonspecific abdominal pain, anemia, or acute gastrointestinal bleeding (see Chapter 37).

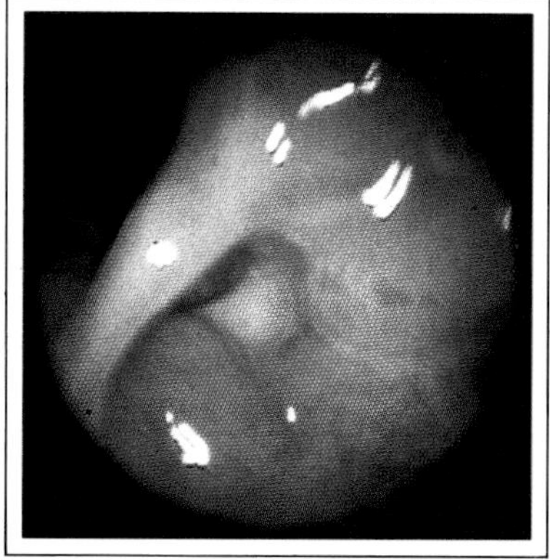

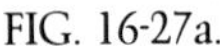

FIG. 16-27a.

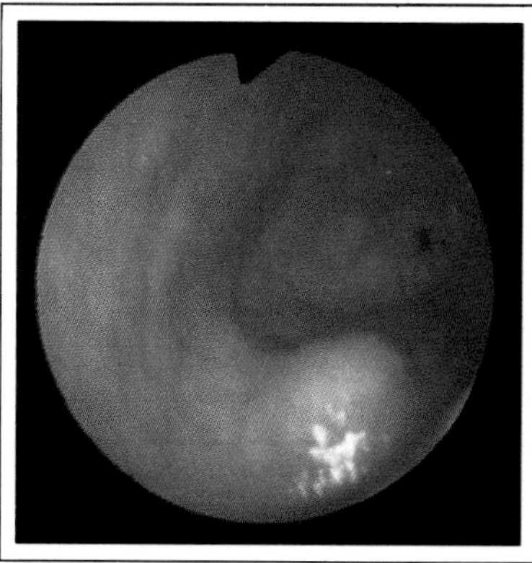

FIG. 16-27b.

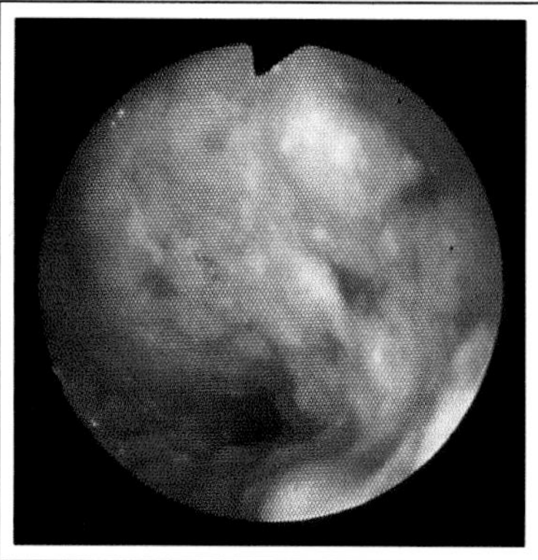

FIG. 16-27c.

FIG. 16-27. a: Metastatic cancer (lung), infiltrated fold. A central ulceration was seen in the upper body in a patient with widespread metastasis. Biopsies showed this gastric lesion to be metastatic. **b:** Metastatic cancer (colon) to the stomach. A submucosal mass of the greater curve (6 o'clock) of the antrum without ulceration. **c:** Metastatic cancer (breast) to the stomach. A linitis plastica appearance with tumor completely replacing the lesser curve of the body.

Appearance

In most cases there is a fairly distinctive appearance of discrete 1- to 2-cm circular mounds of tumor with a central depression or irregular ulceration (Figs. 16-27a and 16-28). This endoscopic finding corresponds to the bull's-eye type radiologic appearance, found in patients with metastasis to the stomach.[30] Some patients have submucosal masses without ulceration or central depression (Fig. 16-27b). Others may have a linitis plastica appearance (Fig. 16-27c), which has been found in particular with breast carcinoma metastasizing to the stomach.[31]

The most immediately recognizable appearance of metastatic cancer of the stomach is that of malignant melanoma[32] in which discrete, dark-brown tumor nodules are seen in the mucosa. However, only smaller implants (<5 mm) appear this way. Larger implants may be seen as yellow-gray plaques with some peripheral pigmentation, or, as even larger masses, they may be entirely amelanotic. Some will appear as submucosal masses with central ulceration and pigmentation within their base (Fig. 16-28).

Biopsy and Cytology

Metastatic carcinoma to the stomach which appears as an ulcerated mass or linitus plastica should be biopsied to document gastric involvement. As the tumor mass represents mucosal breakthrough from the submucosa and serosa, biopsy is often useful.[33] Cytologic study of these lesions plays a subordinate role, especially in cases where technical factors preclude biopsy[33] with the linitis plastica appearance, particularly if superficially ulcerated.

OTHER GASTRIC MALIGNANCIES

Squamous Carcinoma

Our Unit has encountered one case of squamous carcinoma in the setting of squamous metaplasia and tertiary syphilis.[34] The appearance of the carcinoma in this case was that of linitis plastica (Fig. 16-29). The incidental finding of squamous metaplasia in which squamous epithelium is found in the body and fundus is an unusual but important finding in any patient, provoking both a search for evidence for latent syphilis and cancer surveillance. True squamous metaplasia, however, must be differentiated from the appearance of squamous epithelium within a hiatus hernia seen in a retroflexed view of the cardia. In the case of a large hiatus hernia, one may actually see several centimeters of distal esophagus.

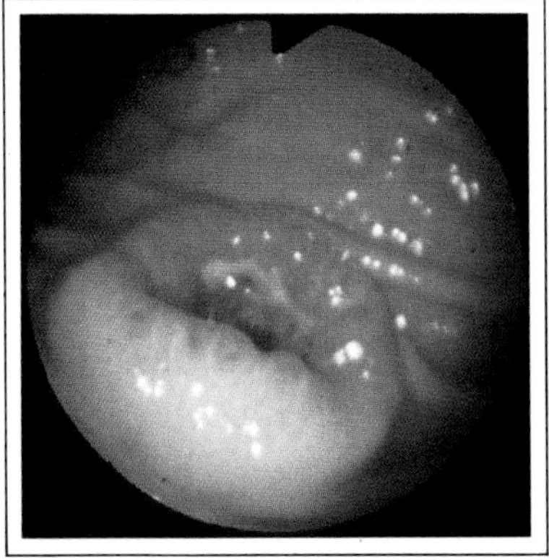

FIG. 16-28.

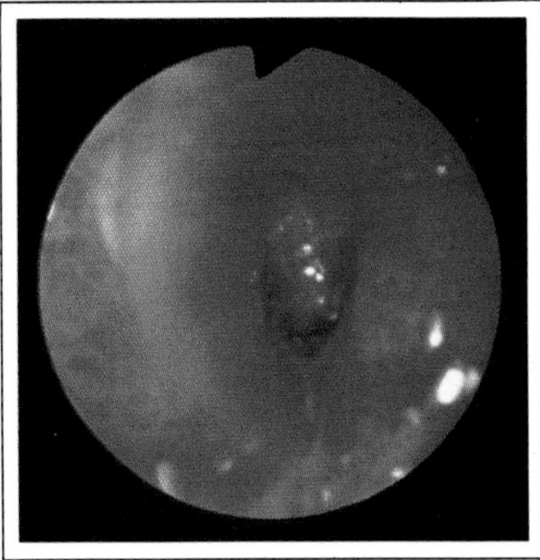

FIG. 16-29.

FIG. 16-28. Metastatic melanoma (to the stomach) with a large tumor implant. One of many large, submucosal masses with central ulceration in which dark (melanin) pigmentation can be identified.

FIG. 16-29. Squamous carcinoma of the stomach. Diffusely erythematous, friable mucosa with marked luminal narrowing was found in a patient with known luetic linitis plastica. Biopsy and brushing cytology were negative, but at surgery well-differentiated squamous carcinoma was found arising from mucosa showing squamous metaplasia.[34]

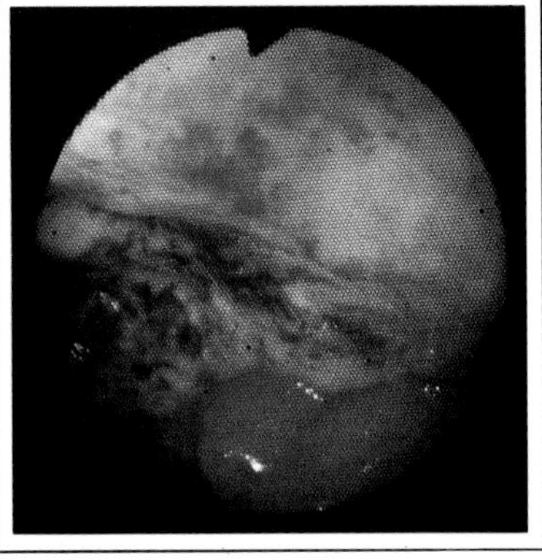

FIG. 16-30.

FIG. 16-30. Leiomyosarcoma in the fundus: a large (4×5 cm) submucosal mass with central ulceration. Except for its size, it is indistinguishable from a typical leiomyoma (see Chapter 17).

Sarcoma

We have already discussed lymphosarcoma, the most common sarcomatous lesion of the stomach, which accounts for 1 to 2% of gastric malignancies.[2] Nonlymphomatous mesenchymal malignancies are themselves quite rare, the one most frequently seen being leiomyosarcoma. We have seen two such cases over the past 7 years, comprising 2.7% of our cases, which is comparable to other reports.[35] It appears as a large (>5 cm) submucosal mass (Fig. 16-30), often with a center of ulceration which, apart from its size, is indistinguishable from a benign leiomyoma. In fact, the definition of leiomyosarcoma is often purely a histologic one, often based on the presence of multiple (five or more) mitotic figures per high power field.[35]

Other types of soft tissue sarcoma (liposarcoma, leiomyoblastoma, carcinosarcoma) may be encountered rarely. These cannot be differentiated visually from each other or from the more common leiomyosarcoma, as they all appear as large ulcerated submucosal masses.

Biopsy and Cytology

If the sarcoma is ulcerated, obtaining brushings and biopsies from the ulcerated portion often reveals some clue as to the mesenchymal origin of the tumor. In the case of the leiomyosarcoma, either brushings or biopsies from the ulcerated portion may show spindle cells with irregular nuclei and mitoses, which on the basis of their unequal size and shape suggest a malignant tumor of mesenchymal origin.[35]

Kaposi's Sarcoma

Although in the past Kaposi's sarcoma was rarely seen in North America or Europe, it is now being increasingly recognized because of its association with the acquired immune deficiency state (AIDS) in homosexuals.[36] In contrast to the isolated cases of Kaposi's sarcoma in the elderly, where gastrointestinal involvement is observed in only 10%,[37] when it occurs in homosexuals with AIDS, gastric or colonic lesions are seen in up to 50%.[36] In these patients the tumor is present in a more aggressive, disseminated form.[36] Where gastrointestinal involvement has been noted, upper endoscopy (as well as colonoscopy) reveals two types of appearance depending on size. In one (Fig. 16-31a) there are clusters of multiple, tiny (1 to 3 mm), discrete, erythematous nodules.[36] Larger lesions (≥5 mm) are seen as discrete, erythematous polyps, often with a zone of central ulceration (Fig. 16-31b).[38]

The endoscopic appearance of Kaposi's sarcoma is similar to that of gastric lymphoma in several aspects, especially

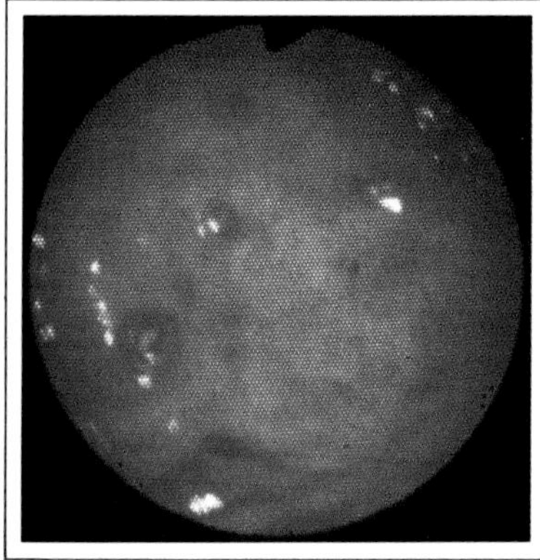

FIG. 16-31a.

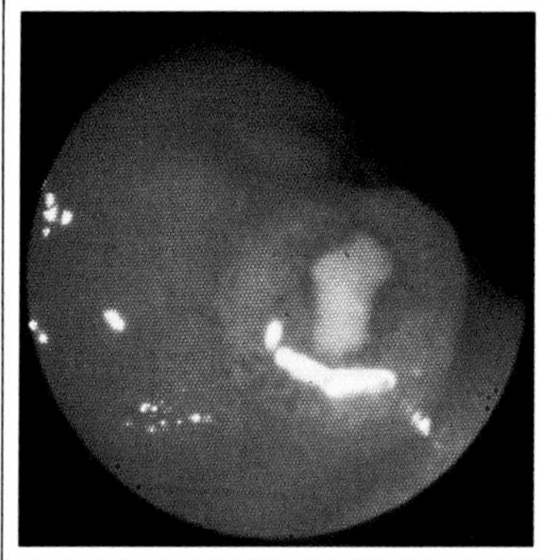

FIG. 16-31b.

FIG. 16-31. Kaposi's sarcoma. In the presence of numerous 2- to 5-mm intensely erythematous nodules (**a**) was a larger 8-mm polypoid mass with central ulceration (**b**). This was observed in an elderly (nonhomosexual) patient with cutaneous involvement. In this setting gastrointestinal lesions may be expected in 10%,[37,38] in contrast to homosexuals where they may be found in 50%.[36]

the presence of the volcano-type lesion, observed as a discrete polypoid mass with central ulcerations[37] (Fig. 16-31b); however, the intensely erythematous character of the smaller lesions (Fig. 16-31a) and the clinical setting with its characteristic cutaneous findings serve to differentiate these two conditions. Moreover, histologic confirmation of Kaposi's sarcoma is readily obtained (see below).

Biopsy

As in the case of lymphoma, the nodule or mass is often composed entirely of tumor cells. Therefore biopsy from any portion of the lesion may be expected to show the typical histologic appearance of spindle cells intermixed with irregular vascular spaces lined with endothelial cells.

REFERENCES

1. Devesa, S. S., and Silverman, D. T. (1978): Cancer incidence and mortality trends in the United States: 1935–1974. *J. Natl. Cancer Inst.*, 60:545–571.
2. Friedman, A. I. (1959): Primary lymphosarcoma of the stomach: a clinical study of seventy-five cases. *Am. J. Med.*, 28:783–796.
3. Adashek, J., Sanger, J., and Longmire, W. P. (1979): Cancer of the stomach: review of consecutive 10 year intervals. *Ann. Surg.*, 189:6–10.
4. Holdstock, G., and Bruce, S. (1981): Endoscopy and gastric cancer. *Gut*, 22:673–676.
5. Winawer, S. J., Posner, G., Lightdale, C. J., Sherlock, P., Melamed, M., and Fortner, J. G. (1975): Endoscopic diagnosis of advanced gastric cancer: factors influencing yield. *Gastroenterology*, 69:1183–1187.
6. Landres, R. T., and Strum, W. B. (1977): Endoscopic techniques in the diagnosis of gastric adenocarcinoma. *Gastrointest. Endosc.*, 23:203–205.
7. Olearchyk, A. S. (1978): Gastric carcinoma: a critical review of 243 cases. *Am. J. Gastroenterol.*, 70:25–45.
8. Cady, B., Ramsden, D. A., Stein, A., and Haggitt, R. C. (1977): Gastric cancer, contemporary aspects. *Am. J. Surg.*, 133:423–429.
9. Webb, J. N., and Busuttil, A. (1978): Adenocarcinoma of the oesophagus and at the oesophago-gastric junction. *Br. J. Surg.*, 65:475–479.
10. Koehler, R. E., Hanelin, L. G., Laing, F. C., Montgomery, C. K., and Margulis, A. R. (1977): Invasion of the duodenum by carcinoma of the stomach. *Am. J. Roentgenol.*, 128:201–205.
11. Menuck, L. (1978): Transpyloric extension of gastric carcinoma. *Am. J. Dig. Dis.*, 23:269–274.
12. Hatfield, A. R. W., Slavin, G., Segal, A. W., and Levi, A. J. (1975): Importance of the site of endoscopic gastric biopsy in ulcerating lesions of the stomach. *Gut*, 16:884–886.
13. Witzel, L., Halter, F., Gretillat, P. A., Scheuer, U., and Keller, M. (1976): Evaluation of specific value of endoscopic biopsies and brush cytology for malignancy of the oesophagus and stomach. *Gut*, 17:375–377.
14. Sancho-Poch, F. J., Balanzo, J., Ocana, J., Presa, E., Sala-Cladera, E., Cusso, X., and Vilardell, F. (1978): An evaluation of gastric biopsy in the diagnosis of gastric cancer. *Gastrointest. Endosc.*, 24:281–282.
15. Dekker W., and Tytgat, G. N. (1977): Diagnostic accuracy of fiberendoscopy in the detection of upper intestinal malignancy: a followup analysis. *Gastroenterology*, 73:710–714.
16. Green, P. H. R., O'Toole, K. M., Weinberg, L. M., and Goldfarb, J. P. (1981): Early gastric cancer. *Gastroenterology*, 81:247–256.
17. Johansen, A. A. (1976): Early gastric cancer. In: *Pathology of the Gastrointestinal Tract. Current Topics in Pathology*, edited by B. C. Morson, pp. 1–47, Springer-Verlag, New York.
17a. Kaneko, E., Nakamura, T., Umeda, N., Fujino, M., and Niwa, H. (1977): Outcome of gastric carcinoma detected by gastric mass survey in Japan. *Gut*, 18:626–630.
17b. Kohli, Y., Kawai, K., and Fujita, S. (1981): Analytic studies on growth of human gastric cancer. *J. Clin. Gastroenterol.*, 3:129–133.
18. Hisamichi, S., Shirane, A., Sugawara, N., Asaki, S., Yanbe, T., Ito, S., Funada, K., Hatori, S., Ikeda, T., Ito, Y., Masuda, Y., and Ooshiba, S. (1978): Early endoscopic features of stomach cancer and its mode of growth. *Tohoku J. Exp. Med.*, 126:239–246.
19. Koybayashi, S., Sugiura, H., and Kasugai, T. (1972): Reliability of endoscopic observation in diagnosis of early gastric carcinoma of the stomach. *Endoscopy*, 4:61–65.
20. Ito, Y., Blackstone, M. O., Riddell, R. H., and Kirsner, J. B. (1979): The endoscopic diagnosis of early gastric cancer. *Gastrointest. Endosc.*, 25:96–101.
21. Elder, J. B., Ganguli, P. C., and Gillespie, I. E. (1979): Cimetidine and gastric cancer. *Lancet*, 1:1005–1006.
22. Sakita, T., Oguro, Y., Takusu, S., Fukutomi, H., Miwa, T., and Yoshimori, M. (1971): Observations of the healing of ulcerations in early gastric cancer: the life cycle of the malignant ulcer. *Gastroenterology*, 60:835–844.
23. Kobayashi, S., Kusagai, T., and Yomazaki, H. (1979): Endoscopic differentiation of early gastric cancer from benign peptic ulcer. *Gastrointest. Endosc.*, 25:55–57.
24. Evans, D. M. D., Craven, J. L., Murphy, F., and Cleary, B. K. (1978): Comparison of "early gastric cancer" in Britain and Japan. *Gut*, 19:1–9.
25. Bjork, J. T., Geenen, J. E., Soergel, K. H., Parker, H. W., Leinicke, J. A., and Komorowski, R. A. (1977): Endoscopic evaluation of large gastric folds: a comparison of biopsy techniques. *Gastrointest. Endosc.*, 24:22–23.
26. Koga, S., Kishimoto, H., Tanaka, K., and Kawaguchi, H. (1978): Clinical and pathologic evaluation of patients with recurrence of gastric cancer more than five years postoperatively. *Am. J. Surg.*, 136:317–321.

27. Bucholtz, T. W., Welch, C. E., and Malt, R. A. (1978): Clinical correlates of resectability and survival in gastric carcinoma. *Ann. Surg.*, 188:711–715.
28. Nelson, R. S., and Lanza, F. L. (1974): The endoscopic diagnosis of gastric lymphoma: gross characteristics and histology. *Gastrointest. Endosc.*, 21:66–68.
29. Posner, G., Lightdale, C. J., Cooper, M., Sherlock, P., and Winawer, S. J. (1975): Reappraisal of endoscopic tissue diagnosis in secondary gastric lymphoma. *Gastrointest. Endosc.*, 21:123–125.
29a. Prolla, J. C., and Kirsner, J. B. (1964): The gastrointestinal lesions and complications of the leukemias. *Ann. Intern. Med.*, 61:1084–1103.
29b. Bynum, T. E. (1970): Gastroscopic appearance of multiple gastric ulcers associated with lymphatic leukemia. *Gastrointest. Endosc.*, 17:38–40.
30. Menuck, L. S., and Amberg, J. R. (1975): Metastatic disease involving the stomach. *Am. J. Dig. Dis.*, 20:903–914.
31. Cormer, W. J., Gaffey, T. A., Welch, J. M., Welch, J. S., and Edmonson, J. H. (1980): Linitis plastica caused by metastatic lobular carcinoma of the breast. *Mayo Clin. Proc.*, 55:747–753.
32. Nelson, R. S., and Lanza, F. (1978): Malignant melanoma metastatic to the upper gastrointestinal tract. *Gastrointest. Endosc.*, 24:156–158.
33. Coughlin, G. P., Bourne, A. J., and Grant, A. K. (1977): Endoscopic diagnosis of metastatic disease of the stomach and duodenum. *Aust. N.Z. J. Med.*, 7:52–57.
34. Vaughan, W. P., Straus, F. H., and Paloyan, D. (1977): Squamous carcinoma of the stomach after luetic linitis plastica. *Gastroenterology*, 72:945–948.
35. Cabre-Fiol, V., Vilardell, F., Sala-Cladera, E., and Mota, A. P. (1975): Preoperative cytological diagnosis of gastric leiomyosarcoma. *Gastroenterology*, 68:563–566.
36. Friedman-Kien, A. E., Laubenstein, L. J., Rubinstein, P., Buimovici-Klein, E., Marmor, M., Stahl, R., Spigland, I., Kim, K. S., and Zolla-Pazner, S. (1982): Disseminated Kaposi's sarcoma in homosexual men. *Ann. Intern. Med.*, 96:693–699.
37. Ahmed, N., Nelson, R. S., Goldstein, H. M., and Sinkovics, J. G. (1975): Kaposi's sarcoma of the stomach and duodenum: endoscopic and roentgenologic correlations. *Gastrointest. Endosc.*, 21:149–152.
38. Port, J. H., Traube, J., and Winans C. S. (1982): The visceral manifestations of Kaposi's sarcoma. *Gastrointest. Endosc.*, 28:179–181.

17

GASTRIC POLYPS

Gastric polyps are found in approximately 2% of endoscopic examinations of the stomach.[1] We, for example, found 125 among 5,000 examinations (2.5%) performed over a 7-year period (Table 17-1), or one case per 50 examinations. This experience contrasts with the finding of polyps in 0.15% of a combined series of 74,823 autopsy reports.[2] The higher percent of polyps found at endoscopy is explained by the fact that patients are often selected for this examination specifically because of suggestive radiographic findings.

EPITHELIAL POLYPS

The majority of gastric polyps are epithelial, i.e., arise from the mucosa itself. We find these to be five times (Table 17-1) more common than submucosal polyps, which arise from mesenchymal elements within the wall of the stomach.

The majority of epithelial polyps are incidental findings at endoscopic examinations performed for nonspecific symptoms. Larger polyps (>1.5 cm) may be associated with chronic blood loss and iron deficiency anemia caused by their eroded or ulcerated surfaces.[3] An extremely rare presentation, even for large polyps of the prepyloric antrum, is prolapse into the duodenal bulb and intermittent obstruction resulting in episodic vomiting and pain.[4]

Epithelial polyps may be classified as either hyperplastic or adenomatous, where "hyperplastic" is synonymous with nonneoplastic and "adenomatous" designates the polyp as a true neoplasm.[5]

TABLE 17-1. *Gastric polyps—125 cases (1974–1980)*

	Number		Percent	
Type of polyp	For individual type	For group as a whole	For individual type	For group as a whole
Epithelial	—	103	—	82.4
Hyperplastic	89	—	71.2	—
Adenomatous	14	—	11.2	—
Submucosal	—	22	—	17.6
Leiomyoma	8	—	6.4	—
Pancreatic rest	2	—	1.6	—
Carcinoid	2	—	1.6	—
Myoepithelial hamartoma	2	—	1.6	—
Peutz-Jeghers polyp	1	—	0.8	—
Eosinophilic granuloma	1	—	0.8	—
No histologic diagnosis	6	—	4.8	—
Patients with polyps	—	125	100	
Total patients examined	—	5,000	2.5*	

* Percent of total patients examined with gastric polyps.

Hyperplastic Polyps

Hyperplastic polyps occur more commonly than other types of gastric polyp. In recent reports of consecutive gastric polypectomies, where the entire polyp is submitted for histologic examination, these were three[3] to 15[1] times commoner than adenomatous polyps. Among 103 epithelial polyps observed by us over a 7-year period, sampled by both forceps biopsy (87%) and polypectomy (13%), we found hyperplastic polyps to be six times commoner than the adenomatous variety (Table 17-1).

The histologic appearance of a hyperplastic polyp has been used to subdivide them into those showing foveolar (gastric pit) proliferation alone, termed "foveolar hyperplasia," a second group showing "gastric gland hyperplasia," and a combined (foveolar and glandular) type, designated as "hyperplasiogenous."[5] Polyps with glandular hyperplasia histologically may have a cystic appearance, in which case the term "gastric glandular cyst" has been used.[6] Finally, in cases where there is a striking inflammatory component, the term "inflammatory polyp" is sometimes employed. Often we find that the inflammatory polyp is simply a hyperplastic polyp which is associated with superficial mucosal ulceration.

Association With Atrophic Gastritis

For single as well as multiple (but fewer than five) hyperplastic polyps, we find the mucosa from which they arise to be either normal or to have nonspecific acute and chronic inflammatory changes. In these cases atrophic gastritis is found in only 7.5% (Table 17-2), similar to its overall incidence in patients coming to endoscopy (10%).[6a] However, where there are more than five hyperplastic polyps, and especially more than 10, the incidence of atrophic gastritis is much higher, 20 to 30% (Table 17-2), a fact which may have a bearing on the increased cancer risk for patients with multiple polyps (see below).

Malignant Potential

The risk of malignancy in patients with hyperplastic polyps is uncertain. Rather than relating to the polyp itself, the cancer risk in these patients may ultimately depend on the state of the gastric mucosa from which they arise, especially whether atrophic gastritis is present, which itself increases the likelihood of cancer.[7] In a study of hyperplastic polyps removed at surgery, Tomasulo found the incidence of cancer to be 28%, where 79% of the specimens showed atrophic gastritis in the adjoining mucosa.[8] This high percentage of atrophic gastritis contrasts with the 11% found at endoscopy in our patients (Table 17-2). This lower percentage of atrophic gastritis in patients with hyperplastic polyps found at endoscopy may explain an only 1 to 2% incidence of cancer found in one large series subsequent to endoscopic removal of hyperplastic polyps.[1]

Another determinant of cancer risk may be the type of hyperplastic polyp, as some cancers arise within the polyp itself.[9] Because of a similarity in the branching architecture of the hyperplasiogenous polyp and adenomas,[5] this polyp has been suspected as being an intermediate form between hyperplastic polyps and adenomas.[5] As cancer has been reported to arise from within a hyperplasiogenous polyp,[10] an increased malignant potential specifically for this type of hyperplastic polyp has been postulated. In one series, cancer found after removal of hyperplastic polyps was noted almost exclusively in cases where this type of polyp had been present.[1]

Based on an apparent risk of cancer—up to 3.5% in patients in whom any type of hyperplastic polyp is discovered at endoscopy[11]—we recommend that such patients have periodic examinations, at least every 2 years, for cancer screening, especially if atrophic gastritis is present. This would be for all patients, even if the original polyp was removed, because the cancers which arise in these patients usually do so at some distance from the original polyp.[11] The finding of dysplasia, especially if it is severe (i.e., with cytologic features which suggest that neoplastic transformation has occurred appearing as cancer *in situ* or to a degree just short of this), in biopsies obtained on two separate examinations, or any definite dyplasias from a discrete, raised area would be a strong indication for surgery.

Appearance

The appearance of these lesions varies. About half occur as single lesions (Table 17-3) which are equally divided

TABLE 17-2. *Hyperplastic polyps in relation to atrophic gastritis*

Parameter	Single polyp	Multiple polyps <5	Multiple polyps 5–10	Multiple polyps >10	Multiple polyps Total	All polyps
No. of cases	40	27	6	16	49	89
No. with histologic atrophic gastritis	3	2	2	3	7	10
% With atrophic gastritis	7.5	7.4	33.0	18.0	14.0	11.0
% With histologic atrophic gastritis in patients coming to endoscopy[6a]	10	—	—	—	—	—

TABLE 17-3. *Location of 89 hyperplastic polyps*

Location	Single polyp	Multiple polyps <5	5–10	>10
Cardia	1	2	—	—
Fundus	4	1	1	2
Body	14	15	3	8
Antrum	21	8	2	—
Body and antrum	—	1	—	6
Total	40	27	6	16

between an antral and a more proximal (body or cardiofundic) location. Single hyperplastic polyps are either tiny (<5 mm) mucosal excrescence-type lesions or are of a more substantial size (>5 mm but <2 cm). Although constituting only a minority of hyperplastic polyps, we find about 15% to be 2 cm or greater in size (Table 17-4).

Slightly less common than the single hyperplastic polyp are those which are multiple but number less than five. We find them constituting almost a third of the cases, with their most frequent location being the body (Table 17-3). Finally, in 25% of our cases (see "Multiple Gastric Polyps," this chapter) the number of hyperplastic polyps exceeds five and especially 10.

A common appearance for the single hyperplastic polyp of the antrum is that of a 5-mm lesion whose surface epithelium is indistinguishable from the mucosa surrounding the polyp (Fig. 17-1a). We find that with larger polyps (>5 mm) the mucosa of the polyp is erythematous (Fig. 17-1b) or eroded (superficially ulcerated) (Fig. 17-1c). Hyperplastic polyps are usually sessile; however, they may be pedunculated (Fig. 17-2a), in some cases having a long pedicle and thereby closely resembling tubular adenomas of the colon (see Chapter 41). A minority (15% or less) of hyperplastic polyps achieve a significant size and appear as fungating masses which are mistaken for either villous adenomas or even carcinoma (Fig. 17-2b).

Biopsy and Polypectomy

As we have already discussed (see "Malignant Potential," this chapter), the cancer risk in these patients is in the mucosa, rather than in the polyp itself. It remains for the endoscopist to establish, first, that the polyp is hyperplastic, and, second, that the surrounding mucosa is histologically atrophic. We believe that for small polyps (<1 cm) discovered as incidental findings forceps biopsies of the polyp and surrounding mucosa are sufficient, given the rarity of carcinoma arising in hyperplastic polyps[9,10] as well as the marginal impact of polypectomy, even for the hyperplasiogenous type, on the risk of cancer. For the larger polyps (>1 cm, especially those between 1.5 and 2 cm), the clinical presentation of the polyp as a cause of occult or even frank gastrointestinal bleeding, intermittent outlet obstruction, etc. may make removal of the polyp desirable. For such polyps we consider endoscopic electrosurgical removal,[13] although often basing our final decision on the histologic characterization of the polyp obtained from forceps biopsies. Although such biopsies cannot exclude small neoplastic foci within a large exophytic polyp, we would not wish to subject an elderly patient who may have a variety of medical problems to the (4%) risk of hemorrhage which might require surgery[3] to remove a nonneoplastic polyp with a risk of cancer of 1% or less and where the indication for therapy is the presence of the polyp alone.

Adenomatous Polyps

True adenomatous polyps are uncommon. The 14 observed by us over a 7-year period accounted for only 11% of our cases of gastric polyps while being found in 4.7[1] and 7.4%[12] in two large gastric polypectomy series. The adenomatous polyps were largely incidental findings in our cases. In a polypectomy series where 25% of the polyps were adenomatous, symptoms or anemia prompted evaluation in 65%, and 81% of the polyps removed were 1 cm or more in size.[3] This suggests that a higher percentage of larger polyps removed from symptomatic patients may be adenomatous than we and others[1,12] have observed.

Predisposing Conditions

Like hyperplastic polyps, most adenomatous polyps arise spontaneously in either normal mucosa or that showing nonspecific chronic inflammation. For only three of the 14 cases was there a predisposing condition (Table 17-5). In two (14%) this was atrophic gastritis,[7] and in the remaining case multiple gastric adenomas were found as part of a familial polyposis syndrome.[13]

Malignant Potential

As adenomatous polyps represent true neoplasms, an even stronger association with gastric malignancy has been reported than for hyperplastic polyps, with cancer being found

TABLE 17-4. *Size of hyperplastic polyps*

Size (mm)	Single polyps	Multiple polyps[a] <5	5–10	>10
<5	18	20	4	12
5–10	10	4	1	2
10–20	6	2	1	1
>20	6	1	—	1
Total	40	27	6	16

[a] Largest polyp.

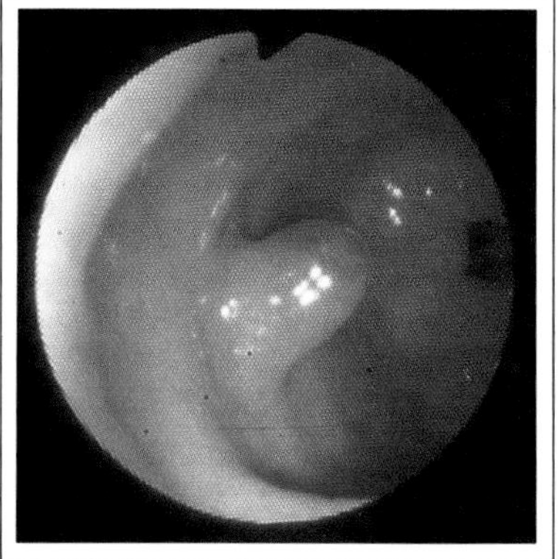

FIG. 17-1a.

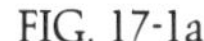

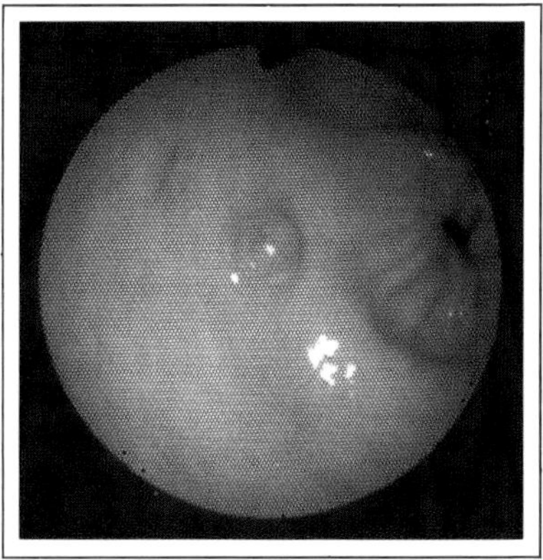

FIG. 17-1b.

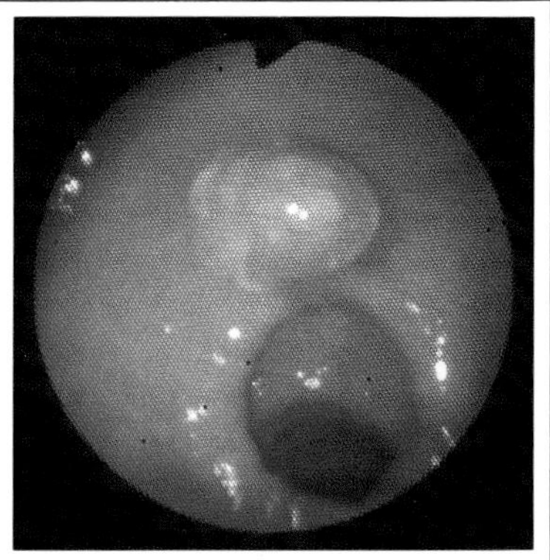

FIG. 17-1c.

FIG. 17-1. a: Hyperplastic polyp. Except for minimal friability (ease of bleeding), the overall surface appearance is indistinguishable from that of its surroundings. **b:** Hyperplastic polyp. The surface mucosa appears erythematous. Biopsy, however, was identical to that in (a). **c:** Hyperplastic (inflammatory) polyp. The surface appears eroded (superficially ulcerated), where biopsy showed acute and chronic inflammation. The histology of the excised polyp indicated it to be hyperplastic with an ulcerated surface.

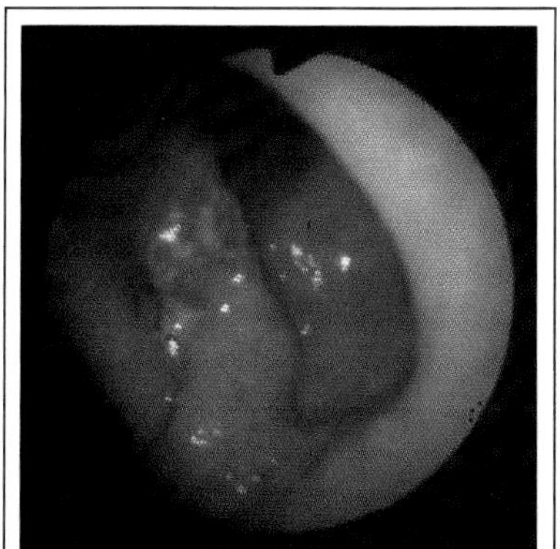

FIG. 17-2a.

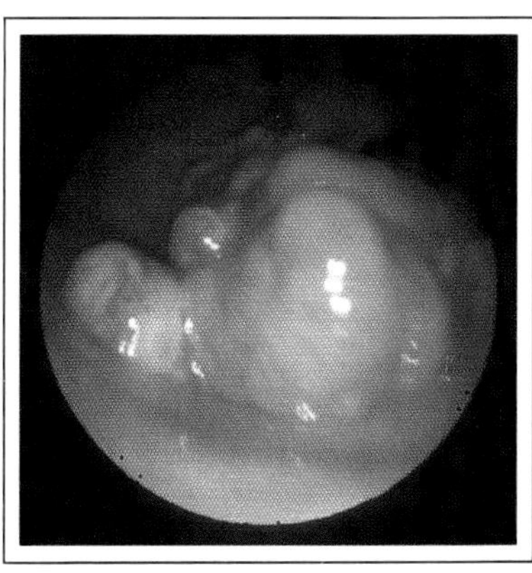

FIG. 17-2b.

FIG. 17-2. a: Hyperplastic polyp. This polyp has a long pedicle, and its appearance resembles a tubular adenoma of the colon. Nevertheless, histology of the excised lesion was that of a hyperplastic polyp. **b:** Giant hyperplastic polyp. This lesion measured over 2 cm. Because of its size and surface nodularity, it was mistaken for a villous adenoma.

in association in up to 59%.[8] In some of these a polyp was admittedly a finding incidental to the cancer for which the patient underwent surgical exploration. However, in a polypectomy series in which the results of 48 consecutive procedures were reported, ReMine et al.[3] found focal malignant changes in 17% of the 12 adenomatous polyps discovered. In none was actual invasive cancer found; moreover, the smallest of these was 1 cm with the average size 1.5 cm.

TABLE 17-5. *Predisposing conditions for 14 adenomatous polyps*

Condition	No. of cases	%
Histologic atrophic gastritis	2	14
Familial polyposis	1	7
No predisposing condition	11	79

As in the case of hyperplastic polyps, the cancer risk may be more directly related to the mucosa, i.e., whether atrophic gastritis is found, in that the strongest association with malignancy (59% of the cases being cancer) was found in a series where 94% had atrophic gastritis.[8] Contributing

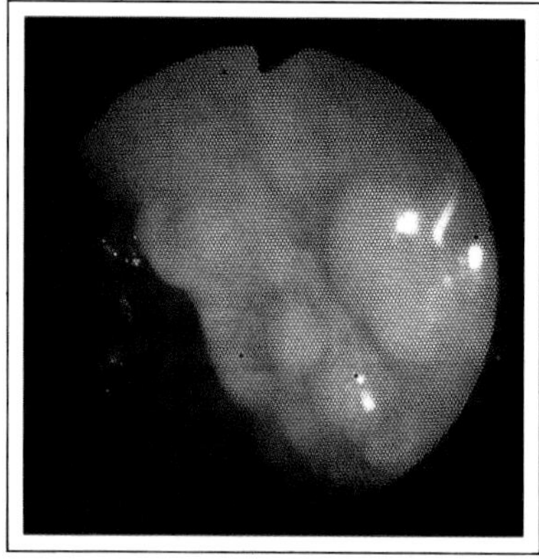

FIG. 17-3a.

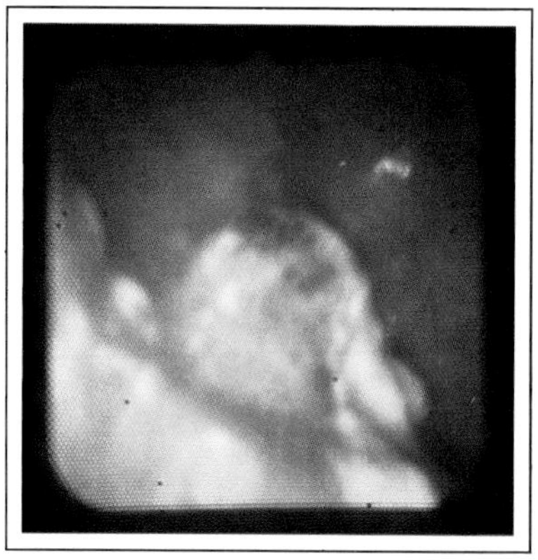

FIG. 17-3b.

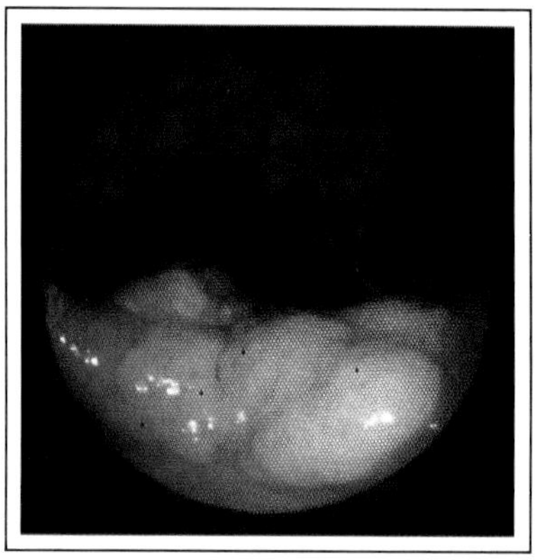

FIG. 17-3c.

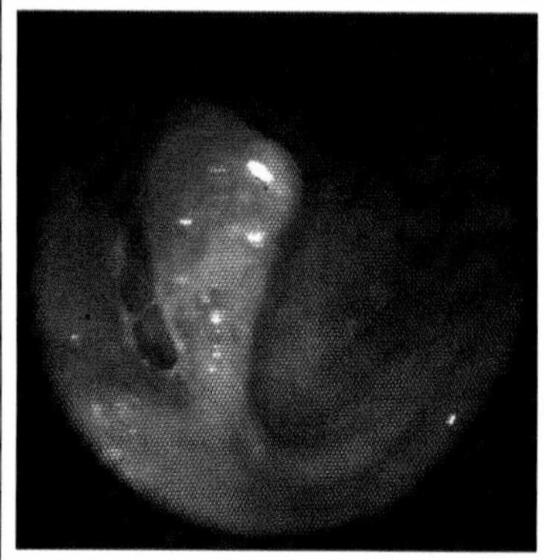

FIG. 17-3d.

FIG. 17-3. a: Sessile (1 to 5 cm) adenomatous polyp. As in this case, adenomas tend to be large (>1 cm)[3] but without features which consistently differentiate them from hyperplastic polyps. In this particular case, the surface was more irregular (nodular) than is usually seen with hyperplastic polyps (Fig. 17-1a). **b:** Adenomatous polyp. We find about half to be between 5 and 10 mm in size. In this case there was possibly more nonspecific surface irregularity than one would see in a hyperplastic polyp of comparable size (Fig. 17-1a). **c:** Adenomatous polyp with malignant transformation. Except for the central ulceration (toward 12 o'clock), the polyp has an appearance similar to that of a sessile adenoma. Forceps biopsies showed only adenomatous tissue, but at surgery invasive cancer was found within the ulcerated portion. **d:** Adenomatous polyp, pedunculated. This appearance is indistinguishable from that of a pedunculated hyperplastic polyp (Fig. 17-2).

to the cancer risk, of course, is the adenomatous polyp itself, which if larger than 1 cm appears to carry an almost 20% risk of focal malignant change already present.[3]

Appearance

We have not found any feature which successfully differentiates adenomatous from hyperplastic polyps. Although adenomas are usually larger than 1 cm (Table 17-6), this is true of only 15 to 20% of hyperplastic polyps (Table 17-4). Moreover, at least one-third of adenomatous polyps are less than 1 cm, within the expected size range of hyperplastic polyps (Table 17-4). The surface of adenomatous polyps may be relatively smooth (Fig. 17-3a) or eroded (Fig. 17-3b).

The presence of a central ulceration is a particularly worrisome feature for any adenomatous polyp, especially one which is sessile, in that it indicates a high likelihood of malignant transformation (Fig. 17-3c). Some adenomatous polyps have a pedicle (Fig. 17-3d), but this does not distinguish them from hyperplastic polyps (Fig. 17-2a). As in the case of single hyperplastic polyps (Table 17-3), adenomatous polyps are equally divided in location between the body and the antrum (Table 17-7).

TABLE 17-6. *Size of 14 adenomatous polyps*

Size (mm)	Single polyp	Multiple polyps[a]
<5	—	—
5–10	5	2
>10–20	7	—

[a] Largest polyp.

TABLE 17-7. *Location of 14 adenomatous polyps*

Location	Single polyp	Multiple polyps
Fundus	1	—
Body	6	1
Antrum	5	—
Body and antrum	—	1
Total	12	2

Biopsy and Polypectomy

Because adenomatous polyps are neoplasms and capable of malignant degeneration, it is desirable that they be removed. Although the technique of gastric polypectomy is now well established,[1,12] it must be remembered that removal of a large gastric polyp is more demanding than that of a similar size colonic polyp because of the higher incidence of bleeding.[3] A 2 to 4% risk of bleeding for lesions

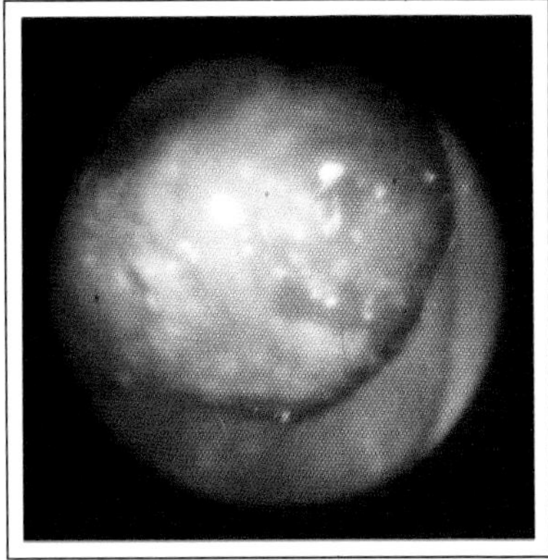

FIG. 17-4.

FIG. 17-4. Villous adenoma. A large (3 cm) polypoid mass with irregular, eroded surface mucosa was seen to prolapse across the pyloric channel (at 12 o'clock).

of the stomach 1 cm or larger must be kept in mind when making a decision concerning any gastric polyp. For this reason we first obtain a forceps biopsy of the polyp itself so as to base a decision concerning endoscopic removal on its histology as well as other factors, e.g., its size and location. For example, if forceps biopsy shows that histologically the polyp is an adenoma, in some patients, especially where the lesion exceeds 2 cm, it still may be safer to excise the lesions surgically than risk the possibility of bleeding from an endoscopic polypectomy.[3] In other high-risk patients, the preferred course may be to observe the patient and the polyp rather than to risk either endoscopic or surgical removal.

For patients in whom endoscopic or surgical polypectomy has been performed for an adenomatous polyp, because of the risk of subsequent cancer being at least as great as that for hyperplasiogenous polyps, i.e., 1 to 3%,[1] continued endoscopic surveillance at 1- to 2-year intervals seems desirable.

Villous Adenomas

Villous adenomas are exceedingly rare. One may expect 1 per 100 polyps and only 1 per 1,500 gastric examinations. We encountered only one villous adenoma out of 125 cases of gastric polyps.

Villous adenomas tend to be large, with 80% being greater than 2 cm and 50% greater than 4 cm.[14] Their size plus prepyloric antral location predisposes them to prolapse across the pyloric channel and to intermittently obstruct it, as was the case for the villous adenoma we encountered (Fig. 17-4). Another case similar to this has also been reported.[4] In addition to symptoms suggesting intermittent gastric outlet obstruction, anemia is a frequent finding because of chronic blood loss from the eroded tumor surface.

The malignant potential of villous adenomas has been stated to be 25 to 75%, being related to size, with malignant degeneration more frequently associated with larger tumors.[4] Like adenomatous polyps, villous adenomas may be associated with carcinomas elsewhere in the stomach.[4]

Appearance

These lesions are encountered as single, large (>2 cm), sessile tumors with broad papillary projections. The surface epithelium is usually eroded or ulcerated (Fig. 17-4). The finding of a large, polypoid lesion of the antrum is suggestive of a villous adenoma, but one should always keep in mind the possibility of a giant hyperplastic polyp (Fig. 17-2b). A forceps biopsy in such a case serves to differentiate these entities.

Biopsy and Polypectomy

Generally, the clinical presentation of a large antral polyp, i.e., anemia, occult blood loss, or intermittent obstruction, argues for resection. As in the case of adenoma, the choice between the endoscopic and surgical route is based on surgical risk on the one hand and the location of the polyp as well as the technical ability of the endoscopist on the other.

Multiple Gastric Polyps (Gastric Polyposis)

As in the case of single polyps, most of the multiple type are hyperplastic. In fact, of 51 cases with multiple polyps out of 103 of the epithelial type, only two were adenomatous, with 49 being hyperplastic (Table 17-8).

Of the hyperplastic type, in half the cases the number is less than five, whereas in only one-third are there 10

TABLE 17-8. *Types of multiple epithelial polyps in 51 cases*

Type	No.
Hyperplastic	45
Mixed: hyperplastic-"adenomatous" (Hyperplasiogenous)	4
Adenomatous	2
Total	51

polyps (gastric polyposis) (Table 17-3). In contrast to single hyperplastic polyps where half the cases occur in the antrum, only a third of the cases of multiple polyps occur in this location (Table 17-3); of the cases of gastric polyposis of the hyperplastic type we encountered, none exclusively involved the antrum.

For most hyperplastic polyps, the histologic examination reveals simple foveolar hyperplasia.[15] For a small, but as yet uncertain percentage, the histologic picture is that of a mixed hyperplastic-adenomatous polyp.[16]

Predisposing Conditions

The most common predisposing condition to hyperplastic polyps is atrophic gastritis. With five or more hyperplastic polyps, we found the incidence of atrophic gastritis to be 22% (Table 17-2) in contrast to 7% for single hyperplastic polyps or where they were multiple but fewer than five. Familial polyposis coli[17] predisposes to multiple adenomatous or hyperplastic polyps, whereas multiple hyperplastic polyps are found in the Cronkhite-Canada syndrome[18] and Cowden's disease (gastrointestinal polyposis with orocutaneous hamartomas).[19]

Malignant Potential

Hyperplastic polyps.

In cases where atrophic gastritis is found in association with hyperplastic polyps, a significant cancer risk exists which cumulatively may approach 10%.[7] In cases where atrophic gastritis is absent the risk may still be substantially greater than that in the general population, and it may approach that for the hyperplasiogenous polyps, which ranges between 1 and 3%.[1] Unfortunately, no prospective studies have been reported for hyperplastic polyps in the absence of atrophic gastritis to establish the malignant potential of the mucosa that gives rise to these lesions. For patients with multiple polyps, especially in the face of atrophic gastritis, periodic screening endoscopy seems highly desirable. At the same time multiple biopsies would be obtained to be examined for evidence of dysplasia, especially severe dysplasia (see above), with the hope that cancer arising in this setting would be detected while it is still treatable rather than in an already advanced stage (Fig. 17-7b, below).

Adenomatous polyps.

The association of multiple adenomatous polyps with malignancy is high, especially in cases of familial polyposis, where gastric carcinoma is said to occur in 33 to 59%.[13] This would make yearly screening mandatory with surgical intervention (i.e., total gastrectomy) if cancer were detected in a polyp or if dysplasia, particularly if severe (see above), is found in representative biopsies of flat mucosa.

Appearance of Multiple Gastric Polyps

The commonest finding at endoscopy is that of several polyps (fewer than five), seen as 2- to 4-mm excrescences which are generally indistinguishable from the surrounding mucosa (Fig. 17-5a). In one-third of the cases, especially in association with atrophic gastritis, multiple polyps of this size can be seen, especially in the body (Fig. 17-5b). Larger polyps (5 to 10 mm) may have intact mucosa (Fig. 17-6a), or the mucosa may appear erythematous and eroded (Fig. 17-6b).

In cases where multiple hyperplastic polyps are associated with large gastric folds (Fig. 17-7a), the term "polypoid gastritis" has been used,[15] a condition which may represent a hyperplastic or growth phase in the natural history of atrophic gastritis and may be a premalignant condition.[15] In a small percentage of these cases, cancer is found at the initial examination (Fig. 17-7b).

In rare instances (1 of 49 cases), multiple hyperplastic polyps are both large (>1.5 cm) and numerous (>10). Some of the larger of these hyperplastic polyps simulate villous adenomas (Fig. 17-2b).

Biopsy and Polypectomy for Multiple Gastric Polyps

We find that 95% of the cases of gastric polyps which occur multiply are hyperplastic (Table 17-8). In a large polypectomy series, Deyhle[1] had no cases of multiple adenomatous polyps. In neither of the two cases of multiple adenomatous polyps we observed were there more than five polyps, and in one it was found in a patient with familial polyposis where multiple gastric adenomas have been described.[13] Multiple gastric adenomatous polyps (exceeding five) must be exceedingly rare, except in patients with familial polyposis, and so it seems unnecessary to remove electrosurgically or by fulguration 10 or more polyps for fear of their being adenomatous or of missing a single polyp having both hyperplastic and adenomatous features. Furthermore, the cancer risk is not clearly lowered even if one such polyp were removed. In these cases[1] as well as in cases where polyps are not removed, the cancer risk remains between 1 and 4%.[1,11]

We believe the most reasonable approach to a patient with multiple gastric polyps is simply to obtain biopsies of representative polyps, as well as larger or otherwise atypical-appearing polyps, to confirm their hyperplastic nature. In some cases the endoscopist may wish to remove one or several larger polyps electrosurgically to determine if the polyp is of the hyperplasiogenous type because of the possible increased cancer risk for patients with this type of polyp,[1] or if it is a hyperplastic polyp with a true adenomatous focus within it. It is also important to determine if atrophic gastritis is present in biopsies taken from flat mucosa, which

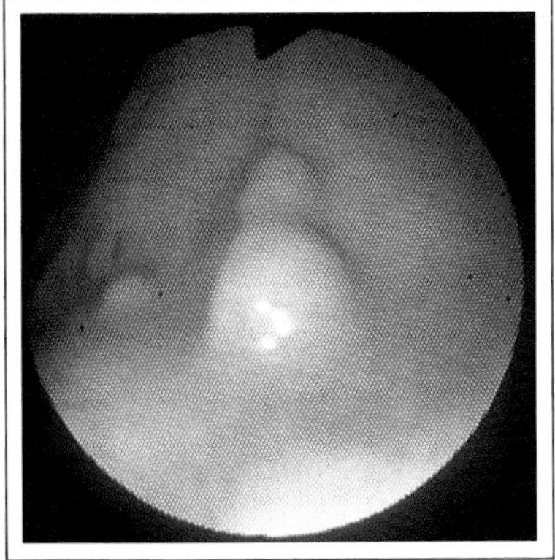

FIG. 17-5a.

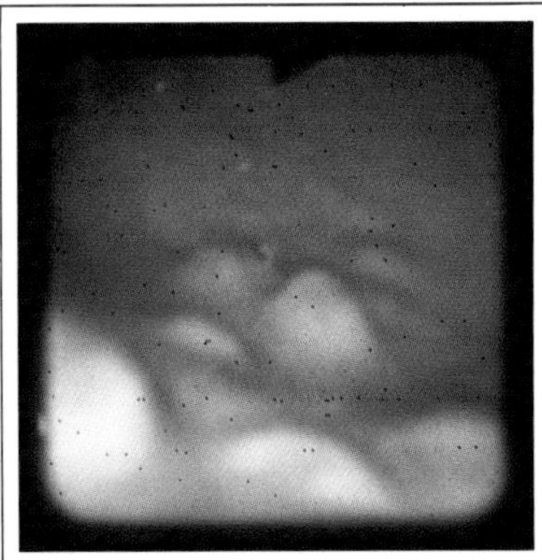

FIG. 17-5b.

FIG. 17-5. a: Multiple hyperplastic polyps in the antrum. Several polyps are noted in the upper body. Two are sessile (9 and 12 o'clock) and have a mucosal appearance which is indistinguishable from that surrounding the polyp. **b:** Multiple hyperplastic polyps associated with pernicious anemia. The lower body is studded with 4- to 5-mm sessile polyps.

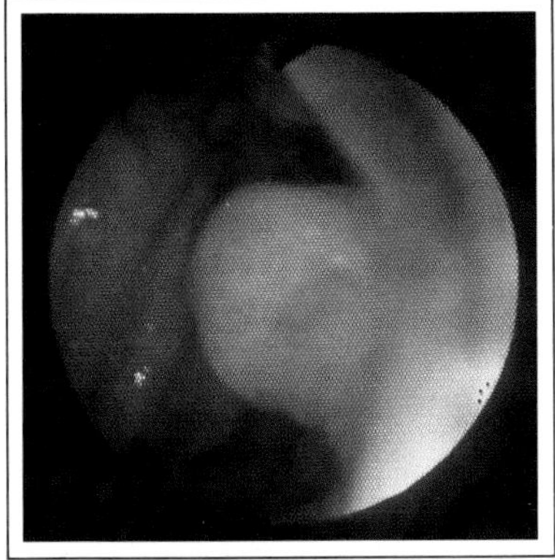

FIG. 17-6a.

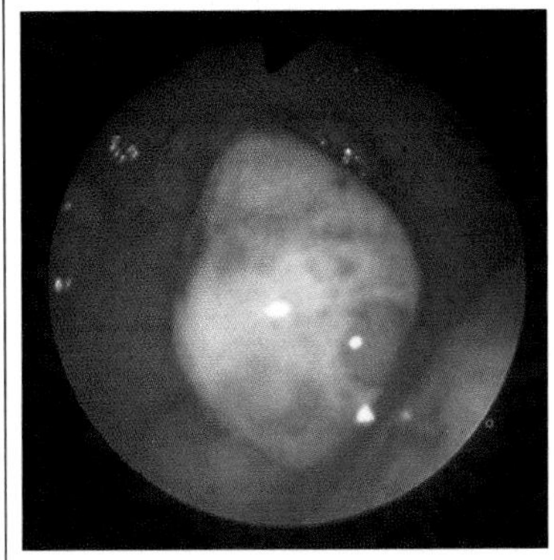

FIG. 17-6b.

FIG. 17-6. a: Hyperplastic polyps, 7.5 mm. One of several polyps of the lower body showing a smooth, regular surface mucosal appearance. **b:** Hyperplastic polyp, 1.2 cm. This larger polyp with an eroded mucosal surface was found among numerous larger polyps of the distal body (see Fig. 17-7a) and large rugal folds. The histology of this polyp was of the mixed (hyperplastic-"adenomatous") type also referred to as hyperplasiogenous.[5]

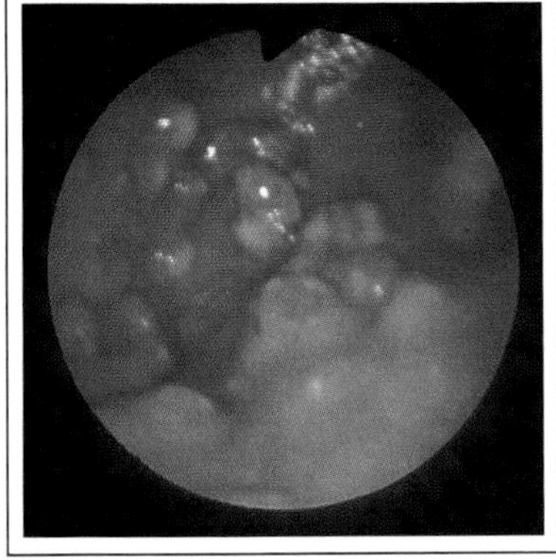

FIG. 17-7a.

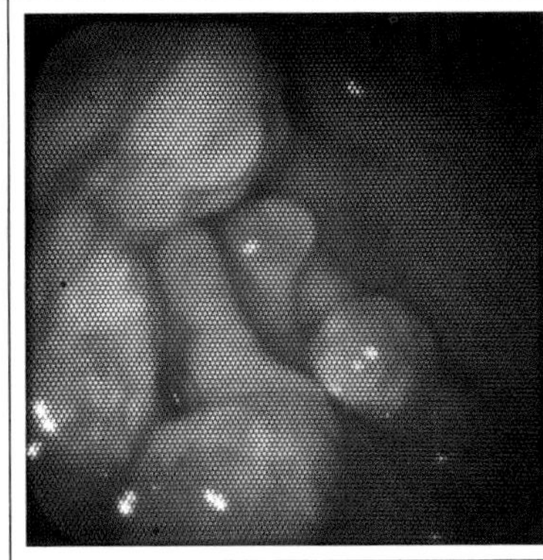

FIG. 17-7b.

FIG. 17-7. a: Multiple hyperplastic polyps with prominent gastric folds (polypoid gastritis). Numerous polyps of the distal body are seen having a variety of shapes and sizes. In addition, prominent gastric folds are noted whose mucosa on biopsy showed atrophic gastritis. Because of a history of weight loss, wedge resection of the polyps and adjacent greater curve was performed. Malignancy was not present. **b:** Multiple hyperplastic polyps with infiltrating carcinoma. Several hyperplastic polyps are seen adjacent to nodular, raised, superficially ulcerated folds. Biopsies from these (but not from the hyperplastic polyps) showed adenocarcinoma. At surgery the cancer proved to be metastatic.

would be another reason for advising periodic follow-up examinations. Finally, at the time of polypectomy, one may wish to perform a large-particle biopsy (see Chapter 1) of prominent rugal folds, especially in symptomatic patients with weight loss, to exclude cancer already present.[15] An alternative approach, one we have employed in some symptomatic patients with multiple polyps and large gastric folds, is to advocate surgical wedge resection of the polyp-bearing surface and adjacent folds so as to provide definite information concerning the nature of the polyps as well as to assure the absence of infiltrating malignancy within the large folds. In either case, long-term follow-up is essential because of the increased cancer risk in these patients.[15]

SUBMUCOSAL POLYPS

Only one-fifth as common as epithelial polyps are those arising from submucosal elements. We found 22 such polyps, contrasted with 103 epithelial polyps, among 5,000 examinations performed over a 7-year period (Table 17-1). Of these 22 polyps, the leiomyoma was the commonest, being found in eight cases, and was representative of all submucosal polyps. Like epithelial polyps, the commonest presentation at endoscopy is as an incidental finding noted on a radiographic study of the stomach. Most often this examination is prompted by complaints having nothing to do with the polyp, so it is not surprising that in 10 to 20% of these cases the polyp is not confirmed at endoscopy.[20] Among patients with leiomyomas, about 20% have iron deficiency anemia or frank gastrointestinal hemorrhage related to the presence of the polyp.[21]

Appearance

The submucosal polyp itself, especially its smaller lesions (<1 cm) have the same general shape as hyperplastic polyps of comparable size (Figs. 17-8a and 17-1a). The most helpful endoscopic feature which denotes their submucosal origin is the presence of "bridging folds" (Fig. 17-8a). For the leiomyoma, these are the result of attachments of the tumor itself to the gastric wall. Bridging folds are generally two in number and may be distinguished from the pedicle (Fig. 17-8b), which constitutes the single attachment of an epithelial polyp to the surrounding mucosa. A second endoscopic feature which suggests a submucosal origin is the presence of a central depression (umbilication) or frank ulceration (Fig. 17-9) within a small, abruptly elevated mass with a perfectly intact mucosa. Whereas a hyperplastic polyp may be eroded (superficially ulcerated), the erosion occurs diffusely (Fig. 17-6b) rather than as one deep central ulceration in the submucosal polyp (Fig. 17-9).

Biopsy

After establishing a high index of suspicion that the polyp is submucosal, one may biopsy repeatedly at a point on the head of the polyp—"pecking"[22]—or from the central ulcer where biopsies as well as brushings occasionally reveal the mesenchymal origin of the polyp.[23] Removal of submucosal polyps, e.g., leiomyomas, is feasible but technically demanding and, unless the entire polyp and its attachments were removed, of uncertain clinical benefit. For submucosal polyps discovered as incidental findings, a conservative approach seems reasonable unless the polyp itself displayed suspicious features (see below). For patients with larger polyps associated with iron deficiency or gastrointestinal bleeding, surgery may be the wisest course unless the general medical condition of the patient precludes it, in which case a decision for endoscopic polypectomy would be based on the usual considerations of benefit versus risk.

Endoscopic Features of Specific Submucosal Polyps

Leiomyomas

Leiomyomas are most commonly found in the fundus and upper body.[21] They range in size from 5 to 15 mm (Fig. 17-9) to greater than 3 cm (Fig. 17-10). Typically, they have a clearly defined attachment to the gastric wall which is seen as a bridging fold (Fig. 17-8a). The overlying mucosa of the polyp itself is loosely adherent so that it can be easily tented (Fig. 17-10b). A central umbilication is common (Fig. 17-10c), especially for lesions >1.5 cm, but is not invariably found. For patients who present with gastric intestinal bleeding, acute or chronic, the central umbilication may in fact be replaced by a deep ulceration (Fig. 17-10d).

Pancreatic Rests

The pancreatic rest, a rare tumor composed of ectopic pancreatic tissue, has an appearance similar to that of the leiomyoma.[24] Like leiomyomas, pancreatic rests may have a central umbilication (Fig. 17-11). They are encountered much less frequently, as in only two cases in our series in contrast with eight leiomyomas observed over the same time period. In contrast to leiomyomas, which favor the fundus and body, these lesions are almost always found in the antrum. Also in contrast to leiomyomas, they rarely achieve a size greater than 1 cm. Bridging folds are almost never seen unless the pancreas rest is unusually large. For the most part, size (≥1.5 cm) and location (fundus and upper body) serve to differentiate the leiomyoma from the

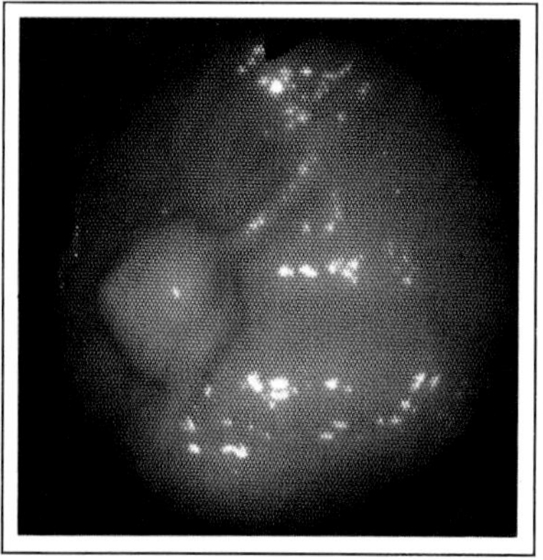

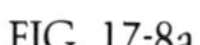

FIG. 17-8a.

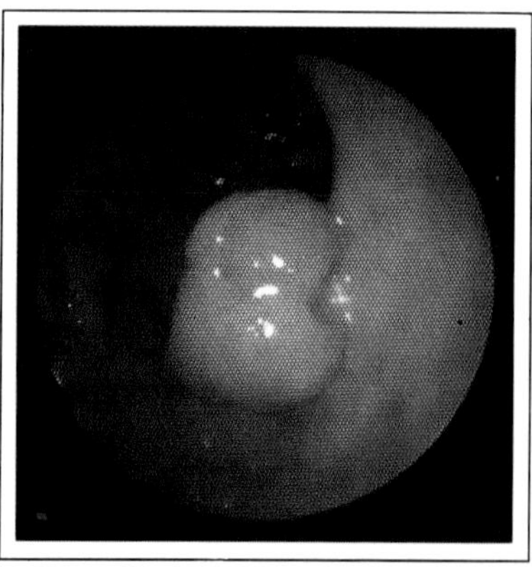

FIG. 17-8b.

FIG. 17-8. a: Submucosal polyp with bridging folds. The polyp appears to be attached to the submucosa by means of two bridging folds (at 3 and 7 o'clock). **b:** Hyperplastic polyp, pedunculated. In this case there is a single attachment, the pedicle, to the surrounding mucosa.

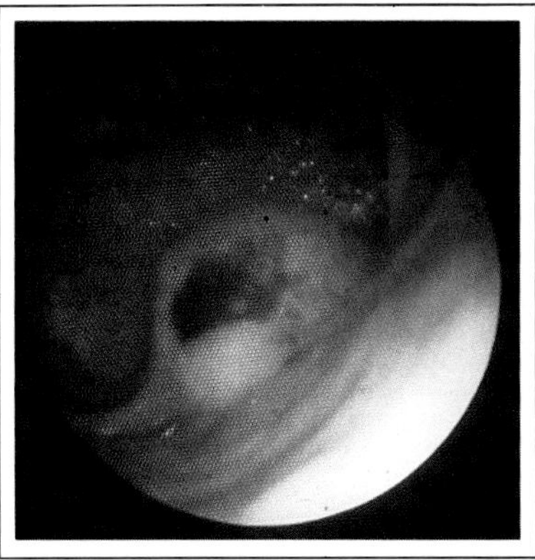

FIG. 17-9.

FIG. 17-9. Leiomyoma with central ulceration. A 1.5-cm sessile lesion on the greater curve of the body with a bridging fold at 8 o'clock with central ulceration (and blood clot) in a patient presenting with upper gastrointestinal hemorrhage.

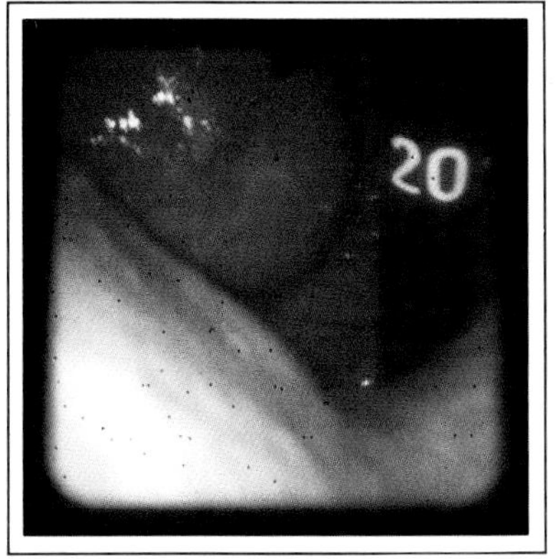

FIG. 17-10a.

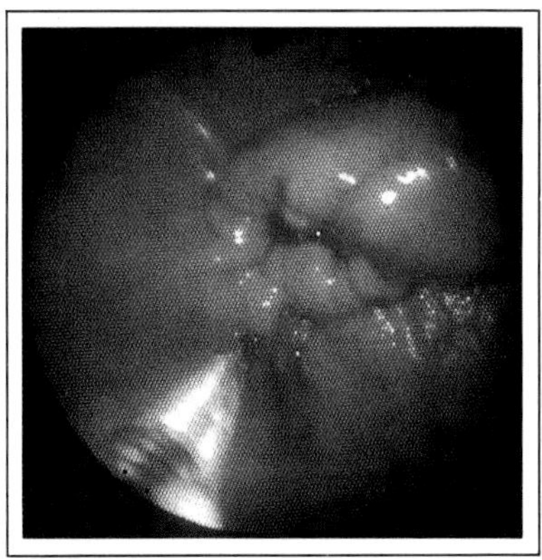

FIG. 17-10b.

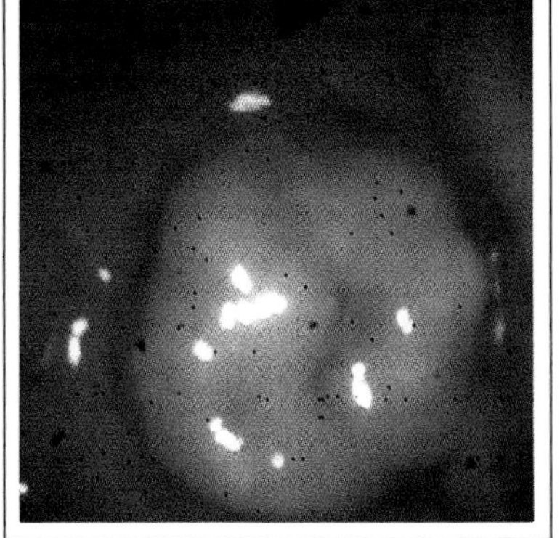

FIG. 17-10c.

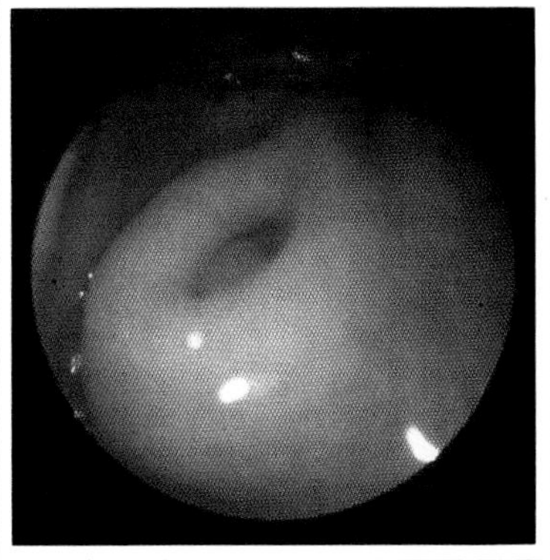

FIG. 17-10d.

FIG. 17-10. a: Leiomyoma in the fundus. A large 3-cm lesion was noted in the retroflexed view of the fundus, a common location for leiomyomas. **b:** Leiomyoma in the body. The overlying mucosa is loosely adherent to the muscle tumor and can be tented somewhat. **c:** Leiomyoma in the fundus. In this case the tumor has a prominent central umbilication. **d:** Leiomyoma with central ulceration located where an umbilication presumably had been. This patient, who was actively bleeding at the time of endoscopy, was admitted with profound iron deficiency anemia.

FIG. 17-11.

FIG. 17-11. Pancreatic rest. The antral location and size (<1 cm) serve to differentiate this lesion from the leiomyoma, which is larger (>1 cm) and is usually found more proximally (Fig. 17-10c).

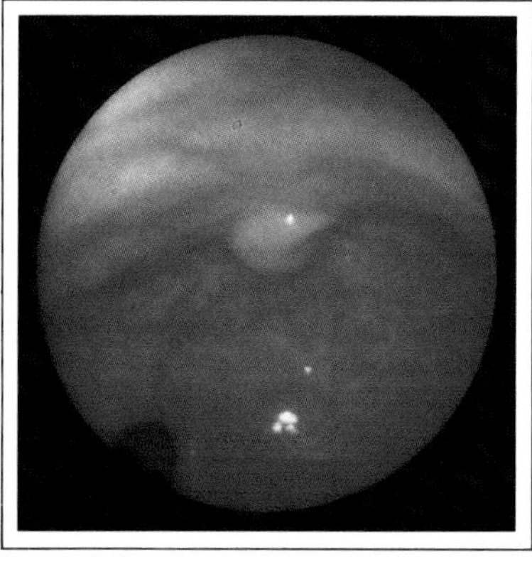

FIG. 17-12.

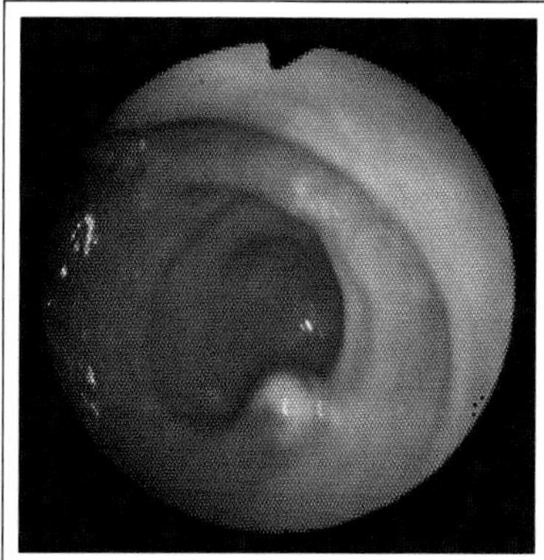

FIG. 17-13.

FIG. 17-12. Myoepithelial hamartoma (gastric adenomyoma). This small antral polyp was thought initially to be hyperplastic. However, histologic examination showed it to be a myoepithelial hamartoma. This was completely excised electrosurgically.

FIG. 17-13. Peutz-Jeghers gastric polyp. A small gastric polyp with an eroded mucosal surface in a patient with known Peutz-Jeghers polyposis.

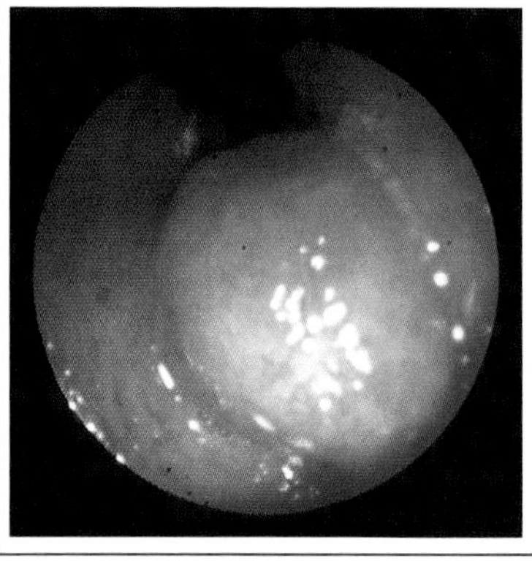

FIG. 17-14a.

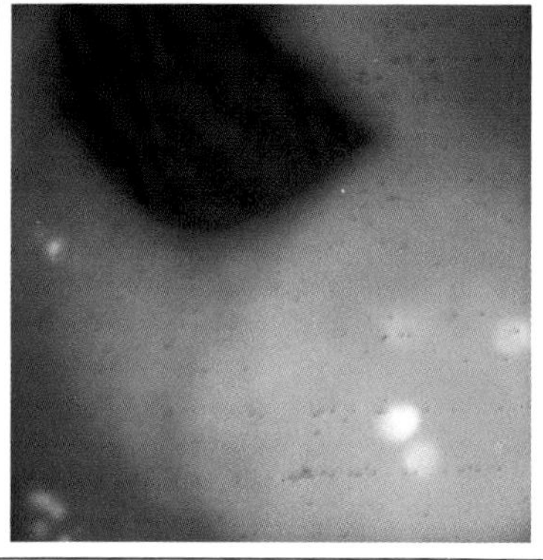

FIG. 17-14b.

FIG. 17-14. a: Gastric carcinoid in the cardia. A submucosal mass with intact mucosa was seen on the posterior wall of the cardia. Surgery in this symptomatic patient with weight loss revealed the mass to be a carcinoid. No other lesions were found. **b:** Gastric carcinoid in the prepyloric antrum. A masslike deformity is seen in the 5 o'clock position of the posterior wall of the prepyloric antrum. This patient was explored because of weight loss and was found to have metastatic carcinoid.

pancreatic rest. For smaller lesions of the antrum, such differentiation is not possible on visual findings alone.[24]

Myoepithelial (Gastric Adenomyoma) and Peutz-Jeghers Hamartomas

We found two cases of myoepithelial hamartoma among 22 submucosal polyps observed over a 7-year period. In both cases the lesion was thought to represent an epithelial polyp and was removed electrosurgically (Fig. 17-12) with the histologic finding of smooth muscle, cysts, and glandular structures coming as a surprise. Both polyps were located in the antrum. The fact that we could observe two cases over a 7-year period probably indicates that these lesions are more common than has been previously reported.[25] Two-thirds of these lesions are true myoepithelial hamartomas; the remaining third contain, in addition, pancreatic acinar tissue for which the term gastric adenomyoma is used.[25]

The lesions range in size from 5 mm to 1.5 cm, being both sessile and pedunculated. The overlying mucosa of the polyp itself may be intact (Fig. 17-12) or eroded.

At endoscopy, gastric hamartomas which occur as part of the Peutz-Jeghers syndrome[26] are indistinguishable from myoepithelial hamartomas or other small polyps of the stomach (Fig. 17-13).

Gastric Carcinoids

The finding of a submucosal polyp is always somewhat worrisome because of the possibility that it could be a gastric carcinoid with its malignant potential. Fortunately, gastric carcinoids are uncommon, accounting for less than 5% of all gastric polyps and 10% or less of submucosal polyps.[27] During the past 7 years, we have encountered only two cases among 125 with gastric polyps. Deyhle[1] reported an even lower incidence of gastric carcinoids in polypectomy material, the figure being only 1.4% of all polyps and 3% of submucosal lesions. The patient with a gastric carcinoid usually has only nonspecific symptoms, prompting investigation. The carcinoid syndrome is unusual,[27a] and such laboratory tests as urinary levels of tryptophan metabolites are for the most part unhelpful as the majority of gastric carcinoids will not have metastasized at the time they are first discovered.[27a]

Gastric carcinoids are typically located on either end of the stomach, with the cardiofundic (Fig. 17-14a) area and the prepyloric antrum (Fig. 17-14b) being the major sites of origin. A smooth submucosa of the cardia or prepyloric antrum would be a typical appearance. Other less common appearances include multiple tiny polyps which are seen as mucosal excrescences[27] or focal raised ulcerated areas resembling the type IIa appearance of early gastric cancer (see Chapter 15).[27]

For a lesion suspected of being a gastric carcinoid, we advise close endoscopic follow-up, at which time additional biopsies may be obtained or the lesion removed electrosurgically. Even in a case where the carcinoid has been removed, continued follow-up is indicated for 2 to 3 years thereafter to look for the appearance of other lesions. For large submucosal polyps (>2 cm) where the diagnosis has been established electrosurgically but the lesion has not been removed, surgery should be strongly considered, as it should in symptomatic patients, especially with unexplained weight loss, to determine if malignant carcinoid is present (Fig. 17-14b). This is especially true for lesions with atypical histologic features.[27]

Other Submucosal Polyps

Less than 10% of submucosal polyps are lipomas, neurofibromas, or other types.[28] In the case of a neurofibroma, although it may represent an isolated finding, it is more likely to occur as part of generalized neurofibromatosis (von Recklinghausen's disease) where the stomach constitutes the second commonest site of involvement.[29] In such a case the presence of a neurofibroma is suggested by its hard, indurated consistency as well as the pattern of reticular brown pigmentation.[30]

Lipomas are also distinctive in that they are said to have a yellowish cast when transilluminated; moreover, when biopsied they exude a greasy yellow material, as in the case of colonic lipomas (see Chapter 41).

A rare type of submucosal polyp which accounted for one of our 22 cases was an eosinophilic granuloma of the stomach. This had a fundic location and umbilicated appearance similar to that of a leiomyoma.[31]

For the less common types of submucosal polyps, performing multiple biopsies ("pecking") at the same site, large-particle biopsy, or needle aspiration cytology (see Chapter 1) may yield representative samples of the specific mesenchymal element which denotes the type of polyp.[22]

REFERENCES

1. Deyhle, P. (1980): Results of endoscopic polypectomy in the gastrointestinal tract. *Endoscopy (Suppl. 1)*, 35–46.
2. Marshak, R. H., and Feldman, F. (1965): Gastric polyps. *Am. J. Dig. Dis.*, 10:909–935.
3. ReMine, S. G., Hughes, R. W., and Weiland, L. H. (1981): Endoscopic gastric polypectomies. *Mayo Clin. Proc.*, 56:371–375.
4. Mark, L. K., and Samter, T. (1975): Villous adenomas of the stomach. *Am. J. Gastroenterol.*, 64:127–139.
5. Elster, K. (1976): Histologic classification of gastric polyps. In: *Pathology of the Gastrointestinal Tract. Current Topics in Pathology*, edited by B. C. Morson, pp. 77–93. Springer-Verlag, New York.
6. Humphries, T. J. (1981): Gastric glandular cysts: uncommon or unrecognized? *Gastrointest. Endosc.*, 27:123.

6a. Taor, R. E., Fox, B., and Johnson, A. G. (1975): Gastritis—gastroscopic and microscopic. *Endoscopy*, 7:209–215.

7. Cheli, R., Santi, L., Ciancamerla, G., and Canciani, G. (1973): A clinical and statistical follow-up study of atrophic gastritis. *Am. J. Dig. Dis.*, 18:1061–1066.
8. Tomasulo, J. (1971): Gastric polyps: histologic types and their relationship to gastric carcinoma. *Cancer*, 27:1346–1355.
9. Papp, J. P., and Joseph, J. I. (1976): Adenocarcinoma occurring in a hyperplastic gastric polyp: removal by electrosurgical polypectomy. *Gastrointest. Endosc.*, 23:38–39.
10. Remmnele, W., and Kolb, E. F. (1978): Malignant transformation of hyperplasiogenic polyps of the stomach. *Endoscopy*, 10:63–65.
11. Mizuno, H., Kobayashi, S., and Kasuqai, T. (1975): Endoscopic followup of gastric polyps. *Gastrointest. Endosc.*, 23:38–39.
12. Singer, M., Busse, R., Seib, H.-J., Elster, K., and Ottenjann, R. (1975): Endoscopic polypectomy in the upper gastrointestinal tract. *Endoscopy*, 7:216–221.
13. Watanabe, H., Enjoji, M., Yao, T., and Ohsato, K. (1978): Gastric lesions in familial adenomatosis coli: their incidence and histologic analysis. *Hum. Pathol.*, 9:269–283.
14. Walk, L. (1951): Villous tumors of the stomach: clinical review and report of two cases. *Arch. Intern. Med.*, 87:560–569.
15. Sanner, C. J., Saltzman, D. A., and Mueller, J. C. (1978): Polypoid gastritis: report of a case associated with gastric carcinoma and review of the literature. *Am. J. Dig. Dis. (Suppl.)*, 23:560–569.
16. Weaver, G. A., and Kleinman, M. S. (1978): Gastric polyposis due to multiple hyperplastic adenomatous polyps. *Am. J. Dig. Dis.*, 23:346–352.
17. Ranzi, T., Castagnone, D., Velio, P., Bianchi, P., and Polli, E. E. (1981): Gastric and duodenal polyps in familial polyposis coli. *Gut*, 22:363–367.
18. Rubin, M., Tuthill, R. J., Rosato, E. F., and Cohen, S. (1980): Cronkhite-Canada syndrome: report of an unusual case. *Gastroenterology*, 79:737–741.
19. Weinstock, J. V., and Kawanishi, H. (1978): Gastrointestinal polyposis with orocutaneous hamartomas (Cowden's disease). *Gastroenterology*, 74:890–895.
20. Gordon, R., Laufer, I., and Kressel, H. Y. (1980): Gastric polyps found in routine double contrast examination of the stomach. *Radiology*, 134:27–30.
21. Das, B. C., Laing, R. R., Dunn, G. D., and Klotz, A. P. (1970): Endoscopic findings in gastric leiomyomas. *Gastrointest. Endosc.*, 16:152–155.
22. Seifert, E. (1981): Endoscopic diagnosis of nonepithelial tumors of the stomach: relevant technique and pitfalls. *Gastrointest. Endosc.*, 26:128.
23. Cabre-Fiol, V., Vilardell, F., Sala-Cladera, E., and Mota, A. P. (1975): Preoperative cytologic diagnosis of gastric leiomyosarcoma: a report of three cases. *Gastroenterology*, 68:563–566.
24. Perrillo, R. P., Zuckerman, G. R., and Shatz, B. A. (1977): Aberrant pancreas and leiomyoma of the stomach: indistinguishable radiological and endoscopic features. *Gastrointest. Endosc.*, 23:162–163.
25. Lasser, A., and Kaufman, W. B. (1977): Adenomyoma of the stomach. *Am. J. Dig. Dis.*, 22:965–970.
26. McKittrick, J. E., Lewis, W. M., Doane, W. A., and Gerwig, W. H. (1971): The Peutz-Jeghers syndrome. *Arch. Surg.*, 103:57–62.
27. Seifert, E., and Elster, K. (1977): Carcinoids of the stomach: report of two cases. *Am. J. Gastrointest.*, 68:372–378.

27a. Feldman, A. J., Weinberg, M., Raess, D., Richardson, M. L., and Fry, W. J. (1981): Gastric carcinoid tumor. *Arch. Surg.*, 116:118–121.

28. Seifert, E., and Elster, K. (1975): Gastric polypectomy. *Am. J. Gastroenterol.*, 66:451–456.
29. Hochberg, F. H., Dasilva, A. B., Galdabini, J., and Richardson, E. P. (1974): Gastrointestinal involvement in von Recklinghausen's neurofibromatosis. *Neurology*, 24:1144–1151.
30. Rutgeerts, P., Hendrickx, K., Geboes, K., Ponette, E., Broeckaert, L., and Vantrappen, G. (1981): Involvement of the upper digestive tract by systemic neurofibromatosis. *Gastrointest. Endosc.*, 27:22–25.
31. Eshchar, J., Kimerling, J. J., and Gilboa, J. (1973): Eosinophilic granuloma of the stomach simulating leiomyoma. *Gastrointest. Endosc.*, 20:72.

18

ALTERATIONS IN THE SHAPE OF THE GASTRIC LUMEN

During examination of the stomach, the endoscopist continually inspects the gastric lumen, his roadway. Typically, it appears as a perfectly symmetrical cylindrical channel, extending directly from a point just beyond the entry in the upper body to the pylorus (Fig. 18-1a).

There are three types of abnormality discussed in this chapter which alter the cylindrical appearance of the gastric lumen. These are: (a) anatomic variations in the shape of the stomach; (b) ulcer scar deformity which involves the mucosal folds and the lumen; and (c) extrinsic compression.

ANATOMIC VARIATION IN THE SHAPE OF THE STOMACH

Variation in the shape of the stomach has long been appreciated by radiologists.[1] These have been designated "steerhorn," "fishhook," and "cascade." In each case there is either disproportionate enlargement of some part of the stomach, e.g., the fundus in the case of the cascade stomach (Fig. 18-1b), or an alteration in the angulation between the body and antrum, either increased as in the fishhook shape or decreased (or absent) in the case of the steerhorn shape.[1]

Of these, the one most likely to alter the appearance of the lumen is the cascade shape, where the fundus is disproportionately enlarged and is seen directly on entry into the stomach (Fig. 18-1c). If the relatively small communication point between the large fundus and smaller body is not observed (Fig. 18-1c), the endoscope tip is repeatedly retroflexed into the cavernous fundus (Fig. 18-1d). Ultimately, when the communication point is found, the lumen appears relatively narrowed because of the oversized fundus (Fig. 18-1c).

In the case of the steerhorn shape, the usual angulation of the antrum in relation to the body is lost, so that the prepyloric antrum appears to be projecting downward from the body.

Finally, in the fishhook type of appearance, the angulation between the body and antrum is accentuated so that the usual site of the antrum continuing just beyond the body is lost, with the antrum not being seen at this point. Sometimes with this stomach shape the antrum must be entered blindly. This is facilitated by aligning the tip in the midline of the lower body and following its passage across what seems to be the angulus, advancing it with maximum "up" deflection.

ULCER SCAR DEFORMITY

The healing of a gastric ulcer (Fig. 18-2a), especially one that is more than 1 cm in diameter and has a depth of more than 3 mm, may be accompanied by submucosal fibrosis, which has the effect of pulling the surrounding mucosa to the site of the ulcer crater. This results in the characteristic endoscopic appearance of converging folds (Fig. 18-2b). Although this generally causes a distorted appearance of the involved portion of the gastric wall with little if any effect on the lumen (Fig. 18-3a), in 10 to 20% of cases there may be distortion of the lumen as well (Fig. 18-3b).

We find the ulcer scar deformity in approximately 2% of examinations, a figure comparable to that found in a radiography series where this pattern has been noted in up to 4% of cases, particularly in patients with prior endoscopic demonstration of gastric ulcers.[2]

When found at endoscopy, especially when performed for the evaluation of ulcer symptoms, the importance of the ulcer scar deformity appearance is that it both suggests previous peptic ulcer disease and signals an area requiring careful examination to exclude an active ulcer (Fig. 18-3c).

Appearance

Body

Previous ulceration in this portion of the stomach distorts the parallelism of the rugal folds (Fig. 18-2a) at a point,

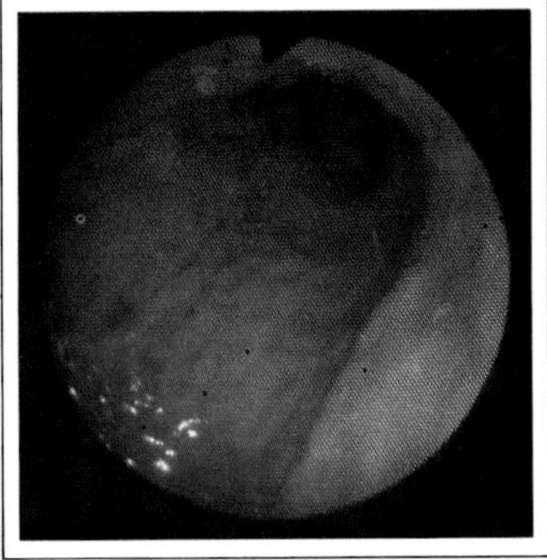

FIG. 18-1a.

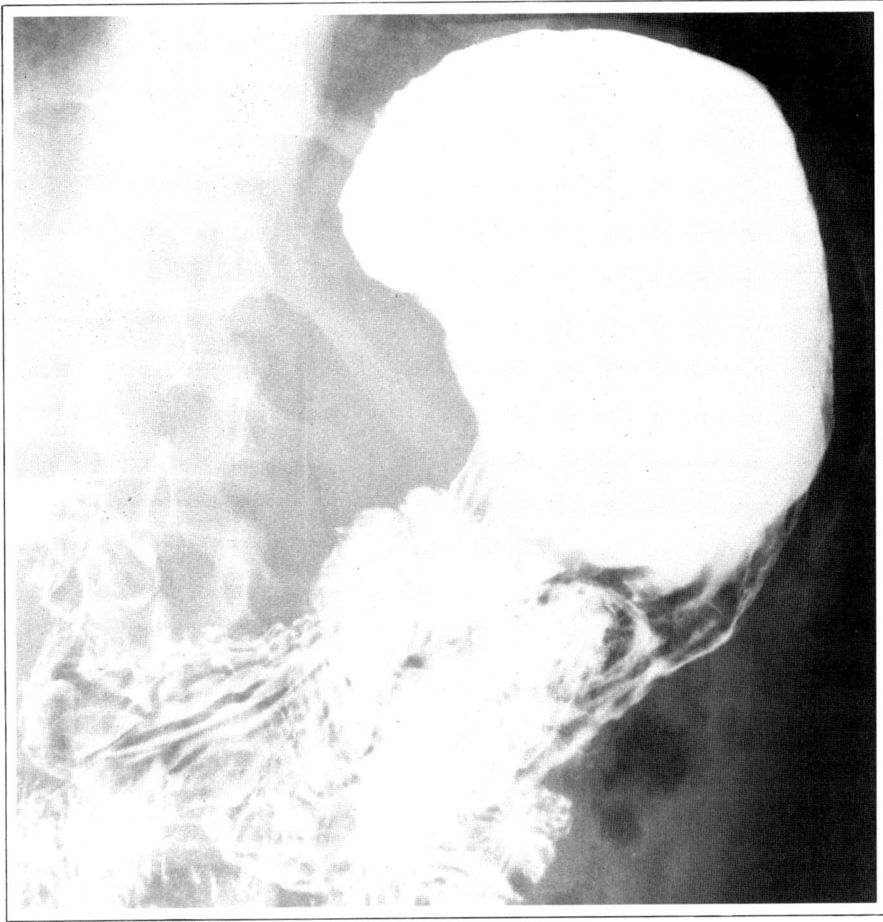

FIG. 18-1b.

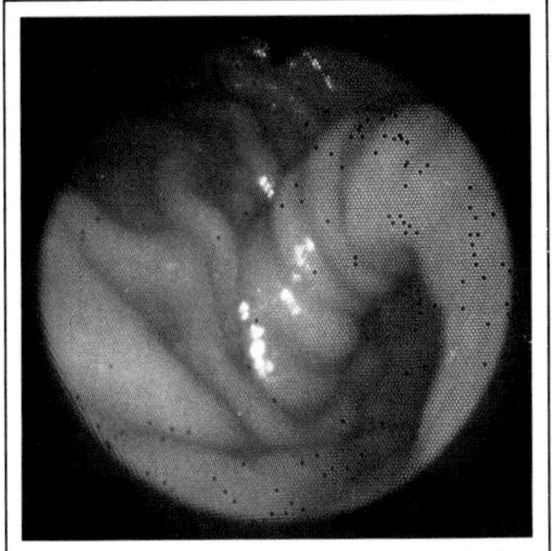

FIG. 18-1c.

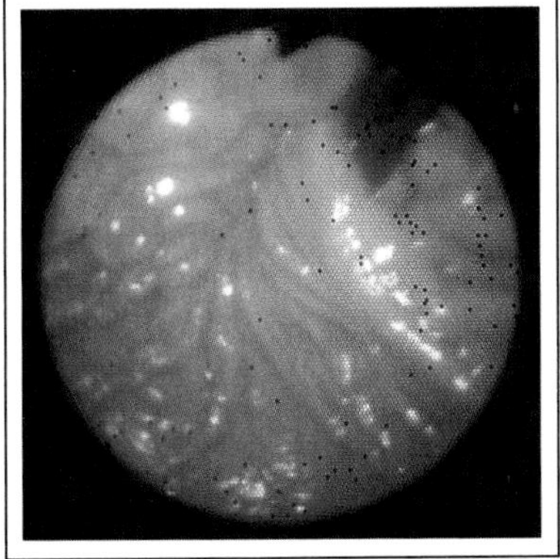

FIG. 18-1d.

FIG. 18-1. a: Gastric lumen, body, and antrum. The typical symmetrical tubular shape of the gastric lumen is apparent. **b:** Radiographic appearance of the cascade stomach, with its disproportionately large fundus. **c:** Gastric lumen, cascade stomach. With this anatomic shape, the fundus has a cavernous, rather than a tubular, appearance. **d:** Fundus, cascade stomach. Because of the disproportionate end of the fundus, it is repeatedly entered unless its relatively narrow communication with the body is identified (c). In a U-type retroflexion, its lumen appears cavernous.

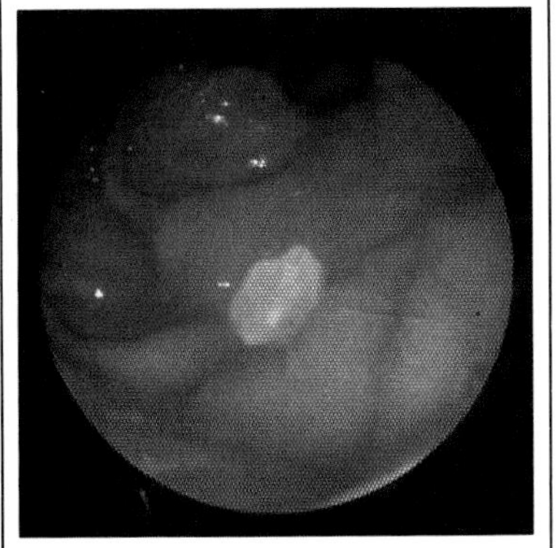

FIG. 18-2a.

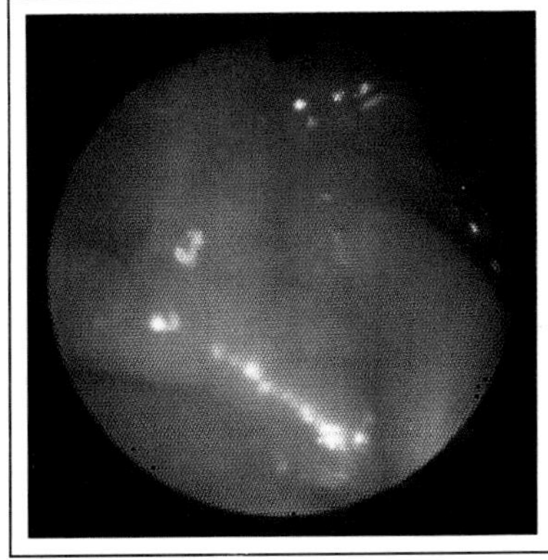

FIG. 18-2b.

FIG. 18-2. a: Gastric ulcer, active. A discrete 0.75-cm punched-out ulcer base is observed on the posterior wall of the body with surrounding folds running into the margin. **b:** Gastric ulcer scar after healing of a previous active ulcer (a). The folds from 9 and 11 o'clock converge at a central point, the site of previous ulceration. The converging folds distort the expected parallelism of the rugal folds.

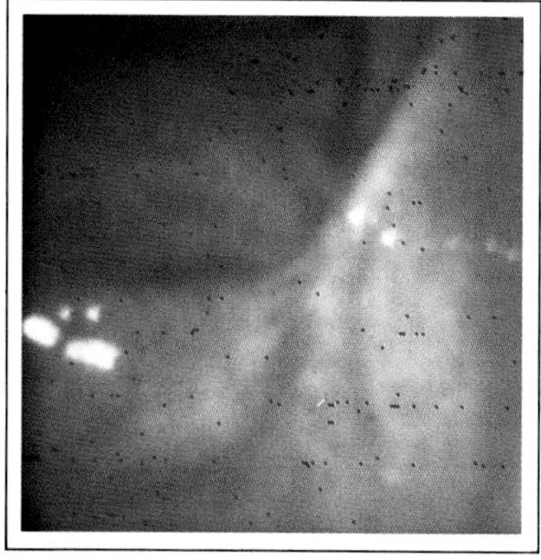

FIG. 18-3a.

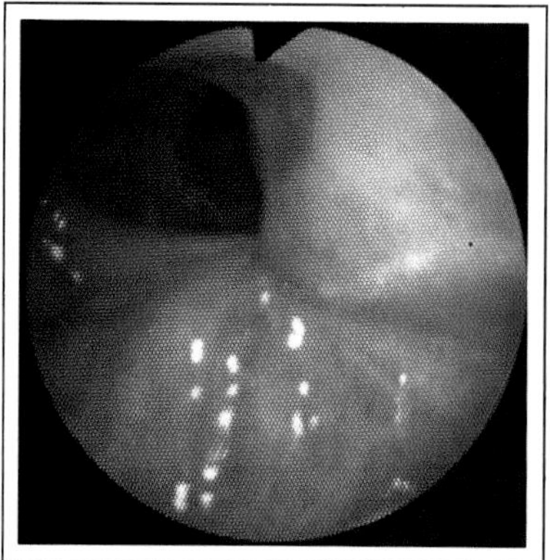

FIG. 18-3b.

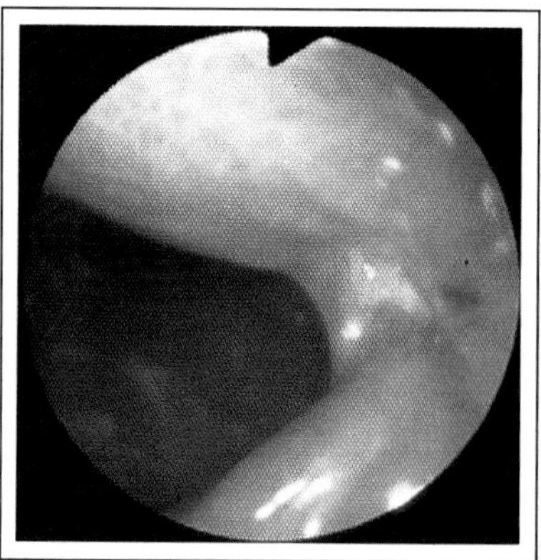

FIG. 18-3c.

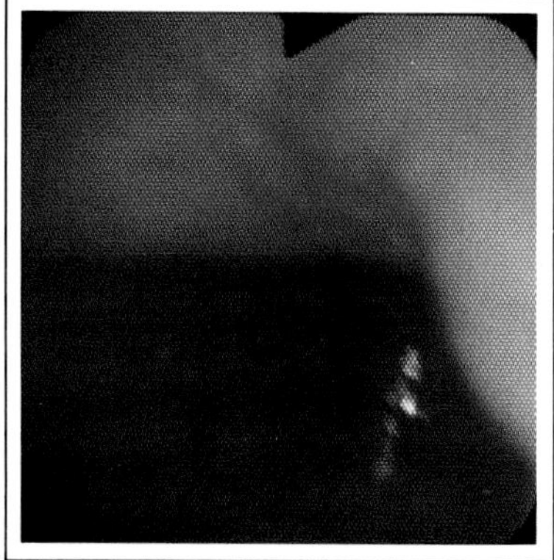

FIG. 18-4a.

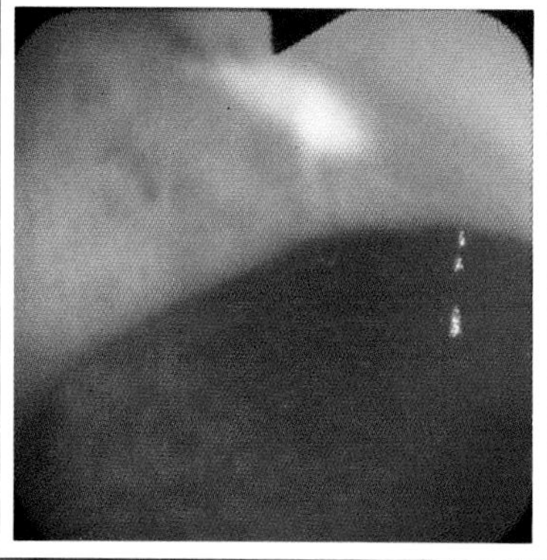

FIG. 18-4b.

FIG. 18-3. Gastric ulcer scar in the body. **a:** Converging folds are seen with minimal distortion of the lumen. **b:** Converging folds (from 6 and 9 o'clock) occur with marked narrowing of the lumen. **c:** Within an ulcer scar. Just beyond the proximal margin of the area of scar deformity (c) is an 8-mm ulceration.

FIG. 18-4. a: Gastric ulcer scar in the angle (Henning sign). The angle is no longer crescent-shaped but is sharply angulated in its midline. The erythema and deformity suggest that an active ulcer may be present. **b:** Gastric ulcer scar, single, with an active ulcer. Careful inspection of the erythematous, depressed area of the gastric angle (a) revealed an active ulcer.

presumably, where there has been recurrent ulceration and healing. The commonest location within the body for ulcer scars would be the posterior aspect of the lesser curve (in the mid-body), the most frequent location for ulcers of this portion of the stomach. In cases where scarification is marked, there may be a striking distortion of the luminal appearance (Fig. 18-3b). In such cases, especially, one inspects carefully for evidence of an active ulcer (Fig. 18-3c).

Angle

At the angle, the "point" effect of ulcer scarring produces the so-called Henning or "V" sign in which the angle loses its perfect crescent shape (see Chapter 11) and becomes sharply angulated or arched (Fig. 18-4a). As in the case of ulcer scar deformity of the body, one must carefully inspect the area within an angular deformity for evidence of an active ulcer (Fig. 18-4b).

Antrum

In the antrum, previous peptic ulcer disease produces converging folds (Fig. 18-5a), which should signal the same need for scrutiny as in other areas where ulcer scar deformity is found. In the antrum, however, prominent folds may be present which because of their size appear to converge (Fig. 18-5b). Not all converging folds of the antrum, therefore, can be taken as evidence of previous peptic disease.

One type of scar deformity peculiar to the antrum is that in which there is involvement of both anterior and posterior walls, which appear to link up, resulting in a circumferential deformity called the pseudopylorus (Fig. 18-5c) similar to congenital antral mucosal diaphragms (webs) already discussed (see Chapter 13). As in other areas of the stomach where scar-type deformity is found (Fig. 18-6a), those of the antrum must be carefully inspected for hidden active ulcers (Fig. 18-6).

Ulcer Scar Deformity and Gastric Cancer

Although one might expect any ulcer associated with scar deformity to be benign, either in the active (Fig. 18-7a) or the healing (Fig. 18-7b) phase, this is not invariably the case. Prior ulceration and scarification does not reduce the likelihood of gastric malignancy. Some investigators in fact believe that the cancer risk is slightly increased over that in the general population.[3] The mucosal appearance within any area of scar deformity must be judged on its own regardless of the question of malignancy. An ulcer within a ulcer scar should have a uniform base and regular margins (Fig. 18-7a), whereas one in the late stages of healing shows focal or linear erythema (Fig. 18-7b). Cases where

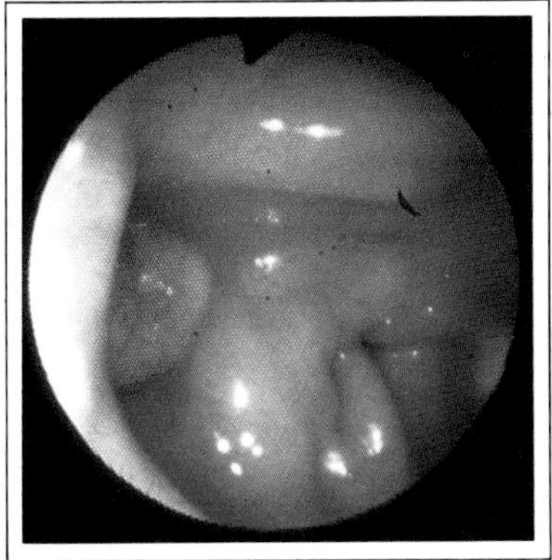

FIG. 18-5a.

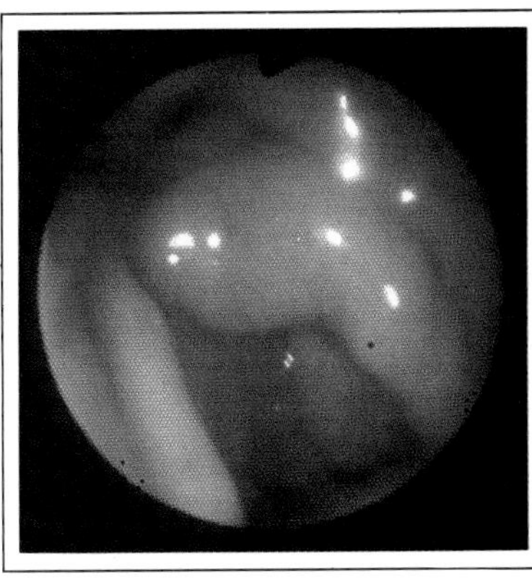

FIG. 18-5b.

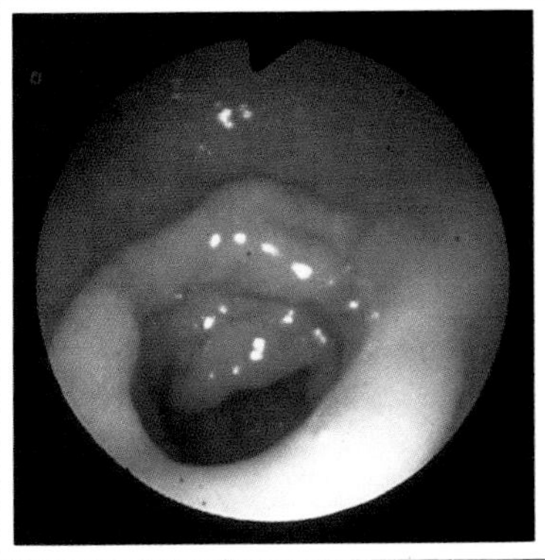

FIG. 18-5c.

FIG. 18-5. a: Gastric ulcer scar in the antrum with an active ulcer. An area of converging folds on the anterior wall of the mid-antrum is noted within which is an active 7.5-mm ulcer. **b:** Prominent prepyloric antral folds simulating an ulcer scar deformity. Multiple large prepyloric folds appear in this asymptomatic patient, examined as part of a work-up for anemia. No history of peptic ulcer disease or ulcer-type symptoms could be elicited in this case. **c:** Gastric ulcer scar in the antrum with a pseudopylorus-type deformity. The scar deformity of the anterior and posterior walls link up by means of a transverse fold. This creates a narrowing just proximal to the pyloric channel giving the appearance of a second pylorus, or pseudopylorus.

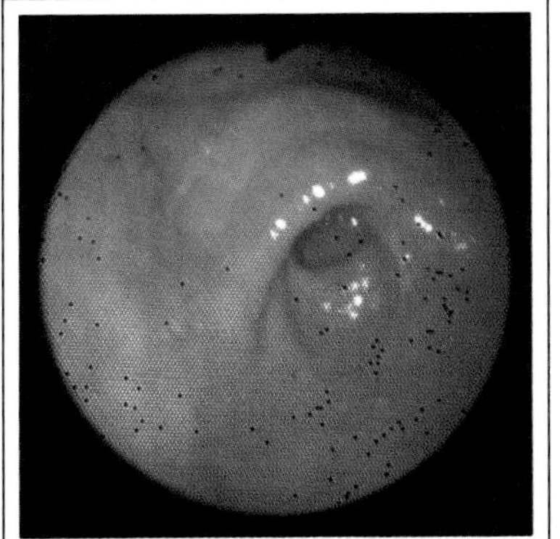

FIG. 18-6a.

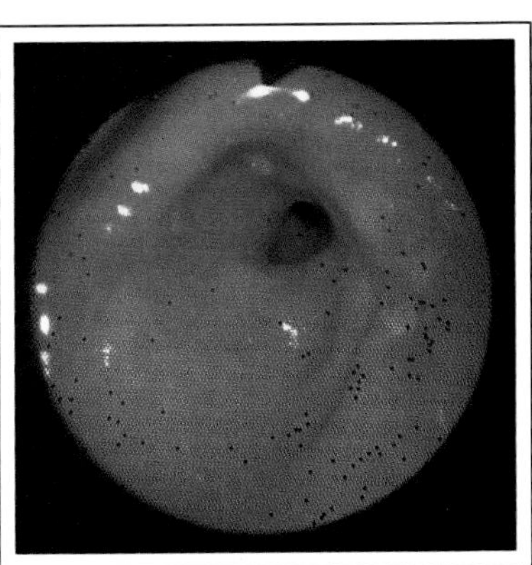

FIG. 18-6b.

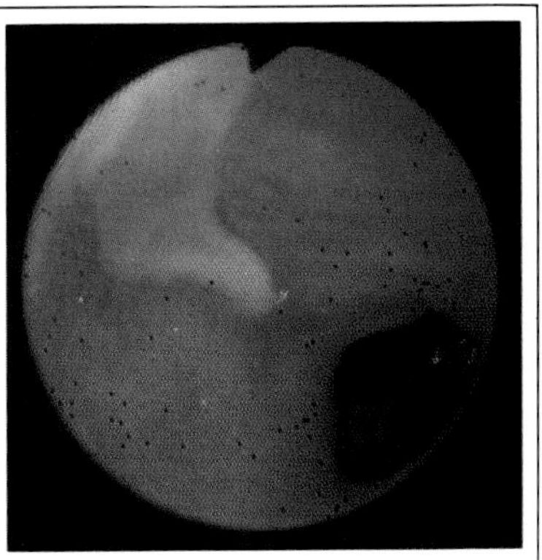

FIG. 18-6c.

FIG. 18-6. Gastric ulcer scar in the prepyloric antrum. **a:** Two converging folds of the greater curve and anterior wall create an asymmetrical appearance for the area just proximal to the pyloric channel. **b:** With active ulceration. Closer inspection of a prepyloric scar deformity (a) suggests an active ulcer. **c:** Even closer inspection of the scar deformity demonstrates a large (5 × 10 mm) active ulcer.

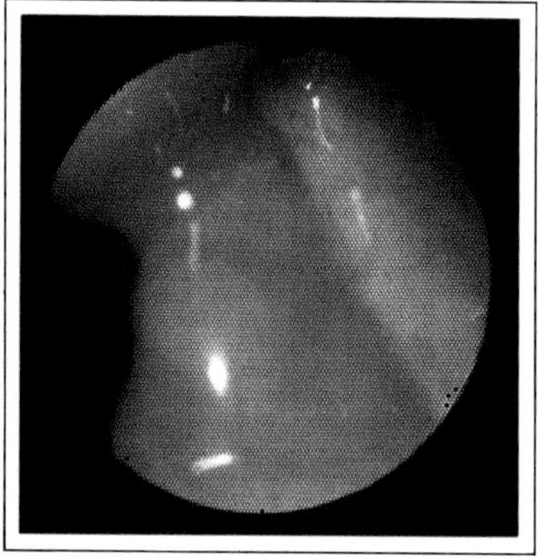

FIG. 18-7a.

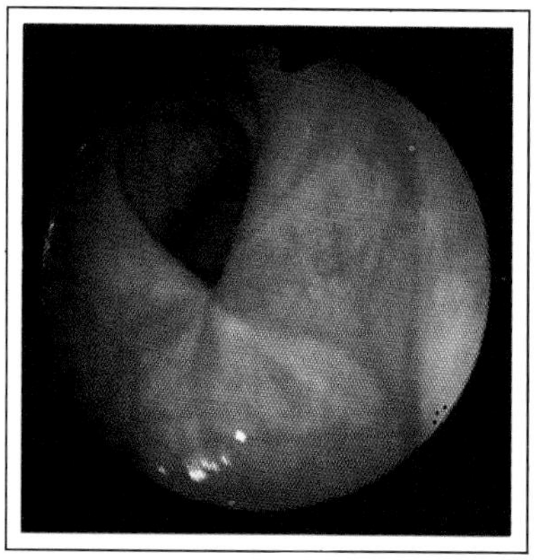

FIG. 18-7b.

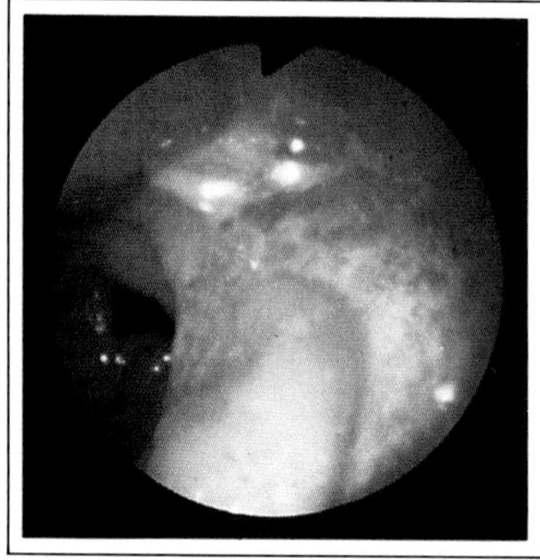

FIG. 18-7c.

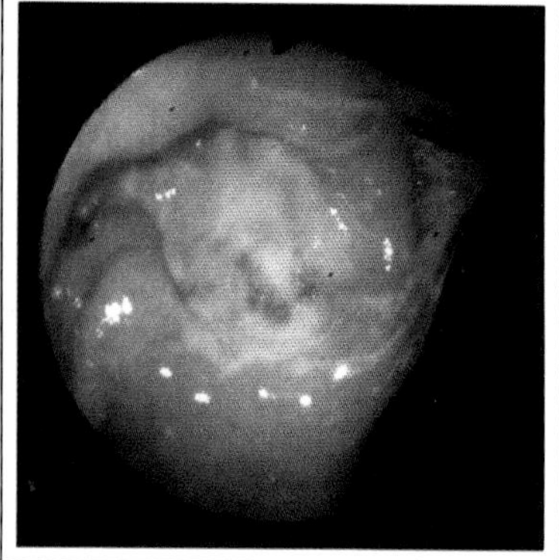

FIG. 18-7d.

FIG. 18-7. a: Ulcer scar deformity in the prepyloric antrum with active ulceration. This is a large ulcer with benign features. **b:** Ulcer scar deformity with an almost healed ulcer (late red scar stage—see Chapter 15). **c:** Ulcer scar deformity with gastric cancer. In this case the mucosa within the scar deformity, adjacent to the ulceration, has an atypical appearance with erythema being broken up by larger areas of gray-white mucosa. **d:** Ulcer scar deformity with gastric cancer. An ulcer is set in a prepyloric deformity with converging folds at 6 and 8 o'clock. Even though previous ulceration had been noted in the same area radiographically several years before, the irregular appearance of the base, especially at its interface with the margin (at 6 o'clock), was regarded by the endoscopist as a highly suspicious feature.

the margin (Fig. 18-7c) or the base, especially at its interface with the margin (Fig. 18-7d), has an atypical appearance should be viewed as highly suspicious and cause the endoscopist to pursue biopsies vigorously (obtaining eight or more specimens) as he would in the case of an ulcer whose appearance was considered malignant (see Chapter 15).

EXTRINSIC COMPRESSION

We already considered alterations in the appearance of the gastric lumen from anatomic variation in the shape of the stomach and as a result of peptic ulcer disease and scarring; these types of alterations we may consider as intrinsic. A third cause of an altered appearance comes from extrinsic sources, i.e., compression from structures which lay adjacent to the stomach. The circumstances in which compression occur are varied, but we may consider them as two main types: (a) nonpathologic, where the organ compressing the stomach is not diseased; and (b) pathologic, where the organ is diseased.

Non-Pathologic Extrinsic Compression

The stomach lies in intimate relation to the spleen and colon. Usually these structures are not apparent when the stomach is distended with air, but from time to time they are evident simply because of the particular relation they bear to the stomach. The appearance of extrinsic compression from these organs, therefore, does not necessarily imply a pathologic condition.

Spleen

One may see in a retroflexed view an elevation of the posterior aspect of the fundus, beginning just adjacent to the cardia and running toward the anterior wall (9 o'clock) aspect (Fig. 18-5). In some cases the raised mucosa takes on a blue-gray cast.

The question which naturally arises in patients with extrinsic compression from the spleen is whether it is from a normal-sized or an enlarged organ. No specific figure can be cited for the upper limits of a "normal" splenic impression. It is our belief that the impression made by a normal-sized spleen rarely runs more than 3 cm in either the anterior (9 o'clock) or the distal (6 o'clock) direction. When the impression exceeds 5 cm (Fig. 18-8) or involves the entire fundus, one should expect splenomegaly.

Colon

Generally, the transverse colon is separated from the stomach by the transverse mesocolon. A distended colon

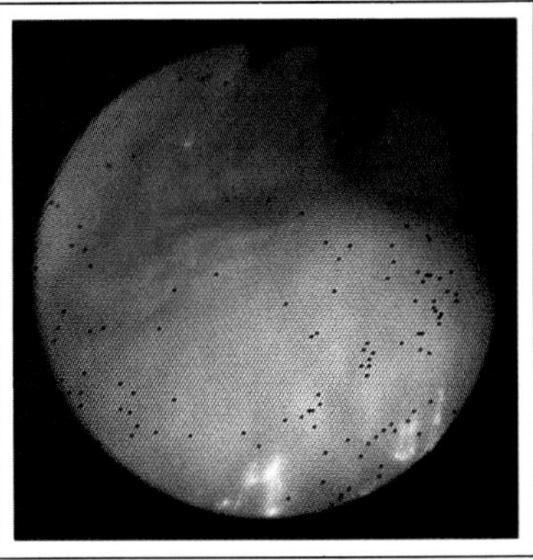

FIG. 18-8.

FIG. 18-8. Extrinsic compression caused by an enlarged spleen. In this patient with massive splenomegaly, extrinsic compression by the spleen involves much of the posterior wall and greater curve aspect of the fundus.

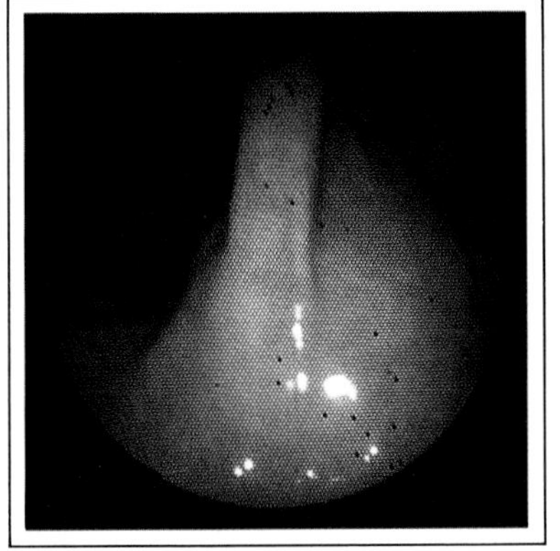

FIG. 18-9a.

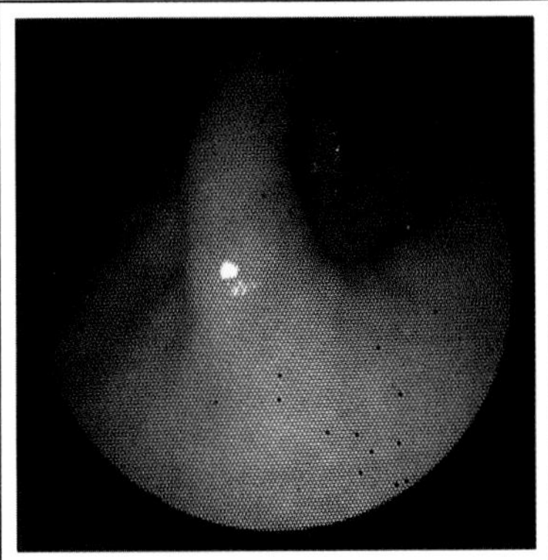

FIG. 18-9b.

FIG. 18-9. Extrinsic compression from the colon. **a:** A submucosal mass of the anterior wall of the gastric angle. **b:** Within 30 sec the submucosal mass (a) has disappeared, most likely as a result of colonic peristalsis.

or one full of feces may produce extrinsic compression of the greater curve of the antrum or lower body and give rise to the endoscopic appearance of a submucosal mass or masses on the anterior wall aspect of the greater curve (Fig. 18-9a). These vary in size and shape with antral as well as colonic peristalsis (Fig. 18-9b). Furthermore, the application of a biopsy forceps to the "mass" generally causes it to disappear, an immediate sign that it is extrinsic to the stomach.

Extrinsic Compression in Pathologic States

One might expect extrinsic compression from an enlarged liver, either with cirrhosis or metastatic disease, or from pancreatic enlargement either with chronic pancreatitis or carcinoma to be relatively common in patients examined at a referral center such as ours. Surprisingly, we find extrinsic compression to be uncommon. We have, in fact, encountered only 20 such cases out of 5,000 examinations performed over a 7-year period. Five of these were found with liver involvement with the remainder being pancreatic, either from carcinoma (10 cases) or chronic pancreatitis (with inflammatory mass or pseudocyst in 5 cases).

Liver Disease

Extrinsic compression from hepatomegaly either from cirrhosis or metastatic carcinoma most commonly involves either the body or antrum. As the liver enlarges, because of its anatomic relation to the stomach, it will compress the lesser curve and anterior wall. In some cases of metastatic liver disease, one may see discrete submucosal masses corresponding to the "gastric cannonball" appearance described radiographically.[4]

Pancreatic Disease

Pancreatic cancer is, in our experience, the most common cause of extrinsic compression of the body or antrum. Because most pancreatic cancers arise from the head of the pancreas, adjacent to the descending duodenum, the extrinsic compression produced will generally be along the greater curve of the antrum, from its posterior wall aspect (Fig. 18-10a). Occasionally, advanced pancreatic cancer is associated with mesenteric or omental spread so that the tumor mass compresses the anterior wall. For carcinomas of the pancreas arising in other locations, there may be extrinsic compression of the posterior wall of either the body or the fundus (Fig. 18-10b).

With marked enlargement of the pancreas and lesser sac in pancreatitis associated with phlegmon or pseudocyst formation, there is extrinsic compression of the posterior wall in the greater curve of the antrum or body. In some cases where the antrum is involved, this results in complete

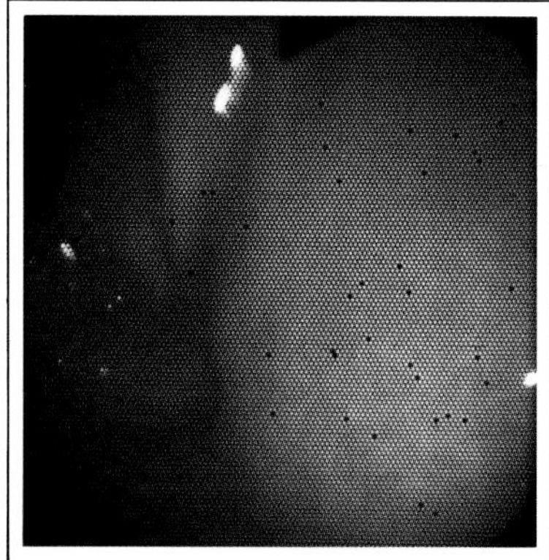

FIG. 18-10a.

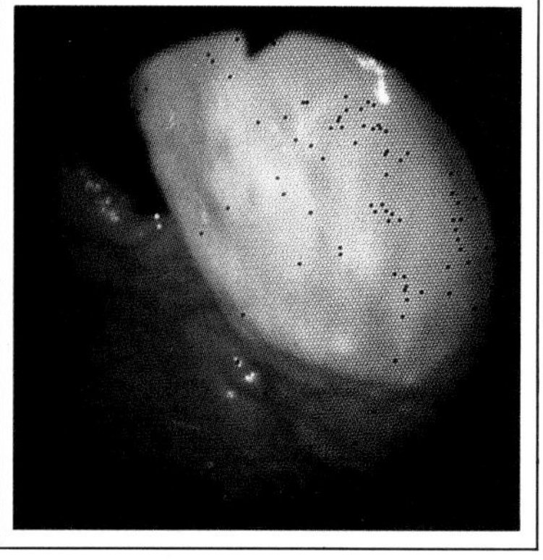

FIG. 18-10b.

FIG. 18-10. a: Extrinsic compression on the antrum from a pancreatic carcinoma (head). Extrinsic compression, deforming the lumen of the antrum, is noted from the posterior wall aspect of the antrum. **b:** Extrinsic compression of the upper body from a pancreatic carcinoma (tail). With U-type retroflexion, extrinsic compression of the cardia, the posterior wall of the fundus, and the lesser curve (toward 12 o'clock) was noted. At surgery a large tumor mass was found to be impinging on the stomach in this area.

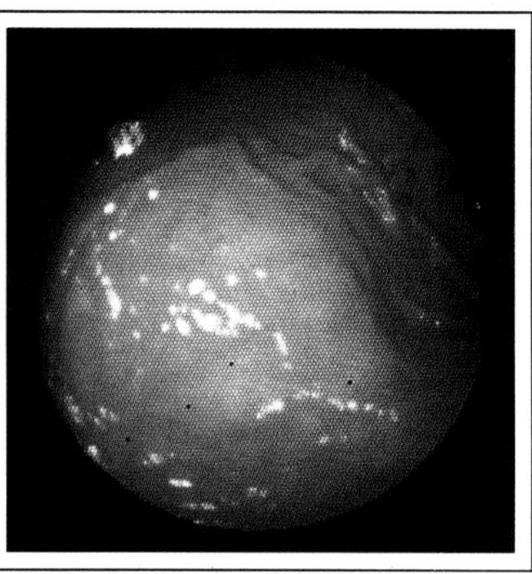

FIG. 18-11.

FIG. 18-11. Extrinsic compression on the upper body, greater curve, from a large pseudocyst of the body of the pancreas.

gastric outlet obstruction. As in the case of duodenal compression (see Chapter 28), extrinsic compression of the stomach may be associated with erythema, sometimes marked, in the setting of acute pancreatitis.

With chronic pancreatitis, inflammatory masses, especially pseudocysts of the body and tail, produce extrinsic compression of the proximal stomach (Fig. 18-11). Rarely, there is spontaneous perforation of pseudocysts to the stomach, where at endoscopy an opening (of 1 cm or more) into the pseudocyst is seen.[5]

REFERENCES

1. Meschan, I., Landsman, H., and Regnier, G. (1953): The normal radiographic adult stomach and duodenum. *South. Med. J.*, 46:878–885.
2. Gelfand, D. W., and Ott, D. J. (1981): Gastric ulcer scars. ***Radiology***, 140:37–43.
3. Montgomery, R. D., and Richardson, B. P. (1975): Gastric ulcer and cancer. *Q. J. Med.*, 46:591–599.
4. Doss, J. C., and Ferucci, J. T. (1974): Gastric cannonballs: a roentgen sign of hepatic metastasis. ***Gastroenterology***, 67:519–520.
5. Bretholz, A., Lammli, P., Corrodi, P., and Knoblauch, M. (1978): Ruptured pancreatic pseudocysts: diagnosis of endoscopy. ***Endoscopy***, 10:19–23.

19

POSTSURGICAL APPEARANCES OF THE STOMACH

Endoscopy is often requested for patients who have had previous gastric surgery. In our practice these cases account for 10 to 15% of the total. Because of the diversity of postsurgical appearances, the endoscopic examinations are some of the most difficult for the endoscopist to perform, providing many technical as well as interpretive challenges. We have organized this chapter in a way which we believe enables the reader to anticipate and better understand the appearances he will encounter in patients with prior gastric surgery.

As peptic ulcer disease is the commonest indication for gastric surgery, the chapter begins with a consideration of the typical anatomic arrangements the endoscopist encounters as a consequence of surgical treatment. Following this, we provide a more detailed account of specific stomal and gastric mucosal appearances. Finally, we briefly consider appearances which are the result of other (nonulcer) surgical procedures.

COMMON APPEARANCES AFTER ULCER SURGERY

In this section, we review the expected appearances for the common ulcer operations, mainly from the standpoint of their general anatomy, reserving for a separate treatment the range of mucosal appearances, especially erythema, which though striking may be found without associated histologic change in asymptomatic patients.[1]

Pyloroplasty

One frequently performed operation for peptic ulcer disease is vagotomy coupled with a Heineke-Mikulicz pyloroplasty.[2] This operation produces the characteristic appearance of a gaping pyloric ring with a concentric second ring just beyond (Fig. 19-1a). This double-ring appearance results from the vertical closure of an incision made along the longitudinal axis of the pyloric channel.[2] In practice, both rings as well as the intervening depression between them are carefully inspected in search of a recurrent ulcer (see below). The mucosa of the first ring is gastric while that of the second ring (which is the site of the original channel) is either gastric or duodenal.

A less common type of pyloroplasty is the Finney or Jaboulay type. Both are in reality a gastroduodenostomy with an anastomotic opening created between the antrum and the descending duodenum, just below an often stenosed pyloric channel (Fig. 19-1b). The distinction between the Finney and Jaboulay types of pyloroplasty has to do with how the gastroduodenal anastomosis is created,[3] but this does not bear on the endoscopic appearance. The gastroduodenostomy stoma, located just below the true pylorus, creates the endoscopic appearance of a double pylorus. This must not be confused with a true double pylorus, which results from a penetrating ulcer having formed a gastroduodenal fistula (Fig. 19-1c). In the true double pylorus (see Chapter 22) both channels generally enter the duodenal bulb, whereas in the Finney or Jaboulay pyloroplasty the gastroduodenal anastomosis is always joined to the descending duodenum and is recognized by the finding of typical Kerckring folds (see Chapter 24).

Billroth II (Hemigastrectomy With Gastrojejunal) Anastomosis

A hemigastrectomy is more often performed with a gastrojejunal (Billroth II) than a gastroduodenal (Billroth I) anastomosis.[3] Technical factors make the Billroth II anastomosis easier to perform. The endoscopist recognizes the Billroth II anatomy by two findings. The first of these is the termination of rugal folds and lumen in a position where one would have expected the antrum (Fig. 19-2a).

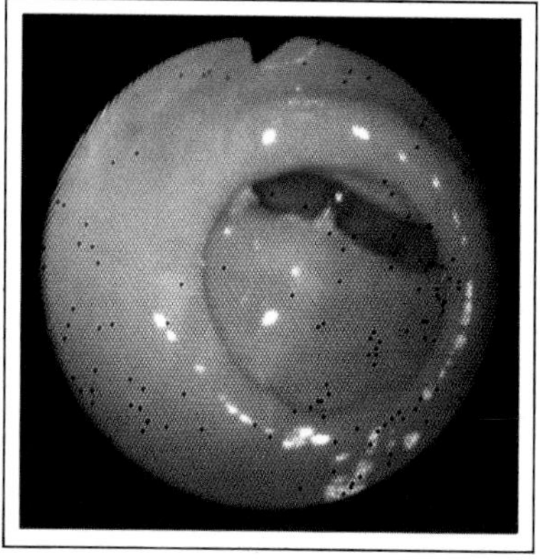

FIG. 19-1a.

FIG. 19-1b.

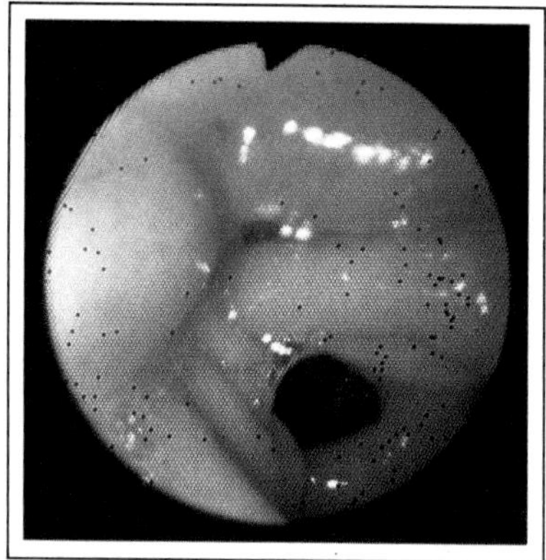

FIG. 19-1c.

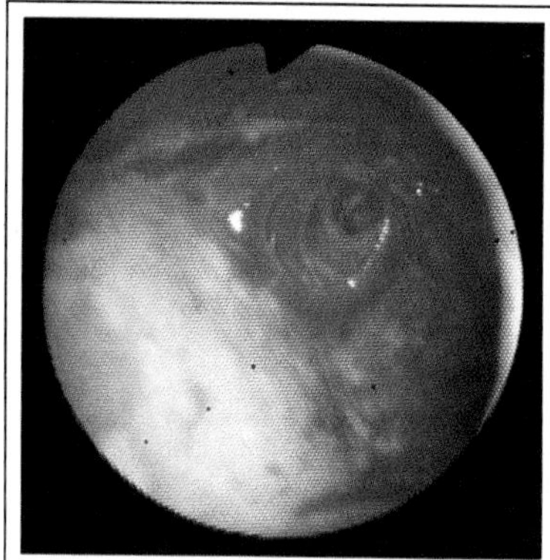

FIG. 19-2a.

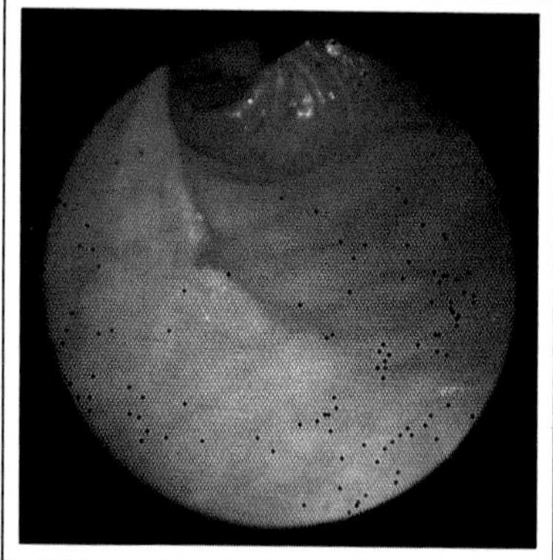

FIG. 19-2b.

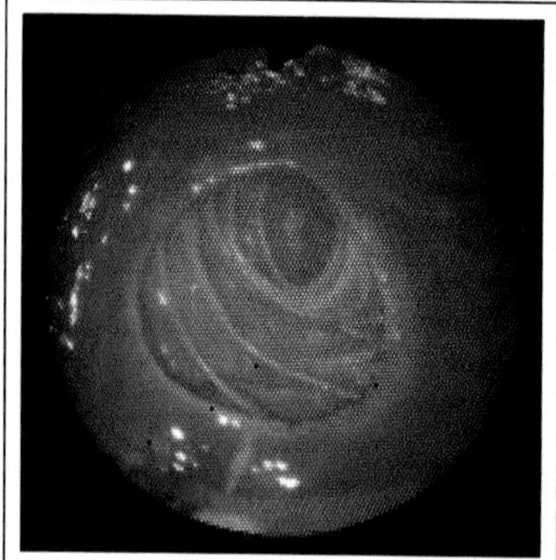

FIG. 19-2c.

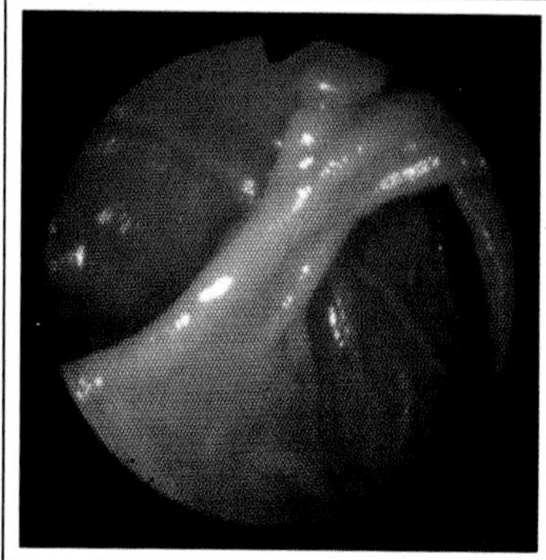

FIG. 19-2d.

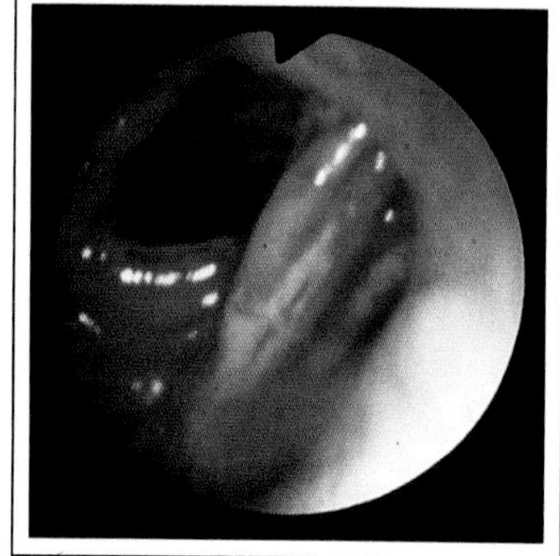

FIG. 19-2e.

FIG. 19-1. a: Heineke-Mikulicz pyloroplasty. This is recognized by the characteristic double-ring pyloric deformity. **b:** Finney pyloroplasty. A gastroduodenostomy (6 o'clock) has been created just below a stenosed pyloric channel. **c:** Acquired double pylorus deformity. In contrast to the Finney-type pyloroplasty, a gastroduodenal fistula is found just above the true pylorus. This deformity is a result of peptic ulcer disease (see Chapter 22).

FIG. 19-2. a: Billroth II hemigastrectomy, antecolic-type anastomosis. The gastrojejunostomy stoma is seen on the anterior wall of the greater curve. **b:** Billroth II hemigastrectomy, retrocolic-type anastomosis. The gastrojejunostomy stoma comes off the posterior wall just beyond the closure line (termination point) of the gastric remnant (9 o'clock). **c:** Billroth II hemigastrectomy, gastrojejunal anastomosis. A demarcation (at 9 o'clock) is seen between the more erythematous gastric mucosa and yellow-gray jejunal mucosa. **d:** Billroth II hemigastrectomy, reversed afferent and efferent loop positions. The afferent loop, which is bile-filled (at 9 o'clock), is located more proximally (higher on the greater curve), and the efferent loop (at 3 o'clock) occupies a more distal position (lower on the greater curve). This is the opposite of their expected positions (see text). **e:** Billroth II hemigastrectomy, with expected positions of the afferent and efferent loop. In this case the afferent loop (marked by bile-stained mucus) takes off from a more distal point on the greater curve (at 3 o'clock), and the efferent loop (at 9 o'clock) occupies the more proximal position as would be expected from only anatomic considerations (see text).

The second finding is that of a gastrojejunostomy stoma located along the greater curve (Fig. 19-2b). Whether the location of the gastrojejunostomy is closer to the anterior wall (Fig. 19-2a) or the posterior wall (Fig. 19-2b) is related to whether the anastomosis was constructed anterior or posterior to the transverse mesocolon. The location of the stoma is generally 15 to 20 cm below the gastroesophageal (GE) junction, usually just beyond the gastric lake.

Within the stomal opening, one can easily define the junction between orange-red gastric mucosa and the yellow-gray jejunal mucosa (Fig. 19-2c). Approximately 1 cm beyond the junctional point is the bridging fold separating the openings of the afferent and efferent loops (Fig. 19-2d). These loops may be distinguished from each other (Fig. 19-2d) based on whether bile is present (afferent loop) or not (efferent loop). As a practical point, the examiner will generally find the efferent loop to have the larger opening and have the more direct lie in relation to gastric lumen (Fig. 19-2e).

As the stoma is entered with the tip perpendicular to the longitudinal axis of the stomach, the 9 o'clock position would be proximal and the 3 o'clock distal. One would therefore expect that the afferent loop coming from the right hand (distal) side would always meet the greater curve distally in the 3 o'clock position (Fig. 19-2e), whereas the efferent loop should always be located more proximally in the 9 o'clock position. Actually, in many cases the reverse is true. The afferent loop is placed more proximally (Fig. 19-2d) and the efferent more distally so as to give this loop the most dependent position and thus facilitate emptying of the gastric remnant by gravity, and by the same token, to avoid postprandial filling of the afferent loop with ingested matter.

The loops themselves can be traversed for a variable distance. In some cases this is considerable. For example, the afferent loop can be traversed in its entirety up to and including the duodenal bulb stump which often terminates in a characteristic 2 to 3 cm mass-like deformity with corrugated surface, formed as a consequence of the standard surgical method of closure using interrupted sutures. Moreover, the duodenal papilla can be visualized for radiologic studies of the pancreas and biliary systems.[4] The efferent loop can be traversed for a similar distance, 20 to 30 cm more. However, failure to traverse a given length beyond 5 cm is not taken as evidence of obstruction. Although there is a great temptation to probe the afferent and efferent loops for a considerable distance looking for hidden ulcers, it should be remembered that the location of most such ulcers is in and around the stomal margin (between gastric and jejunal mucosa) and on the bridging fold between the openings of the afferent and efferent loops.[5] It is these areas which must be examined with particular care.

Billroth II With Roux-en-Y Jejunostomy

In some patients with a Billroth II type anatomy, an opening for the afferent loop does not appear as part of the stoma but is actually located some 25 to 50 cm down the efferent loop. Some of these patients will have had revision of a previous Billroth II anastomosis in order to divert bile and intestinal contents away from the stomach because of symptomatic alkaline reflux gastritis (see below). Endoscopic clues (Fig. 19-3a) to a Roux-en-Y type anastomosis are: (a) the absence of bile in the stomach; (b) the absence of significant peristomal erythema; and (c) the presence of only one loop at the stoma (Fig. 19-3a). Occasionally, one finds a blind pouch marking the prior location of the afferent loop (Fig. 19-3a).

Billroth I (Hemigastrectomy With Gastroduodenal) Anastomosis

The Billroth I procedure is performed less often than the Billroth II anastomosis because technically it is more difficult to do after substantial gastric resection has been performed (on the order of 35 to 55%, as is done in an ulcer operation).[2]

With the Billroth II anatomy the endoscopist typically sees rugal folds which terminate circumferentially around the stoma (Fig. 19-3b). Within the stoma is the junction of erythematous gastric and gray-pink flat duodenal mucosa (Fig. 19-3b).

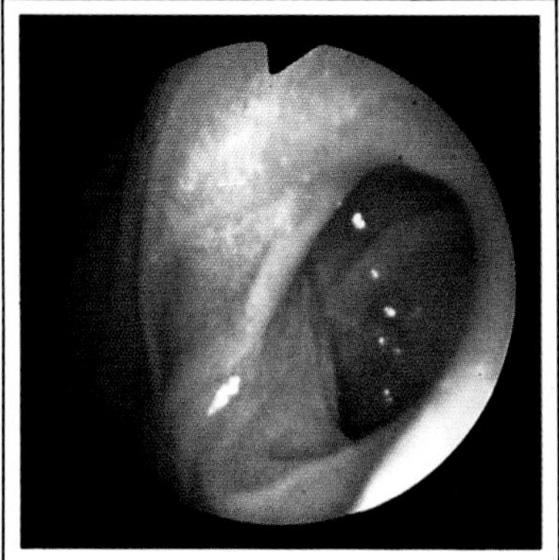

FIG. 19-3a.

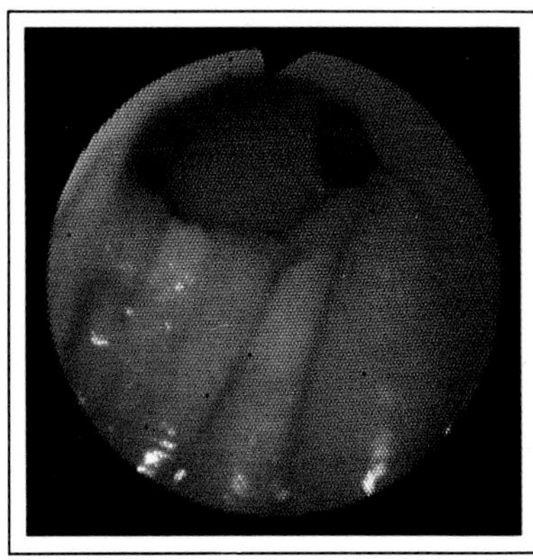

FIG. 19-3b.

FIG. 19-3. a: Billroth II hemigastrectomy after a Roux-en-Y jejunojejunostomy. The efferent loop runs toward 5 o'clock as would be expected with it being in a reversed position, whereas the takeoff point for the afferent loop (just off 2 o'clock) ends as a blind passage. **b:** Billroth I hemigastrectomy, gastroduodenal anastomosis. The stoma is formed by the termination of rugal folds. Beyond this is the duodenal bulb.

Simple Gastrojejunostomy

Simple gastrojejunostomy may be performed for peptic ulcer disease in a compromised patient as an emergency measure or to bypass duodenal obstruction, as in the case of pancreatic carcinoma. The appearance of the stoma would be identical to that of the Billroth II (Fig. 19-4), but the presence of the antrum and the pyloric channel indicates that the operation was a gastrojejunostomy and not a Billroth II, the latter term implying an antral resection.

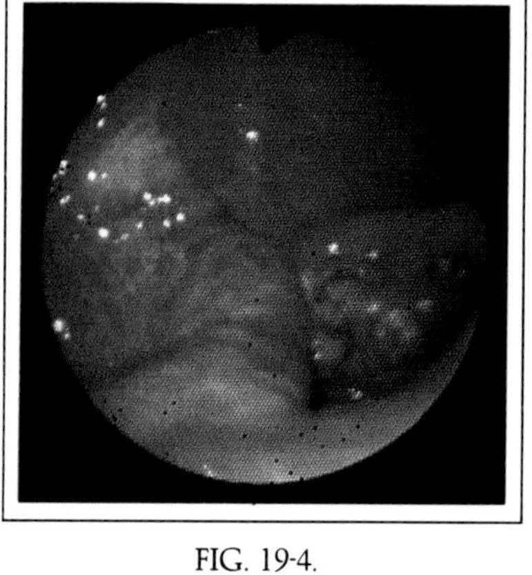

FIG. 19-4.

FIG. 19-4. Simple gastrojejunostomy without resection. The antrum distal to the stoma is visualized and found to be intact, indicating that no resection was performed. The mucosa displays erythema. However, this is of uncertain clinical significance (see "Postoperative Gastric Mucosal Appearance: Alkaline Reflux Gastritis," this chapter).

POSTOPERATIVE STOMA

Nonspecific Appearances

There is great variation in stomal appearance, making it impossible to state what is normal or atypical. Short of ulceration, stenosis, or frank malignant change (see below), the examiner correctly regards any stomal abnormality as nonspecific.

Elevation

There is a great variation in the height of the gastric portion of the stoma. It may be altogether flat (Fig. 19-5a), heaped up (Fig. 19-5b), or in between (Fig. 19-5c), depending on how the stoma was constructed. Even with heaped-up stoma, the rugal folds forming the stoma are sharp and the mucosa is generally pliant (Fig. 19-5b). In some of these cases the mucosa tents poorly and seems "tacked down," especially in the area of the anastomotic line, yet can be

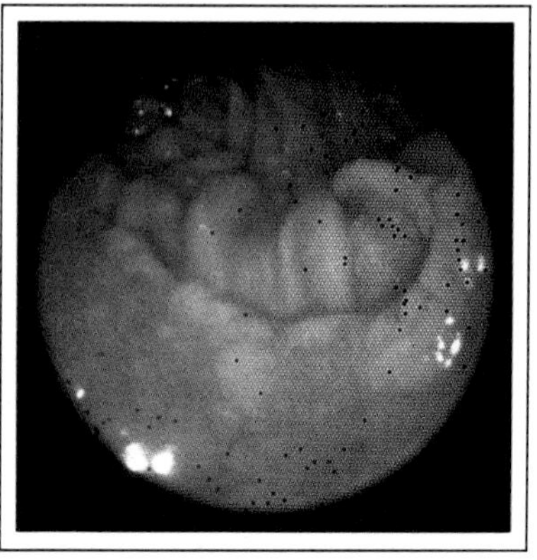

FIG. 19-5a.

FIG. 19-5b.

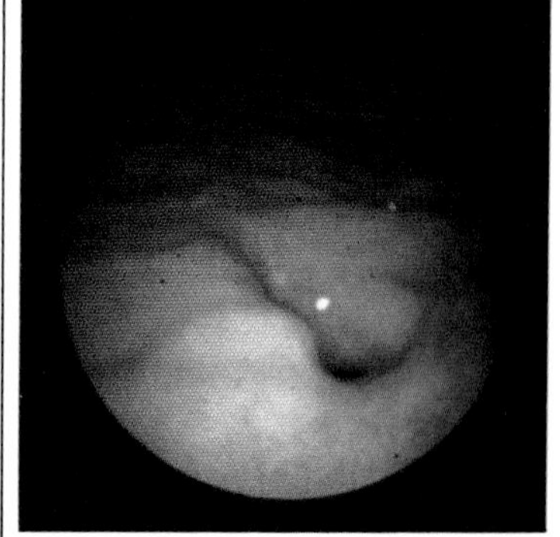

FIG. 19-5c.

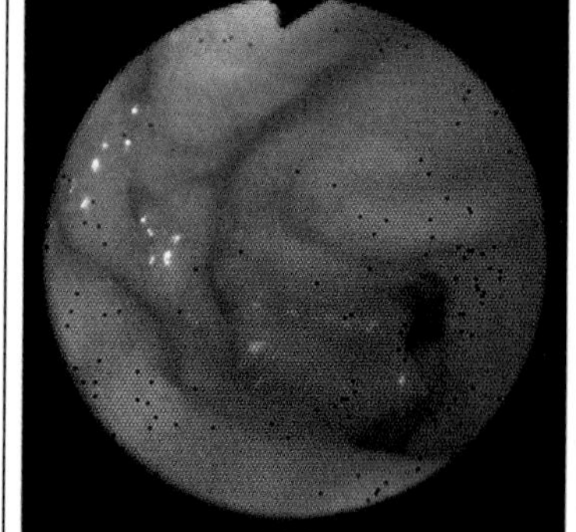

FIG. 19-5d.

FIG. 19-5. a: Gastroenterostomy stoma, flat. A widely patent stomal opening is present with a clear demarcation between erythematous gastric and gray jejunal mucosa. **b:** Gastroenterostomy stoma, raised. The margin is heaped up and the stomal opening appears narrow; yet this easily admitted an intermediate-sized (11 mm) instrument. **c:** Gastroenterostomy stoma, slightly raised. The fact that the stoma is slightly raised causes it to be incompletely seen and thus appear narrow. Still, an 11-mm instrument was easily passed across the stoma in this asymptomatic patient. **d:** Gastric remnant (stump) cancer in a patient with a slightly raised stoma. The stomal appearance (just off 3 o'clock) is unremarkable. The rugal folds running down to the stoma, however, were both prominent (>10 mm) and rigid with fixed overlying mucosa. These appearances, rather than that of the stoma, were clues to the presence of an infiltrating malignancy.

normal. Still, lack of pliancy proximal to the stoma (Fig. 19-5d), should cause the endoscopist to seriously consider an infiltrating malignancy, especially in patients having had the surgery 15 years or more previously [see "Gastric Remnant (Stump) Carcinoma," this chapter].

Erythema

Some stomal erythema (Fig. 19-6a) is found in up to 15% of both symptomatic and asymptomatic patients who have had prior gastric surgery.[1] The findings therefore cannot be considered necessarily abnormal, and the endoscopist should resist the temptation to interpret this appearance as such. In our practice we use the term "nonspecific stomal erythema" to describe this appearance rather than a term such as "stomatitis," which might be construed as a definite abnormality.

The erythema itself resembles nonspecific gastric erythema of the unoperated stomach (see Chapter 12). On close inspection one can make out innumerable red islands (Fig. 19-6b) which, we believe, represent the areae gastricae with interconnecting linear areas, the lineae gastricae. Because of the mucosal capillary dilatation which may be found histologically in association with this appearance, the endoscopist often encounters some degree of mucosal friability as the endoscope is passed across the stoma (Fig. 19-6c). Some use the finding of mucosal friability as evidence of stomatitis, a term which, for the reasons stated above, we prefer not to use.

Another interpretive problem arising in connection with stomal erythema and marked friability is to what extent this appearance may account for iron deficiency anemia found in postgastrectomy patients.[6] Although marked stomal friability may be an explanation for anemia, this should always be a diagnosis of exclusion and not accepted until at least a careful double-contrast radiographic examination of the colon, or possibly even colonoscopy, has been performed. We have observed at least one case of cecal carcinoma discovered 6 months after an endoscopic diagnosis of "stomatitis" was accepted as the explanation for his iron deficiency anemia.

Even though the finding of stomal erythema is nonspecific, if it is present the endoscopist should examine the stoma very carefully for ulcerations, especially in cases where the erythema is seen on the jejunal side. Unlike stomal erythema involving gastric mucosa alone, we find that the erythema which involves the jejunum is often associated with ulceration (Fig. 19-6d).

Stomal Nodules

Three types of nonneoplastic nodules may be encountered during examination of the stoma. First, especially in the

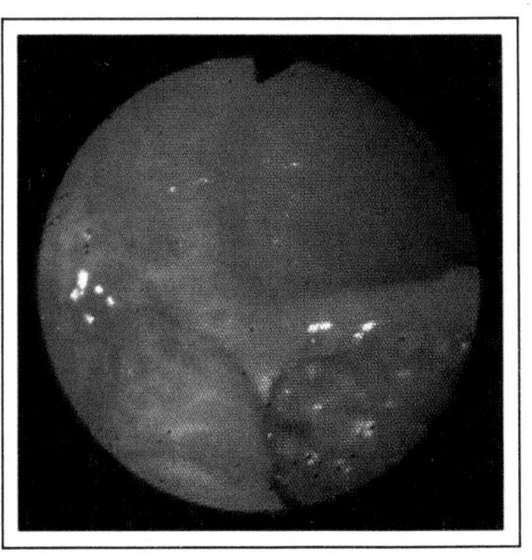

FIG. 19-6a.

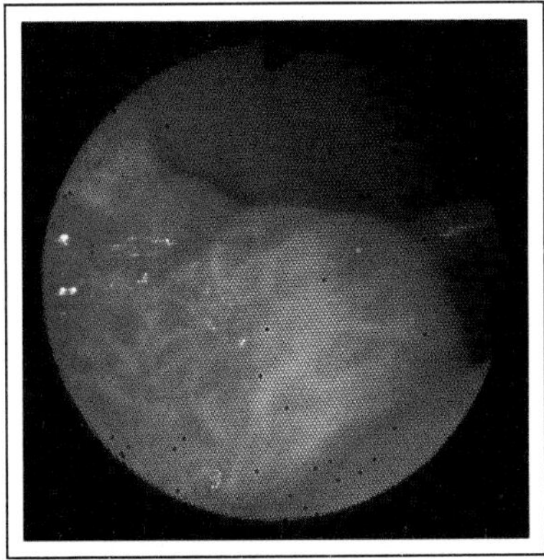

FIG. 19-6b.

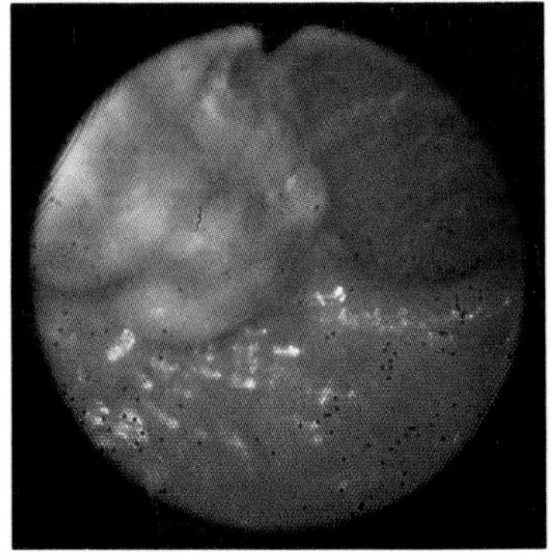

FIG. 19-6c.

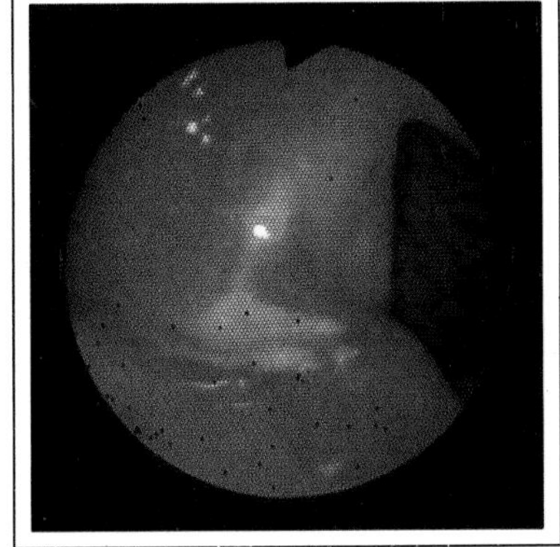

FIG. 19-6d.

FIG. 19-6. a: Stomal erythema. The mucosa of the stoma and adjacent area is erythematous. Even at 5 cm from the mucosa, white lines (i.e., lineae gastricae) can be seen breaking up the erythema. **b:** Stomal erythema, close-up view. The erythema is easily seen to consist of multiple red dots, which we believe are the areae gastricae, broken up by intervening pale linear areas, the lineae gastricae, similar to nonspecific gastric erythema in the unoperated stomach (see Chapter 12). **c:** "Stomatitis." The stoma is composed of enlarged folds with erythematous, friable mucosa. Some inflammatory exudate is seen as well. Despite this appearance, the patient was asymptomatic with endoscopy performed because of anemia. **d:** Stomal erythema adjacent to an ulcer. Erythema involving the jejunum should always cause one to look carefully for an ulcer.

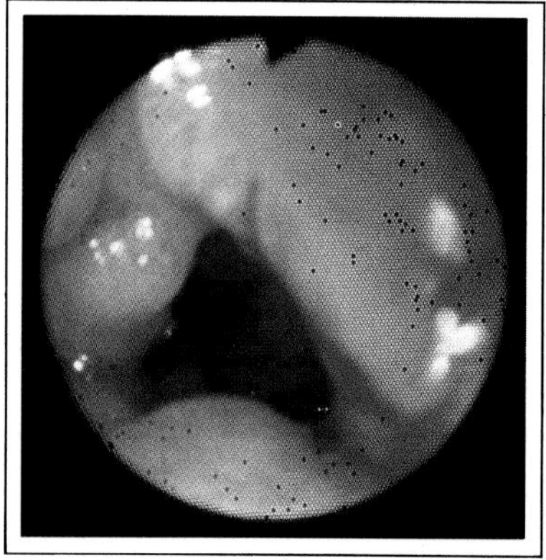

FIG. 19-7a.

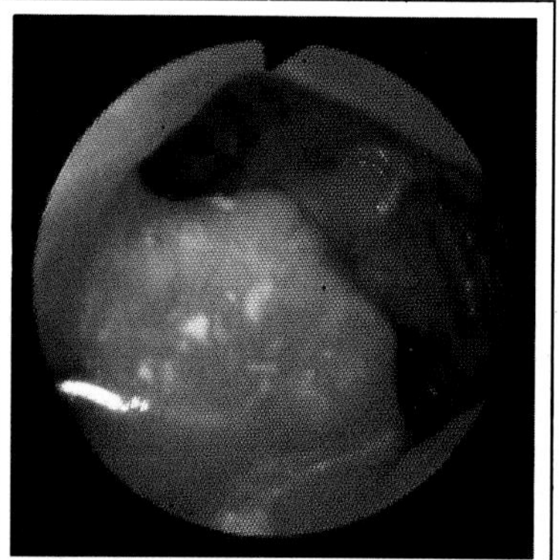

FIG. 19-7b.

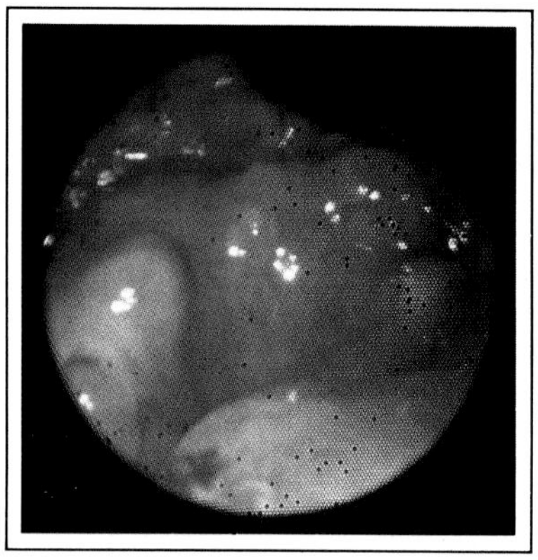

FIG. 19-7. a: Stomal nodularity caused by the termination of prominent rugal folds within the stoma. **b:** Stomal hyperplastic polyp. One of several large (1.5 cm) polyps noted to be separate from rugal folds in a patient presenting with recurrent upper gastrointestinal bleeding. The mucosa of the polyp was more erythematous, granular, and friable than the surrounding mucosa. Biopsy, however, showed only nonspecific inflammation. **c:** Gastric remnant (stump) carcinoma. An indurated 2-cm mass was found adjacent to the stoma (about 3 o'clock). Its nodular, indurated appearance allows it to be differentiated from the hyperplastic polyp (b). **d:** Lipid islands. These are xanthomas (especially at 12 o'clock) which appear on the gastric side of the anastomosis 5 years or more after surgery. Biopsy in this case showed characteristic lipid-filled histiocytes.

FIG. 19-7c.

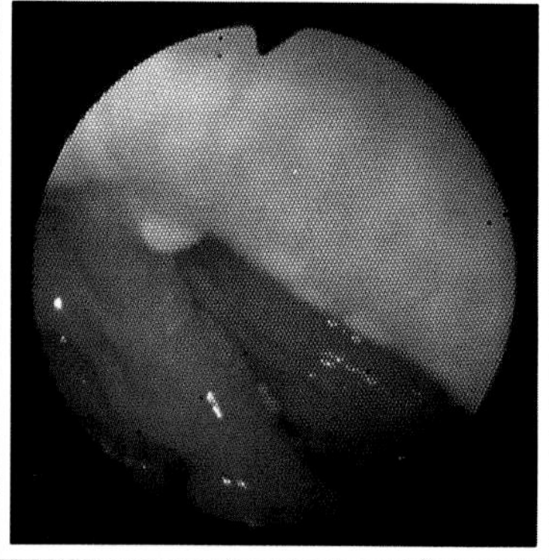

FIG. 19-7d.

case of the Billroth I anastomosis, the rugal folds terminate abruptly, giving the appearance of nodules at their termination (Fig. 19-7a). The mucosa of these nodules is identical to that surrounding the stoma, and their width exceeds that of a rugal fold.

A second type is the hyperplastic polyp (Fig. 19-7b). These are similar in appearance to terminations in rugal folds but larger, more erythematous, and often eroded (superficially ulcerated). These are in fact similar in all respects to hyperplastic polyps appearing in unoperated stomachs (see Chapter 17). Some hyperplastic polyps may be quite large and associated with bleeding, which prompts endoscopy. In most cases, however, a variety of nonspecific symptoms causes the examination to be performed. In cases where hyperplastic polyps are found, a Billroth II anastomosis will have been present for 5 and often 10 years.[7] In patients having had gastric surgery performed 15 years or more before, hyperplastic polyps must be differentiated from gastric remnant carcinoma (Fig. 19-7c).

A third type, distinct from prominent rugal folds or hyperplastic polyps, is the stomal xanthoma, also called the "lipid island" (Fig. 19-7d).[8] These are also found in patients having had gastric surgery 5 years or more prior to the endoscopic examination.[8] They are similar to gastric xanthomas encountered in the unoperated stomach (see Chapter 20). Generally, they are seen as groups of two to five yellow-white mucosal excrescences, ranging in size from 2 to 4 mm. The lesions are entirely incidental findings; however, they do serve as a marker for the gastroenteric anastomosis of 5 years or more duration.[8]

Stomal Ulceration

Ulcer surgery is associated with recurrence in 5% of cases.[9] We find most of these to be located within 2 cm on either side of the surgical stoma, although others have reported 60% of recurrences to be more proximal.[5] We believe the diagnosis of stomal ulceration requires the definite identification of an ulcer. We would not accept an erythematous and friable stoma as a stomal ulcer "equivalent" (Fig. 19-8a). In this regard, care must be taken not to confuse apparent bile or bile-stained mucus (Fig. 19-8a) with true ulceration (Fig. 19-8b) with its depressed yellow-white base. In those cases where the endoscopist is uncertain about the nature of the "yellow-white exudate" (Fig. 19-8c), the presumed ulcer base should be biopsied. The histologic finding of granulation tissue would confirm that the "exudate" is the base of an ulcer.

Once the presence of an ulcer is established, one carefully notes its location on the stoma, as this may be a clue to

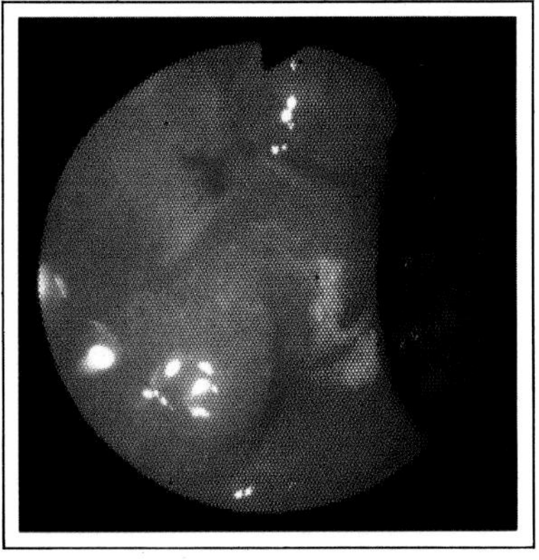

FIG. 19-8a.

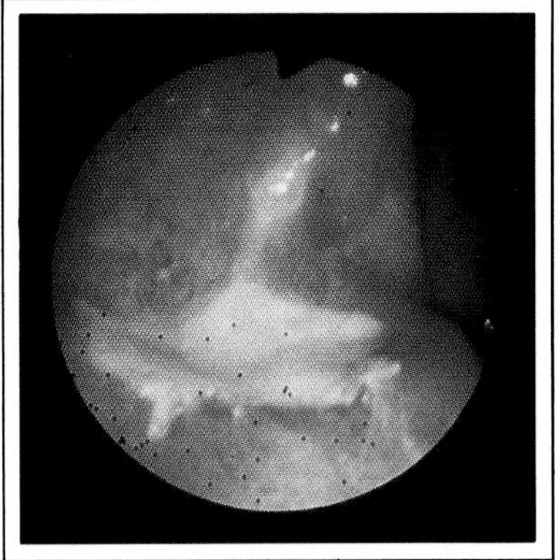

FIG. 19-8b.

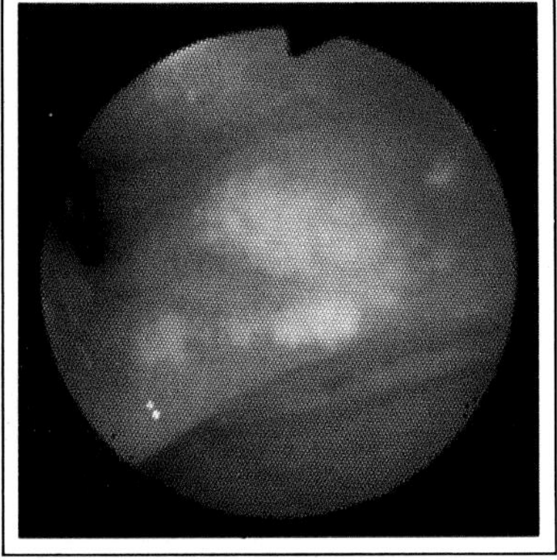

FIG. 19-8c.

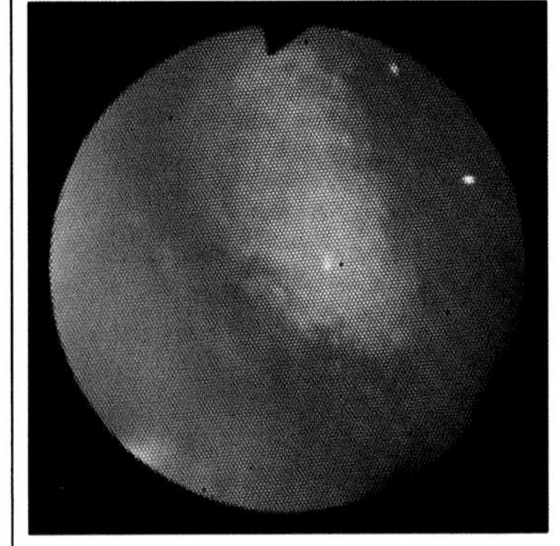

FIG. 19-8d.

FIG. 19-8. a: Stomal erythema with adherent bile but no ulceration. **b:** Stomal ulceration. This ulcer is easily recognized by the definite depression of its base. **c:** Stomal ulcer, superficial. This ulcer lacks a depressed base. For this reason it is difficult to differentiate from simply adherent foreign material. Biopsies, however, showed granulation tissue, indicating it to be a definite ulcer. **d:** Stomal ulcer, jejunal side, in a patient with an incomplete vagotomy.

its pathogenesis. An ulcer entirely within intestinal mucosa (Fig. 19-8d) often means that a component of gastric hypersecretion is present. If maximally stimulated gastric acid secretion is measured, it may be expected to be greater than 15 mEq/hr, a value associated with recurrence[9] (Fig. 19-9a). In such cases one would consider hypersecretion from either: (a) an incomplete vagotomy; or (b) a situation in which the initially high level of acid secretion was only partially corrected by vagotomy and resection was performed. Much less often such patients may have retained gastric antrum as part of the duodenal stump in a Billroth II operation or, rarely, the Zollinger-Ellison syndrome. Not all cases of jejunal ulcers, however, are associated with hypersecretion. In fact, many are found with appropriately low values; in these cases one must consider other, as yet poorly defined, factors that affect mucosal resistance as being causative (Fig. 19-9a).

Ulceration of the gastric side of the stomach (Fig. 19-9b) is analogous to the primary gastric ulcer, which is not typically associated with a high acid output. In these cases of stomal ulcers involving gastric mucosa, the low acid outputs suggest a pathogenetic mechanism involving the loss of stomal mucosal resistance rather than continued gastric hypersecretion, as in the case of ulceration of the intestinal side. We have in fact encountered patients with recurrent ulceration of the gastric side of the stoma (Fig. 19-9b) who have repeated determinations of stimulated acid output of 2 mEq/hr or less!

Single or multiple ulcers involving both intestinal and gastric mucosa (Fig. 19-9c) probably have several pathogenetic mechanisms. Here the intestinal component may be primary and produce reactive changes which compromise stomal emptying, leading to the retention of acid or other injurious luminal contents, e.g., bile salts or active pancreatic enzymes, which result in ulceration of gastric mucosa.

As in the case of gastric ulcers in unoperated patients (see Chapter 15), it is incumbent on the endoscopist to attempt to elicit a history of ingesting aspirin or other nonsteroidal analgesic agent. As in the case of ulcers in general, the endoscopist, after finding a stomal ulcer, is in a unique position to focus directly on the issue of such ingestion. Others may have asked only in a general way about aspirin or other medications without going through a specific prepared list of common aspirin-containing medications and other nonsteroidal analgesics such as is presented in Chapter 14. To miss the opportunity of discovering the ingestion of a significant ulcerogenic agent would be as unfortunate as missing the stomal ulcer itself. Such a patient, without the additional history, could be adjudged a failure of medical management and in need of remedial surgery when he may only have needed education about the deleterious effects of the analgesic agents he uses.

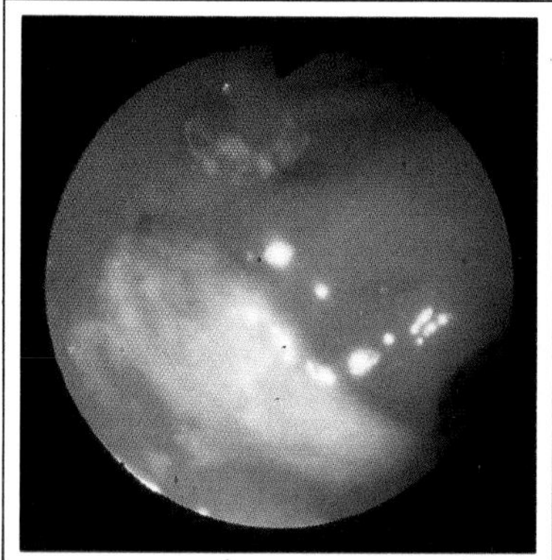

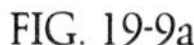

FIG. 19-9a.

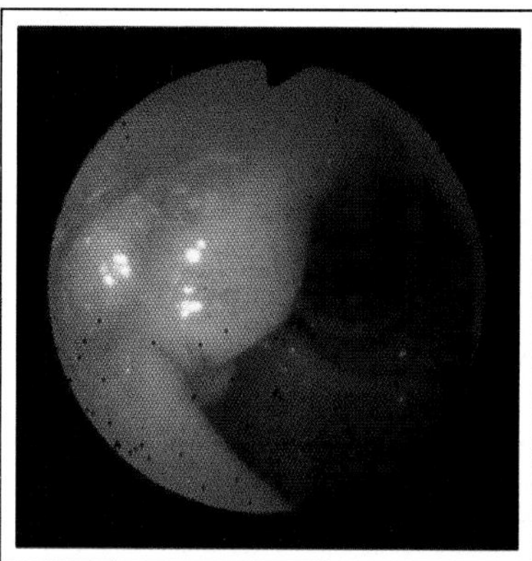

FIG. 19-9b.

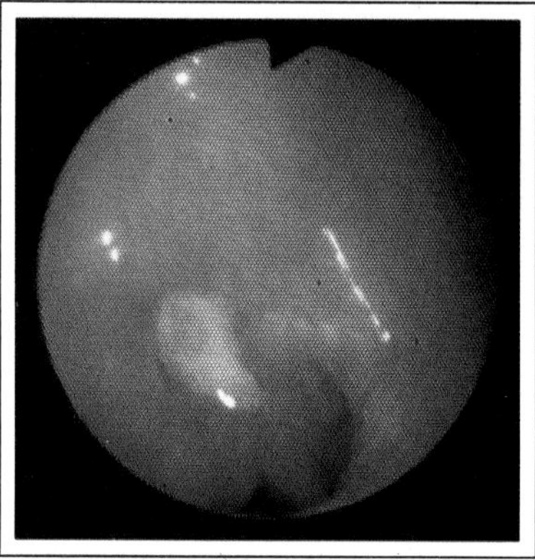

FIG. 19-9c.

FIG. 19-9. a: Stomal ulcer, jejunal side, 5 years after conversion of a Billroth II to a Roux-en-Y jejunojejunostomy for alkaline reflux gastritis. This ulcer had resisted attempts at medical management for 1 year. **b:** Stomal ulcer, gastric side, after Billroth II surgery. In this case no factors predisposing to recurrence, e.g., residual hypersecretion, were found, suggesting that diminished mucosal resistance rather than continued hypersecretion may have been the important pathogenetic mechanism. **c:** Stomal ulcer, anastomotic margin. Such ulcers may be secondary to both continued hypersecretion leading to ulceration of the intestinal mucosa, with secondary stomal changes resulting in ulceration on the gastric side.

Stomal Strictures

Stomal stricture is said to occur after 1 to 5% of gastric resections.[10] The endoscopic test for patency is the successful passage of an instrument of at least 11 mm. This corresponds roughly to the test for patency performed by the surgeon when the stoma is constructed—which is the passage of his index finger.[10] We take the failure to pass an 11-mm instrument across the stoma as suggestive, although not conclusive, evidence of stenosis, as an occasional stoma is constructed with an unusual angle, which prevents passage across the stoma. We therefore require any endoscopic suggestion of stenosis to be corroborated by radiographic studies of the stoma before a patient is considered for surgery. Conversely, should a radiographic study suggest stenosis, but this is not confirmed endoscopically (in that an 11-mm endoscope can be easily passed), functional obstruction with gastric atony is suspected.[10]

Stomal stenosis of a Billroth I anastomosis generally affects the gastric portion alone, whereas that involving a Billroth II affects the gastric side of the stoma as well as either or both jejunal loops (Fig. 19-10a). In addition, in the case of a Billroth II anastomosis one can see mechanical obstruction of either the afferent or efferent loop at a distance of 5 cm or more from the stoma. It is therefore necessary to examine both loops for a distance of at least 5 cm before concluding that mechanical obstruction is not present (Fig. 19-10b). Generally, though, when obstruction occurs it is present within 2 cm of the stomal anastomosis.

In the case of a Billroth II or simple gastrojejunostomy, the afferent loop alone may be intermittently obstructed (Fig. 19-10a) causing the patient to present with the characteristic symptom of afferent loop syndrome[11]; which is intermittent postprandial pain experienced 20 to 40 min after meals that is relieved by vomiting. In such patients, failure to enter the afferent loop at endoscopy raises the suspicion of afferent loop obstruction; functional assessment of the afferent loop with radionuclide studies, now available at many centers, is then performed.[12] A delay in the clearance of the radionuclide secreted into the afferent loop beyond 2 hr is suggestive of some degree of obstruction and confirms the endoscopic impression of stomal narrowing that involves the afferent loop (Fig. 19-10a).

Benign stomal obstruction (Fig. 19-10a) must be differentiated from that caused by malignancy (Fig. 19-11a), especially in those patients having had gastric surgery 10 years or more before (see below). This is often difficult because of the wide range of appearances for a stoma associated with benign stricture especially when the stricture is accompanied by ulceration or nonspecific stomatitis and appears erythematous and even nodular (Fig. 19-11b). Generally with benign obstruction, though, the stomal mucosa

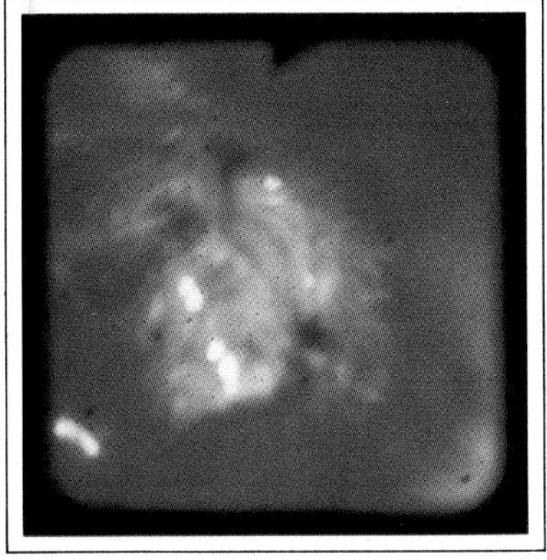

FIG. 19-10a.

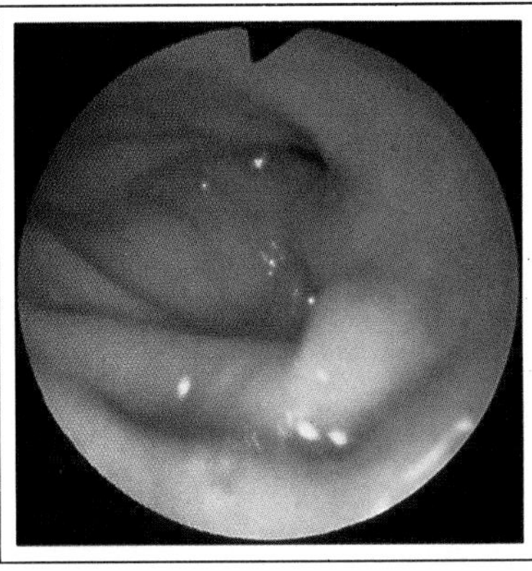

FIG. 19-10b.

FIG. 19-10. a: Stomal stenosis, Billroth II anastomosis. The gastric as well as the jejunal side of the stoma are markedly narrowed. Most striking are the pinpoint openings to the afferent and efferent loops. The stenosis of the afferent loop resulted in the syndrome of intermittent afferent loop obstruction (see text). **b:** Efferent loop obstruction, from peristomal adhesions. The narrowed portion of the efferent loop (seen at 12 o'clock) was found 6 cm from the stoma.

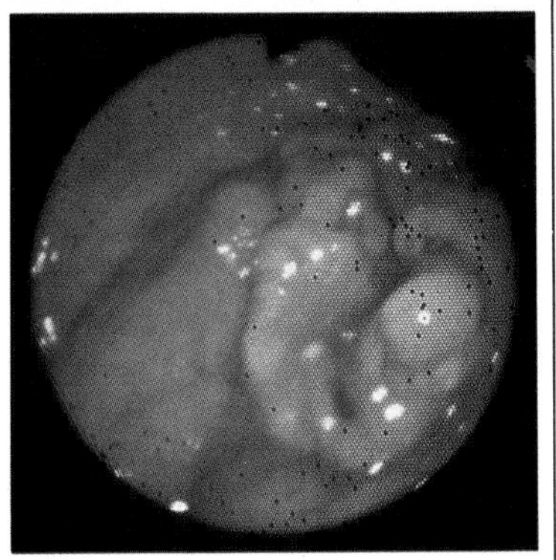

FIG. 19-11a.

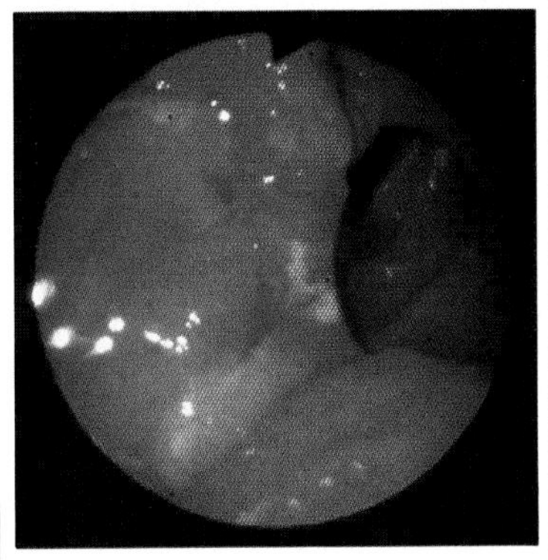

FIG. 19-11b.

FIG. 19-11. a: Malignant obstruction of a Billroth II stoma from a gastric remnant (stump) carcinoma. The polypoid mass at 3 o'clock completely occludes the gastric stoma. **b:** Billroth II anastomosis with stomal erythema and some narrowing.

continues to display erythema consisting of tiny red dots or islands, what we believe represents the areae gastricae, with intervening pale linear areas, the lineae gastricae (Fig. 19-11b). With malignant obstruction, the stomal mucosa consists of tumor nodules (Fig. 19-11a).

For some patients with stomal strictures who are not candidates for additional surgery, endoscopic dilatation can be considered[13], a measure that has been utilized for benign as well as malignant strictures. For other patients, especially those with malignant strictures, stents have been placed across the stoma.[14]

Stomal (Retrograde-Intragastric) Intussusception

Stomal intussusception is a rare but serious complication of a gastroenteric anastomosis of the Billroth II or simple gastrojejunostomy procedure. We have seen only three cases out of more than 300 examinations involving stomas. Two were patients having had a total pancreatectomy for cancer with a Billroth II and Roux-en-Y anastomosis. Intussusception may involve the efferent loop (most frequently reported), the afferent loop (less often reported), or a combination which is the least common of all types reported.[15] Most occur within 5 years of the surgery, with some as an immediate postoperative complication, making this diagnosis one which should always be considered in patients with acute nonfunctioning stomas.

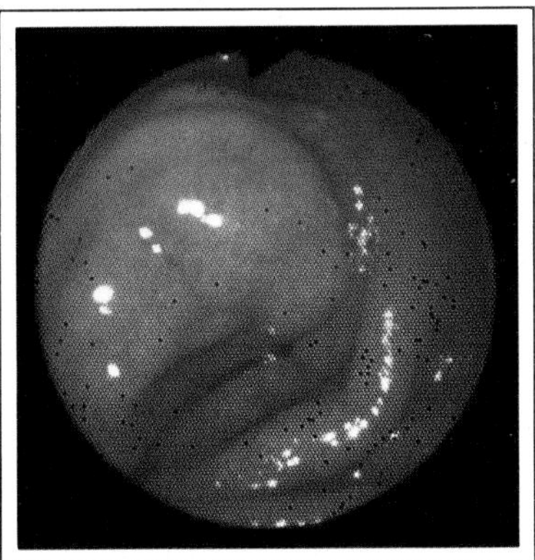

FIG. 19-12.

FIG. 19-12. Stomal intussusception. A mass consisting of Kerckring folds—in fact the afferent loop projects into the lumen at 10 o'clock, having the appearance of a single-loop intussusception.

Endoscopically, one observes the stoma to be compromised by an erythematous mass projecting into the lumen which contains jejunal rather than gastric mucosa. In these cases the jejunal mucosa is apparent by virtue of the appearance of Kerckring folds (Fig. 19-12). In the case of a combined intussusception, twin stomal masses of protruding, erythematous jejunal mucosa can be identified.[15]

POSTOPERATIVE GASTRIC MUCOSAL APPEARANCE: ALKALINE REFLUX GASTRITIS

A variety of symptoms may prompt endoscopy in patients who have had previous surgery. These include postprandial or constant burning epigastric pain, nausea, vomiting, bloating, and weight loss. These collectively have been referred to as the syndrome of "alkaline" (bile) reflux gastritis.[16,17] Endoscopy in such patients may reveal varying amounts of gastric mucosal erythema and bile in the gastric lake, which when marked some regard as highly significant.[18] However, as both symptomatic and asymptomatic patients may have identical findings,[1,18] the significance of such an observation is questionable. Even when one chooses to regard symptomatic patients as only those with postprandial pain relieved by bilious vomiting, which is the classic alkaline reflux gastritis symptom,[16,17] in no study has there been any more than a trend suggested for marked and extensive gastric erythema, along with the presence of bile, to be associated with such symptoms.[1] However, even in a study where a trend was suggested, the converse was also true, in that a third of the patients with severe and extensive erythema were asymptomatic! Also of interest in this study was the fact that no bile was observed in the gastric lake in half of those considered symptomatic.[1] Furthermore, there was no association between symptoms and the result of biopsies taken either around the stoma or elsewhere. For the majority of symptomatic patients, the histologic appearance was indistinguishable from that of patients without symptoms.[1]

Unlike endoscopic and histologic findings, a clearer separation between symptomatic and asymptomatic patients has been achieved using radionuclide studies to measure enterogastric reflux,[19] the bile acid content of intestinal secretions,[17] the potential of intestinal secretions for producing symptoms,[17] and finally studies of gastric emptying.[20] However, even though these studies can separate symptomatic from asymptomatic patients, no study to date has been reported suggesting that any of the modalities can predict whether a given symptomatic patient will benefit from surgery aimed at diverting bile and intestinal contents away from the stomach by means of a Roux-en-Y jejunojejunostomy. It should not be surprising therefore that visual assessment of the mucosa endoscopically or histologically which does not effectively separate symptomatic from asymptomatic patients does not predict whether surgery will be successful, even when the endoscopic appearance is considered severe and diffuse.[21] It therefore seems that neither visual assessment at endoscopy nor any histologic material obtained can select either patients who have symptomatic alkaline reflux gastritis or which symptomatic patients would benefit from surgery.[21]

Appearance

At least half the patient with previous gastric surgery show some degree of mucosal erythema (Fig. 19-13a) as well as bile staining of the gastric lake (Fig. 19-13b). These findings tend to be more extensive in patients with Billroth II anatomy (Fig. 19-13c), often involving the fundus, than in those with Billroth I or pyloroplasty, where they tend to be confined to the peristomal region (Fig. 19-13d).

The erythema may have either a diffuse or linear (Fig. 19-13a) appearance, which in the latter case has been referred to as "tiger stripes,"[22] especially when the erythema is seen to run along the crests of rugal folds. The explanation for this may be that this mucosa is exposed longer to an injurious agent in the refluxed intestinal secretion than the mucosa between the folds, causing a sequence of injury with resultant mucosal regeneration accompanied by mucin depletion and capillary dilatation, changes associated with the appearance of gastric erythema in the unoperated stomach (see Chapter 12).

GASTRIC BEZOARS

Bezoars are masses of solidified foreign material which do not readily pass out of the stomach. In most cases bezoars form as a result of surgical removal of the antrum,[23] which is normally responsible for "grinding up" such material. In occasional cases the cause of ineffective antral motor function is either diabetic gastroparesis (see Chapter 20)[22] or obstruction from peptic ulcer[23] or carcinoma.[24] Although bezoars are uncommon, being found in only 1 to 2% of endoscopic examinations overall, we find them in 10 to 25% of patients with prior antrectomy who are endoscoped because of symptoms. These symptoms are usually intermittent and nonspecific, e.g., nausea, vomiting, early satiety, and weight loss.

There are three types of bezoar based on composition: (a) phytobezoar—largely cellulose; (b) mucobezoar—essentially mucus; and (c) trichobezoar—hair. In the postgastrectomy patient the most common type is the phytobezoar.[25] In these cases we find the most common offending ingested material to be apple skins and orange and grapefruit rinds. Traditionally associated foods, e.g., persimmons, we and others[25] rarely if ever find to be the cause. In many patients improper mastication because of ill-fitting dentures is an important contributing factor.

Phytobezoars

The phytobezoar is typically recognized as a yellow-green solid or semisolid mass which fills the gastric lake (Fig. 19-14a) or obstructs the stoma (Fig. 19-14b). Parts of the bezoar may project out from its surface (Fig. 19-14a), giving it an irregular appearance. Usually the bezoar is loosely constructed so that it may be probed with a biopsy forceps or polyethylene cannula. The latter may be used to instill enzymes or water directly into the bezoar to break it up. In some cases this occurs spontaneously, so that fragments are observed in the small bowel (Fig. 19-14c).

Often dissolution of the bezoar can be accomplished with a combination of dietary restriction of fiber, improved mas-

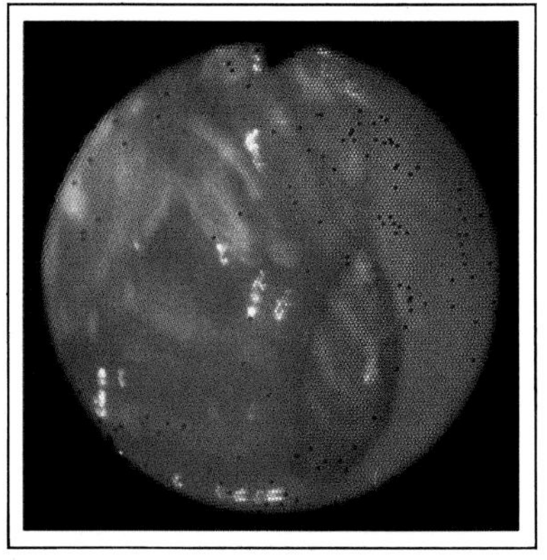
FIG. 19-13a.

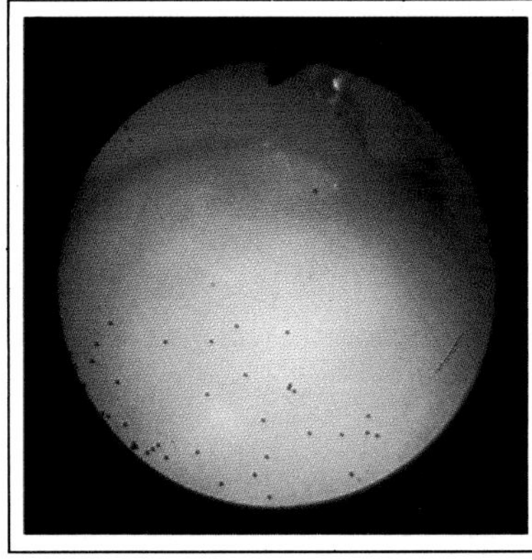
FIG. 19-13b.

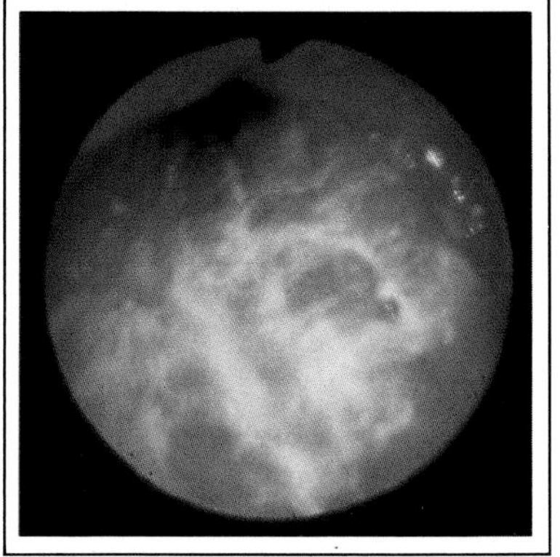
FIG. 19-13c.

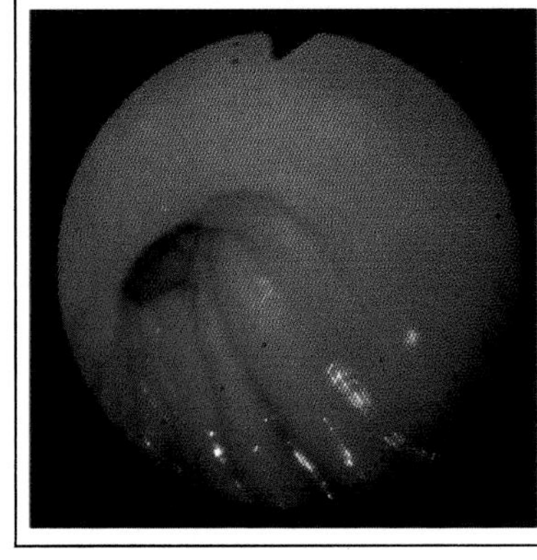
FIG. 19-13d.

FIG. 19-13. Billroth II hemigastrectomy. **a:** Nonspecific mucosal erythema. The tips of the rugal folds appear more erythematous than the intervening mucosa, producing the "tiger stripe" appearance. Bile is also present (at 9 o'clock). **b:** With bile and nonspecific gastric erythema present. A large amount of bile was found in the gastric lake of this asymptomatic patient. Nonspecific gastric erythema is also noted in the adjacent mucosa. **c:** Bile and nonspecific gastric erythema appear. Copious amounts of bile and nonspecific erythema, similar to those in (b), were found in a patient with postprandial bile vomiting suggestive of alkaline reflux gastritis. **d:** Nonspecific peristomal erythema. Although erythema is generally less marked and less extensive in Billroth I patients as compared with those having the Billroth II procedure, it may be as extensive as was true in this case. Despite this appearance, the patient was entirely asymptomatic.

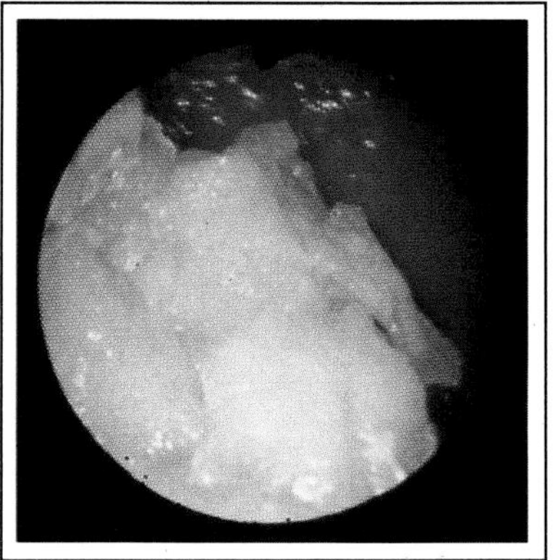
FIG. 19-14a.

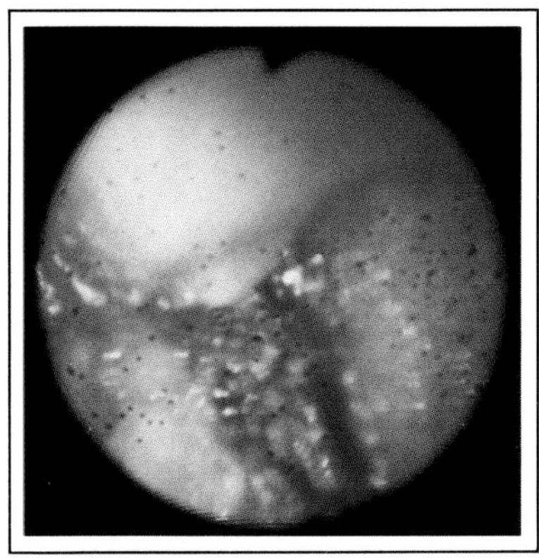
FIG. 19-14b.

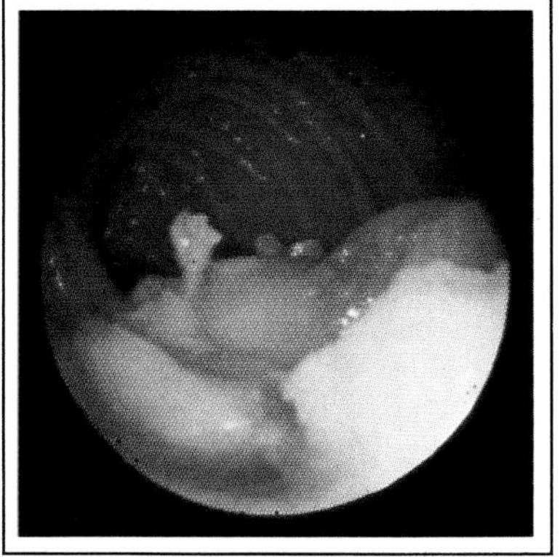
FIG. 19-14c.

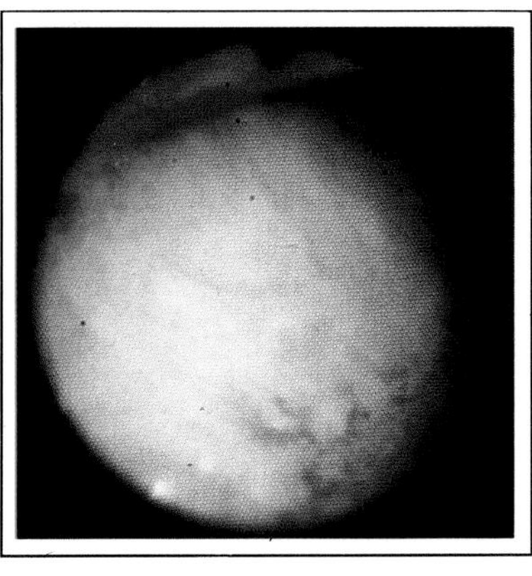
FIG. 19-14d.

FIG. 19-14. a: Phytobezoar. A large bezoar was found in a patient with a Billroth I anastomosis and ill-fitting dentures. The patient admitted to difficulty chewing and a penchant for roughage. **b:** Phytobezoar. The mass has moved into and is obviously blocking the stoma in a patient with symptoms of intermittent gastric outlet obstruction. **c:** Phytobezoar in the efferent loop. Large pieces may break off and produce symptoms suggestive of intermittent intestinal obstruction. **d:** Mucobezoar. A loosely constructed, semisolid amorphous mass occupying an extensive area of the greater curve.

tication, and the use of oral preparations of cellulase.[26] For those bezoars which prove refractory to such treatment, endoscopy may be utilized for breaking up the bezoar using: (a) the Water Pik technique[27] for instillation of enzyme directly into the bezoar; or (b) the recently developed "overtube" technique allowing for repeated passage of the endoscope into the stomach and removal of large pieces of the bezoar.[28]

Mucobezoars

A mucobezoar is suggested by the appearance of a semisolid mass having a loose construction such that it readily comes apart on contact (Fig. 19-14d). For dissolution of these, Adolph's Meat Tenderizer (papase) has been found to be effective, as has Mucomist (acetylcysteine).[26]

Trichobezoars

Trichobezoars are seen almost exclusively in children who ingest hair,[29] although very occasionally they are seen in psychotic adults. The appearance is unmistakable: a mass of dark sticky material with a tar-like consistency. In general, trichobezoars have been resistant to medical efforts at dissolution, although the endoscopic overtube may provide an alternative to surgery in selected patients.[28]

GASTRIC REMNANT (STUMP) CARCINOMA

Carcinoma in patients having had previous gastric surgery has been recognized throughout the world since the 1950s but especially in more recent Scandinavian studies where an incidence has been noted ranging from 0.8%[30] to 5%[31] and as high as 8.9%.[32] In these studies the patients at highest risk are those in whom gastric surgery, especially partial resection, had been performed 10 to 20 years previously,[33] with a risk of gastric cancer in these patients as much as 12 times that of others in the general population, for countries where the yearly risk of cancer in the general population is already high, approaching 400 per 100,000 in some areas.[34] The risk for similar patients in the United States compared to the general population is unclear. With the lower overall risk of gastric cancer in the general population (10 per 100,000)[35] one might expect the comparative risk for patients with prior surgery to also be reduced. However, to date no study has been reported from the United States from which the true cancer risk in these patients can be precisely determined, although a recent study has suggested an incidence of 6.1%,[35a] similar to that found in Scandinavian reports.[30-32]

Several factors may predispose patients with prior surgery to gastric cancer. First, atrophic gastritis with intestinalization is a common sequela of vagotomy and hemigastrectomy, where vagal innervation and antral gastrin both exert important trophic effects on the parietal mucosa. The absence of both predictably leads to atrophic gastritis in more than 50% of patients within 2 years.[36] For patients with atrophic gastritis there is a cumulative incidence of gastric cancer which approaches 10% in some series.[37]

Second, there is significant bile reflux in patients with a hemigastrectomy, even in those who are asymptomatic. This critical role of bile was suggested in a recent experimental study in which gastric carcinoma occurred in rats following a variety of gastric operations, with the highest incidence of cancer associated with a gastroenterostomy (70%), and lower incidences with Billroth II (30%) and Billroth I (10%) type operations. Of importance was the fact that the cancer risk in these animals could be entirely abolished by diverting bile away from the stomach by means of a Roux-en-Y jejunojejunostomy for the afferent loop.

Finally, with reduced acid secretion within a gastric remnant, there is the potential for bacterial overgrowth. These bacteria, especially the anaerobes, have the capability of converting cholic acid to deoxycholic acid, which promotes large bowel cancer in experimental animals.[38] Furthermore, other bacteria may emerge which are capable of converting dietary nitrates and tertiary amines to nitrites and N-nitroso compounds, the latter being potential carcinogens.[39]

Length of Time from Ulcer Surgery

Reports of carcinoma occurring in patients with previous gastric surgery indicate the vulnerable period to be 10 to 25 years afterward, with the greatest risk being between 20 and 25 years.[34] In one Norwegian study of 108 patients having endoscopy who had undergone partial gastrectomy 20 to 25 years earlier, four were found to have invasive carcinoma and three others had cancer *in situ,* making the incidence of cancer (invasive or *in situ*) 7%. This was 20 to 40 times the incidence of carcinoma in the general adult Norwegian population.[31]

A somewhat earlier onset of remnant cancer has been observed in patients having had prior resection and radiation for gastric lymphoma, where half the reported cases occurred between 5 and 16 years following surgery.[39a]

Only one study has been reported from the United States similar to those from Scandinavian centers where follow-up endoscopy was performed in a group of patients having had surgery 20 to 25 years earlier.[35a] Among a group of 66 patients who underwent endoscopy after a mean of 22.2 years from surgery, 6% (4 of 66) had cancer. Also noteworthy was an additional 14.4% with either atypia (4.5%) or adenomas (9.9%).

This study suggested that the rate of gastric cancer in the United States for patients with prior subtotal gastrectomy was similar to that of the Scandinavian countries, where the incidence of gastric cancer in the general population approaches 100 to 200 per 100,000 (10 times that seen in the United States). However, much larger numbers of patients must be studied before the cancer risk and the role of endoscopic surveillance can be precisely defined.

Type of Operation Performed

It had been thought that the type of anastomosis performed had a bearing on the cancer risk, with the Billroth II type being more predisposed to malignant transformation. However, recent studies suggest that this may have been simply an artifact of the greater prevalence of Billroth II operations. When a group of patients having had previous Billroth I surgery 10 years or more before was examined, the incidence of gastric carcinoma was found to be as high as that in comparable patients with a Billroth II anastomosis.[40] Similarly, cancer may follow in patients having had a simple gastrojejunostomy without antral resection, although the true incidence of malignancy in this group of patients is unknown.[41] Gastric carcinoma, however, rarely occurs in patients with a pyloroplasty.

Appearance

As with gastric cancer in general (see Chapter 16), there are early and advanced type lesions, each with its own distinctive appearance. For the most part, early lesions are only found in asymptomatic patients having endoscopy performed because of gastric surgery done 15 years or more previously (see below). Virtually all symptomatic patients will have advanced lesions. Unlike patients with early cancers for whom surgery may be curative, patients with advanced lesions are virtually always unresectable. In these patients, suspicion of cancer will derive from new weight loss, subxiphoid pain, anorexia, or early satiety as well as a change in the shape of the radiographic appearance of the gastric remnant.

Early Gastric Cancer

These lesions have been described with the Billroth I[42] and Billroth II[43] anatomy and may account for up to one-third of the gastric remnant cancer discovered, especially when asymptomatic patients having screening endoscopy are included.[42] The commonest appearance has been that of a small polypoid mass (Fig. 19-15a) of the type I or IIa variety. Less commonly, the endoscopist may recognize focal mucosal discoloration and/or depression as evidence of malignancy, although it would be extremely difficult or impossible to differentiate these appearanees from other nonspecific mucosal changes. Surprisingly, the ulcer type of early gastric cancer has yet to be reported in patients with early gastric remnant carcinoma.

Although these lesions may arise anywhere within the remnant and are in some cases multicentric, the mucosa with 2 cm of the stomal anastomosis is the commonest location. Because early gastric cancer of the stoma could easily be confused with other stomal findings, e.g., hyperplastic polyps (Fig. 19-15b), multiple biopsies must be obtained whenever the diagnosis is suspected.

Advanced Gastric Cancer

At least 70%,[42] and in our experience 95%+, of gastric remnant carcinomas are seen as advanced cancers with the appearance of a polypoid mass (Fig. 19-15c) or infiltrating lesion (Fig. 19-15d), involving the stoma and extending for variable distances into the remnant. Some cases with the linitis plastica appearance involving the entire remnant show submucosal extension above the GE junction. Despite the extensive involvement, histologic confirmation may still be problematic, as is true of any infiltrating malignancy (see Chapter 16). Biopsy therefore needs to be aggressively pursued along with cytology, with the latter especially useful in cases where either the rugal folds are diffusely ulcerated or areas likely to represent mucosal breakthrough of tumor (see Chapter 16) cannot be biopsied because of technical factors. The newer techniques of large-particle biopsy and needle aspiration cytology (see Chapter 1) may be especially useful in cases with an infiltrating appearance, but without apparent mucosal breakthrough of tumor.

Screening for Gastric Remnant Cancer

As patients with previous gastric surgery are at increased risk for malignancy after 15 years, and especially 20 years, we recommend routine screening for visual inspection and multiple biopsies.[31] However, because the yield from screening is low, at best only 6%,[35a] the policy of routine screening for this group has been questioned. Nonetheless, we are impressed by the cure rate of 70% for patients whose cancers were detected by screening contrasted with one of only 5% for those presenting with symptoms,[43a] and continue to feel that surveillance is justified. While the ideal frequency of endoscopy has not been determined we believe that a 2-year interval between examinations is reasonable. We would obtain at least four biopsies from around the stoma and four others from areas above. Should biopsies show dysplasia, but be short of cancer *in situ,* we would reendoscope the patient at 6 months to 1 year. The finding of cancer *in situ* (severe dysplasia) with or without macroscopic lesion would constitute a strong indication for surgery.[31]

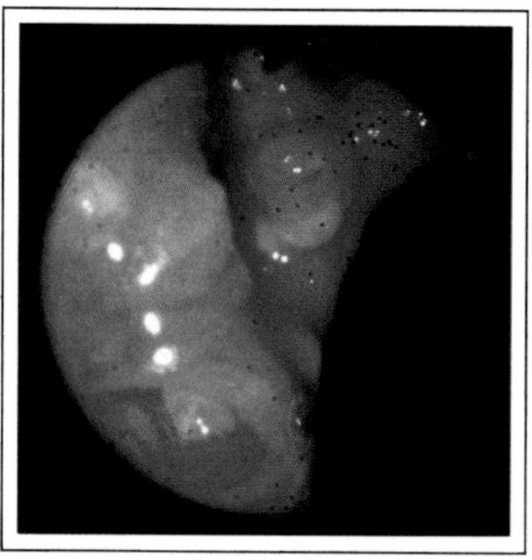

FIG. 19-15a.

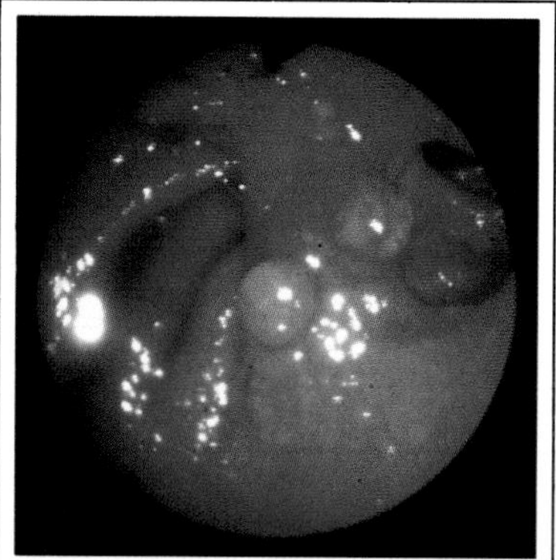

FIG. 19-15b.

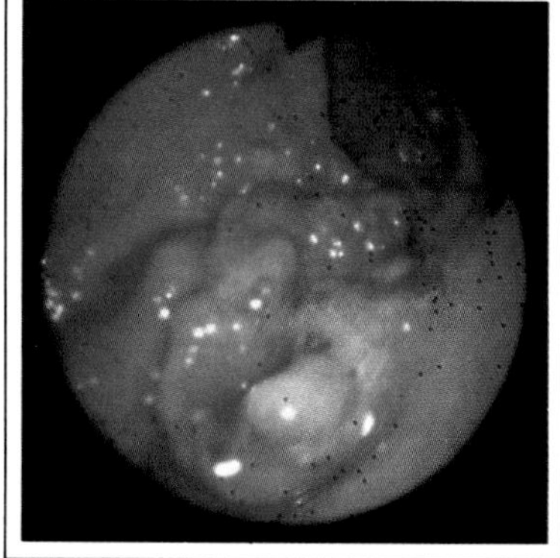

FIG. 19-15c.

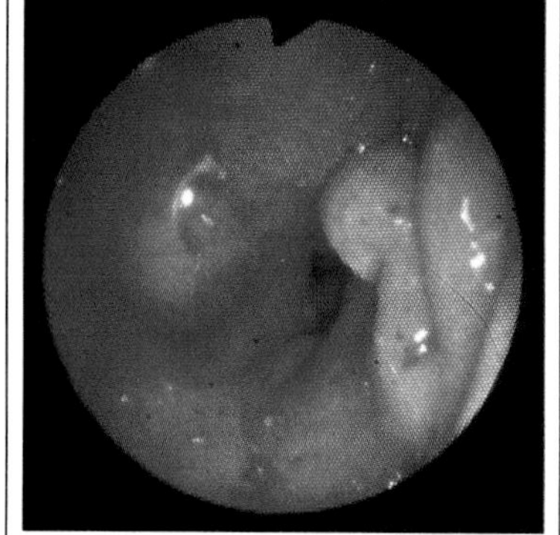

FIG. 19-15d.

FIG. 19-15. a: Gastric remnant (stump) cancer, early (IIa) type. A small raised nodule is seen on the stomal margin, having an appearance similar to that of a hyperplastic polyp (b). A biopsy, however, showed this to be a focus of invasive carcinoma. **b:** Stomal hyperplastic polyps. Multiple small nodular lesions are seen on the stomal margin which simulate the IIa appearance (a). Biopsy, however, serves to differentiate these two appearances. **c:** Gastric remnant carcinoma, advanced (Borrmann I) type. A large polypoid mass was found adjacent to the stoma in a patient having had previous hemigastrectomy and Billroth II anastomosis 25 years previously. **d:** Gastric remnant carcinoma, advanced (Borrmann IV) type. Infiltrated folds extend from the stoma throughout most of the gastric remnant in a patient having had an antral resection and irradiation for lymphoma 9 years before. Both irradiation and the previous gastric malignancy may have predisposed to the earlier (<10 years) development of carcinoma.[39a]

OTHER POSTSURGICAL APPEARANCES

Suture Appearances

Single or multiple sutures may be seen either along the line of closure where resection has been performed or at an anastomosis. These characteristically appear as tiny, yellow-green, raised areas (Fig. 19-16a). On closer examination, the individual suture will easily be recognized. There may be a tiny, yellowish, loosely adherent exudate which in part may be tissue reaction but generally contains simply cellular detritus and adherent foreign material (Fig. 19-16a). Less commonly, the mucosa around the suture breaks down and a frank ulceration appears (Fig. 19-16a). In these cases one observes an actual ulcer base.

As sutures themselves are rarely the cause of symptoms, it is unnecessary for the most part to attempt to remove them. If they are to be removed because of an associated ulcer (Fig. 19-16b) or a suture granuloma (see below), this is not attempted with a standard biopsy forceps as there is a real danger of these forceps becoming enmeshed in the suture once the forceps has been closed—which to rectify may require pulling off the suture and thereby risking bleeding. One therefore attempts to remove a suture with a forceps only after cutting it with endoscopic surgical scissors (FS3L, Olympus Corporation of America, New Hyde Park, New York).

In addition to ulcers, suture granulomas may be encountered (Fig. 19-16c). These are submucosal masses resulting from a marked inflammatory reaction to the suture material itself. In some patients they become large enough to actually obstruct the gastric outlet.[44] Suture granulomas tend to deform the stoma in an asymmetrical fashion (Fig. 19-16c) and can be differentiated from the more symmetrical, nonspecific stomal deformity in which a suture is an incidental finding. In cases where a suture granuloma is present and considered a cause of symptoms, endoscopic suture removal in the manner described for suture ulcers (see above) could be attempted.

Gastrostomy Tube

A gastrostomy tube in place has a very characteristic appearance (Fig. 19-17a). It cannot be mistaken for a foreign body once the diagnosis is considered. Usually the referring physician advises the endoscopist about a gastrostomy tube or visual inspection of the abdomen suggests that the patient has one in place, but neither is always the case. Therefore the endoscopist must recall its appearance when confronted with a "foreign body" in a patient with recent abdominal surgery.

In patients with gastrostomy tubes in place, one actually sees the tube (Fig. 19-17a), which has a yellow-green col-

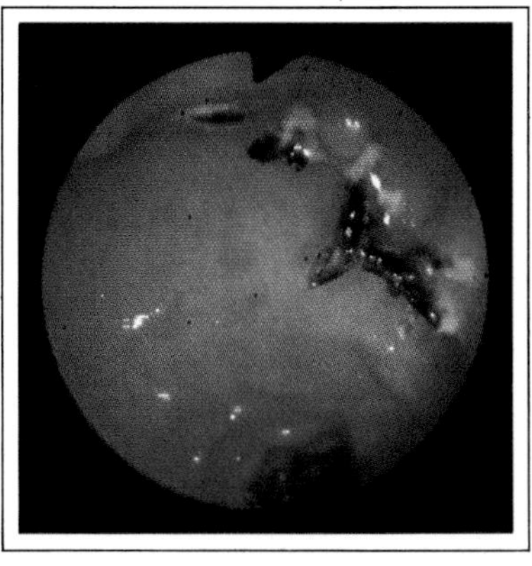

FIG. 19-16a.

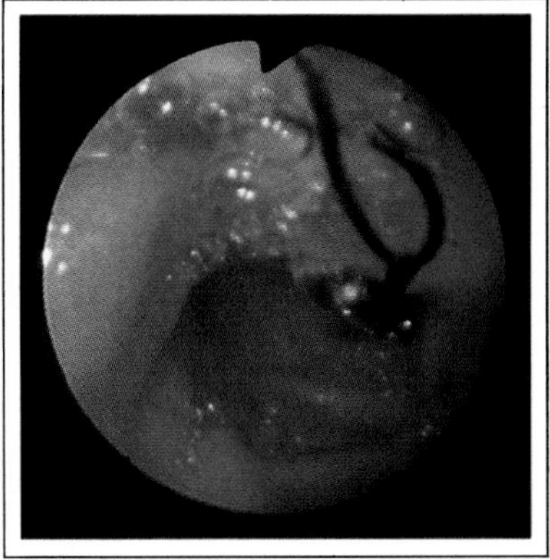

FIG. 19-16b.

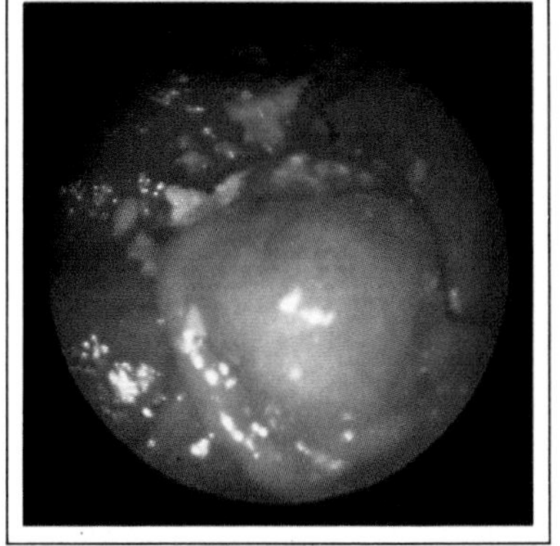

FIG. 19-16c.

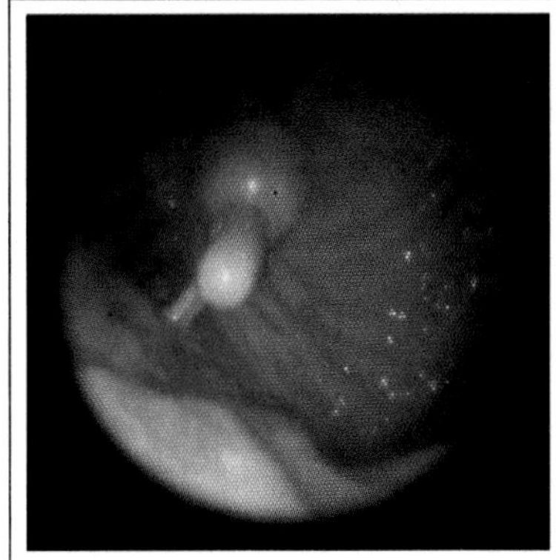

FIG. 19-17a.

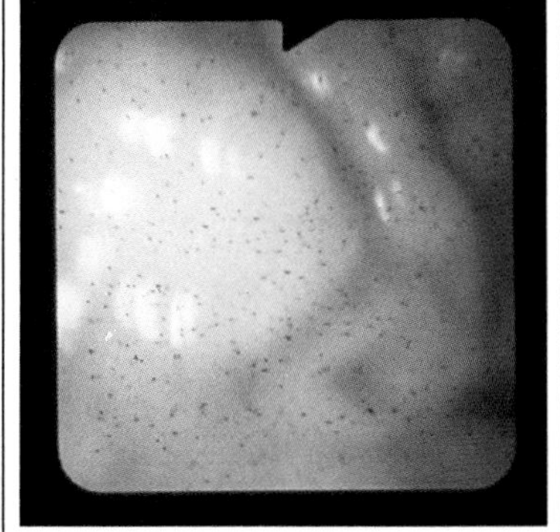

FIG. 19-17b.

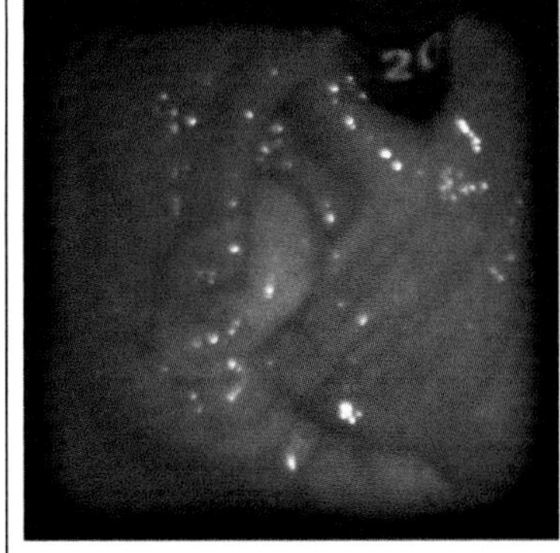

FIG. 19-18.

FIG. 19-16. a: Billroth I stoma with a retained suture. A white exudate is found around the green-black suture. This consists of some acute inflammatory exudate, but most of it is adhering foreign material. This appearance, even with the exudate, is rarely a cause of symptoms. **b:** Billroth I stoma with a suture and recurrent ulcer. The suture was in the base of the ulcer and suggests a role in the pathogenesis of the ulcer. One can remove such a suture by means of an endoscopic accessory, surgical scissors. **c:** Suture granuloma. In this case there is an asymmetrical mass deformity from the jejunal side of the stoma. Suture material could be identified within the mass (not shown).

FIG. 19-17. a: Gastrostomy tube. This green balloon-tipped tube is observed to enter the stomach from the anterior wall at the junction of the fundus (at 9 o'clock) and the body (at 3 o'clock). **b:** Gastrostomy tube, scar deformity. A mass-like deformity is seen on the anterior wall 1 year after removal of the gastrostomy tube. The central depression within the mass marks the exact position of the tube.

FIG. 19-18. Wedge resection deformity. A confluence of folds around a central point (just off 9 o'clock) was noted 1 year after wedge resection of a leiomyosarcoma. This mass-like deformity changed in shape with air insufflation and tented well, evidence against recurrence.

oration, projecting out from the anterior wall. If the tube is followed to its termination, its balloon tip will be seen (Fig. 19-17a). After withdrawal of the gastrostomy tube, scarring occurs, with the central dimple marking the site of the tube, along with radiation of surrounding folds to this point (Fig. 19-17b).

Wedge Resection Deformity

After wedge resection of lesions—generally large epithelial and submucosal polyps—scar deformity is present at the site of the resection. In these cases prominent, heaped-up folds appear to converge on a central point (Fig. 19-18). In some cases the deformity suggests recurrence, especially if the original tumor was submucosal and had malignant potential, such as would be the case of a gastric carcinoid. Any question of recurrence would be difficult to resolve without a full-thickness surgical biopsy of the gastric wall. However, features which favor postsurgical deformity rather than tumor recurrence are: (a) the mass itself consists of folds; (b) there is a change in the shape of the folds with air insufflation; and (c) there is a central depression below the level of the surrounding mucosa (Fig. 19-18).

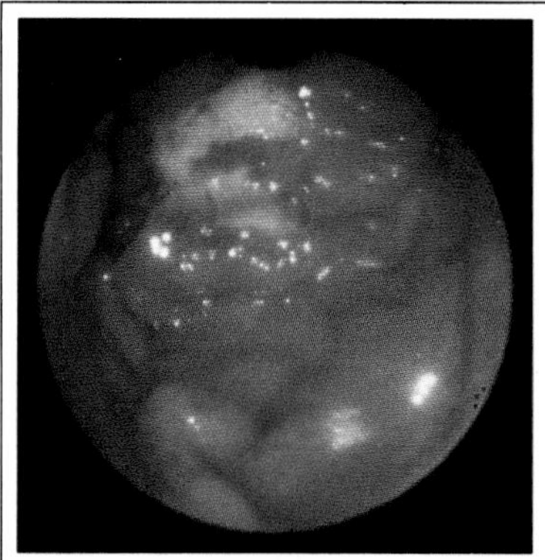

FIG. 19-19a.

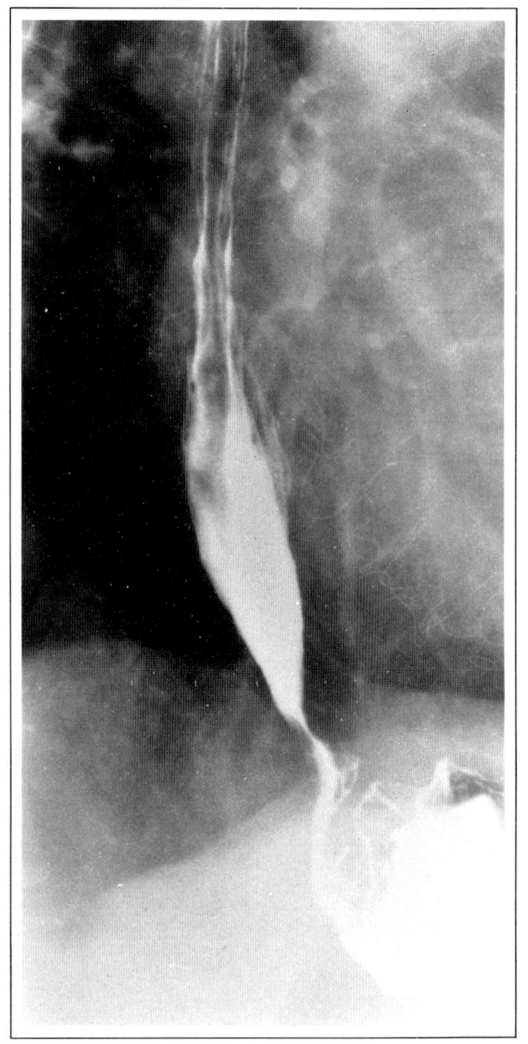

FIG. 19-19b.

FIG. 19-19. a: Fundoplication. The surgery produces an extremely pliant cardia when viewed by means of U-type retroflexion (with the endoscope just seen at 12 o'clock). The cardial fold can be mistaken for a mass or infiltrating lesion, especially when the history of antireflux surgery is obtained. **b:** Fundoplication, radiographic appearance. A mass lesion of the cardia was suggested without the history of a previous fundoplication.

Fundoplication Deformity

In fundoplication, a common operation for peptic esophagitis, the fundus is wrapped around the distal esophagus and they are sutured together just below the diaphragm for about 5 cm.[45] This produces a deformity of the cardia which is observed when a retroflexed (U-type) view is achieved. Here one sees an enlarged cardia, usually 1.5 to 2 times its normal size (Fig. 19-19a). This may be mistaken for a submucosal tumor, especially when this possibility has been suggested radiographically (Fig. 19-19b). Unlike an infiltrating lesion or mass of the cardia, with a fundoplication deformity the cardia is seen as prominent but entirely symmetrical with extremely pliant folds which are easily tented (Fig. 19-19a). The history of previous antireflux surgery is important, however, as without it one would still need to seriously consider the possibility of infiltrating malignancy.

Gastric Surgery for Obesity

Because morbid obesity is a serious medical problem but one which is generally refractory to nonsurgical management, a variety of operations have been utilized. The disenchantment with jejunoileal bypass because of its many long-term complications has led to a greater utilization of gastric surgery for obesity. These operations have revolved around a gastric partitioning technique to create a proximal fundic pouch which limits the amount that can be ingested at a given time. As partitioning alone fails to achieve significant weight reduction in up to 20% and is associated with dissatisfaction for this and other reasons in over half the cases, the original operation has been modified so that the proximal pouch has a volume of only 50 cc and empties by way of a Roux-en-Y loop of jejunum.[46] Another modification has been the creation of a stoma between the proximal and distal stomach.[47] As in the case of the gastrojejunostomy

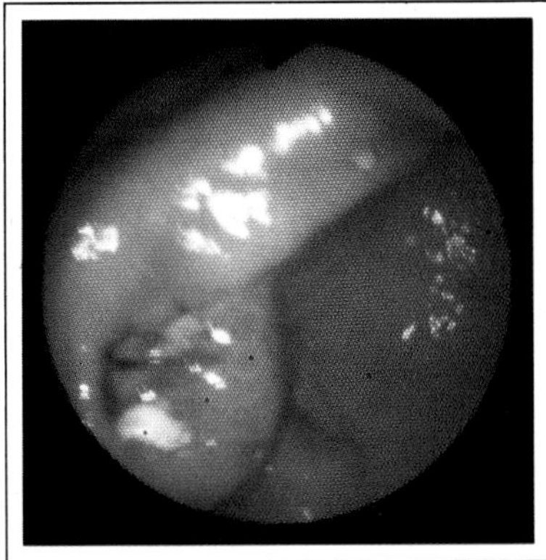

FIG. 19-20.

FIG. 19-20. Gastric partitioning operation for obesity with gastrogastrostomy stoma. The ridge-like fold, formed as a result of the stapling procedure, was found approximately 5 cm from the gastroesophageal junction, creating the proximal pouch. On the fold is a stomal opening to the remainder of the stomach.

modification, this also allows for the creation of a smaller proximal pouch so that there is greater weight reduction while lowering the incidence of postsurgical nausea and vomiting.[47]

In patients having had gastric surgery for obesity, endoscopy is requested to evaluate persistent nausea and vomiting, which can be expected in at least 10%,[46,47] as well as for persistent epigastric pain in order to exclude the possibility of stomal ulcers, which have been reported after gastric bypass.[48]

Appearance

The striking feature on entering the stomach is that of the ridge-like fold which separates the proximal pouch (Fig. 19-20) from the remainder of the stomach. In addition, there may be a stoma, which is just above the fold if a gastric bypass has been performed with a Roux-en-Y loop or on the fold itself if it connects with the distal stomach as a gastrogastrostomy (Fig. 19-20).

REFERENCES

1. Hoare, A. M., Jones, E. L., Alexander-Williams, J., and Hawkins, C. F. (1977): Symptomatic significance of gastric mucosal changes after surgery for peptic ulcer. *Gut,* 18:295–300.
2. Pemberton, J. H., and Van Heerden, J. (1980): Vagotomy and pyloroplasty in the treatment of duodenal ulceration: long-term results. *Mayo Clin. Proc.,* 55:14–18.
3. Hubert, J. P., Kiernan, P. D., Beahrs, O. H., and ReMine, W. H. (1980): Truncal vagotomy and resection in the treatment of duodenal ulcer. *Mayo Clin. Proc.,* 55:19–24.
4. Osnes, M., and Myren, J. (1975): Endoscopic retrograde cholangiopancreatography (ERCP) in patients with Billroth II partial gastrectomies. *Endoscopy,* 7:227–232.
5. Sharaiha, Z., Graham, D. Y., Smith, J. L., Schwartz, J. T., and Cain, G. D. (1981): Location and presentation of recurrent ulcers after peptic ulcer surgery: a modern assessment. *Gastroenterology,* 80:1281.
6. Baird, I. M., St. John, D. J. B., and Nasser, S. S. (1970): Role of occult blood loss in anemia after gastrectomy. *Gut,* 11:55–61.
7. Joffe, N., Goldman, H., and Antonioli, D. A. (1978): Recurring hyperplastic gastric polyps following subtotal gastrectomy. *Am. J. Roentgenol.,* 130:301–305.
8. Domellof, L., Eriksson, S., Helander, H. F., and Janunger, K.-G. (1977): Lipid islands in the gastric mucosa after resection for benign ulcer disease. *Gastroenterology,* 72:14–18.
9. Stabile, B. E., and Passaro, E. (1976): Recurrent peptic ulcer. *Gastroenterology,* 70:124–135.
10. Jordan, G., and Walker, L. L. (1973): Severe problems with gastric emptying after gastric surgery. *Ann. Surg.,* 177:660–668.
11. Dahlgren, S. (1964): The afferent loop syndrome. *Acta Chir. Scand. [Suppl.],* 327:1–149.
12. Rosenthal, L., Fonseca, C., Arzoumanian, A., Hernandez, M., and Greenberg, D. (1979): ^{99m}Tc-IDA hepatobiliary imaging following upper abdominal surgery. *Radiology,* 130:735–739.
13. Mauer, H. G., and Goodale, R. L. (1977): Endoscopic dilatation of a gastric anastomotic stricture. *Arch. Surg.,* 112:312–313.
14. Den Hartog Jager, F. C. A., Bartelsman, J. F. W. M., and Tytgat, G. N. W. (1979): Palliative treatment of obstructing esophagogastric malignancy by endoscopic positioning of a plastic prosthesis. *Gastroenterology,* 77:1008–1014.
15. Woodward, J. C., Mainz, D. L., and Webster, P. D. (1973): Afferent-efferent loop intragastric intussusception: diagnosed by gastroscopy. *Gastroenterology,* 64:170–177.
16. Scudamore, H. H., Eckstam, E. E., Fencil, W. J., and Jaramillo, C. A. (1973): Bile reflux gastritis. *Am. J. Gastroenterol.,* 60:9–22.
17. Meskinpour, H., Marks, J. W., Schoenfield, L. J., Bonnoris, G. G., and Carter, S. (1980): Reflux gastritis syndrome: mechanism of symptoms. *Gastroenterology,* 79:1283–1287.
18. Keighley, M. R. B., Asquith, P., and Alexander-Williams, J. (1975): Duodenogastric reflux: a cause of gastric mucosal hyperaemia and symptoms after operations for peptic ulceration. *Gut,* 16:28–32.
19. Tolin, R. D., Malmud, L. S., Stelzer, F., Menin, R., Makler, P. T., Applegate, G., and Fisher, R. (1979): Enterogastric reflux in normal subjects and patients with Billroth II gastroenterostomy: measurement of enterogastric reflux. *Gastroenterology,* 77:1027–1033.
20. Ludwig, S., and Ippoliti, A. (1979): Objective evaluation of symptomatic bile reflux after antrectomy. *Gastroenterology,* 76:1189.
21. Boren, C. H., and Way, L. W. (1980): Alkaline reflux gastritis: a reevaluation. *Am. J. Surg.,* 140:40–46.
22. Burbige, E. J., French, S. W., Tarder, G., and Belber, J. P. (1979): Correlation between gross appearance and histologic findings in the post-operative stomach. *Gastrointest. Endosc.,* 25:3–5.
23. Brady, P. G. (1978): Gastric phytobezoars consequent to delayed gastric emptying. *Gastrointest. Endosc.,* 24:159–161.
24. Van Thiel, D. H., DeBelle, R. C., Painter, T. D., McMillan, W. B., and Haradin, A. R. (1975): Phytobezoar occurring as a complication of gastric carcinoma. *Gastroenterology,* 68:1291–1296.
25. Amjad, H., Kumar, G. K., and McCaughery, R. (1975): Postgastrectomy bezoars. *Am. J. Gastroenterol.,* 64:327–331.
26. Zarling, E. J., and Moeler, D. D. (1981): Bezoar therapy: complications using Adolph's Meat Tenderizer and alternatives from literature review. *Arch. Intern. Med.,* 141:1669–1670.
27. Madsen, R., Skibba, R. M., Galvan, A., Striplin, C., and Scott, P. (1978):

Gastric bezoars: a technique of endoscopic removal. *Am. J. Dig. Dis.*, 23:23.

28. Rogers, B. H. G. (1979): A new method for extraction of impacted meat from the esophagus utilizing a flexible fiberoptic endoscope and an overtube. *Gastrointest. Endosc.*, 25:47.
29. Harris, V. J., and Hanley, G. (1975): Unusual features and complications of bezoars in children. *Am. J. Roentgenol.*, 123:742–745.
30. Ewerth, S., Bergstrand, O., Hellers, G., and Ost, A. (1978): The incidence of carcinoma in the gastric remnant after resection for benign ulcer disease. *Acta Chir. Scand. [Suppl. 482]*, 2–5.
31. Schrumpf, E., Stadaas, J., Myren, J., Serck-Hanssen, A., Aune, S., and Osnes, M. (1977): Mucosal changes in the gastric stump 20–25 years after partial gastrectomy. *Lancet*, 2:467–469.
32. Domellof, L., Eriksson, S., and Janunger, K.-G. (1977): Carcinoma and possible precancerous changes of the gastric stump after Billroth II resection. *Gastroenterology*, 73:462–468.
33. Geboes, K., Rutgerts, P., Broeckhaert, L., VanTrappen, G., and Desmet, V. (1980): Histologic appearances of endoscopic gastric mucosal biopsies 10–20 years after partial gastrectomy. *Ann. Surg.*, 192:179–182.
34. Domellof, L., and Janunger, K.-G. (1977): The risk of gastric carcinoma after partial gastrectomy. *Am. J. Surg.*, 134:581–584.
35. Devesa, S. S., and Silverman, D. T. (1978): Cancer incidence and mortality trends in the United States: 1935–1974. *J. Natl. Cancer Inst.*, 60:545–571.

35a. Hiltz, S. W., and Schuman, B. M. (1982): The occurrence of gastric stump cancer in a U.S. population. *Gastrointest. Endosc.*, 28:133.

36. Pulimood, B. M., Knudsen, A., and Coghill, N. F. (1976): Gastric mucosa after partial gastrectomy. *Gut*, 17:463–470.
37. Cheli, R., Santi, L., Ciancameria, G., and Cancianoui, G. (1973): A clinical and statistical followup study of atrophic gastritis. *Am. J. Dig. Dis.*, 18:1061–1066.

37a. Langhans, P., Heger, R. A., Hohenstein, J., and Bünte, H. (1981): Operation-sequel carcinoma: an experimental study. *Hepato-Gastroenterol.*, 28:34–37.

38. Lowenfels, A. B. (1978): Does bile promote extra-colonic cancer? *Lancet*, 2:239–241.
39. Schlag, H., Ulrich, H., Merkle, P., Bockler, R., Peter, M., and Herfarth, C. (1980): Are nitrite and N-nitroso compounds in gastric juice factors for carcinoma in the operated stomach? *Lancet*, 1:727–729.

39a. Sellin, J., Levin, B., Reckard, C., and Riddell, R. (1980): Gastric adenocarcinoma following gastric lymphoma. Role of partial gastrectomy. *Cancer*, 45:996–1000.

40. Domellof, L., Eriksson, S., and Janunger, K.-G. (1976): Late precancerous changes and carcinoma of the gastric stump after Billroth I resection. *Am. J. Surg.*, 132:26–31.
41. Kobayashi, S., Prolla, J., and Kirsner, J. B. (1970): Late gastric carcinoma developing after surgery for benign conditions: endoscopic and histologic studies of the anastomosis and diagnostic problems. *Am. J. Dig. Dis.*, 15:905–912.
42. Miederer, S. E., Muller, R., Kutz, K., Wobser, E., and Elster, K. (1977): Multicentric early gastric carcinoma mimicking type I (10 years after B-1 surgery). *Endoscopy*, 9:50–53.
43. Osnes, M., Lotveit, T., Myren, J., and Serck-Hanssen, A. (1977): Early gastric carcinoma in patients with a Billroth II partial gastrectomy. *Endoscopy*, 9:47–49.

43a. Tytgat, G. N. J., Offerhaus, G. J. A., van der Stadt, J., Huibregtse, K., de Boer, J., Verhoeven, T., and van Olffen, G. H. (1983): Longstanding partial gastrectomy, a premalignant condition? *Gastroenterology*, 84:1338.

44. Gueller, R., Shapiro, H. A., Nelson, J. A., and Bush, R. (1976): Suture granuloma simulating tumors: a preventable postgastrectomy complication. *Am. J. Dig. Dis.*, 21:223–228.
45. Skucas, J., Mangla, J. C., Adams, J. T., and Cutcliff, W. (1976): An evaluation of the Nissen fundoplication. *Radiology*, 118:539–543.
46. Pories, W. J., Flickinger, E. G., Meelheim, D., Van Rij, A. M., and Thomas, F. T. (1982): The effectiveness of gastric bypass over gastric partition in morbid obesity: consequence of distal gastric and duodenal exclusion. *Ann. Surg.*, 196:389–399.
47. Smith, L. B. (1981): Modification of the gastric partitioning operation for morbid obesity. *Am. J. Surg.*, 142:725–730.
48. Printen, J. J., Scott, D., and Mason, E. E. (1980): Stomal ulcers after gastric bypass. *Arch. Surg.*, 115:525–527.

20

UNCOMMON GASTRIC APPEARANCES

The conditions considered in this chapter are of three types: (a) primary gastric disorders; (b) gastric involvement in selected disorders involving the gastrointestinal tract; and (c) opportunistic infections of the stomach and syphilis.

PRIMARY GASTRIC DISORDERS

Gastric Xanthoma (Xanthelasma)

Gastric xanthomas are rare throughout the world except in Japan where they are said to be found in up to 1% of endoscopic examinations.[1] We have encountered only five cases (0.1%) out of 5,000 examinations performed over a 7-year period. Xanthomas are always an incidental finding at endoscopy. They are rarely large enough to be demonstrated radiographically and in themselves cause no symptoms. They bear no definite relationship to hyperlipidemia.[2] At endoscopy they range in size between 1 and 5 mm (Fig. 20-1a) and are typically seen as tiny, yellow mucosal excrescences.[1,2] The antrum is the commonest location, but some are found in the cardiofundic area. Larger lesions appear as yellow-white sessile nodules (Fig. 20-1b). Biopsy of these lesions confirms the visual impression of gastric xanthoma with the finding of lipid-filled histiocytes.

Gastric Candida

Candida is sometimes found in the base of gastric ulcers.[3] We in fact found four such cases among 219 patients with gastric ulcers examined over a 5-year period. The fact that *Candida* is found within the base of an ulcer might seem surprising in view of the fact that acid suppresses the growth of *Candida* at least *in vitro*. However, gastric ulcers can be found in patients with very low acid output, even achlorhydria. In cases where *Candida* is found, the presence of hypoacidity may allow for any swallowed *Candida* to become established within the base of a chronic ulcer.[3] Generally in these cases there are none of the usual predisposing conditions for *Candida*, e.g., diabetes, an immunocompromised state, or prior antibiotic usage. However, in some reported cases underlying conditions have been noted, e.g., alcoholism and hematologic and other malignancies.[4] Other cases have been described in association with a large hiatus

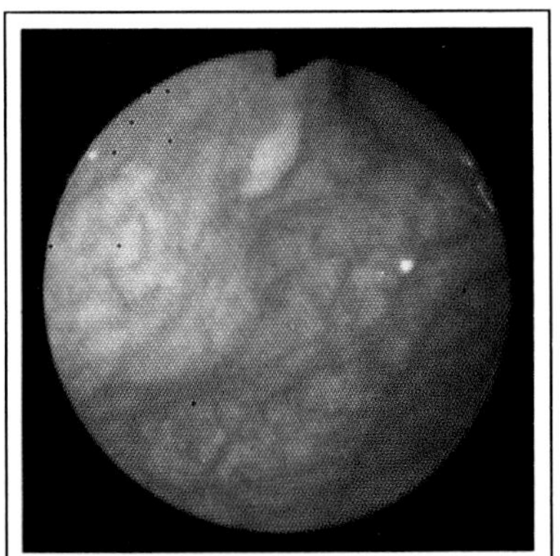

FIG. 20-1a.

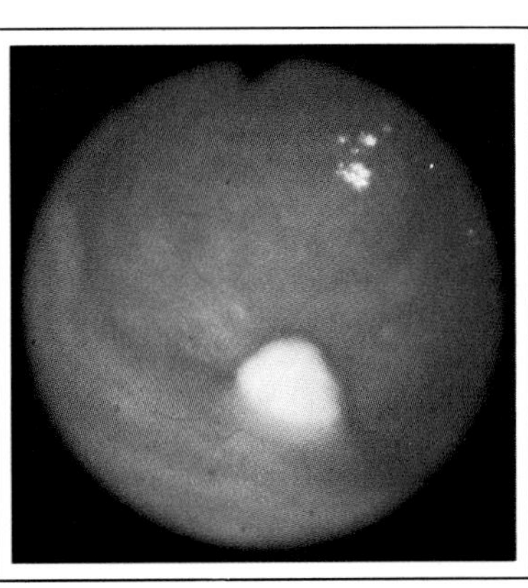

FIG. 20-1b.

FIG. 20-1. Gastric xanthoma. **a:** A characteristic 3-mm raised yellow-white polyp. **b:** A large (6 mm) yellow-white sessile polyp of the distal antrum.

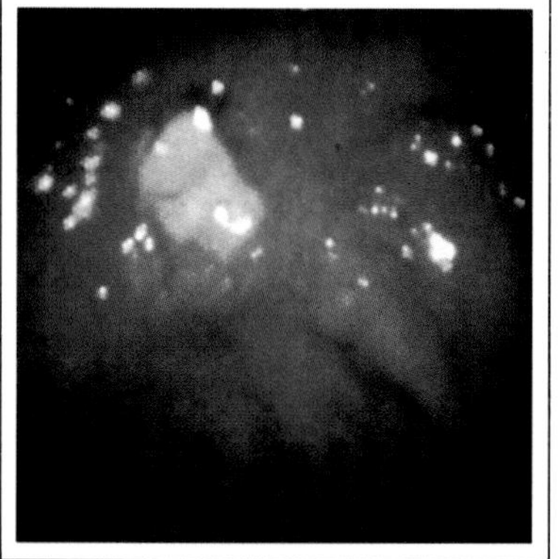

FIG. 20-2a.

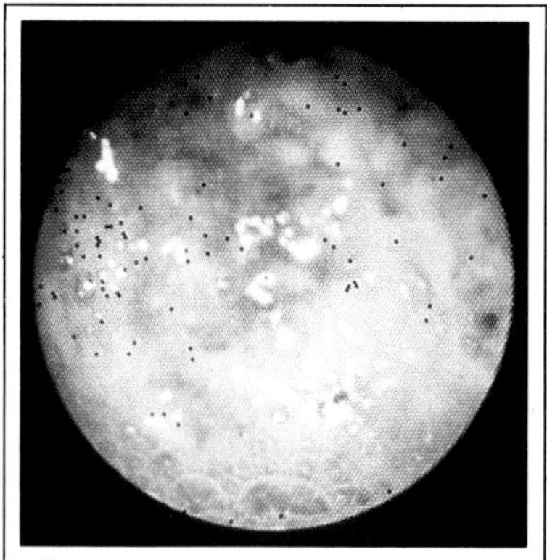

FIG. 20-2b.

FIG. 20-2. a: Gastric *Candida* (in a benign ulcer base). A fundic ulcer in an elderly patient was biopsied and found to contain hyphae and budding yeast in its base suggestive of *Candida*. **b:** Gastric *Candida* in a malignant ulcer base. The base was noted to be irregular with mounds of granulation tissue, a feature suggesting *Candida*. At autopsy an adenocarcinoma was present just below the *Candida* in this patient with disseminated lymphoma.

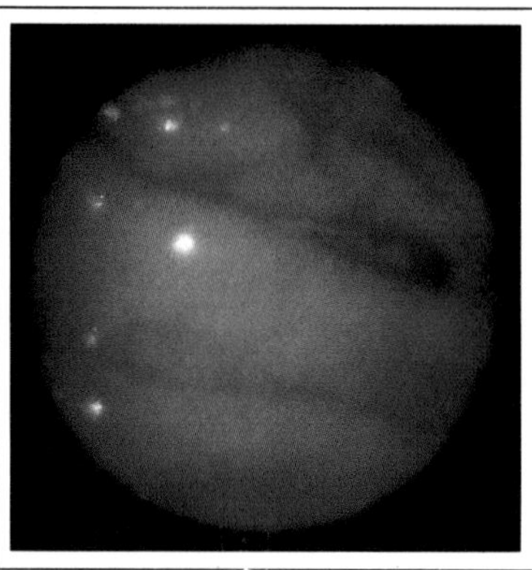

FIG. 20-3.

FIG. 20-3. Foreign body (dental probe) hidden between two rugal folds (toward 3 o'clock).

hernia[5] and in patients who had gastric surgery up to 25 years before.[6]

Patients with gastric *Candida* may present with typical ulcer symptoms or nonspecific complaints, e.g., nausea, vomiting, or upper gastrointestinal (GI) bleeding. Double-contrast gastric radiography may reveal aphthous ulcers as the earliest findings.[7] The most common radiographic finding is that of a deep ulcer with marked irregularity of the base.[3,5] Often the appearance suggests carcinoma. When tested for maximum stimulated gastric acidity, this has been found to be less than 5 mEq/hr.[3] Gastric *Candida*, in addition, has been noted to be a risk factor for massive GI bleeding in these ulcers as well as a port of entry for systemic candidiasis.[4]

Appearance

Typically, this is a discrete punched-out ulcer, usually 1 cm or larger with an irregular yellow base, projecting out into the lumen (Fig. 20-2a). When viewed closely, especially if the ulcer is large, the base appears to have an irregular, cheesy consistency (Fig. 20-2b). Even though the base is irregular, in most cases the candidal ulcer is benign. In the occasional case where there is underlying malignancy (Fig. 20-2b), there are no features related to *Candida* to suggest this.

Another appearance that has been described is that of multiple ulcerated papules[8] which would correspond to an appearance noted radiographically as aphthoid ulcerations.[7] The endoscopic appearance of multiple ulcerated papules has been suggested as the earliest appearance of gastric *Candida*.[8] In patients with previous gastric surgery, the gastric *Candida* may form a yeast bezoar and appear as a single amorphous mass or multiple masses.[6]

Foreign Bodies

A wide variety of objects have been observed in the stomach, including coins, spoons, paperclips, toothpicks, and needles.[9] We have ourselves observed the tip of a dental probe which was broken off during the course of an examination and swallowed (Fig. 20-3). The distinctive appearance of most foreign objects means that they are rarely confused with other gastric pathology. The problem, however, is finding them. The fundus may be a potential hiding place, as the patient may have been supine prior to the examination, allowing the object to "fall" into the fundus.

To find an object, a careful search must be instituted with the patient both on his left side and in the prone position at which time the anterior wall would be examined with particular care. U-type retroflexion needs to be performed as part of the examination in both positions. Need-

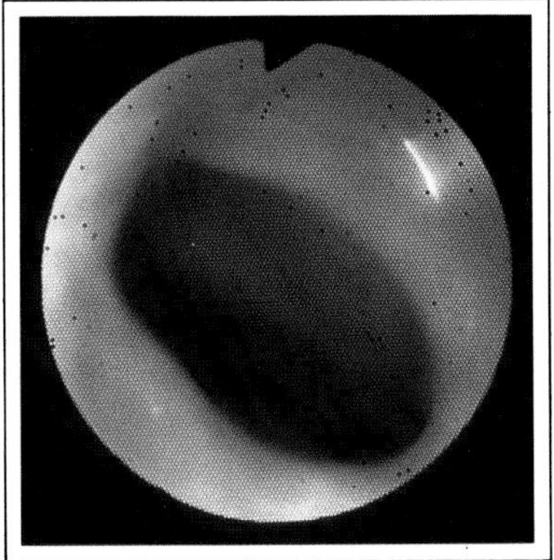

FIG. 20-4a.

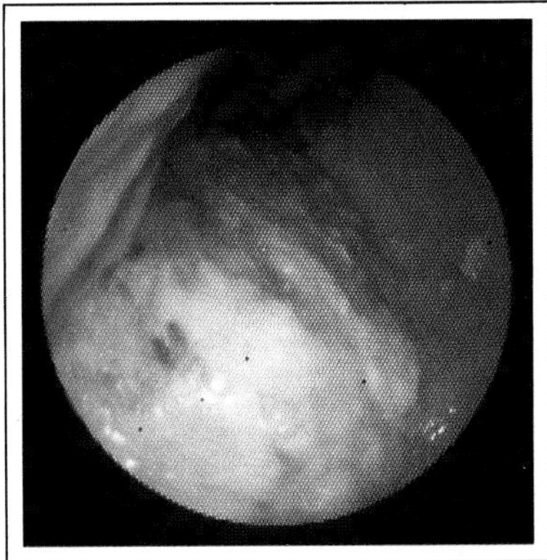

FIG. 20-4b.

FIG. 20-4. Diabetic gastroparesis. **a:** The pyloric channel is widely patent in this case, although gastric emptying is markedly delayed, as evidenced by the presence of a large bezoar (b). **b:** A large bezoar was found in this patient with a partially patent pylorus as evidence of antral motor failure.

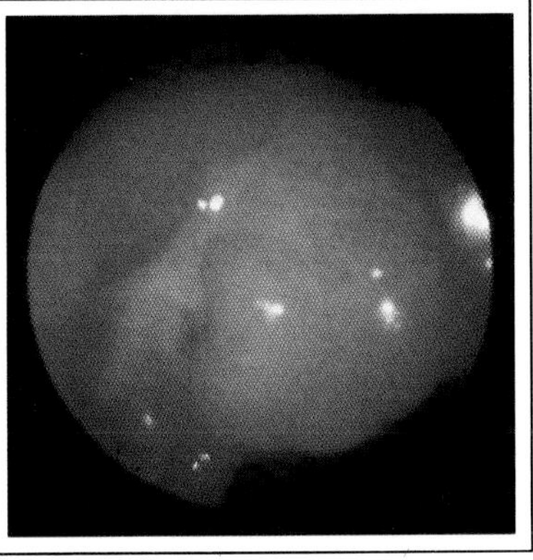

FIG. 20-5.

FIG. 20-5. Gastric pseudolymphoma. A deeply penetrating ulcer set within a mass-like deformity was thought at endoscopy to be suspicious for malignancy. At examination of the surgically resected specimen, pseudolymphoma was revealed within the deeply penetrating ulcer.

less to say, having a recent plain abdominal radiograph would be a great help, as it would determine if the object is still in the stomach.

Various techniques for extracting foreign bodies have been described, the most common one being by means of snares.[10] Recently, an overtube has been utilized to facilitate extraction.[11]

Diabetic Gastroparesis

Although antral motor dysfunction may occur in up to 30% of patients with insulin-dependent diabetes,[12] only one-third of these have symptoms suggestive of gastric outlet obstruction. With an incidence of insulin-dependent diabetes in the general population of only 1 to 2%, the endoscopist can expect to encounter diabetic gastroparesis in only one or two cases per 1,000 examinations (0.1 to 0.2% of cases).

Recent studies suggest that gastroparesis is a form of neuropathy with functionally intact antral smooth muscle.[13] The effect of this neuropathy in an insulin-dependent diabetic, however, is that of antral motor failure leading to symptoms which suggest gastric outlet obstruction and radiographic findings of gastric retention.

At endoscopy, no organic obstruction of the pyloric channel is demonstrated with free passage of an 11- or 13-mm endoscope (Fig. 20-4a). The presence of a gastric bezoar (Fig. 20-4b) or other retained foreign material in the space of a patent pyloric channel should immediately suggest this diagnosis in an insulin-dependent diabetic.

GASTRIC PSEUDOLYMPHOMA

Gastric pseudolymphoma is a rare condition in which a nodular or ulcerating mass lesion (Fig. 20-5) is found in the body or antrum,[14] prompting the diagnosis of malignancy although biopsies show only an infiltrate of mature lymphocytes along with a mixture of inflammatory cells. If the biopsy is deep enough, the lymphoid follicles with germinal centers are also seen.[15]

We have encountered only one case out of 5,000 examinations performed over a 7-year period. In this case a gastric mass was observed along with a deep gastric ulcer (Fig. 20-5). As in other reported cases, a pleomorphic lymphoid infiltrate was found on initial forceps biopsies.[14,15] Because of this suspicious appearance of the lesion, even with the "benign" lymphoid elements found on biopsy, the temptation to remove this lesion proved irresistable. At surgery, pseudolymphoma in association with a deeply penetrating benign gastric ulcer as well as an ulcer scar deformity was found. The finding of pseudolymphoma in many cases in association with benign ulcers, especially ones which

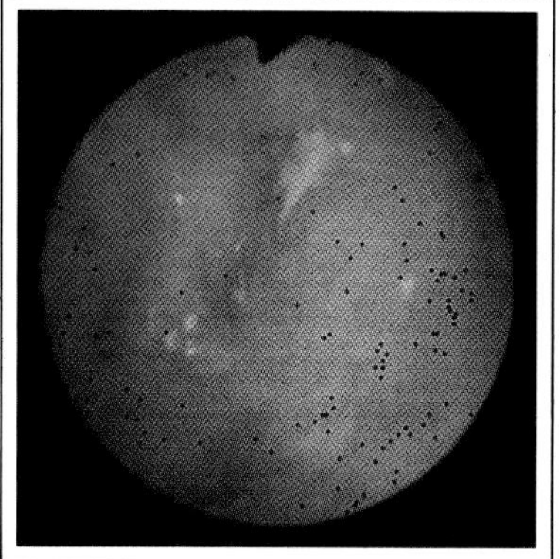

FIG. 20-6a.

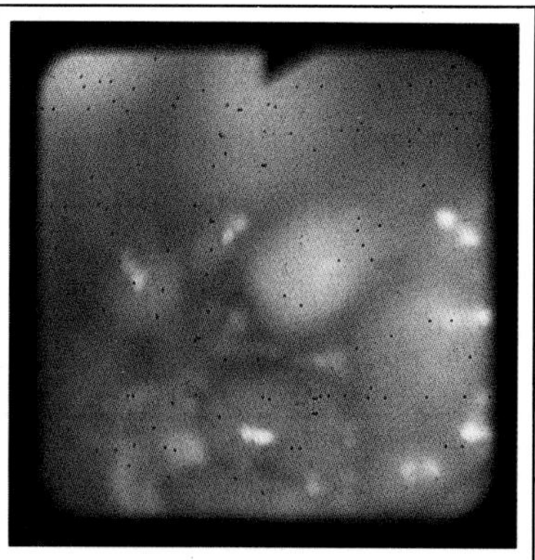

FIG. 20-6b.

FIG. 20-6. a: Gastric Crohn's disease. Scattered superficial (aphthoid) ulcerations in the prepyloric antrum. The adjacent mucosa appears uninvolved. **b:** Gastric Crohn's disease aphthoid ulcerations of the prepyloric antrum appear with intervening nodular mucosa, creating a cobblestone appearance.

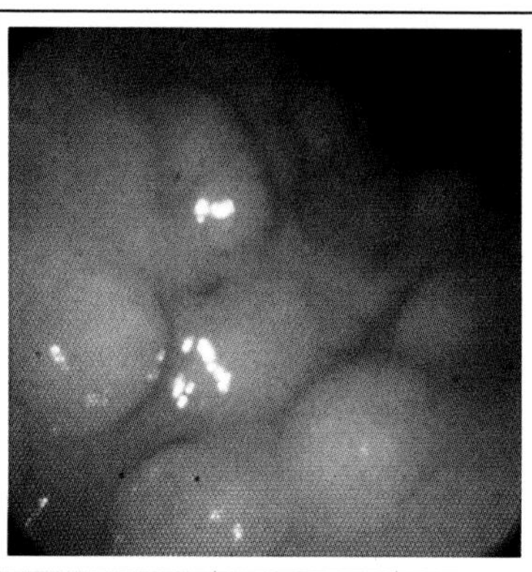

FIG. 20-7.

FIG. 20-7. Gastric Crohn's disease, hyperplastic polyps of the body. By themselves, these are a nonspecific finding in a patient with Crohn's disease elsewhere in the GI tract.

are deep, suggests that pseudolymphoma in these cases may simply represent a more extreme lymphoreticular response to the presence of an ulcer than that which ordinarily occurs in peptic ulcer disease, but to a lesser degree.[16]

GASTRIC INVOLVEMENT IN SELECTED DISORDERS INVOLVING THE GI TRACT

Gastric Crohn's Disease

Only 1% of patients with Crohn's disease have gastric involvement.[17] It is therefore rarely seen. Even at a center such as ours, specializing in the care of patients with inflammatory bowel disease, on the average only one case per year (1 per 500 to 700 examinations) is seen.

When the stomach is involved, the antrum, in particular the prepyloric antrum, is the usual site, giving rise to obstructive symptoms such as nausea, vomiting, early satiety, and weight loss.[18] This presentation prompts endoscopy,[18] as would ulcer-type pain or an abnormal radiographic appearance.[18]

Appearance

The endoscopic appearance is similar to that seen in the colon (see Chapter 43). Typically, superficial or "aphthoid" ulcers (Fig. 20-6a) are seen focally in the prepyloric antrum with the intervening mucosa appearing uninvolved. In some cases the mucosa between ulcerations becomes nodular or polypoid, often referred to as the cobblestone appearance (Fig. 20-6b). Along with areas of ulceration and the cobblestone appearance, there is considerable scarring and deformity of the antrum.

The body may also show evidence of involvement with Crohn's disease if the antrum is narrowed; the body may appear dilated, especially if the pyloric channel is obstructed. In addition, hyperplastic polyps (Fig. 20-7) may be found diffusely. As in the distal stomach, aphthoid ulcerations set in otherwise normal mucosa are found. Occasionally large ulcers are seen with a serpiginous shape.[18] In some patients with gastric Crohn's disease in whom gastrojejunostomy was performed because of pyloric obstruction, the disease is particularly prone to appear on the stoma as multiple, aphthous-type ulcerations, along with stomal narrowing, and nonspecific stomatitis (Fig. 20-8).

Differentiation from Peptic Ulcer Disease

The appearance of gastric ulcers in a patient with Crohn's disease still requires differentiation from those of peptic ulcer disease, especially as the incidence of the latter may be increased in patients with Crohn's disease.[19] Particularly

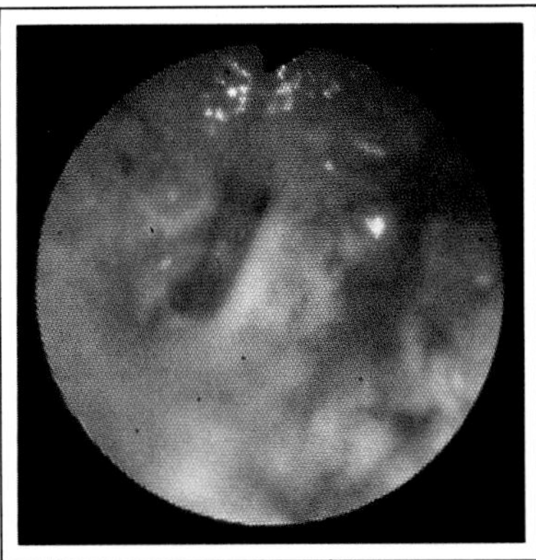

FIG. 20-8.

FIG. 20-8. Gastric Crohn's disease in a patient having had previous gastrojejunostomy. Ulcerations around a narrowed stoma suggest Crohn's disease involving the anastomosis.

important in this regard is the finding of multiple superficial or aphthoid ulcers of the antrum. While these certainly could be consistent with gastric Crohn's disease, their presence still should always prompt the endoscopist to question the patient about his use of aspirin or other nonsteroidal agents which could give rise to a similar if not identical endoscopic appearance (see Chapter 14). If there is no such usage, multiple prepyloric antral ulcers in a patient with known Crohn's disease favors the diagnosis of gastric involvement, especially if they are found in association with nodularity (cobblestone appearance) of the surrounding mucosa. Single ulcers in flat, erythematous mucosa or with converging folds suggesting scar deformity favor the diagnosis of peptic ulcer.[18]

Biopsy

Biopsy specimens may be taken with the hope of demonstrating typical granulomas of Crohn's disease. Although the chances of demonstrating these lesions are increased if the biopsy specimens are taken from an ulcer base,[18] granulomas are nonetheless found in only a minority of patients—in one series in only two of nine patients.[18] The low yield from biopsy as far as granulomas are concerned accords with our own experience, where these were found in one of seven patients examined over a 7-year period. More often (in 4 of 10 cases) we found microscopic "skip" areas with a focus of inflammation next to an area of normal or hyperplastic-appearing mucosa which we believe is highly suggestive of gastric involvement with Crohn's disease, as it would be if found in biopsies taken from other locations in the GI tract.

Eosinophilic Gastroenteritis

Gastric involvement may be found in up to half of the cases of eosinophilic gastroenteritis, a rare condition.[20] Often food and other allergic manifestations are present in association with a peripheral eosinophilia and elevations of IgE. Patients with gastric involvement will often present with symptoms of gastric outlet obstruction, as the most common area involved is the prepyloric antrum and pyloric channel.[20] The smooth muscle layers of these areas may become infiltrated with the eosinophils without gross mucosal involvement,[20] although in cases where this condition is suspected, mucosal biopsies should be performed which may show increased numbers of eosinophils. When the mucosa is involved directly, nodularity and ulceration may be present and may suggest either Crohn's disease (see above) or infiltrating malignancy (see Chapter 16).

Eosinophilic gastroenteritis with stomach involvement classically differs from an eosinophilic granuloma of the stomach where there is a focal submucosal mass composed of a dense eosinophilic infiltrate, but without a peripheral eosinophilia.[20]

However, we have encountered a case where there was both submucosal mass (eosinophilic granuloma) and peripheral eosinophilia. In this patient, the mass involved the cardiofundic area, causing gastric inlet obstruction with dysphagia which was initially treated surgically. While the resected specimen was felt to be consistent with an eosinophilic granuloma, the peripheral eosinophilia remained and the lesion reoccurred in the same location two years later, finally disappearing after a course of steroids, similar to eosinophilic gastroenteritis.[23]

Radiation Therapy

Radiation doses of up to 4,500 rads are generally well tolerated by the stomach.[21] Doses in excess of this may be associated with symptoms of nausea, vomiting, early satiety, and hematemesis,[21] which prompt endoscopy.

Appearance

In symptomatic patients, one may see antral narrowing (Fig. 20-9a), where the mucosal folds appear thickened and the mucosa itself is erythematous and friable. The mucosal erythema at close range (Fig. 20-9b) is actually found to consist of multiple red islands (areae gastricae) with inner

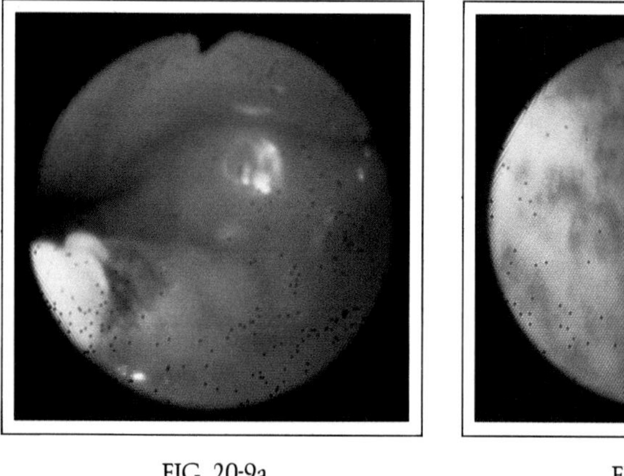

FIG. 20-9a.

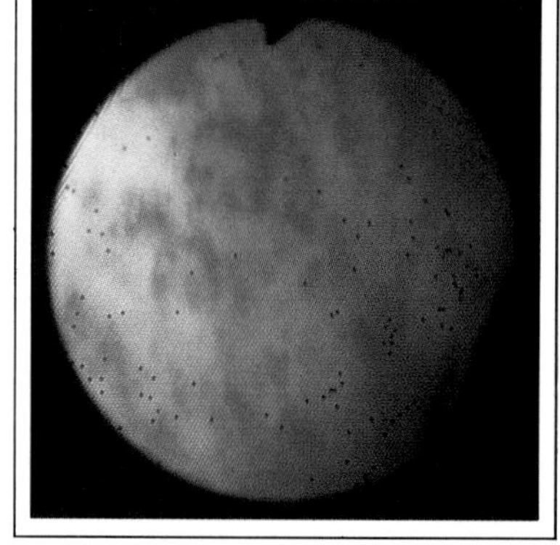

FIG. 20-9b.

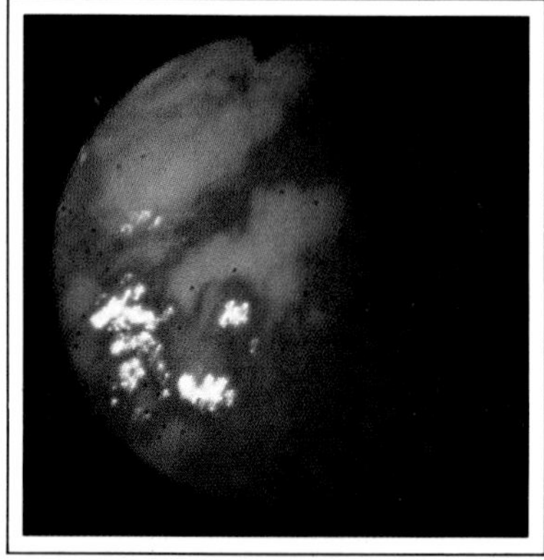

FIG. 20-9c.

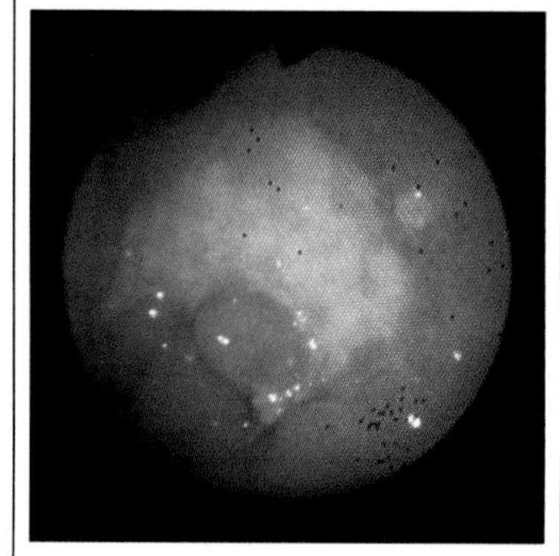

FIG. 20-10a.

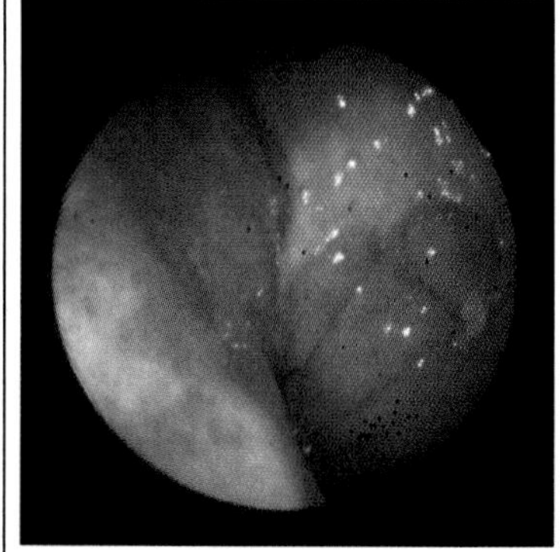

FIG. 20-10b.

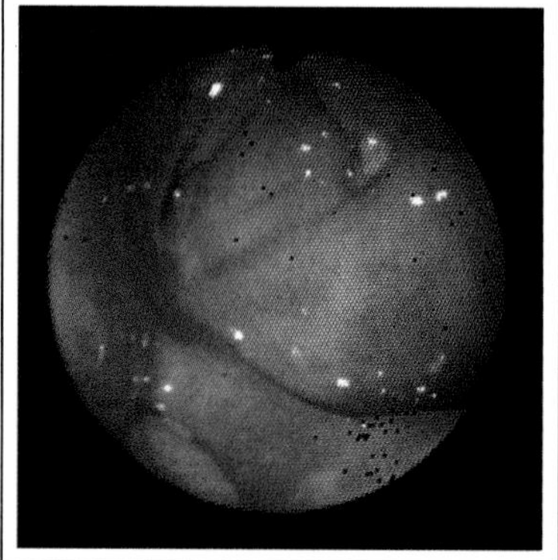

FIG. 20-10c.

FIG. 20-9. a: Gastric irradiation of the body after resection of a cardial carcinoma. The enlarged, indurated folds tented poorly, making it impossible to exclude recurrent carcinoma (see Chapter 16). **b:** Gastric irradiation, nonspecific gastric erythema. In this case there is punctate erythema with intervening linear areas. **c:** Gastric irradiation, large gastric telangiectasia. An extensive area of intense erythema appeared on the anterior wall of the antrum. The capillary projections (best seen toward 9 o'clock) indicate the nature of this to be a large vascular malformation which has occurred as a response to irradiation.

FIG. 20-10. a: Radiation ulcer. A 1.5-cm antral ulcer in a patient having previously received radiation for gastric lymphoma. **b:** Radiation ulcer associated with antral deformity. At a distance from the radiation ulcer (a), one notes thickening of the adjacent prepyloric folds which continue on into the prepyloric antrum. The deformity along with the deep ulceration created the impression of recurrent lymphoma. This, however, was not borne out by the biopsies taken or the patient's subsequent course. **c:** Prepyloric antral deformity associated with a radiation ulcer (a and b). Note the marked deformity of the pyloric channel, which is now found in an eccentric position at 9 o'clock.

connecting pale linear areas (lineae gastricae). Along with this, one may see telangiectasia (Fig. 20-9c) similar to that encountered with radiation changes of the rectosigmoid colon (see Chapter 44). Ulcerations may also be seen,[20,23] usually superficial but on occasion deep (Fig. 20-10a); they heal slowly and are associated with scar deformity (Fig. 20-10b), obstruction (Fig. 20-10c), or perforation.[21]

Relation of Radiation Changes to Symptoms

For the majority of patients in whom we see radiation changes, the symptoms are either nonspecific or relate to the underlying malignancy for which the radiation was administered. Generally these patients have mucosal changes alone, rather than ulcerations and/or outlet obstruction in which the symptoms are more obviously related to radiation injury.

Differentiation from Recurrent Malignancy

For patients with lymphoma or gastric carcinoma who receive radiation, the endoscopist may be called on to differentiate radiation change from recurrent tumor (Fig. 20-10). This is difficult because of the variety of appearances

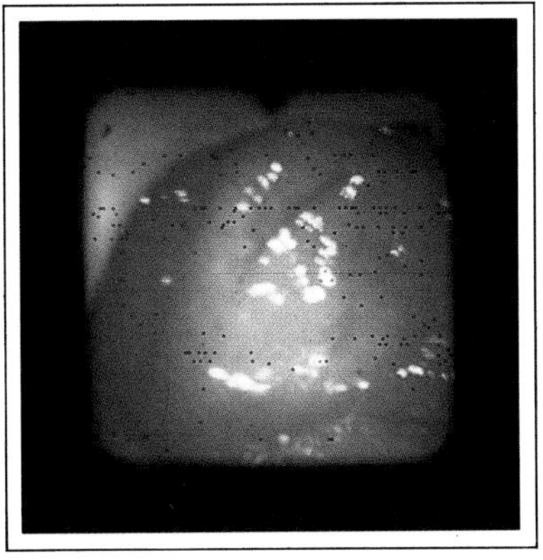

FIG. 20-11.

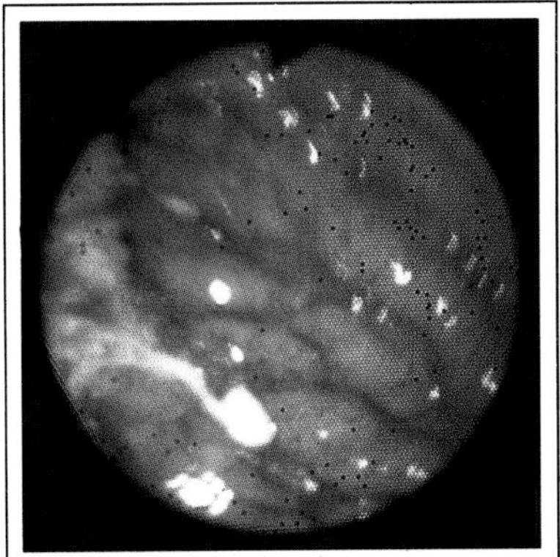

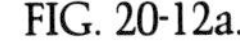

FIG. 20-12a.

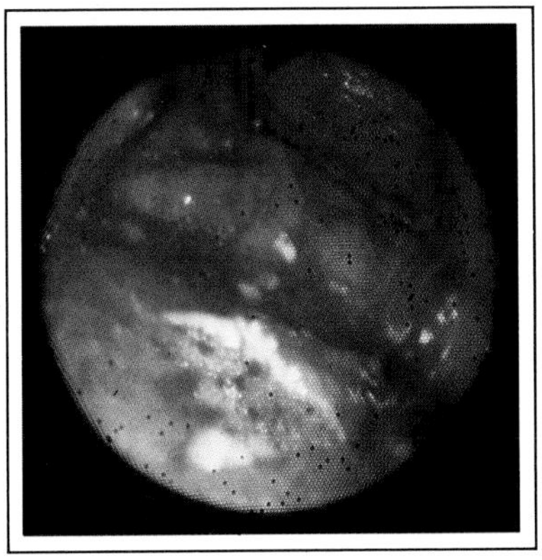

FIG. 20-12b.

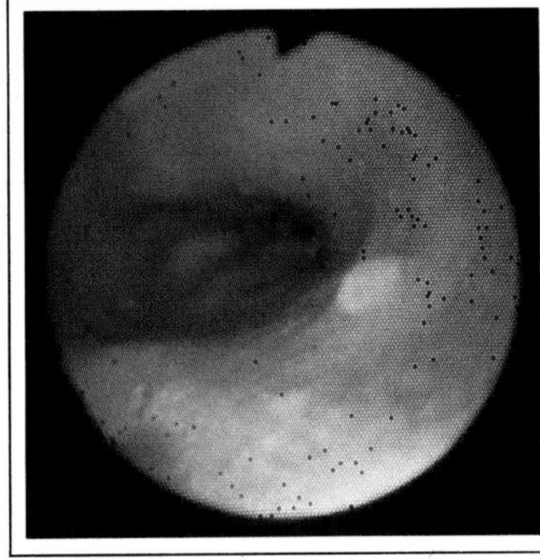

FIG. 20-12c.

FIG. 20-11. Gastric sarcoid appearing as an antral deformity. Biopsy from the depressed area within the converging folds revealed noncaseating granulomas consistent with sarcoid in a patient with multisystem involvement.

FIG. 20-12. Gastroduodenal amyloid. **a:** Biopsies of the prominent rugal folds of the lower body were positive for amyloid in a patient with multisystem involvement. **b:** Proximal to prominent rugal folds of the lower body (Fig. 20-12a), retained gastric secretion and bezoar formation were noted as evidence of impaired gastric emptying in a patient with amyloid and profound autonomic neuropathy. **c:** Nonspecific erythema of the bulb was noted along with the 4-mm duodenal polyp. Biopsies taken from the polyp as well as the adjacent flat mucosa showed amyloid.

seen after irradiation which overlap those of recurrent malignancy (see Chapter 16). Endoscopic features such as prominent rubbery ulcerated folds where the mucosa is fixed to the submucosa and does not tent up are findings which are common to both.[22] Moreover, superficial punch biopsies cannot exclude recurrence, which may be confined to the deeper mucosa or submucosa (see Chapter 16). In some cases large-particle snare biopsy or needle aspiration cytology (see Chapter 1) may be useful, although yield from these techniques in this particular context has not been established. Where additional treatment would follow a definite diagnosis of recurrence, in the face of equivocal or unrevealing endoscopic biopsies, surgery may ultimately be required.

Sarcoidosis

Sarcoidosis has been reported only occasionally and in our experience is an exceedingly rare finding. The patient may present for endoscopy with nonspecific complaints or with symptoms and radiographic studies suggestive of gastric outlet obstruction.[24] We have seen only one case[25] where gastric changes were found along with multisystem involvement (lung, liver, bone marrow, and parotid glands). Endoscopy in this case revealed an antral deformity (Fig. 20-11) in which a biopsy showed noncaseating granulomas. In our case and in other reports,[24] the antrum is the most common site of involvement, with prominent antral folds and ulcerations the most often described finding. The lack of distensibility of the mucosa and the presence of nodules present an endoscopic appearance which simulates an infiltrating malignancy. However, in a patient with sarcoid involving other organ systems, sarcoid of the stomach would be a principal diagnostic consideration.

Amyloidosis

Gastrointestinal involvement in systemic amyloidosis results in motility disturbances, malabsorption, or vascular insufficiency,[26] with amyloid deposited in and around the walls of blood vessels within the GI tract. Common sites of gastrointestinal involvement are the distal stomach, pyloroduodenal junction, and duodenal bulb.[27] With involvement of these areas, one may find prominent, nondistensible gastric folds (Fig. 20-12a). These may be so indurated as to suggest infiltrating carcinoma.[27] In addition, there may be bezoar formation from delayed gastric emptying because of antral motor dysfunction from infiltration or autonomic neuropathy (Fig. 20-12b).[28] Other findings include mucosal ulceration of the antrum and duodenal bulb, and the presence of duodenal erythema and polyps (Fig. 20-12c). Biopsy specimens from involved areas displaying any of these findings often show amyloid deposits.[28]

OPPORTUNISTIC INFECTIONS OF THE STOMACH AND SYPHILIS

Opportunistic Infections of the Stomach

Rare cases of opportunistic infection involving the stomach have been reported in immunologically compromised patients. These have occurred with herpes simplex,[29,30] cytomegalovirus,[31–33] and *Histoplasma.*[34–36]

Herpes Simplex

Herpes simplex has been reported both in association with herpetic esophagitis[29] and as an isolated finding. In either case, the typical appearance is that of diffuse, tiny, papular, ulcerating lesions.[29,30] Biopsies demonstrate characteristic eosinophilic intranuclear inclusion bodies of the herpes virus. In one case brushing cytology was diagnostic, showing typical "ground-glass" nuclei and intranuclear inclusion bodies.[30]

Cytomegalovirus

Two types of appearance have been described for cytomegalovirus (CMV) involving the stomach. One of these, multiple white-based erosions,[31] resembles that of herpes simplex, described above. Another appearance in immunosuppressed patients after a kidney transplant is that of a large ulcer and multiple gastric erosions.[32] In this case biopsies taken from the edge of the ulcer revealed intranuclear inclusions typical of CMV.[32] Finally, a case of CMV-associated gastric ulcer has been reported in a patient with posttransfusion CMV mononucleosis.[33]

Histoplasma

Although the stomach is one of the least common sites of gastrointestinal involvement with *Histoplasma,*[34] rare cases may be encountered. Two types of appearance have been reported, one where there is focal narrowing[35] and a second where there are giant (hypertrophic) gastric folds.[36] In the latter case, where the endoscopic appearance was reported,[36] the folds were described as "enlarged and reddened . . . [with] the mucosa . . . pliable." It is important to be aware of this appearance because of its similarity to that of infiltrating gastric lymphoma, a condition which may predispose to disseminated histoplasmosis.[36] Endoscopic biopsies from enlarged folds[32] and presumably other types of involvement[35] show typical *Histoplasma* organisms.

Gastric Syphilis

Involvement of the stomach by syphilis has been known since the nineteenth century. In the exceptional patient, symptoms of gastric outlet obstruction may be the first manifestation which brings the disease to the attention of the physician.[37,38] In these cases endoscopy reveals a picture of diffusely ulcerated, friable mucosa of the distal stomach (lower body and antrum).[37,38] Once the diagnosis is suspected, fresh biopsy material crushed in saline and immediately examined with darkfield and phase-contrast microscopy may show motile spirochetes.[37] In addition, one may perform special stains (Warthin-Starry) on formalin-fixed material, as well as immunofluorescence studies.[37] The key, however, would be a high index of suspicion in a homosexual male patient manifesting with symptoms suggestive of gastric outlet obstruction.

Longstanding syphilitic involvement of the stomach may result in a linitis plastica appearance. In such cases squamous metaplasia may be noted as well. We have observed squamous carcinoma with linitis plastica in a patient with congenital syphilis and squamous metaplasia.[39]

REFERENCES

1. Javdan, P., Pitman, E., and Schwartz, I. S. (1974): Gastric xanthelasma: endoscopic recognition. *Gastroenterology,* 67:1006–1010.
2. Mast, A., Elewaut, A., Mortier, G., Quatacker, J., Defloor, E., Roels, H., and Barbier, F. (1976): Gastric xanthoma. *Am. J. Gastroenterol.,* 65:311–317.
3. Mohtashemi, H., and Davidson, F. Z. (1973): Candidiasis and gastric ulcer. *Am. J. Dig. Dis.,* 18:915–919.
4. Peters, M., Weiner, J., and Whelan, G. (1980): Fungal infection associated with gastroduodenal ulceration: endoscopic and pathologic appearances. *Gastroenterology,* 78:350–354.
5. Binder, R. J., and Nelson, J. A. (1975): Candida albicans ulcer within hiatus hernia sac presenting as an ulcerated mass. *Gastroenterology,* 68:587–590.
6. Konok, G., Haddad, H., and Strom, B. (1980): Postoperative gastric mycosis. *Surg. Gynecol. Obstet.,* 150:337–341.
7. Cronan, J., Burrell, M., and Trepeta, R. (1980): Aphthoid ulcerations in gastric candidiasis. *Radiology,* 134:607–611.
8. Nelson, R. S., Bruni, H., and Goldstein, H. M. (1975): Primary gastric candidiasis in uncompromised subjects. *Gastrointest. Endosc.,* 22:92–94.
9. McCaffery, T. D., and Lilly, J. O. (1975): The management of the foreign affairs of the GI tract. *Am. J. Dig. Dis.,* 20:1210–1226.
10. DeGerome, J. H. (1973): Snare extraction of a gastric foreign body. *Gastrointest. Endosc.,* 20:73–75.
11. Rogers, B. H. G. (1979): A new method for extraction of impacted meat from the esophagus utilizing a flexible fiberoptic endoscope and overtube. *Gastrointest. Endosc.,* 25:47.
12. Goyal, R. K., and Spiro, H. M. (1971): Gastrointestinal manifestations of diabetes mellitus. *Med. Clin. North Am.,* 55:1031–1044.
13. Behar, J., and Fox, J. (1980): Pathogenesis of diabetic gastroparesis: a pharmacologic study. *Gastroenterology,* 78:757–763.
14. Mattingly, S. S., Cibull, M. L., Ram, M. D., Hagihara, P., and Griffen, W. O. (1981): Pseudolymphoma of the stomach: a diagnostic and therapeutic dilemma. *Arch. Surg.,* 116:25–29.
15. Stroehlein, J. R., Weiland, L. H., Hoffman, H. N., and Judd, E. S. (1977): Untreated gastric pseudolymphoma. *Am. J. Dig. Dis.,* 22:465–470.
16. Faris, T. D., and Saltzstein, S. L. (1964): Gastric lymphoid hyperplasia: a lesion confused with lymphosarcoma. *Cancer,* 17:207–212.
17. Tottla, F., Lucas, R. J., Bernacki, E. G., and Tabor, H. (1976): Endoscopic features of gastroduodenal Crohn's disease. *Gastroenterology,* 70:9–13.
18. Danzi, J. T., Farmer, R. G., Sullivan, B. H., and Rankin, G. B. (1976): Endoscopic features of gastrointestinal Crohn's disease. *Gastroenterology,* 70:9–13.

19. Sanders, M., and Schmimmel, E. M. (1972): The relationship between granulomatous bowel disease and duodenal ulcer. *Am. J. Dig. Dis.*, 17:1100–1108.
20. Cello, J. F. (1979): Eosinophilic gastroenteritis—a complex disease entity. *Am. J. Med.*, 67:1097–1104.
21. Kellum, J. M., Jaffe, B. M., Calhoun, T. R., and Ballinger, W. F. (1977): Gastric complications after radiotherapy for Hodgkin's disease and other lymphomas. *Am. J. Surg.*, 134:314–317.
22. Novak, J. M., Collins, J. T., Donowitz, M., Farman, J., Sheahan, D. G., and Spiro, H. M. (1979): Effects of radiation on the human gastrointestinal tract. *J. Clin. Gastroenterol.*, 1:9–39.
23. DeSagher, L. I., VandenHeule, B., VanHoutte, P., Engelholm, L., Balikdjan, D., and Bleiberg, H. (1979): Endoscopic appearance of irradiated gastric mucosa. *Endoscopy*, 3:163–165.
24. Berens, D. L., and Montes, M. (1975): Gastric sarcoidosis. *N.Y. State J. Med.*, 75:1290–1293.
25. Blackstone, M. O., Dhar, G. J., Mizuno, H., and Para, M. F. (1976): Gastric sarcoidosis, presenting as antral scarring. *Gastrointest. Endosc.*, 22:211–212.
26. Chernenkoff, R. M., Costopoulous, L. B., and Bain, G. O. (1972): Gastrointestinal manifestations of primary amyloidosis. *Can. Med. Assoc. J.*, 106:567–579.
27. Ikeda, K., and Murayama, H. (1978): A case of amyloid tumor of the stomach. *Endoscopy*, 10:54–58.
28. Coughlin, G. P., Reiner, R. G., and Grant, A. K. (1980): Endoscopic diagnosis of amyloidosis. *Gastrointest. Endosc.*, 26:154–155.
29. Howiler, W., and Goldberg, H. I. (1976): Gastroesophageal involvement in herpes simplex. *Gastroenterology*, 70:775–778.
30. Speling, H. V., and Reed, W. G. (1977): Herpetic gastritis. *Am. J. Dig. Dis.*, 22:1033–1034.
31. Ayulo, M., Aisner, S., Margolis, K., and Moravec, C. (1980): Cytomegalovirus-associated gastritis in a compromised host. *JAMA*, 243:1364.
32. Allen, J. I., Silvis, S. E., Sumner, H. W., and McClain, C. (1981): Cytomegalic inclusion disease diagnosed endoscopically. *Am. J. Dig. Dis.*, 26:133–135.
33. Campbell, D. A., Piercey, J. R. A., Shnitka, T. K., Goldsand, G., Devine, R. D. O., and Weinstein, W. (1977): Cytomegalovirus-associated gastric ulcer. *Gastroenterology*, 72:535–555.
34. Miller, D. P., and Everett, E. D. (1979): Gastrointestinal histoplasmosis. *J. Clin. Gastroenterol.*, 1:233–236.
35. Nudelman, H. L., and Rakatansky, H. (1966): Gastric histoplasmosis: a case report. *JAMA*, 195:134–136.
36. Fisher, J. R., and Sanowski, R. A. (1978): Disseminated histoplasmosis producing hypertrophic gastric folds. *Am. J. Dig. Dis.*, 23:282–285.
37. Sachar, D. B., Klein, R. S., Swerdlow, F., Bottone, E., Khilnani, M., Waye, J. D., and Wisniewski, M. (1974): Erosive syphilitic gastritis: dark field and immunofluorescent diagnosis from biopsy specimen. *Ann. Intern. Med.*, 80:512–515.
38. Reisman, T. N., Leverett, F. L., Hudson, J. R., and Kalser, M. H. (1975): Syphilitic gastropathy. *Am. J. Dig. Dis.*, 20:588–593.
39. Vaughan, W. P., Straus, F. H., and Paloyan, D. (1977): Squamous carcinoma of the stomach after luetic linitis plastica. *Gastroenterology*, 72:945–948.

21

PYLORIC CHANNEL—TECHNIQUE OF EXAMINATION AND NORMAL APPEARANCE

INTUBATION

With a forward-viewing instrument, once the pylorus is found in the course of intubating the antrum (see Chapter 11), it may be entered directly, providing the endoscope tip is in reasonably correct alignment. Prior to making any attempts at entering the pyloric channel, an effort is made to change the tip position from one which is eccentric to the channel (Fig. 21-1a) to one which is better aligned (Fig. 21-1b). At this point one is in a better position to pass the endoscope across the channel into the duodenal bulb. Rather than attempting to "push across," we believe it is easier to first lodge the tip within the channel (Fig. 21-1c) and realign, if necessary (Fig. 21-1d), before advancing. This is necessary because of the extreme flexibility of the tip, especially if the narrow-caliber (9 mm) instrument is used. After an adjustment while the tip is lodged within the pyloric channel, the tip controls, especially the left-right control, are

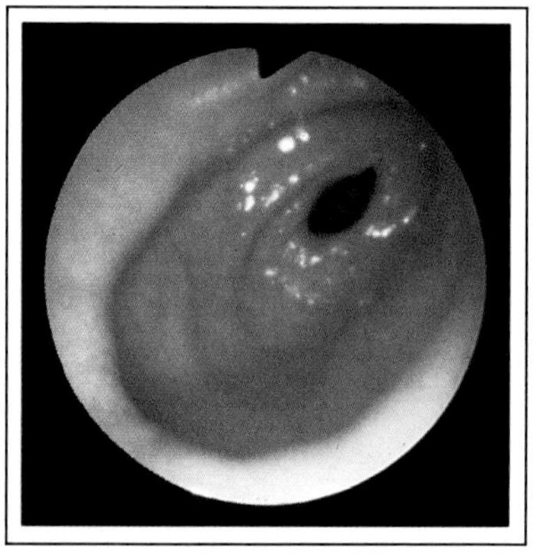

FIG. 21-1a.

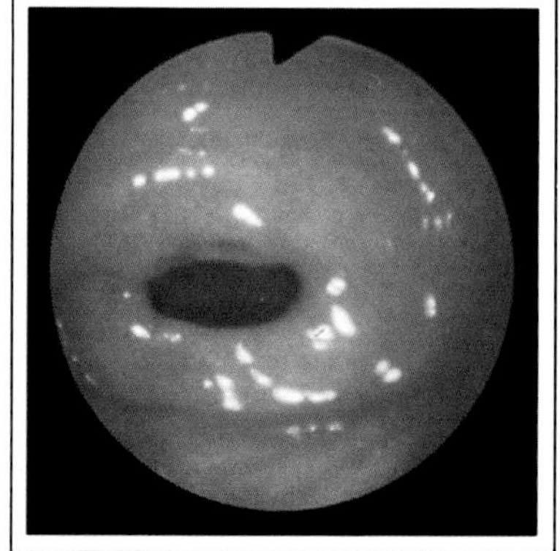

FIG. 21-1b.

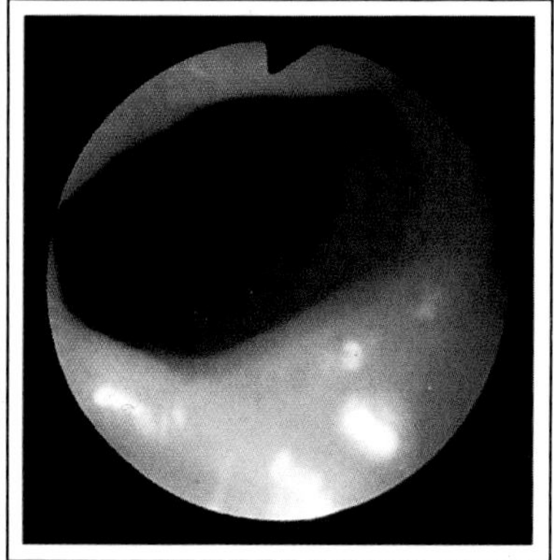

FIG. 21-1c.

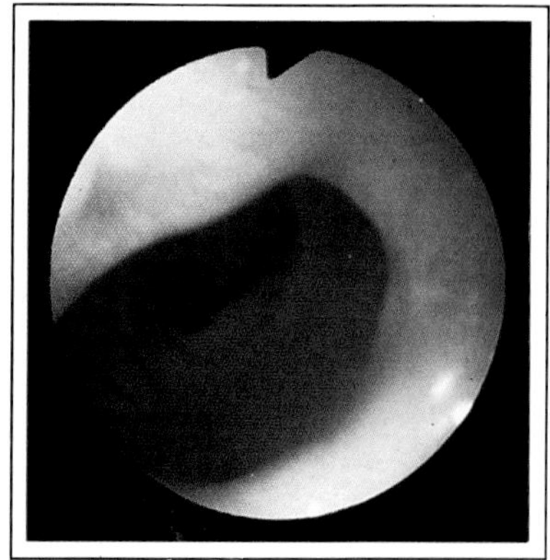

FIG. 21-1d.

FIG. 21-1. Pyloric channel. **a:** The direction of the tip toward the anterior wall causes the pylorus to appear eccentrically placed (off the posterior wall). **b:** The tip has now been properly aligned, and the channel appears in the midline. **c:** Partially intubated. The endoscope tip is lodged within the channel prior to being advanced into the duodenal bulb just beyond. **d:** In the course of gentle advancement across the channel, the tip has partially slipped out and deviates posteriorly (toward 3 o'clock).

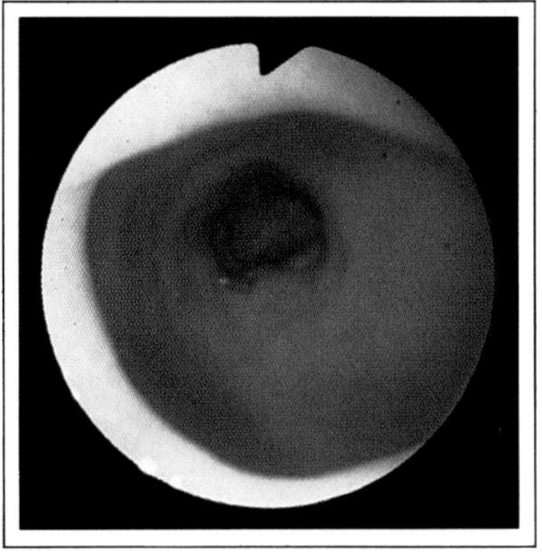

FIG. 21-2.

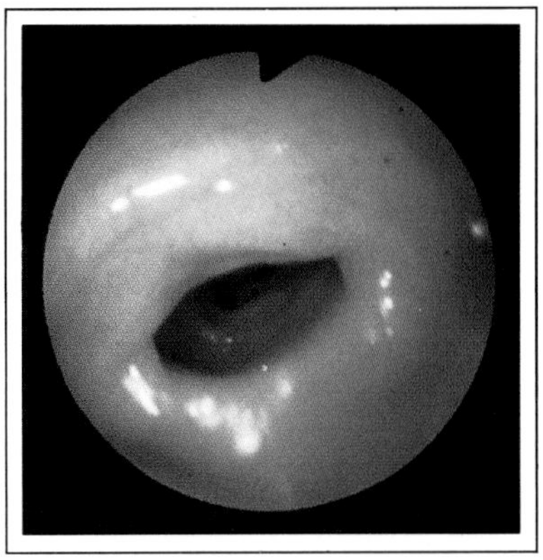

FIG. 21-3a.

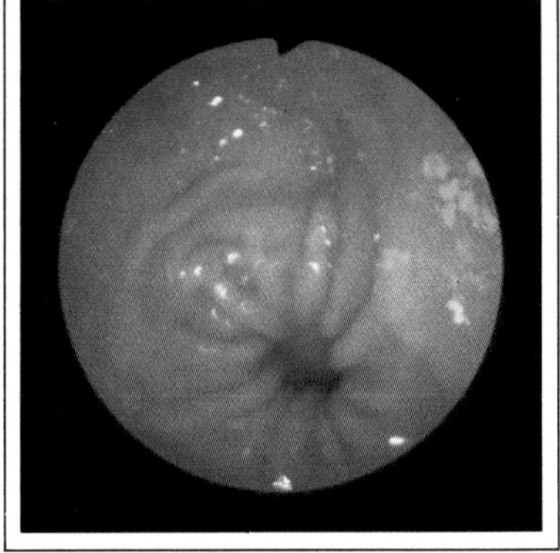

FIG. 21-3b.

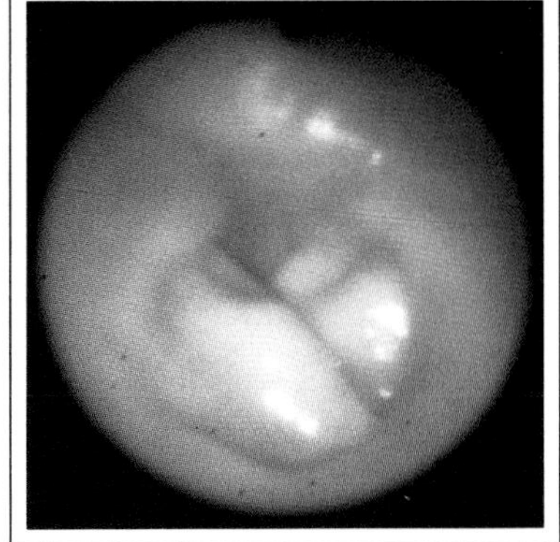

FIG. 21-4.

FIG. 21-2. Pyloric channel, almost completely intubated. The tip is now securely placed within the channel and can be advanced directly into the bulb with its lumen fully in view.

FIG. 21-3. a: Pyloric channel set in flat mucosa. **b:** Pyloric channel associated with prominent though symmetrical prepyloric folds.

FIG. 21-4. Pyloric channel, associated with prominent though somewhat eccentric-appearing prepyloric folds, especially those from the greater curve.

locked. Finally, with the tip secured within the channel, it is gently encouraged across, ideally with the lumen of the duodenal bulb fully in view (Fig. 21-2).

ENDOSCOPIC EXAMINATION

The pyloric channel is, in effect, a very short tubular structure, generally less than 1 cm in length. Because of this, effective examination of it remains a continuing challenge to the endoscopist. It should not be rushed; therefore we believe it is best performed after the duodenal bulb and descending duodenum are entered and examined rather than at the time it is being entered. In cases where peptic ulcer disease is expected (see Chapter 22), we require six passes as a minimum, with each quadrant being examined at least once so as not to miss a recessed or otherwise hidden channel (see Chapter 22).

NORMAL APPEARANCES OF THE PYLORIC CHANNEL

The expected endoscopic finding for the pyloric channel is that of a perfectly round, tubular opening, 5 mm long which with air insufflation becomes 1 to 1.5 cm wide (Fig. 21-1b). It may be set in flat mucosa (Fig. 21-3a) or be associated with prominent raised folds radiating out for 2 cm or more (Fig. 21-3b).

Rather than any "typical" appearance for the pyloric channel, which would be found probably in only one-third of cases, we believe it is more realistic to view the pylorus as having numerous variations in shape, location, and size in entirely asymptomatic patients in whom no disease of the pyloric channel is ever found. Because of this we refer to these as normal variations in pyloric channel appearance.

Normal Variations in Pyloric Channel Appearance

Shape

The perfectly round appearance of the channel is often distorted by prepyloric folds which give it a wave-like appearance (Fig. 21-4). Sometimes this causes the normally rounded channel to appear square, elliptical, or even rectangular. For us, the deciding factor in regarding this as a normal variation, rather than a pathologic appearance, is the presence of symmetry. If the distortion is similar for both sides of the channel (Fig. 21-4), it is unlikely to present the effects of peptic ulcer scarring, which should affect one side or the other but not both in exactly the same manner. An example of a distorted appearance of the channel which is in reality a normal variation is the presence of a prepyloric roof-like fold which lies over the pyloric channel, located exactly at its midpoint (Fig. 21-3b). Although this distorts the appearance of the channel, the channel itself is perfectly symmetrical, indicating this to be a normal variation.

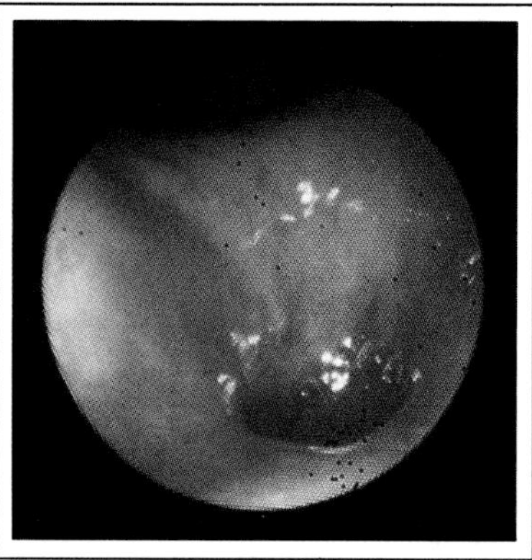

FIG. 21-5.

FIG. 21-5. Pyloric channel, eccentrically placed. This is a normal variation in a patient with a steerhorn-shaped stomach (see Chapter 18).

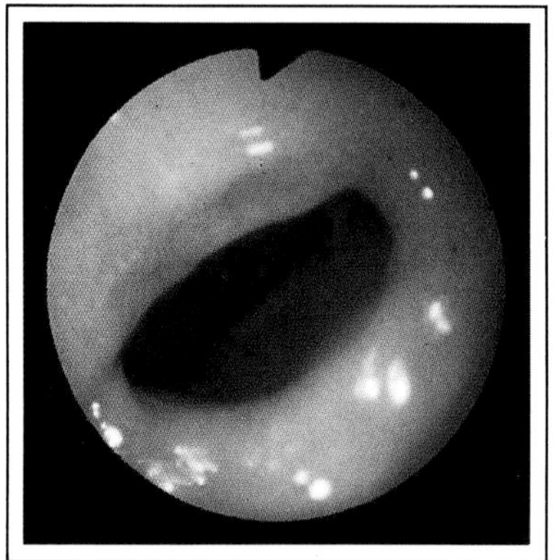

FIG. 21-6a.

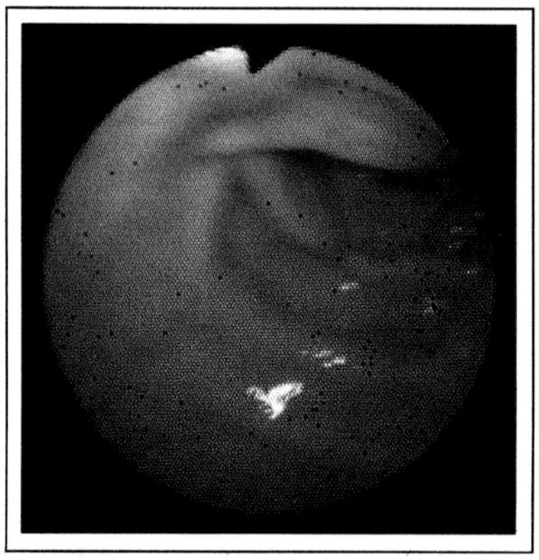

FIG. 21-6b.

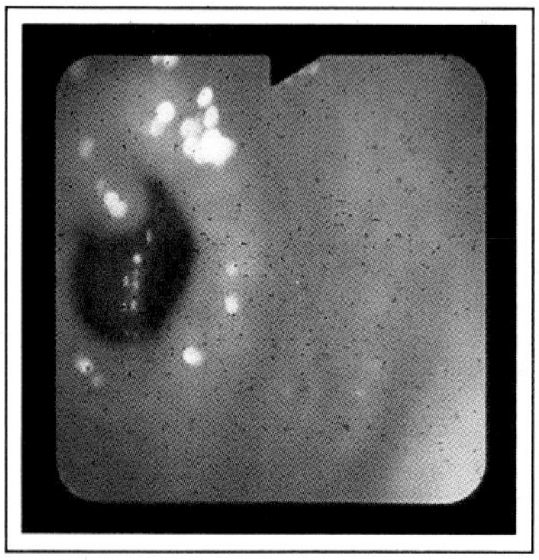

FIG. 21-6c.

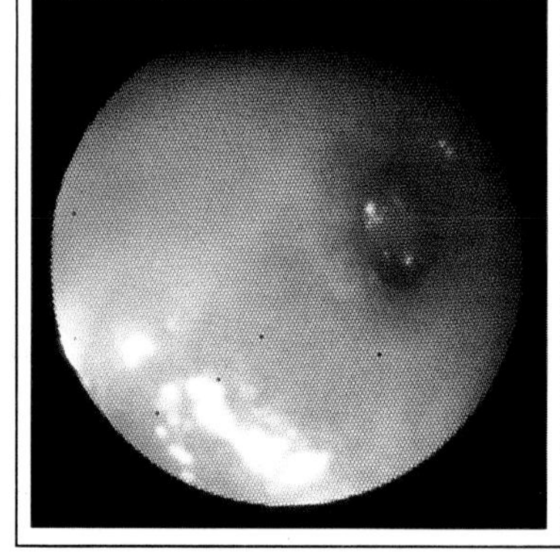

FIG. 21-6d.

FIG. 21-6. a: Pyloric channel, normal size. This usually dilates enough to easily admit an endoscope with an 11- or 13-mm diameter. **b:** Pyloric channel, patulous. There is virtually no barrier between the duodenal bulb and the stomach. Nevertheless, the patient was entirely asymptomatic. **c:** Pyloric channel, possibly narrow. In this case a 13-mm endoscope could not be passed across the channel, although the significance of this is uncertain. **d:** Pyloric channel, narrowed. In this case the channel would not admit even a 9-mm instrument. This is highly suggestive of pyloric stenosis (see Chapter 23).

Location

The pyloric channel may not lie in the center of the distal antrum. Not infrequently it is shifted to lie just off the greater (Fig. 21-5) or lesser curves. These locations relate to the configuration of the stomach (see Chapter 18). In this case, where the antrum occupies the position where it is sharply angulated in relation to the body, one may expect a "high" takeoff point for the pyloric channel just off the lesser curve; conversely, if the antrum is not angulated or actually is directed caudally in relation to the body, one expects the pylorus to be found just off the greater curve (Fig. 21-5).

Size

Normally, after air insufflation alone the pyloric channel has a diameter between 1 and 1.5 cm (Fig. 21-6a). When the diameter is in excess of 1.5 cm the channel is often described as patulous (Fig. 21-6b). The term patulous implies that the appearance is abnormal, yet, in truth, the significance of this finding is unknown. One may see in association with the patulous pyloric channel the reflux of bile or other intestinal constituents with antral or generalized gastric erythema and bile in the gastric lake—all nonspecific findings (see Chapter 12). As no particular symptom or symptom complex at present can be attributed to a patulous pylorus, we regard it as simply an incidental finding.

In contrast to the patulous pylorus, we presume the narrow pyloric channel (<1 cm) to be abnormal (Fig. 21-6d), whereas those between 11 and 13 mm are of uncertain significance. The failure to pass such an endoscope across any pyloric channel (Fig. 21-6c) might cause the endoscopist to believe that the channel is abnormal, although it may simply reflect inadequacy of the endoscopist's technique in finding, centering, or stabilizing the tip before attempting to cross the channel (see above). In experienced hands, such a finding of a "tight" channel (Fig. 21-6d) is one in which the passage of the endoscope was either difficult or impossible. One study has suggested a fivefold increase in the prevalence of peptic ulcer disease and a sixfold increase in true antral deformity for such patients contrasted with others having endoscopy.[1] Although the range of pyloric diameters for the study was not given, we accept the concept that with true pyloric channel deformity there is a loss of compliance of the channel which precludes passage of the larger endoscopes across it. Because this endoscopic test is crude, however, it is necessary to secure other studies in order to determine the significance of a tight pyloric channel if a peptic ulcer is not found (see Chapter 22).

REFERENCE

1. Fisher, R. W., and Kleinman, M. S. (1977): Significance of endoscopically-observed pyloric stenosis in adults. *Gastrointest. Endosc.*, 23:227.

22

PEPTIC ULCER DISEASE OF THE PYLORIC CHANNEL

The commonest abnormalities of the pyloric channel relate to peptic ulcer disease. We found pyloric channel ulcers in 1.5% of 5,000 cases examined over a 7-year period. This was about one-third the frequency of gastric ulcers but only one-sixth that of duodenal ulcers. Pyloric channel deformity of the ulcer scar type (see below) was found in an additional 1.4% of cases, an incidence similar to that of active ulcers.

PYLORIC CHANNEL ULCERS

The difficulty the endoscopist has with ulcers in the pyloric channel is not so much in interpretation as in the demonstration of a lesion. As already stated (see Chapter 21), the channel is not adequately examined unless it is done separately and repeatedly, rather than only once or twice, either on the way into the duodenum or back into the stomach. The difficulty in finding channel ulcers is compounded if the wider-caliber (11 to 13 mm) instruments are used, especially if the channel is deformed. Although these instruments can be pushed across a deformed channel, they do not allow a detailed examination because of their size.

To minimize the chance of missing a pyloric channel ulcer suspected because of either a suggestive radiographic study or a previous endoscopic examination, ideally one uses a narrow-caliber (9 mm) pediatric-type instrument. This is because of the ease of passing it across most pyloric channels, even those which are deformed, as well as its shorter "turning length," which facilitates examination of recessed areas within a deformed channel, generally the site of an active ulcer.

Appearance

One occasionally encounters a deep ulcer (Fig. 22-1a) within a channel which shows no abnormality apart from the ulcer. More often, the ulcer is set in a channel which has been deformed by a pyloroduodenal junctional fold (Fig. 22-1b), with the ulcer being recessed between the opening of the channel and the fold itself.

From an interpretive standpoint, two questions must be answered: (1) Is the ulcer real? (2) Is it benign or malignant?

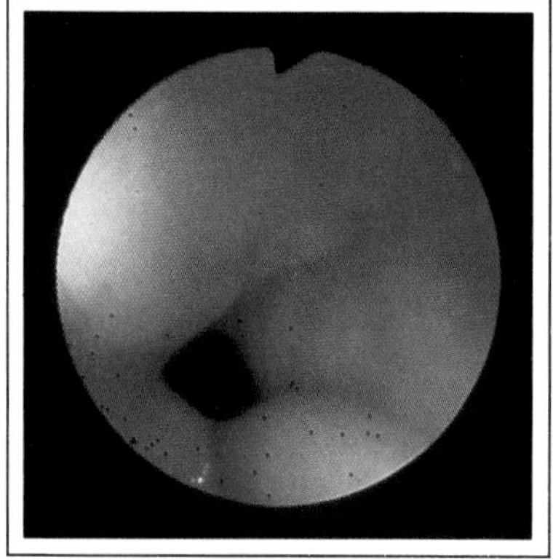

FIG. 22-1a.

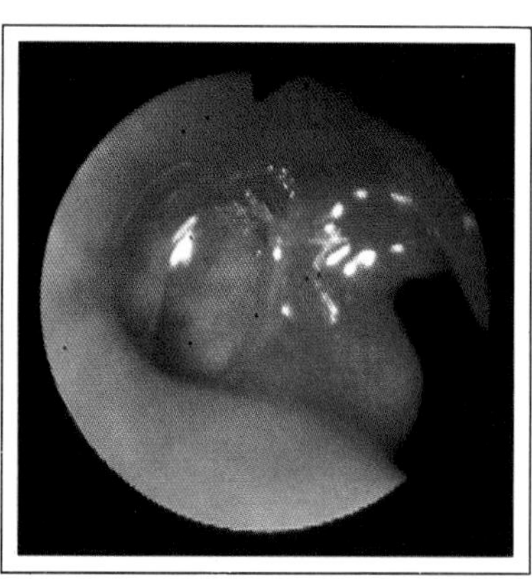

FIG. 22-1b.

FIG. 22-1. a: Pyloric channel ulcer, without deformity. A 5-mm ulcer is set within an otherwise normal-appearing channel. **b:** Pyloric channel ulcer, with marked deformity. This 1-cm ulcer is recessed within an area of marked pyloroduodenal junctional deformity, evidenced by a distal transverse junctional fold.

Ulcer or Mucus?

In practice, the answer as to whether the abnormality seen is an ulcer or simple mucus may be more difficult than one would think for the following reasons. The endoscopist on his way to examining the duodenal bulb does not always carefully examine the pylorus. Passage across a deformed ring may be forceful, resulting in traumatic erythema and intramucosal hemorrhage of the ring, which may be first observed only when returning from the duodenal bulb. Because the erythema may not be uniform it may, in conjunction with adherent mucus, create an ulcer-like appearance (Fig. 22-2). When in doubt, biopsies should be taken of the suspected ulcer base (Fig. 22-2). If an ulcer is present, these biopsies should show granulation tissue. The absence of this finding would be considered strong evidence against the presence of an ulcer.

Benign or Malignant Ulcer?

With regard to the question of whether an ulcer is benign or malignant, the same criteria apply to channel ulcers as they do for ulcers elsewhere in the stomach (see Chapter 16). Special care must be taken to examine the margin of an ulcer in relation to the prepyloric antral folds. Because of the presence of prominent pyloric folds (Fig. 22-3a), the margin of a benign channel ulcer may appear nodular or mass-like (Fig. 22-3b), especially if the pyloric channel ulcer is deep (Fig. 22-3c). Still, in these cases the intactness of the mucosa itself continues to be a useful differential feature. An ulcer margin which, while being irregular or heaped-up, has a sharp interface with the ulcer base along with intact mucosa that shows a regenerative pattern with intact areae and lineae gastricae (see Chapter 15) suggests that the ulcer is benign. Although the absence of these features does not necessarily indicate malignancy, one would regard the status of such an ulcer as "indeterminate" (see Chapter 16). In such cases, at least 10 biopsies are taken from the margin along with several brushings for cytology from within the channel. In addition, endoscopic follow-up at 4 to 6 weeks is strongly recommended.

ULCER SCAR DEFORMITY

As a result of scarring from previous pyloric channel ulcers, the channel may narrow (Fig. 22-4), have an atypical location (Fig. 22-5, a and b), or have an ulcer scar appearance with a transverse pyloroduodenal junctional fold connecting the anterior wall of the channel with the posterior wall of the duodenal bulb (Fig. 22-6). Of these, the pyloroduodenal junctional fold represents for us the most specific finding indicative of ulcer scar deformity as this fold is often seen as the distal margin of a recurrent ulcer within a deformed channel (Fig. 22-5b).

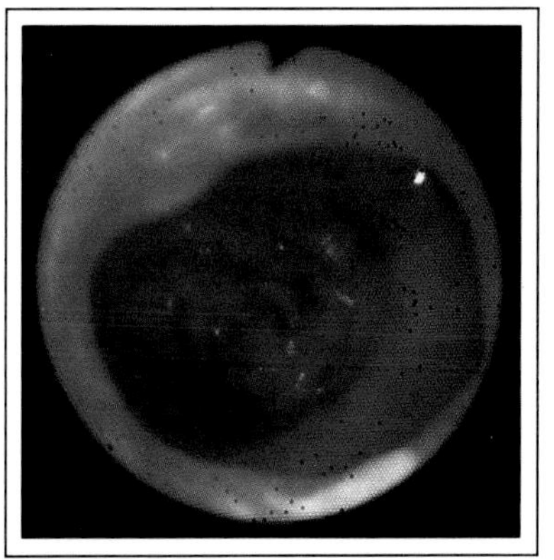

FIG. 22-2.

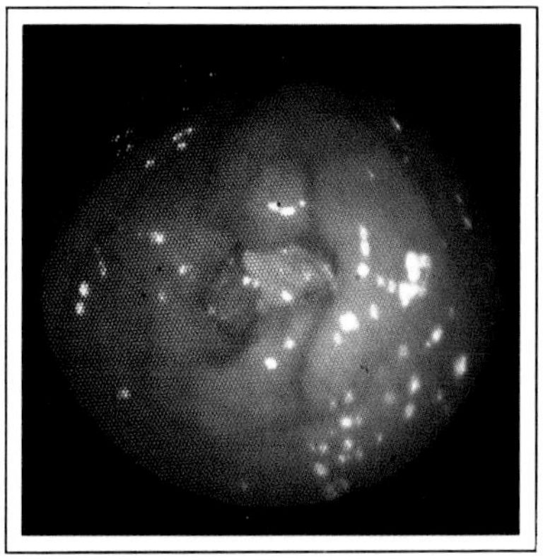

FIG. 22-3a.

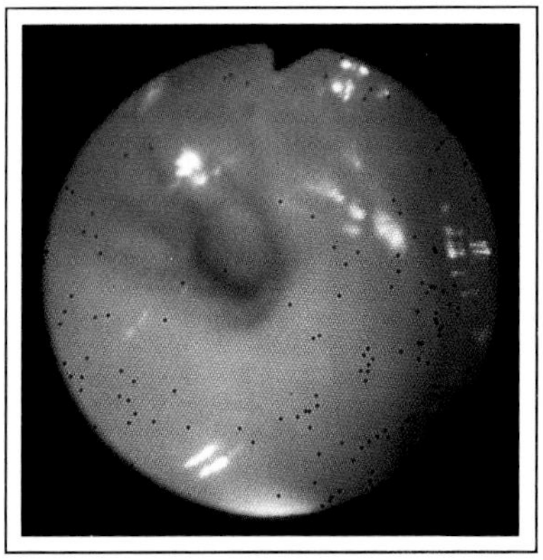

FIG. 22-3b.

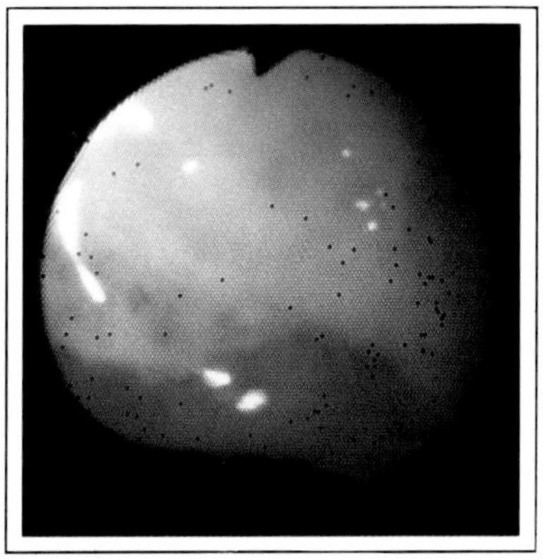

FIG. 22-3c.

FIG. 22-2. Pyloric channel erythema with possible superficial ulceration. The erythema is from a difficult passage across the channel. The whitish linear area at 12 o'clock is either mucus or an ulceration. In this case, a biopsy proved it to be a linear ulcer.

FIG. 22-3. a: Pyloric channel ulcer with a prepyloric (nodular) deformity. The degree of nodularity associated with this appearance raised the question of a malignant process. **b:** Pyloric channel deformity with a prepyloric mass-like deformity. In this case a deep channel ulcer (c), found at surgery to be penetrating, has given rise to this mass-like appearance. **c:** Large (3 cm) pyloric channel ulcer found with a mass-like deformity (b). The entire pyloric channel is replaced by a penetrating ulcer.

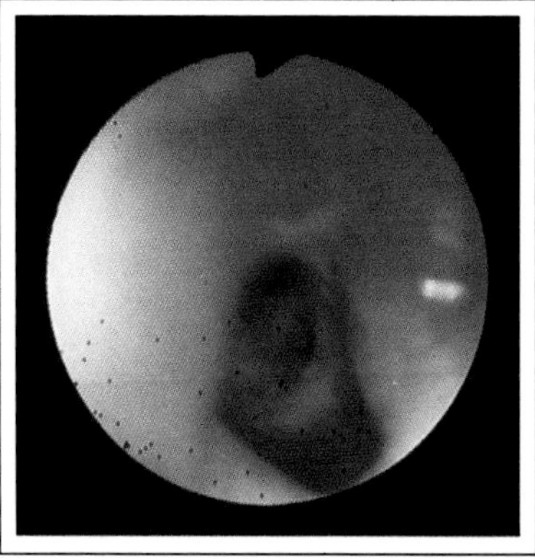

FIG. 22-4.

FIG. 22-4. Pyloric channel scar deformity with narrowing. An active ulcer was found within the channel; however, the narrowing persisted even after complete ulcer healing.

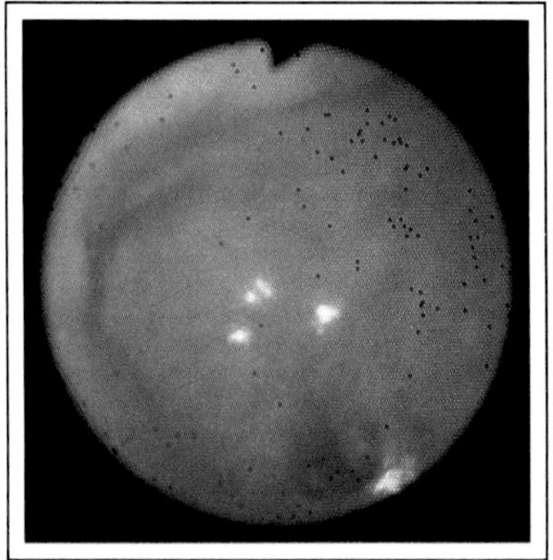

FIG. 22-5a.

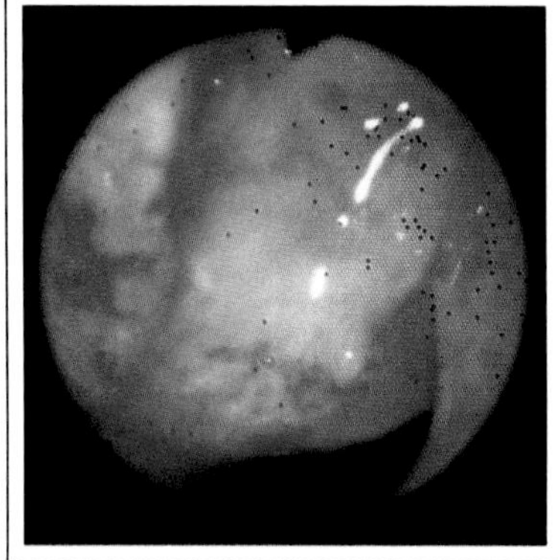

FIG. 22-5b.

FIG. 22-5. a: Pyloric channel, scar deformity, eccentric position. The pyloric channel was found in an atypical location, off the greater curve and posteriorly (at 5 o'clock). By itself, this atypical location is a nonspecific finding but would prompt an especially careful examination of the channel. **b:** Pyloric channel ulcer within a pyloric channel having an atypical location (a). An examination of the pylorus reveals a large channel ulcer.

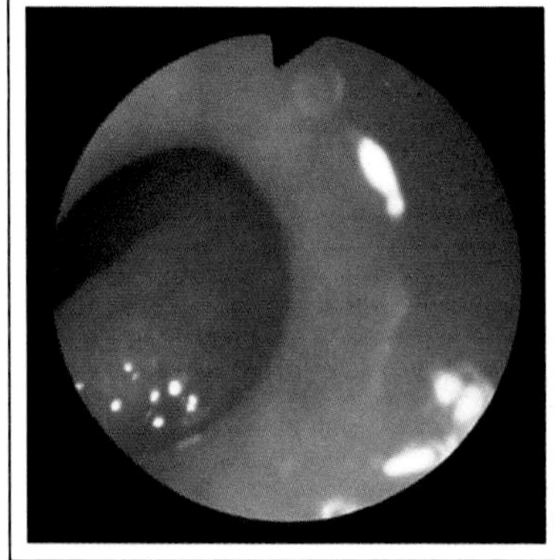

FIG. 22-6.

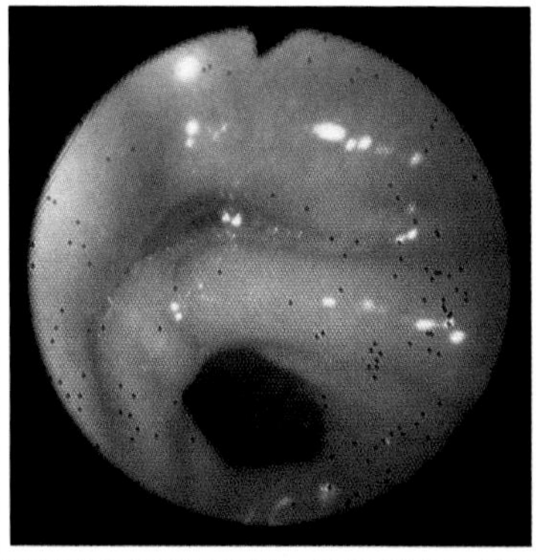

FIG. 22-7.

FIG. 22-6. Pyloric channel deformity with junctional fold. The fold running from the anterior wall of the pylorus (at 7 o'clock) toward the posterior wall of the bulb (at 3 o'clock) suggests deformity of the ulcer scar type.

FIG. 22-7. Double pylorus. The true pylorus is at 6 o'clock with an acquired channel (Fig. 22-8) just off 9 o'clock.

DOUBLE PYLORUS

An unusual type of pyloric channel deformity is the double pylorus (Fig. 22-7); we have seen only four such cases. In most reported cases,[1-3] as is true in our own experience, it is acquired rather than congenital, occurring where a penetrating ulcer has caused a fistula to form from the prepyloric antrum (Fig. 22-8a) to the duodenal bulb (Fig. 22-8b).[1-3] Most often this is located above the pyloric channel (Fig. 22-8a). When it occurs below the pylorus, the appearance resembles the surgically created Finney or Jaboulay pyloroplasty (see Chapter 19).[4] The fistulous tract as it forms is composed entirely of granulation tissue (Fig. 22-8), but it may completely re-epithelialize to become a second pyloric channel.[5] This is vulnerable mucosa, however, and a site for recurrent ulceration which occurs close to the lumen of the stomach or duodenum.

A second type of acquired double pylorus (Fig. 22-9) is for a gastrogastric rather than a gastroduodenal communication of the fistulous tract. Such a case has been reported from our Unit in a patient with deeply penetrating ulcers associated with prolonged heavy aspirin usage.[6]

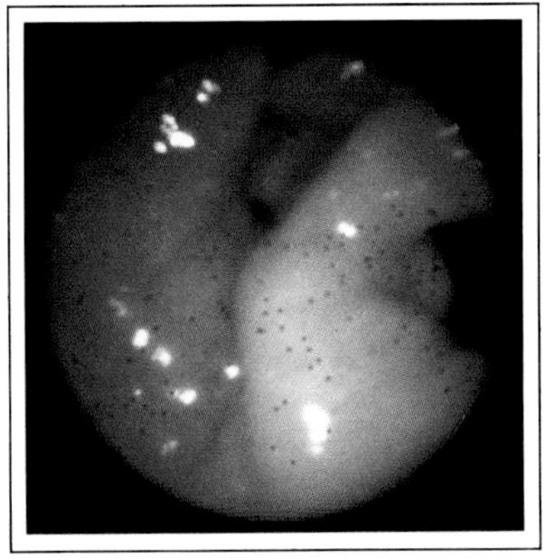

FIG. 22-8a.

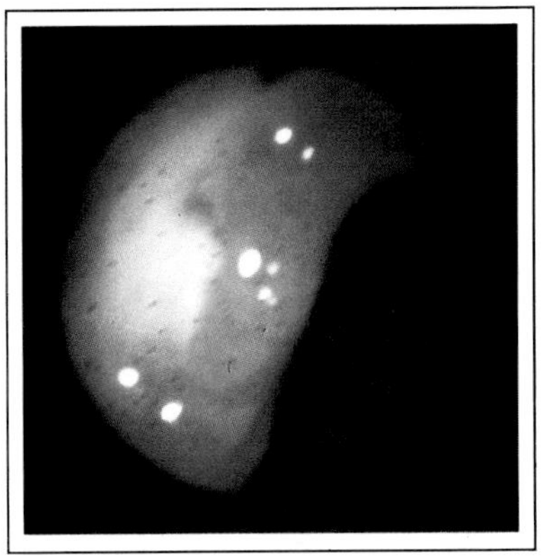

FIG. 22-8b.

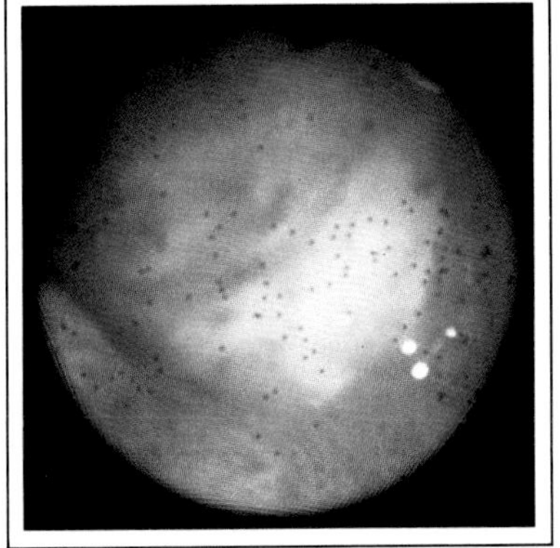

FIG. 22-8c.

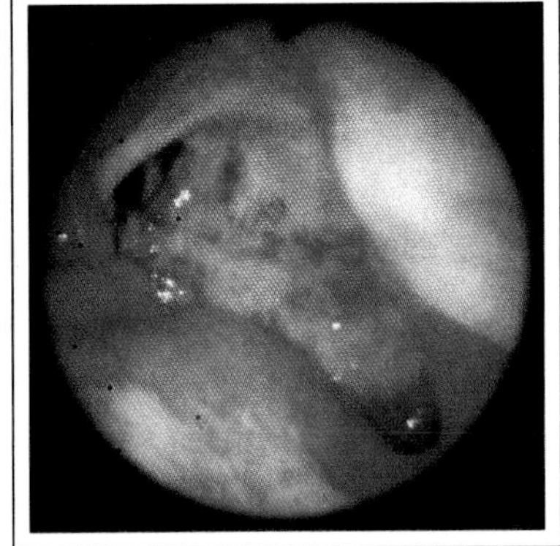

FIG. 22-9a.

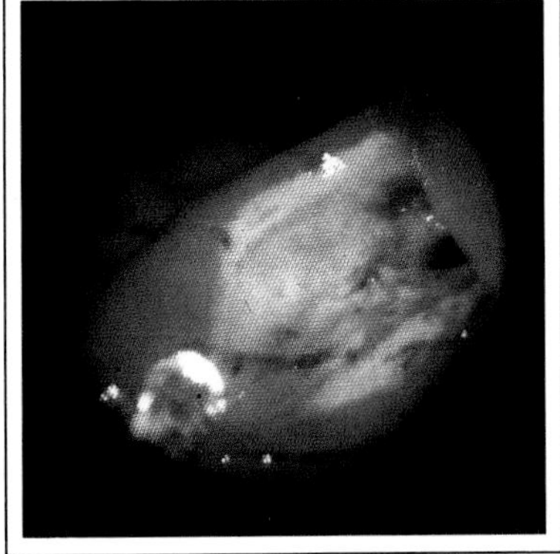

FIG. 22-9b.

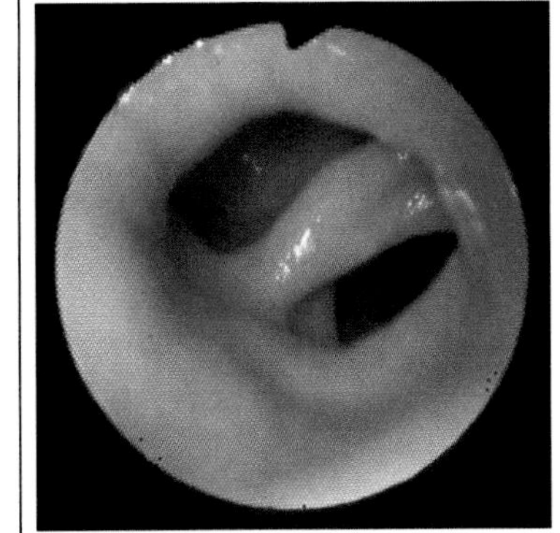

FIG. 22-10.

FIG. 22-8. Double pylorus with a gastroduodenal fistula. **a:** This occurred in a patient ingesting large amounts of aspirin (also on corticosteroids) and convalescing from recent surgery for Crohn's disease. A biopsy suggested peptic ulcer disease rather than Crohn's disease. **b:** The duodenal aspect of the fistula is noted with the duodenal lumen itself off to 3 o'clock. **c:** The duodenal aspect of the gastroduodenal fistula is composed entirely of granulation tissue. Over the next 3 months it was entirely epithelialized (Fig. 22-7).

FIG. 22-9. a: Double pylorus with a gastrogastric fistula. The acquired channel (at 10 o'clock) within this deep ulcer is continuous with another large ulcer of the gastric angle in a patient using large amounts of aspirin (a). **b:** Deep aspirin ulcer of the gastric angle forming a gastrogastric fistula and double pylorus (a). The opening to the fistulous tract can be seen at 3 o'clock.

FIG. 22-10. Double pylorus, possibly congenital, in a patient with no history of peptic ulcer disease.

Some cases of the double pylorus appearance may be congenital[7] as in a patient we observed without ulcer symptoms in whom the double pylorus was an incidental finding (Fig. 22-10).

REFERENCES

1. Farack, U. M., Goresky, G. A., Jabbari, M., and Kinnear, D. G. (1974): Double pylorus: a hypothesis concerning its pathogenesis. *Gastroenterology*, 66:596–600.
2. Minoli, G., Terruzzi, V., Levi, C., Pezzi, W. L., and Rossini, A. (1981): Acquired double pylorus or gastroduodenal fistula: report of a case and review of the literature. *Digestion*, 21:1–5.
3. Ghahremani, G. G., Gore, R. M., and Fields, W. R. (1980): Acquired double pylorus due to gastroduodenal fistula complicating peptic ulceration. *Arch. Surg.*, 115:194–198.
4. Goldstein, W. B. (1981): Unusual periduodenal fistulas in peptic ulcer disease. *J. Clin. Gastroenterol.*, 3:185–188.
5. Kelly, M. E., Mohlashemi, H., Patel, S., and Gupta, R. (1979): Report of a case of double pylorus. *Dig. Dis. Sci.*, 24:807–810.
6. Ito, Y., Blackstone, M. O., and Hatfield, G. E. (1978): A gastro-gastric fistula linking two penetrating ulcers: report of a case. *Gastrointest. Endosc.*, 24:247–248.
7. Gupta, A., and Hollander, D. (1977): Duplication of the pylorus found concomitantly with achalasia: congenital or peptic etiology? *Am. J. Dig. Dis.*, 22:829–830.

23

PYLORIC STENOSIS

The causes of pyloric stenosis to be discussed in this chapter are: (a) peptic ulcer disease; (b) gastric malignancy involving the pylorus; and (c) adult hypertrophic pyloric stenosis. Patients with significant pyloric stenosis present with symptoms of repeated postprandial vomiting, weight loss, and a succussion splash on physical examination, as well as evidence of gastric retention on upper gastrointestinal radiographic studies. Because these findings are common to pyloric stenosis from any cause, endoscopy is requested to determine the specific cause.

PYLORIC STENOSIS ASSOCIATED WITH PEPTIC ULCER DISEASE

In patients with pyloric stenosis producing symptoms and other findings of gastric outlet obstruction, there is usually no doubt about the diagnosis visually, with the channel often less than 6 mm in diameter and sometimes on the order of 3 mm (Fig. 23-1a). In the latter case, the pylorus may be so small it is difficult to identify. Once found, however, the diagnosis of pyloric stenosis is obvious (Fig. 23-1a) because of the diameter of the pylorus (≤10 mm) and the inability to pass even a pediatric-caliber instrument (9 mm) across. In some cases, rather than marked stenosis alone, there is an ulcer just proximal to, within, or distal to the already compromised channel (Fig. 23-1b). The addition of the ulcer with its associated acute inflammation and edema (Fig. 23-1c) can convert a stenosed yet working pyloric channel into one which is functionally obstructed.

In addition to attempting to find evidence of an active ulcer within the narrowed pyloric channel, the endoscopist must carefully examine the mucosa of the prepyloric antrum, as this bears on the differentiation of benign ulcer stenosis from that caused by malignancy (see below). The finding of a smooth, perfectly symmetrical prepyloric antrum with intact mucosa points to benign ulcer stenosis (Fig. 23-1a), whereas an asymmetrical appearance or an ulcer with atypical features raises the question of malignancy (Fig. 23-2), even if the stenotic channel itself appears benign.

In most cases, however, rather than mucosal changes, one observes a structural abnormality in relation to pyloric stenosis from peptic ulcer disease. The commonest of these is the mass-like ulcer scar deformity (Fig. 23-3a). Although intact overlying mucosa is reassuring, it does not exclude malignancy (Fig. 23-3d). Conversely, an atypical appearance to the mucosa (Fig. 23-3b) does not prove malignant pyloric stenosis (Fig. 23-3c). In cases where some atypical feature is present, either structural or mucosal, one regards the appearance as indeterminate and vigorously pursues biopsies and especially brushing cytology from within the stenosed pyloric channel. Even in a case where the overlying mucosa is intact, with an appreciable mass-like deformity associated with pyloric stenosis (Fig. 23-3d) the appearance is regarded as suspicious and biopsies and brushings are vigorously pursued both at the time of initial observation and at 4 to 6 weeks to provide the maximum opportunity for detecting malignant change.

PYLORIC STENOSIS ASSOCIATED WITH MALIGNANCY

Gastric cancer is an infrequent cause of pyloric channel obstruction, occurring much less often than pyloric stenosis from peptic ulcer disease. In our Unit over a 7-year period, 14 cases of benign pyloric stenosis from ulcer disease were observed in contrast to only three cases of pyloric stenosis from malignancy. The reason for this was twofold. First, the pyloric channel itself appears to be an uncommon site of origin of gastric cancer. Second, gastric cancer arising elsewhere in the stomach crosses the pylorus in no more than 20% of the cases and obstructs it in less than one-third.[1]

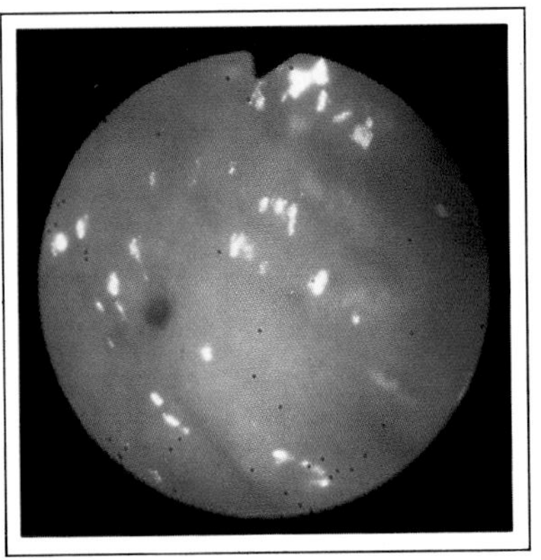

FIG. 23-1a.

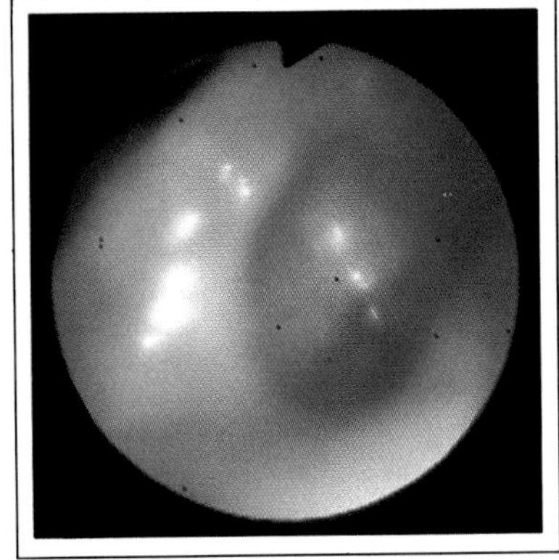

FIG. 23-1b.

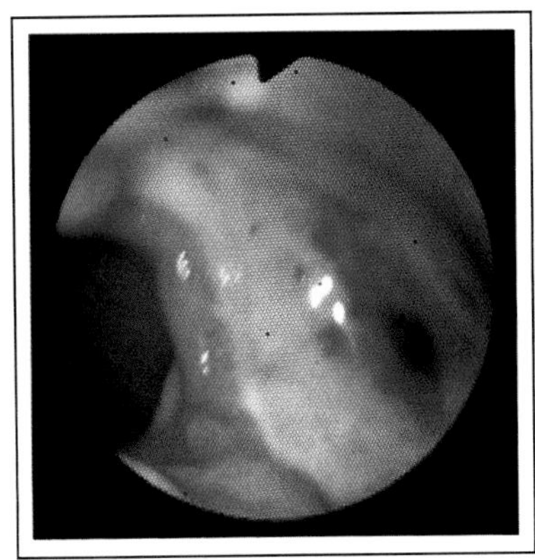

FIG. 23-1c.

FIG. 23-1. a: Pyloric channel stenosis, peptic. A pinpoint (2 to 3 mm) pyloric channel is seen just off the anterior wall (9 o'clock aspect). **b:** Pyloric channel stenosis with an active channel ulcer (c). **c:** Pyloric channel ulcer associated with pyloric stenosis (b). Acute inflammation and edema of the ulcer margin further compromised an already narrowed channel.

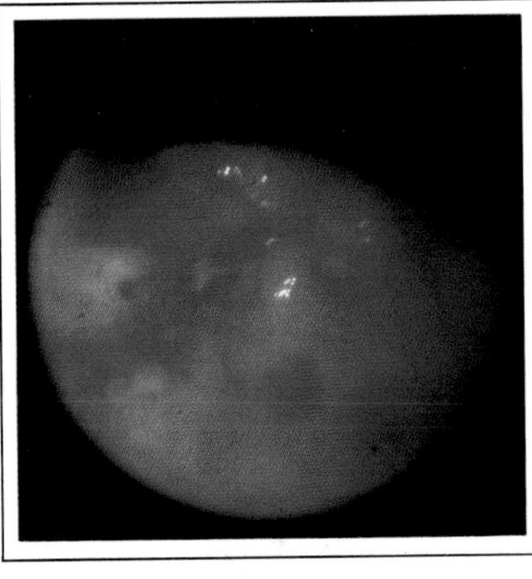

FIG. 23-2.

FIG. 23-2. Pyloric channel stenosis with atypical-appearing ulcerations (9 o'clock). The irregular, indistinct margin of the ulcer was a clue to a correct diagnosis of gastric cancer which in this case proved to be of the early type (see Chapter 16).

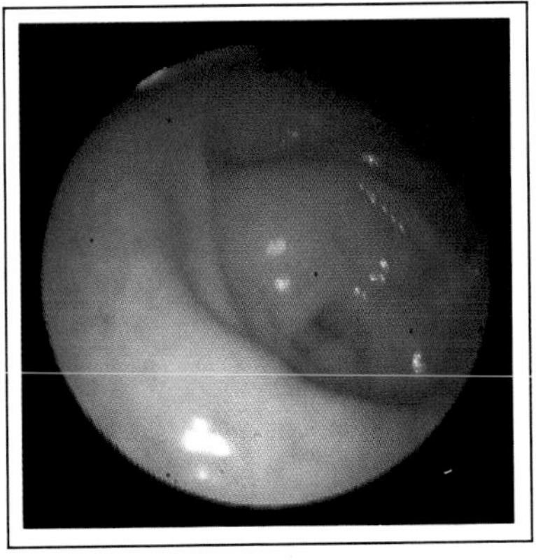

FIG. 23-3a.

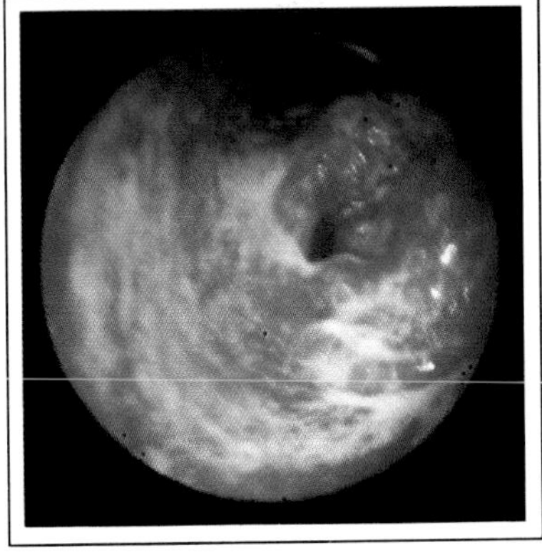

FIG. 23-3b.

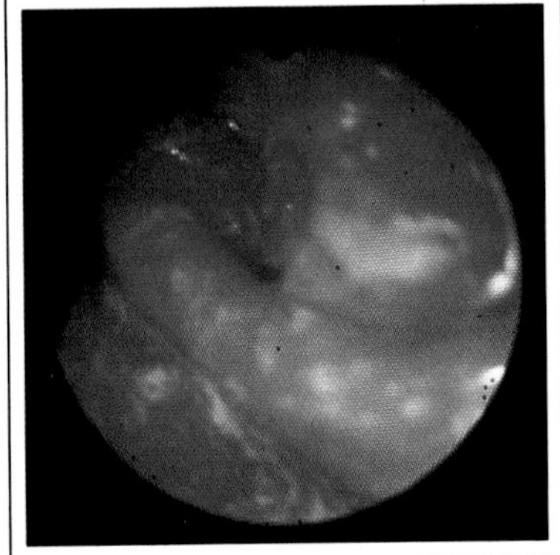

FIG. 23-3c.

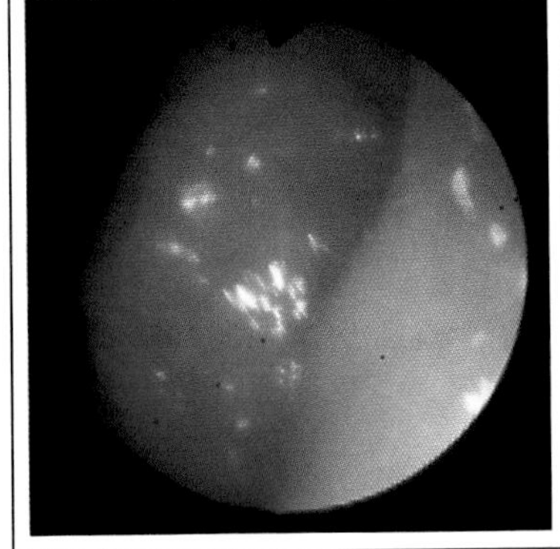

FIG. 23-3d.

FIG. 23-3. a: Pyloric channel stenosis, benign. Peptic ulcer with prepyloric mass deformity. The pyloric channel itself is a pinpoint (2 to 3 mm) just off 5 o'clock. **b:** Pyloric channel stenosis, indeterminate. The retained gastric secretions (in this case barium) give the mass-like deformity a superficially ulcerated appearance. At surgery this was proved benign. **c:** Pyloric channel stenosis, indeterminate. A close-up view of (b) suggests an irregularly ulcerated mucosa. For this reason, the appearance was called indeterminate. Mucosal biopsies were negative, and brushing cytology unfortunately was not performed. At surgery carcinoma was found to arise within the channel and extend into the duodenal bulb. **d:** Pyloric stenosis, indeterminate. The mucosa is smooth and glistening, suggesting it to be intact. Still, the mass-like appearance of the folds, especially at 9 o'clock, caused one to regard this as suspicious. Infiltrating carcinoma was found at surgery.

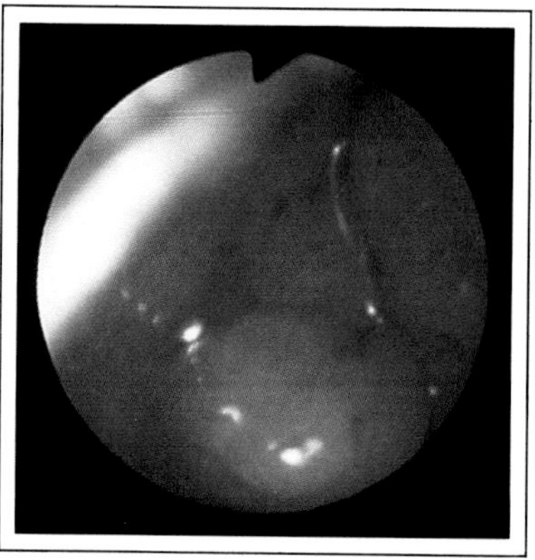

FIG. 23-4a.

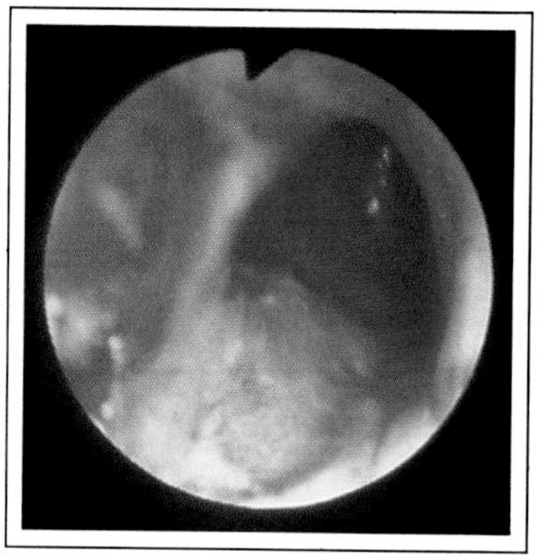

FIG. 23-4b.

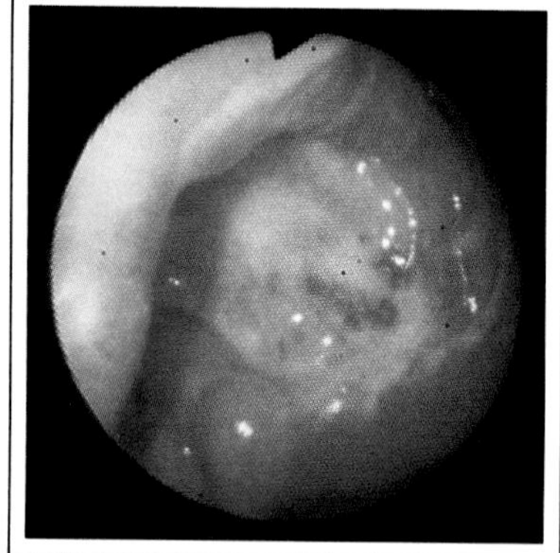

FIG. 23-4c.

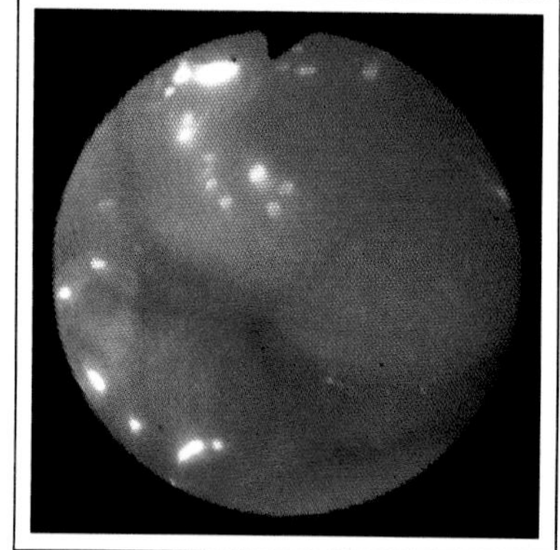

FIG. 23-4d.

FIG. 23-4. Pyloric stenosis, malignant. **a:** Large indurated folds radiate to a stenotic pyloric channel. Multiple biopsies were negative, however. Brushing cytology through the channel was positive, emphasizing the importance of cytology when malignant pyloric stenosis is suspected. **b:** A mass is seen to form and narrow the pyloric channel. In this case biopsies from the mass were positive. **c:** The ulcer adjacent to a narrow pyloric channel has a somewhat irregular base with an irregular-appearing interface of the base and the ulcer margin. Biopsies in this case showed the ulcer to be malignant. **d:** The infiltrating carcinoma was confined to the pyloric channel and appeared as enlarged, indurated folds. Biopsies were not helpful, but brushing cytology was positive.

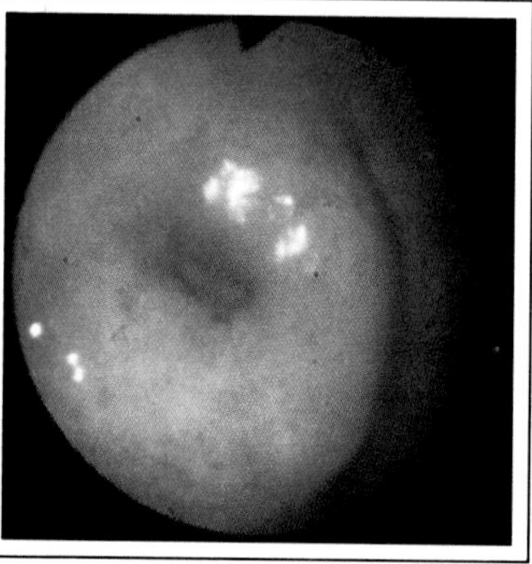

FIG. 23-5.

FIG. 23-5. Hypertrophic pyloric stenosis. A smooth, raised circumferential prepyloric fold abuts out into the lumen. This, in addition to elongation of the channel, suggests hypertrophic pyloric stenosis. Moreover, the easy passage of a 9-mm instrument suggested the narrowing to be due to muscle hypertrophy, a finding confirmed at surgery.

In malignant pyloric obstruction there is often other evidence of infiltrating malignancy of the antrum with indurated, superficially ulcerated folds (Fig. 23-4a), a polypoid mass involving the channel (Fig. 23-4b), or an ulcerating lesion adjacent to the stenotic pyloric channel (Fig. 23-4c). Rather than there being any antral involvement, the cancer may be entirely confined to the pyloric channel, appearing as indurated folds (Fig. 23-4d). Biopsies of an ulcerated mass or infiltrated mucosa may show evidence of frank malignancy, but brushing through the stenotic pyloric channel may increase the diagnostic yield,[2] especially where the area of tumor breakthrough is not obvious (Fig. 23-4a).

ADULT HYPERTROPHIC PYLORIC STENOSIS

Rarest of all types of pyloric stenosis is the adult hypertrophic form.[3] Of 16 cases of pyloric stenosis encountered among 5,000 examinations, only one was of the adult hypertrophic type. The presentation is similar to that of other types of pyloric stenosis, with nausea, vomiting, and weight loss occurring for the first time even in middle age. Generally patients have been symptomatic 6 to 12 months prior to diagnosis.[3] The pathogenesis of this lesion is unknown.[4] It may not be simply the persistence of infantile pyloric stenosis but may have to do with an irritative phenomenon affecting the pylorus beginning in adulthood which leads to hypertrophy of its smooth muscle.

The appearance at endoscopy is distinctive. There is both elongation (>2 cm) of the pyloric channel as well as a characteristic fixed, circumferential prepyloric fold which causes the pylorus to "pout out" into the lumen (Fig. 23-5), with the mass-like deformity caused by compression of the prepyloric mucosa by the hypertrophic pyloric musculature. In addition to hypertrophic pyloric stenosis involving the channel circumferentially, a focal variant has been described in which the hypertrophy is confined to the lesser curve aspect. Such focal hypertrophic pyloric stenosis has been referred to as torus hyperplasia.[4] The asymmetry of this appearance and its resemblance to malignant pyloric stenosis necessitate an "indeterminate" designation and vigorous pursuit of biopsies and brushing cytology.

REFERENCES

1. Koehler, R. E., Hanelin, L. G., Laing, F. C., Montgomery, C. K., and Margulis, A. R. (1977): Invasion of the duodenum by carcinoma of the stomach. *Am. J. Roentgenol.*, 128:201–205.
2. Witzel, L., Halter, F., Gretillat, P. A., Scheurer, U., and Keller, M. (1976): Evaluation and specific value of endoscopic biopsies and brushing cytology for malignancy of the esophagus and stomach. *Gut*, 17:375–377.
3. Wellmann, K. F., Kagan, A., and Fang, H. (1964): Hypertrophic pyloric stenosis in adults: survey of the literature and report of a case of the localized form (torus hyperplasia). *Gastroenterology*, 46:601–608.
4. Aron, J. M., Newman, A., and Heaton, J. W. (1973): Torus hyperplasia of the pyloric antrum presenting as gastric pseudotumor. *Gastroenterology*, 64:634–636.

Section 3

THE DUODENUM

24

THE DUODENUM—ENDOSCOPIC ORIENTATION, TECHNIQUE OF EXAMINATION, AND NORMAL APPEARANCE

DUODENAL BULB

Endoscopic Orientation

The same endoscopic-anatomic relationships previously described for the stomach (see Chapter 11) pertain to the duodenal bulb (Fig. 24-1). As in the stomach, the anterior and posterior walls are observed in the 9 and 3 o'clock positions of the visual field, respectively. Again, leftward deflection of the tip and a counterclockwise torquing of the endoscope shaft brings the 9 o'clock lens image position more fully into alignment with the anterior wall, whereas rightward deflection and clockwise torquing provide increased visualization of the posterior wall. Because the 12 o'clock lens position is closest to the superior wall of the bulb (Fig. 24-1), this surface is preferentially seen in this position in the visual field whereas the inferior wall is found in the 6 o'clock visual field position. Enhanced visualization of the positions is accomplished with upward (toward the superior wall) and downward (toward the inferior wall) tip deflections, respectively.

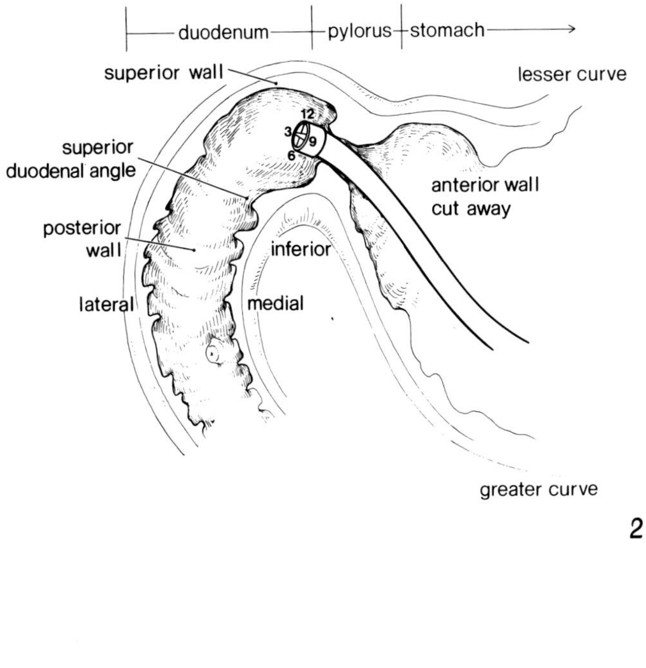

Anatomically, the duodenal bulb is a small, triangular structure, generally 4 to 6 cm long and 2 to 3 cm wide, bridging the more anterior intraperitoneal antrum of the stomach with the more posterior retroperitoneal descending duodenum. The duodenal bulb therefore courses posteriorly, a fact which explains why its most distal point, the apex, appears first in the 3 o'clock (posterior) portion of the visual field (Fig. 24-2a). Conversely, as the endoscope enters the bulb from an immediately adjacent portion of the antrum stomach, the tip tends to look initially at the anterior (9 o'clock) wall (Fig. 24-2b); to advance the tip in the direction of the apex as well as to examine the posterior wall, clockwise torquing and rightward deflection of the tip are necessary (Fig. 24-2c).

Technique of Examination

Because of its small size, the duodenal bulb can be difficult to examine effectively. Certain areas are overlooked unless the bulb as a whole is examined in a careful and systematic

FIG. 24-1. The walls of the duodenum in relation to the image positions of the lens.

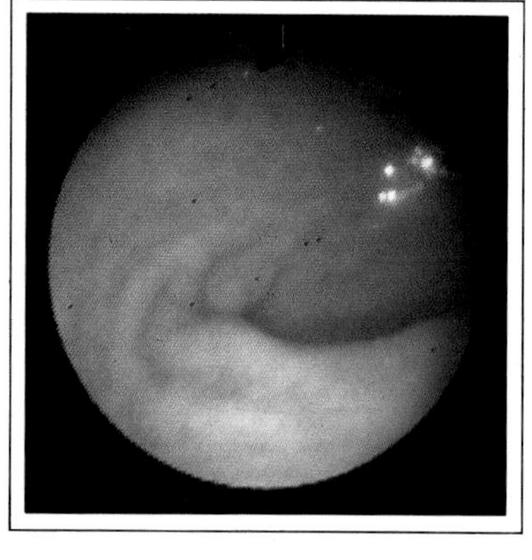

FIG. 24-2a.

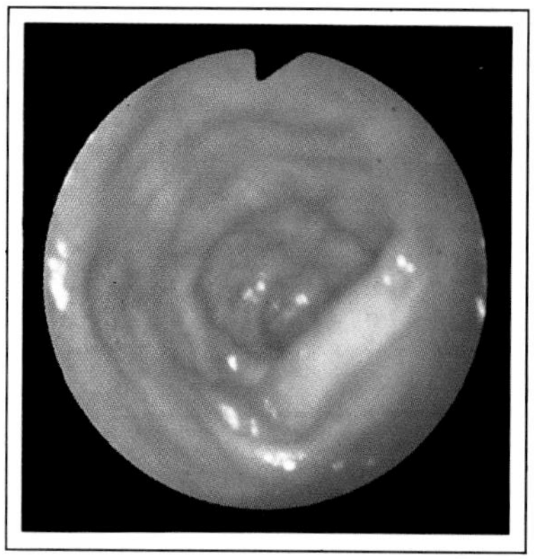

FIG. 24-2b.

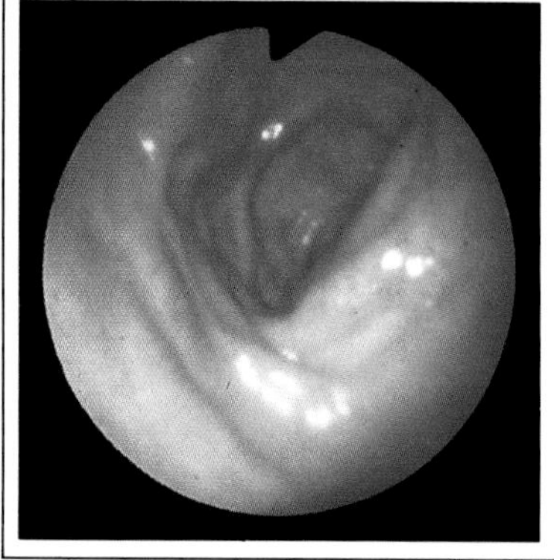

FIG. 24-2c.

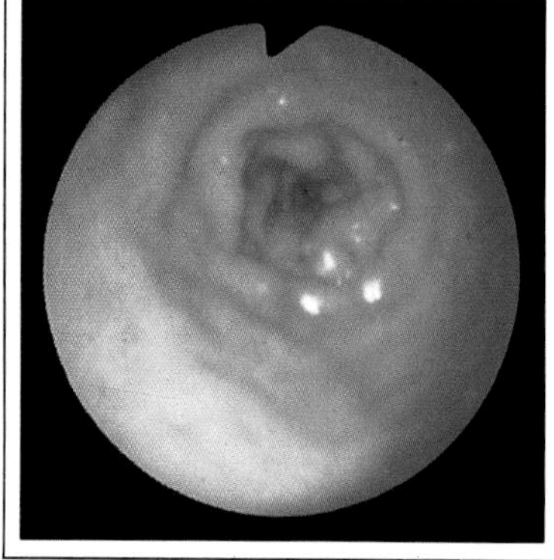

FIG. 24-3.

FIG. 24-2. Duodenal bulb. **a:** The anterior wall is observed at 9 o'clock, and the apex, being posterior, is seen at 3 o'clock. Running from 3 o'clock to 9 o'clock is the superior duodenal angle, the junction of the inferior wall of the bulb and the medial wall of the descending duodenum. **b:** The anterior wall (running from 6 to 10 o'clock) is best seen on entry into the bulb, with the superior wall between 9 and 1 o'clock, and with the apex in the distance just off the posterior wall (running from 2 o'clock to 5 o'clock). **c:** Distal duodenal bulb after a clockwise torquing maneuver. More of the posterior and superior wall (9 to 1 o'clock) is now seen as the tip is turned toward it.

FIG. 24-3. Duodenal bulb on entry. The endoscope tip is positioned just beyond the pyloroduodenal junction, where the inferior wall (between 5 and 8 o'clock) is best seen. The apical folds appeared prominent, but with further insufflation, these largely disappeared.

fashion. In practice, one performs either a screening examination or a detailed one, depending on the clinical index of suspicion.

Screening Examination

In cases where the bulb is not a prime clinical concern, satisfactory screening can be performed if the bulb is inspected twice—on the way to and back from the descending duodenum. This is performed in the following way. Upon entering the proximal bulb from the pyloric channel (see Chapter 21), one stops to wait until sufficient air has been given to inflate the bulb (Fig. 24-3). A clockwise torquing maneuver allows one to direct the tip toward the apex and posterior wall (Fig. 24-2c). With the apex sighted, the tip is advanced in that direction. Within the mid-bulb, the examiner arcs the tip from the anterior to the posterior position, examining these as well as the superior wall. A second arc is made just prior to reaching the apex itself and entering the descending duodenum (see below). Once the descending duodenum has been examined and the endoscope withdrawn back into the bulb, this area is again examined, once at the apical area and again in the mid-bulb. The endoscope is thereupon withdrawn several centimeters proximally while the inferior wall is examined (Fig. 24-3). During the course of this screening examination, the endoscopist makes a special effort to examine the posterior wall of the bulb (Fig. 24-2c), especially the junction of the apex and descending duodenum, the superior duodenal angle (Fig. 24-2a).

Detailed Examination

A high clinical index of suspicion about the bulb calls for more detailed examination. This may be accomplished with a standard adult (11 to 13 mm) endoscope; however, with radiographic evidence or a high clinical suspicion of ulcer disease, one might well consider using a pediatric-type endoscope, which because of its narrow caliber (8 to 9 mm) and shorter turning length (2 cm) often proves to be a more effective examining instrument than endoscopes of larger caliber (11 to 13 mm). As in the screening examination, two or more arcs are made from anterior to posterior as the instrument is advanced toward the apex. In some cases, depending on the difficulty with which the duodenal bulb is entered, a decision must be made as to whether it is wise to continue the examination into the descending duodenum. In cases for example, where there is a definite question to be answered about a bulb which has been entered with great difficulty, one would not wish

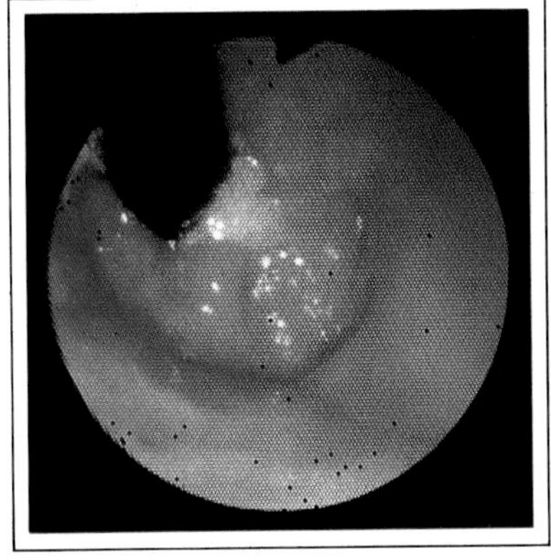

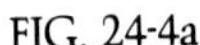

FIG. 24-4a.

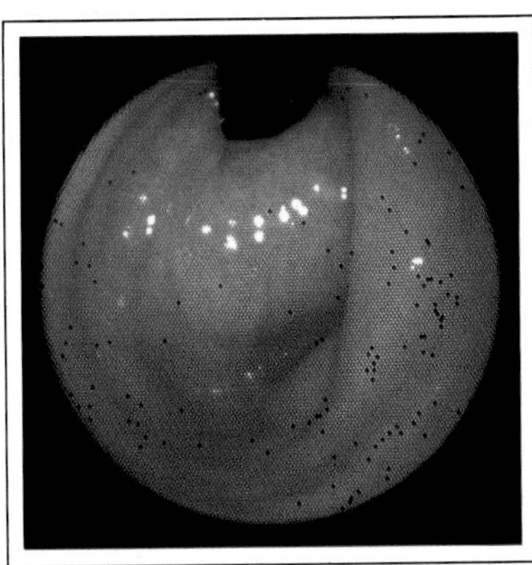

FIG. 24-4b.

FIG. 24-4. Duodenal bulb, retroflexed view of the pyloroduodenal junction. **a:** Because of the retroflexion, the superior and inferior walls are found in reversed positions in the visual field. The endoscope, seen in the 12 o'clock position, actually runs along the inferior wall, with the superior wall being "observed" in the 6 o'clock lens image position. The anterior and posterior walls are still found in their accustomed 9 and 3 o'clock positions, respectively. A small elevation is noted (the pyloroduodenal junction) just as the endoscope emerges. **b:** The posterior fornix. The ring-like pyloroduodenal junction is noted in the 12 o'clock position as the endoscope emerges out onto the inferior wall. Just adjacent to this is its junction with the posterior wall, which makes up the posterior fornix.

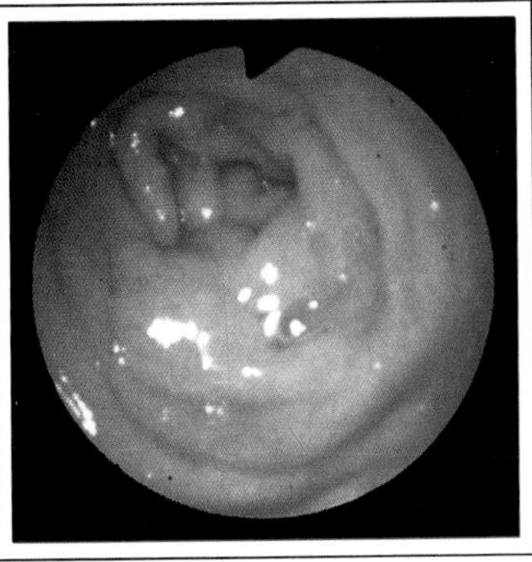

FIG. 24-5.

FIG. 24-5. Pyloroduodenal junction. This is the most distal point of the pyloric channel, which in this case is fairly visible at 6 o'clock. In the midline it is equidistant from the anterior and posterior walls and their respective fornices (their junctions with the inferior wall are seen at 9 and 3 o'clock).

to risk losing the opportunity to examine it in detail because after entry into the descending duodenum the endoscope is suddenly retracted back into the stomach and cannot be reinserted. If the descending duodenum is examined, on return into the bulb at least two additional arcing movements are made in the mid and distal bulb, with special attention to the superior duodenal angle and posterior wall. In addition, an arc is made in the proximal bulb and another as close to the pyloroduodenal junction as possible, this being the commonest site of duodenal ulcers (see Chapter 26).

In select cases, especially if a pediatric-type instrument is used, one may wish to retroflex the tip so that the pyloroduodenal junction (Fig. 24-4a) and fornices (Fig. 24-4b) can be seen from below. Retroflexion is accomplished in the bulb with upward deflection and continued intubation beginning in the mid-bulb (Fig. 24-4a). Although we find this maneuver most readily accomplished with the use of a pediatric-type endoscope, we do not do this routinely, especially in a scarred bulb where we believe there is a small but real chance of perforation.

Finally, even with meticulous examination with a forward-viewing instrument with a short turning length, the lesion in question, especially if located on the posterior superior aspect, can be missed. In cases where there is a strong clinical index of suspicion, one follows the initial examination with a second one using a side-viewing endoscope. The technique for this examination is discussed below (see "Descending Duodenum, Side-Viewing Technique," this chapter).

Normal Appearance of the Duodenal Bulb

Anatomic Features

The duodenal bulb is, in essence, a triangle, the base of which is demarcated by the angular fornices. From these, the anterior and posterior walls extend to a third angular terminal point, the apex. All other landmarks of the bulb may be thought of in terms of its fornices, apex, and anterior and posterior walls.

Pyloroduodenal junction.

The pyloroduodenal junction is identified as the most distal point of the pyloric channel, just before its opening into the lumen of the bulb (Fig. 24-5). It is not normally seen as a separate structure. Typically, it is found at a point equidistant from the anterior and posterior walls (Fig. 24-5). On retroflexion, it may appear as a small ring-like

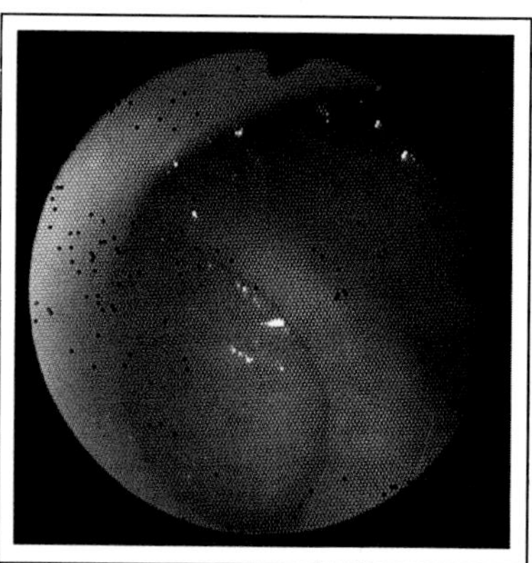

FIG. 24-6.

FIG. 24-6. Deformed pyloroduodenal junction (peptic ulcer disease) with a prominent anterior fornix. The deforming fold runs from the junction at 6 o'clock to the anterior wall at 9 o'clock, accentuating the opening to the fornix.

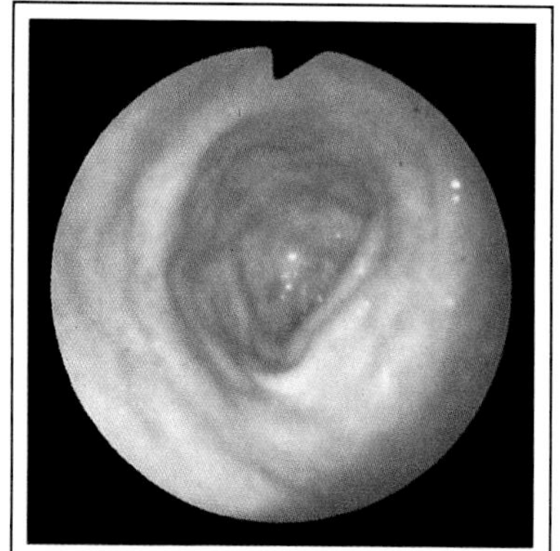

FIG. 24-7a.

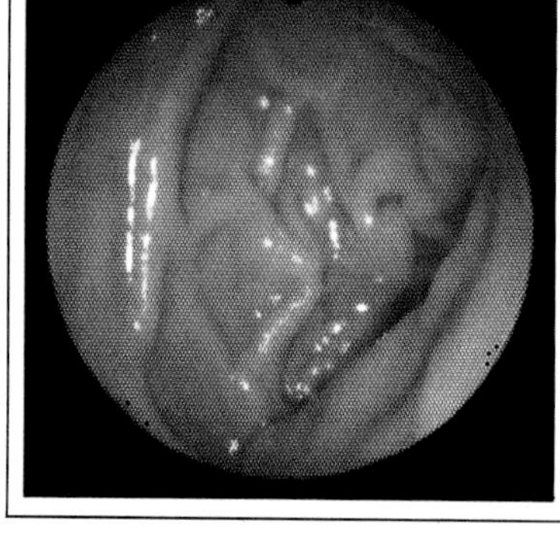

FIG. 24-7b.

FIG. 24-7. Duodenal bulb anterior wall. **a:** The surface, in this case running from 6 to 12 o'clock, is the first structure encountered on entering the bulb because of its anterior location. In most cases it is perfectly flat, allowing full insufflation of the bulb. **b:** With corrugated appearance. Kerckring folds are found in this case proximal to the apex, giving the anterior wall this appearance.

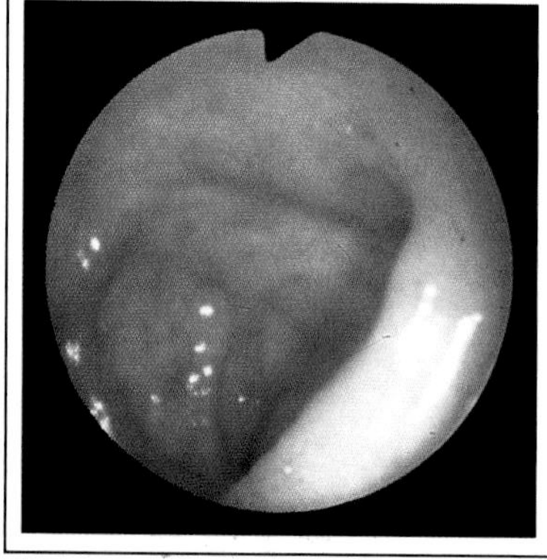

FIG. 24-8a.

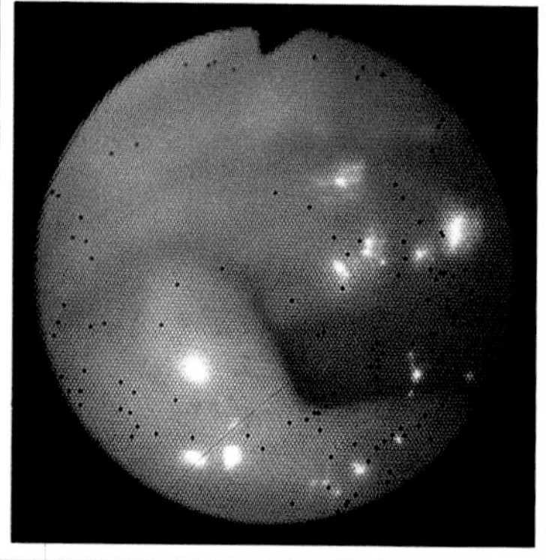

FIG. 24-8b.

FIG. 24-8. Superior duodenal angle. **a:** The junction of the inferoposterior wall of the bulb and medial wall of the descending duodenum is seen here as a single prominent apical fold. **b:** Nodular-appearing. The terminal point approaching the mucosa of the superior duodenal angle as it approaches the anterior wall is redundant and appears nodular, even after complete insufflation.

eminence encircling the endoscope as it emerges from the pyloric channel (Fig. 24-4a).

Fornices.

As one enters the bulb, one may sense the location of the fornices at the points where the pyloroduodenal junction meets the anterior and posterior walls (Fig. 24-5). With retroflexion, they may be identified in the normal bulb (Fig. 24-4b). With pyloroduodenal deformity, the fornix, usually the anterior one, is accentuated by the presence of a fold running from the pyloroduodenal junction to the anterior wall (Fig. 24-6). This type of deformity is discussed in detail elsewhere (see Chapter 26).

Anterior wall.

The anterior wall is seen immediately on entering the bulb (Fig. 24-7a). The wall is perfectly smooth down to the distal bulb and apical area where one sees the beginning of the concentric ring-like Kerckring folds, which continue into the descending duodenum. In some cases these folds

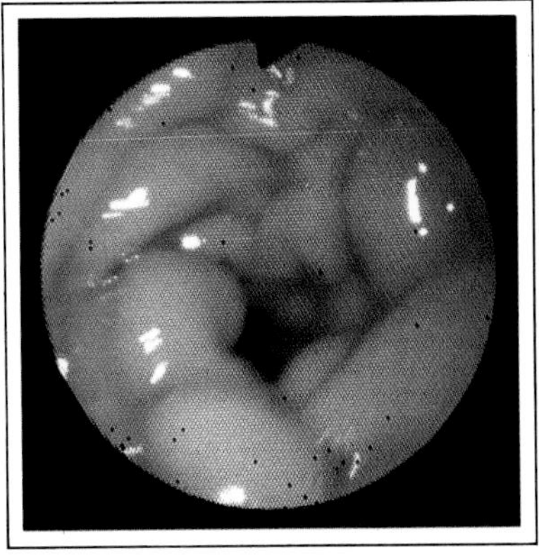

FIG. 24-9.

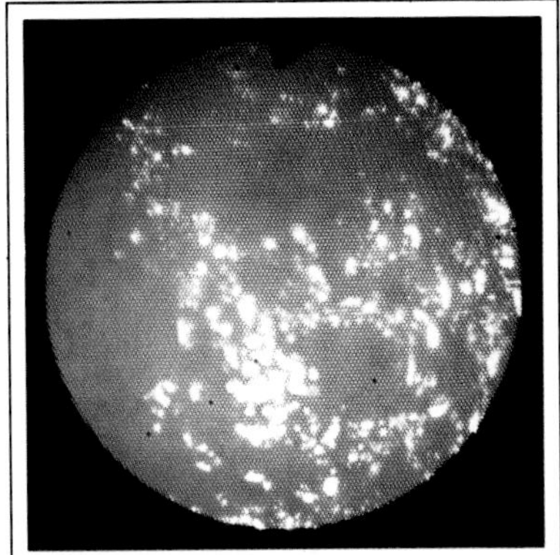

FIG. 24-10a.

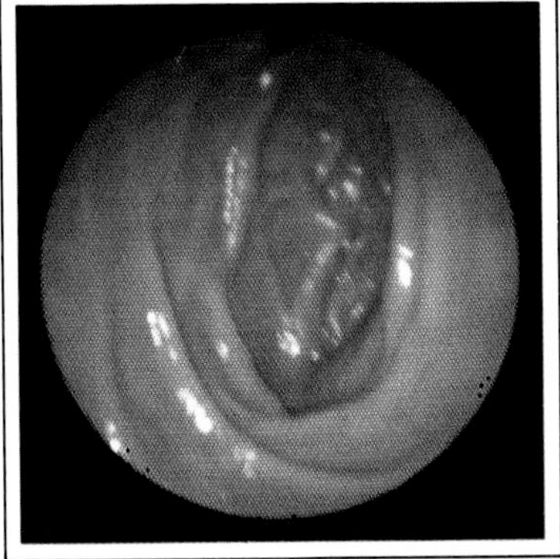

FIG. 24-10b.

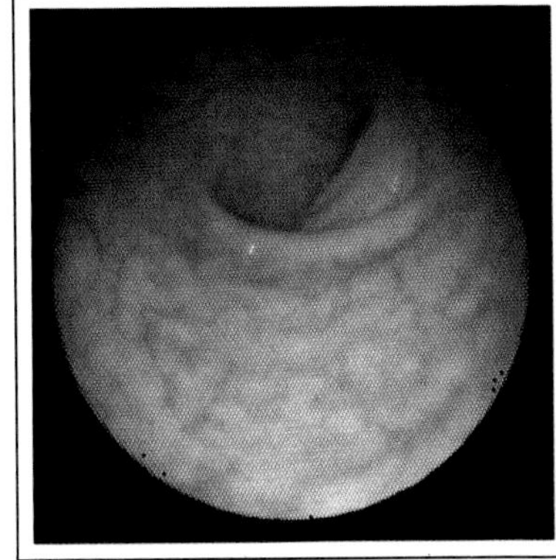

FIG. 24-10c.

FIG. 24-9. Duodenal bulb apex. Here the apical folds are prominent because of redundant mucosa and appear nodular.

FIG. 24-10. a: Duodenal bulb mucosa. The light reflected breaks up in a dot-like fashion because of the villi. This causes the mucosa to appear granular when viewed up close. **b:** Duodenal bulb mucosal coloration. In contrast to the orange-pink color within the stomach, the mucosa of the bulb tends to appear yellow-gray. **c:** Duodenal bulb mucosal vascular pattern. Distinct, short, thin capillaries are characteristic of duodenal bulb mucosa.

may continue into the mid-bulb, giving the anterior wall a corrugated appearance (Fig. 24-7b).

Superior and inferior walls.

The inferior wall, like the anterior wall, is seen directly on entering the bulb (Fig. 24-2a). The superior wall may also be observed in this position (Fig. 24-2b), but may be adequately visualized only after advancing the tip toward the apex, while deflecting upwards (Fig. 24-2c). The superior and inferior walls are for the most part smooth; however, like the anterior wall in the distal bulb, Kerckring folds may be present (Fig. 24-7b).

Posterior wall.

Because of the anterior location of the endoscope tip on entry, the posterior wall is not readily seen unless the tip is moved toward it with a clockwise torquing maneuver and rightward deflection (Fig. 24-2b). Like the anterior wall, it is generally smooth or made to appear corrugated by the presence of Kerckring folds in its terminal portion.

Superior duodenal angle.

The inferoposterior aspect of the bulb joins the medial wall of the descending duodenum at a ridge-like fold in the apex (Fig. 24-8a). This fold, which extends from the posterior wall, marking the terminal point of the inferior wall, is referred to as the superior duodenal angle. This is the landmark for the medial wall of the descending duodenum (Fig. 24-1). The fold is generally flat (Fig. 24-8a), although it may appear heaped-up or mass-like (Fig. 24-8b) even after air insufflation.

Apex.

The apex is the terminal portion of the bulb. It may appear flat or heaped-up (Fig. 24-9) with heaped-up redundant Kerckring mucosal folds which continue into the descending duodenum.

Mucosal Appearance

The mucosa of the duodenal bulb can be distinguished from that of the pyloric region of the stomach by its texture, coloration, and vascular pattern. A knowledge of these features is useful in cases where the exact location of the pyloroduodenal junction is uncertain, providing the endoscopist with a means to ascertain the position as being in the duodenal bulb by careful examination of the mucosa.

Mucosal texture.

From a distance of several centimeters the mucosa appears perfectly smooth; however, with the high-resolution optics of currently available endoscopes, the fine villous texture of the mucosa can be appreciated when inspected at closer range (Fig. 24-10a). At this distance the light reflex has a granular appearance, consisting of tiny dots of light (Fig. 24-10a), resulting from the presence of mucosal villi.

Coloration.

In contrast to the yellow-orange appearance of the stomach, the mucosa of the duodenum is yellow-gray (Fig. 24-10b). The explanation of this color difference is unknown.

Vascular pattern.

There is a characteristic vascular pattern for duodenal mucosa. This consists of the appearance of tiny, thread-like interconnecting capillaries which terminate after running only a short distance (Fig. 24-10c). These vessels are especially well seen with complete air insufflation of the bulb when the mucosa is perfectly flat (Fig. 24-10c).

DESCENDING DUODENUM

Endoscopic Orientation

The endoscopic orientation for the descending duodenum is dependent first on the type of instrument used, i.e., forward-viewing or side-viewing endoscope, and second on the type of intubation technique used. In the case of the forward-viewing instrument, this is either by the direct entry technique, where the apex and descending duodenum are intubated by simple forward advancement, or the indirect technique, where prior to intubation there is a clockwise torquing maneuver performed at the apex.

In this section we consider the orientation for the direct entry and indirect entry techniques for the forward-viewing endoscope, as well as the orientation for intubation using a side-viewing instrument.

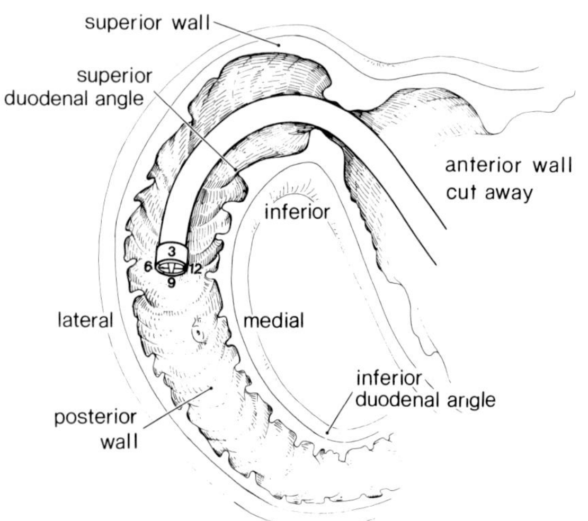

FIG. 24-11. The walls of the descending duodenum in relation to the image positions of the lens after intubation using the direct entry technique (see text).

Intubation by Direct Technique

In approximately 30% of the cases it is possible to intubate the descending duodenum with a forward-viewing instrument by simply following the lumen. This we refer to as the direct entry method. It is accomplished by initial downward deflection of the tip at the apex so that the 12 o'clock lens image position "looks at" the lateral wall and the 6 o'clock position, with further downward deflection, "sees" the medial wall (Fig. 24-11). With this entry technique, the 9 o'clock and 3 o'clock lens positions have the same anterior (9 o'clock) and posterior (3 o'clock) relationship as in the duodenal bulb and stomach (Fig. 24-11). In this orientation, further posterior deflection of the tip (toward 3 o'clock) can be accompanied with counterclockwise torquing of the shaft, as is sometimes necessary for complete intubation of the posterior descending duodenum.

Confirmation of these relationships comes from viewing the inferior duodenal angle, a landmark for the medial wall, found at the point the lumen changes direction from the vertical descending duodenum to the horizontal third portion. If the intubation has been by the direct entry technique, one expects the inferior duodenal angle to be seen in the 6 o'clock position with the lateral wall in the 12 o'clock position (Fig. 24-12).

Intubation by Indirect Technique

We find that in 70% of cases the apex is sharply angulated to the descending duodenum so that the latter cannot be entered under direct vision. We found early in our experience that the apex and proximal descending duodenum could be intubated blindly if the tip became positioned so it would run with forward advancement precisely along the anterior aspect of the medial wall of the descending duodenum. To accomplish this, what is required is an initial clockwise (posterior) torquing movement of the shaft to the tip 90° to 120° in the apex. With additional rightward (posterior) and upward deflection, the tip becomes aligned with the medial wall. Here the 12 o'clock lens image position now comes to look directly at the medial wall (Fig. 24-13). The lateral wall in this orientation is seen in the 6 o'clock position. Because of the initial clockwise rotation of the tip to enter the descending duodenum, the anterior

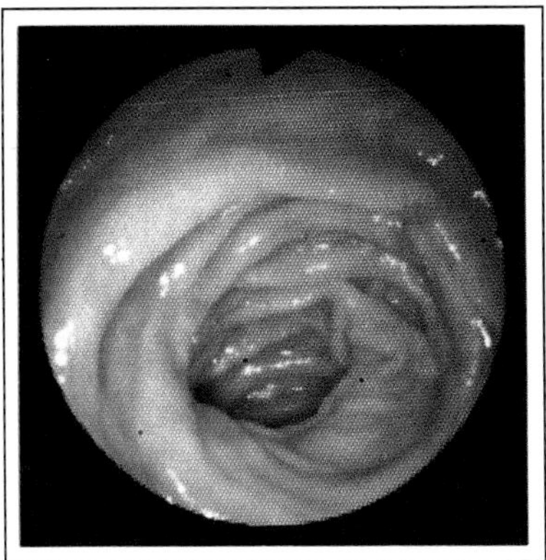

FIG. 24-12.

FIG. 24-12. Descending duodenum after direct entry. The lateral wall is found in the 12 o'clock position, with the anterior and posterior walls in their accustomed 9 and 3 o'clock positions. The medial wall and its landmark, the inferior duodenal angle, are seen in the 6 o'clock position, indicative of direct entry intubation.

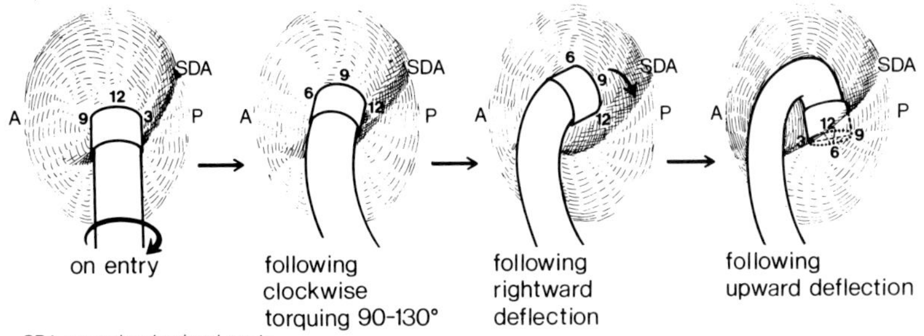

FIG. 24-13. The image positions of the lens for the indirect entry technique in relation to the walls of the duodenal bulb and descending duodenum.

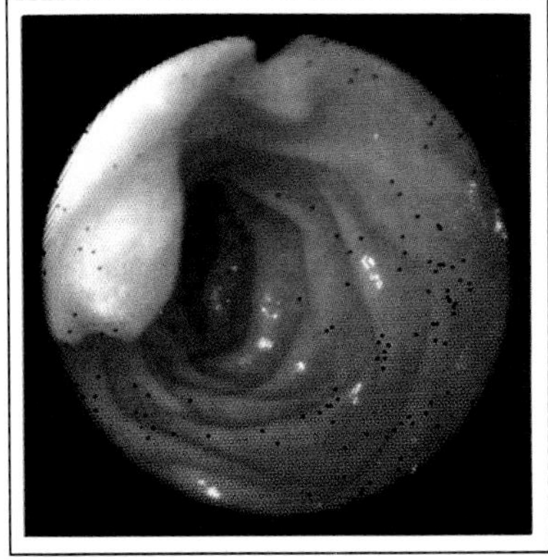

FIG. 24-14.

FIG. 24-14. Descending duodenum after indirect entry intubation. The lumen runs toward the medial wall in the 12 o'clock position. In this orientation the anterior and posterior walls are found to occupy positions in the visual fields opposite from those found in the stomach, with the posterior wall (marked by the major papilla) at 9 o'clock and the anterior wall (with the minor papilla) toward 3 o'clock (see text).

and posterior walls are viewed by the opposite lens positions. In contrast to the stomach and duodenal bulb, the posterior wall is now seen in the 9 o'clock position, and the anterior wall is in the 3 o'clock position (Fig. 24-14). Furthermore, clockwise and counterclockwise torquing produce changes in the tip position just opposite to those produced by the same maneuvers in the stomach. A clockwise torquing maneuver with the indirect entry technique produces anterior (rather than posterior) movement of the tip, and counterclockwise torquing produces posterior (rather than anterior) tip deflection.

Side-Viewing Technique

The orientation of a side-viewing instrument in the stomach and duodenum is simple once one discovers the lens image positions for the side-viewing instrument which correspond to those already known for the forward-viewing endoscope. The side-viewing instrument lens system may be thought of as a forward-viewing lens which has been moved out of the distal tip onto the side immediately adjacent to it, which is also the side closest to the upward deflecting ("upturn") point of the bending portion (Fig. 24-

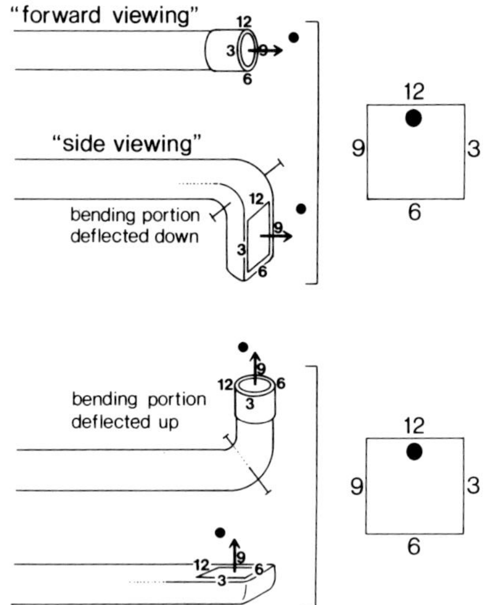

FIG. 24-15. The lens positions of a side-viewing endoscope in relation to those of a forward-viewing instrument.

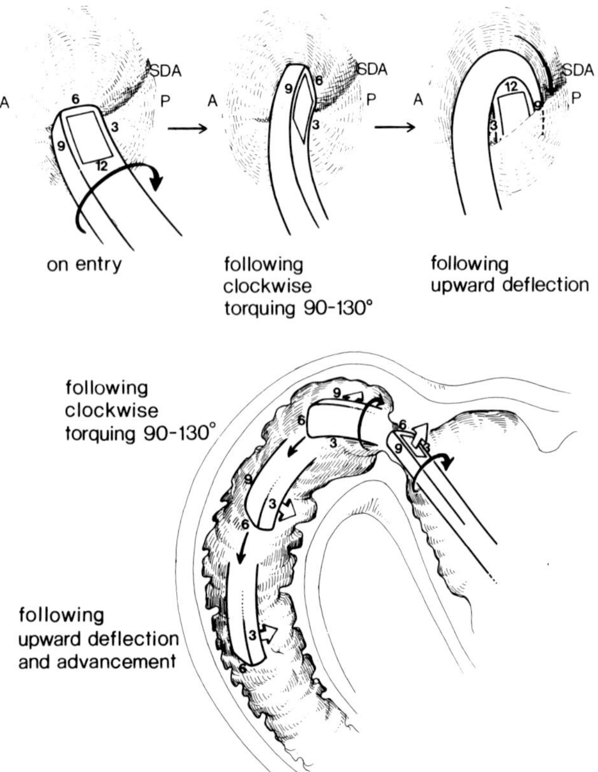

FIG. 24-16. The lens positions of the side-viewing duodenoscope in relation to the walls of the duodenal bulb (upper half) and descending duodenum (lower half) during intubation.

15). The 12 o'clock lens image position of the side-viewing instrument is still the position of the lens closest to this point. The 6 o'clock position is that furthest away from the turning point. Also, as in the case of the forward-viewing instrument, the 9 o'clock and 3 o'clock positions are defined in terms of the left-hand and right-hand sides of the instrument, respectively.

Because the lens system of the side-viewing instrument is 90° out of phase with that of the forward-viewing instrument, to achieve the same view as a forward-viewing instrument in a neutral position the side-viewing instrument must be deflected downward (Fig. 24-15). Conversely, for the forward-viewing instrument to achieve a view comparable to that afforded by the side-viewing instrument, it must be deflected 90° upward (Fig. 24-15). This fact explains why the initial sighting of the pyloric channel with a side-viewing instrument is accomplished with the tip in the downward position; the tip must be elevated to a neutral position (and thus lose the pyloric channel image) for the tip to be into the duodenum (see below).

As the descending duodenum is entered after an initial 120° clockwise torque maneuver (Fig. 24-16), the final orientation within the descending duodenum is the same as that for a forward-viewing instrument where the descending duodenum was intubated using the indirect entry technique. As in this case, the medial wall and inferior duodenal angle would be best seen in the 12 o'clock position with the lateral wall in the 6 o'clock position. As in the case of the indirect entry technique, the anterior and posterior walls are found in positions just opposite to those for the stomach, with the anterior wall being found in the 3 o'clock position and the posterior wall in the 9 o'clock position (Fig. 24-16). As in the case of the indirect entry technique, clockwise torquing and rightward tip deflection produced an anterior change in the tip position (Fig. 24-17, a and b), whereas counterclockwise torquing and leftward deflection produced a change in the tip position toward the posterior direction.

Technique of Examination

Direct Entry Technique

As already mentioned, we find that in about 30% of cases the angle made between the apex and the descending duodenum allows the lumen of the descending duodenum to be seen directly. In these cases the descending duodenum is entered by direct intubation, with the tip deflected down and the endoscope advanced to the most distal point possible (Fig. 24-18a). In some cases where the descending duodenum makes a sharper angulation with the bulb, causing its lumen to be obscured, it still may be entered directly, although blindly, if the tip is placed in the apex and deflected down with the instrument shaft torqued slightly counterclockwise so as to point the tip posteriorly into the descending duodenum.

Once the most distal point which can be intubated directly is reached, it may still be possible to advance the instrument

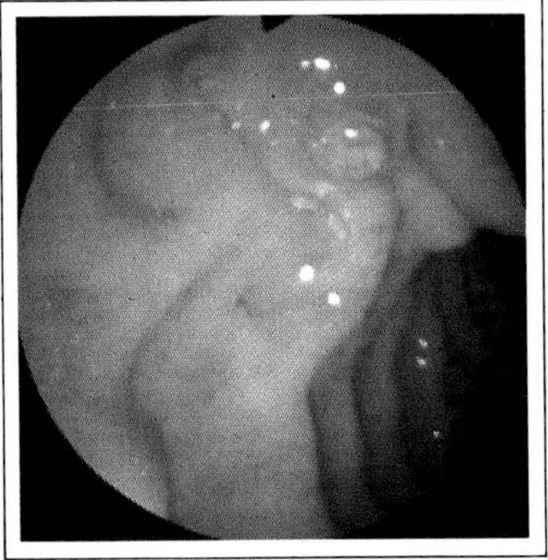

FIG. 24-17a.

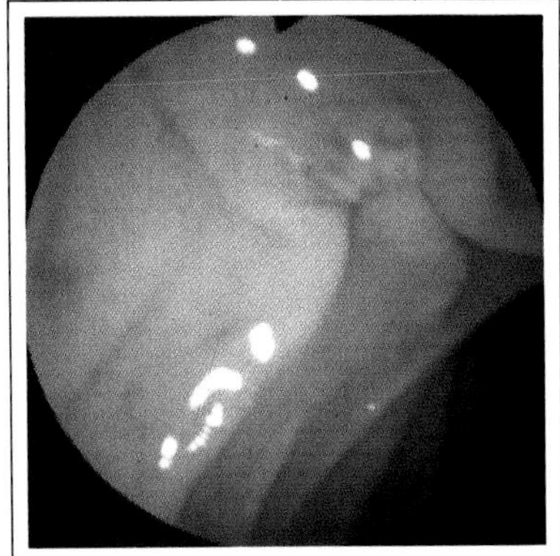

FIG. 24-17b.

FIG. 24-17. a: Descending duodenum, as seen with a side-viewing instrument. The medial wall is denoted by the duodenal papilla, seen at 12 o'clock, with the posterior wall at 9 o'clock. **b:** The posterior wall of the descending duodenum after clockwise rotation. This brings the tip into further alignment with the posterior wall, resulting in the position of the duodenal papilla becoming relatively anterior (at 3 o'clock).

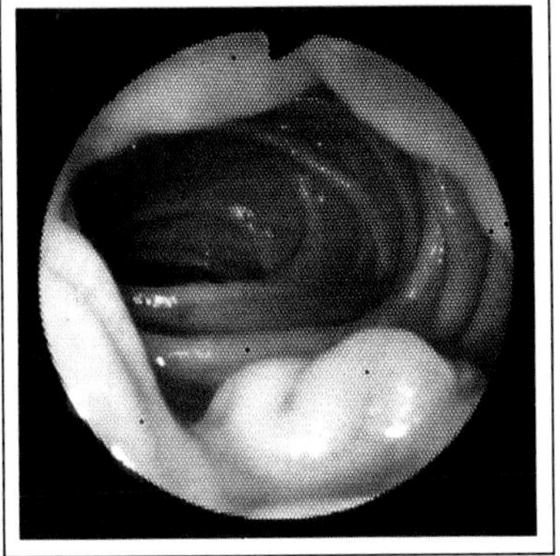

FIG. 24-18a.

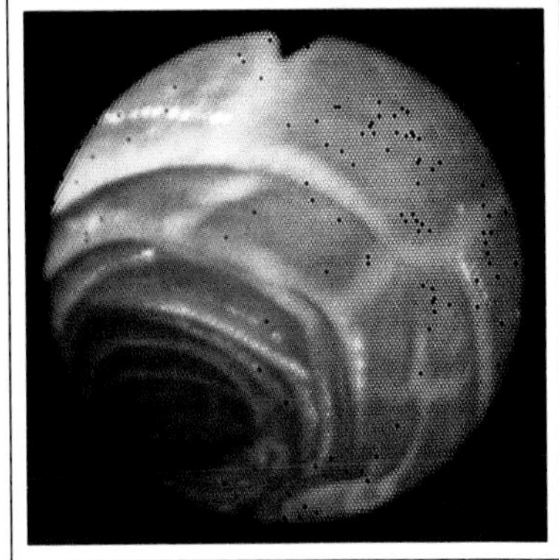

FIG. 24-18b.

FIG. 24-18. a: Mid-descending duodenum after direct entry intubation. This is the most distal point to which the tip could be directly advanced. **b:** Mid-distal descending duodenum after withdrawal and paradoxical advancement.

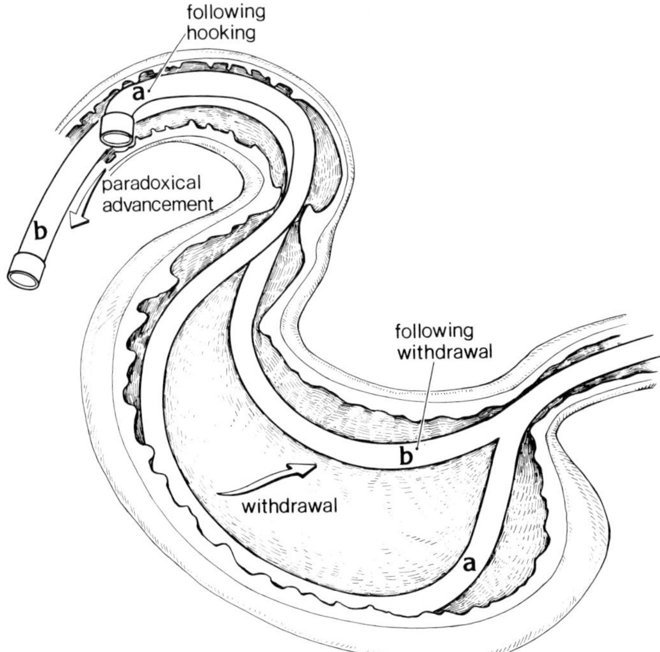

FIG. 24-19. Tip positions in the descending duodenum after withdrawal and paradoxical advancement.

further by paradoxical advancement (Fig. 24-19). This is accomplished by hooking (upward deflection under a fold) and withdrawing the instrument. The paradoxical advancement of the tip in the descending duodenum (Fig. 24-18b) results from reducing the large "bow" which is formed within the stomach on the greater curve in the course of intubating the duodenum (Fig. 24-19). The maneuver succeeds to the extent that the endoscope can be

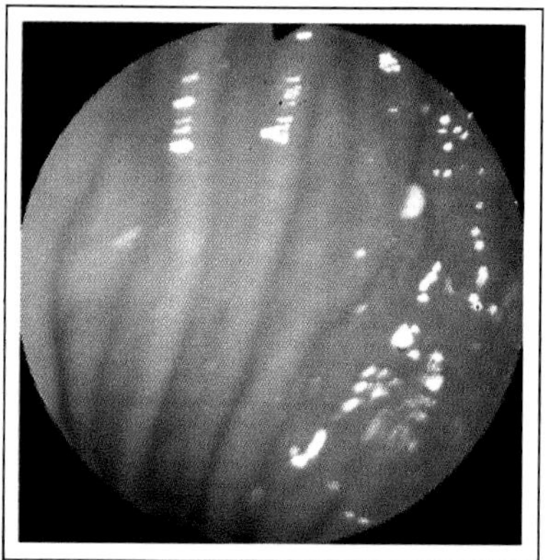

FIG. 24-20a.

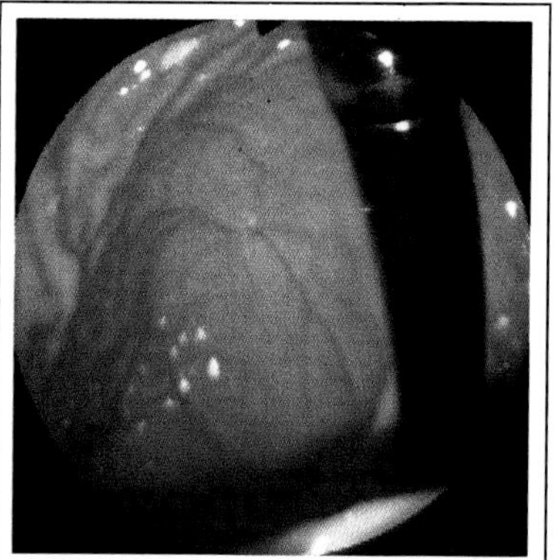

FIG. 24-20b.

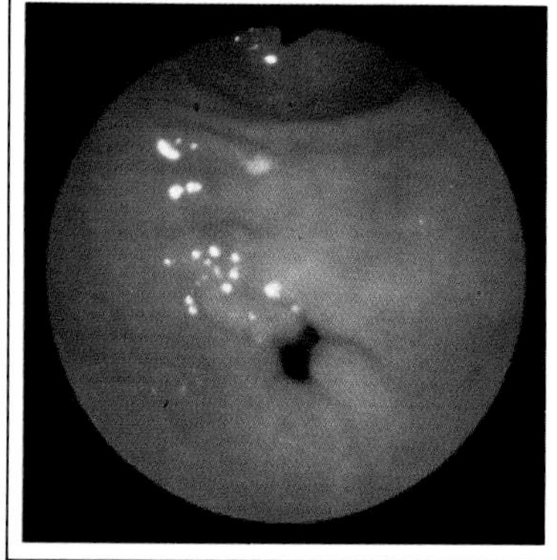

FIG. 24-20c.

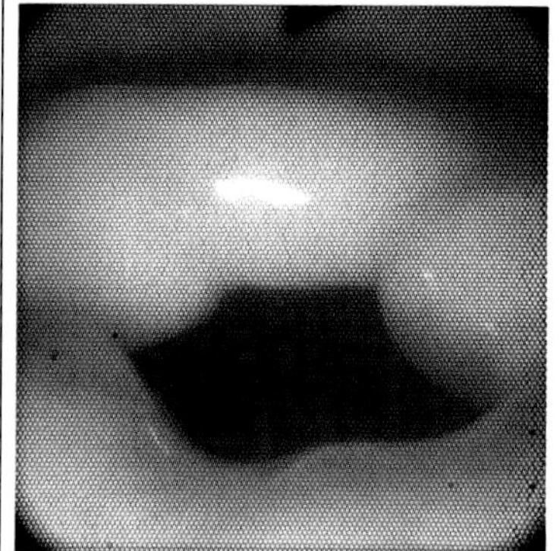

FIG. 24-20d.

FIG. 24-20. a: Lesser curve of the stomach, observed with a side-viewing instrument. After a clockwise torquing maneuver, the lens is directed toward the lumen and greater curve (at 6 o'clock), with the lesser curve seen at 12 o'clock and the anterior and posterior walls in their usual positions (at 9 and 3 o'clock, respectively). **b:** Fundus and cardia as observed with a side-viewing endoscope. Continued upward deflection and forward advancement in a position such as that shown in (a) leads to a J-type retroflexed view of the fundus with the endoscope emerging from the cardia at 5 o'clock and running along the posterior wall. **c:** Antrum and pyloric channel as seen with a side-viewing endoscope. Continued forward advancement with the tip in the "down" direction from a position such as that shown in (a) leads to intubation of the distal body and antrum. **d:** Intubation of the pylorus. The pylorus is still visualized, indicating that the tip is still deflected down (Fig. 24-4). The channel cannot be entered until the tip is deflected up so that it lies *en face* with the pylorus. In this alignment the tip would blindly slide across into the duodenal bulb.

"straightened" in the stomach, i.e., come to lie on the lesser curve (Fig. 24-19).

At the point of furthest advancement, an attempt is made to survey the descending duodenum in two or three arc-like movements at 2- to 3-cm intervals. If there is radiographic suspicion of a lesion, additional arcs are required as well as, in some cases, the use of a side-viewing endoscope (see below).

Indirect Entry Technique

In the majority of cases, because of an acute angulation made with the apex, the descending duodenum must be entered blindly. We have found that this is facilitated by causing the tip to deflect off the posterior lateral wall so as to follow the course of the anterior aspect of the medial wall. This is readily accomplished if the following maneuvers are performed: (a) an initial clockwise (posterior) torquing movement of 90° to 120° at the apex; (b) rightward deflection of the endoscope tip to enter the descending duodenum; and finally (c) upward deflection of the endoscope tip toward the medial wall once the descending duodenum is entered (Fig. 24-13). After these maneuvers, the endoscope is advanced by direct intubation. Once the endoscope is positioned in the distal portion of the descending duodenum, an attempt may be made to enter the third portion using the technique of withdrawal and paradoxical advancement (Fig. 24-19).

Once the point of furthest advancement has been reached, the descending duodenum is examined with two to four arc-like movements beginning posteriorly (9 o'clock) and surveying the medial wall over to its anterior (3 o'clock) position with the lateral wall being seen at 6 o'clock and inspected with downward deflection of the tip (Fig. 24-14).

Side-Viewing Endoscope Technique

The side-viewing endoscope technique has been treated in detail by this author elsewhere.[1] Our purpose here is to present a brief outline of the technique.

The manuevers for introducing the side-viewing endoscope into the hypopharynx are the same as for the forward-viewing instrument (see Chapter 1), with the difference being that one does not attempt to visualize the lumen. Rather, the tip is advanced blindly to the cricopharyngeus, causing the patient to swallow; just afterward the instrument is gently "pushed" into the esophagus. The instrument is then advanced rapidly through the esophagus with no attempt to visualize the lumen unless there is a question regarding the presence of varices. In this case the tip may be deflected down so that the lumen and mucosa can be viewed.

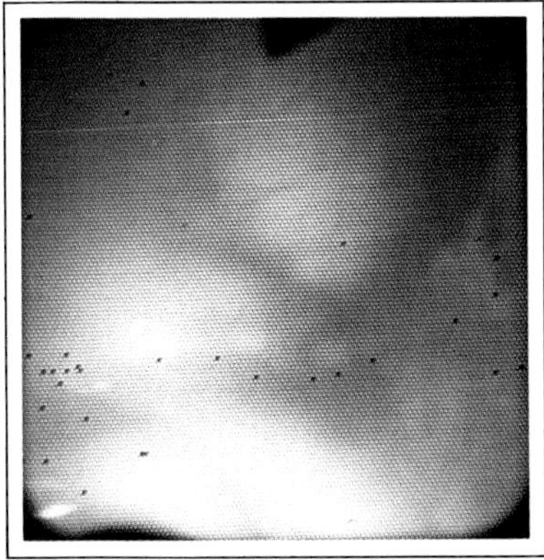

FIG. 24-21a.

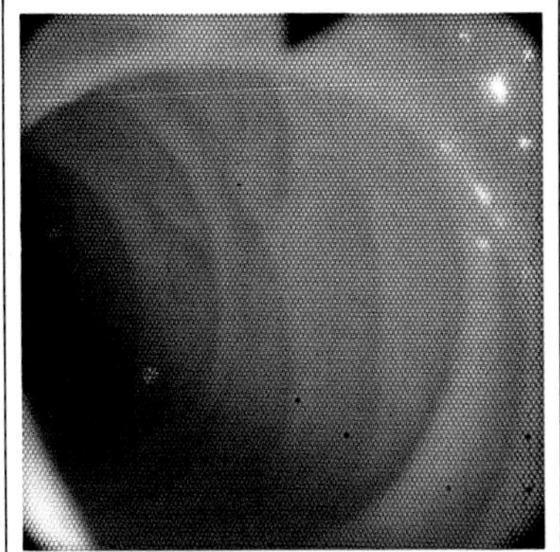

FIG. 24-21b.

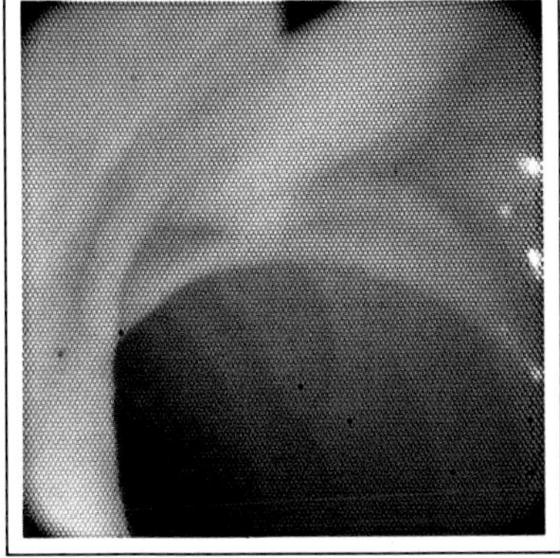

FIG. 24-21c.

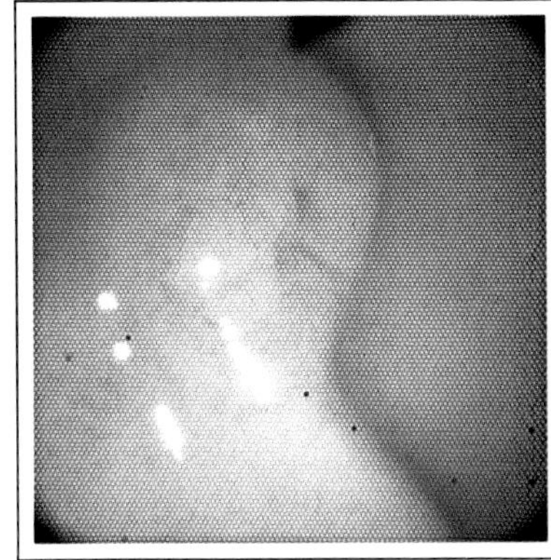

FIG. 24-21d.

FIG. 24-21. a: Apex of the bulb as seen with a side-viewing endoscope. The superior duodenal angle is sensed (but not seen) to be at 3 o'clock as the instrument is torqued clockwise by 120° to 150°. **b:** Medial wall of the descending duodenum as observed with a side-viewing endoscope. After passage across the apex and upward deflection of the tip (Fig. 24-16), the endoscope is blindly advanced down the descending duodenum into the third portion. This is marked by the presence of the duodenal papilla at 12 o'clock. **c:** Duodenal papilla, longitudinal fold (toward 12 o'clock). This may be the first part of the papilla to be recognized, especially if the endoscope has been passed distal to it. **d:** Duodenal papilla located just proximal to the junction of the second and third portions.

Entry into the stomach is made by the same counterclockwise torquing maneuver and upward deflection of the tip as for the forward-viewing instrument (see Chapter 11). Upon entering the stomach, the endoscope tip is turned posteriorly toward the antrum with clockwise torquing of the shaft. Downward deflection of the tip in the stomach permits a complete view of the distal stomach (Fig. 24-20a) and avoids retroflexion into the proximal stomach (Fig. 24-20b), which would be contrary to the desired distal advancement. The endoscopist, however, may wish to take advantage of the side-viewing capability within the stomach to provide the best possible views of the lesser curve, especially of the lower body (Fig. 24-20a), gastric angulus, and antrum. With forward advancement within the antrum, continued downward deflection of the tip is necessary to bring the pyloric channel into view (Fig. 24-20c). Once it is found and the tip is perfectly aligned with the channel, the tip must be deflected up, just as the channel is entered (Fig. 24-20) with the pyloric ring traversed in a blind fashion.

Once in the bulb, the side-viewing endoscope looks directly at the superior wall. Counterclockwise torquing brings the anterior wall into better view, whereas clockwise torquing allows for better definition of the posterior wall.

After entry and the desired examination of the bulb, a 90° to 150° clockwise torquing movement of the shaft is necessary to bring the tip into alignment into the apex (Fig. 24-21a). The apex is entered, and with upward deflection of the tip the descending duodenum is entered (Fig. 24-16). With entry, the lumen is viewed fleetingly; however, it is not desirable to intubate the descending duodenum looking directly at its lumen as this tends to retard forward advancement of the tip. With clockwise torquing and upward deflection off the posterior lateral wall (Fig. 24-16), the tip becomes aligned with the anterior aspect of the medial wall as the descending duodenum is entered. Because of the tendency of the tip to deflect excessively toward the anterior wall during intubation of the descending duodenum, one must correct for this with constant counterclockwise (posterior) torquing. In this way, the tip can generally be advanced into the distal portion of the descending duodenum (Fig. 24-21b) and often into the third portion. In some cases, it is desirable to reduce the bow which forms in the stomach so as to provide further advancement of the tip as well as greater tip control. As with the forward-viewing endoscope, this is best accomplished if the tip can be hooked into the third portion (Fig. 24-19) and withdrawn, with the instrument having been torqued in a clockwise fashion so as to fix the shaft in the stomach up against the posterior wall.

By far the major reason for employing a side-viewing endoscope is to locate and cannulate the duodenal papilla in order to carry out radiographic studies of the pancreas

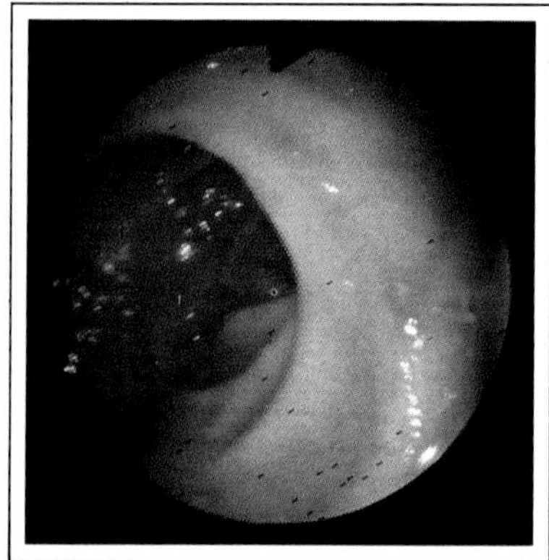

FIG. 24-22a.

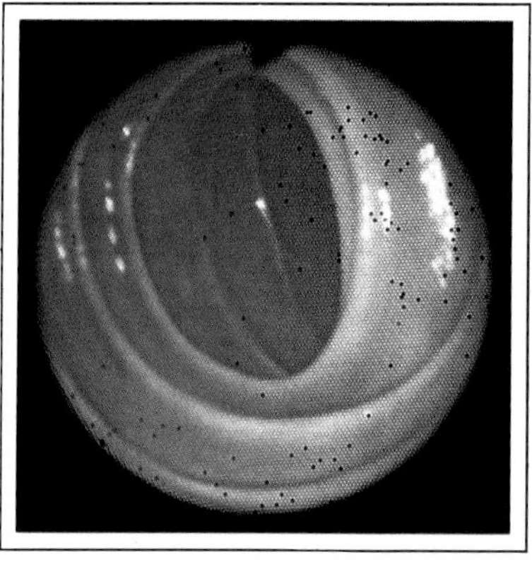

FIG. 24-22b.

FIG. 24-22. Inferior duodenal angle. **a:** Seen as a single mucosal fold. **b:** Seen as the conjunction of two mucosal folds.

and biliary system.[1] This is possible because the medial wall is observed in greater detail than is possible with a forward-viewing instrument. To find the duodenal papilla with a side-viewing instrument, several sweeping arcs are made systematically beginning at the junction of the second and third portions (inferior duodenal angle) in the 9 o'clock (posterior) aspect, moving toward the midline at 12 o'clock and finally on to the anterior aspect at 3 o'clock. Most often, the longitudinal (bifid) fold (see below and Fig. 24-21c) is found first, especially when the tip has been first advanced to a point distal to the papilla. This is first seen in the 12 o'clock (proximal) lens image position [the most proximal portion for the lens (Fig. 24-15)]. As the tip is further withdrawn, the longitudinal fold moves down to the 6 o'clock (distal) position (Fig. 24-21d). After the longitudinal fold, one sees the papillary orifice moving "down" the lens followed by the hooded fold in the 12 o'clock position, at which point the entire duodenal papilla is visualized (Fig. 24-21d).

Normal Appearance of the Descending Duodenum

Anatomic Features

The descending duodenum may be thought of as a cylindrical tube, approximately 10 cm long and 3 to 5 cm wide, bound by the superior duodenal angle above and the inferior duodenal angle below. On inspection, the descending duodenum is seen to be made up of concentric rings of mucosa, the Kerckring folds, which connect the anterior and posterior walls with their medial and lateral aspects. Finally, on the medial wall, generally within 3 cm of its midpoint, one finds the main (Wirsung's) duodenal papilla, and 2 cm proximal and anterior to this is the accessory (Santorini's) papilla. These anatomic features are considered in this section.

Superior duodenal angle.

We have previously discussed the superior duodenal angle in the context of the anatomic landmarks of the duodenal bulb (see above). It marks the junction of the posterior inferior wall of the bulb (at the apex) and the beginning of the medial wall of the descending duodenum (Fig. 24-8a). It is of variable thickness and prominence. In most cases its thickness is that of a typical Kerckring fold (Fig. 24-10b). In about 30% of the cases it is not seen at all (Fig. 24-12), in which case there is a continuous channel between the bulb and the descending duodenum.

Inferior duodenal angle.

The inferior duodenal angle is formed by the medial wall of the descending duodenum and its counterpart, the superior aspect, of the third portion. As such, it is a medial wall landmark. It is viewed in the 12 o'clock position (Fig. 24-22a) if the endoscope was first turned 180° toward the medial wall prior to entry into the descending duodenum (indirect entry technique) or in the 6 o'clock position if the descending duodenum was intubated directly with the 12 o'clock lens position "looking at" the lateral wall.

The appearance of the inferior duodenal angle may be identical with that of other Kerckring folds, the angle itself appearing as simply a Kerckring fold. In other cases the angle is more prominent, being formed by the confluence of several Kerckring folds (Fig. 24-22b).

Kerckring folds.

Kerckring folds are the most prominent structural feature of the descending duodenum and are highly variable in appearance. They are entirely concentric, ring-like mucosal folds, 1 to 2 mm thick and 2 to 4 mm tall (Fig. 24-23a), although their apparent height and thickness may vary with the amount of insufflation of the descending duodenum (Fig. 24-23b). Even after adequate insufflation, however, they may appear taller (4 mm) and thicker (2 mm) than is usually the case, but they are still considered "normal" (Fig. 24-23c). Irrespective of variations in height and thickness, the folds are sharply demarcated, being spaced apart by approximately 2 to 4 mm, sometimes even more widely. They are extremely pliant and can be easily raised (tented) with a biopsy forceps.

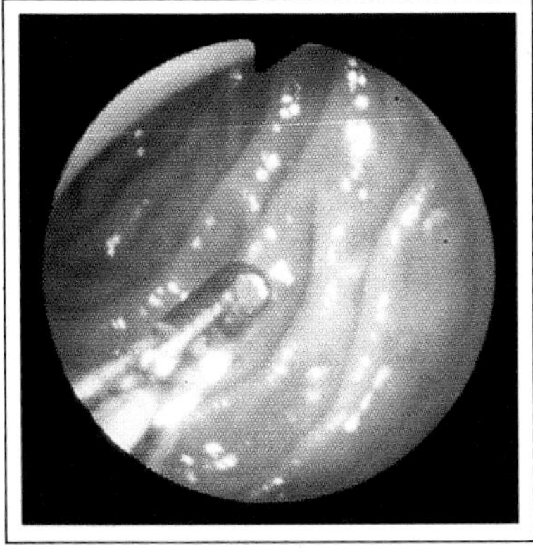

FIG. 24-23a.

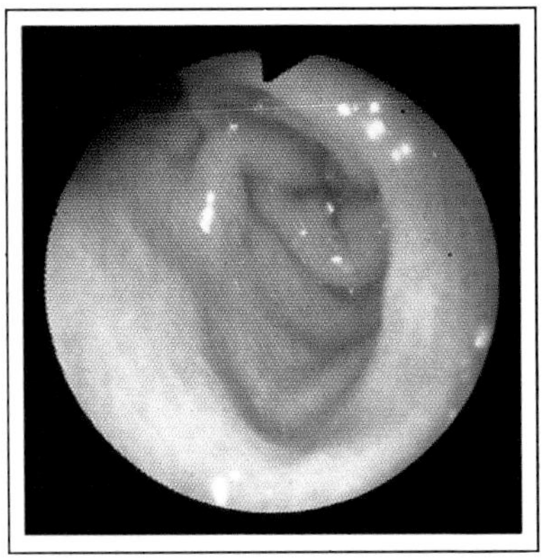

FIG. 24-23b.

FIG. 24-23. Duodenal mucosal (Kerckring) folds. **a:** The forceps open bite width is 5 mm, making the height of both these folds approximately 2 mm. This is one-half of the open bite width. **b:** This is the same case as in (a), but the folds appear thicker because insufflation is not complete. **c:** These are thicker and taller than those in (a) but are still normal.

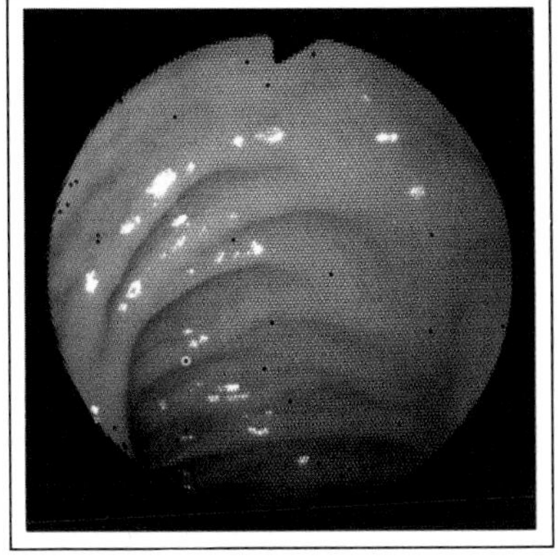

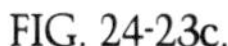

FIG. 24-23c.

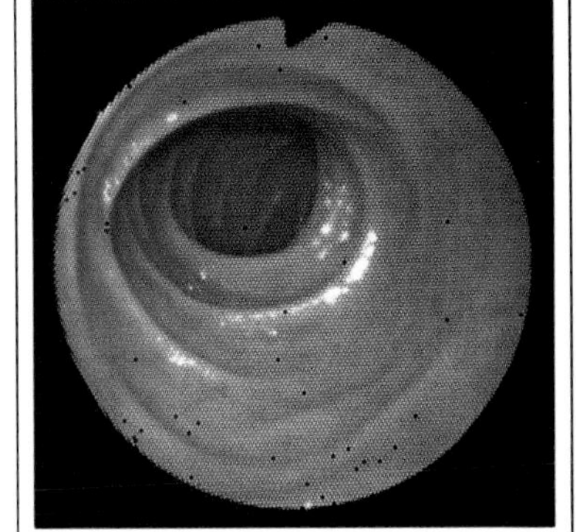

FIG. 24-24.

FIG. 24-24. Luminal diameter of the descending duodenum. The diameter in this case was estimated to be 3.5 cm, which is well within the expected range of the descending duodenum.

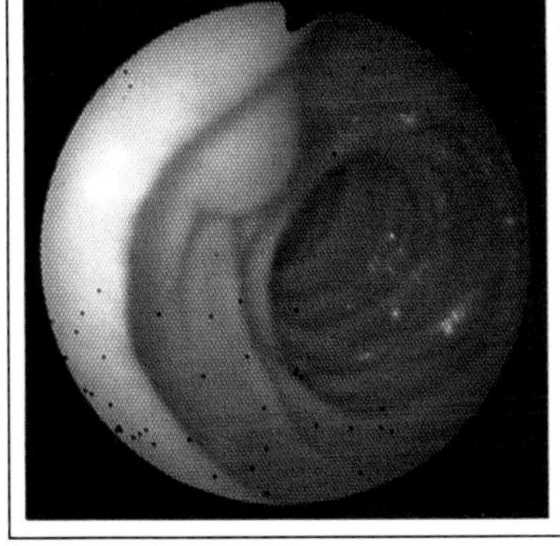

FIG. 24-25a.

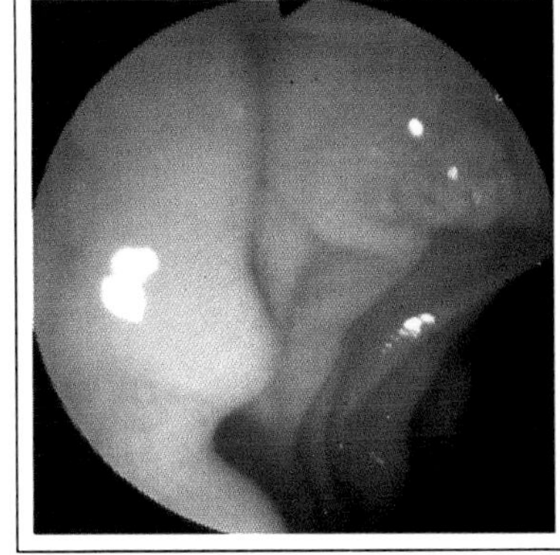

FIG. 24-25b.

FIG. 24-25. a: Duodenal papilla, as observed with a forward-viewing instrument. In this case a tangential view of the hooded fold only (at 11 o'clock) is obtained. **b:** Duodenal papilla as observed with a side-viewing duodenoscope. An *en face* view of Fig. 24-23a was obtained with an instrument designed especially for examining this structure.

Luminal diameter.

The maximum diameter of the descending duodenum varies greatly but is usually between 3 and 4.5 cm, depending on the amount of air insufflation (Fig. 24-24). A descending duodenum having a diameter of greater than 5 cm is considered dilated, although this does not necessarily have any pathologic significance (see Chapter 25).

Duodenal papilla.

The larger (13 mm diameter) forward-viewing endoscope with a turning length of 5 cm or more rarely views the duodenal papilla. However, the currently popular smaller-caliber (9 to 11 mm diameter) instruments with turning lengths of 3 cm or less can provide a reasonable view of the duodenal papilla (Fig. 24-25a), although not with the same definition provided by a side-viewing endoscope specifically developed for viewing this structure in detail (Fig. 24-25b).

If a side-viewing endoscope is employed, one may observe three components (Fig. 24-26a). These are: (a) the hooded fold, which appears as a prominent fold-like eminence just above the orifice; (b) the orifice, consisting of concentric erythematous and granular ring-like folds; and (c) a single or bifid longitudinal fold coming in just below the orifice.

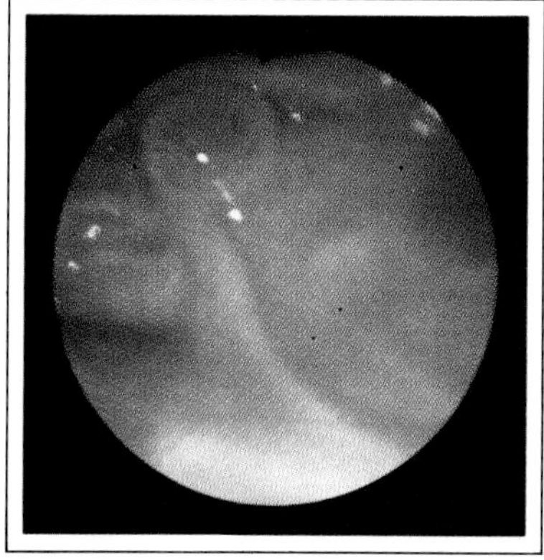

FIG. 24-26a.

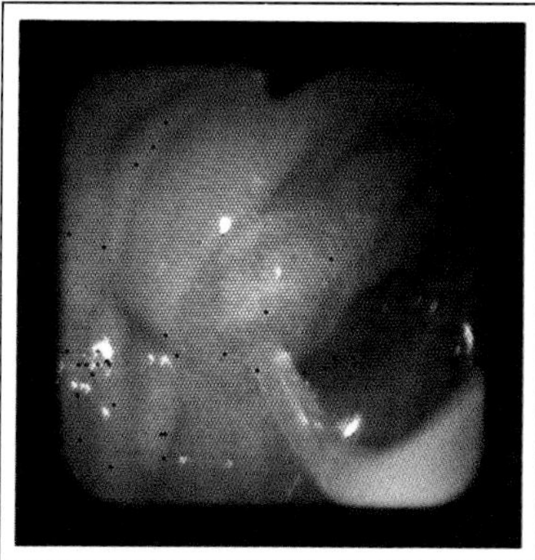

FIG. 24-26b.

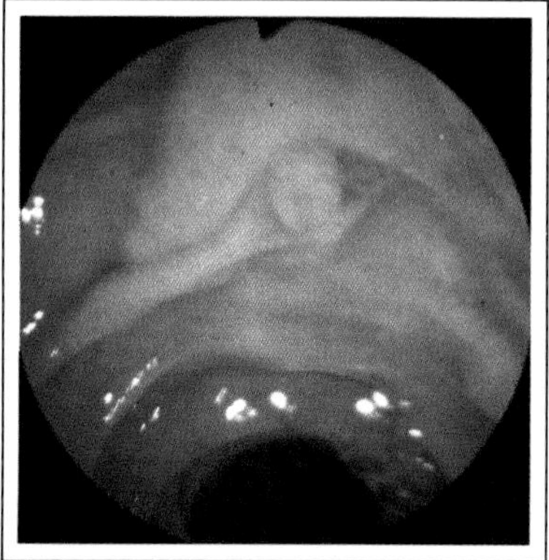

FIG. 24-26c.

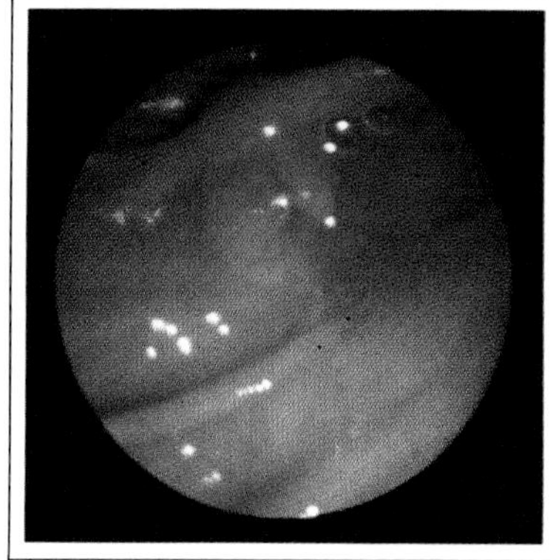

FIG. 24-26d.

FIG. 24-26. a: Duodenal papilla, papillary type. The hooded fold is proximal (at 12 o'clock) and has a diameter of approximately 7.5 mm, which is equal to that of the orifice which appears just below, being erythematous and granular in the center of the field. Just below this is the bifid longitudinal fold at 6 o'clock. **b:** Duodenal papilla, hemispherical type. The hooded fold at 12 o'clock measured approximately 1.5 cm, which is considerably greater than the diameter of the orifice (here cannulated with a polyethylene tube for radiologic studies of the biliary and pancreatic duct systems). **c:** Duodenal papilla, hemispherical type with a recessed orifice. The prominent hooded fold in this example largely obscures the orifice. **d:** Duodenal papilla, flat. A hooded fold was not apparent. The orifice, not well visualized, was seen to be almost flush with the surrounding duodenal mucosa.

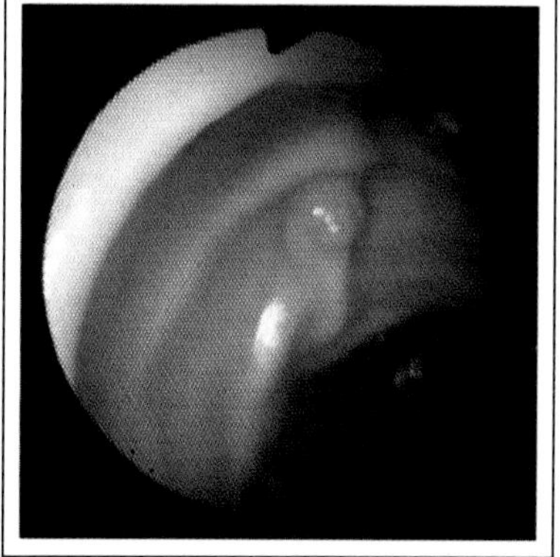

FIG. 24-27a.

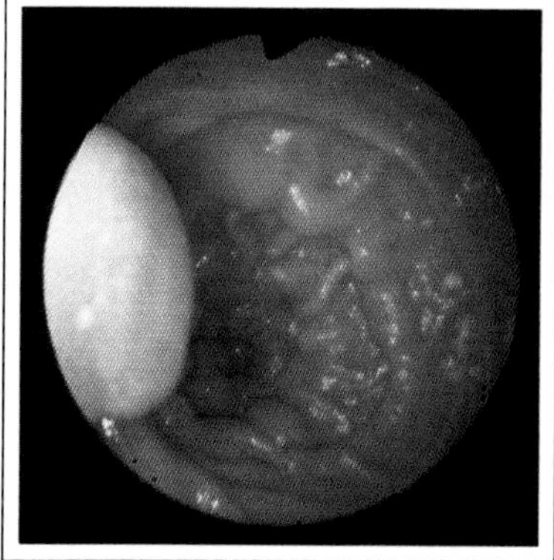

FIG. 24-27b.

FIG. 24-27. a: Duodenal papilla, accessory. A tiny papilla is seen with a forward-viewing instrument. The main papilla was posterior (toward 9 o'clock) and 2 cm distal (b). **b:** Duodenal papilla, hemispheric type as seen with a forward-viewing instrument. In this case the papilla is viewed at 9 o'clock after intubation using the direct entry technique.

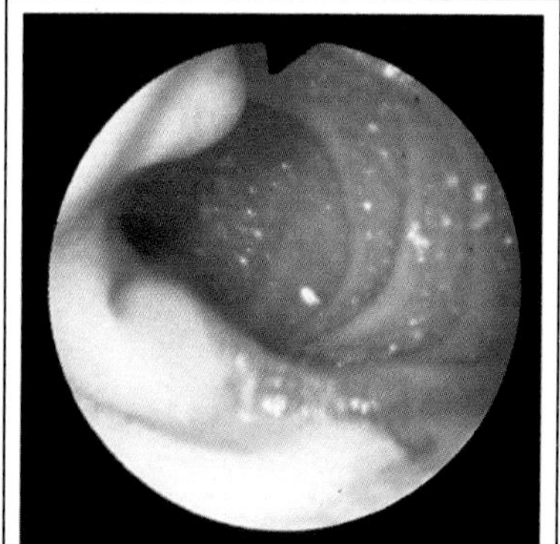

FIG. 24-28a.

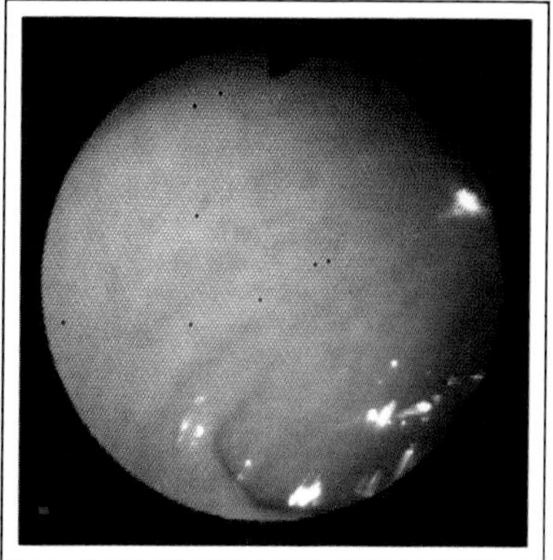

FIG. 24-28b.

FIG. 24-28. a: Descending duodenum with a yellow-orange coloration. This is in contrast to the color of the duodenal bulb (b). **b:** Duodenal bulb, mucosal coloration. The more gray-white coloration of the bulb stands in contrast to the yellow-orange of the descending duodenum.

Based on the appearance of the hooded fold, one can define three types of papilla: (a) the papillary papilla, where the diameter of the hooded fold does not greatly exceed that of the orifice, being less than 10 mm (Fig. 24-26a); (b) the hemispherical papilla, where the diameter of the hooded fold greatly exceeds that of the orifice, being 10 to 15 mm or larger (Fig. 24-26, b and c); and (c) the flat papilla, where the hooded fold is rudimentary (<4 mm) or absent (Fig. 24-26d). We and others[2] find approximately 60% of papillas to be of the hemispherical type, with 30% being papillary and 10% flat.

Even using a forward-viewing endoscope, one may observe the minor papilla as a 1- to 3-mm sessile polyp-like structure in the proximal to mid descending duodenum (Fig. 24-27a). If a forward-viewing endoscope has been introduced using the indirect entry technique, which would preferentially view the medial wall, the minor papilla would be expected in the 3 o'clock (anterior) position of the visual field, 2 cm proximal to the major papilla. This is found by continued counterclockwise torquing and distal intubation for approximately 2 cm (Fig. 24-27b). The relationship of this structure to the major papilla helps differentiate it from a duodenal polyp (see Chapter 30).

Mucosal Appearance

One would expect the mucosal appearance of the descending duodenum to closely resemble that of the duodenal bulb. Histologically, they are virtually identical, yet endoscopically there are differences which are probably related to the optical properties of these two very different anatomic structures. For example, the descending duodenum, as a long cylinder containing bile, tends to diffuse light, causing the mucosa to take on a yellow-orange coloration (Fig. 24-28a) rather than the gray-white appearance of the duodenal bulb (Fig. 24-28b). The increased surface area of the descending duodenum, caused by the presence of the Kercking folds, may be another factor which tends to dissipate light and to give the mucosa a red-orange coloration. Yet another factor may be the presence of bile causing an alteration in light transmission, and the appearance of "redness" similar to its effect when present in the stomach (see Chapter 12). In addition to the difference in the color of descending duodenal mucosa contrasted to that of the bulb is the absence of a mucosal vascular pattern (Fig. 24-28b) in histologically normal mucosa.

REFERENCES

1. Blackstone, M. O. (1980): Endoscopic retrograde cholangiopancreatography in the diagnosis of pancreatic tumors. In: *Tumors of the Pancreas*, edited by A. R. Moossa, pp. 307–353. Williams & Wilkins, Baltimore.
2. Kasugai, T., Kuno, N., Aoki, I., Kizu, M., and Kobayashi, S. (1971): Fiberduodenoscopy: analysis of 353 examinations. *Gastrointest. Endosc.*, 18:9–15.

25

THE DUODENUM—VARIATIONS FROM THE NORMAL APPEARANCE

DUODENAL BULB

Appearances are found in the examination of the duodenal bulb in terms of shape and mucosal detail which are different enough from those usually encountered to suggest an abnormality yet which are of uncertain significance. In this section we consider these under two main headings; the first consideration is structural, i.e., variations in shape, and the second concerns the alterations in mucosal appearance referred to as duodenitis.

Variations in Shape

We consider here two common variations in shape: (a) foreshortening of the bulb; and (b) prominent apical folds, including those which appear mass-like.

Foreshortening of the Bulb

In the course of recurrent peptic ulcer disease, the bulb may contract in size as a result of scarification of the anterior and posterior walls (see Chapter 26). However, we do not regard a "short" bulb (Fig. 25-1) alone as evidence of peptic ulcer disease but simply as a variation of shape.

Prominent Apical Folds

There is great variability in the appearance of the ring-like folds of the apex, from a single fold (Fig. 25-2a) to several slightly elevated apical folds (Fig. 25-2b) and finally to multiple raised (2 to 4 mm) prominent folds (Fig. 25-3c). We have already seen that Kerckring folds may extend several centimeters into the distal bulb or even the mid-bulb (see Chapter 24), giving the mucosa a corrugated texture. Because the finding of prominent duodenal bulb and apical folds (along with that occurring in the descending duodenum) is similar radiologically and endoscopically in patients with Zollinger-Ellison syndrome,[1,2] some endoscopists interpret this as a definite abnormality and suggest the possibility of gastric hypersecretion on the basis of this alone. However, we find prominent apical folds in 30 to 40% of all patients examined, the majority of whom have no findings or history suggestive of ulcer disease. To date, no study has been reported which suggests any association of the presence of Kerckring folds of the mid or distal duodenal bulb with gastric hypersecretion. For the present, therefore, large folds of the apex or those which extend proximally into the bulb must be regarded simply as a variation in the appearance of the duodenal bulb without any direct relation to gastric hypersecretion or peptic ulcer disease.

Mass-like Deformity

A discrete area may be found within the bulb, but especially at the apex (Fig. 25-3), which takes on the appearance of a submucosal mass. These have been recognized radiologically as "flexural pseudolesions."[3] Biopsy of these "masses" reveals normal tissue or shows nonspecific histologic changes.[4] However, the concern raised by radiographic study or endoscopy may cause the endoscopist to suspect a submucosal tumor. Large-particle biopsy (see Chapter 1) or complete electrosurgical excision may be thought desirable for any polypoid mass of the duodenum, but successful execution of this technique in the apical area is particularly difficult and potentially dangerous, with perforation and hemorrhage as potential complications.

The endoscopist may take some comfort in the fact that the large majority of polyps of the duodenal bulb are non-neoplastic.[4] Even for a polyp of the apex having a diameter of 1 cm or more, we find that there is a 30 to 40% chance that a definitive examination (snare biopsy or surgical excision) will reveal it to be only a mass-like deformity, espe-

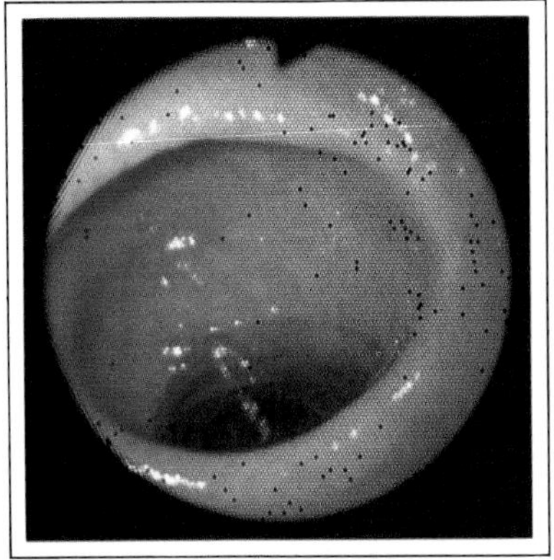

FIG. 25-1.

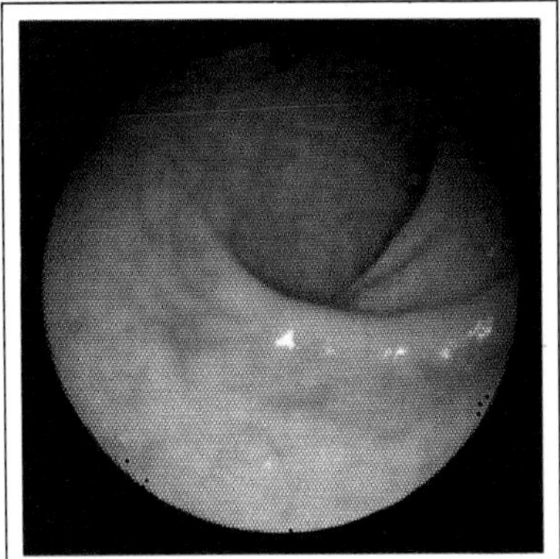

FIG. 25-2a.

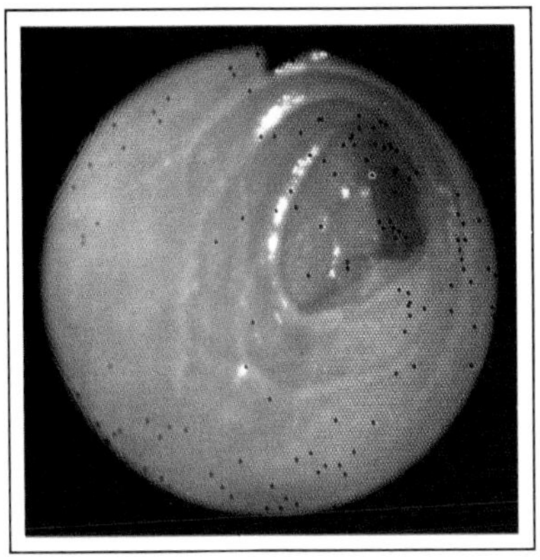

FIG. 25-2b.

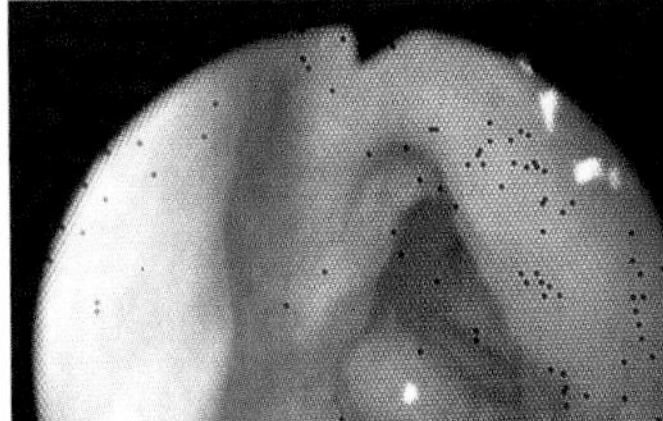

FIG. 25-2c.

FIG. 25-1. Foreshortened duodenal bulb. The apex is seen within 2 cm of the pyloric ring in a patient with no symptoms to suggest peptic ulcer disease.

FIG. 25-2. a: Apical folds, flat appearance. A single apical fold is present along with the superior duodenal angle beginning at 2 o'clock. **b:** Apical folds extending into the mid-bulb. The Kerckring folds of the descending duodenum extend into the mid-bulb. **c:** Apical folds, enlarged. These are both tall (3 to 4 mm) and thick (2 to 3 mm) in contrast to those in (a).

cially if the mucosa can be easily tented (Fig. 25-3b). Of five patients with polyps (the apex exceeding 1 cm) in whom over a 5-year period surgical excision or large-particle biopsy was performed, only two had malignant potential (one carcinoid and one leiomyoma); a lipoma was found in one other patient and normal mucosa in the remaining two (Fig. 25-3c).

Variations in Mucosal Appearance—Duodenitis

In 1 to 3% of examinations performed by us, a nonspecific alteration in mucosal appearance of the duodenal bulb is the principal endoscopic finding. In these cases we find the mucosa to be focally erythematous (Fig. 25-4a), diffusely so (Fig. 25-4b), or nodular (Fig. 25-4c). Others have found these alone or in combination in up to 20% of the patients endoscoped.[5] In cases where these appearances are present, the term "duodenitis" is used with the justification that in up to 50% of such patients the endoscopic appearance is associated with histologic findings of acute inflammation (the presence of polymorphonuclear leukocytes), which is rarely found in biopsies taken from endoscopically normal mucosa.[6] For the remainder (up to 50%[6]), chronic inflammation, gastric metaplasia, or eosinophilic infiltrates are present—findings which occur in only 30% of those with endoscopically normal duodenal mucosa.[6]

The endoscopic finding of duodenitis in the mucosa surrounding ulcers (Fig. 25-5), which on biopsy shows acute inflammation, has given rise to the notion that duodenitis found by itself is an ulcer-equivalent, especially in patients with ulcer-like symptoms.[7] Indeed, in one prospective study of 14 symptomatic patients[7] where the sole endoscopic finding was duodenitis, six of eight whose symptoms persisted had ulcers at subsequent endoscopy; six became asymptomatic on treatment, with the duodenitis disappearing in five. Further support for the concept of duodenitis as an ulcer equivalent was a report of a controlled trial showing symptomatic and endoscopic improvement with cimetidine in comparison to placebo treatment.[7a] Cotton et al.,[6] however, followed 21 patients with ulcer-like symptoms who had only duodenitis, with the biopsies showing acute changes; they found that the symptoms persisted in 11 despite standard ulcer management. In only two of eight who had a second endoscopy were ulcers actually found. In the remainder, the finding was again duodenitis.[6]

Others have found no relationship between the symptoms and the presence or severity of duodenitis.[5] In one study where the course of 50 patients with duodenitis was reviewed 6 months after endoscopy and compared with a control group having a "normal"-appearing bulb, no differences were found between the two groups regarding continuing symptoms or antacid use.[5] Palmer advised against attaching any clinical importance to duodenitis except for acute gastrointestinal bleeding (see Chapter 38).[8]

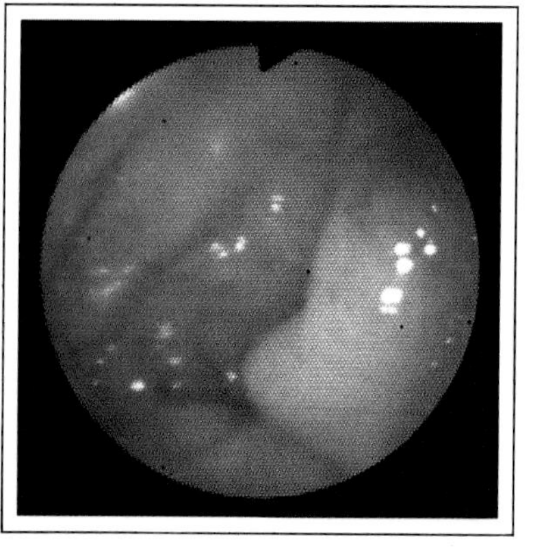

FIG. 25-3a.

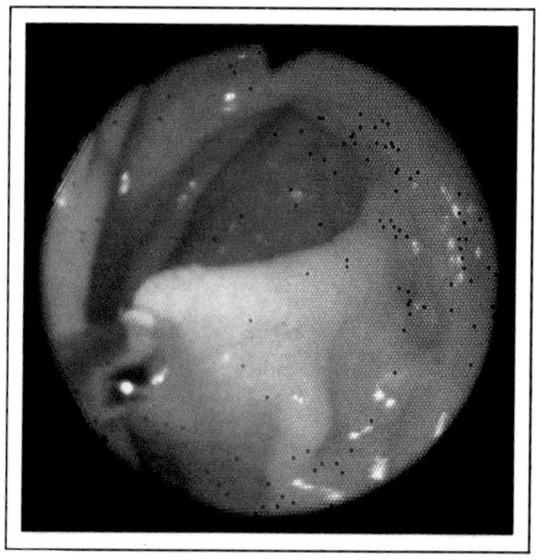

FIG. 25-3b.

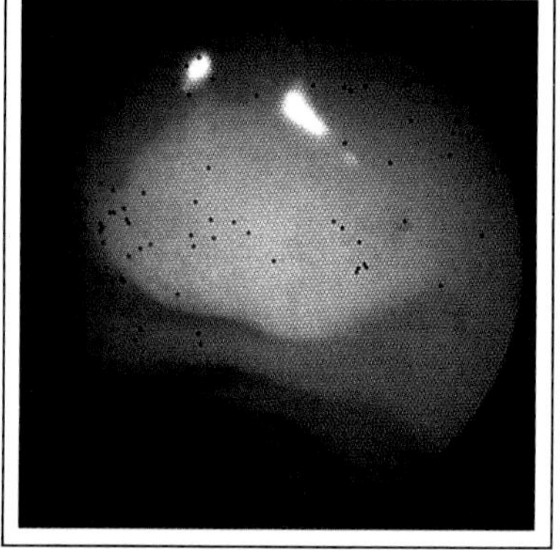

FIG. 25-3c.

FIG. 25-3. Apical mass-like deformity. **a:** A single mass-like fold at the apex stands out from the rest. **b:** The mucosa of the prominent mass-like apical fold in (a) is easily tented, i.e., raised up with a biopsy forceps, suggesting that it is not a submucosal tumor. **c:** "Mass" of redundant mucosa, surgically proven. The patient was explored because of the finding of this apical "mass." A wedge resection, however, revealed only normal mucosa.

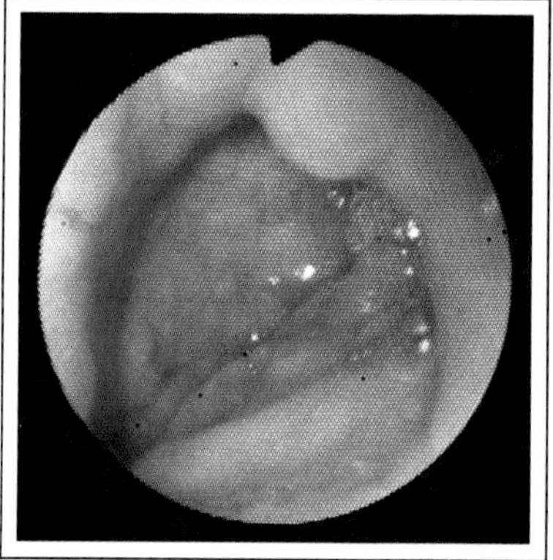

FIG. 25-4a.

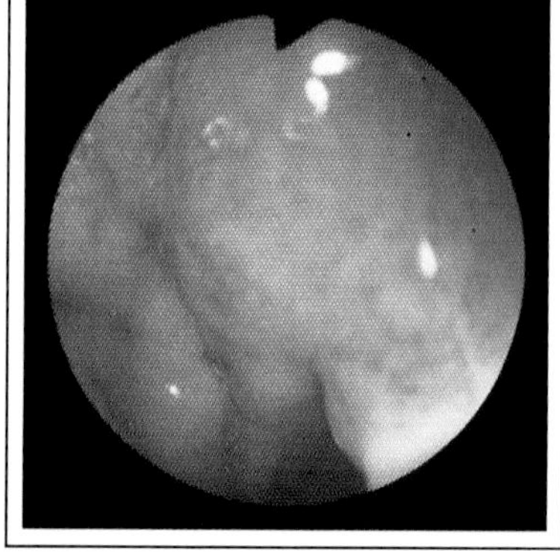

FIG. 25-4b.

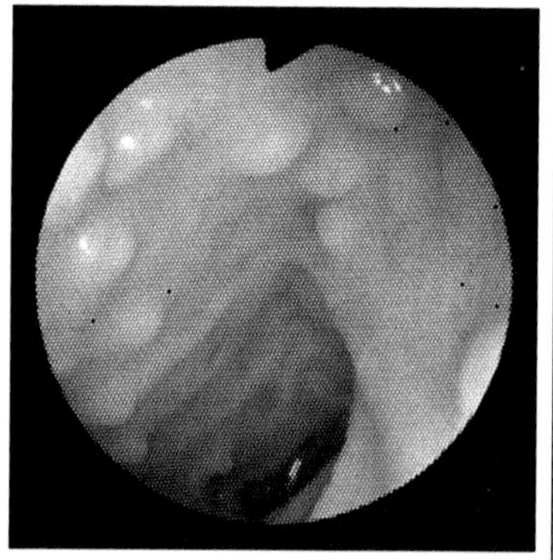

FIG. 25-4c.

FIG. 25-4. a: Duodenitis with focal erythema of the bulb (apical area). Biopsies of this area showed acute and chronic inflammation. **b:** Duodenitis with diffuse bulb erythema. A close-up view of the mucosa shows a characteristic punctate erythema or what has been termed the salt and pepper appearance. Biopsy in this case showed acute and chronic inflammation. **c:** Duodenitis with mucosal nodularity. Biopsy showed chronic inflammation only.

Based on available evidence, one may wish to regard duodenitis that is seen as focal or diffuse erythema as a possible "ulcer-equivalent," especially if associated histologically with the acute inflammatory changes found in many patients with unequivocal duodenal ulcers.[7,9] Still, this would be reasonable only for symptoms typical of peptic ulcer disease. Even for typical ulcer symptoms the chance of medical management succeeding is no more than 75%,[7a] and in our experience only about 50%. For patients with other symptoms, especially in the absence of acute inflammation histologically, we find no predictable response to medical therapy.

Appearance

The endoscopist may expect one of three appearances in patients with duodenitis, although all may coexist. These are: (a) confluent or patchy erythema; (b) erosions; and (c) nodularity.

Erythema.

Erythema is the commonest finding, being either patchy (Fig. 25-4a) or diffuse (Fig. 25-4b). In our cases of duodenitis and in the experience of others,[10,11] approximately two-thirds of the cases recognized at endoscopy have erythema

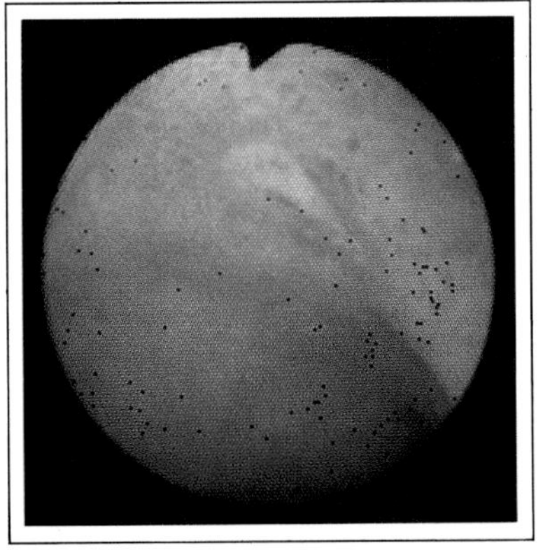

FIG. 25-5.

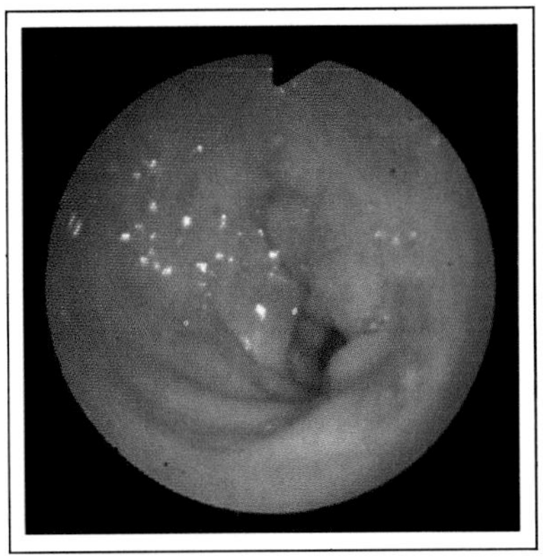

FIG. 25-6a.

FIG. 25-5. Duodenitis surrounding an active peptic ulcer. This has a punctate appearance similar to the salt and pepper type of duodenitis found in Fig. 25-4b.

FIG. 25-6. a: Duodenitis appearing as focal erosions of the apex. **b:** Duodenitis appearing as focal erythema with white exudates (exudative duodenitis). Biopsy showed these exudates to consist of granulation tissue, suggesting that this finding is an intermediate between focal (red) erosions alone (a) and the duodenitis surrounding active ulcers (c). **c:** Duodenal ulcer with duodenitis of the surrounding mucosa. In addition to erythema, focal inflammatory exudates were present on the opposite wall (b).

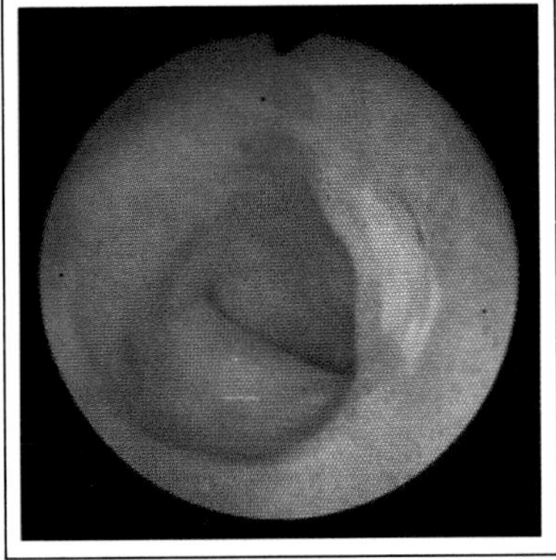

FIG. 25-6b.

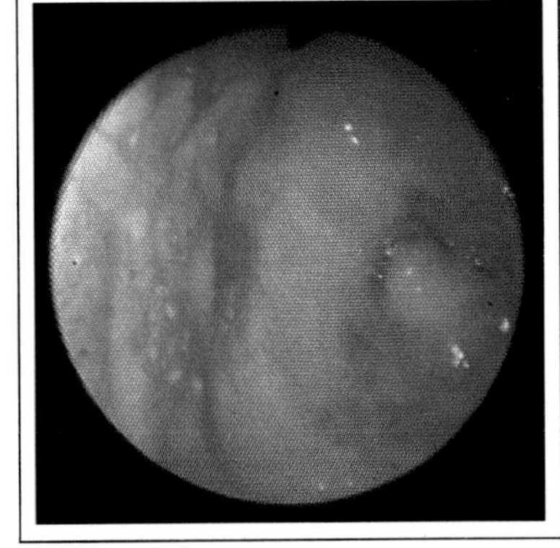

FIG. 25-6c.

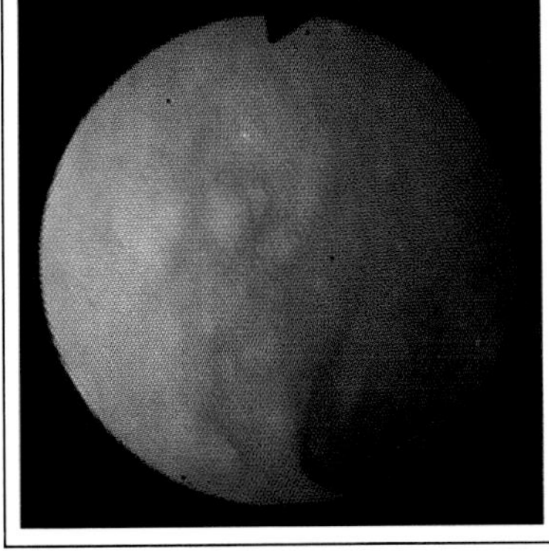

FIG. 25-7a.

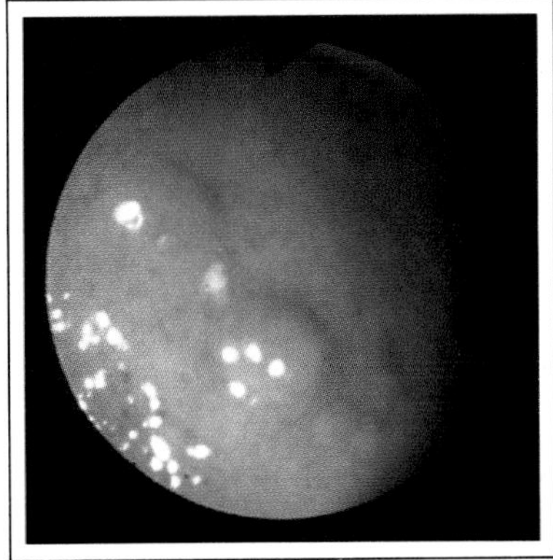

FIG. 25-7b.

FIG. 25-7. Nodular duodenitis. **a:** Mucosal nodularity with 1- to 3-mm excrescences running from the duodenal bulb to the descending duodenum. Biopsy showed chronic inflammation only. **b:** Larger mucosal nodules (3 to 4 mm) were found in the bulb. Some erythema of their surface mucosa was also noted. Biopsies nevertheless showed chronic inflammation only.

either as focal (.3 to 1.5 cm) zones or as diffuse reddening of the entire bulb. In patients in whom the erythema is confined to small (1 to 3 mm) areas with intervening pale ones, the term "salt and pepper" appearance has been used (Fig. 25-4b). Histologically, acute inflammation with polymorphonuclear leukocytes has been found in about 50%.[6,10]

Erosions.

Discrete, focal erosions are a predominant feature in about 20% of our cases (Fig. 25-6a). These are either simple erosions which consist of focal red spots (1 to 5 mm) or exudative erosions, generally 1 to 3 mm which appear as white adherent inflammatory exudates (Fig. 25-6b) but are occasionally larger (Fig. 25-6c). Histologically, about 75% of erosions show acute changes, especially with erosions of the exudative type.[11] For this reason we regard focal erosions, especially those of the exudative type, as the duodenitis appearance most likely to be an ulcer-equivalent.

Nodularity.

Mucosal nodules (excrescences) are found in 10% or less of the cases endoscopically called duodenitis.[11] These range in size from 1 to 3 mm (Fig. 25-7a) and are generally confined to the duodenal bulb, although they may continue into

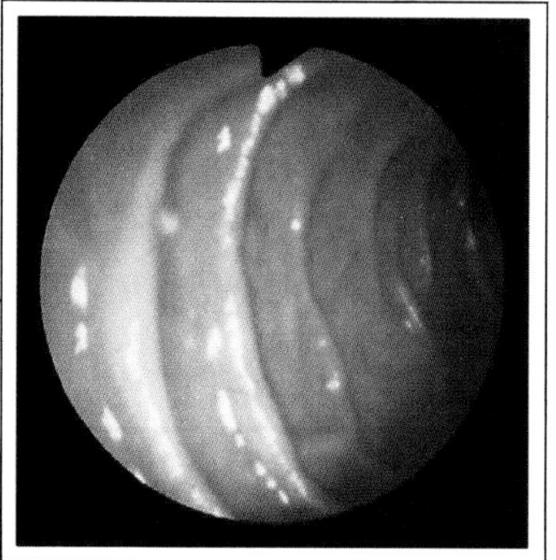

FIG. 25-8a.

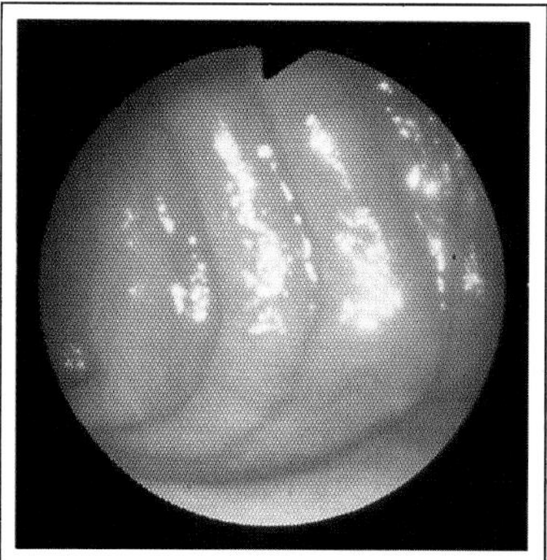

FIG. 25-8b.

FIG. 25-8. a: Normal Kerckring folds of the descending duodenum, 1 to 3 mm tall and 1 to 2 mm thick. **b:** Thickened Kerckring folds, 3 to 5 mm tall and 2 to 4 mm thick. Biopsies, however, were entirely normal.

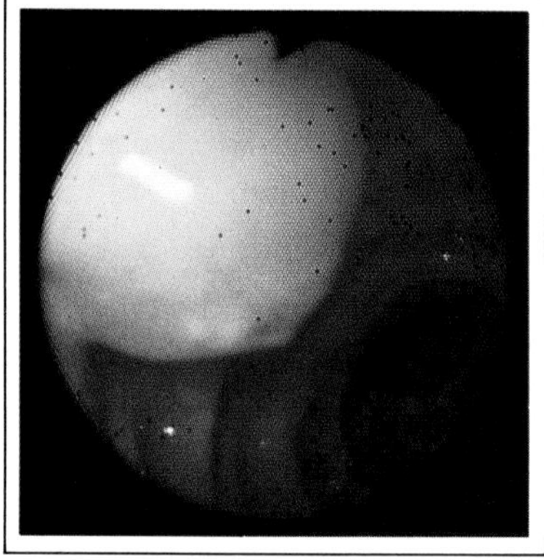

FIG. 25-9a.

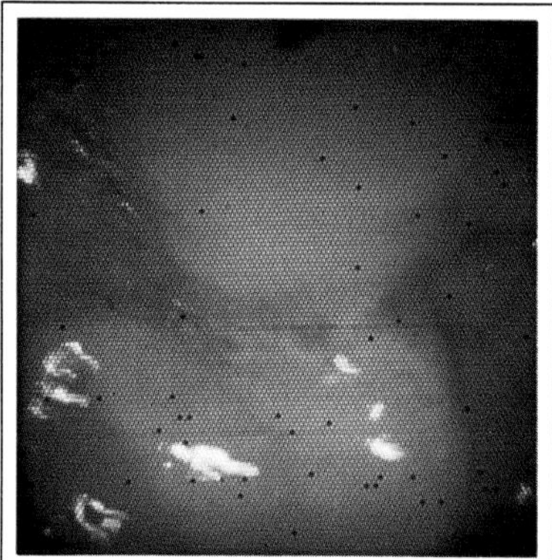

FIG. 25-9b.

FIG. 25-9. a: Prominent duodenal papilla seen with a forward-viewing endoscope. The hooded fold in this case was estimated to be 1.5 by 2 cm, projecting out to nearly half the diameter of the lumen in a patient without pancreatic or biliary disease. **b:** A prominent duodenal papilla seen with a side-viewing endoscope. In this case the prominent hooded fold is seen along with a large longitudinal fold in a patient with a common bile duct stone.

the descending duodenum. The mucosal folds of the apex, in the presence of this nodularity, are normal or slightly increased in thickness; however, mucosal coloration is usually normal. In some cases, however, this may verge on erythema (Fig. 25-7b). Histologically, there is generally an increased cellularity of the lamina propria, but acute changes are uncommon.[11] For this reason, this appearance is the one least expected to be correlated with ulcer-like symptoms. It may be that the mucosal appearance represents an altered growth pattern associated with a chronic inflammatory infiltrate, similar to the tiny mucosal excrescences which one may see in patients with atrophic gastritis (see Chapter 14). In other patients with nodular duodenitis, biopsy shows the 2- to 4-mm nodules to consist of heterotopic gastric mucosa (see Chapter 30).

DESCENDING DUODENUM

Like the duodenal bulb, there are both structural and mucosal appearances which can be classified definitely as either normal or abnormal. The structural appearances falling into this gray area are: (a) prominence or thickening of the Kerckring folds; (b) enlargement of the duodenal papilla; and (c) dilatation of the lumen. The troublesome mucosal appearances of the descending duodenum which also must be considered are: (a) erythema; (b) nodularity; and (c) granularity, as in the "snow-white" duodenum.

Structural Variations

Prominence or Thickening of the Kerckring Folds

Generally, Kerckring folds range up to 3 to 4 mm in height and 2 to 3 mm in width (Fig. 25-8a). Folds of greater than 3 mm in either dimension may strike the examiner as prominent or thickened (Fig. 25-8b). We find that in nearly all of these cases there is no associated disorder, e.g., gastric hypersecretion, to account for this finding; hence it must be regarded as a nonspecific appearance.

Enlarged Duodenal Papilla

Even with a forward-viewing endoscope, enlargement of the duodenal papilla, especially one of the hemispherical type (see Chapter 24), may be noted. This can exceed 1.5 cm and occasionally 2 cm (Fig. 25-9a). There is probably no upper limit of normal for the hooded fold, which merges into surrounding Kerckring folds and thus gives the impression of enlargement beyond any actually present. Although enlargement of the duodenal papilla is the commonest finding in patients with pancreatic carcinoma (see Chapter 29) and can be seen in pancreatitis and biliary calculus disease involving the common bile duct (Fig. 25-9b), because it is nonspecific this appearance alone in the absence of other clinical findings should not cause one to embark on an investigation of a patient for these conditions.

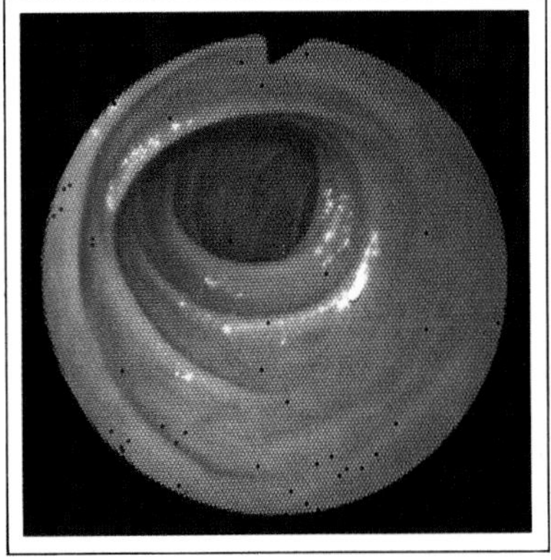

FIG. 25-10a.

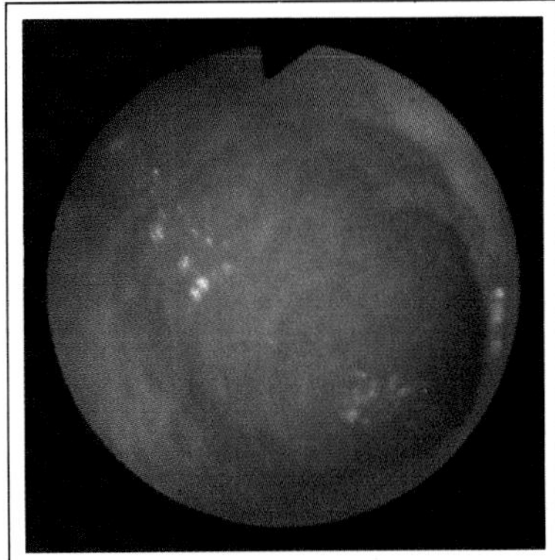

FIG. 25-10b.

FIG. 25-10. a: Descending duodenum, normal luminal diameter. This was estimated to be 3.5 cm. The Kerckring fold pattern is strikingly evident. **b:** Dilated-appearing descending duodenum in a patient with a profound recent weight loss from anorexia nervosa. Starvation with profound weight loss in these cases may result in thinning of the muscle layer, causing the descending duodenum to appear dilated. Consistent with this is the loss of Kerckring folds [in contrast to (a)]. Despite the degree of luminal dilatation, one need not see either mechanical obstruction or a motor disorder, e.g., scleroderma (see Chapter 27).

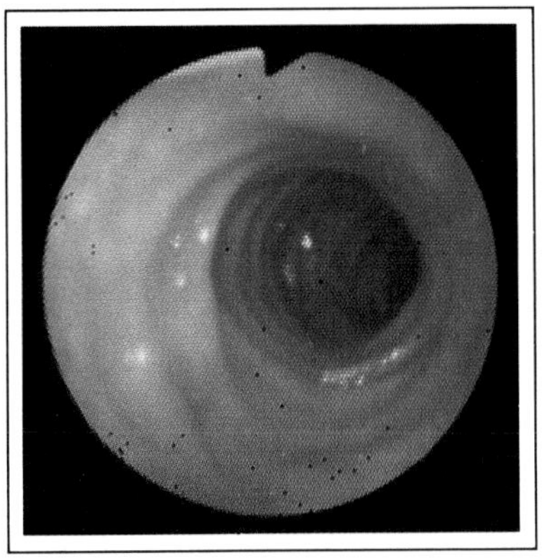

FIG. 25-11a.

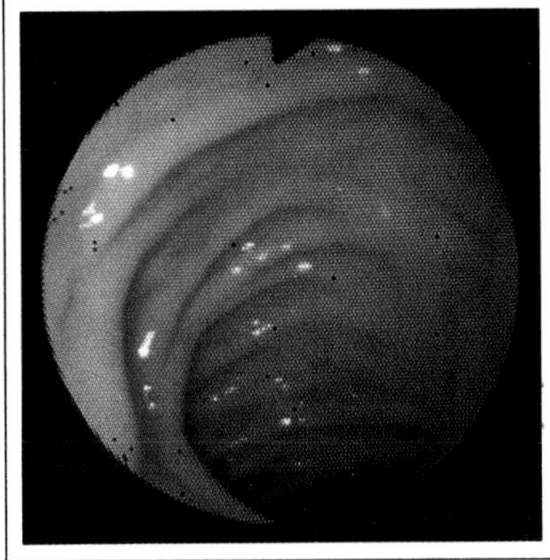

FIG. 25-11b.

FIG. 25-11. a: Descending duodenum with slight mucosal erythema. Biopsies were negative, and the patient had nonspecific abdominal complaints. **b:** Descending duodenum with a more typical coloration.

Dilatation

If one estimates the maximum diameter of the descending duodenum using the open bite width method (see Chapter 15), most cases would fall in the range of 3 to 5 cm (Fig. 25-10a). A diameter in excess of 5 cm is not necessarily the result of mechanical obstruction or a motor disorder, e.g., scleroderma (see Chapter 27). We have seen nonspecific dilatation in thin patients, especially those with recent substantial weight loss, as in anorexia nervosa. We believe that this may occur as a result of thinning of the muscle layer of the descending duodenum, possibly accounting for its tendency to balloon up with air and thus appear dilated (Fig. 25-10b). We therefore regard dilatation itself as a nonspecific finding.

Variations in Mucosal Appearance

Erythema

Mucosal coloration varies greatly, especially along the tips of Kerckring folds (Fig. 25-11). One may see mucosa as pink-gray or even orange-red (Fig. 25-11a) rather than the more usual yellow-gray (Fig. 25-11b). These color changes occur in both asymptomatic patients and those with a variety of nonspecific gastrointestinal complaints. Biopsies of mucosa showing some reddening, or erythema, may be normal or have a nonspecific increase in chronic inflammatory cells.

The significance of erythema of the descending duodenum is even less clear than that of the duodenal bulb, already discussed as duodenitis (see above). First, the long cylindrical shape of the descending duodenum and the presence of bile may affect the way light is reflected from the mucosal surface, giving the impression of redness, even though the mucosa is histologically normal (Fig. 25-11a). Even in cases where the erythema is not an artifact, being associated with a histologic abnormality, the clinical significance of this relating to specific symptoms and their response to treatment is entirely unknown.

We therefore regard the appearance of erythema of the descending duodenum, especially when found in the context of Kerckring folds of normal height and width, to be entirely nonspecific and refer to it as simply erythema. Some choose to call this duodenitis, especially if the biopsy shows inflammatory change. Whatever one calls it, we believe it is unwise to attribute any symptoms to it, regarding this as a variation of normal mucosal appearance.

Nodularity

Rather than a smooth mucosal appearance, the endoscopist may encounter in the descending duodenum discrete, tiny (2 to 4 mm) excrescences (Fig. 25-12a) or larger (5 to

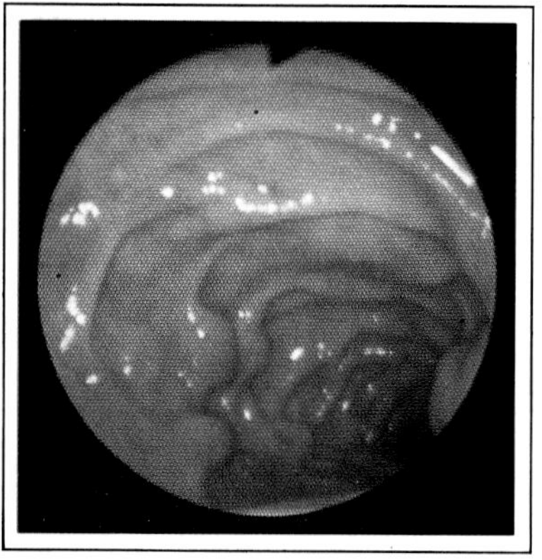

FIG. 25-12a.

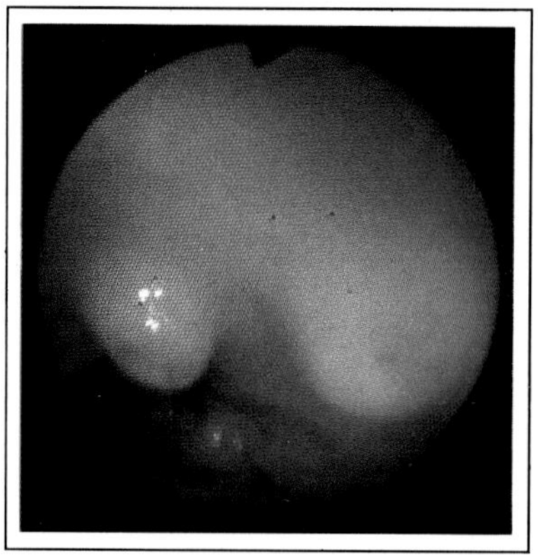

FIG. 25-12b.

FIG. 25-12. a: Nodular duodenitis of the descending duodenum. In this case biopsy of representative 2- to 4-mm nodules showed chronic inflammation. **b:** Brunner gland hyperplasia of the descending duodenum. There are 5-mm nodules throughout. Biopsies showed an increased number of Brunner glands within the specimen suggestive of Brunner gland hyperplasia. **c:** Brunner gland hyperplasia. In a case where endoscopy was performed for nonspecific symptoms, 1- to 3-mm nodules were found in both the duodenal bulb and the descending duodenum. Biopsies showed Brunner gland hyperplasia.

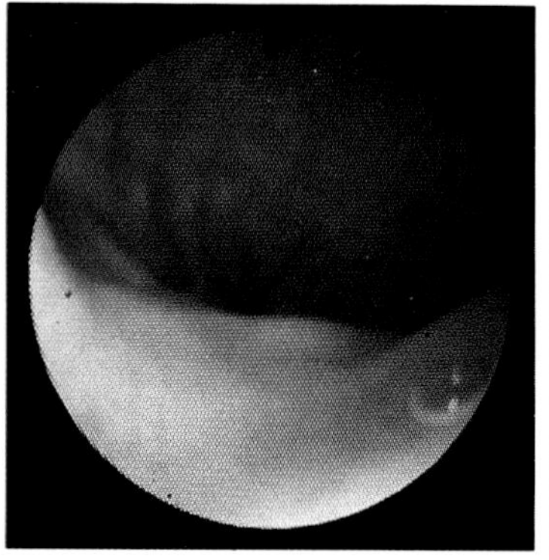

FIG. 25-12c.

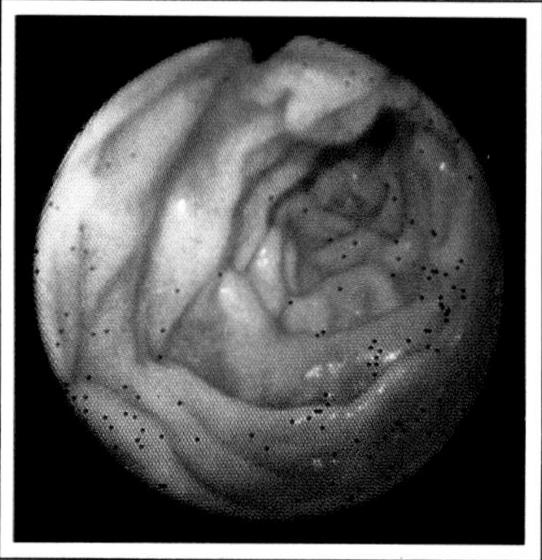

FIG. 25-13.

FIG. 25-13. Granularity of the descending duodenum. The mucosa has a gray-white appearance with a diffusely irregular texture, giving the impression of granularity. This appearance may be due to mucosal adsorption of antacids.

10 mm) nodules (Fig. 25-12b). These may be accompanied by an increase in the thickness of Kerckring folds (Fig. 25-12a). In two-thirds of the cases, biopsies may show nonspecific inflammatory changes, causing the term nodular duodenitis to be used to describe this appearance, as it was for a similar appearance of the duodenal bulb.[11] In fact, one may see fine nodularity (1 to 3 mm) beginning in the duodenal bulb and continuing throughout most of the descending duodenum (Fig. 25-12c). As is true of nodularity confined to the bulb (see above), we regard its appearance in the descending duodenum as entirely nonspecific, without any relationship to the symptoms which may have prompted endoscopy.

Brunner Gland Hyperplasia

In 30% of the cases of nodularity of the descending duodenum, biopsy of a nodule shows it to consist largely of Brunner (submucosal mucosa) glands; hence the term Brunner gland hyperplasia (see also Chapter 30) is used for the associated endoscopic appearance.[12] In most cases of Brunner gland hyperplasia, the descending duodenum is involved exclusively (Fig. 25-12b). In 20 to 30%, the duodenal bulb is involved as well (Fig. 25-12c), whereas the involvement of the duodenal bulb alone occurs in less than 20% of the cases.

While Brunner gland hyperplasia is seen in association with gastric hypersecretion, we have not found it exclusively in such patients or others with a history of peptic ulcer disease, though in one study, 6 of 11 patients with Brunner gland hyperplasia had ulcer-like symptoms, whereas none of 30 asymptomatic controls had Brunner gland hyperplasia.[12] Among our cases, the majority of patients with Brunner gland hyperplasia have neither ulcer symptoms nor gastric hypersecretion; hence we do not regard it as an indication of peptic ulcer disease.

In addition to nodular duodenitis and Brunner gland hyperplasia, an occasional (about 5% incidence) cause of a nodular descending duodenum is nodular lymphoid hyperplasia, which we consider elsewhere (see Chapter 28).

Granularity

The usual smooth, yellow-gray mucosal appearance is occasionally replaced by a coarsened texture, appearing almost as a chalky white exudate. For this we use the term granularity (Fig. 25-13). Neither the cause nor the significance of this term has been determined. Biopsies show a nonspecific increase in chronic and inflammatory cells or somewhat blunted villi, but nothing to account for the whitish appearance of the mucosa. Often we see this pattern in patients who have been treated for peptic ulcer disease, and a possible explanation for this appearance could be the adsorption of antacid, which may both accentuate the villi as well as provide a basis for the chalky white coloration.

REFERENCES

1. Isenberg, J., Walsh, J. H., and Grossman, M. I. (1973): Zollinger-Ellison syndrome. *Gastroenterology,* 65:140–165.
2. Regan, P. T., and Malagelada, J.-R. (1978): A reappraisal of clinical roentgenographic and endoscopic features of the Zollinger-Ellison syndrome. *Mayo Clin. Proc.,* 53:19–23.
3. Burrell, M., and Toffler, R. (1976): Flexural pseudolesions of the duodenum. *Radiology,* 120:313–315.
4. Reddy, R. R., Schuman, B. M., and Priest, R. J. (1981): Duodenal polyps: diagnosis and management. *J. Clin. Gastroenterol.,* 3:139–145.
5. Holdstock, G. E., Smith, C. L., and Isaacson, P. (1980): Prevalence and significance of duodenitis in patients undergoing endoscopy. *Gut,* 21:902A.
6. Cotton, P. B., Price, A. B., Tighe, J. R., and Beales, J. S. M. (1973): Preliminary evaluation of "duodenitis" by endoscopy and biopsy. *Br. Med. J.,* 3:430–433.
7. Thomson, W. O., Joffe, S. N., Robertson, A. G., Lee, F. D., Imrie, C. W., and Blumgart, L. H. (1977): Is duodenitis a dyspeptic myth? *Lancet,* 1:1197–1198.

7a. MacKinnon, M., Willing, R. L., and Whitehead, R. (1982): Cimetidine in the management of symptomatic patients with duodenitis. A double-blind controlled trial. *Dig. Dis. Sci.,* 27:217–219.

8. Palmer, E. D. (1974): Common duodenitis—of any clinical import? *JAMA,* 230:599.
9. Hasan, M., Sircus, W., and Ferguson, A. (1981): Duodenal mucosal architecture in non-specific and ulcer associated duodenitis. *Gut,* 22:637–641.
10. McCallum, R. W., Singh, D., and Wollman, J. (1979): Endoscopic and histologic correlations of the duodenal bulb: the spectrum of duodenitis. *Arch. Pathol. Lab. Med.,* 103:169–172.
11. Fontan, A. N., Rapaport, M., Celener, D., Piskorz, E., Paralta, C. G., and Rubio, H. H. (1978): Chronic nonspecific duodenitis (bulbitis). *Endoscopy,* 10:94–98.
12. Maratka, Z., Kocianova, J., Kudrmann, J., Jirko, P., and Pirk, F. (1979): Hyperplasia of Brunner's glands: radiology, endoscopy and biopsy findings in 11 cases of diffuse, nodular, and adenomatous form. *Acta Hepatogastroenterol. (Stuttg.),* 26:64–69.

26

PEPTIC ULCER DISEASE

One of the commonest indications for both endoscopy and specifically an examination of the duodenum is to determine if an active ulcer is present. This is particularly important in a number of instances, for example, in patients with symptoms suggestive of peptic ulcer disease but negative or equivocal radiographic studies. Here endoscopy may reveal an ulcer in up to 10%[1] and in 20 to 30%[1,2] if duodenal bulb deformity is present (Fig. 26-1). In patients with atypical symptoms and/or an incomplete response to prior ulcer therapy, endoscopy is crucial for rational management because in many cases no ulcer is actually present. Finally for patients being considered for ulcer surgery on the basis of symptoms refractory to medical management and radiologic findings alone, endoscopy is sought to confirm the presence of ulcer because of the lower accuracy of a radiologic diagnosis. This is especially true with the radiologic finding of an ulcer and bulb deformity (Fig. 26-2a), where at endoscopy either a completely normal bulb or one with deformity but no ulcer (Fig. 26-2b) may be found in up to 20% of cases diagnosed radiologically as having a duodenal ulcer.[1,2]

Endoscopy is therefore a powerful tool for evaluating patients thought to have peptic ulcer disease, particularly those with atypical symptoms or an incomplete response to medical treatment. While endoscopic interpretation in these cases is usually straightforward, difficulties arise when dealing with some of the less common ulcer appearances, especially in the setting of ulcer scar type deformity. The

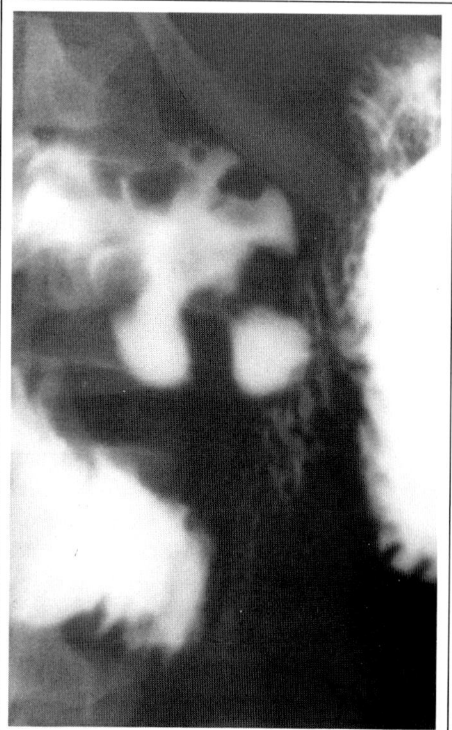

FIG. 26-1a.

FIG. 26-1. a: Duodenal bulb deformity found radiographically in a patient with peptic ulcer-like symptoms. A definite ulcer could not be confidently diagnosed from this study. **b:** At endoscopy an ulcer was seen within the deformed duodenal bulb noted radiographically in (a).

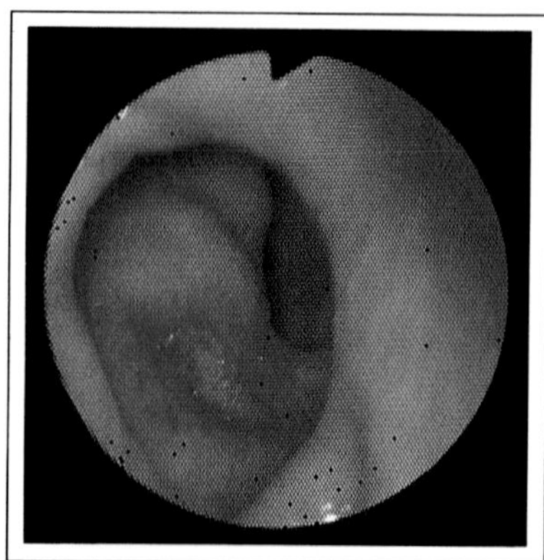

FIG. 26-1b.

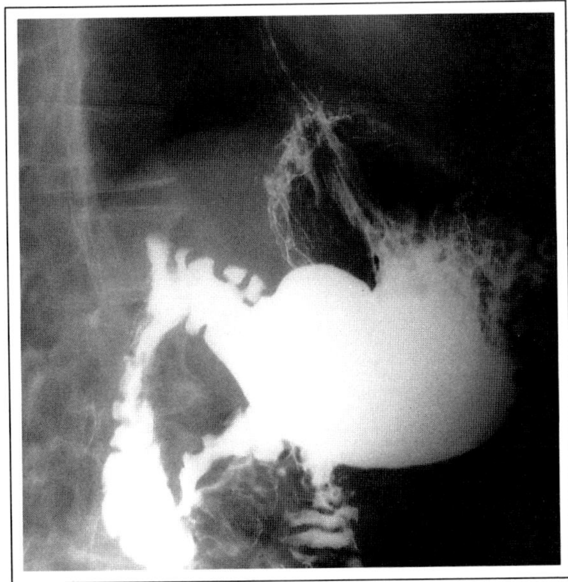

FIG. 26-2a.

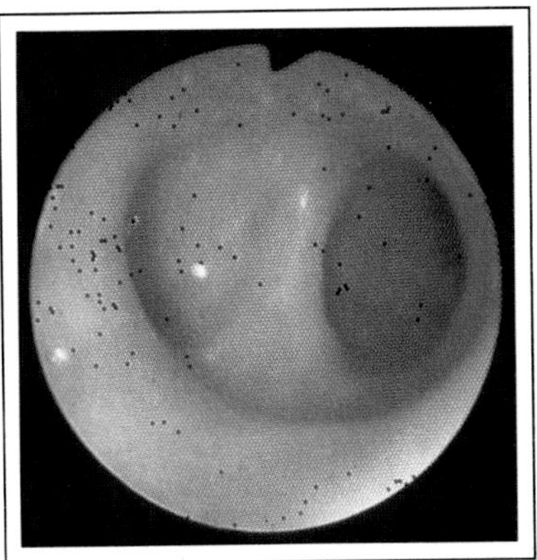

FIG. 26-2b.

FIG. 26-2. a: Duodenal bulb ulcer found radiographically in a patient with atypical symptoms, e.g., continuous abdominal pain and bloating. **b:** Duodenal bulb deformity (pseudodiverticulum) found at endoscopy in a patient with atypical symptoms but with a radiographic study suggesting an active ulcer (a). The radiographic "ulcer" was probably barium collecting in the pseudodiverticulum.

plan of this chapter is therefore first to consider the typical appearance of single ulcers, then that of less common multiple ulcers and the uncommon giant duodenal ulcer, and finally the appearance of ulcers in the rare Zollinger-Ellison syndrome. We then describe findings associated with ulcer healing. We conclude the chapter with a discussion of ulcer scar deformity in relation to the endoscopic appearance of ulcers, the problem of their recognition, and finally the significance of deformity and duodenitis in the absence of an ulcer.

ACTIVE ULCERS

Location

Anterior Wall

The commonest location for ulcers of the duodenal bulb is the anterior wall (Fig. 26-3). A proportion of ulcers in this location has been reported in the range of 30 to 55% of cases,[3] which agrees with our own experience (Table 26-1), where over a 7-year period 43% were located on the anterior wall. Most of these occur 1 to 2 cm from the pyloric channel (Fig. 26-3). The precise explanation for this predominance of proximal anterior wall ulcers is unknown. We believe that it occurs because of the location of the anterior wall in line with the antrum, predisposing it to receive the brunt of increased acid from the stomach commonly found in patients with duodenal ulcers.[4]

TABLE 26-1. *Location of 300 duodenal (bulb) ulcers seen over a 7-year period (1974–1980)*

Location	No.	%
Anterior wall	129	43
Posterior wall	117	39
Superior wall	9	3
Inferior wall	21	7
Apex	24	8
Total	300	100

Posterior Wall

We find ulcers on the posterior wall (Fig. 26-4) just slightly less commonly than those on the anterior wall (Table 26-1), with an incidence of 39%. Others have found a somewhat lower incidence of posterior wall ulcers (23 to 26%[3]), although these studies were largely from the early and mid-1970s when large-caliber instruments (13 mm) with relatively long turning lengths (>3 cm) were used, so that some ulcers of the posterior wall may have gone undetected. By contrast, we largely use a narrow-caliber (9 mm), pediatric-type instrument with a short turning length, which is better suited to examine the relatively inaccessible posterior wall.

Superior and Inferior Walls

Together, the surfaces of the superior and inferior walls accounted for only 10% of duodenal ulcers in our series, but for 27 to 35% in others.[3] Of the two locations, we find the inferior wall to be the more common, which alone accounted for 7% and in other series for up to 26%.[3] As with anterior wall ulcers, most of these are located within 1 to 2 cm of the pyloroduodenal junction (Fig. 26-5). We find an inferior wall site particularly in patients with pyloroduodenal junction deformity (Fig. 26-5). Despite the fact that the endoscopist has a direct view of this area, the deformity itself may cause him, especially if his examination is cursory, to overlook the active ulcer.

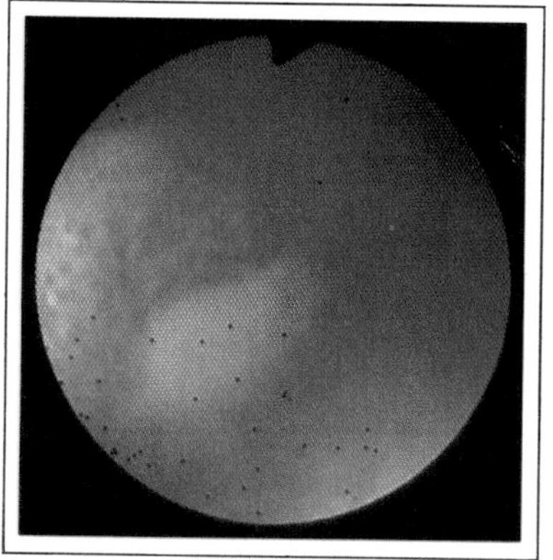

FIG. 26-3.

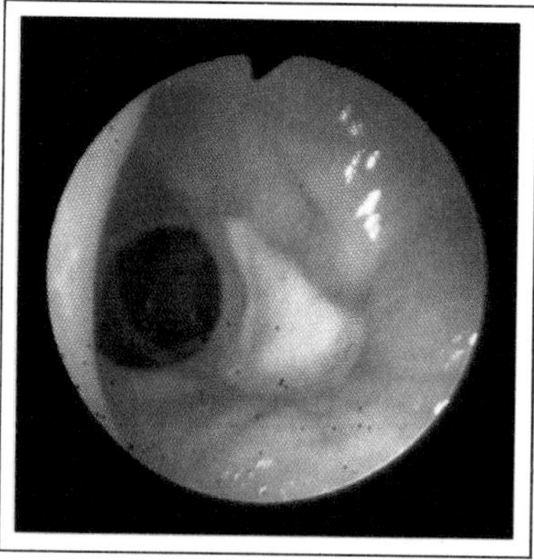

FIG. 26-4.

FIG. 26-3. Duodenal ulcer on the anterior wall. A 4-mm ulcer is seen in the mid-bulb.

FIG. 26-4. Duodenal ulcer on the posterior wall. A 1.5 × 1 cm ulcer was observed just beyond the pyloric channel.

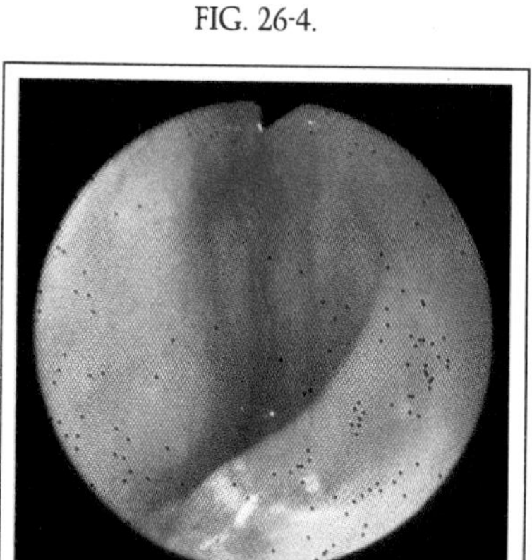

FIG. 26-5.

FIG. 26-5. Duodenal ulcer on the inferior wall. Part of a 0.5 × 1.0 cm ulcer is seen just beyond the pyloroduodenal junction.

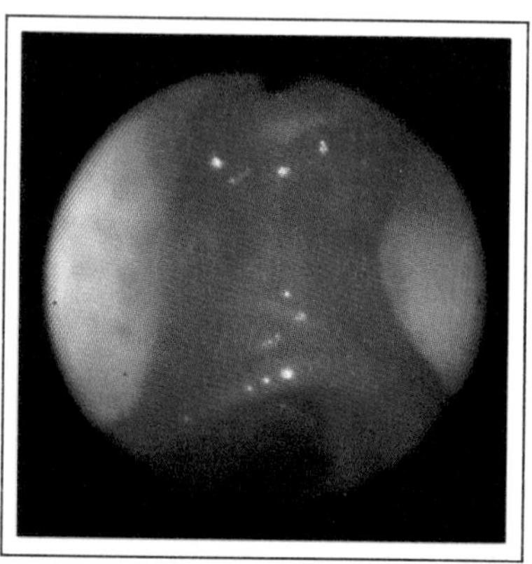

FIG. 26-6a.

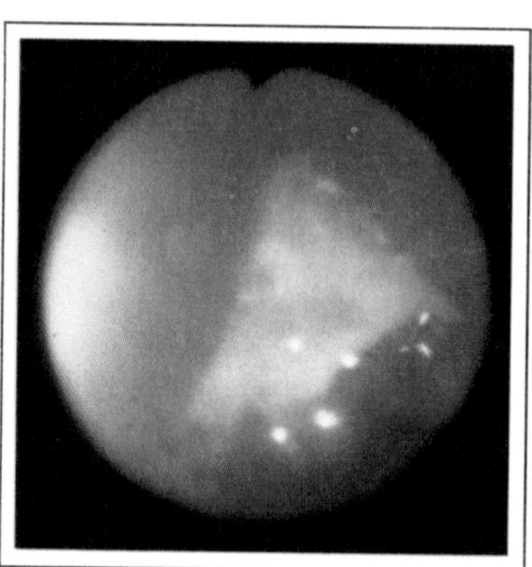

FIG. 26-6b.

FIG. 26-6. Duodenal ulcer on the superior wall. **a:** A large (1.5 cm) ulcer is just seen at 12 o'clock. **b:** Because a narrow-caliber (8.8 mm) endoscope has been employed within a (<3 cm) turning length, sufficient upward deflection was obtained for a better view of the ulcer.

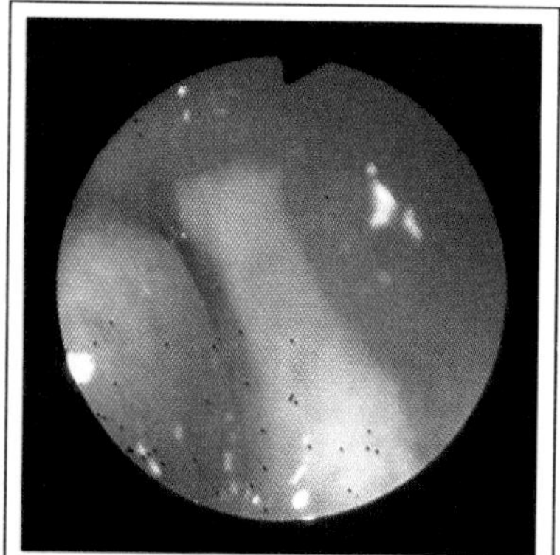

FIG. 26-7.

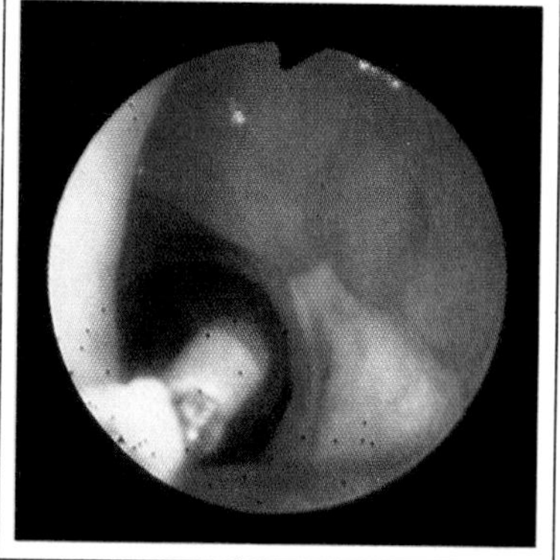

FIG. 26-8.

FIG. 26-7. Duodenal ulcer on the apex. A 0.7 × 1.0 cm ulcer is set between two prominent converging apical folds suggesting ulcer scar deformity.

FIG. 26-8. Duodenal ulcer, measured. The open bite width of the forceps is 9 mm. The dimensions of this triangular ulcer measure one bite width in one dimension and 1.5 bite widths in the other, or approximately 0.9 × 1.4 cm.

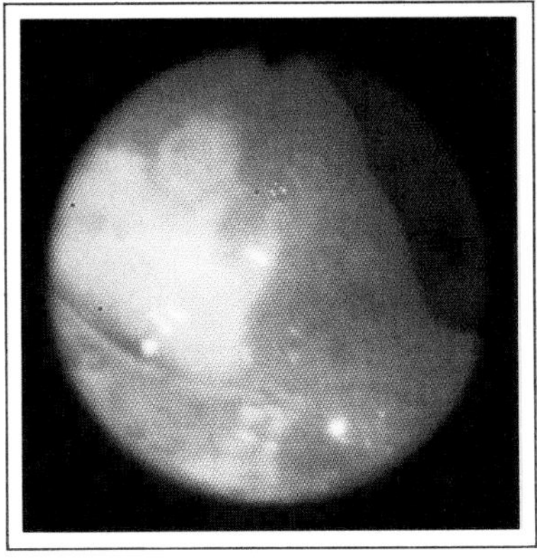
FIG. 26-9a.

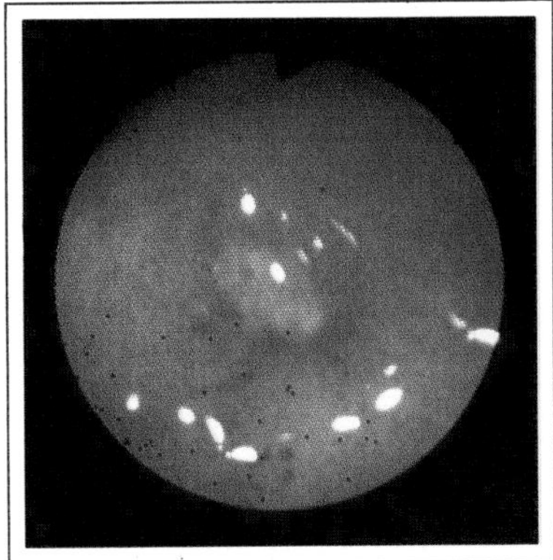
FIG. 26-9b.

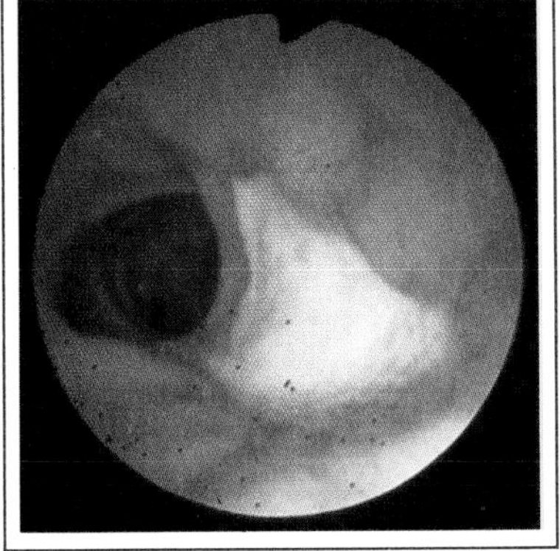
FIG. 26-9c.

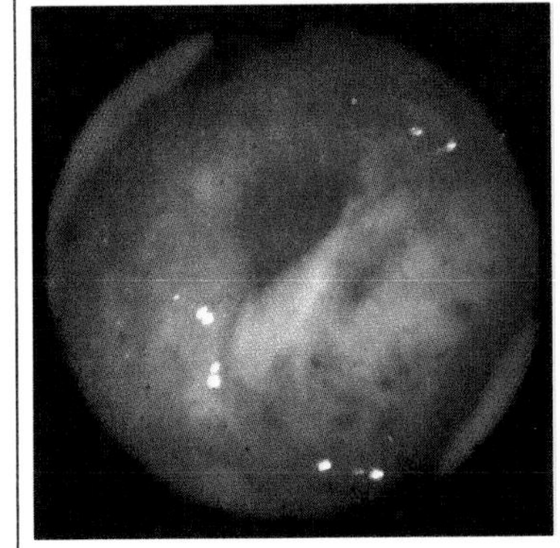
FIG. 26-9d.

FIG. 26-9. a: Duodenal ulcer, 8 mm maximum dimension. We find 50% of duodenal ulcers with a maximum dimension between 5 and 9 mm (Table 26-2). **b:** Duodenal ulcer, 4 mm. Twenty percent of duodenal ulcers are small (<5 mm), as in this case. **c:** Large duodenal ulcer with a maximum dimension of 1.4 cm (same ulcer as in Fig. 26-8). **d:** Giant duodenal ulcer with a maximum dimension of 2.5 cm. This ulcer largely replaced the anterior and superior walls of a somewhat shortened bulb.

Decidedly uncommon are superior wall ulcers, accounting for only 3% in our series and a maximum of only 10% in that of others.[3] Possibly this low incidence reflects a major problem (Fig. 26-6a) in examining the superior wall with a forward-viewing endoscope, even one with a short turning length (Fig. 26-6b), i.e., the difficulty of achieving an *en face* view of this surface, especially the proximal portion where ulcers are most likely to occur. Because of this, one must examine this surface with a side-viewing instrument when the suspicion of an ulcer of this location has been raised radiologically.

TABLE 26-2. *Size of 300 duodenal ulcers seen over a 7-year period (1974–1980)*

Maximum dimension (mm)	No.	%
>2–5	60	20
>5–9	150	50
>9–14	45	15
>14–20	30	10
>20	15	5
Total	300	100

Apex

An ulcer on the apex is also relatively uncommon, accounting for only 8% of our cases and a similar percent in other series.[3] Often ulcers of this location are associated with prominent apical folds and show features of scar deformity (Fig. 26-7) (see below).

Ulcer Size

With practice, we feel the endoscopist can correctly estimate the size of a given ulcer, surprisingly within the true dimensions found at surgery. Generally the error is on the side of underestimation. Rather than a "guesstimate" which may have an error rate of 10 to 20% or more, the endoscopist may wish to provide a more precise measurement, especially in cases where serial endoscopy may be anticipated, as for large (>1.5 cm) ulcers and those whose presentation involve a complication, e.g., bleeding. A more precise estimation can be achieved with the use of either the open forceps (Fig. 26-8) method already discussed for gastric ulcers (see Chapter 15) or the use of a calibrated probe.[3]

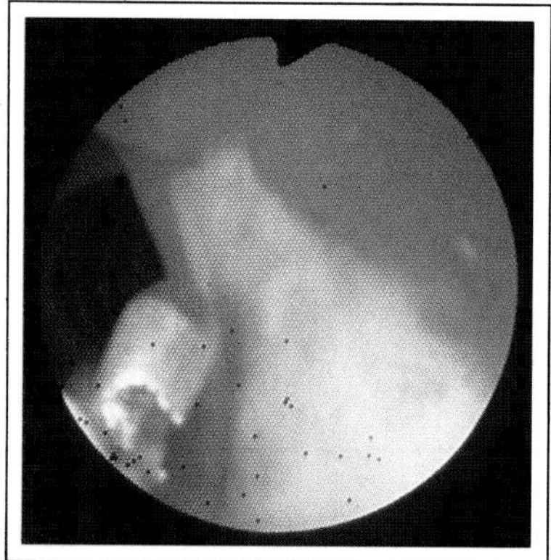

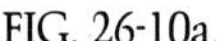

FIG. 26-10a.

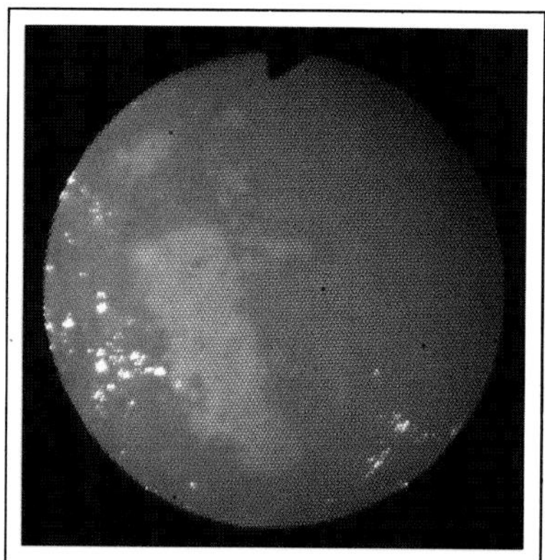

FIG. 26-10b.

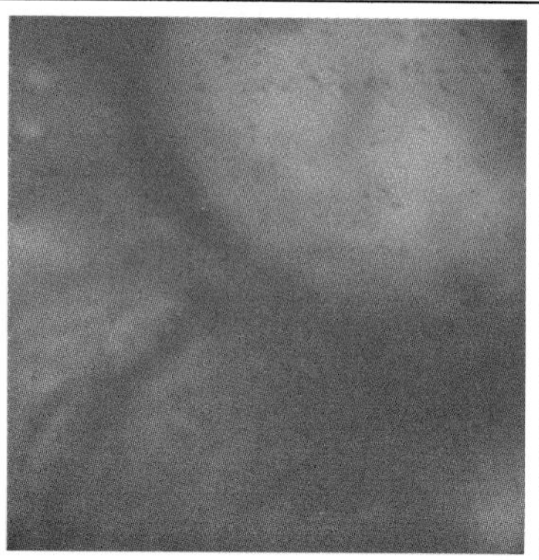

FIG. 26-10c.

FIG. 26-10. a: Duodenal ulcer, depth. The maximum depth is approximately one-fourth of the open bite width, or 2 mm. **b:** Superficial duodenal ulcer. The depth of this ulcer is barely appreciated. **c:** Deep duodenal ulcer. The depth of this posterior wall ulcer was estimated to be 5 mm. At surgery the ulcer was found to have penetrated into the pancreas.

Range of Ulcer Size

We find that the majority of duodenal bulb ulcers are under 1 cm in their greatest dimension (Table 26-2). We consistently find 50% in the 5 to 9 mm range (Fig. 26-9a), with 20% less than 5 mm (Fig. 26-9b). In only 25% of ulcers the size ranges between 10 and 20 mm (Fig. 26-9c), with the majority of these (15% of the total) being between 10 and 14 mm. Only 5% of ulcers exceed 2 cm (Fig. 26-9d).

Depth of Ulceration

The depth of a duodenal ulcer (depression from the luminal surface) ranges in most cases between 1 and 3 mm, with about two-thirds between 1 and 2 mm (Fig. 26-10a). Many examiners do not specifically comment on the depth of ulcers falling within this range. Other ulcers are designated as either superficial or deep to indicate that their depth is outside the expected range. The term superficial is used to denote an ulcer whose depth is barely appreciable, if at all (Fig. 26-10b). The term deep is used to indicate a depth which exceeds the normal range, i.e., greater than 3 mm (Fig. 26-10c).

The depth of an ulcer is important as it may be of prognostic significance. Somewhat surprisingly, superficial ulcers, especially if multiple, may have an unpredictable response to medical management, often showing greatly delayed healing. In this regard they are similar to the exudative-type duodenitis (see Chapter 25). Actually, there may be only a shade of difference between what the endoscopist calls a superficial ulceration or a (white-based or exudative) erosion (Fig. 26-10b).

Deep ulcers, even those which are relatively small (Fig. 26-10c) seem also to have a much slower rate of healing than other ulcers of comparable size but usual depth.

Appearance

In addition to size, the single most striking visual feature of an ulcer is its shape. Although most duodenal ulcers have a punched-out, rounded appearance, there are actually five types,[3] classified as the: (a) round type; (b) irregular type; (c) linear type; (d) patchy or salami type; and (e) mixed type. An awareness of the different shapes of duodenal ulcers is important not only because it facilitates recognition of the less common types but also because the shape of an ulcer may have important bearing on its response to medical management.[3]

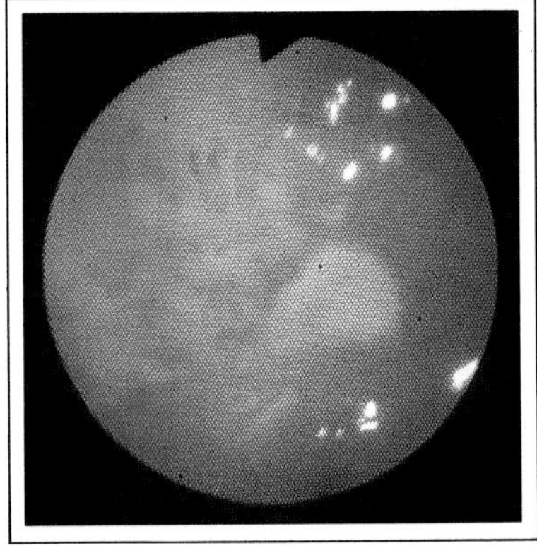

FIG. 26-11a.

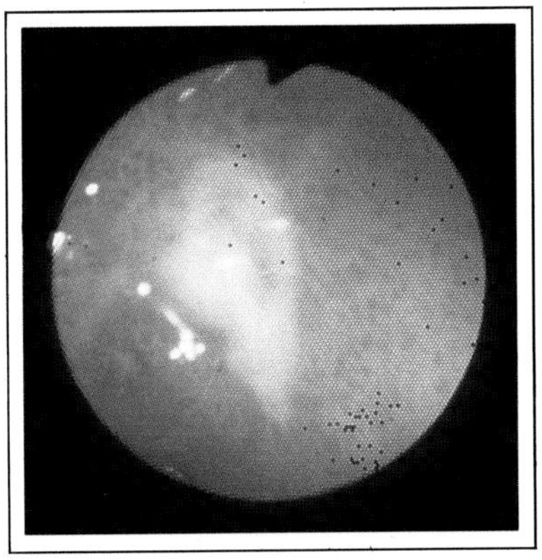

FIG. 26-11b.

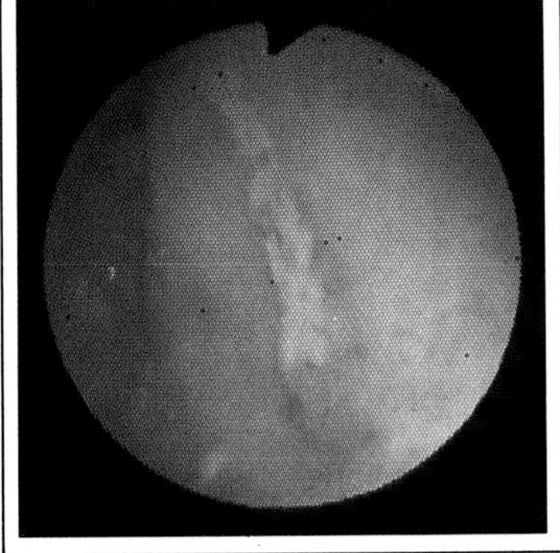

FIG. 26-11c.

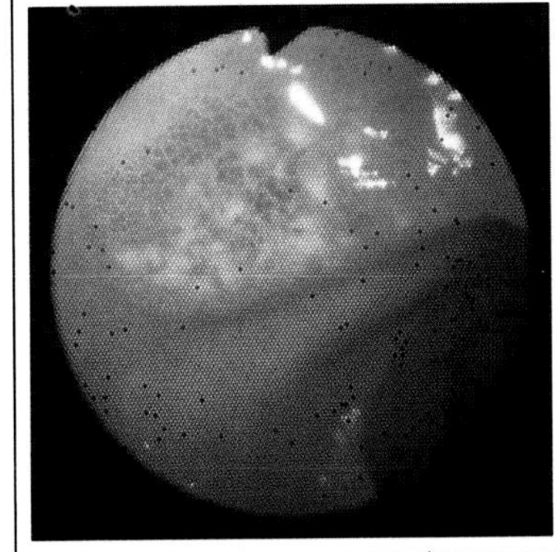

FIG. 26-11d.

FIG. 26-11. Duodenal ulcer. **a:** Round appearance. This is the most common appearance for an ulcer, representing about 60% in which the shape is circular or oval. **b:** Irregular appearance. About 5 to 10% of ulcers have a shape somewhere between a circle and a square. **c:** Linear appearance. For up to 20% the appearance is simply that of a line of ulceration. **d:** Salami appearance. For 5% the appearance consists of multiple tiny ulcerations or exudates set in a background of erythema, thereby resembling salami.

Round Type

The round ulcer represents the most common appearance, accounting for 60 to 70% in series specifically noting ulcer shape.[3] As is true of duodenal ulcers in general, the majority are between 5 and 10 mm (Fig. 26-11a). There may be a circumferential 2- to 4-mm rim of erythema which on histologic examination appears as acute duodenitis. This may be regarded as a zone of active regeneration, similar to the rim of erythema found as part of the appearance of gastric ulcers in the healing phase (see Chapter 15). Ulcers having the round appearance show the most predictable response to medical treatment,[3] with a high proportion (60%+) being healed at the end of 4 weeks of therapy.

Irregular Type

About 5 to 10% of duodenal ulcers have irregular margins (Fig. 26-11b); these are found especially in association with scar deformity, which contributes to the irregular appearance. It may be that scarification causes differential rates of healing within the ulcer, also giving rise to an irregular shape, thus a less predictable response to treatment, as in one study with only 20% healed at 4 weeks.[3]

Linear Type

For 10 to 20% of ulcers, the appearance is simply a line of ulceration (Fig. 26-11c). As was true of the irregular type, linear ulcers are commonly associated with scar deformity. In these cases the ulcer is typically found along the ridges of one or more of the deforming folds. In addition to the ulcer, one notes duodenitis (patchy erythema) (Fig. 26-11c). This type of ulcer has been associated with the least predictable response to treatment with less than 10% healed at 4 weeks.[3]

Patchy or Salami Type

The patchy (salami) appearance is distinctly uncommon, representing less than 5% of the total in reported series.[3] The principal feature is that of a discrete area of multiple tiny ulcerations on a background of intense erythema (Fig. 26-11d). This appearance of white dots set on a red background has been likened to cut salami, hence the term salami ulcer.[3] These ulcers are generally less than 1 cm and often less than 5 mm. Despite their modest size, they are among the slowest ulcers to heal and have high rates of recurrence, often in the setting of normal or even low-

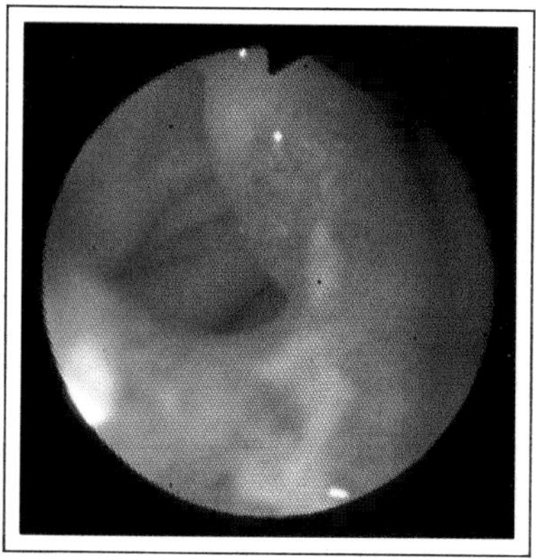

FIG. 26-12.

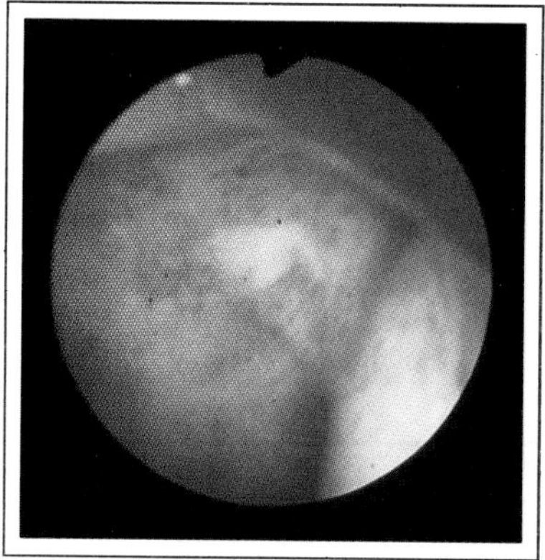

FIG. 26-13.

FIG. 26-12. Duodenal ulcer, mixed appearance. For less than 5%, there is a combination of types, most often a round or irregular appearance combined with a linear appearance, as in the present case. This latter appearance has been given the designation "racket" ulcer.[3]

FIG. 26-13. Duodenal ulcer versus mucus. In this case a biopsy from the central white spot showed granulation tissue and therefore indicated an ulcer rather than mucus or antacid.

normal gastric secretion. One suspects in cases where ulcers of this type are present that a primary mucosal defect may be present.

Mixed Type

In about 5 to 10% the ulcer appearance is a combination of two or more of the above, generally the round and linear types. In our experience these are most commonly found associated with scar deformity (Fig. 26-12), and as such may have an unpredictable response to treatment, similar to that of the linear type ulcers.

Biopsy

Usually the endoscopist can be relatively confident about his impression of an active ulcer. Because of the negligible incidence of primary carcinomas arising in the duodenal bulb, even sizable ulcers with irregular margins are not routinely biopsied. Moreover, in patients presenting with complications of peptic ulcer disease (e.g., obstruction or bleeding), a biopsy could lead to recurrent bleeding or complete obstruction.

Biopsy, however, is indicated when there is a question about the nature of the appearance as representing, rather than an ulcer, adherent mucus, antacid, or even barium from a recent radiographic study (Fig. 26-13). In these cases the endoscopist first attempts to remove the material with washing. However, if the picture is still confusing, biopsy of the suspected ulcer is indicated. The absence of granulation tissue histologically would be evidence against an ulcer.

SPECIAL TYPES OF DUODENAL ULCERS

Multiple Duodenal Ulcers

In up to 30% of cases a second ulcer is found usually within a short distance from the main ulcer (Fig. 26-14a). Generally, multiple duodenal ulcers are located at common ulcer sites, e.g., the pyloroduodenal junction, the mid-bulb (anterior or posterior wall), or the apex. When ulcers are located at the same site but on opposite walls, the term "kissing ulcer" is used (Fig. 26-14b). In rare cases the bulb is literally teeming with ulcers (Fig. 26-14c). The significance of multiple ulcers lies in their tendency to display delayed healing and prompt recurrence after termination of medical therapy.[3]

Giant Duodenal Ulcers

Ulcers of the duodenal bulb that are greater than 2.5 cm are considered giant (Fig. 26-15a). These represent, generally, 2 to 5% of duodenal ulcers. Their significance lies in their poor prognosis for healing as well as their increased complication rate, especially bleeding and intractability.[5,6]

Most giant ulcers are found on the anterior wall within 2 cm of the pyloroduodenal junction (Fig. 26-15a). They have a round overall shape, but their margins may be angulated, causing one to see them as irregular. Because of their depth, they may not be entirely appreciated, having a greater surface area than may be seen endoscopically, especially if a large-caliber (11 to 13 mm) instrument is used with its long turning length.

As with large gastric ulcers (>2 cm), the margin may appear nodular (Fig. 26-15b) because of inflammatory changes within. This may give the margin an appearance indistinguishable from that of "indeterminate" gastric ulcers. In such cases the endoscopist may consider biopsy; however, as duodenal malignancies as a whole are rare, constituting only 3% of gastrointestinal neoplasms, and the bulb is the least common site,[7] biopsy is not indicated. This is particularly true because of the potential in these cases for a biopsy complication, especially perforation if the anterior wall is involved.

Zollinger-Ellison Ulcers

Duodenal ulcers are found in patients with pancreatic and extrapancreatic gastrinomas or antral gastrin cell hyperplasia causing gastric hypersecretion,[8,9] but their precise

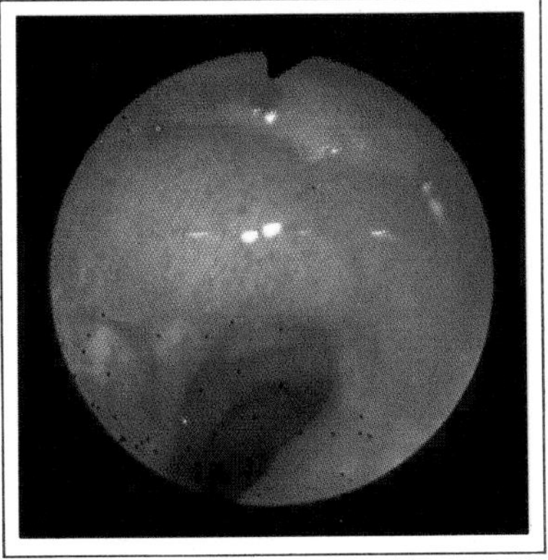

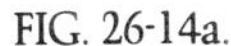

FIG. 26-14a.

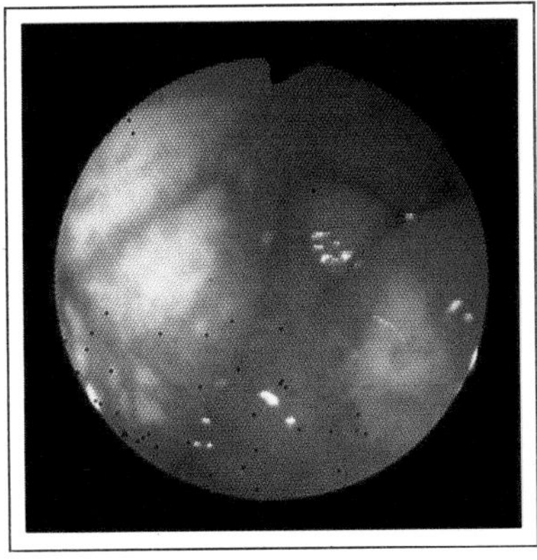

FIG. 26-14b.

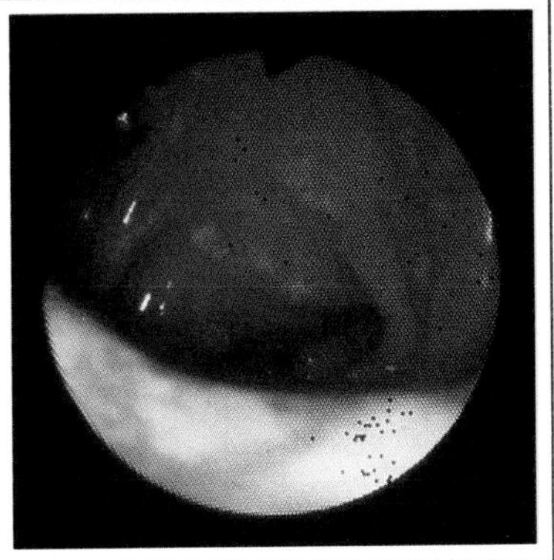

FIG. 26-14c.

FIG. 26-14. Multiple duodenal ulcers. **a:** A salami appearance was noted just proximal to an apical scar deformity (stenosis), with a second larger "regular" ulcer on the superior wall at 12 o'clock. **b:** "Kissing." Two ulcers are found in the mid-bulb on opposite walls of the duodenum. **c:** These cover an extensive area of the bulb, including the apex and superior posterior and inferior walls.

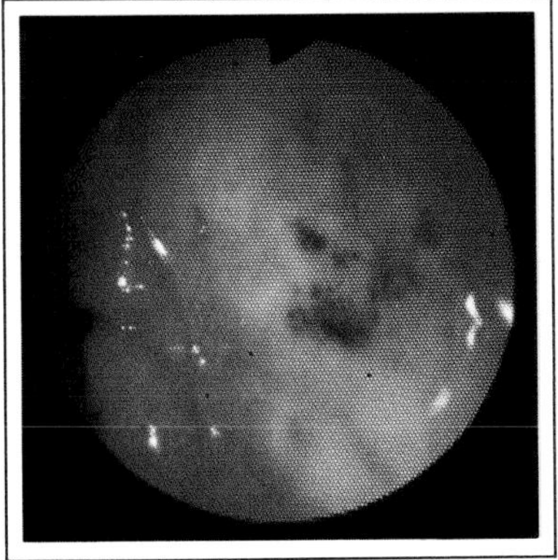

FIG. 26-15a.

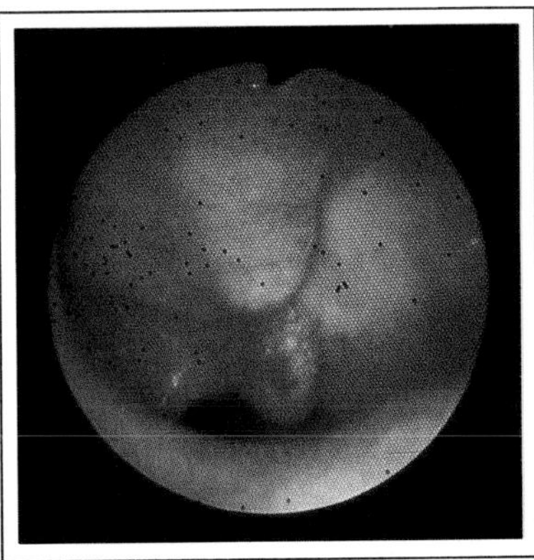

FIG. 26-15b.

FIG. 26-15. Giant duodenal ulcer. **a:** A 2.5-cm ulcer replaces the entire anterior and superior walls of the bulb. **b:** Mass effect. A 2.5-cm deep ulcer of the posterior wall of the bulb at 3 o'clock whose margin at 12 o'clock appears mass-like.

pathogenesis is uncertain. Just the amount of acid secreted (>2 liters 0.1 NHCl per day) over a 24-hr period may be enough to produce an aggressive ulcer diathesis.[8] However, mucosal factors must also play a role, because in some cases of Zollinger-Ellison gastric hypersecretion (up to 7%) mucosal integrity is so well maintained that ulcers do not occur, with diarrhea rather than ulceration as the clinical presentation.[10]

Appearance

The duodenal bulb is the commonest site of ulceration.[9] These ulcers do not differ from other duodenal ulcers (Fig. 26-16a), being mainly single and located in the pyloroduodenal junction. Also as in common duodenal ulcers, the surrounding mucosa of the bulb shows evidence of acute duodenitis with erythema, friability, and erosions. In one study[9] duodenitis was found in 15 of 17 patients with Zollinger-Ellison syndrome; in eight it was associated with an ulcer, whereas in seven it appeared as a single finding and was the commonest endoscopic finding in this series. We have observed what we believe to be a more specific endoscopic finding for Zollinger-Ellison syndrome, i.e., the appearance of multiple ulcers of the duodenal bulb (Fig. 26-16b) and descending duodenum. These ulcerations,

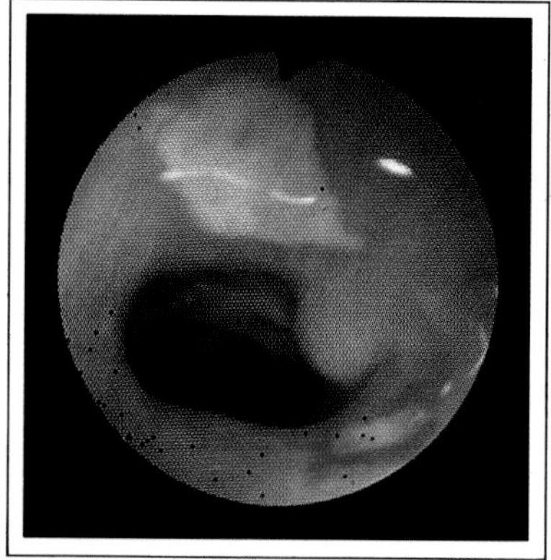

FIG. 26-16a.

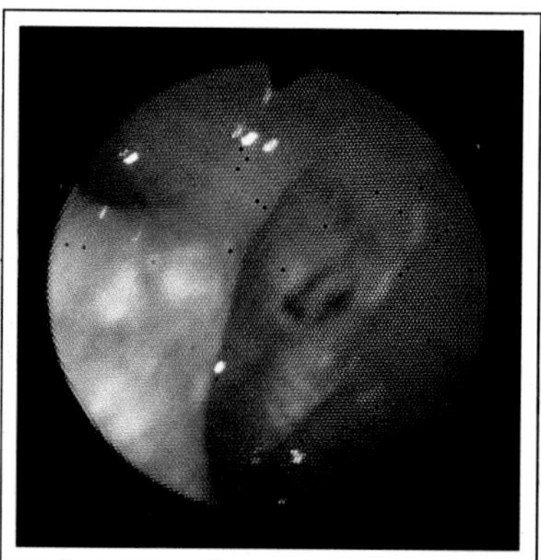

FIG. 26-16b.

FIG. 26-16. Zollinger-Ellison ulcer. **a:** This patient with proved Zollinger-Ellison ulcer syndrome has one irregularly shapped 7.5-mm ulcer of the superior wall and a second smaller ulcer on the opposite wall, indistinguishable from other duodenal ulcers. **b:** Multiple superficial ulcers of the apex and descending duodenum are a characteristic Zollinger-Ellison type appearance.

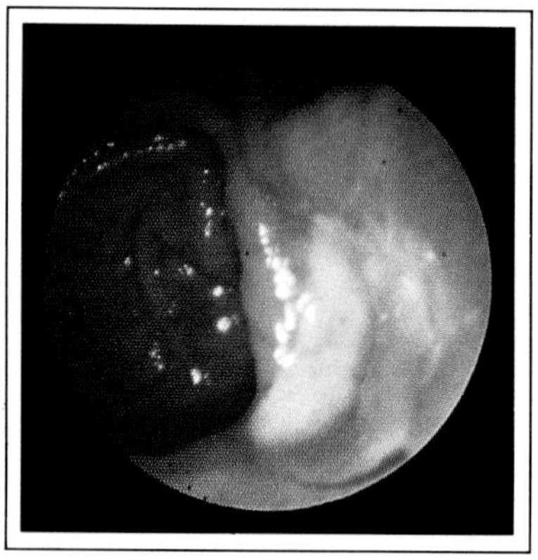

FIG. 26-17a.

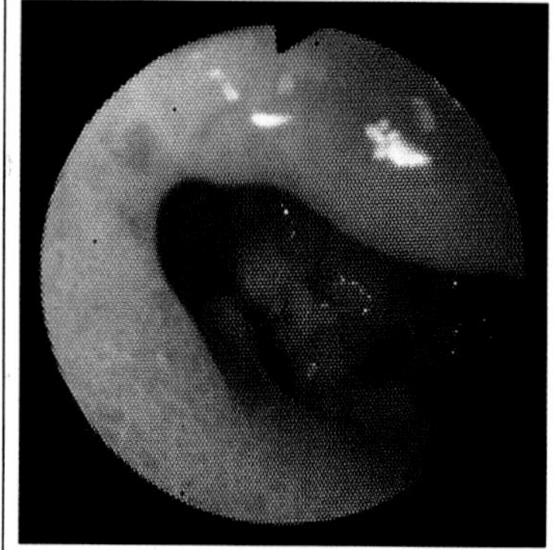

FIG. 26-17b.

FIG. 26-17. a: Gastric ulcer in a patient with a duodenal ulcer. A large prepyloric antral ulcer is observed along with prepyloric antral deformity. The ulcer's size as well as its irregular margin caused it to be judged "indeterminate" (see Chapter 15). Gastric ulcers coexisting with those of the duodenum must be judged on their own merits as to whether they are benign, malignant, or indeterminate. **b:** Duodenal ulcer found with a large gastric ulcer (a).

which for the most part are superficial, appear on the uppermost portions of prominent Kerckring folds (Fig. 26-16b). As these ulcers are generally less than 5 mm in greatest dimension, with little or no depth, they are easily missed on standard radiographic studies. In the absence of Crohn's disease, which could produce an identical appearance (see Chapter 28), the presence of superficial ulcers of the descending duodenum should always make one suspect Zollinger-Ellison syndrome.

Active Ulcers of the Duodenum and Stomach

Gastric ulcers may also be found in patients with peptic ulcer disease of the bulb. These are called "secondary" gastric ulcers to distinguish them from the "primary" gastric ulcers found in patients with a normal duodenal bulb whose acid secretory status is normal or low compared with the higher acid outputs associated with duodenal ulcer disease.

Use of Aspirin or Other Nonsteroidal Analgesics

Aspirin and other nonsteroidal agents, although less strongly associated with duodenal ulcers than those of the stomach (see Chapter 15), may affect duodenal ulcers, especially in regard to the response to treatment. The endoscopist should therefore inquire as to the use of these agents in any patient with a duodenal ulcer, but especially in those patients with gastric ulcers, so as not to miss the opportunity of making a significant contribution to the patient's chances of complete ulcer healing. In addition, a positive history will materially aid the examiner in his interpretation of any atypical or indeterminate gastric ulcer appearance (see Chapter 15).

Location

Typically, these ulcers are found in the prepyloric antrum adjacent to or within 2 cm of the pyloric channel (Fig. 26-17a). Ulcers found in this location should always cause the endoscopist to perform a detailed examination of the duodenal bulb (see Chapter 24) in search of others. Another common location for "secondary" gastric ulcers is the gastric angle, adjacent to the lesser curve.

Appearance

Gastric ulcers associated with peptic disease of the duodenum are indistinguishable from primary ulcers of the stomach. Those which occur in the prepyloric antrum may be associated with considerable scarring of the duodenal bulb (Fig. 26-17b), the pyloroduodenal junction, and the antrum itself (Fig. 26-17a). The antrum may be diffusely erythematous and contain foreign material when the degree of obstruction produced by the ulcer and prior scarring is functionally significant. In addition, a mass-like deformity of the antrum may be present with the result that the ulcer may have an indeterminate appearance as to whether it is benign or malignant (see Chapter 15). The large majority of indeterminate ulcers are in fact benign, but in our experience up to 20% are malignant (see Chapter 15). The presence of peptic disease of the duodenum as evidenced by scarring or even active ulcers is no assurance as to the benignity of an indeterminate gastric ulcer. In fact, the incidence of gastric carcinoma in patients with previous peptic disease may be increased over that in the general population.[11,12] The coexistence of gastric carcinoma and an active duodenal ulcer, although rare, is not unknown, so that the presence of an active duodenal ulcer by no means excludes a gastric ulcer's being malignant.[12]

Biopsy and Brushing

Any gastric ulcer must be judged on its own appearance as to whether it is benign, malignant, or indeterminate (see Chapter 15). Any ulcer with a suspicious appearance should be aggressively biopsied (at least six and ideally nine samples taken), even though an active duodenal ulcer may be present.

ULCER HEALING

A duodenal ulcer heals essentially by re-epithelialization from the periphery with gradual replacement of the granulation tissue comprising the ulcer base similar to gastric ulcers. One does not observe healing endoscopically for duodenal ulcers as readily as for gastric ulcers (see Chapter 15)—where one often can find a halo of histologically immature, regenerative-type mucosa surrounding the ulcer which, if followed sequentially, may be seen ultimately to be replaced by mature epithelium indistinguishable from its surroundings. In the case of duodenal ulcer healing, this progression is not observed for several reasons. First, because duodenal ulcers tend to be smaller, they tend to heal faster than gastric ulcers and may have healed completely within the 4- to 6-week period before endoscopy is performed again. Second, the ulcer itself may be set in a mucosal matrix which will chronically display duodenitis both visually and histologically.[13,14] Such changes may not progress to a truly healed stage but may persist as abnormal-appearing mucosa. This seems to be especially the case with ulcers having a salami, linear, or irregular type appearance all associated with delayed clinical resolution and a high recurrence rate.[3] In these cases, persistent duodenitis may be indicative of a defective type of re-epithelialization which may never allow for complete healing.

Rates of Ulcer Healing

We find that duodenal ulcers tend to heal with a reduction in their maximum dimension of approximately 1 to 4 mm per week.[3] Even without specific medication[15] a 50% reduction in the surface area of the ulcer has been observed within 3 weeks and complete healing by 6 weeks for nearly 75%. With treatment with cimetidine complete healing at 6 weeks has been found in up to 90%.[15a]

Apart from size, another factor found by Lambert et al.[3] to bear on the rate of ulcer healing is its initial appearance (see above), with round ulcers tending to heal the fastest and those of the regular, linear, or salami appearance having slower rates. In one study, 60% of the round ulcers healed within 1 month compared with only 20% of irregular, 18% of salami, and only 7% of linear ulcers showing healing in this period of time.[16] Others, however, found no difference in the healing rate for round compared with irregular ulcers, but did find slower rates of healing associated with marked scar deformity (stenosis) of the bulb.[16a] It is our impression that scar deformity slows the healing rate for any ulcer found, and that those ulcers present are more likely to have one of the appearances (i.e., irregular, linear, or salami) associated with the slowest rates of healing (less than 1 mm per week in the maximum dimension).[3]

Appearance of Healing Ulcers

Two patterns of ulcer healing may be observed: (a) rapid (spontaneous) healing; and (b) delayed healing.

Rapid (Spontaneous) Healing

The healing of duodenal ulcers even of large size (Fig. 26-18a) is usually rapid, especially for those having the round configuration. In these cases 60% may have healed within 4 weeks,[16] especially for ulcers less than 1 cm. For larger round ulcers 6 to 8 weeks may be required (Fig. 26-18b). In other cases the healing is slightly less rapid, with substantial but incomplete healing occurring over the same time period. In these cases one notes a marked reduction in the surface area but with some residual granulation tissue within the area of the previous ulcer base (Fig. 26-18c).

Delayed Healing

For as many as 40% of duodenal ulcers complete healing may not be present after 8 weeks.[16a] In those cases associated with scar deformity, complete healing may not occur for months. Where delayed healing is observed the initial shape of the ulcer is likely to have been other than round. Even for a round ulcer, healing may be delayed, especially in the presence of scar deformity (Fig. 26-19a). In these cases

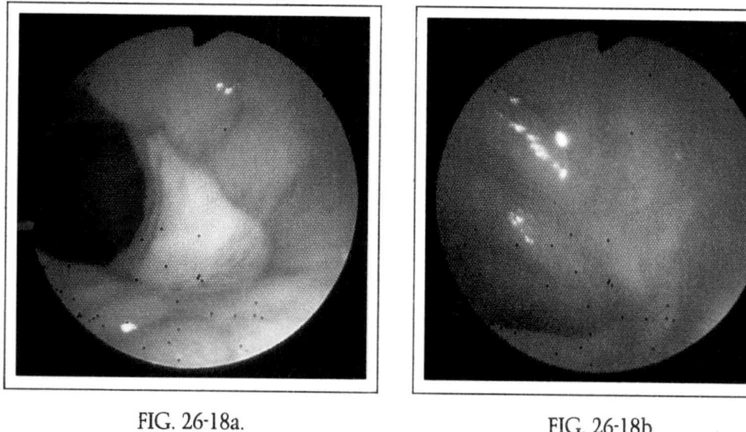

FIG. 26-18a.

FIG. 26-18b.

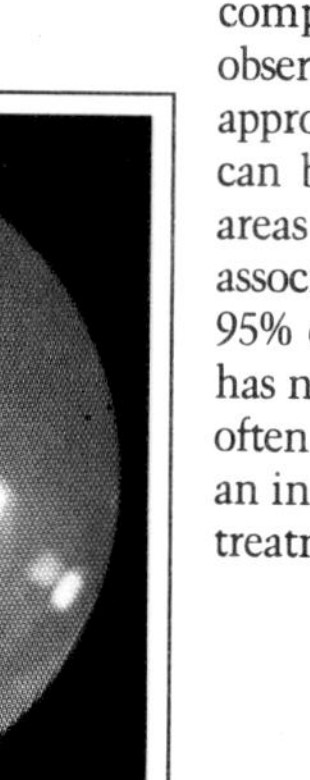

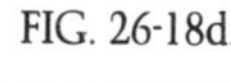

FIG. 26-18c.

FIG. 26-18d.

FIG. 26-18. a: Large duodenal ulcer, active. A 1.4 × 0.9 cm ulcer was noted on the posterior wall just beyond the pyloroduodenal junction. **b:** Duodenal ulcer, healed. At repeat endoscopy 6 weeks later, complete healing with re-epithelialization of a large ulcer base (a) has occurred. **c:** Duodenal ulcer, incomplete healing. An ulcer similar to that in (a) is observed at 8 weeks. The size of the base has decreased approximately 50%. In addition, reddish pink areas can be seen within the base itself which represent areas of re-epithelialization. **d:** Slow ulcer healing associated with scar deformity. At 16 weeks, when 95% of duodenal ulcers will have healed, this ulcer has not completely re-epithelialized. Delayed healing, often seen in association with scar deformity, indicates an increased likelihood of symptom recurrence once treatment is stopped.

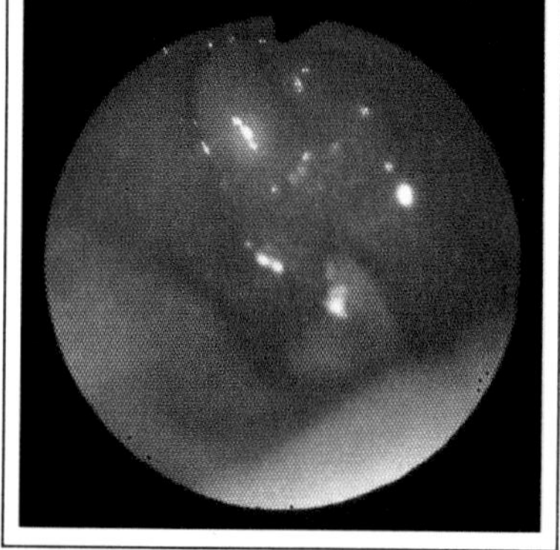

FIG. 26-19a.

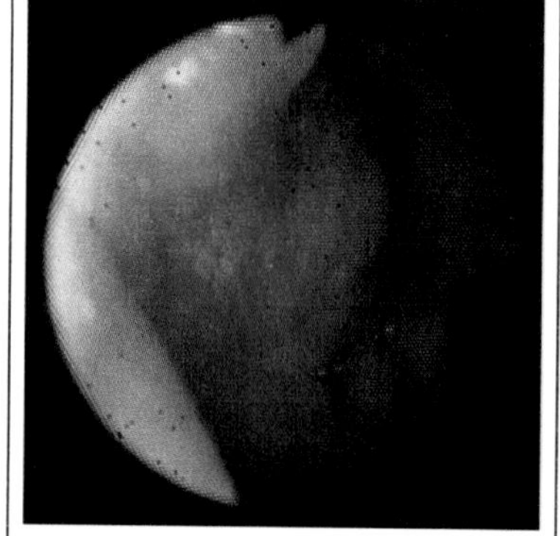

FIG. 26-19b.

FIG. 26-19. Duodenal ulcer. **a:** Active. A 5-mm round ulcer is noted in the mid-body anterior wall. **b:** Incompletely healed. At endoscopy performed 6 weeks later because of an incomplete response to medical treatment, tiny islands of acute inflammatory exudate are noted between erythematous areas representing mucosal regeneration. With the healing which has occurred, an ulcer scar deformity of the anterior wall can be appreciated. Note the similarity in appearance of the incompletely healed ulcer to that of the salami ulcer (Fig. 26-11d).

the area initially showing the ulcer base continues to show tiny zones of ulceration on a red background of presumably regenerating epithelium, an appearance which resembles the salami-type ulcer (Fig. 26-11d), which itself is associated with delayed healing. We find patients with ulcers having the delayed appearance tend to respond symptomatically less well to medical management than those who undergo spontaneous healing. Furthermore, it is our impression that these ulcers have a greater tendency to reulcerate over the next 6 to 12 months in comparison to those which have entirely healed (as seen by endoscopy) within 3 to 6 weeks.

The propensity for delayed healing to be associated with an increased likelihood of recurrence may be attributable to an abnormality of duodenal mucosa, either present from the outset or which develops as a result of ulcer scarring.[16]

ULCER RECURRENCE

Endoscopic studies of patients where ulcer healing occurred while receiving either antacids or cimetidine (Tagamet),[17,18] indicate that the majority (75%+), when the

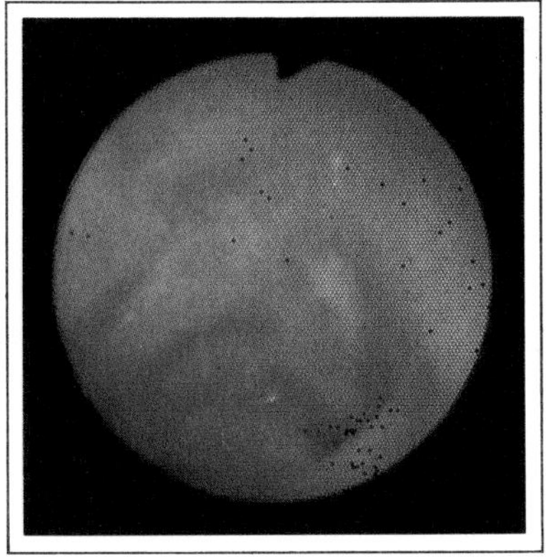

FIG. 26-20a.

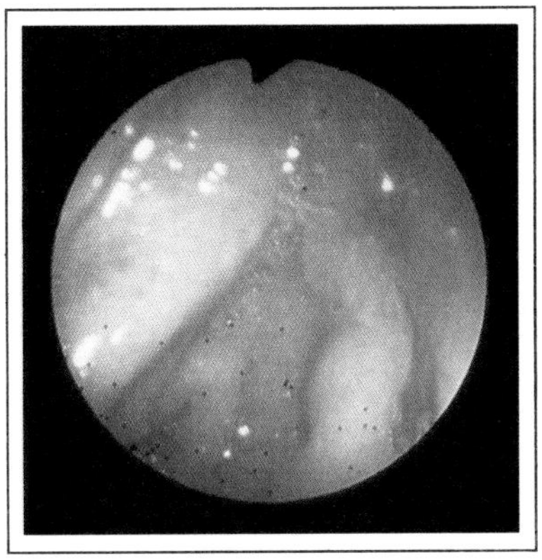

FIG. 26-20b.

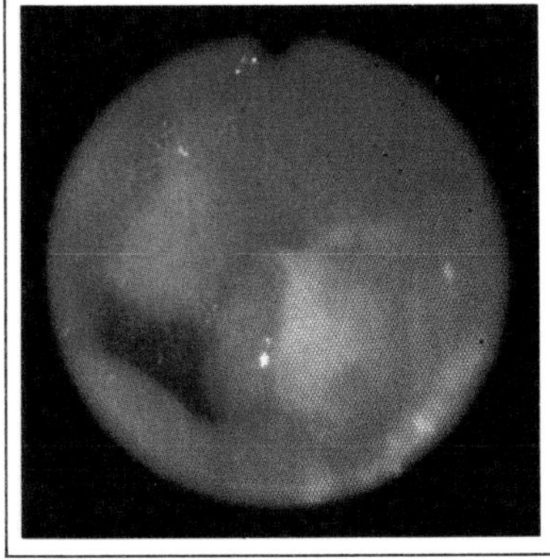

FIG. 26-20c.

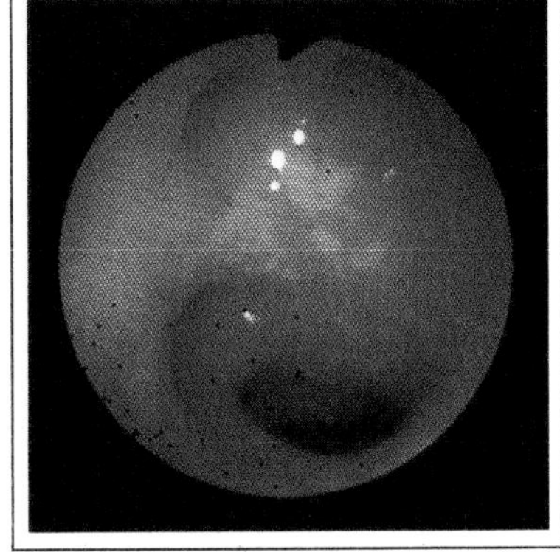

FIG. 26-21.

FIG. 26-20. a: Duodenal ulcer in the apex. The erythema around the ulcer may in part reflect ongoing healing. **b:** Healed duodenal ulcer in the apex after 6 weeks of medical treatment which included cimetidine (Tagamet). **c:** Recurrent apical ulcer 8 months after discontinuation of treatment.

FIG. 26-21. Duodenal ulcer in the mid-bulb, salami appearance. An 8-week course of antacids and Tagamet was associated with complete symptomatic relief and endoscopic improvement (but not disappearance of the ulcer) over a 10-week period; however, both symptoms and the ulcer itself recurred within 3 months after discontinuing treatment.

treatment is discontinued, will reulcerate within a 12-month period (Fig. 26-20a). The recurrent ulcer is usually found in areas of scar deformity (Fig. 26-20b), precisely at the same point as the original (Fig. 26-20c). That there is a cyclical pattern of ulceration and healing with reulceration after healing[16] accords with the clinical observation of symptomatic recurrence once or twice a year ("spring and fall" recurrence pattern).[3]

Although 75%+ of ulcers recur, the tendency of a specific ulcer to do so depends, we find, on its shape. In our experience, only 50% of ulcers of the round type recur, whereas nearly all of those which are not round (i.e., linear, salami, or irregular types) do so. The fact that these shapes are associated with delayed healing[3] as well as scar deformity (Fig. 26-21) suggests an underlying mucosal defect which may be the result of scar deformity, which gives rise to a shape, other than round, as well as delayed healing, and invariable reulceration.

ULCER SCAR DEFORMITY

True ulcer scar deformity may be considered a marker for peptic ulcer disease. Its presence radiologically in symptomatic patients, even in those where an ulcer cannot be demonstrated, indicates the likelihood of an ulcer being found at endoscopy in 30 to 40%,[1] contrasted in our Unit with the 10% incidence of duodenal ulcers for endoscopy patients in general. Because of the high association between scar deformity and active ulceration, findings at endoscopy suggestive of ulcer scarring must indicate to the endoscopist the need for a careful search for an active ulcer.

As has already been mentioned, the presence of scar deformity affects the shape of the ulcer, predisposing the non-round type to delayed healing as well as an increased tendency to recurrence.[16] The manner in which scar deformity occurs is unsettled. That the majority of duodenal ulcers recur within 1 year of their initial healing at the same location suggests that scarification is a result of repeated injury at the same location, causing submucosal and mucosal fibrosis with some muscle hypertrophy around the site of ulceration radiating out from the ulcer base. The combination of fibrosis and muscle hypertrophy, over time, would tend to pull the adjacent mucosa and submucosa toward the point of recurrent ulceration, producing the characteristic feature of ulcer scarring, i.e., converging (Fig. 26-22a) or projecting (Fig. 26-22b) folds.

Appearance

The principal locations for scar deformity are those of the duodenal ulcers themselves, i.e., the pyloroduodenal junction, the mid-bulb, and the apex. When deformity of

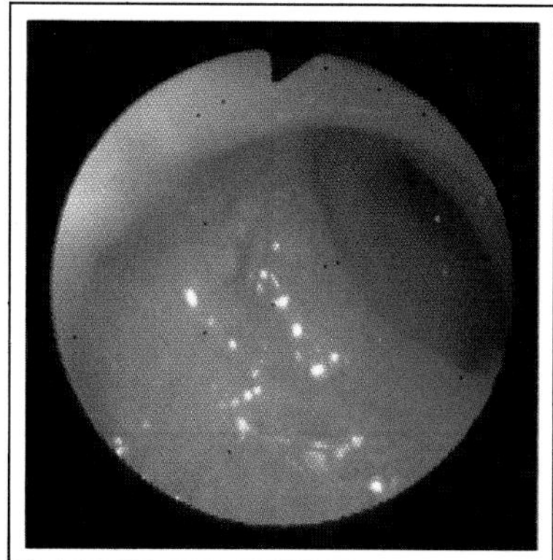

FIG. 26-22a.

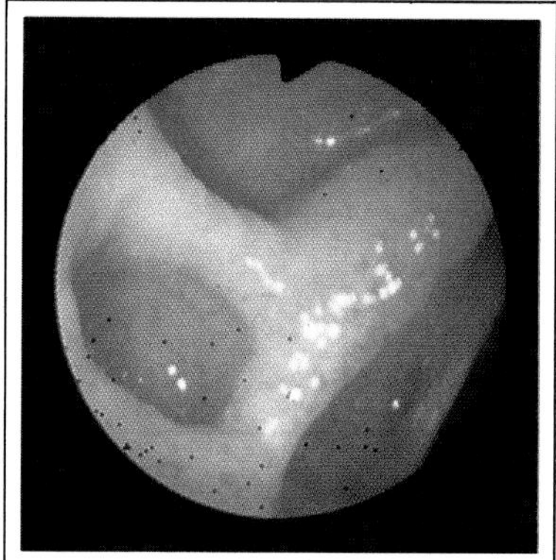

FIG. 26-22b.

FIG. 26-22. Ulcer scar deformity. **a:** With converging folds of the pyloroduodenal junction. Just beyond the channel a fold is seen extending out onto the anterior wall in a patient with a long ulcer history. **b:** With projecting folds of the mid-bulb. Several folds project out into the lumen and converge onto a single apical fold. Beyond (at 3 o'clock) is the descending duodenum. Between the folds are pseudodiverticula formed possibly as a result of a pulsion effect on the uninvolved portion of the duodenal wall.

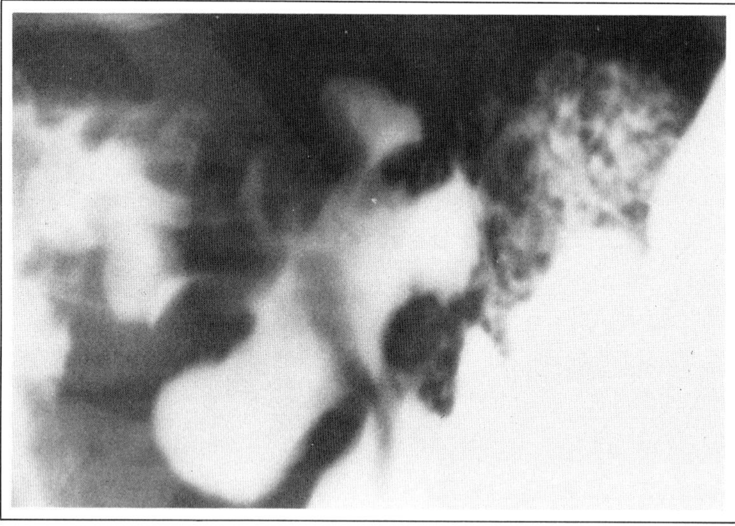

FIG. 26-23.

FIG. 26-23. Cloverleaf radiographic appearance. A combination of apical and mid-bulb ulcer scar deformity (as in Fig. 26-24a) produces this appearance.

these sites is combined, the characteristic radiographic appearance of ulcer scarring, the "cloverleaf" appearance, can be demonstrated (Fig. 26-23). In this section, we consider the distinctive features of scarring in these locations, alone and in combination. In addition, we consider foreshortening of the bulb and pseudodiverticula formation, which also occurs with the other appearances of scar deformity.

Pyloroduodenal Junction Deformity

On entering the pyloric channel, the pyloroduodenal junction deformity is usually evident as an extension from the inferior wall onto the anterior-posterior side walls (Fig. 26-22a). It is common to see pyloroduodenal junction deformity in association with pyloric channel deformity (see Chapter 22).

Mid-Bulb Deformity

Mid-bulb deformity is a common type of scar formation that generally involves the anterior wall; it is seen immediately on entering the bulb as a fold protruding into the lumen (Fig. 26-24a). The fold may be narrow or broad, but in some cases it is prominent enough to partially compromise the lumen. It may be single or composed of several converging folds from either the superior or the inferior wall (Fig. 26-24a).

Apical Deformity

At the apex the deformity appears as stenosis. Within the apex the mucosal folds are effaced and the lumen is narrowed (Fig. 26-24b). Combined deformity—pyloroduodenal, mid-bulb, and apical—appears radiographically as the cloverleaf type of deformity because of focal narrowing of the bulb in its mid-portion and apex with dilatation of the relatively uninvolved fornices and mid-distal portion (Fig. 26-23). Further dilatation of one of these uninvolved areas leads to the pseudodiverticulum appearance (see below).

Foreshortening of the Bulb

Mid-bulb or apical deformity alone or in combination may be sufficient to contract the bulb, giving it a length of less than 3 cm. This appearance is referred to as fore-

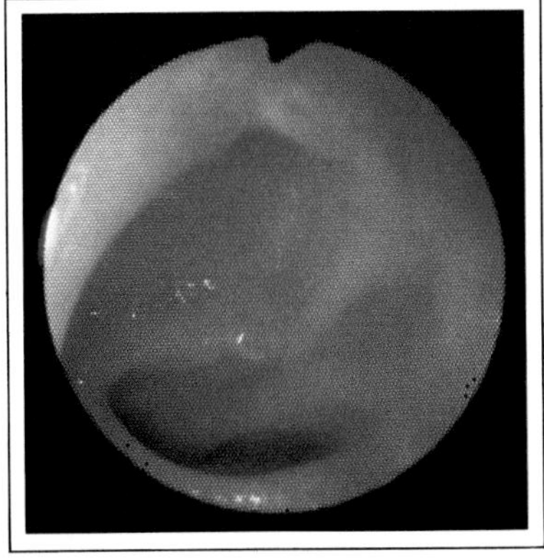

FIG. 26-24a.

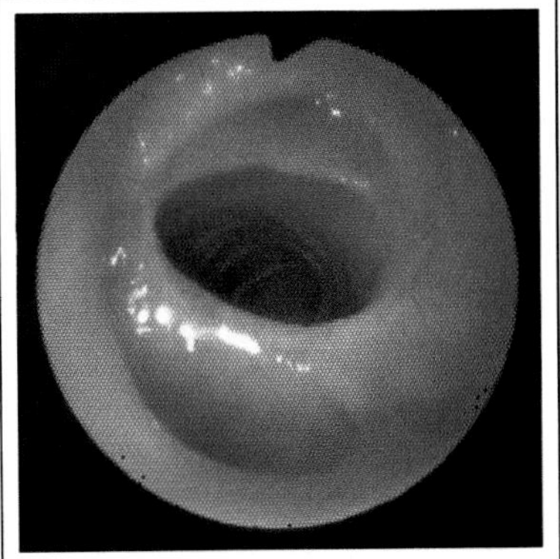

FIG. 26-24b.

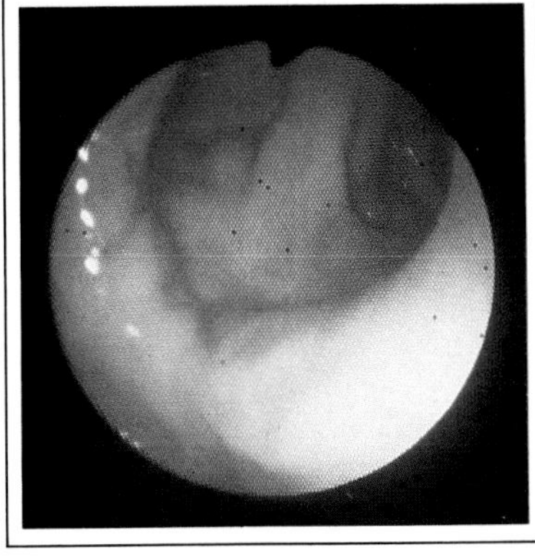

FIG. 26-24c.

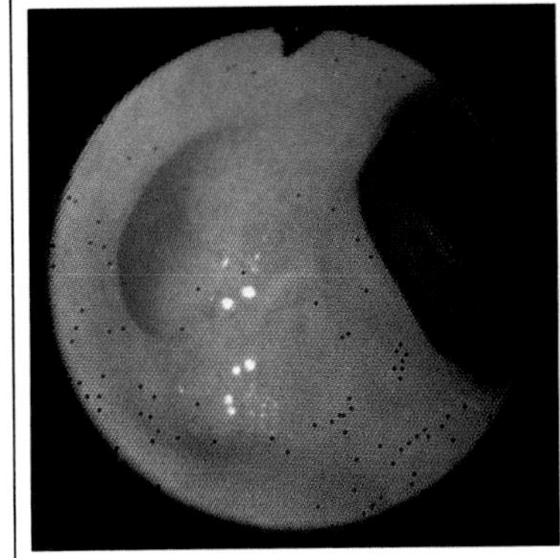

FIG. 26-24d.

FIG. 26-24. a: Ulcer scar deformity in the mid-bulb and apex. There are apparent strut-like deforming folds at the anterior and posterior walls of the mid-bulb (9 to 2 o'clock). A second fold connects the anterior and posterior walls at the apex (at 6 o'clock). In between is a large pseudodiverticulum (going off toward 11 o'clock). **b:** Ulcer scar deformity in the apex and mid-bulb with foreshortening. The apical deformity appears ring-like, whereas the mid-bulb deformity is seen as a second fold running from 6 to 9 o'clock. Between these areas of deformity are several pseudodiverticula. **c:** Ulcer scar deformity with foreshortening and a pseudodiverticulum. The apex at 3 o'clock can be seen from the pyloric channel, indicating marked foreshortening of the bulb. In addition, a pseudodiverticulum is seen adjacent to a raised deformed apical fold. **d:** Ulcer scar deformity with a pseudodiverticulum encompassing the anterior fornix. A prominent deforming fold runs from the inferior pyloroduodenal junction to the anterior wall which has led to the conversion of the anterior fornix into a pseudodiverticulum.

shortening (Fig. 26-24c). However, foreshortening in the absence of other evidence of scar deformity cannot be properly regarded as a marker for peptic ulcer disease but is probably a normal variant (see Chapter 25).

Pseudodiverticula

Pseudodiverticula may be thought of as single or multiple outpouchings within the bulb between cones of scar deformity (Fig. 26-24d). The term pseudodiverticulum is used to distinguish these outpouchings from others of the descending duodenum which occur as a result of primary defects in the wall (see Chapter 27).

The usual locations for the pseudodiverticulum to occur are the fornices (Fig. 26-24d) and the mid-distal portion of the bulb (Fig. 26-24c). The precise mechanism by which the pseudodiverticula occur is uncertain, but they may simply be the result of a stretching effect of the uninvolved wall by material entering the bulb between fixed points of scarring.

Appearance of Active Ulcers in Areas of Scar Deformity

Pyloroduodenal Junction Deformity

The deforming fold of the pyloroduodenal junction deformity is the distal margin for an ulcer scar set within the distal portion of the pyloric channel. Recurrent ulceration of the round or irregular type tends to be located within this depression (Fig. 26-25a). Recognition of the pyloroduodenal deforming fold in a symptomatic patient requires careful examination, particularly of this area.

Mid-Bulb Deformity

Any of the four types of ulcer appearance may be seen with mid-bulb deformity. Round or irregular ulcers may be set within converging folds making up the deformity (Fig. 26-25b). In other cases, linear-type ulcers may run along the peaks of the folds themselves (Fig. 26-25c). Finally, a mixed type of ulcer may be present with either the round, irregular, or salami ulcer found within the depressed area between converging folds of the ulcer scar joining up with one of a linear type running along the tip of a fold itself (Fig. 26-25d).

Apical Deformity

The ulcers associated with this type of deformity are generally of the linear or irregular type (Fig. 26-26a), usually located just at or within the stenotic area.

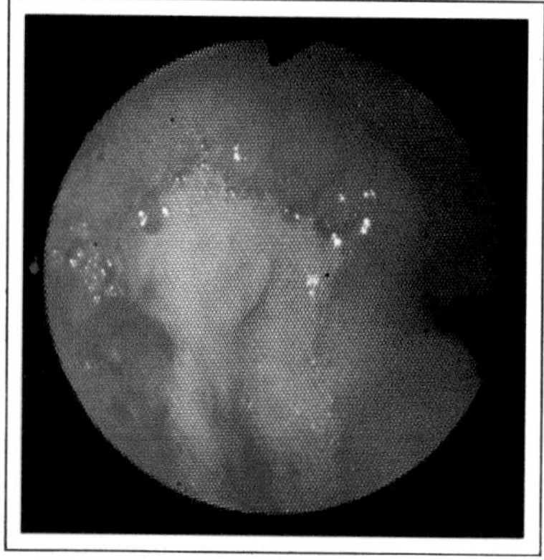

FIG. 26-25a.

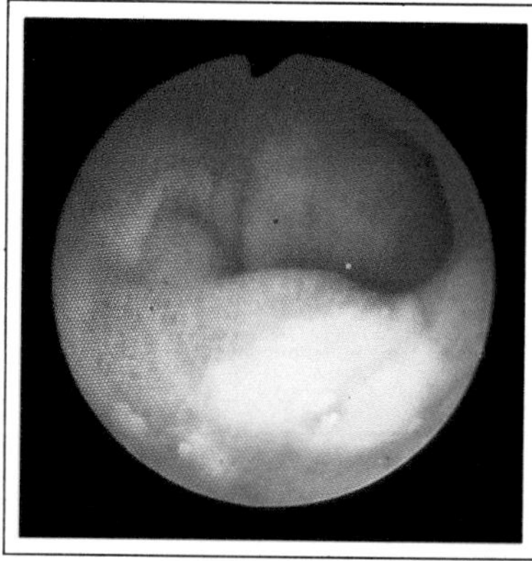

FIG. 26-25b.

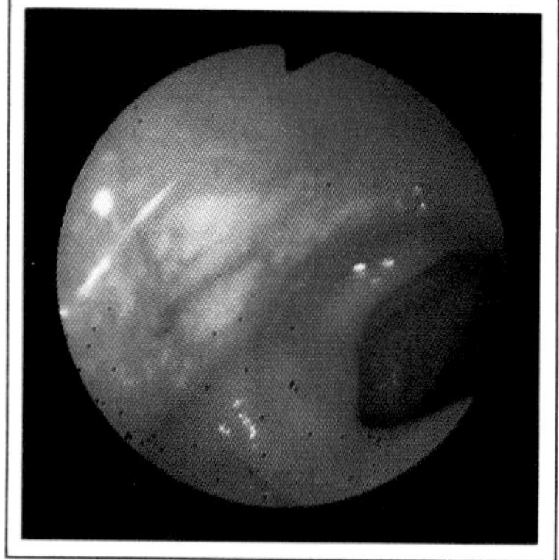

FIG. 26-25c.

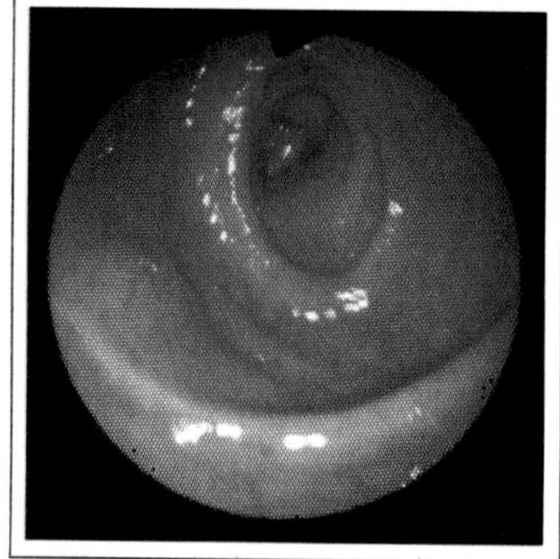

FIG. 26-25d.

FIG. 26-25. a: Pyloroduodenal junction scar deformity with a large (1 cm) irregular ulcer. The scar deformity here is similar to that shown in Fig. 26-14a. **b:** Mid-bulb scar deformity with multiple ulcers. On the inferior wall there is a round ulcer, and on the anterior wall a second ulcer is found with an irregular shape (see text). **c:** Mid-bulb deformity with a linear ulcer. A ring-like deforming inferior wall fold is seen on which is situated a linear ulcer. **d:** Mid-bulb scar deformity with ulcers of a mixed appearance. A salami appearance was found next to a round ulcer (not shown) just proximal and joining with a linear ulcer running along a ridge of the deforming fold (shown).

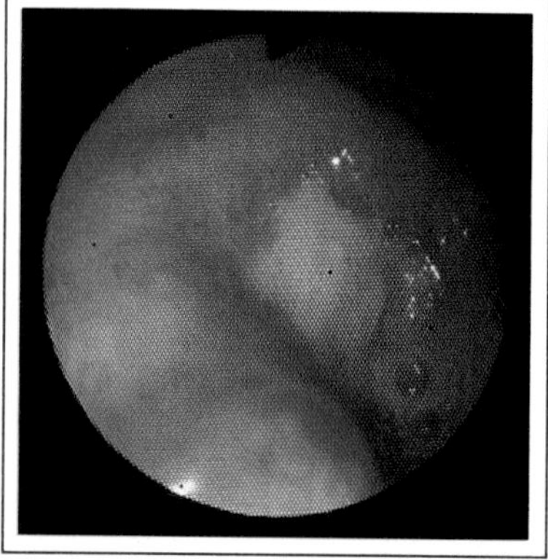

FIG. 26-26a.

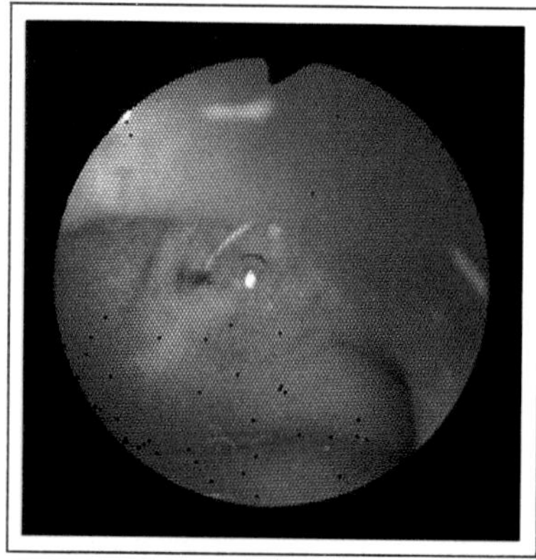

FIG. 26-26b.

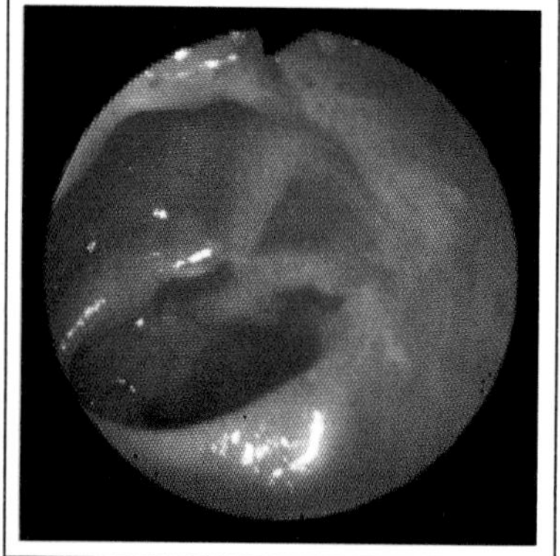

FIG. 26-26c.

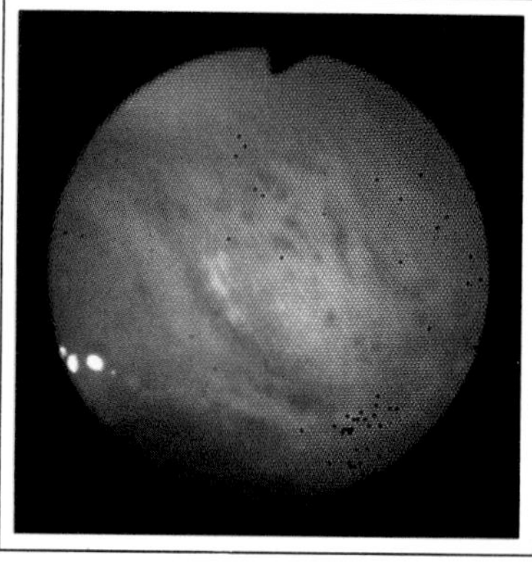

FIG. 26-26d.

FIG. 26-26. a: Apical deformity with a 1-cm irregular ulcer. **b:** Pseudodiverticulum deformity (off to 9 o'clock) with an ulcer set at the edge but not within. **c:** Apical and mid-bulb deformity with acute duodenitis. Discrete zones of erythema are seen in the apex of a patient with ulcer-like symptoms, without a definite ulcer identified. This appearance may constitute an ulcer-equivalent. **d:** Apical deformity with acute duodenitis. This salt and pepper appearance (red and white dots) resembles that of the salami ulcer (Fig. 26-11d). This finding in a patient with an ulcer scar deformity may constitute an ulcer-equivalent, but the symptomatic and endoscopic response to treatment is altogether unpredictable.

Pseudodiverticula

Although it might be thought that the pseudodiverticulum is in some way more vulnerable, ulcers rarely if ever are situated within it but are found just adjacent to it (Fig. 26-26b).

Ulcer Scar Deformity and Duodenitis: An Ulcer-Equivalent?

Patients with typical ulcer symptoms may be found at endoscopy to have an ulcer scar deformity and duodenitis but to lack an ulcer, even after careful examination. The duodenitis in these cases is present especially in the mucosa of the deforming fold and appears as patchy or focal erythema (Fig. 26-26c) or as a salt and pepper appearance with 1-mm whitish areas on a reddened background (Fig. 26-26d). Both appearances, but especially the salt and pepper type because of its resemblance to the salami ulceration (Fig. 26-11d), cause one to consider this appearance as an ulcer-equivalent. Moreover, as biopsies often show acute inflammation or even microscopic ulceration, it seems reasonable to regard this as an ulcer-equivalent, especially for a patient with symptoms suggestive of ulcer disease, and to regard the appearance as an explanation for the symptoms as well as an indication for medical management.[19]

Another reason causing one to regard the finding of bulb deformity and duodenitis as an ulcer-equivalent is the low, but appreciable, number of symptomatic patients, 7% in one series,[2] where despite an ulcer being demonstrated on x-ray, at endoscopy because of deformity of the bulb or other reasons, only duodenitis will be found. One expects this to be true even in cases where small-caliber (8 to 9 mm) instruments have been used.

While patients with duodenitis without ulceration may respond to ulcer treatment[19a] in the absence of scarring, with deformity, in our experience this is unpredictable even in patients with ulceration present histologically. In one series, 50% of patients with duodenitis with histologic changes continued to be symptomatic despite an intensive ulcer regimen, and had unpredictable response to conventional ulcer surgery.[20] While scar deformity and duodenitis may be an ulcer-equivalent, it may actually be more indicative of an underlying mucosal defect, one which may not be improved with simple reduction of acid secretion and neutralization. Moreover, as an ulcer-equivalent, this appearance may be more closely akin to the salami type of ulcer, with its tendency toward slow healing and a high recurrence rate, rather than the more easily treated round type for which rapid healing and a lower recurrence rate are characteristic.[3]

REFERENCES

1. Cameron, A. J., and Ott, B. J. (1977): The value of gastroscopy in clinical diagnosis: a computer-assisted study. *Mayo Clin. Proc.*, 52:806–808.
2. Bianchi Porro, G., Petrillo, M., and Raschi, P. (1975): Endoscopic examination of the duodenal bulb: a comparison with x-ray. *Aktual. Gastrol.*, 4:173–174.
3. Lambert, R., Mainguet, P., and Moulinier, B. (1978): Endoscopy in the management of duodenal ulcers. *Digestion*, 18:110–124.
4. Dubois, A., and Castell, D. O. (1981): Abnormal gastric emptying response to Pentagastrin in duodenal ulcer disease. *Dig. Dis. Sci.*, 26:292–296.
5. Klamer, T. W., and Mahr, M. M. (1978): Giant duodenal ulcer: a dangerous variant of a common illness. *Am. J. Surg.*, 135:760–762.
6. Lumsden, K., MacLarnon, J. C., and Dawson, J. (1970): Giant duodenal ulcer, *Gut*, 11:592–599.
7. Kerremans, R. P., Lerut, J., and Penninckx, F. M. (1979): Malignant duodenal tumors. *Ann. Surg.*, 190:179–182.
8. Isenberg, J. I., Walsh, J. H., and Grossman, M. I. (1973): Zollinger-Ellison syndrome. *Gastroenterology*, 65:140–165.
9. Regan, P. T., and Malagelada, J.-R. (1978): A reappraisal of clinical, roentgenographic, and endoscopic features of the Zollinger-Ellison syndrome. *Mayo Clin. Proc.*, 53:19–23.
10. Fang, M., Ginsberg, A. L., Glassman, L., Glassman, L., McCarthy, D. M., Cohen, P., Geelhoed, G. W., and Dobbins, W. O. (1979): Zollinger-Ellison syndrome with diarrhea as the predominant clinical feature. *Gastroenterology*, 76:378–387.
11. Ellis, D. J., Kingston, R. D., Brooks, V. S., and Waterhouse, J. A. H. (1974): Gastric carcinoma and previous peptic ulceration. *Br. J. Surg.*, 66:117–119.
12. Burns, G. P., and Taubman, J. (1967): The association of gastric carcinoma with duodenal ulcer. *Br. J. Surg.*, 54:174–176.
13. Branson, C. J., Boxer, M. E., Palmer, K. R., Clark, J. C., Underwood, J. C. E., and Duthie, H. L. (1981): Mucosal cell proliferation in duodenal ulcer and duodenitis. *Gut*, 22:277–282.
14. Hasan, M., Sircus, W., and Ferguson, A. (1981): Duodenal mucosal architecture in non-specific and ulcer-associated duodenitis. *Gut*, 22:637–641.
15. Scheurer, U., Witzel, L., Halter, F., Keller, H.-M., Huber, R., and Galeazzi, R. (1977): Gastric and duodenal ulcer healing under placebo treatment. *Gastroenterology*, 72:838–841.

15a. Chuong, J. J. H., and Spiro, H. M. (1982): Cimetidine duodenal ulcers: an analysis of methodologic problems in randomized controlled trials. *J. Clin. Gastroenterol.*, 4:311–320.

16. Kohli, Y., Misaki, F., and Kawai, K. (1972): Endoscopical follow up observation of duodenal ulcer. *Endoscopy*, 4:202–208.

16a. Massarrat, S., and Eisenmann, A. (1981): Factors affecting the healing rate of duodenal and pyloric ulcers with low-dose antacid treatment. *Gut*, 22:97–102.

17. Dronfield, M. W., Batchelor, A. J., Larkworthy, W., and Langman, M. J. S. (1979): Controlled trial of maintenance cimetidine treatment in healed duodenal ulcer: short and long-term effects. *Gut*, 20:526–530.
18. Korrman, M., Hetzel, D. J., Hansky, J., Shearman, D. J. C., and Don, G. (1980): Relapse rate of duodenal ulcer after cessation of long-term cimetidine treatment: a double-blind control study. *Dig. Dis. Sci.*, 25:88–91.
19. Greenlaw, R., Sheahan, D. G., Deluca, V. A., Miller, D., Myerson, D., and Myerson, P. (1980): Gastroduodenitis: a broader concept of peptic ulcer disease. *Dig. Dis. Sci.*, 25:660–672.

19a. MacKinnon, M., Willing, R. L., and Whitehead, R. (1982): Cimetidine in the management of symptomatic patients with duodenitis. A double-bind controlled trial. *Dig. Dis. Sci.*, 27:217–220.

20. Cotton, P. B., Price, A. B., Tighe, J. R., and Beales, J. S. M. (1973): Preliminary evaluation of "duodenitis" by endoscopy and biopsy. *Br. Med. J.*, 3:430–433.

27

STRUCTURAL ABNORMALITIES OF THE DUODENUM

Structural abnormalities of the duodenum appear for the most part as alterations in the shape of the lumen. In the two previous chapters we considered altered structural appearances which are either variations of normal (see Chapter 25) or related to peptic ulcer disease (see Chapter 26). In this chapter we consider other types of abnormalities, including those which result from extrinsic compression, surgery, mechanical obstruction, motor disorders, and anatomic defects, e.g., duodenal diverticula.

DUODENAL BULB

We have already discussed the most frequently encountered structural abnormalities of the duodenal bulb, i.e., ulcer scar deformity (see Chapter 26), as well as other common variations of normal appearance, e.g., foreshortening of the bulb (see Chapter 25). We now consider less common appearances, which include: (a) extrinsic compression of the bulb; (b) dilatation; and (c) postsurgical (nonpeptic) deformity.

Extrinsic Compression

The pancreas, liver, and extrahepatic biliary system (bile duct and gallbladder) bear a close anatomic relationship to the duodenal bulb. Enlargement of any of these structures may impinge on the duodenal bulb and alter its shape.

Pancreas

Enlargement of the head of the pancreas by cancer or pancreatitis, although more commonly distorting the appearance of the descending duodenum (see below), can also deform the duodenal bulb at its apex and along the inferior wall (Fig. 27-1a).[1] In our experience this occurs more often in patients ultimately proved to have chronic pancreatitis, especially in the presence of pseudocysts of the head of the pancreas (Fig. 27-1a). The mucosa with either pancreatitis or carcinoma may be normal or show nonspecific erythema and enlargement of the mucosal folds (Fig. 27-1b), although the latter are more commonly found in patients with pancreatitis[2] (see Chapter 28).

Liver

Despite the frequency with which patients with liver enlargement undergo endoscopy, it is somewhat surprising that extrinsic compression of the bulb is seldom observed. The reason for this lack of involvement is unknown but may bear on the fact that the liver is largely anterior to the bulb and could enlarge without involving it at all. In cases where it is involved either from benign (Fig. 27-2a) or malignant (Fig. 27-2b) causes, one sees compromise of the lumen by a mass-like deformity, generally from the anterior superior aspect (Fig. 27-2b), although occasionally this may be posterior (Fig. 27-2a).

Bile Ducts and Gallbladder

Massive dilatation of the common bile duct may lead to posterior compression of the bulb at or just beyond the apex (Fig. 27-3). In patients with as yet unexplained jaundice, the endoscopist may provide an important clue to the jaundice being secondary to extrahepatic obstruction. In cases where the gallbladder fossa of the liver is contiguous with the duodenal bulb, gallbladder enlargement from extrahepatic obstruction or gallbladder malignancy itself (Fig. 27-4a) produces deformity of the anterior aspect of the bulb (Fig. 27-4b).

Dilatation

In cases of dilatation, the lumen of the bulb has an increased diameter, possibly exceeding 5 to 6 cm (Fig. 27-5a) with normal being 3 cm (Fig. 27-5b). One sees di-

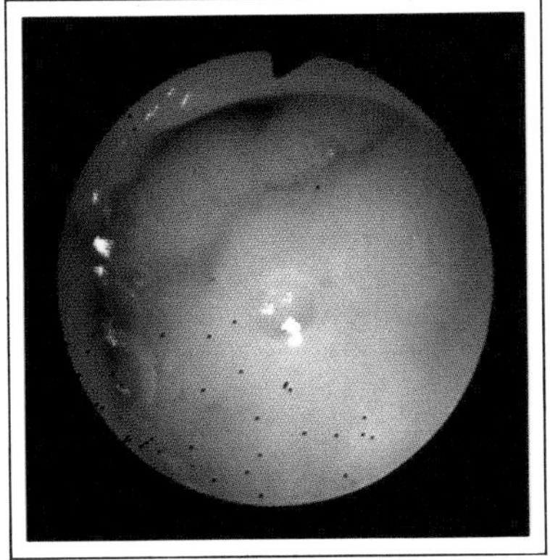

FIG. 27-1a.

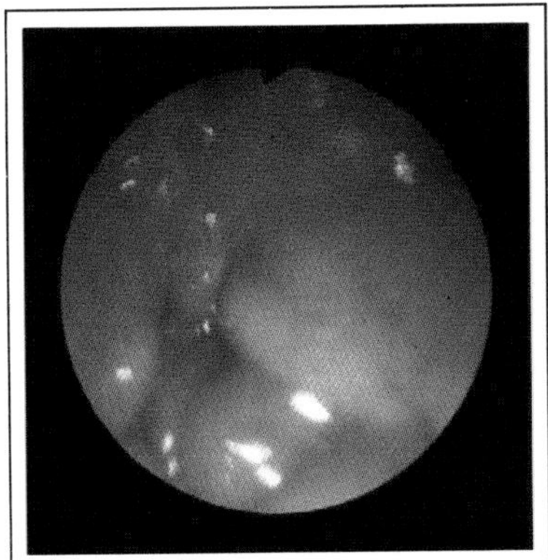

FIG. 27-1b.

FIG. 27-1. Extrinsic compression of the duodenal bulb in a patient with chronic pancreatitis. **a:** Enlargement of the head of the pancreas from pseudocysts produced extrinsic compression of the inferior wall and apex of the duodenal bulb. The mucosa itself is unremarkable. **b:** The mucosa folds appeared enlarged, but soft, and displayed focal erythema.

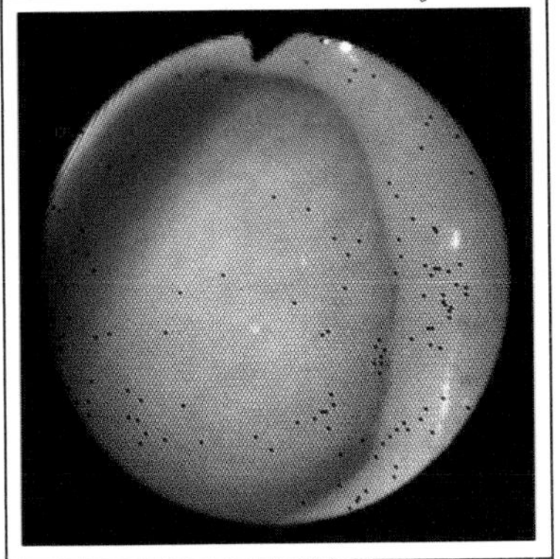

FIG. 27-2a.

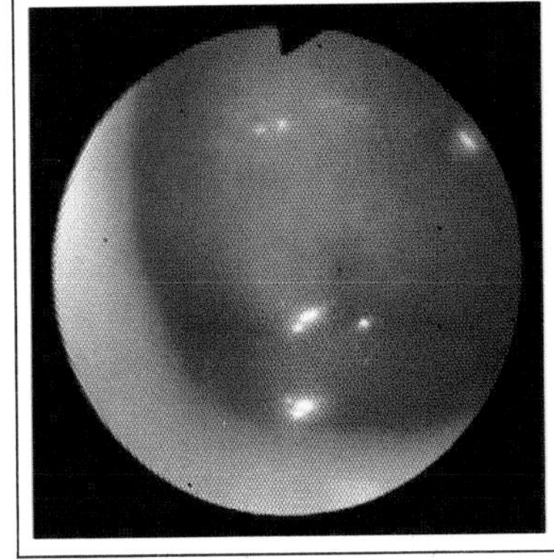

FIG. 27-2b.

FIG. 27-2. Extrinsic compression of the duodenal bulb. **a:** In a patient with hepatomegaly from primary biliary cirrhosis. The massive enlargement of the liver produced compression of the inferior and posterior walls. **b:** In a patient with metastatic liver disease. The superior wall as seen from the pyloric channel shows a fixed indentation probably from compression by a metastatic hepatic tumor mass.

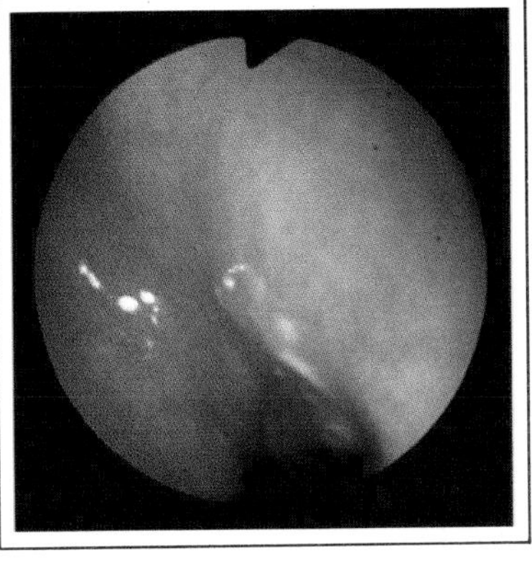

FIG. 27-3.

FIG. 27-3. Extrinsic compression of the apex by a dilated common bile duct showing indentation from the posterior wall.

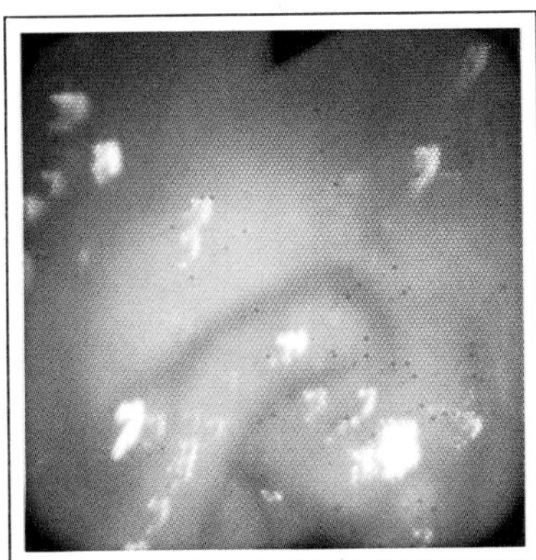

FIG. 27-4a.

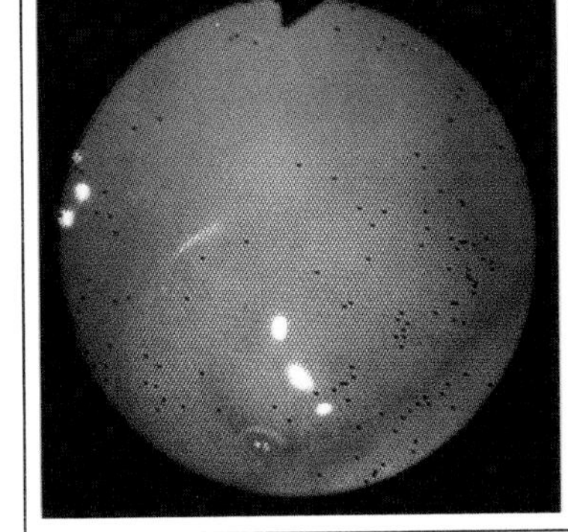

FIG. 27-4b.

FIG. 27-4. a: Extrinsic compression of the bulb in a patient with bile duct carcinoma. A nodular fold from the posterior-superior aspect of the bulb corresponds to the location of the carcinoma demonstrated cholangiographically. **b:** Extrinsic compression of the anterior wall of the bulb by a gallbladder carcinoma.

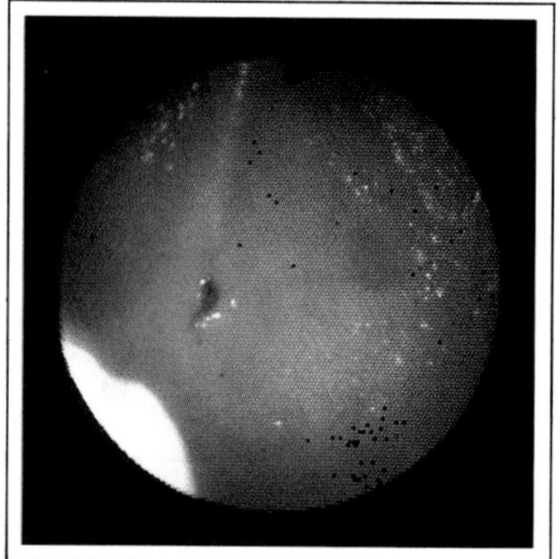

FIG. 27-5a.

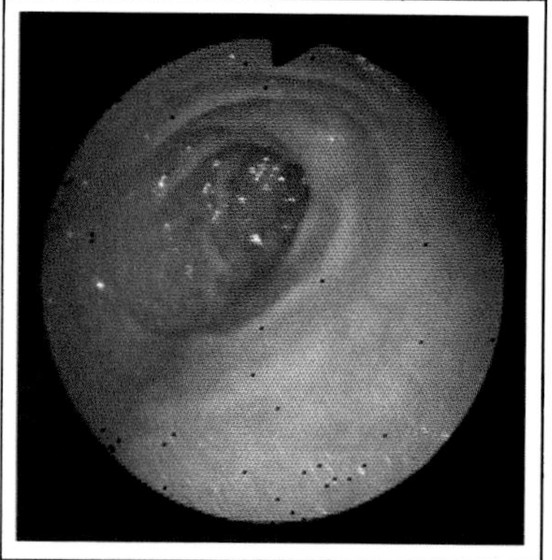

FIG. 27-5b.

FIG. 27-5. a: Dilated duodenal bulb in a patient with longstanding apical obstruction from chronic pancreatitis. The bulb appears cavernous in contrast to one of normal diameter (b). **b:** Duodenal bulb with a normal luminal diameter.

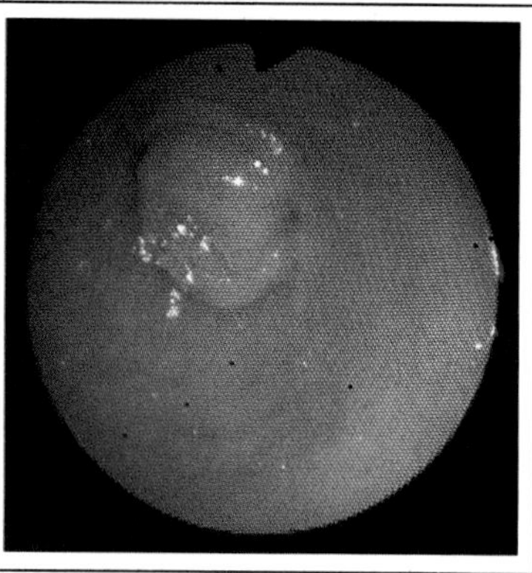

FIG. 27-6.

FIG. 27-6. Apical stenosis in a patient with longstanding peptic ulcer disease. The apex has a puckered appearance with a pinpoint opening from which bile is bubbling (toward 9 o'clock). The overlying mucosa is intact, favoring a benign cause for the obstruction; this does not exclude carcinoma, however, which may produce a similar appearance (Fig. 27-7b).

latation in two main settings: mechanical obstruction and motor disorders.

Mechanical Obstruction

Peptic ulcer disease.

Although it is a much less common complication of peptic ulcer disease than pyloroduodenal obstruction, peptic ulcer disease is occasionally encountered (Fig. 27-6). The dilatation of the bulb is seen with tight stenotic deformity of the apex resulting in complete or total obstruction. At endoscopy one sees typical apical deformity with a pinpoint lumen but no other deformity in the bulb. The mucosa overlying the obstruction is generally intact (Fig. 27-6). Although this appearance is consistent with benign obstruction, an identical appearance may be seen with malignant obstruction (see below).

Malignant obstruction of the apex.

Carcinoma arising from the head of the pancreas, duodenum, or common bile duct may rarely spread locally to involve the apex. Rather than seeing a pinpoint stenotic lesion in these cases, the endoscopist more often sees simply extrinsic compression from the anterior aspect of the distal duodenal bulb with a mass-like deformity which obstructs the lumen at the apex (Fig. 27-7a). The duodenum proximal to this appears dilated. The eccentric appearance of apical obstruction, especially if present with an irregular mass-like deformity from the inferior wall, strongly suggests the possibility of malignancy. In some cases, however, the obstruction appears more circumferential with intact mucosa, thus simulating the appearance of peptic ulcer disease (Fig. 27-7b).

Congenital abnormalities.

One may on rare occasions encounter a patient with an annular pancreas occluding the descending duodenum just below the apex (see Chapter 31). Another congenital lesion we have seen producing massive dilatation of the duodenal bulb (Fig. 27-8) is congenital atresia of the descending duodenum that was surgically corrected during infancy. In this case there was still partial outlet obstruction accompanied by massive dilatation of the bulb.

Motor Disorder

Scleroderma alone or as a mixed connective tissue disorder produces dilatation of the duodenal bulb and descending duodenum (see below). In some cases duodenal bulb dilatation is the most striking feature (Fig. 27-9). In contrast

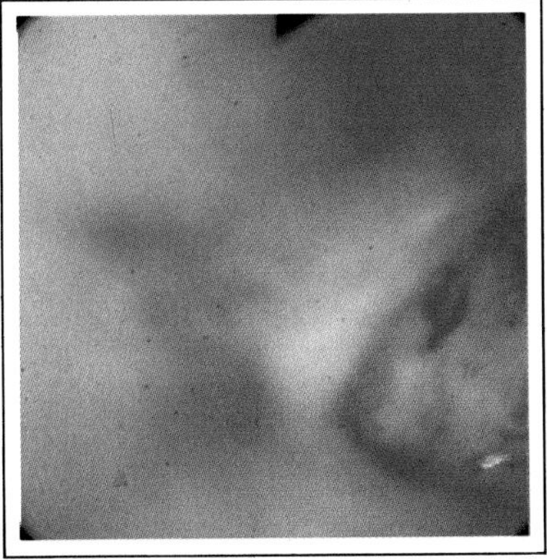

FIG. 27-7a.

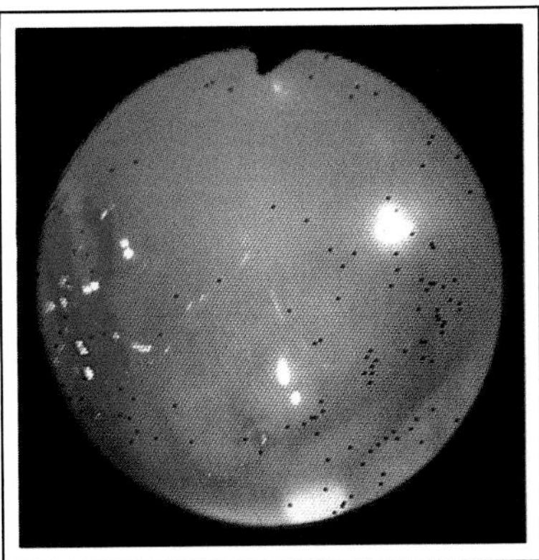

FIG. 27-7b.

FIG. 27-7. Apical obstruction. **a:** From a pancreatic carcinoma. A nodular, ulcerated lesion is seen invading the duodenum just below the apex. **b:** From a bile duct carcinoma. Extrinsic compression from this lesion, because of its anatomic position, produces apical obstruction. The intactness of the mucosa simulates obstruction from peptic ulcer disease (Fig. 27-6).

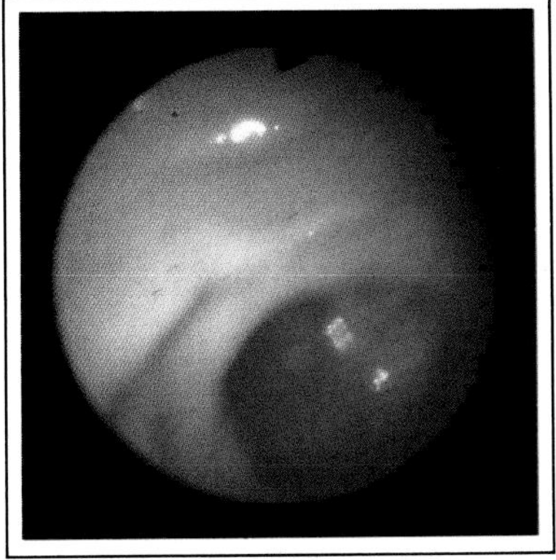

FIG. 27-8.

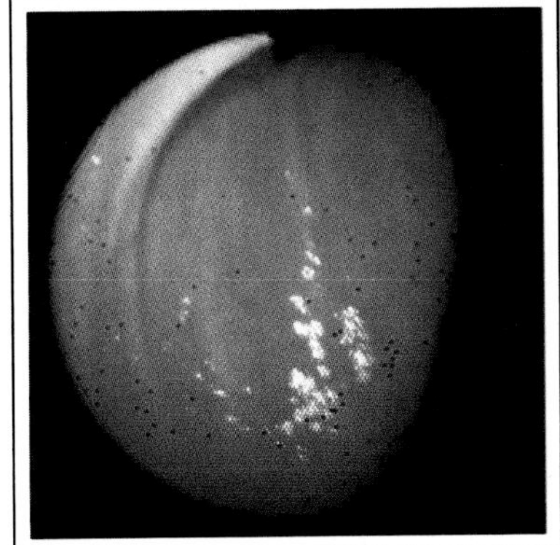

FIG. 27-9.

FIG. 27-8. Massive dilatation of the duodenal bulb in a 21-year-old patient with atresia of the descending duodenum that had been treated during infancy with a gastrojejunostomy.

FIG. 27-9. A dilated duodenal bulb in a patient with scleroderma. The luminal diameter is increased approximately twice normal, exceeding (by estimation) 5 cm.

to the mechanical obstruction, the apex in these cases is widely patent (Fig. 27-9).

Postsurgical Deformity

We have already considered the most common type of postsurgical deformity—that from ulcer surgery (see Chapter 19). The endoscopist may also encounter an altered appearance of the duodenal bulb in patients after biliary surgery, most often cholecystectomy but occasionally a bile duct anastomosis into the posterior wall of the duodenal bulb.

Postcholecystectomy Appearance

For the most part, prior gallbladder surgery does not affect the appearance of the duodenum. One can, however, observe extrinsic compression from scarring along the anterior superior aspect of the bulb or inferior wall (Fig. 27-10). In these cases the mucosa of the wall which projects into the lumen is either normal (Fig. 27-10) or shows nonspecific erythema. Probing the mass-like deformity (Fig. 27-10) which the surgical scarring produces shows it to be relatively fixed, not affected by air insufflation or gentle manipulation. As such, this appearance is indistinguishable from that produced by extrinsic compression from carcinoma (Fig. 27-4b).

Postcholedochoduodenostomy Appearance

During choledochoduodenostomy the common bile duct is anastomosed to the posterior wall of the duodenal bulb. The endoscopist generally sees converging folds on the posterior wall aspect of the apex (Fig. 27-11). In some cases surgical sutures themselves mark the anastomotic point, as well as the appearance of bile draining from this area. If the endoscopist is unaware of the history of previous biliary surgery, he may mistake this appearance for the extremely rare posterior wall ulcer which penetrates into the common bile duct.[3] Additional features (e.g., the irregular appearance of the stoma, erythema, and adherent bile and foreign material) may be confusing to the endoscopist who is unaware of the patient's previous biliary surgery.

DESCENDING DUODENUM

Four types of structural change leading to an abnormal appearance of the descending duodenum are considered here. The commonest is an altered appearance of the lumen and medial wall from extrinsic compression by an enlarged head of the pancreas or common bile duct. Less common appearances are those from duodenal diverticula, dilatation, and finally postsurgical deformity, especially that involving the duodenal papilla.

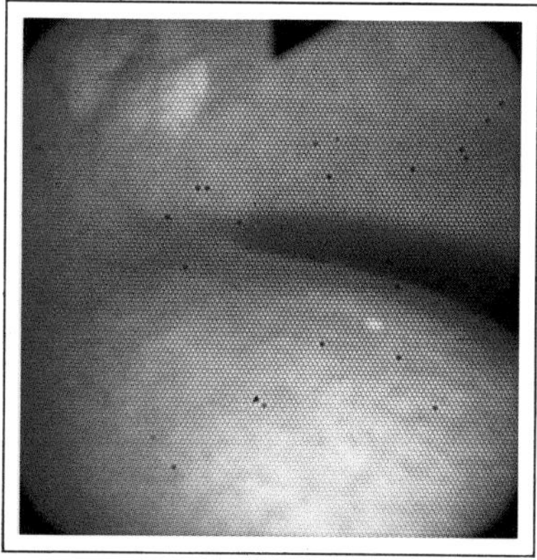

FIG. 27-10.

FIG. 27-11.

FIG. 27-10. Extrinsic compression of the duodenal bulb and apex from previous gallbladder surgery. On gentle probing, the indentation of the inferior wall at 6 o'clock appeared fixed.

FIG. 27-11. Scar deformity of the apex of the duodenal bulb from choledochoduodenostomy. The anastomosis of the common bile duct to the posterior wall of the bulb has an appearance similar to that of ulcer scar deformity (see Chapter 26). In the absence of a history of previous surgery, this appearance could be mistaken for a rare choledochoduodenal fistula from a penetrating ulcer.[3]

FIG. 27-12a.

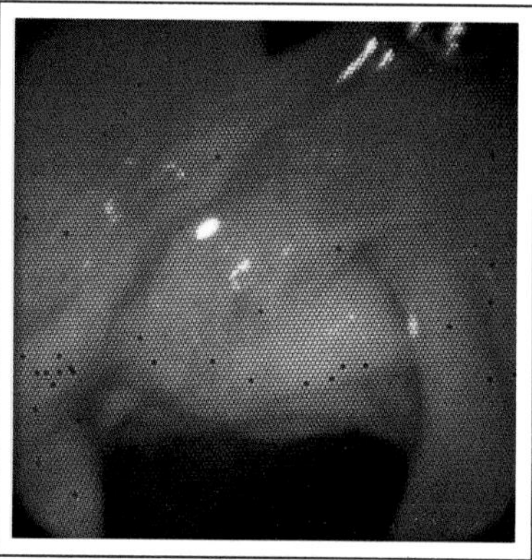

FIG. 27-12b.

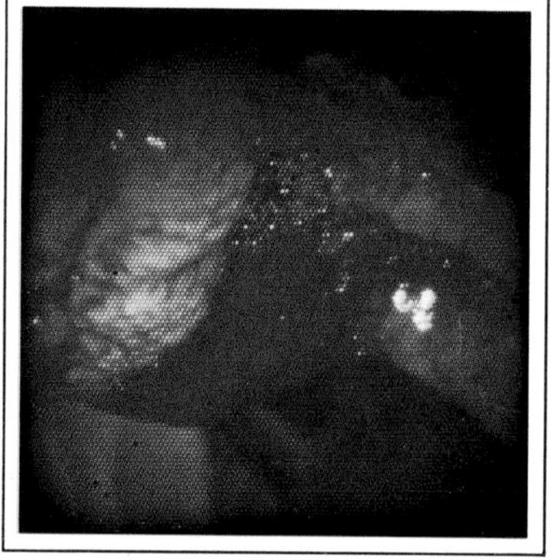

FIG. 27-12c.

FIG. 27-12. Extrinsic compression of the descending duodenum from pancreatic carcinoma. **a:** Although there is enlargement of the Kerckring folds and duodenal papilla (pictured here), in the surgically resected specimen the tumor was not found invading the duodenum. **b:** The medial wall (at 12 o'clock) projects into the lumen and compromises it. Despite the enlargement of the mucosal folds and erythema, biopsies were negative. Moreover, the resected specimen showed no histologic evidence of invasion. **c:** With mucosal invasion. In addition to the extrinsic compression from the medial wall, nodular, friable tumor masses are present. Biopsies and brushings were both positive for malignancy.

Extrinsic Compression

Pancreatic Disease

Pancreatic carcinoma.

In our experience, extrinsic compression of the descending duodenum occurs in approximately 20% of patients with pancreatic carcinoma (see Chapter 29). Most commonly it occurs in patients in whom the site of origin of the malignancy is within 2 cm of the ampulla, i.e., periampullary cancers. In these cases the mucosa may be either unaffected or show nonspecific changes, e.g., increased size of the Kerckring folds at the ampulla (Fig. 27-12a) and/or nonspecific erythema (Fig. 27-12b). These changes do not correlate well with the presence of invasion in surgically resected specimens, being found in only 30 to 40% of such patients. They should not, therefore, be interpreted as evidence of local tumor spread, as would the presence of frank malignancy within the wall of the duodenum (Fig. 27-12c).

Pancreatitis.

Acute and/or chronic pancreatitis may cause enlargement of the head of the pancreas to an extent which compromises the medial wall of the duodenum (Fig. 27-13a). It is unknown, however, in what percent of the cases this actually occurs because the large majority of patients are not en-

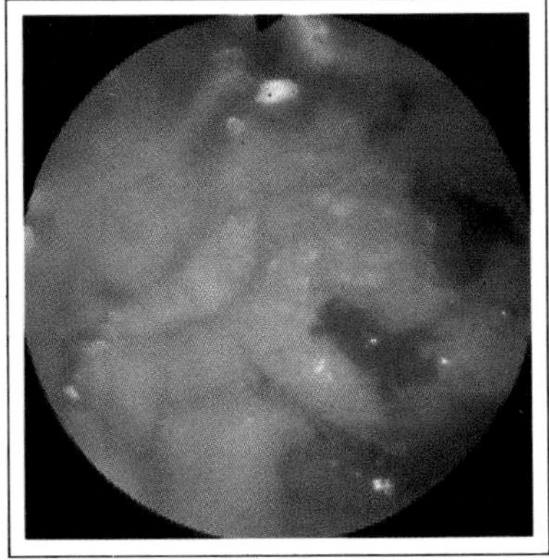

FIG. 27-13a.

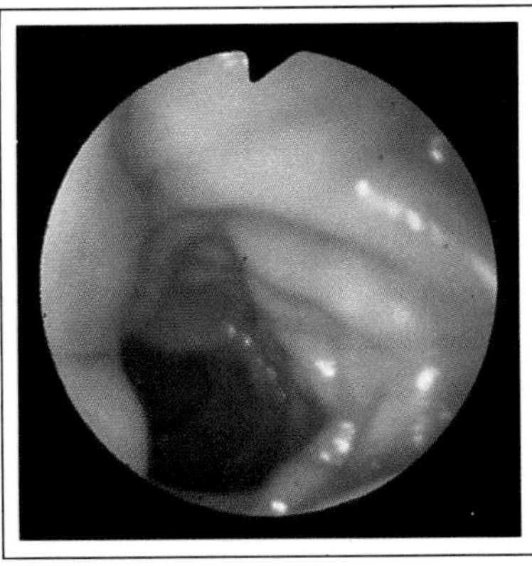

FIG. 27-13b.

FIG. 27-13. a: Extrinsic compression of the descending duodenum in a patient with chronic pancreatitis. The folds are enlarged with nonspecific mucosal erythema similar to that found in patients with pancreatic carcinoma (Fig. 27-12b). **b:** Extrinsic compression (localized to the apex) in a patient with chronic pancreatitis and a probable pseudocyst involving the duodenal wall. This effect is most prominent in the posterior (9 o'clock) position after intubation using the indirect technique (see Chapter 24).

doscoped. It is our impression that, although changes such as enlargement of the Kerckring folds and nonspecific erythema are observed rather frequently in patients endoscoped for pancreatitis, significant extrinsic compression where the lumen is compromised by more than 50% (Fig. 27-13a) is uncommon. When it does occur, there is often a pseudocyst either in the contiguous portion of the pancreas[4] or extending into the wall of the duodenum itself.[4,5] In the latter case, one may observe localized extrinsic compression at or just below the apex (Fig. 27-13b). Unlike the extrinsic compression associated with pancreatic carcinoma, which may be associated with little or no mucosal effect (Fig. 29-12a), that associated with pancreatitis is often found with intense (reactive) mucosal changes, particularly those of marked erythema and thickening of the Kerckring folds. Because striking nodularity may be present, the appearance may be mistaken for invasive carcinoma (Fig. 27-13a).[4]

Common Bile Duct Dilatation

A characteristic tubular indentation of the medial wall may be observed with bile duct obstruction, especially that associated with pancreatic carcinoma where massively dilated bile ducts (>2 cm) are common. We find this appearance in 15 to 20% of patients with pancreatic cancer whose presentation is jaundice. With this appearance, one sees a 2- to 3-cm tubular impression beginning at and encompassing hooded folds of the duodenal papilla and extending up the medial wall from this point (Fig. 27-14a). The Kerckring folds which overlie the tubular indentation are decreased in size or entirely effaced (Fig. 27-14a) from the greatly enlarged bile duct (Fig. 27-14b). As the carcinoma in most cases does not invade the duodenal papilla directly or its orifice, these structures, despite the striking tubular impression above, may appear entirely normal (Fig. 27-14c).

Duodenal Diverticula

Although radiologists regard duodenal diverticula as being relatively common, being demonstrated in 1 to 5% of upper gastrointestinal (GI) series,[6] they are encountered much less frequently at endoscopy. We observed only 15 cases in a series of 5,000 examinations, an incidence of 0.3%. The infrequency with which these may be found at endoscopy is probably related to the fact that the majority are small and would have required the use of a side-viewing instrument if they were to have been seen, and possibly not even then (Fig. 27-15a). The endoscopist, however, can easily observe larger diverticula, especially in the mid-portion of the descending duodenum on the medial aspect within 2 cm of the duodenal papilla. In most of these cases endoscopy would have been requested for nonspecific symptoms. A few with diverticula may have a presentation suggestive of biliary calculus disease with which there is an increased incidence,[7] while yet other rare patients may present with obstructive jaundice secondary to impaction with foreign material or with the diverticulum as the site of upper GI bleeding.[8] The endoscopist performing endoscopic retrograde cholangiopancreatography (ERCP) must be aware of the presence of periampullary diverticula as he searches for the duodenal papilla, which has an altered relationship to the descending duodenum, being partly within the diverticulum.[9]

Appearance

Characteristically, a diverticulum is seen as an abrupt termination on the medial wall of the Kerckring folds (Fig. 27-15a) ending in a blind, foldless pouch. In cases where the diverticulum is large, it freely admits the endoscope, allowing one to observe flat mucosa with a prominent vascular pattern (Fig. 27-15b). In addition, one may find formed foreign material (Fig. 27-15c). When the duodenal papilla is present within the diverticulum, if the 12 o'clock tip position is oriented toward the medial wall the hooded fold and orifice are found on the inferior (6 o'clock) wall aspect directed toward the posterior (9 o'clock) wall side (Fig. 27-15d).

Intraluminal Duodenal Diverticula

Recently an exceedingly rare type of diverticulum was described: intraluminal duodenal diverticulum. In these

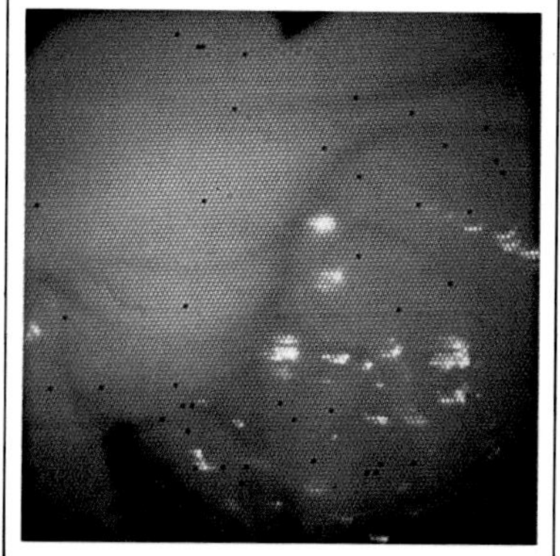

FIG. 27-14a.

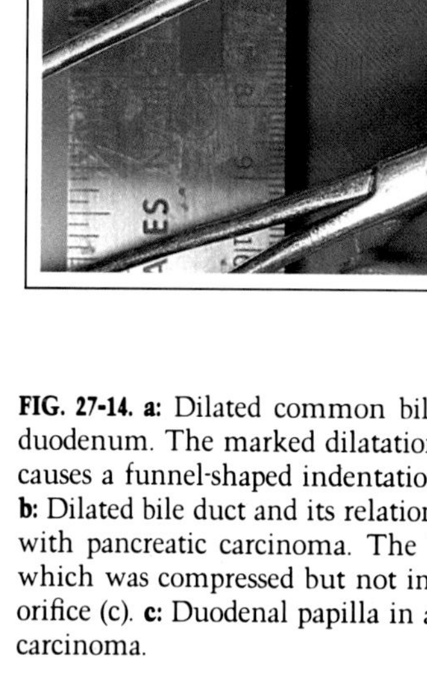

FIG. 27-14b.

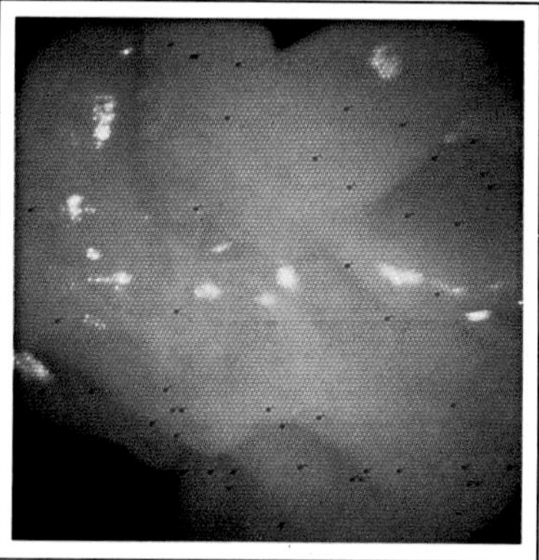

FIG. 27-14c.

FIG. 27-14. a: Dilated common bile duct compression on the medial wall of the descending duodenum. The marked dilatation of the bile duct (b) in a patient with pancreatic carcinoma causes a funnel-shaped indentation on the medial wall to run from the apex to the ampulla. **b:** Dilated bile duct and its relationship to the duodenum in the resected specimen of a patient with pancreatic carcinoma. The bile duct is markedly dilated (>2 cm) above the ampulla, which was compressed but not invaded, accounting for the intact appearance of the capillary orifice (c). **c:** Duodenal papilla in a patient with massive bile duct obstruction from pancreatic carcinoma.

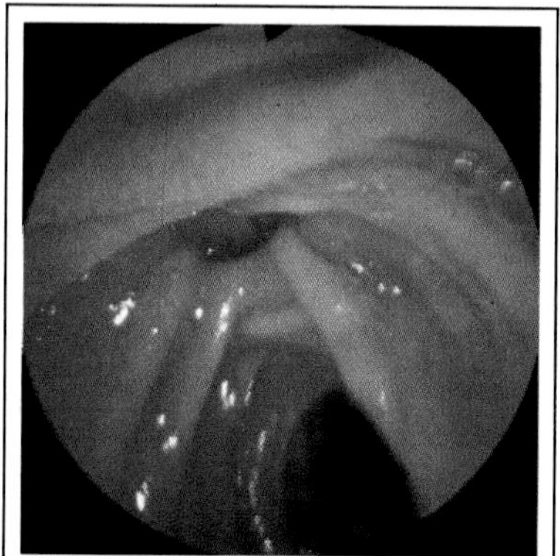

FIG. 27-15a.

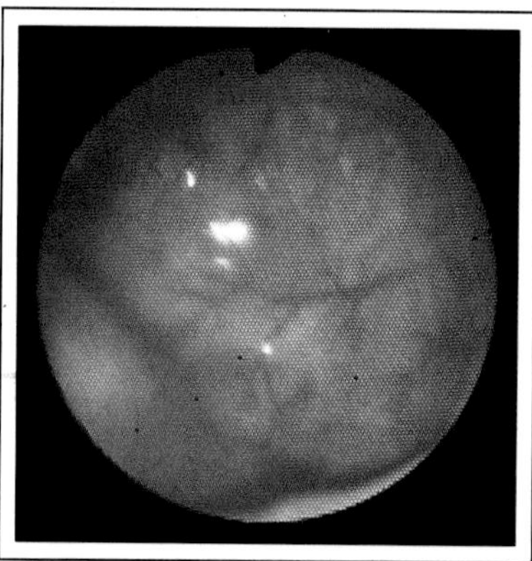

FIG. 27-15b.

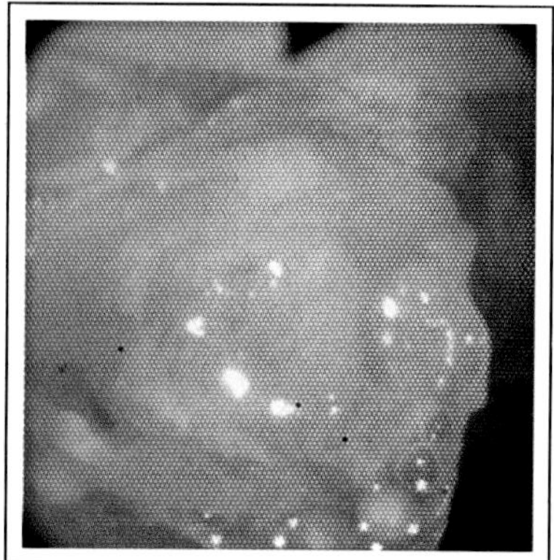

FIG. 27-15c.

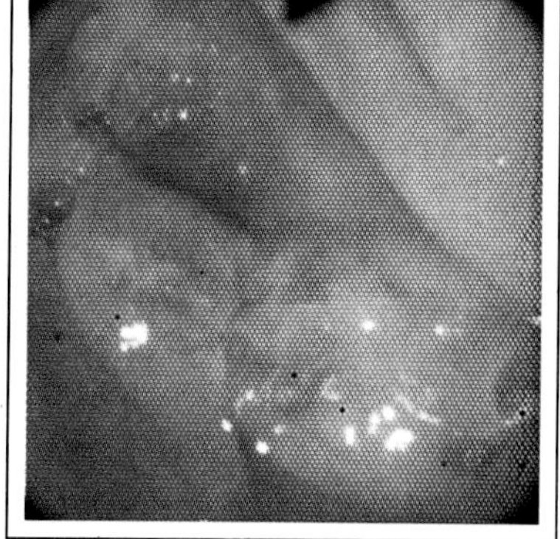

FIG. 27-15d.

FIG. 27-15. a: Duodenal diverticulum. The surrounding Kerckring folds radiate into a small opening at 10 o'clock where they terminate abruptly. This appearance, rather than that of concentrically arranged, continuous folds (as in the case of the lumen at 6 o'clock) suggests the mouth of a diverticulum. **b:** Large duodenal diverticulum. Because of its size, the endoscope tip may enter and display a foldless interior along with a prominent vascular pattern of its mucosa. **c:** Bezoar in large duodenal (periampullary) diverticulum. The bezoar entirely fills the diverticulum and projects into the lumen. **d:** Large duodenal diverticulum [same as in (c)]. Once the bezoar was removed, the papilla was observed in its characteristic location within a diverticulum, the posterior (9 o'clock) aspect of the inferior wall.

cases the opening of the diverticulum is seen adjacent to and running in the same direction as the lumen itself.[10] Patients with an intraluminal diverticulum may present with nonspecific symptoms. In some patients obstruction of the duodenum itself has been reported as the diverticulum fills with foreign material,[11] and in other patients bleeding and pancreatitis have been found.[12]

Dilatation

As in the duodenal bulb (see above), dilatation of the descending duodenum (Fig. 27-16a) may occur because of the presence of mechanical obstruction of the third or fourth portion (Fig. 27-16b) or with sclerodermatous involvement of the small bowel (Fig. 27-16c). The lumen may be enlarged to 7 cm (1.5 times its normal maximal diameter). With dilatation, the Kerckring folds are generally decreased in height (Fig. 27-16c) or entirely effaced (Fig. 27-16d).

It may be impossible to tell from endoscopy whether the cause of dilatation is mechanical obstruction or a motor disorder. Good radiographic studies of the third and fourth portion of the duodenum are therefore necessary; they may suggest to the endoscopist whether the dilatation is caused by a motor disorder (Fig. 27-17a) or mechanical obstruction (Fig. 27-17b), and, if the latter, whether it is (Fig. 27-17c) or is not (Fig. 27-17b) within the reach of a conventional (105 cm) forward-viewing endoscope. In cases where an obstructing lesion is within reach, fluoroscopy may be employed as an aid to increase the depth of insertion using the technique of paradoxical advancement (see Chapter 24). In cases where this cannot be done, a longer side-viewing duodenoscope (135 cm) may be used, although it is often more difficult to biopsy an obstructing lesion with this instrument. In many instances, however, the endoscopist cannot reach the obstruction with any instrument, so that the diagnosis may have to await exploratory laparotomy (Fig. 27-17b).

Postsurgical Deformity

Postsurgical Appearances of the Duodenal Papilla

The commonest surgical procedure performed involving the descending duodenum is a transduodenal sphincteroplasty.[12] In this operation, an incision is made across the oddic sphincter and a stoma is fashioned that has a longitudinal dimension of 1.5 cm or more. Endoscopically, one sees a slit-like opening in what anatomically would correspond to the hooded fold (Fig. 27-18a) instead of the expected orifice (see Chapter 24). In cases where a distal

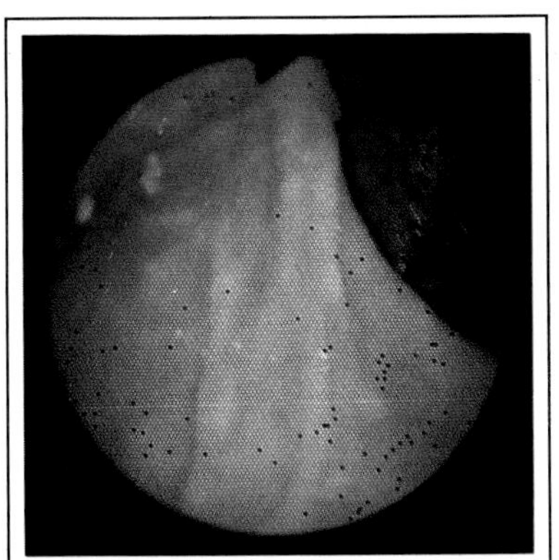

FIG. 27-16a.

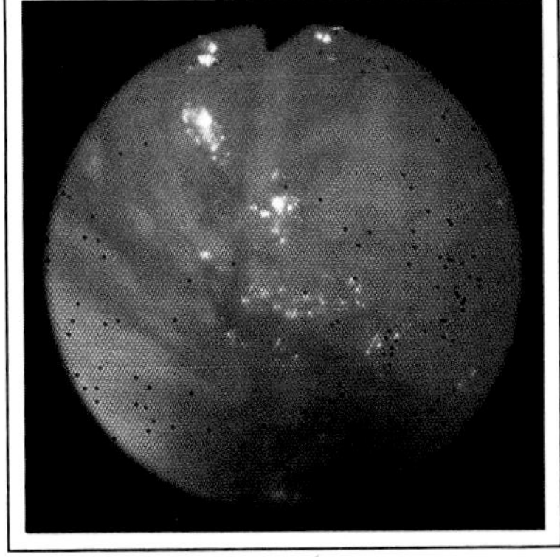

FIG. 27-16b.

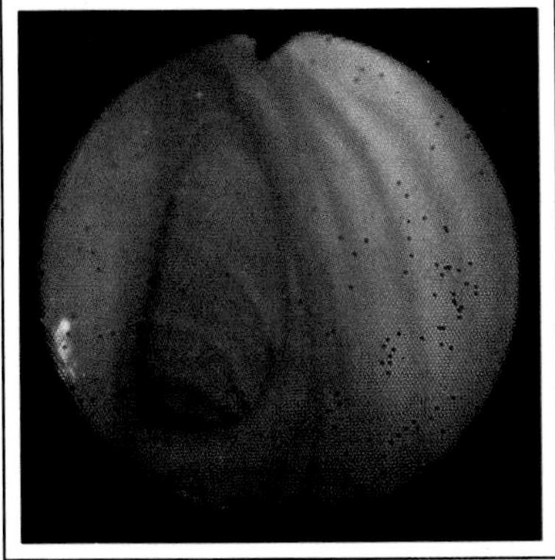

FIG. 27-16c.

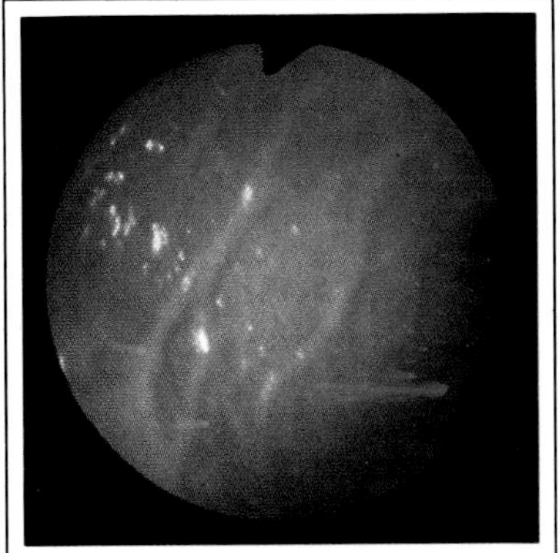

FIG. 27-16d.

FIG. 27-16. a: Dilatation of the descending duodenum and third portion. A retroflexed view of the descending duodenum is obtained (with the endoscope lying along the lateral wall at 2 o'clock) with the tip at the junction of the second and third portion. The diameter of both descending duodenum and third portion is estimated to be 6 to 7 cm. The Kerckring folds are almost completely effaced. **b:** Mechanical obstruction of the third portion of the duodenum from Crohn's disease. The lumen ends just above the bile pool at 6 o'clock, the pinpoint stenosis surrounded by raised erythematous areas. The degree of dilatation proximally causes a loss of the expected Kerckring folds. **c:** Dilatation of the third portion in a patient with scleroderma. The dilatation of the duodenal bulb and descending duodenum allow for intubation using the direct technique (see Chapter 24) with the medial wall at 6 o'clock. On entering the third portion, extrinsic compression from the anterior-lying superior mesenteric artery and vein is seen at 9 o'clock. In addition, because of the marked dilatation, the Kerckring folds are diminished in size. **d:** Dilatation of the descending duodenum with effaced Kerckring folds. Because of the dilatation from longstanding mechanical obstruction, the Kerckring folds are barely visible.

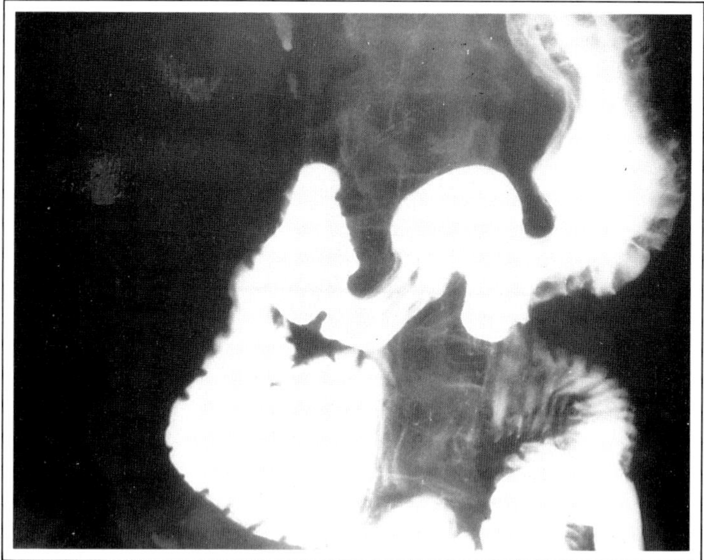

FIG. 27-17a.

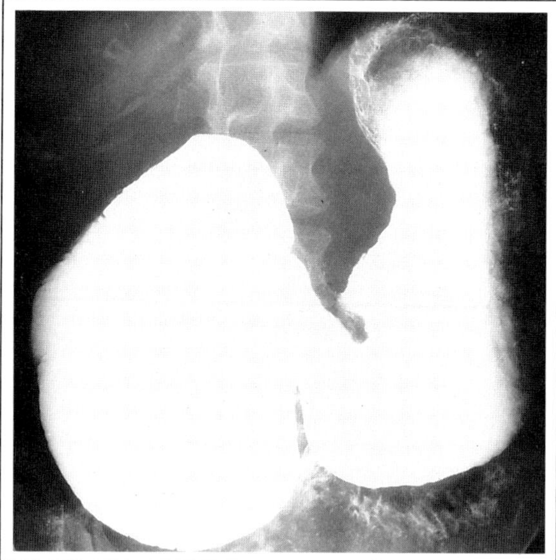

FIG. 27-17b.

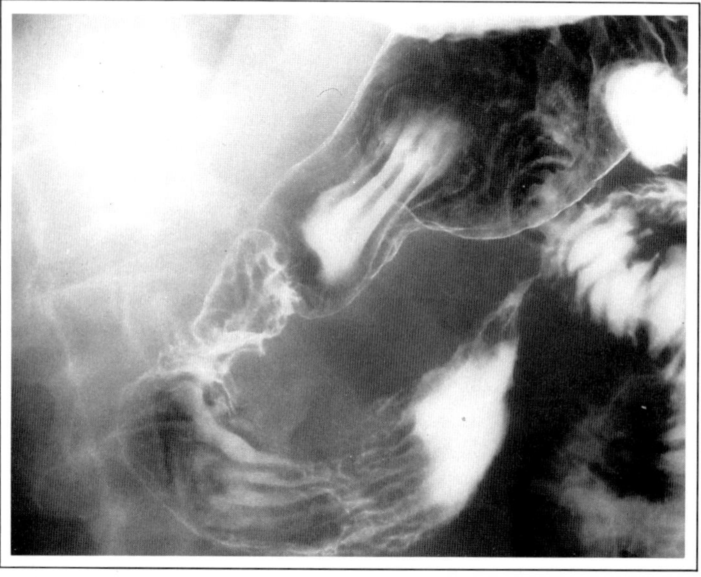

FIG. 27-17c.

FIG. 27-17. a: Marked dilatation of the duodenum, especially its third portion, is demonstrated radiographically in a patient with scleroderma. The apparent cutoff in the third portion is from the crossing of the superior mesenteric artery and vein (Fig. 27-16c). Dilatation elsewhere in the small bowel suggests that no obstruction will be found at endoscopy. **b:** Duodenal dilatation demonstrated radiographically in a patient with obstructing carcinoma of the fourth portion. In this case the absence of small bowel dilatation was a clue to mechanical obstruction. Furthermore, its location was one unlikely to have been reached by a conventional forward-viewing endoscope. **c:** A dilated duodenum is demonstrated radiographically in a patient with Crohn's disease in the third portion. The relatively short descending duodenum suggested that the obstruction might be within reach of the endoscope (Fig. 27-16b).

choledochoduodenostomy was performed instead, the duodenal papilla is intact, with the surgically created stomal orifice just proximal and posterior (Fig. 27-18b). The substantial (>1.5 cm) diameter of the stoma can be appreciated as it is gently probed with a polyethylene cannula (Fig. 27-18c).

Pancreatic Cystoduodenostomy Appearance

Pseudocysts of the head of the pancreas may be drained by way of a surgical anastomosis created between them and the descending duodenum. If endoscopy is subsequently performed in these patients, the endoscopist may encounter a mass-like deformity consisting of multiple folds radiating to a central point. As there is generally prompt involution of the pseudocyst once it is effectively drained, one would expect there to be no residual opening after 2 to 3 months. The appearance of a widely patent anastomosis 6 months or more after surgery, especially one where mucoid material is seen extruding from the orifice (Fig. 27-19), makes one suspect that a cystodenoma or cystadenocarcinoma is present rather than an inflammatory pseudocyst.[13]

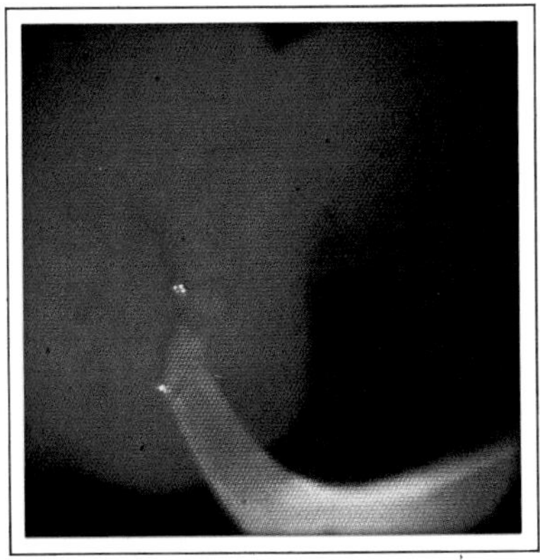

FIG. 27-18a.

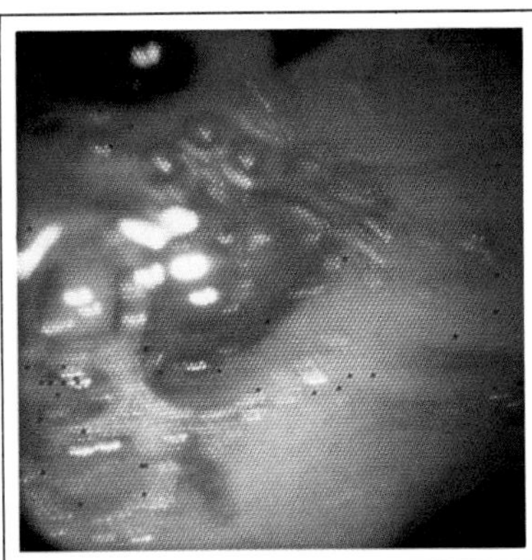

FIG. 27-18b.

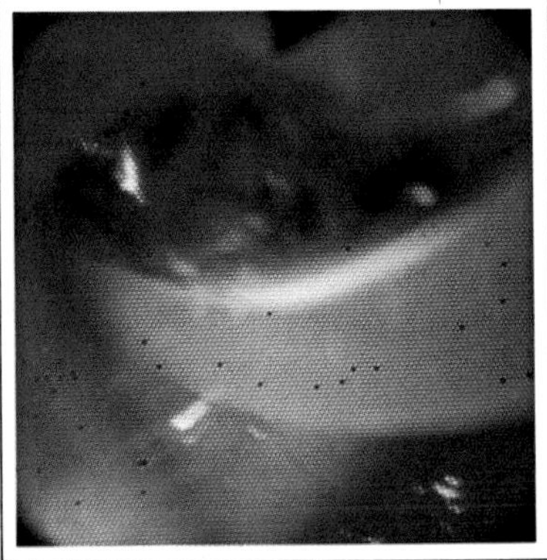

FIG. 27-18c.

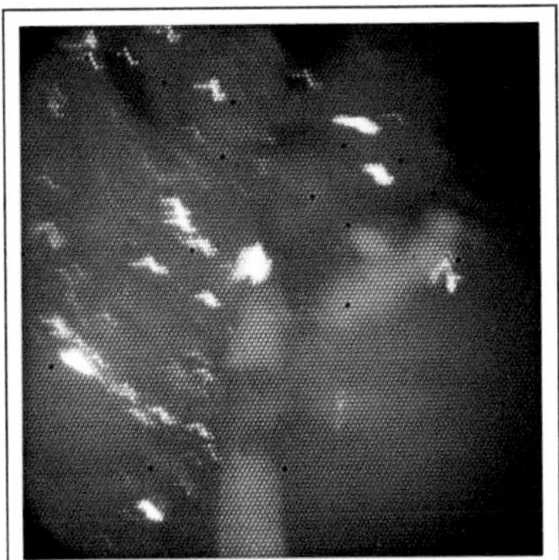

FIG. 27-19.

FIG. 27-18. a: Duodenal papilla 1 year after surgical sphincteroplasty. A slit-like opening of approximately 1 to 1.5 cm was seen in the area corresponding to the papillary orifice (see Chapter 24). The 1.8-mm polyethylene cannula which has been passed into the bile duct proves the orifice to be widely patent. **b:** Distal choledochoduodenostomy stoma just posterior (9 o'clock) to the ampulla and slightly above the level of its orifice. A 1.5-cm widely patent circular opening is noted here. **c:** Distal choledochoduodenostomy stoma with a cannula inserted into the bile duct. Probing the stoma with a 1.8-mm cannula suggests its effective diameter to be between 1 and 1.5 cm (five to six cannula widths at the point of entry).

FIG. 27-19. Cystoduodenostomy stoma in a patient with surgically proved cystadenocarcinoma. The stoma into which a polyethylene cannula has been inserted was fashioned 1.5 years before. The presence of an open cystoduodenostomy stoma 6 months or more after surgery should cause one to suspect the presence of a cystic neoplasm of the pancreas (cystadenoma or cystadenocarcinoma).[13]

REFERENCES

1. Eaton, S. B., and Ferrucci, J. T. (1973): *Radiology of the Pancreas and Duodenum,* pp. 113–119. Saunders, Philadelphia.
2. Belber, J. B. (1974): Bulbar duodenoscopy, techniques and pathology. In: *Gastrointestinal Pan-Endoscopy,* edited by L. H. Berry, pp. 371–378. Charles C Thomas, Springfield, Illinois.
3. Feller, E. R., Warshaw, A. L., and Shapiro, R. H. (1980): Observations on management of choledochoduodenal fistula due to penetrating peptic ulcer. *Gastroenterology,* 78:126–136.
4. Blackstone, M. O., and Mizuno, H. (1977): Reactive duodenal changes in chronic pancreatitis simulating the contiguous spread of pancreatic carcinoma. *Am. J. Dig. Dis.,* 22:658–661.
5. Bellon, E., George, C. R., Schreiber, H., and Marshall, J. B. (1979): Pancreatic pseudocysts of the duodenum. *Am. J. Roentgenol.,* 133:827–831.
6. Margulis, A. R., and Burhenne, H. J. (1967): *Alimentary Tract Roentgenology,* p. 110. Mosby, St. Louis.
7. Leinkram, C., Roberts-Thomson, I. C., and Kune, G. A. (1980): Juxtapapillary duodenal diverticula: association with gall stones and pancreatitis. *Med. J. Aust.,* 1:209–210.
8. Ghahremani, G. G., and Hietala, S.-O. (1977): Arteriography of a bleeding duodenal diverticulum. *Am. J. Dig. Dis.,* 22:445–448.
9. Nelson, J. A., and Burhenne, H. J. (1976): Anomalous biliary and pancreatic duct insertion into duodenal diverticula. *Radiology,* 120:49–52.
10. Mathieu, B., Salducci, J., Ramacle, J.-P., Pin, G., and Monges, H. (1978): Intraluminal duodenal diverticulum: report of a case investigated by fiberoptic endoscopy. *Am. J. Dig. Dis. (Suppl.),* 23:1S–4S.
11. Economides, N. G., McBurney, R. P., and Hamilton, F. H. (1977): Intraluminal duodenal diverticulum in the adult. *Ann. Surg.,* 185:147–152.
12. Rutledge, R. (1976): Sphincteroplasty and choledochoduodenostomy for benign biliary obstructions. *Ann. Surg.,* 183:476–486.
13. Ito, Y., and Blackstone, M. O. (1977): Mucinous biliary obstruction associated with a cystic adenocarcinoma of the pancreas. *Gastroenterology,* 73:1410–1412.

28

MUCOSAL APPEARANCE OF THE DUODENUM IN SELECTED BENIGN DISORDERS

We considered elsewhere (Chapter 26) the spectrum of appearances for the commonest disorder to involve duodenal mucosal peptic ulcer disease. Other less frequently observed conditions not generally thought of in connection with the duodenum may nevertheless alter its mucosal appearance. Crohn's disease is such a case. Although this condition is usually thought of in connection with the colon or ileum, the duodenum may be involved as a primary site or in association with the involvement in other more common locations. Celiac sprue and immunoglobulin deficiency states may also produce duodenal mucosal abnormalities which may be observed endoscopically in association with that observed radiographically in the jejunum. Pancreatitis, especially if acute, may be found in association with reactive changes of the mucosa, especially within the contiguous portions of the duodenal bulb and descending duodenum. Finally, patients with renal failure or radiation injury may have a variety of endoscopic findings in the duodenum in addition to those already noted for these conditions in the stomach. In this chapter we consider the endoscopic appearances of these selected conditions.

CROHN'S DISEASE OF THE DUODENUM

As in the case of the stomach (see Chapter 20), symptomatic duodenal involvement is said to be rare, occurring in only 1 to 2% of patients with Crohn's disease.[1] This figure is derived from studies in which symptoms (e.g., ulcer-like pain, nausea, vomiting, and weight loss) occurring alone or in combination prompted radiologic as well as endoscopic evaluation.[1] The percentage of patients without symptoms suggestive of ulcer disease or duodenal obstruction who would nevertheless have endoscopic findings compatible with duodenal Crohn's disease is unknown, although it is our impression that this might be on the order of 5 to 10%.

The site of duodenal Crohn's disease involvement is generally the duodenal bulb in conjunction with the descending duodenum or prepyloric antrum.[2] For example, ulceration of the duodenal bulb alone without similar involvement of the prepyloric antrum or remainder of the duodenum would be unusual and should raise the suspicion of peptic ulcer disease. The two anatomic patterns of duodenal Crohn's disease involvement discussed below are: (a) gastroduodenal involvement; and (b) involvement of the distal bulb and/or remainder of the duodenum.

Gastroduodenal Involvement

The commonest appearance of Crohn's disease in the duodenum is that which involves both the prepyloric antrum (Fig. 28-1a) and the proximal or entire duodenum (Fig. 28-1b) with discrete aphthous (superficial) ulcerations (Fig. 28-1b). Surrounding these ulcerations is a halo of erythema; however, between the ulcerations the mucosa appears uninvolved (Fig. 28-1c). When the intervening mucosa is raised in the form of mucosal (hyperplastic) polyps, one refers to this as the cobblestone appearance (Fig. 28-2). The cobblestone appearance is common in symptomatic patients, occurring in one series in 13 of 14 patients with duodenal Crohn's disease who were symptomatic at the time of endoscopy. In addition, in symptomatic patients, there may be long, even, deep serpiginous ulcerations (Fig. 28-3) within areas displaying the cobblestone appearance and in areas of normal mucosa. In rare cases, discrete ulcers (Fig. 28-4a) may form the mouth of a fistula (Fig. 28-4b).

In contrast to findings such as ulceration and the cobblestone appearance, which are "definite" involvement with Crohn's disease, we find nonspecific, acute duodenitis (Fig. 28-5a) in approximately 5 to 10% of patients with Crohn's disease elsewhere in the gastrointestinal (GI) tract. These patients had endoscopy for symptoms other than peptic ulcer disease or obstruction. As in the case of acute duodenitis itself (see Chapter 25), we regard the appearance of focally discrete erythema (Fig. 28-5a), nodular duodenitis

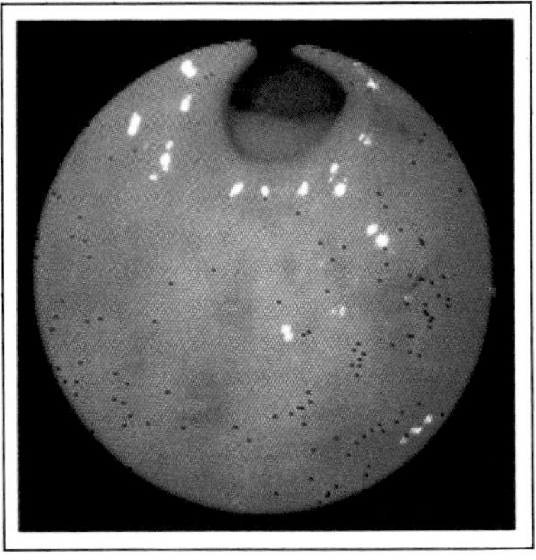

FIG. 28-1a.

FIG. 28-1b.

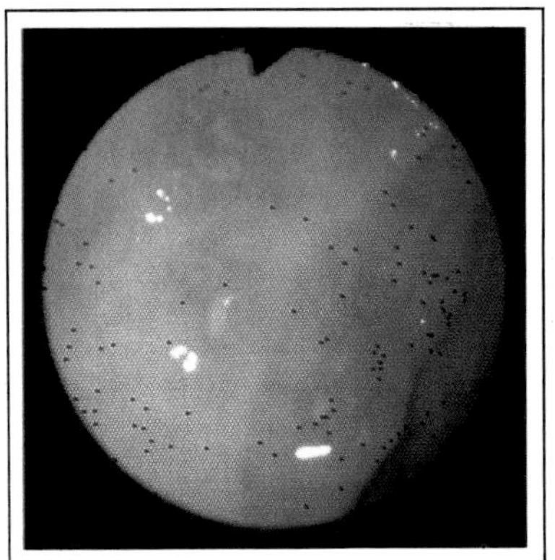

FIG. 28-1c.

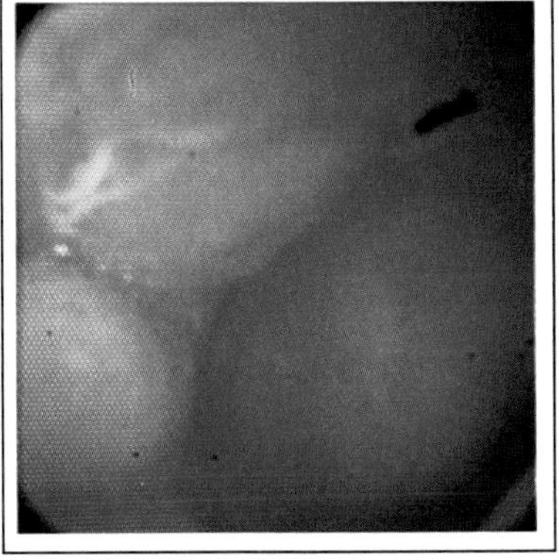

FIG. 28-2.

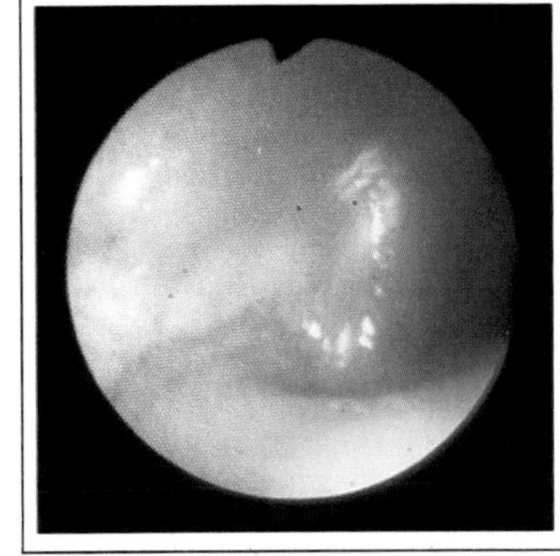

FIG. 28-3.

FIG. 28-1. a: Crohn's disease with gastroduodenal involvement. In this case evidence of involvement was first noted in the prepyloric antrum with the appearance of aphthous ulcers having erythematous margins but intact mucosa in between. **b:** Crohn's disease with gastroduodenal involvement in a case with prepyloric antral involvement. Aphthous ulcerations were seen in the mid-portion and apical area of the bulb. They did not continue into the descending duodenum. **c:** Aphthous ulcerations of the duodenal bulb in a patient with Crohn's disease. The ulcer is set on a background of erythematous mucosa, but elsewhere it appears intact. Histologically, skip areas[3] were present.

FIG. 28-2. Crohn's disease of the duodenal bulb with the cobblestone appearance. Ulcerations are found on the tips or between polypoid masses of hyperplastic mucosa. In this case linear ulcerations can be seen on the tips of hyperplastic nodules of mucosa.

FIG. 28-3. Crohn's disease of the duodenal bulb with a long, serpiginous ulceration.

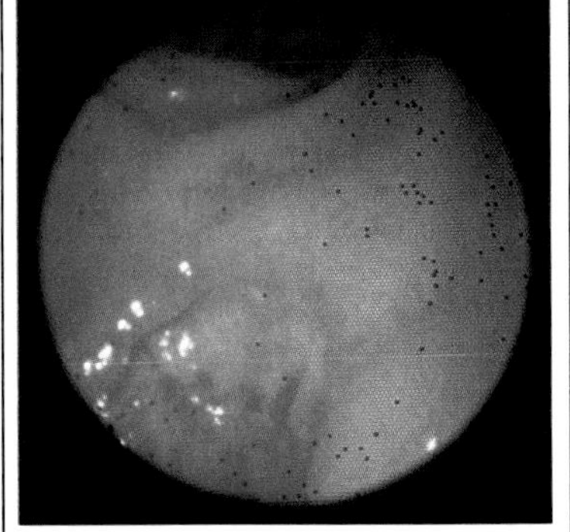

FIG. 28-4a.

FIG. 28-4. Crohn's disease of the duodenum. **a:** With an ulcer as the mouth of a fistulous tract. A deep inferior wall was noted at 6 o'clock which was, in fact, the mouth of a long fistulous tract demonstrated radiographically (b). **b:** With a fistulous tract to the hepatic flexure, noted radiographically.

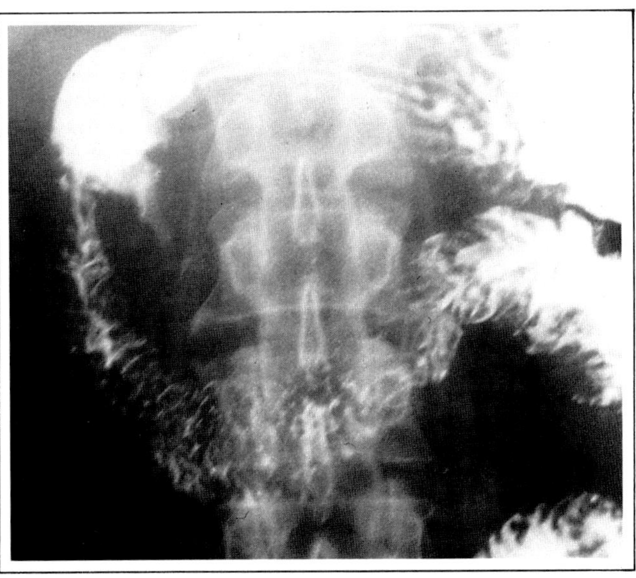

FIG. 28-4b.

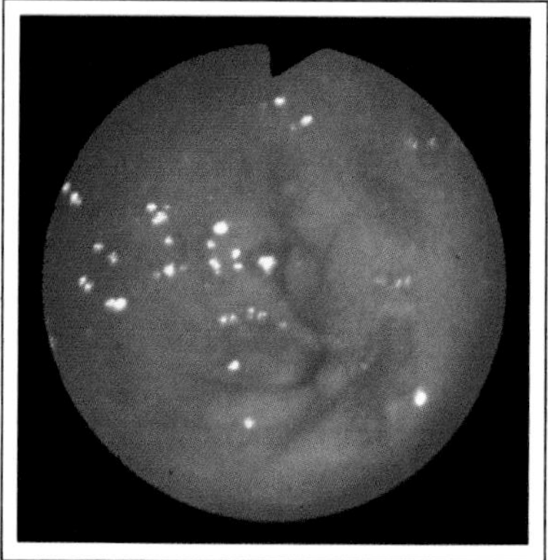

FIG. 28-5a.

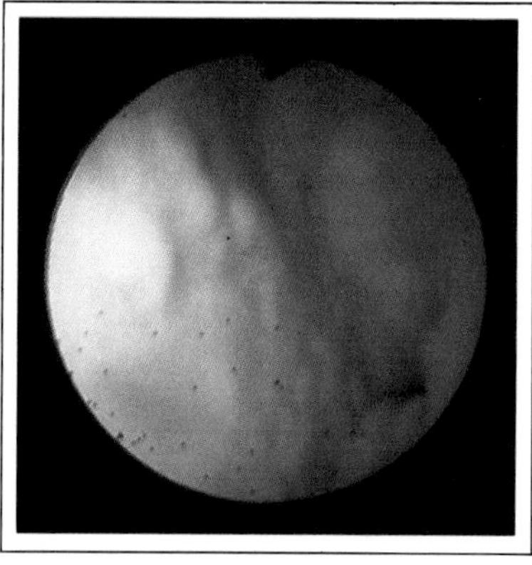

FIG. 28-5b.

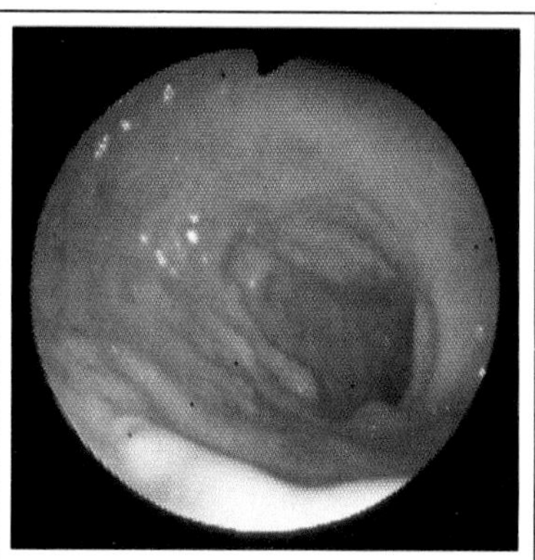

FIG. 28-5c.

FIG. 28-5. a: Nonspecific acute duodenitis in a patient with Crohn's colitis. In this case multiple focal areas of erythema are seen in the mid-bulb and apex. Like other patients with nonspecific acute duodenitis, the significance of this finding is unknown. **b:** Nonspecific nodular duodenitis in a patient with inactive ileocolic Crohn's disease and occasional postprandial pain. **c:** Nonspecific acute and nodular duodenitis of the descending duodenum in a patient with Crohn's disease of the terminal ileum, episodic pain, and diarrhea.

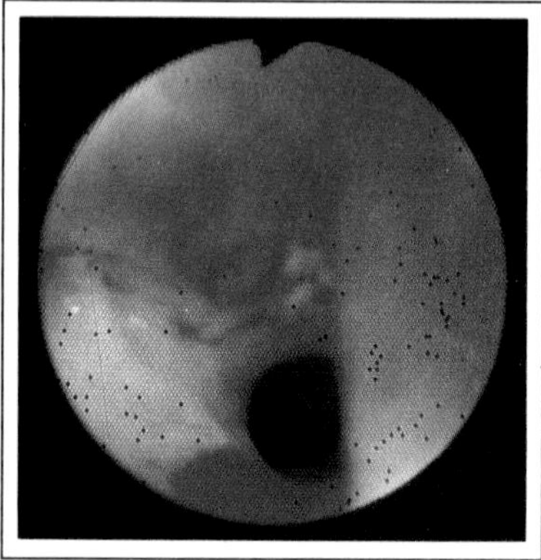

FIG. 28-6a.

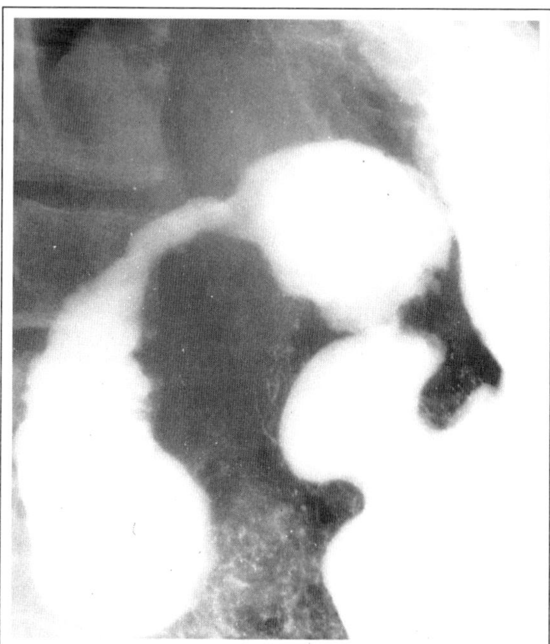

Fig. 28-6b.

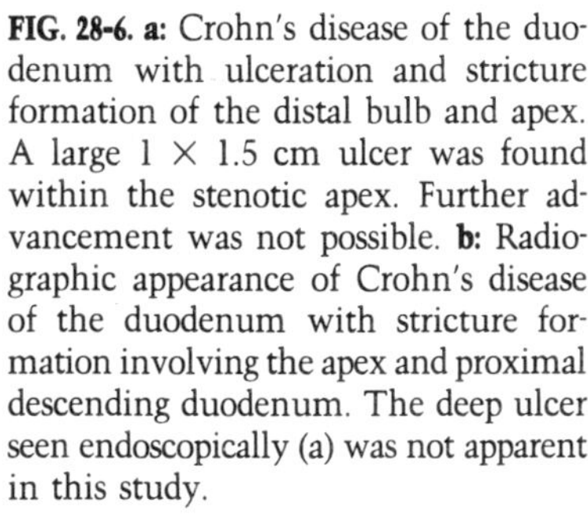

FIG. 28-6. a: Crohn's disease of the duodenum with ulceration and stricture formation of the distal bulb and apex. A large 1 × 1.5 cm ulcer was found within the stenotic apex. Further advancement was not possible. **b:** Radiographic appearance of Crohn's disease of the duodenum with stricture formation involving the apex and proximal descending duodenum. The deep ulcer seen endoscopically (a) was not apparent in this study.

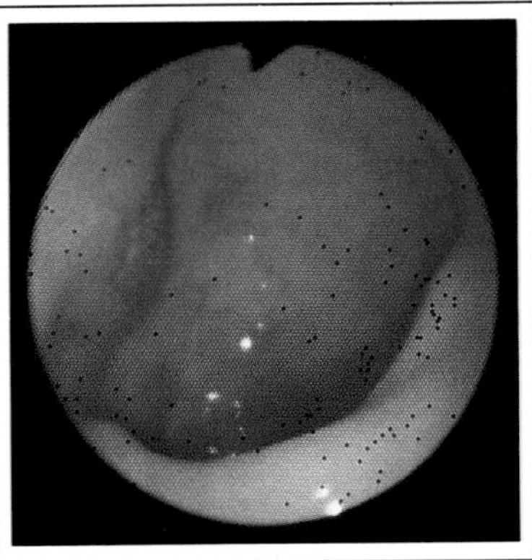

FIG. 28-7.

FIG. 28-7. Nonspecific acute duodenitis with aphthous ulceration of the descending duodenum in a patient with nonspecific abdominal pain 15 years after proctocolectomy for Crohn's colitis. Biopsies showed focal ulceration with microscopic skip areas suggestive of Crohn's disease.[3]

(Fig. 28-5b), or a combination of the two (Fig. 28-5c) as having uncertain significance, especially in regard to symptoms, even if biopsies (see below) show microscopic skip areas suggestive of Crohn's disease.[3] It may be, however, that such areas result from the presence of Crohn's disease in a subclinical form throughout the entire GI tract.[4]

Involvement of the Distal Bulb and/or Remainder of the Duodenum

In cases where the distal bulb and/or the rest of the duodenum are involved, the involvement generally begins at the apex of the duodenal bulb and extends into the descending duodenum for a variable distance. The apex itself may be ulcerated and stenotic, an appearance indistinguishable from that of peptic ulcer disease (Fig. 28-6a). However, this lesion extends into the descending duodenum, often involving the proximal mid-portion (Fig. 28-6b), a distribution which would be unusual for peptic ulcer disease. In other cases the mucosa of the descending duodenum appears focally nodular and ulcerated (Fig. 28-7). In patients with stenotic lesions of the second or third portion, the lumen appears dilated both radiographically (Fig. 28-8a) and endoscopically (Fig. 28-8b). The stenotic area itself (Fig. 28-8c) appears narrowed or even pinpoint, with activity in the form of erosions and ulcerations in and around the point of obstruction (Fig. 28-8c). Although the endoscopist may not be able to examine within the stricture, he may inspect the mouth and note its characteristic nodular, ulcerated mucosa. In cases where the ulcers are deep, episodes of bleeding may be associated (see Chapter 38).

Biopsy

As in the stomach (see Chapter 20), biopsy most often shows only nonspecific inflammatory changes. Granulomas are found in only a minority of the cases, in one series in less than 10%.[2] Histologic skip areas (of entirely normal mucosa) adjacent to microscopic or macroscopic ulcerations are, we find, a more common finding to suggest duodenal involvement. The same skip areas found in association with a nonspecific endoscopic appearance, e.g., acute duodenitis or nodular duodenitis, also suggest the presence of Crohn's disease, although the clinical relevance of this finding is uncertain, especially in the absence of ulcer or obstructive-type symptoms.

CELIAC SPRUE

A diagnosis of celiac sprue is suggested by a clinical picture of weight loss, abdominal distention, and diarrhea in a patient with evidence of malabsorption. The conventional means of obtaining histologic confirmation has been intestinal biopsy capsule or tube.

Recently several groups have utilized endoscopic biopsies of the duodenum as a means of establishing histologically the diagnosis of celiac sprue.[5,6] As a result of these studies, a characteristic endoscopic appearance for this condition has emerged.[5,6] In a study of 19 patients in whom celiac sprue was suspected, the diagnosis was established in all 19 with biopsies taken from the duodenum[5]; moreover, visually, villous atrophy could be anticipated by observing the mucosa at close range (see below). After institution of a gluten-free diet, a normal mucosal appearance was observed endoscopically and confirmed by biopsy. In another study,[6] biopsies taken from the duodenal bulb show a degree of villous atrophy similar to that observed in histologic material obtained from the jejunum, the ligament of Treitz. In addition, the presence of villous atrophy could be easily demonstrated visually using an indigo carmine dye scattering technique.[7]

It may be anticipated that an endoscopist will be called on more frequently in the future to provide histologic material in patients suspected of celiac sprue, thus obviating the need for the often extremely time-consuming intestinal capsule tube technique. As histologic involvement can be patchy,[8] the endoscopist may wish to biopsy those areas that display a suggestive mucosal appearance.

Appearance

The most identifiable mucosal feature, which is observed without the dye scattering technique (see above), is the loss

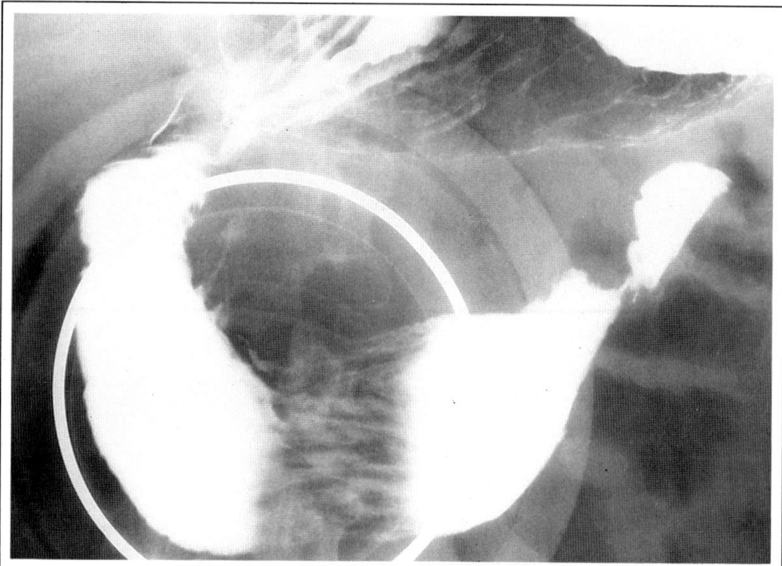

FIG. 28-8a.

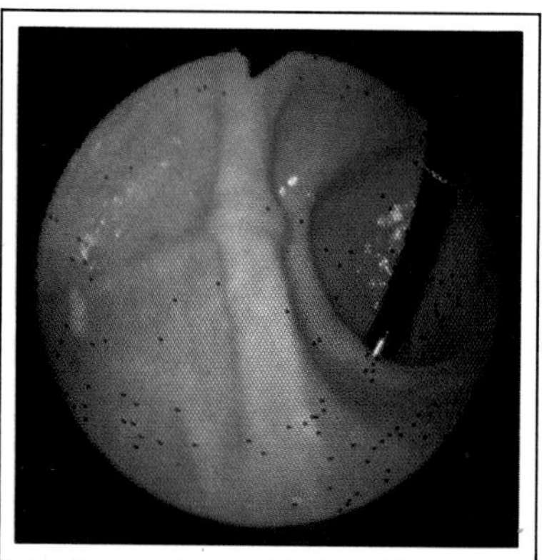

FIG. 28-8b.

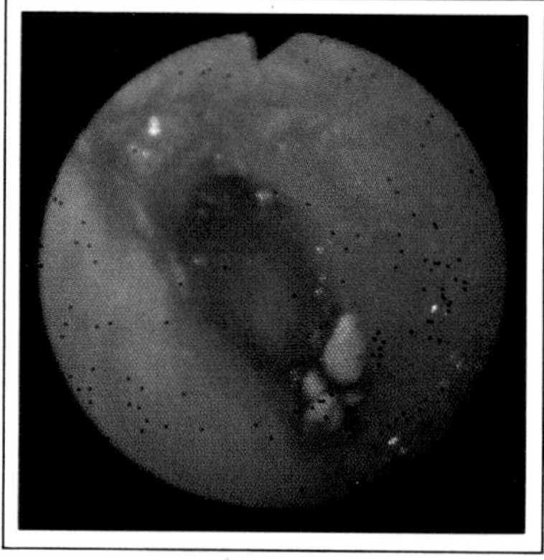

FIG. 28-8c.

FIG. 28-8. a: Crohn's disease with stenosis of the distal duodenum (third portion) and marked proximal dilatation demonstrated radiographically. **b:** Same case as in (a). The dilatation is so pronounced that retroflexion of the tip is easily accomplished at the inferior duodenal angle. (This endoscope is seen running from 12 to 16 o'clock.) The stenotic area is just distal at 9 o'clock. **c:** Crohn's disease of the distal duodenum (third portion). The stenotic area surrounded by nodular ulcerated mucosa is at 9 o'clock, with marked dilatation in the remainder of this segment causing bile and foreign material to accumulate along the 6 o'clock surface.

of the expected coarsened mucosal appearance and granularity seen especially in the duodenal bulb on close inspection (Fig. 28-9a). This occurs as a result of villous atrophy and causes the mucosa to appear smooth and shiny (Fig. 28-9b), reminiscent of that in the antrum. Another feature noted by one group[6] was a decrease in mucosal contact bleeding, especially in the presence of mucosal erythema where it would be expected.

Within the descending duodenum, the Kerckring folds tend to be prominent, possibly as a result of mucosal edema, especially when found in patients with a low serum albumin level (Fig. 28-9b). From preliminary studies it appears that well-oriented biopsies can be diagnostic in the majority of cases of celiac sprue.[5,6] Areas of the duodenal bulb or the descending duodenum that have a smooth, shiny appearance, a normal or somewhat reddened (erythema) mucosal coloration, and no discernible villous type of light reflex are especially worth biopsying in patients whose clinical presentation suggests celiac sprue.[5,6]

IMMUNOGLOBULIN DEFICIENCY—NODULAR LYMPHOID HYPERPLASIA

Common variable, late-onset, immunoglobulin deficiency, especially immunoglobulin A (IgA), can be associated with malabsorption, diarrhea, *Giardia lamblia* infestation, and the histologic appearance of subtotal villous atrophy.[9] Patients with immunoglobulin deficiency and a clinical picture of enteropathy may be referred for endoscopy along with those with IgA deficiency without malabsorption who have a history of only respiratory or sinus infections and nonspecific upper abdominal complaints.[9,10] In either case, at endoscopy the key finding is that of nodular lymphoid hyperplasia.[11]

Appearance

The striking endoscopic feature is that of raised, 2- to 5-mm nodules which appear in the descending duodenum, almost in a carpet-like fashion (Fig. 28-10). The Kerckring folds may be normal or appear thickened because of the nodules themselves, and in some cases may be associated with hypoproteinemia.

Biopsy

Biopsies taken from the nodules themselves may demonstrate lymphoid follicles.[10] The overlying mucosa is either normal or shows a variable degree of villous atrophy in cases where malabsorption is clinically suspected. In all

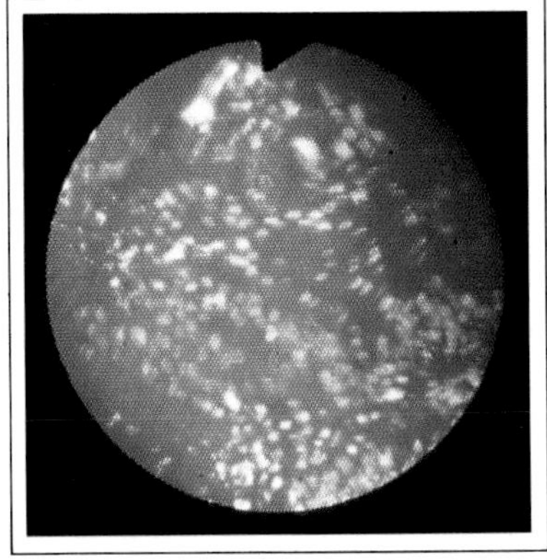

FIG. 28-9a.

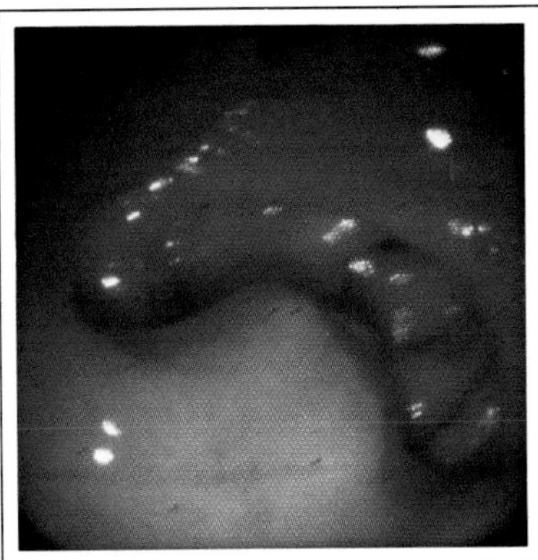

FIG. 28-9b.

FIG. 28-9. a: Duodenal mucosa, close-up view with normal light reflex. The granular pattern seen as a myriad of dots of light is created by the normal mucosal villous pattern. **b:** Celiac disease in the apex of the bulb and the descending duodenum. The duodenal mucosa is strikingly smooth, without a granular-type appearance, as histologically the villi are flat. The Kerckring folds in this case were enlarged because of associated hypoproteinemia. This gave the impression of a polypoid mass at the apex. Well-oriented biopsies from this area were diagnostic of celiac sprue.

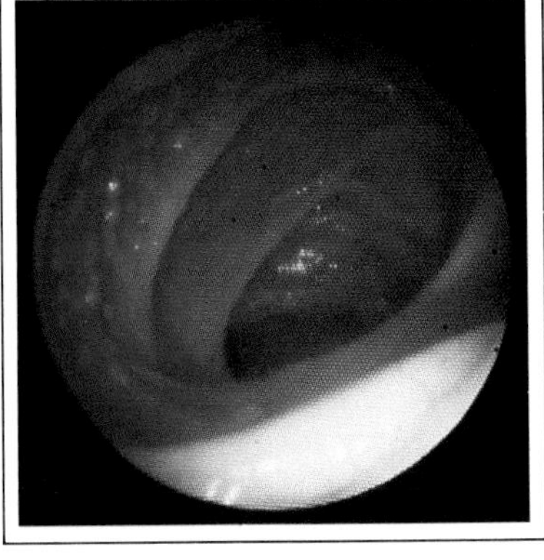

FIG. 28-10a.

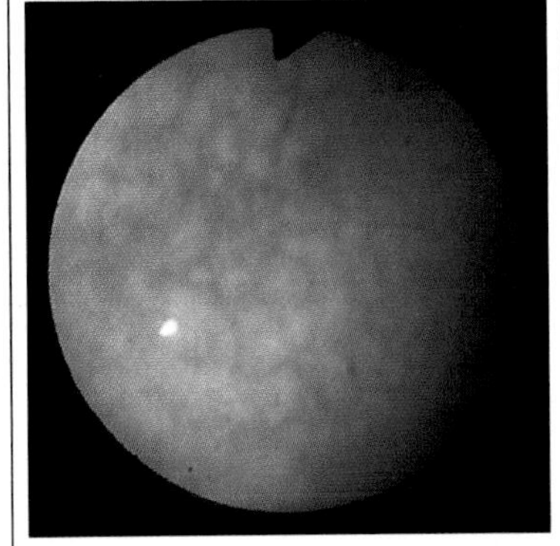

FIG. 28-10b.

FIG. 28-10. a: Nodular lymphoid hyperplasia. Multiple 2- to 4-mm nodules are found in a patient with hypogammaglobulinemia, diarrhea, and weight loss. Biopsies showed *Giardia lamblia* along with nodular lymphoid hyperplasia. **b:** Lymphoid hyperplasia as a variant of nonspecific duodenitis. Tiny (2 to 4 mm) pale mucosal polyps were noted in a patient with chronic epigastric pain. Biopsies showed lymphoid hyperplasia.

cases, a careful search should be made for *Giardia,*[11] especially if partial or subtotal villous atrophy is present.[12]

PANCREATITIS

The head of the pancreas lies in direct contact with the medial wall of the descending duodenum. Both acute and chronic inflammation of the pancreas may, by extension, involve this wall, leading to an altered mucosal appearance. The mechanism by which this occurs is uncertain but possibly involves serosal inflammation and lymphatic obstruction leading to further inflammatory changes and edema of the entire medial wall.[13] Whatever the mechanism, one frequently encounters an altered mucosal appearance in patients with both acute and chronic pancreatitis. The endoscopist needs to be mindful of these so as not to be misled into a diagnosis of malignancy because of the resemblance of these appearances to malignant changes (see Chapter 29).

Acute Pancreatitis

We have noted an altered mucosal appearance in approximately 30 to 40% of patients endoscoped within the first 7 to 14 days of an episode of acute pancreatitis. A similar number (25%) have been found to have duodenal abnormalities if upper GI radiographic studies were performed during the same period.[13] Although serial studies have not been performed, it is our impression that many of these patients who are subsequently examined do not show persistence of these changes, suggesting that in part they are "reactive" to the acute episode. In other patients, nonspecific thickening of the Kerckring folds are found on subsequent examination, possibly indicating a mucosal response (chronic pancreatitis).

The striking endoscopic finding observed in patients with acute pancreatitis is the increased size of the Kerckring folds and associated patchy erythema of the mucosa (Fig. 28-11a), beginning at the apex (Fig. 28-11b) and extending distally, often with striking changes in the appearance of the papilla (Fig. 28-11c). Here one sees marked papillary enlargement, as well as intense erythema of the mucosa of the hooded fold and the orifice (Fig. 28-11c). In cases of acute gallstone pancreatitis, where the episode is thought to be the result of a gallstone migrating across the papilla,[14] one may see evidence of "papillitis" as disproportionate erythema and enlargement of the papilla (Fig. 28-11d) in contrast to the medial wall. In rare cases, a combination of extrinsic compression and enlargement of the Kerckring folds leads to marked compromise of the lumen or even complete obstruction.[13] The cases of obstruction in the setting of acute pancreatitis tend to be reversible,[13] in contrast to those occurring with chronic pancreatitis (see below).

Smooth or nodular masses (Fig. 28-12a) covered by either normal or erythematous mucosa may be found in patients

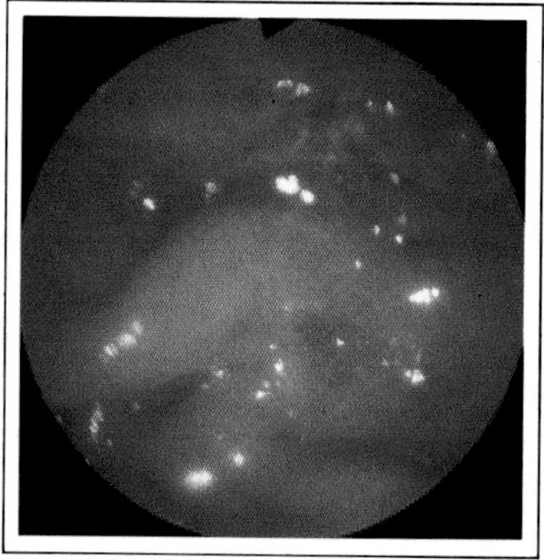

FIG. 28-11a.

FIG. 28-11b.

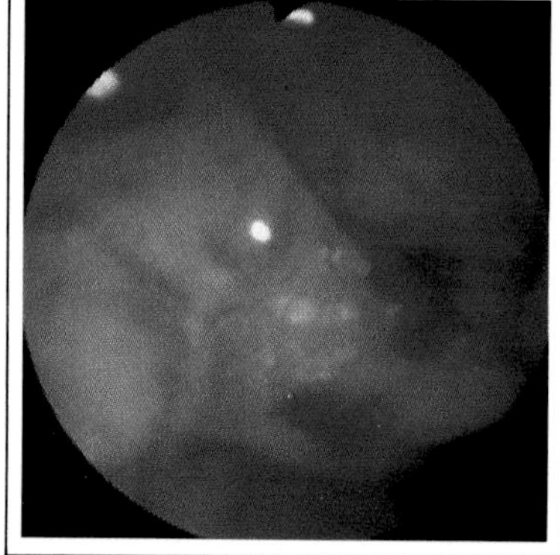

FIG. 28-11c.

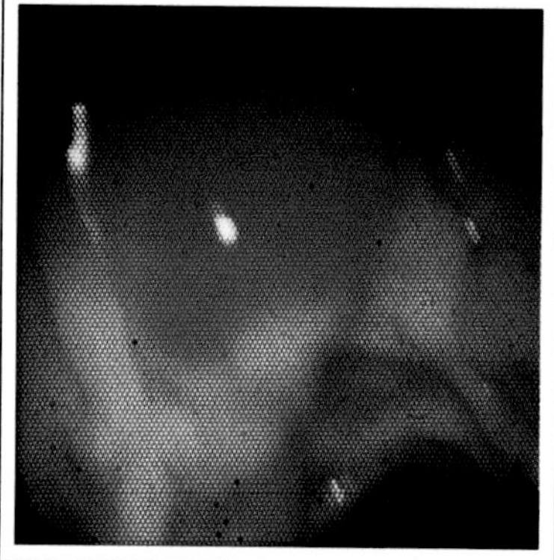

FIG. 28-11d.

FIG. 28-11. a: Descending duodenal mucosa in acute alcoholic pancreatitis. The Kerckring folds appear enlarged and erythematous probably secondary to reactive edema and acute inflammation. We find this appearance in up to 20% of patients with acute pancreatitis. **b:** Duodenal bulb, apex, in acute pancreatitis [same patient as in (a)]. The mucosa is erythematous with enlarged (edematous) mucosal folds. **c:** Duodenal papilla in acute pancreatitis. As with the rest of the medial wall, there is marked enlargement of the hooded and longitudinal folds as well as intense erythema and friability of the orifice (see at 2 o'clock). **d:** Duodenal papilla in acute gallstone pancreatitis. The papilla is erythematous and slightly enlarged, possibly from injury induced by the passage of a gallstone into the duodenum, but the enlargement of the papilla and surrounding Kerckring folds is less than is found in alcoholic pancreatitis (c).

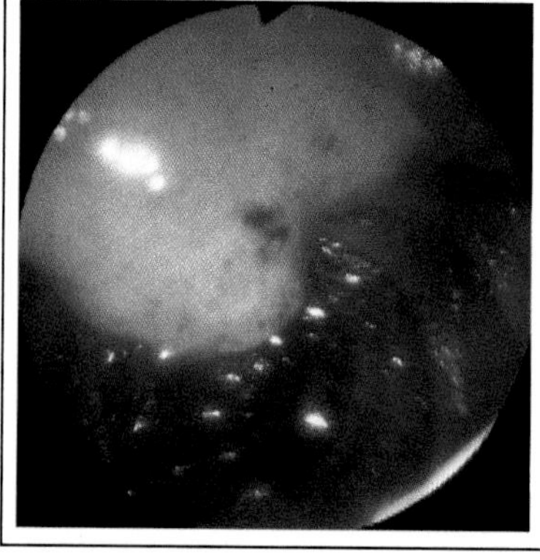

FIG. 28-12a.

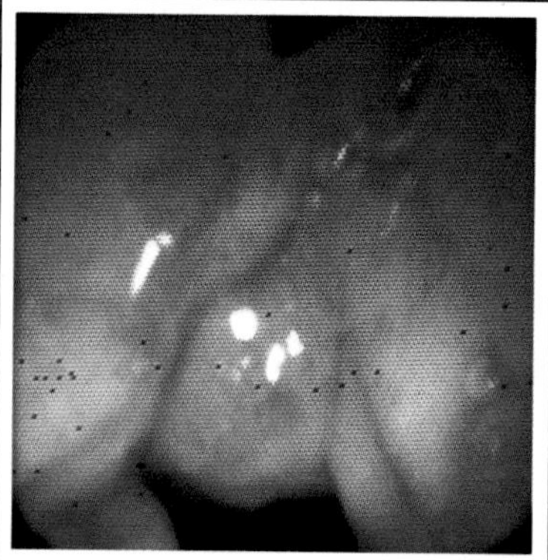

FIG. 28-12b.

FIG. 28-12. a: Duodenal submucosal mass in alcoholic pancreatitis. There is extrinsic compression of the lumen with a 2- to 3-cm mass. At surgery, chronic pancreatitis with a pseudocyst within the wall of the duodenum was found to account for the mass. **b:** Duodenal mass-like deformity in pancreatic carcinoma. Endoscopically this appearance is similar to the mass-like deformity associated with chronic pancreatitis and pseudocysts (a).

with acute pancreatitis, especially those with pseudocysts, with the mass itself a pseudocyst embedded in the wall of the duodenum.[15] Because of the mass-like appearance and extrinsic compression, one may be tempted to consider a diagnosis of pancreatic malignancy because of the similarity in appearance (Fig. 28-12b).[16] Although pancreatic cancer can present as acute pancreatitis,[17] virtually all masses (Fig. 28-12a) observed in the setting of acute pancreatitis are inflammatory.

Chronic Pancreatitis

Endoscopy in patients with chronic pancreatitis may show an entirely normal appearance of the duodenum or only a nonspecific enlargement of the Kerckring folds (Fig. 28-13a). Focal or diffuse erythema would be expected in patients with a recent acute clinical episode (see above). As in patients with acute pancreatitis (see above), those with extrinsic compression and submucosal masses (Fig. 28-13b) are likely to have pseudocysts adjacent to or embedded in the wall of the duodenum (Fig. 28-13c). Also found in rare cases of patients with chronic pancreatitis is complete duodenal obstruction (Fig. 28-14). Unlike the reversible type of obstruction found with acute pancreatitis, obstruction in patients with chronic pancreatitis is often irreversible, generally with involvement of the entire descending duodenum in a fibrous inflammatory mass.[13]

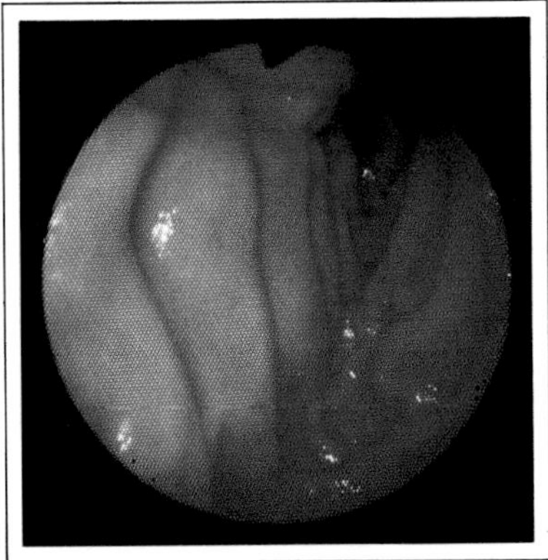

FIG. 28-13a.

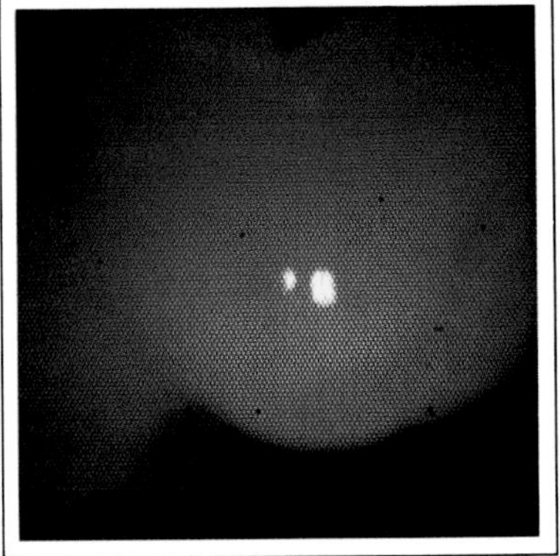

FIG. 28-13b.

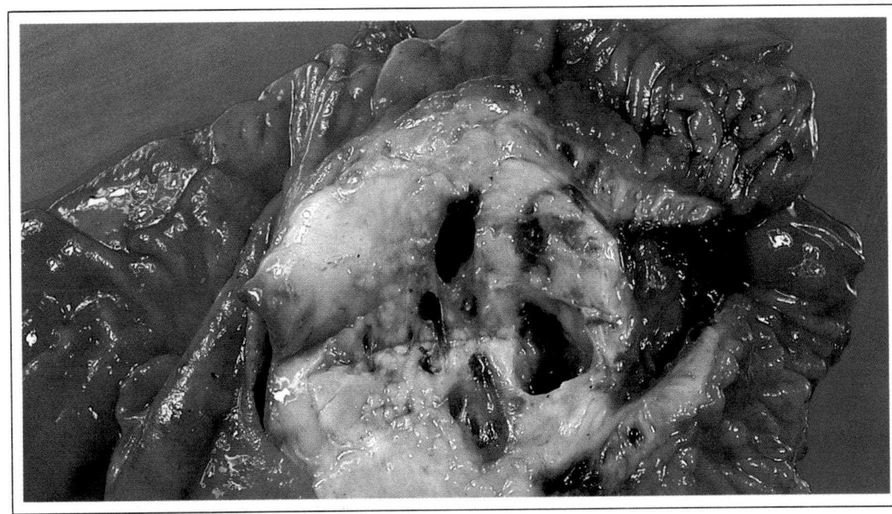

FIG. 28-13c.

FIG. 28-13. a: Enlarged Kerckring folds with extrinsic compression in a patient with chronic pancreatitis. **b:** Mass-like deformity of the medial wall just above the duodenal papilla in a patient with chronic pancreatitis with a pseudocyst, presenting with jaundice. This appearance, as well as the patient's weight loss, raised the clinical suspicion of pancreatic carcinoma.[17] **c:** Resected specimen in chronic pancreatitis with fibrocystic replacement of the head of the pancreas. In this case the "mass" (b) consisted of inflammatory changes from a contiguous pseudocyst embedded in the wall of the duodenum.

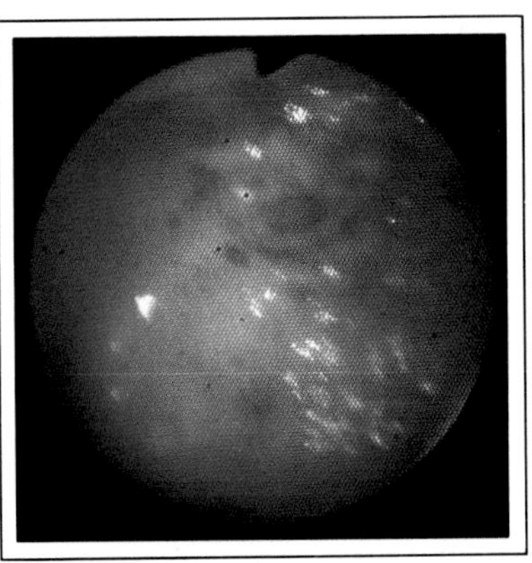

FIG. 28-14.

FIG. 28-14. Complete duodenal obstruction in a patient with chronic pancreatitis. The lumen terminates at 3 o'clock in an erythematous pinpoint stricture.

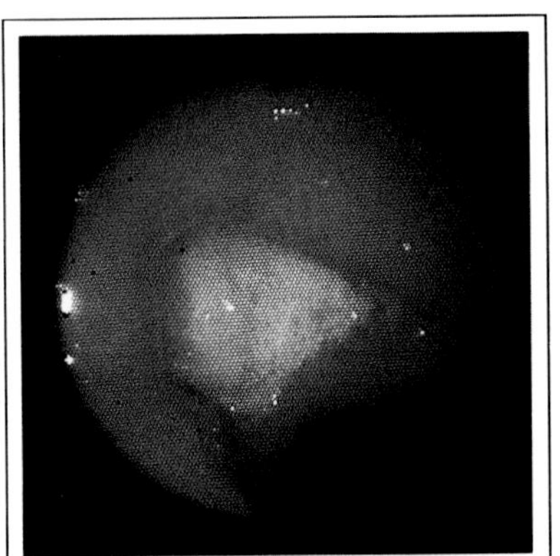

FIG. 28-15a.

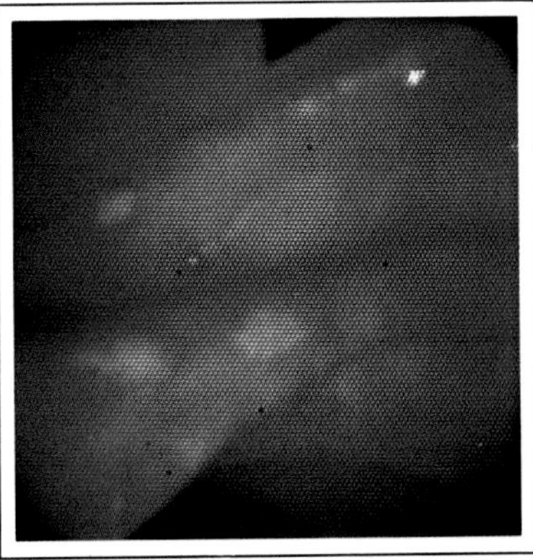

FIG. 28-15b.

FIG. 28-15. a: Pyloric channel ulcer in a patient with chronic pancreatitis. Such patients may be predisposed to ulcer disease because of a decreased buffering capacity of the duodenal bulb consequent to a low bicarbonate output from the pancreas as well as gastric hypersecretion, which can also occur. **b:** Scattered aphthous ulcerations in the descending duodenum in a patient with chronic pancreatitis. These may be part of the spectrum of nonspecific acute duodenitis (see Chapter 25). Whether they should be considered an ulcer-equivalent is unsettled.

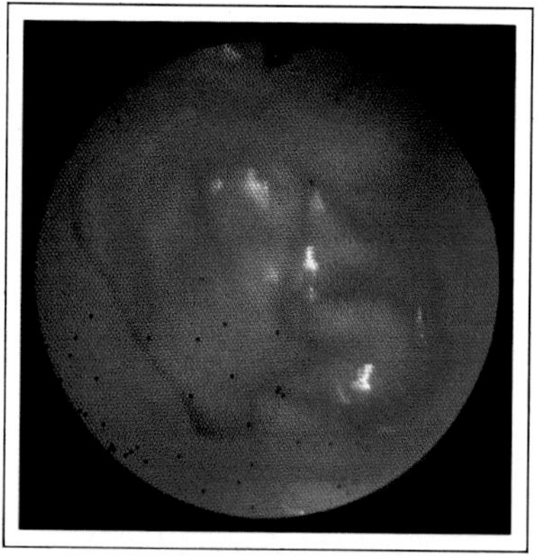

FIG. 28-16a.

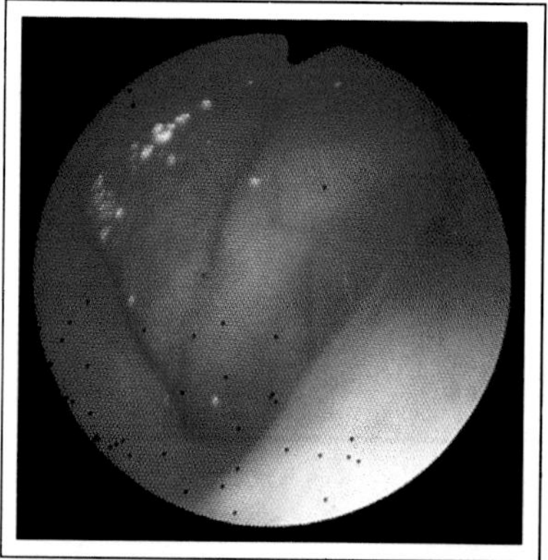

FIG. 28-16b.

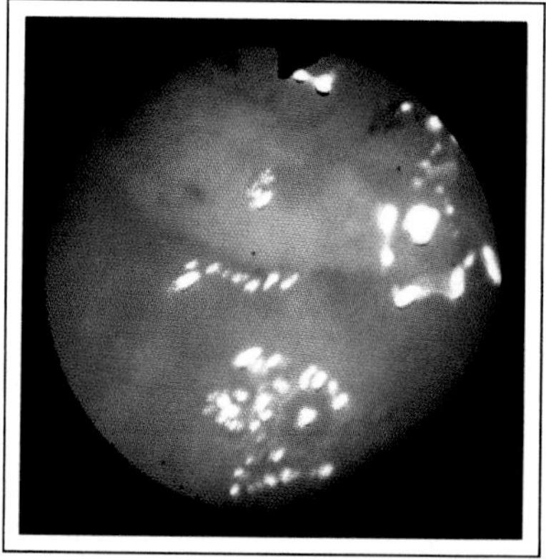

FIG. 28-16c.

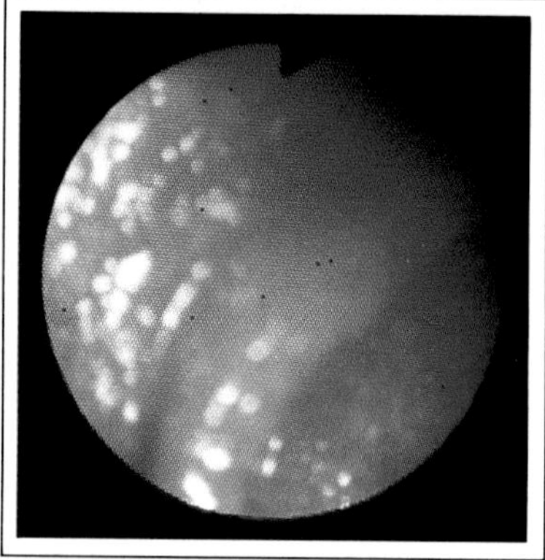

FIG. 28-17a.

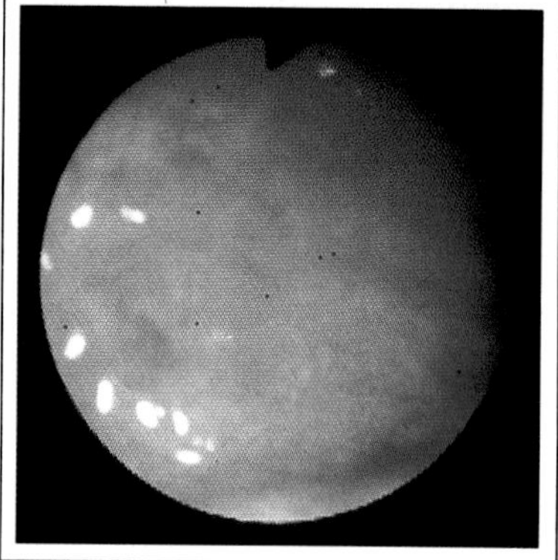

FIG. 28-17b.

FIG. 28-16. a: Duodenal bulb mucosa in chronic renal failure. The folds are enlarged and erythematous. The origin of these changes is unknown. **b:** Duodenal bulb mucosa in chronic renal failure. The Kerckring folds are greatly enlarged, a change which continues into the descending duodenum. **c:** Acute ulceration in a patient with chronic renal failure. The absence of any ulcer scarring in this patient with longstanding renal failure suggests that the ulceration was of recent onset. In this case it may have been related to a period of hypotension (stress-related duodenitis—see Chapter 38) or the use a nonsteroidal analgesic agent (Motrin).

FIG. 28-17. Radiation effect. **a:** The mucosal folds of the descending duodenum are enlarged 6 months after the patient received 4,000 rads to the abdomen for Hodgkin's disease. **b:** The mucosa of the duodenal bulb and apex [same patient as in (a)] shows focal nonspecific erythema.

Finally, one may encounter peptic ulcers in patients with chronic pancreatitis. Whether there actually is an increase of peptic ulcer disease in patients with chronic pancreatitis is unsettled.[18] Nevertheless, peptic ulcers occur either as single, discrete, often deep ulcers (Fig. 28-15a) or as multiple superficial ulcers of the duodenal bulb and descending duodenum (Fig. 28-15b). Single ulcers are more likely to be found in patients with pain which we have seen incorrectly attributed to the chronic pancreatitis but which disappears promptly once ulcer treatment is instituted. Multiple ulcers, on the other hand, occur with a variety of symptoms and may be themselves a form of nonspecific acute duodenitis (see Chapter 25) caused by reactive mucosal changes from the pancreatitis. The symptoms associated with these have an unpredictable response to ulcer treatment.

RENAL FAILURE

As in the stomach (see Chapter 14), the appearance of the duodenal mucosa is altered in chronic renal failure, especially in cases requiring dialysis. In patients with chronic renal failure, endoscopy may be prompted by nonspecific symptoms, e.g., nausea, vomiting, and upper abdominal pain, as well as symptoms suggestive of esophageal reflux. Prior to endoscopy, upper GI radiologic studies may show large folds of the duodenal bulb or descending duodenum in almost half the cases.[19]

Appearance

Erythema and nodularity of the duodenal bulb are commonly observed at endoscopy and are indistinguishable from that seen in nonspecific duodenitis (Fig. 28-16a). Large folds are common, being found especially at the apex (Fig. 28-16a) and extending into the descending duodenum (Fig. 28-16c) corresponding to those observed by radiographic studies. These changes were noted in 60% of patients with chronic renal failure in one endoscopic study.[19] As these changes are found in less than 10% of other patients having endoscopy (see Chapter 25), one may legitimately expect that chronic renal failure produces an alteration in the appearance of duodenal mucosa in an as yet unknown fashion.

Associated Peptic Ulcer Disease

The question of whether there is an increase in incidence of peptic ulcer disease among patients with chronic renal failure is controversial.[18] However, in one recent prospective study[19] of 85 patients with chronic renal failure who had endoscopy for reasons other than gastrointestinal bleeding, none had peptic ulcers. The commonest endoscopic finding was nonspecific duodenitis, which was found in 60%. This accords with our own experience, particularly in regard to the rarity of ulcers at endoscopy in patients with renal failure who are not bleeding contrasted with the finding of ulcers in up to 40% of patients who are.[20] In the latter cases, ulcers are of the acute type with no suggestion of scar deformity (Fig. 28-16c) and are most likely to be caused by superimposed stress conditions, e.g., sepsis, or surgery (see Chapter 38), or possibly the ingestion of aspirin or other ulcerogenic drug.

RADIATION

Radiation injury may occur in patients who receive in excess of 4,000 rads to the entire abdominal para-aortic lymph node chain or to the right upper retroperitoneal area.[21] Generally in these cases the radiation had been given for metastatic carcinoma of the cervix, testicular carcinoma, or primary right-sided retroperitoneal tumors.[21]

Appearance

Enlargement of the mucosal folds (Fig. 28-17a) is a common appearance corresponding to the diffuse thickening of the mucosal folds seen radiographically. In addition, there is either focal or diffuse nonspecific erythema (Fig. 28-17b) as well as coarsening of the mucosal villous pattern. Rarely, as in the colon (see Chapter 44), ulceration and stricture formation may be observed.[21]

REFERENCES

1. Nugent, F. W., Richmond, M., and Park, S. K. (1977): Crohn's disease of the duodenum. *Gut,* 18:115–120.
2. Danzi, J. T., Farmer, R. G., Sullivan, B. H., and Rankin, G. B. (1976): Endoscopic features of gastroduodenal Crohn's disease. *Gastroenterology,* 70:9–13.
3. Schuffler, M. D., and Chaffee, R. G. (1979): Small intestinal biopsy in a patient with Crohn's disease of the duodenum: the spectrum of abnormal findings. *Gastroenterology,* 76:1009–1014.
4. Dunne, W. T., Cooke, W. T., and Allan, R. N. (1977): Enzymatic and morphometric evidence for Crohn's disease as a diffuse lesion of the gastrointestinal tract. *Gut,* 18:290–294.
5. Gillberg, R., and Ahren, C. (1977): Coeliac disease diagnosed by means of duodenoscopy and endoscopic duodenal biopsy. *Scand. J. Gastroenterol.,* 12:911–916.
6. Stevens, F. M., and McCarthy, C. F. (1976): The endoscopic demonstration of coeliac disease. *Endoscopy,* 8:177–180.
7. Kohli, Y., Nakajima, M., Ida, K., and Kawai, K. (1974): Minute endoscopic findings using the dye scattering method. *Endoscopy,* 6:1–6.
8. Scott, B. B., and Losowsky, M. S. (1976): Patchiness and duodenal-jejunal variation of mucosal abnormality in coelic disease and dermatitis herpetiformis. *Gut,* 17:984–992.
9. Ament, M. E., Ochs, H. D., and Starkey, D. (1973): Structure and function of the gastrointestinal tract in primary immunodeficiency syndromes: a study of 39 patients. *Medicine,* 52:227–243.
10. Hermans, P. E., Huizenga, K. A., Hoffman, H. N., Brown, A. L., and Markowitz, H. (1966): Dysgammaglobulinemia associated with nodular lymphoid hyperplasia of the small intestine. *Am. J. Med.,* 40:78–89.
11. Saffouri, B., Mishriki, Y., Bartolomeo, R. S., and Fuchs, B. (1980): The value of endoscopy in the diagnosis of lymphoid nodular hyperplasia. *J. Clin. Gastroenterol.,* 2:169–171.
12. Ament, M. E., and Rubin, C. E. (1974): Relation of giardiasis to abnormal intestinal structure and function in gastrointestinal immunodeficiency syndromes. *Gastroenterology,* 62:216–226.
13. Bradley, E. L., and Clements, J. L. (1981): Idiopathic duodenal obstruction: an unappreciated complication of pancreatitis. *Ann. Surg.,* 193:638–648.
14. Acosta, J. M., Pellegrini, C. A., and Skinner, D. B. (1980): Etiology and pathogenesis of acute biliary pancreatitis. *Surgery,* 88:118–125.
15. Bellon, E. M., George, C. R., Schreiber, H., and Marshall, J. B. (1979): Pancreatic pseudocysts of the duodenum. *Am. J. Roentgenol.,* 133:827–831.
16. Blackstone, M. O., and Mizuno, H. (1977): Reactive duodenal changes in chronic pancreatitis simulating the contiguous spread of pancreatic carcinoma. *Am. J. Dig. Dis.,* 22:658–661.
17. Gambill, E. (1971): Pancreatitis associated with pancreatic carcinoma: a study of 26 cases. *Mayo Clin. Proc.,* 46:174–177.
18. Langman, M. J. S., and Cooke, A. R. (1976): Gastric and duodenal ulcer and their associaetd diseases. *Lancet,* 1:680–683.
19. Margolis, D. M., Saylor, J. L., Geisse, G., DeSchryver-Kecskemeti, K., Harter, H. R., and Zuckerman, G. R. (1978): Upper gastrointestinal disease in chronic renal failure: a prospective evaluation. *Arch. Intern. Med.,* 138:1214–1217.
20. Johnston, B., and Boyle, J. M. (1981): Non-variceal upper gastrointestinal hemorrhage in patients with chronic renal insufficiency. *Am. J. Gastroenterol.,* 76:181.
21. Goldstein, H. M., Rogers, L. F., Fletcher, G. H., and Dodd, G. D. (1975): Radiological manifestations of radiation-induced injury to the normal upper gastrointestinal tract. *Radiology,* 117:135–140.

29

DUODENAL MALIGNANCIES

Duodenal malignancies are relatively uncommon. They accounted for only 25 of 211 cases of upper gastrointestinal malignancy studied by our unit over a 7-year period (1974–1980). This contrasts with the 119 gastric and 67 esophageal malignancies seen over the same period.

Malignancy involving the duodenum arises from a variety of sites (Table 29-1), with primary carcinoma of the duodenum or ampulla of Vater representing only a minority (24%). The single commonest cancer of the duodenum is that which arises from the head of the pancreas and involves the duodenum by direct extension (36% of the total). Less often the direct extension is from the bile duct, colon, or liver. Finally, one may have metastatic cancer arising from a distant primary, e.g., the bronchus, or the duodenal involvement may be part of a more generalized abdominal malignant process, e.g., duodenal lymphoma.

TABLE 29-1. *Duodenal malignancies seen over a 7-year period (1974–1980)*

Type	No.	%
Primary	6	24
Duodenal	2	8
Ampullary	4	16
Invading the duodenum	11	44
Pancreatic	9	36
Bile duct	1	4
Colon	1	4
Metastatic	2	8
Breast	1	4
Melanoma	1	4
Other	6	24
Lymphoma	4	16
Sarcoma	1	4
Malignant carcinoid	1	4
Total	25	100

Even though duodenal malignancies are relatively rare, the endoscopist's role can be a crucial one, much more so than for the more common esophageal or gastric malignancies. This is so for two reasons. First, endoscopy in patients with primary duodenal or ampullary carcinomas may allow prompt diagnosis with histologic confirmation and referral for surgery where the percentage in whom curative resection can be performed is high.[1] For patients with primary duodenal carcinoma, the resectability rate is 60% and is even higher (>90%) for ampullary carcinoma,[2] with a 5-year survival of 15% for duodenal carcinoma and 30%+ for ampullary malignancies.[2] This contrasts with the lower 5-year survival rates of 8%[2a] and 4%[2b] for gastric and esophageal malignancies, respectively. Even for pancreatic cancer arising in a periampullary location and invading the duodenum, resection may still be possible in upward of 30%,[3] although with a 5-year survival of at best 15%[4] and generally less than 10%.

For other cancers, especially those metastasizing to the duodenum from a distance, endoscopy allows tissue confirmation of metastatic spread, as well as determining the primary in some cases.

In the sections which follow, we consider first adenocarcinoma arising as a primary process by contiguous spread or as a metastatic lesion from a distant primary. After this we briefly touch on endoscopic aspects of less common duodenal malignancies (e.g., lymphoma), of appearances in leukemia, and of rare sarcomas.

PRIMARY DUODENAL CARCINOMA

Primary duodenal carcinomas are generally found to be rare, representing less than 1% of cancers of the upper gastrointestinal tract.[5] Our own experience confirms this. Out of 211 cancers found at upper gastrointestinal (GI) endoscopy over a 7-year period, only two (1%) were primary duodenal carcinomas. Most are located in the second portion

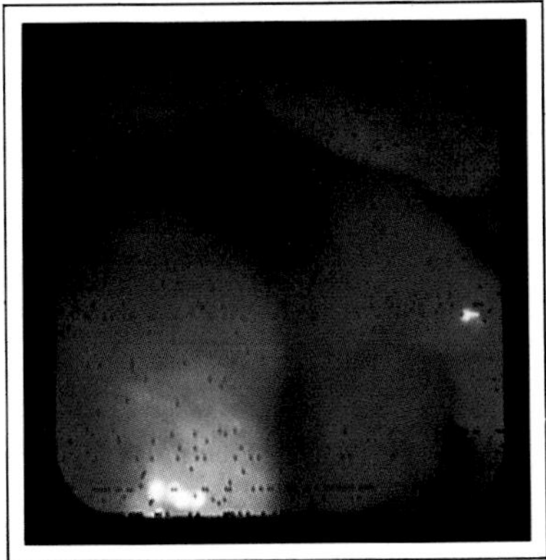

FIG. 29-1a.

FIG. 29-1. Primary carcinoma of the duodenum. **a:** This appeared as a 2 × 3 cm mass with central ulceration in a patient presenting with GI hemorrhage. At the time of endoscopy, bleeding was observed from the excavated portion of the lesion (at 5 o'clock). **b:** Resected specimen [same case as in (a)]. The duodenal papilla is located just proximal (to the 3 o'clock side) of the tumor, indicating the location of the malignancy to be the medial wall.

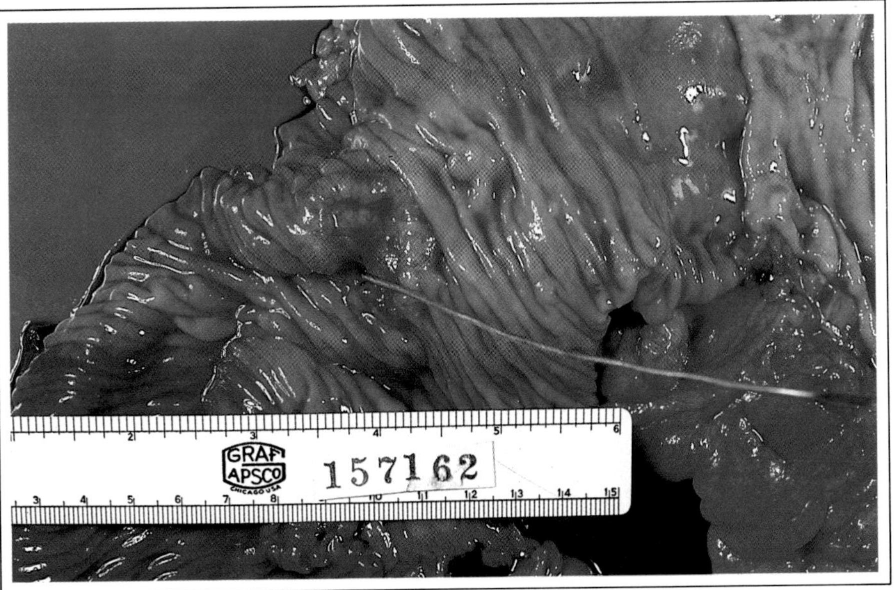

FIG. 29-1b.

of the duodenum—our two cases were within 2 cm of the duodenal papilla—but as many as one-fourth may arise from the third or fourth portion.[5] Characteristically, patients present during the sixth and seventh decades of life with jaundice, pain, and weight loss if the location is periampullary[1] or obstructive symptoms for carcinomas of the third and fourth portions.[1] In about 20% the presentation is upper GI bleeding (Fig. 29-1a).[1]

In spite of the fact that diagnosis may be delayed for more than 3 months from the onset of symptoms, 50% are resectable with a prospect of a 5-year survival rate of 25%,[1,5] about 2.5 times the anticipated 5-year survival rate for pancreatic carcinoma with the same periampullary location.[4] Interestingly, in one series the duration of symptoms prior to diagnosis, whether less or more than 3 months, did not affect the resectability rate or survival.[1]

Appearance

The endoscopist finds the typical duodenal carcinoma as a nodular, ulcerated, polypoid mass (Fig. 29-1a) with a maximum dimension between 3 and 6 cm.[6] In most cases, it appears as a well-circumscribed mass confined to the medial wall (Fig. 29-1b). Rarely, it involves the duodenum in a circumferential fashion or entirely replaces the wall (usually the medial) in which it originates (Fig. 29-2). In these cases with more widespread involvement, the mass may invade and entirely replace the duodenal papilla, which is then seen as simply part of the nodular ulcerated mass lesion of the medial wall (Fig. 29-2). Endoscopically, this appearance is identical to that of the more common duodenal involvement from contiguous spread of pancreatic carcinoma.[7]

Biopsy and Cytology

Primary carcinomas of the duodenum are by nature exophytic, a growth pattern which in other locations such as the stomach (see Chapter 16), is associated with a high yield from endoscopic biopsy and brushing cytology. Multiple brushings should be taken from nodular areas, avoiding the ulcerations which tend, by virtue of the association of the granulation tissue, to be poor sampling sites. Biopsy is the primary modality in these cases, with cytology having a complementary role; the latter is to be used for those lesions which cannot easily be biopsied, e.g., circumferential tumors.

Because of the exophytic nature of duodenal carcinoma, forward-viewing endoscopes usually suffice both to visualize the tumor and for adequate histologic and cytologic sampling. Because of the larger biopsy channel, which allows for a 2.8 mm forceps to be used with its larger bite (see Chapter 1), the larger (11 to 13 mm) caliber forward-viewing instruments have been preferred. However, the new generation of narrow-caliber (8.8 to 9.5 mm) instruments with

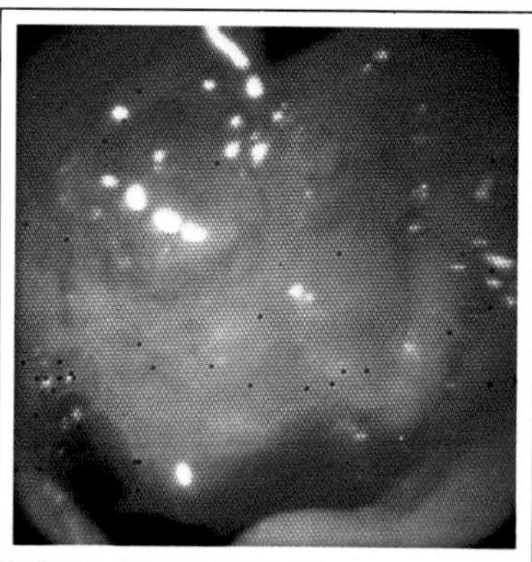

FIG. 29-2.

FIG. 29-2. Primary carcinoma of the duodenum. The entire medial wall has been replaced by a tumor mass that extends from 12 o'clock distally toward 6 o'clock.

a biopsy channel of 2.5+ mm offer an advantage of greater ease with which directed biopsies can be obtained. In cases where the endoscopist believes the lesion is not adequately demonstrated with forward-viewing instruments, he can reinsert a side-viewing duodenoscope.

PRIMARY AMPULLARY CARCINOMA

Carcinoma arising directly from the duodenal papilla is, in our experience, about twice as common as primary carcinoma arising elsewhere in the duodenum. These are still rare lesions, however, constituting less than 2% of carcinomas of the upper GI tract and only 5 to 10% or less of all ampullary malignancies.[8] In fact, we have found the mucosa of the ampulla to be involved with malignancy from the pancreas, bile duct, or duodenum about two to three times as often as primary carcinoma of the ampulla. In many of these cases, however, it is not possible to determine the precise origin of the carcinoma. Still, for cases which endoscopically appear to be ampullary carcinoma and in which the tumor can be resected *en bloc*, the outcome is the same regardless of origin, so long as the specimen is free of nodal metastasis.[8]

The commonest presenting symptom is jaundice,[2,8] but this is variable, occurring in 85% in one series but in only 40% in another. Classically, this is said to be fluctuating, but in one series this pattern was found in only 25%.[8] Other symptoms, e.g., weight loss, pruritus, nausea, and vomiting, are found in less than half the cases.[8] The endoscopist becomes involved in many cases because of performing endoscopic retrograde cholangiopancreatography (ERCP).[9]

The importance of recognizing the appearance of ampullary carcinoma lies in the fact that of all cancers encountered at upper GI endoscopy this has one of the highest rates of resectability, ranging from 60%[8] to 96%,[2] with acceptable mortality and morbidity rates, a 5-year survival in excess of 34%,[2,8] and a 10-year incidence of surgical cure of 20%.[2]

Appearance

At endoscopy one sees the duodenal papilla to be two to three times its normal size, appearing as a cylindrically shaped mass (Fig. 29-3a). Part of this enlargement, particularly within the hooded fold area, is related to extrinsic compression from a dilated bile duct (see Chapter 27), with the remainder of the mass from the carcinoma itself, especially in the position where one expects to find the papillary orifice. Here one sees a characteristic raised tumor mass projecting out from the hooded fold (Fig. 29-3a). In the typical case, the cancer infiltrates circumferentially, causing the peripheral portion of the orifice to become raised in relation to a central depressed area (Fig. 29-3b) giving it an excavated appearance. This is the most recognizable endoscopic feature associated with ampullary cancer. Tumor nodules and ulcerations may be seen within the excavated area, especially if a side-viewing instrument is employed (Fig. 29-3b).

Biopsy and Cytology

In patients with a high index of suspicion of ampullary carcinoma based on endoscopic findings, the endoscopist should vigorously pursue biopsy and/or cytologic confirmation of the presence of carcinoma so that any attempt at surgical resection can proceed directly without requiring additional time for histologic confirmation. Fortunately for the endoscopist, ampullary carcinomas are bulky tumors and usually present no difficulty in obtaining positive histologic and cytologic material, with an expected yield, in our experience, of over 80%.[9] To obtain a positive result, the endoscopist first observes the lesion for the presence of frank tumor nodules which have the highest yield on biopsy. At least five biopsy specimens should be obtained, especially if a small (2 mm) caliber forceps is used. Biopsies are taken from the periphery as well as the excavated portion; extremely ulcerated areas from which only granulation tissue is generally obtained are avoided. If cytology is available, it should be utilized especially to obtain brushings from within the excavated portion of the tumor.

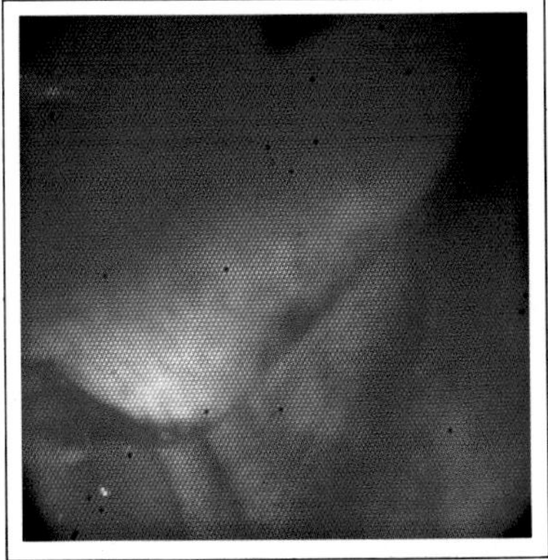

FIG. 29-3a.

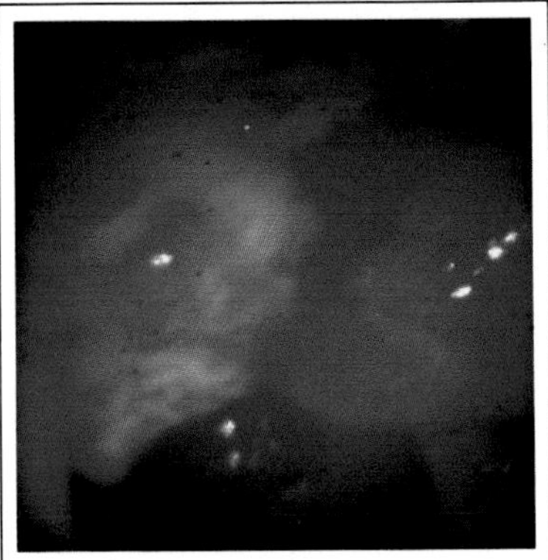

FIG. 29-3b.

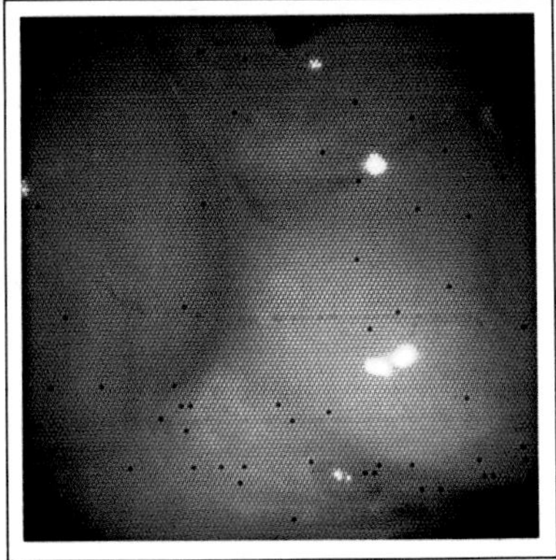

FIG. 29-3c.

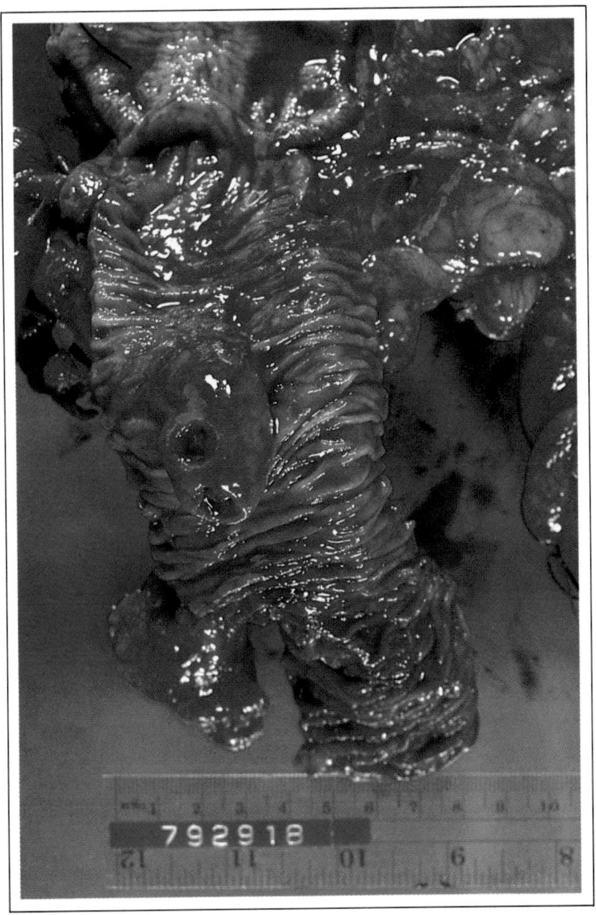

FIG. 29-3d.

FIG. 29-3. a: Primary carcinoma of the ampulla of Vater. The hooded fold is enlarged because of infiltrating tumor, but the overlying mucosa was intact. **b:** Primary carcinoma of the ampulla of Vater. The characteristic appearance is of a central excavation (at 9 o'clock) surrounded by tumor nodules (at 3 o'clock). **c:** Duodenal papilla with impacted stone. Biliary calculus disease, especially with impaction, may be associated with nonspecific enlargement and an altered appearance of the orifice with the potential for being mistaken for ampullary carcinoma. **d:** Primary carcinoma of the ampulla of Vater, resected specimen [same case as in (b)]. The duodenal papilla is grossly enlarged, measuring 2.5 to 3 cm, running proximally (left portion of the field) into a dilated bile duct. The distal end (orifice) has an excavated appearance with an indurated margin. A second excavated area is also apparent resulting from mucosal ulceration from the carcinoma.

CARCINOMA ARISING FROM OTHER PRIMARY SITES

We find that nearly half the cases of carcinoma found in the duodenum have primary sites elsewhere (Table 29-1). Most of these are an extension to the duodenum from carcinoma of the head of the pancreas, with a few cases where it is from either the bile duct or hepatic flexure of the colon. For about 10% we find the carcinoma to be a metastatic implant from a distant primary, e.g., breast, skin (melanoma), bronchus, or kidney (Table 29-1). In this section we consider the types of carcinoma which involve the duodenum from these other primary sites.

Duodenal Involvement by Contiguous Periampullary Malignancies

The commonest type of duodenal malignancy is actually that which arises from the adjacent head of the pancreas or bile duct. Of these, one may expect that all are pancreatic, as this carcinoma is 5 to 10 times more common than carcinoma of the bile duct. In most cases the patient presents

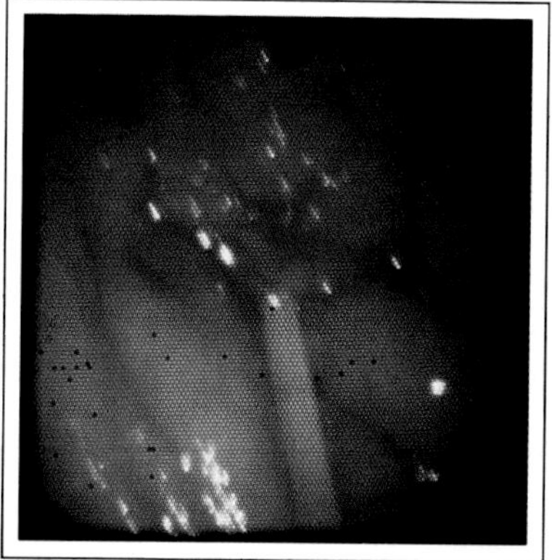

FIG. 29-4a.

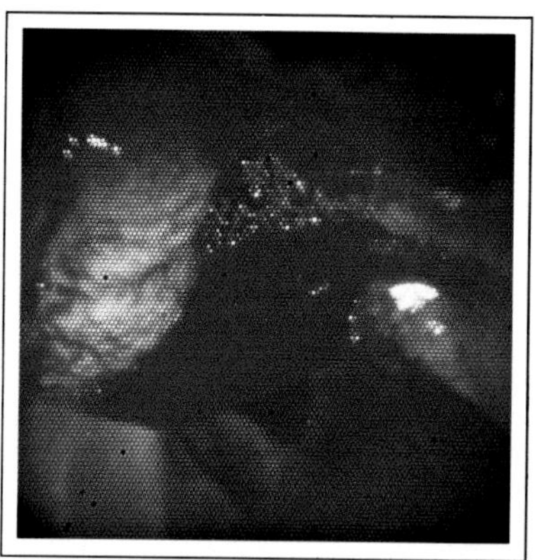

FIG. 29-4b.

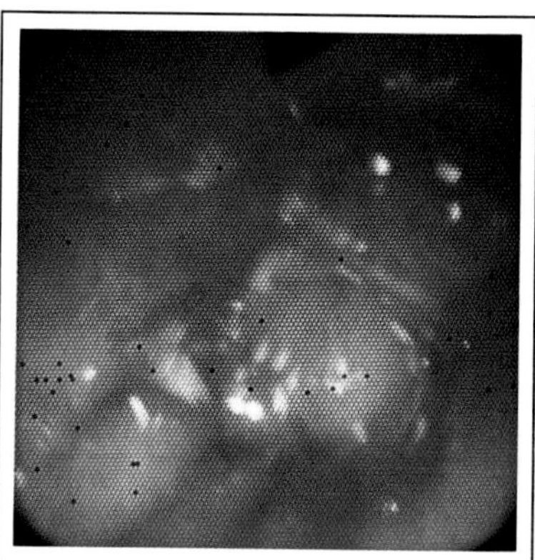

FIG. 29-4c.

FIG. 29-4. a: Secondary carcinoma of the ampulla of Vater, arising from the pancreas. The ampullary orifice is denoted by the polyethylene cannula. The orifice has been entirely replaced by nodular tumor masses. **b:** Secondary carcinoma of the ampulla arising from the pancreas. A central excavated portion surrounded by raised tumor masses has an appearance indistinguishable from primary ampullary carcinoma (Fig. 29-3b). **c:** Secondary carcinoma of the duodenum arising from the head of the pancreas. The entire wall of the descending duodenum was replaced by a friable, nodular tumor mass.

with jaundice, with the carcinoma having been suspected by the presence of a mass demonstrated by ultrasound or computed tomography (CT) scan. This periampullary presentation accounts for 30 to 40% of the patients with pancreatic carcinoma.[3] In our experience, a duodenal and/or ampullary mass may be expected in 10 to 15% of periampullary carcinomas of the pancreas (Table 29-2).

As with ampullary carcinomas themselves, jaundice is the commonest presentation for duodenal involvement by a contiguous periampullary malignancy. Although the presentation may be identical, the resectability rate for periampullary carcinomas arising in the head of the pancreas is lower than that for ampullary carcinoma, being at best 30%[3] with a 5-year survival rate of 10% or less[4] in contrast to the 30%+ 5-year survival rate for resected ampullary carcinoma.[2,8]

Appearance

Using the newer, smaller-caliber endoscopes with their shorter turning lengths, the medial wall of the descending duodenum can be visualized in almost all cases, especially if the indirect entry technique is utilized (see Chapter 24). The best visualization of the medial wall, however, is obtained using a side-viewing duodenoscope (see Chapter 24). The commonest endoscopic finding of contiguous spread is that of an irregular, ill-defined mass of the medial wall. It is often extensive, usually involving the ampulla (Fig. 29-4a) and in some cases replacing the entire medial wall (Fig. 29-4c). In most cases the mass is nodular, with the nodules being 3 to 5 cm and occasionally larger.

An altered appearance of the duodenum occurs in half the patients with pancreatic and bile duct cancers (Table 29-2), with extrinsic compression and ampullary enlargement being the commonest findings and a carcinomatous mass being found in only one-sixth of all patients with duodenal involvement. Of the cases where a definite tumor mass is present, carcinoma is confined to the ampulla in about one-third, appears as a duodenal mass separate from the ampulla in another third, and as a duodenal mass which involves the ampulla in the remainder (Table 29-2).

In cases where only the ampulla is involved, one observes a nodular mass which appears to have replaced the entire

TABLE 29-2. *Duodenal involvement in 92 patients with periampullary cancer over a 7-year period (1974–1980)*

Periampullary cancer		No. with duodenal involvement	Extrinsic compression	Ampullary involvement		Duodenal mass	Ampullary and duodenal mass
				Enlargement	Mass		
Pancreatic	75	39	14	15	3	3	4
Duodenal	2	2	—	—	—	1	1
Ampullary	4	4	—	—	4	—	—
Bile duct	11	4	2	1	—	—	1
Total	92	49	16	16	7	4	6
Pancreatic and bile duct carcinoma	86	43	16	16	3	3	5

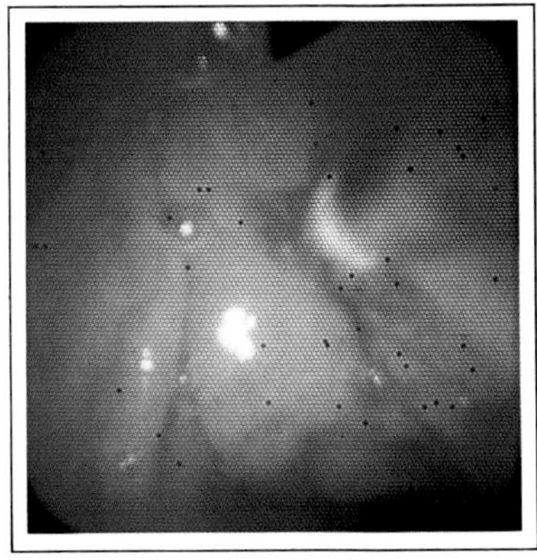

FIG. 29-5a.

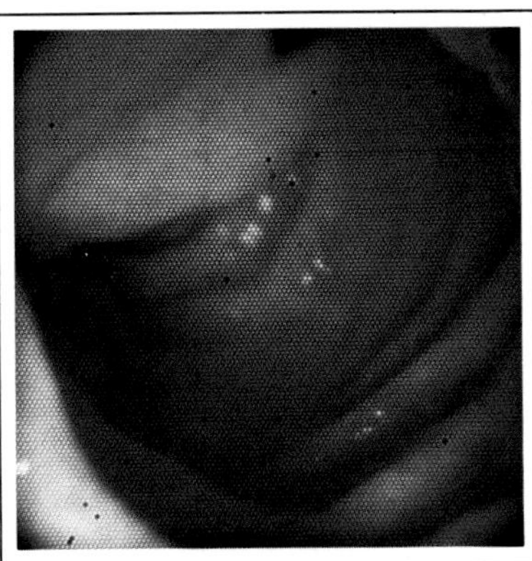

FIG. 29-5b.

FIG. 29-5. Pancreatic carcinoma. **a:** Associated with extrinsic compression of the descending duodenum and nonspecific enlargement of the ampulla. The surgically resected specimen in this case showed no evidence of duodenal or ampullary invasion. **b:** Associated with nonspecific ampullary enlargement. The mucosa is intact, and biopsies were negative. Careful examination of the resected specimens failed to disclose evidence of ampullary invasion.

ampullary structure (Fig. 29-4a). Some of these lesions have an excavated appearance (Fig. 29-4b) and are virtually indistinguishable from primary ampullary carcinoma (Fig. 29-3b). In this regard, it is important to remember that pancreatic carcinoma is a common cause of ampullary malignancy found at endoscopy. Of seven such lesions observed by us over a 7-year period (Table 29-2), four proved to be of ampullary origin, but three were secondary to pancreatic spread. Among our patients with periampullary malignancy, the finding of a duodenal mass, often extensive and with or without ampullary involvement, was seen more commonly as an extension of pancreatic carcinoma than as a primary duodenal carcinoma (Table 29-2).

As we have said, what is more commonly found than the mass with contiguous spread of carcinoma is either extrinsic compression (Fig. 29-5a) and/or ampullary enlargement (Fig. 25-5b). Singly or in combination, these were found in almost 40% of patients endoscoped by us over a 7-year period with a final diagnosis of pancreatic carcinoma (Table 29-2) and account for two-thirds of the cases where an altered duodenal appearance is present. These findings do not imply duodenal invasion, however, which is confirmed histologically in less than half the patients with these findings who undergo surgical resection.

Biopsy and Cytology

Aggressive biopsy and, if available, cytology of an irregular, nodular surface have high yields, especially if multiple biopsies are taken. In such cases, we have found this to be in excess of 75%.[9]

Contiguous Spread of Colonic (Hepatic Flexure) Carcinoma

Although right-sided colon carcinomas are being recognized with increasing frequency, actual contiguous spread from a hepatic flexure location is exceedingly rare, even though three such cases were reported from the same institution.[10] We have seen only one case (Fig. 29-6) where unresectable carcinoma had eroded into the wall of the descending duodenum with formation of a giant tumor cavity.

Metastatic Spread to the Duodenum

Metastasis to the duodenum from a distant primary accounts for less than 10% of duodenal malignancies. The most common is malignant melanoma.[11] Other primary sites include bronchus, breast, kidney,[12] and even the uterine cervix.[13] The routes of spread are peritoneal, hematogenous, and lymphatic.

In patients with metastatic duodenal implants, endoscopy is most often requested because of acute GI bleeding (see Chapter 38). In other cases endoscopy is prompted by clinical problems relating to intraabdominal malignancies such as weight loss and pain.[12] Prior radiologic studies in patients with metastatic implants often show single or multiple filling defects, especially of the descending duodenum.[12]

Appearance

The typical metastatic implant appears as a 1- to 2-cm ulcerated mass (Fig. 29-7). In the case of malignant melanoma, small (5 mm) pigmented lesions are seen (Fig. 29-8a), as well as large (1 cm) lesions in which the central portion is ulcerated with the periphery remaining pigmented (Fig. 29-8b). Metastatic implants are generally set apart from the duodenal papilla, although in one case observed by us a metastatic implant had appeared in the ampulla, causing progressive jaundice (Fig. 29-9). In this case, which came to resection, the histology of the metastatic focus was identical with that from a breast carcinoma that had been removed 16 years earlier.

The finding of a tumor mass (Fig. 29-7) in a patient with a known primary capable of metastasis to the duodenum should always make one suspect this diagnosis. Generally, biopsies taken from the periphery as well as the central portion of the lesion confirm the diagnosis.

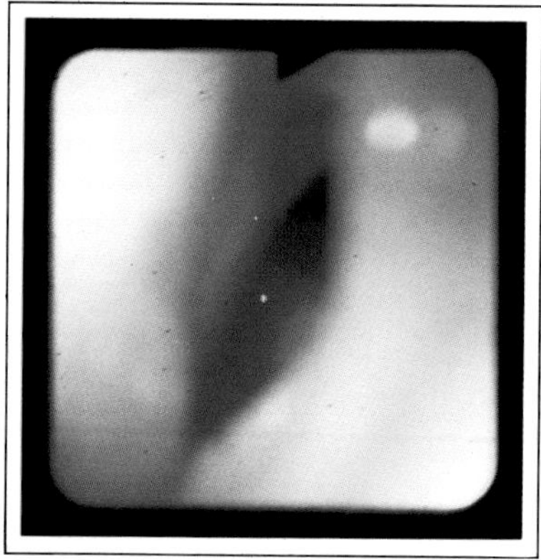

FIG. 29-6.

FIG. 29-7.

FIG. 29-6. Contiguous spread of colonic (hepatic flexure) carcinoma to involve the descending duodenum. The lumen opens into a large tumor cavity.

FIG. 29-7. Metastatic carcinoma to the duodenum from a distant primary. A 2- to 3-cm nodular mass appears in a patient with a known primary carcinoma capable of metastasizing to the duodenum, in this case malignant melanoma. As in the stomach (see Chapter 16), larger implants tend to be amelanotic.

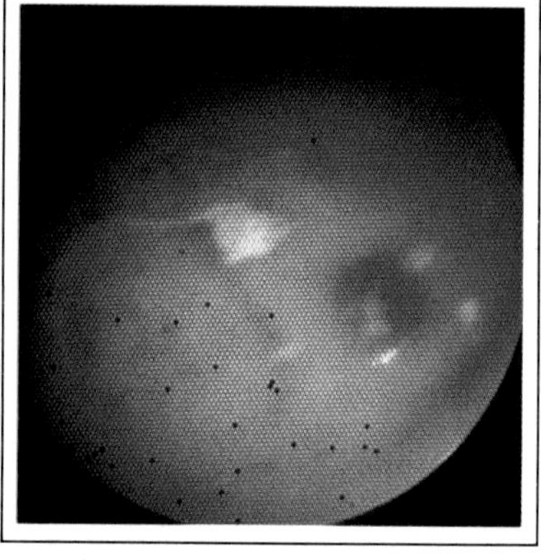

FIG. 29-8a.

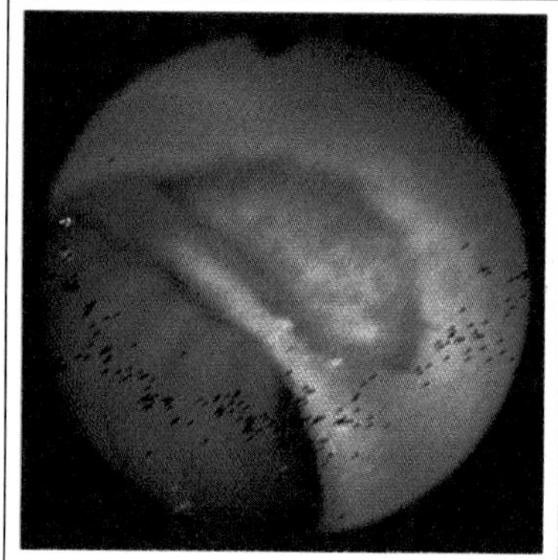

FIG. 29-8b.

FIG. 29-8. Malignant melanoma involving the duodenum. **a:** A small (5 mm) pigmented implant is seen at the apex of the duodenal bulb. **b:** A larger (1.5 cm) lesion is seen within the descending duodenum having a central ulcerated portion with a peripheral brown-black pigmented zone.

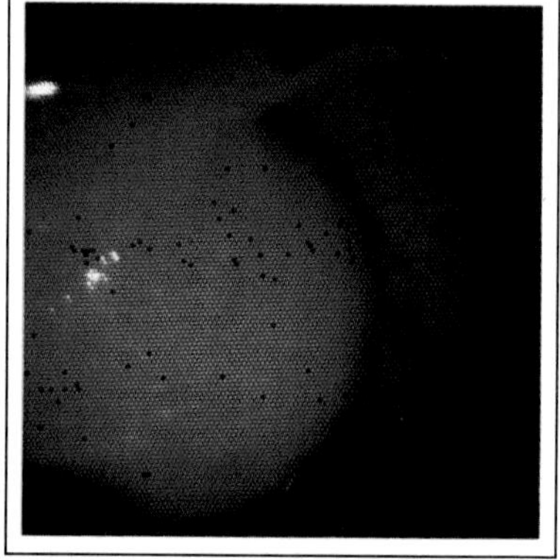

FIG. 29-9a.

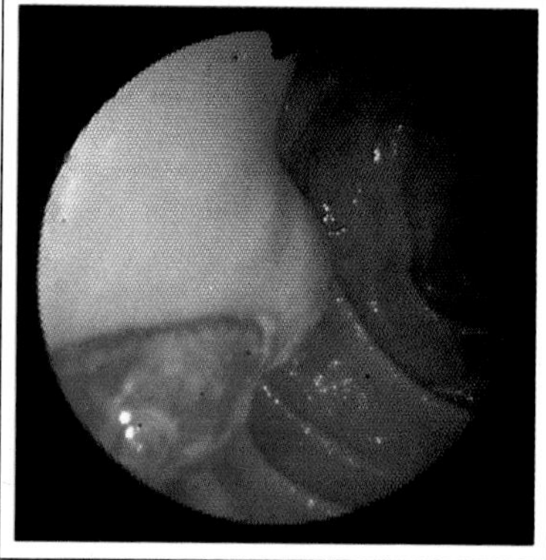

FIG. 29-9b.

FIG. 29-9. a: Breast carcinoma metastatic to the ampulla. The hooded fold is enlarged because of obstructive jaundice as well as the ampulla being the site of metastasis from a breast cancer (proved at surgery). **b:** Renal carcinoma metastatic to the duodenum. A 3-cm submucosal mass with an ulcerated, friable surface was observed on the posterior wall of the descending duodenum. Biopsy showed this to have histology identical to that of a renal carcinoma removed 12 years previously.

DUODENAL LYMPHOMA

Associated With Gastric Lymphoma

Lymphoma accounts for 10 to 20% of duodenal malignancies. Most are found in association with gastric lymphoma.[14,15] In these cases there is transpyloric extension of the lymphoma with duodenal bulb involvement. Less often, the body and fundus are involved, with the antrum apparently spared. In cases where there is gastric involvement, the endoscopist may observe a single ulcerated fungating mass or multiple nodular lesions ranging in size from 5 to 15 mm (Fig. 29-10a) or an even larger (>2 cm) polypoid mass (Fig. 29-10b).

Our experience accords with that reported by others for the association of gastric and duodenal lymphoma.[14,16] In three of 10 patients with gastric lymphoma observed by us over a 7-year period, duodenal involvement was found at endoscopy, surgery, or autopsy, respectively. In all cases the involvement was confined to the duodenal bulb. In one case multiple (5 to 15) polypoid masses were observed (Fig. 29-10a), whereas in a second case a large ulcerated mass had replaced the entire anterior inferior aspect of the bulb (Fig. 29-10b). In the remaining case the mucosa had a diffusely infiltrated appearance with some nodularity but no definite mass.

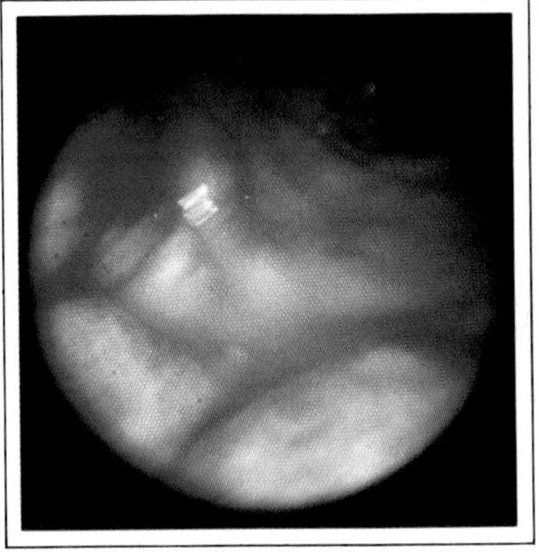

FIG. 29-10a.

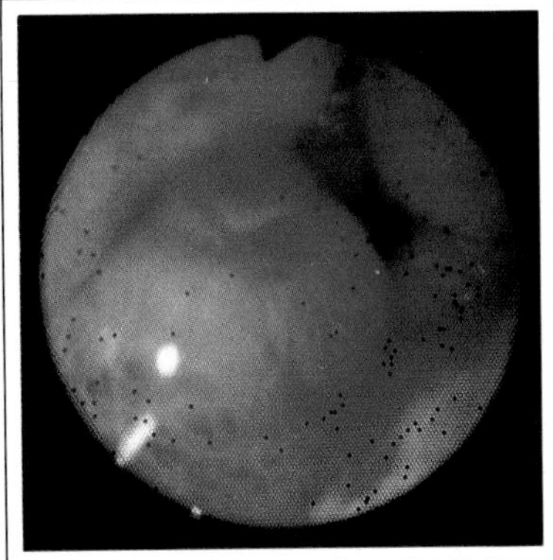

FIG. 29-10b.

FIG. 29-10. a: Lymphoma of the duodenal bulb in a patient with gastric lymphoma. Large gastric rugal folds were found in this patient with 1.5 × 2 cm nodules of the duodenal bulb. Biopsies from both reveal poorly differentiated lymphoma. **b:** Lymphoma of the duodenal bulb in a patient with gastric lymphoma. In this case a large ulcerated polypoid mass is replacing the anterior inferior wall. **c:** Lymphoma of the duodenum, third portion, presenting as GI bleeding. In this case biopsy of the nodular mass at 12 o'clock showed poorly differentiated lymphoma.

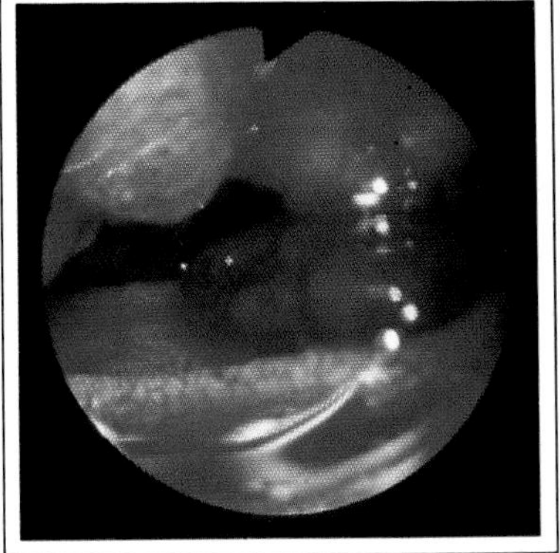

FIG. 29-10c.

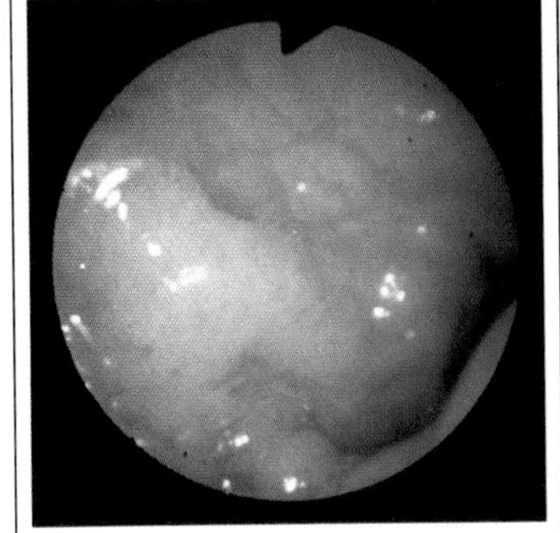

FIG. 29-11.

FIG. 29-11. Nonspecific mucosal changes in abdominal lymphoma. The Kerckring folds appeared enlarged and nodular in this patient with untreated abdominal lymphoma. The biopsy showed only nodular inflammation. At autopsy there was no evidence of duodenal involvement. Nonspecific enlargement of folds should not be interpreted as evidence of involvement.

Primary Duodenal Lymphoma

The lymphoma occurring as a primary process rather than as an extension of gastric involvement is quite rare, as the duodenum is the least common site of primary small bowel lymphoma.[16] Only one of our four cases of duodenal lymphoma was this type. As with lymphoma elsewhere in the small bowel, pain, weight loss, and obstructive symptoms are the commonest presentation[16] along with GI bleeding, the presentation of our patient. In the reported cases of primary duodenal lymphoma the second portion is the most common site,[17] although the third portion, as in our case (Fig. 29-10c), and the fourth portion may also be sites of involvement. In these cases the lymphoma appears as nodular, sessile, ulcerated masses (Fig. 29-10c).

Nonspecific Appearances in Abdominal Lymphoma

A variety of nonspecific appearances may be observed, especially in the descending duodenum, in patients with abdominal lymphoma. These include an increased size of the Kerckring folds, erythema, increased friability of the mucosa, and extrinsic compression (Fig. 29-11). These changes are similar to those observed in patients with pancreatic carcinoma who are ultimately found not to have duodenal invasion. As in the case of pancreatic carcinoma, nonspecific findings should not be taken as evidence of duodenal involvement. Multiple biopsies, however, should be taken from any such questionably involved area.

Biopsy and Cytology

As in the case of gastric lymphoma, biopsies and brushing sites are often successful, even given the infiltrating nature of the lymphoma.[9] Any extensive lesion, especially if associated with polypoid masses or ulcerations, should be aggressively brushed by biopsy with the expectation that in the majority of cases the diagnosis of lymphoma will be confirmed.

DUODENAL APPEARANCES IN LEUKEMIA

Duodenal infiltration occurs in patients with leukemia, similar to that which can be observed in the stomach (see Chapter 16), but apparently less often. In an autopsy series from our institution, leukemic infiltration of the duodenum was found in only 7%, compared with 23% of cases with gastric involvement.[18] The 10 cases of duodenal involvement were either "stem cell" or myelogenous leukemias with one case of the lymphatic type, in contrast to the predominance of this latter type in association with gastric involvement.[18] The cases varied from microscopic involvement alone to the presence of focal gross involvement as "plaque-like thickenings of folds" and finally diffuse involvement with "elevated nodular lesions and polypoid masses," which in one case were found throughout the entire small bowel and colon.[18]

Despite the findings of some duodenal involvement in 7% at autopsy, we failed to recognize duodenal involvement

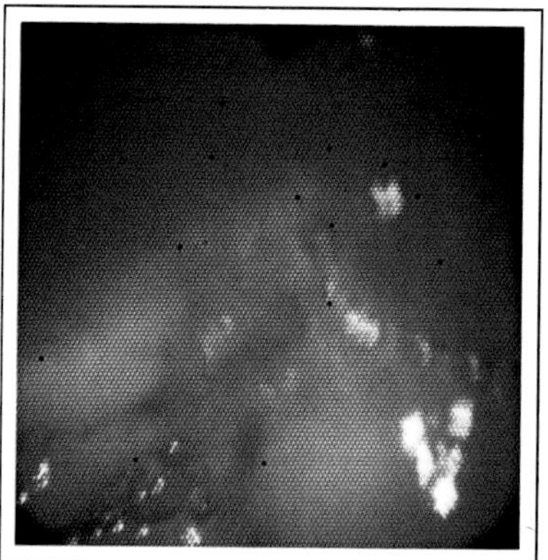

FIG. 29-12.

FIG. 29-12. Retroperitoneal fibromyosarcoma involving the duodenum. There is extrinsic compression and enlargement of the folds of the medial wall. Biopsy suggested a mesenchymal tumor, which was ultimately proven at surgery. The appearance in this case was indistinguishable from that associated with pancreatic carcinoma.

in any of 300 patients with leukemia examined over a 10-year period. Indeed, only one case report since 1970 has appeared in which duodenal leukemia was apparent at endoscopy, a case of chronic lymphocytic leukemia with enlarged, nodular duodenal folds showing histologically evidence of the leukemia.[19]

Rather than leukemic infiltrates, the endoscopist is more likely to encounter nonleukemic acute mucosal injury with hemorrhagic necrosis or mucosal hemorrhages, being three times commoner at autopsy. These cases present as gastrointestinal bleeding similar to that found in association with this appearance with other malignancies (see Chapter 37). An exceedingly rare type of nonleukemic involvement has been reported as peptic ulcer disease with gastric hypersecretion in association with basophilic leukemia. In this case, the gastric hypersecretion, being secondary to histamine release (from leukemic basophils) was entirely suppressed with cimetidine.[20]

RARE DUODENAL MALIGNANCIES

Retroperitoneal sarcoma, other mesenchymal tumors, and malignant carcinoids (see Chapter 30) are occasionally discovered to involve the duodenum.[21] In one case of a fibromyosarcoma studied by us, there was extensive replacement of the wall of the descending duodenum by this tumor. In this case, the endoscopic appearance was indistinguishable from that of pancreatic carcinoma invading the duodenum; however, biopsy revealed the mesenchymal origin of this malignancy (Fig. 29-12).

REFERENCES

1. Kerremans, R. P., Lerut, J., and Penninckx, F. M. (1979): Primary malignant duodenal tumors. *Ann. Surg.*, 19:179–182.
2. Akwari, O. E., van Heerden, J. A., Adson, M. A., and Baggenstass, A. H. (1977): Radical pancreatoduodenectomy for cancer of the papilla of Vater. *Arch. Surg.*, 112:451–456.

2a. Dupont, J. B., Lee, J. R., Burton, G. R., and Cohn, I. (1978): Adenocarcinoma of the stomach: review of 1,497. *Cancer*, 41:941–947.

2b. Earlham, R., and Cunha-Melo, J. R. (1980): Oesophageal squamous cell carcinoma: I. A critical review of surgery. *Br. J. Surg.*, 67:381–390.

3. Moossa, A. R., Lewis, M. H., and Mackie, C. R. (1979): Surgical treatment of pancreatic cancer. *Mayo Clin. Proc.*, 54:468–474.
4. Tepper, J., Nardi, G., and Suit, H. (1976): Carcinoma of the pancreas: review of MGH experience from 1963 to 1973: analysis of surgical failure and implications for radiation therapy. *Cancer*, 37:1519–1524.
5. Spira, I. A., Ghabi, A., and Wolff, W. I. (1977): Primary adenocarcinoma of the duodenum. *Cancer*, 39:1721–1735.
6. Wald, A., and Milligan, F. D. (1975): The role of fiberoptic endoscopy in the diagnosis and management of duodenal neoplasms. *Am. J. Dig. Dis.*, 20:499–505.
7. Kato, O., Kuno, N., Kasugai, T., and Matsuyama, M. (1979): Pancreatic carcinoma difficult to differentiate from duodenal carcinoma. *Am. J. Gastroenterol.*, 71:74–77.
8. Walsh, D. B., Eckhauser, F. E., Cronenwett, J. L., Turcotte, J. G., and Lindenauer, S. M. (1982): Adenocarcinoma of the ampulla of Vater. *Ann. Surg.*, 195:152–156.
9. Hall, T. J., Blackstone, M. O., Cooper, M. J., Hughes, R. G., and Moossa, A. R. (1978): Prospective evaluation of endoscopic retrograde cholangio-pancreatography in the diagnosis of periampullary cancers. *Ann. Surg.*, 187:313–317.
10. Alfonso, A., Morehouse, H., Dallemand, S., Wapnick, S., Suster, B., Farman, J., and Gardner, B. (1979): Local duodenal metastasis from colonic carcinoma. *J. Clin. Gastroenterol.*, 1:149–152.
11. Sivak, M. V., and Sullivan, B. H. (1973): Endoscopic diagnosis of malignant melanoma metastatic to the duodenum. *Gastrointest. Endosc.*, 22:36–38.
12. Theodors, A., Sivak, M. V., and Carey, W. D. (1980): Hypernephroma with metastasis to the duodenum: endoscopic features. *Gastrointest. Endosc.*, 26:48–51.
13. Gurian, L., Ireland, K., Petty, W., and Katon, R. (1981): Carcinoma of the cervix involving the duodenum: case report and review of the literature. *J. Clin. Gastroenterol.*, 3:291–294.
14. Meyers, M. A., Katzen, B., and Alonso, D. R. (1975): Transpyloric extension to the duodenal bulb in gastric lymphoma. *Radiology*, 15:575–580.
15. Hricak, H., Thoeni, R. F., Margulis, A. R., Eyler, W. R., and Francis, I. (1980): Extension of gastric lymphoma into the esophagus and duodenum. *Radiology*, 135:309–312.
16. Loehr, W. J., Mujahed, Z., Zahn, D., Gray, G. F., and Thorbjarnarson, B. (1968): Primary lymphoma of the gastrointestinal tract: a review of 100 cases. *Ann. Surg.*, 170:232–238.
17. Payson, B. A., Weingarten, L., and Pollack, J. (1979): Lymphosarcoma of the duodenum associated with carcinoma of the lung. *Am. J. Gastroenterol.*, 71:295–300.
18. Prolla, J. C., and Kirsner, J. B. (1964): The gastrointestinal lesions and complications of the leukemias. *Ann. Intern. Med.*, 61:1084–1103.
19. Wasser, A. H., and Spector, J. I. (1977): Endoscopic evaluation of small-bowel leukemia. *Am. J. Dig. Dis.*, 22:1028–1032.
20. Swisher, R. W., Mueller, J. M., and Halloran, L. G. (1978): Basophilic leukemia presenting as gastroduodenal ulceration: Effect of H-2-receptor blockade. *Am. J. Dig. Dis.*, 23:952–955.
21. Yassinger, S., Imperato, T. J., Midgly, R., Michas, C., and Bolt, R. J. (1977): Leiomyosarcoma of the duodenum. *Gastrointest. Endosc.*, 24:38–40.

30

DUODENAL POLYPS

Duodenal polyps are present in about 1% of examinations.[1] We noted 64 (1.3%) in 5,000 examinations performed over a 7-year period (Table 30-1). For the large majority (44 cases), the polyp was observed as multiple, small (2 to 6 mm) mucosal nodules (Fig. 30-1a). Whether the endoscopist refers to this appearance as polyps or nodules, mammillations, or nodularity is ultimately a subjective matter. We use the term polyps for an appearance where discrete mucosal elevations are seen because it conforms to a similar usage for this term in the stomach (see Chapter 17) and the colon (see Chapter 41), provided that flat, intervening mucosa between the elevations can be identified (Fig. 30-1a). We do not wish to use the term nodule for the duodenum when the same appearance in the stomach or colon is referred to by the term polyp. In contrast to the appearance of discrete mucosal elevations is the case where there is no flat mucosa between the elevated surfaces (Fig. 30-1b). For this, we use the term nodularity or mammillations.

As a majority of duodenal polyps are less than 5 mm, it is not surprising that most are discovered as incidental findings, where endoscopy was prompted by either nonspecific symptoms or prior radiologic study.[1] Larger single polyps (>1 cm) may be associated with acute or chronic blood loss for which endoscopy is performed.[1-3] Rarely, such a polyp is located at a site that causes intermittent obstruction,[3] or it arises from the duodenal papilla causing jaundice.[1,4]

Like polyps elsewhere in the gastrointestinal (GI) tract, one could consider duodenal polyps based on their origin as either epithelial or submucosal (Table 30-2). Although this is a convenient way to think about duodenal polyps, it is less satisfying from the standpoint of the endoscopist examining them because there is virtually no effective visual feature for distinguishing those of epithelial origin (Fig. 30-1c) from submucosal polyps (Fig. 30-1d). A more useful way of classifying these polyps, we believe, is in regard to their number and size—whether multiple small (<1 cm) polyps or single large (≥1 cm) polyps. We therefore discuss duodenal polyps in two main sections—multiple polyps and single polyps—considering under the latter category the submucosal and adenomatous types.

TABLE 30-1. *Duodenal polyps—64 cases (1974–1980)*

Appearance	No.	%
Single polyp	20	31.3
Multiple polys	44	68.7
Total patients with polyps	64	100
Total patients examined	5,000	1.3*

* With duodenal polyps.

TABLE 30-2. *Histologic classification of duodenal polyps*

- Epithelial polyps
  - Hyperplastic-inflammatory
  - Heterotopic gastric mucosa
  - Lymphoid hyperplasia
  - Adenatomous
    - Simple adenomas
    - Villous adenomas
- Submucosal polyps
  - Brunner gland hyperplasia
    - Diffuse
    - Focal (Brunner gland adenomas)
  - Tumors of mesenchymal origin
    - Leiomyomas
    - Lipomas
    - Carcinoids
    - Rare types, e.g., angiomas, myxomas and others
  - Other submucosal polyps
    - Duplication cysts
    - Pancreatic rests

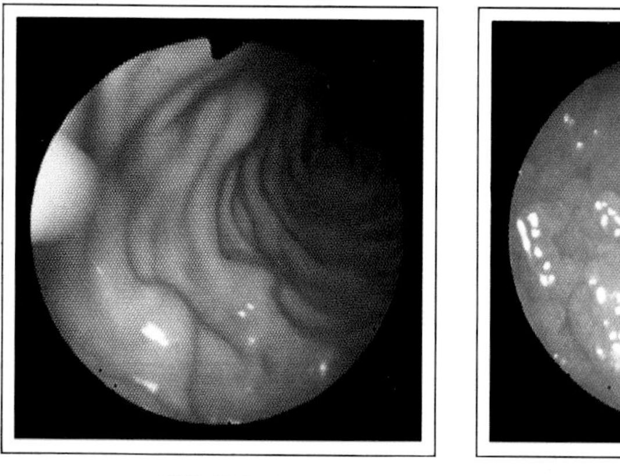

FIG. 30-1a.

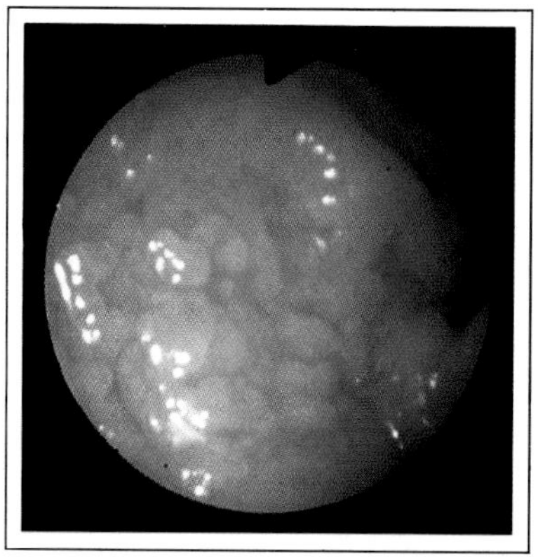

FIG. 30-1b.

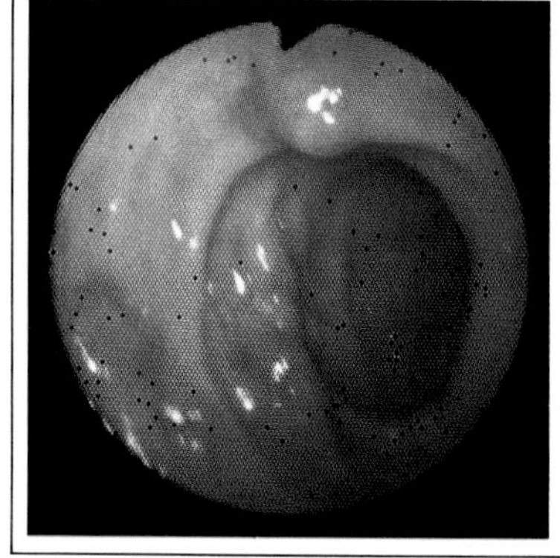

FIG. 30-1c.

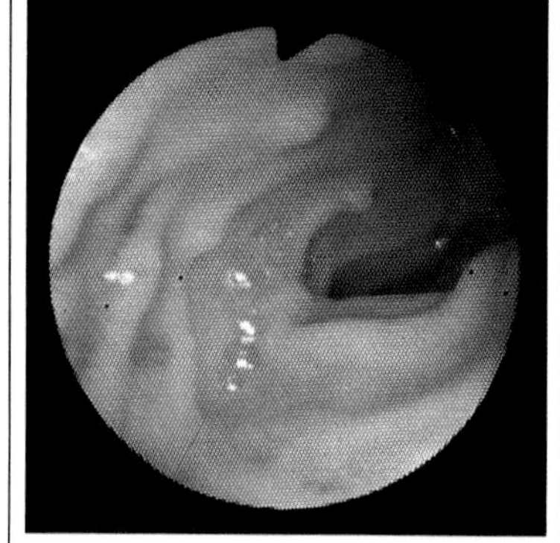

FIG. 30-1d.

FIG. 30-1. a: Multiple polyps. Discrete mucosal elevations are observed in the descending duodenum with flat mucosa in between. **b:** Nodular mucosa. There is no intervening flat mucosa, causing the entire mucosal surface of the duodenal bulb to appear bumpy or nodular. **c:** Nodular duodenitis, appearing as multiple polyps. Biopsies from the polyps as well as surrounding mucosa revealed chronic inflammation. **d:** Brunner gland hyperplasia, appearing as multiple duodenal polyps. Biopsies showed the discrete elevations to be accompanied by an increased number of Brunner glands.

MULTIPLE POLYPS

Multiple polyps commonly are of four types: (a) hyperplastic-inflammatory; (b) heterotopic gastric mucosa; (c) Brunner gland hyperplasia; and (d) lymphoid hyperplasia. We have already considered Brunner gland hyperplasia (see Chapter 25) and lymphoid hyperplasia (see Chapter 28) elsewhere. In this section we concentrate on the hyperplastic-inflammatory type and polyps composed of heterotopic gastric mucosa which together account for over 60% of cases with multiple polyps (Table 30-3).

TABLE 30-3. *Multiple duodenal polyps—44 cases*

Type	No.	% of multiple polyps	% of total cases
Hyperplastic-inflammatory	24	54.6	37.5
Brunner gland hyperplasia	9	20.5	13.8
Lymphoid hyperplasia	6	13.6	8.3
with IgA deficiency	2		
Heterotopic gastric mucosa	4	9.1	7.3
Adenomatous polyps[a]	1	2.2	1.8
Total	44	100	68.7

[a] Patient with Gardner's syndrome (familial polyposis).

Hyperplastic-Inflammatory Polyps

We find hyperplastic-inflammatory polyps to be the commonest type of multiple duodenal polyp, accounting for over half the cases (Table 30-3). These polyps arise from mucosa which is histologically normal or shows nonspecific duodenitis (see Chapter 25). Because biopsies of the polyp often show an inflammatory component, we term them hyperplastic-inflammatory polyps. Some regard the appearance of these polyps as evidence of nodular duodenitis, especially if biopsies reveal chronic inflammation.[5]

At endoscopy the polyps appear as discrete 2- to 6-mm elevations (Fig. 30-2a). They may be confined to the duodenal bulb (Fig. 30-2a) or extend into the descending duodenum (Fig. 30-2b). Less commonly they appear as isolated mucosal elevations of the descending duodenum (Fig. 30-2c).

Generally the mucosa of the polyp is indistinguishable from that of its surroundings (Fig. 30-2c). For larger polyps (>6 mm) this may become erythematous or even superficially ulcerated (Fig. 30-2d). Because of these surface changes, the endoscopist may consider the possibility of their being adenomatous. Based on our experience, in the absence of a known polyposis syndrome (see Chapter 41) we believe that this would be exceedingly rare. Among our 44 cases of multiple polyps (Table 30-3), in only one

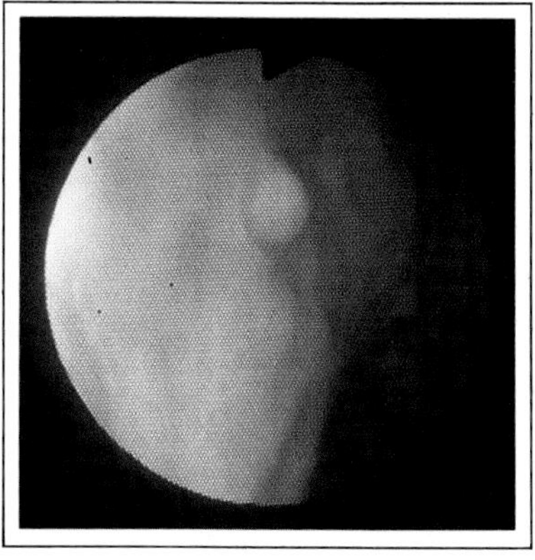

FIG. 30-2a.

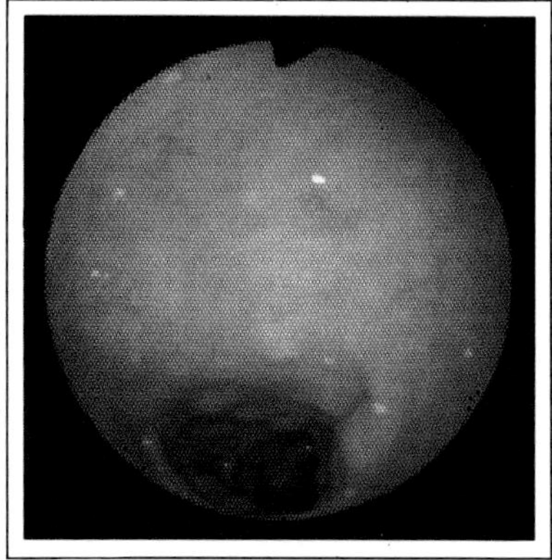

FIG. 30-2b.

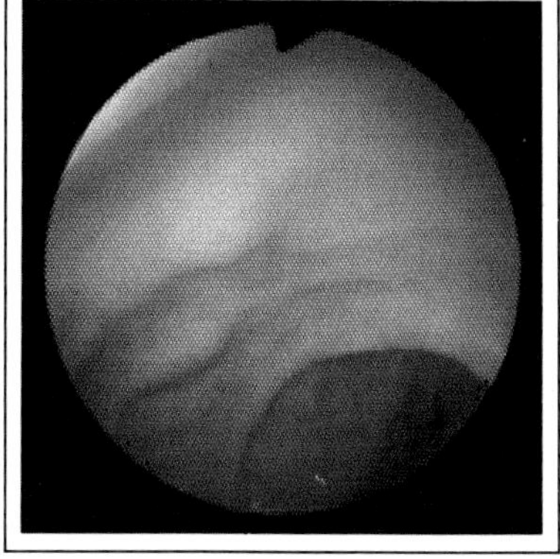

FIG. 30-2c.

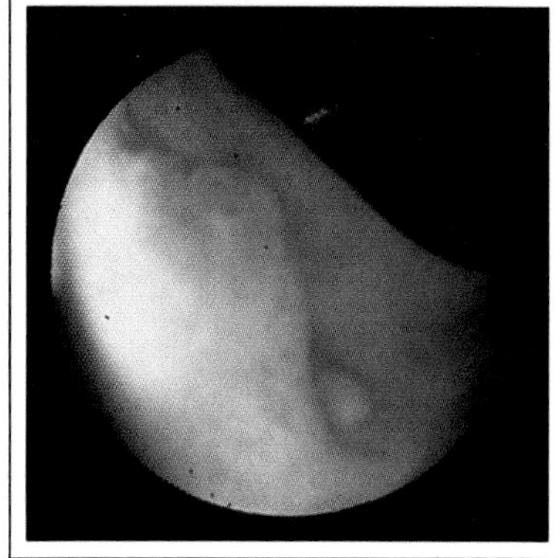

FIG. 30-2d.

FIG. 30-2. a: Hyperplastic-inflammatory polyps. Multiple polyps ranging in size between 3 and 8 mm were found confined to the duodenal bulb. Biopsies showed mild chronic inflammation. **b:** Hyperplastic-inflammatory polyps. Multiple polyps were present in the bulb and descending duodenum. **c:** Hyperplastic-inflammatory polyps of the descending duodenum. In this case there were 2- to 4-mm polyps scattered in the descending duodenum only. **d:** Hyperplastic-inflammatory polyp with erythema and an irregular surface, raising the question of an adenoma. Despite this appearance, a biopsy showed only mild chronic inflammation.

did the polyps prove to be adenomatous (see below), and this was in a patient with familial polyposis (Gardner's syndrome). Although it is probably wise to biopsy any polyp greater than 5 mm (especially one with ulcerated or otherwise atypical mucosa), almost invariably these are nonneoplastic.

Heterotopic Gastric Mucosa Appearing as Multiple Polyps

Less common than hyperplastic polyps, but by no means rare, are polyps which appear to be composed entirely of heterotopic gastric mucosa.[6] Although it has been known for over 50 years that a polypoid mucosal appearance could result from this type of mucosa, only recently has it been recognized radiographically and endoscopically.[6] In that report[6] it was found in up to 2.8% of endoscopic examinations of the bulb. Since this report and our awareness of polyps of this type, we now identify them with the same incidence (i.e., four to six cases per 700 examinations per year) as did others in a recent report.[6a] Their overall low number in our series (only 8 cases out of 5,000) may be a reflection of our lack of awareness of them until 1980.[6]

At endoscopy one may see a diffusely nodular surface with 1- to 6-mm excrescences having no intervening flat mucosa (Fig. 30-3a), discrete smaller polyps (Fig. 30-3b), or larger (>1 cm) single (Fig. 30-3c) or multiple (Fig. 30-3d) polyps. Like hyperplastic polyps, these are mainly confined to the duodenal bulb (Table 30-3).

A clue to the presence of polyps composed of heterotopic mucosa may be a disagreement with the pathologist concerning the location of biopsy site. As the biopsy shows parietal cells with or without chief cells, the pathologist may suspect that the endoscopist is mistaken about the location of his biopsies. If the endoscopist is confident that he has taken his biopsies from a duodenal polyp, however, the diagnosis of heterotopic gastric mucosa should be accepted by all concerned.

Brunner Gland Hyperplasia

Brunner gland hyperplasia accounted for 20% of our cases of multiple duodenal polyps (Table 30-1), which was about twice the incidence of heterotopic gastric mucosa polyps, although as we said the latter type is being increasingly recognized. When Brunner gland hyperplasia is present, the polyps are 2 to 6 cm in size and appear in the duodenal bulb (Fig. 30-4a) as well as the descending duodenum (Fig. 30-4b).[7] Although there is no universal feature to distinguish Brunner gland hyperplasia from the other types, they do

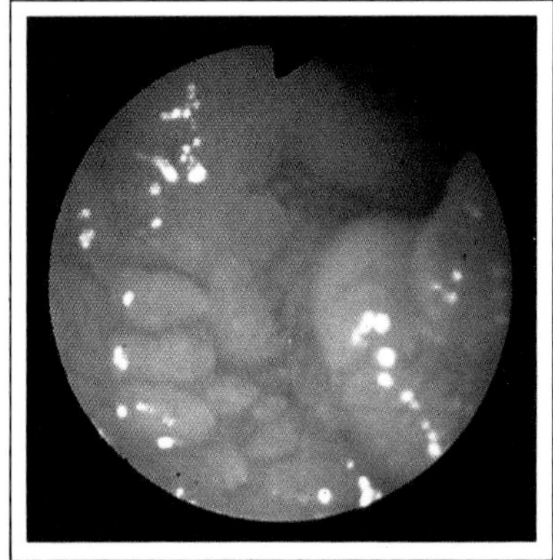
FIG. 30-3a.

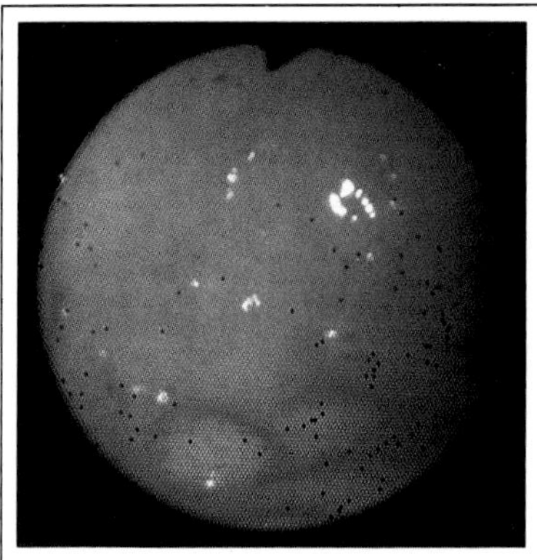
FIG. 30-3b.

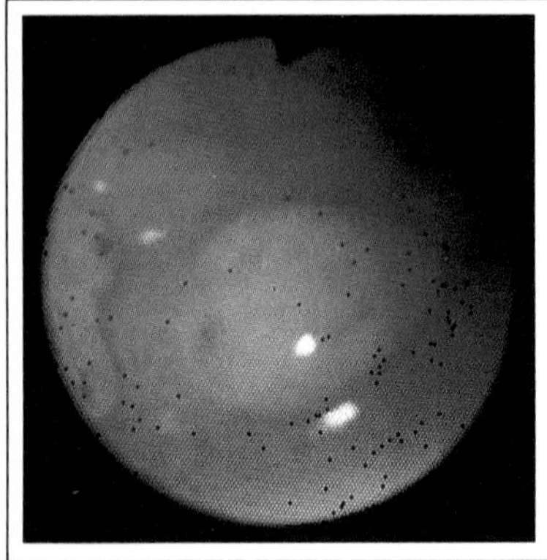
FIG. 30-3c.

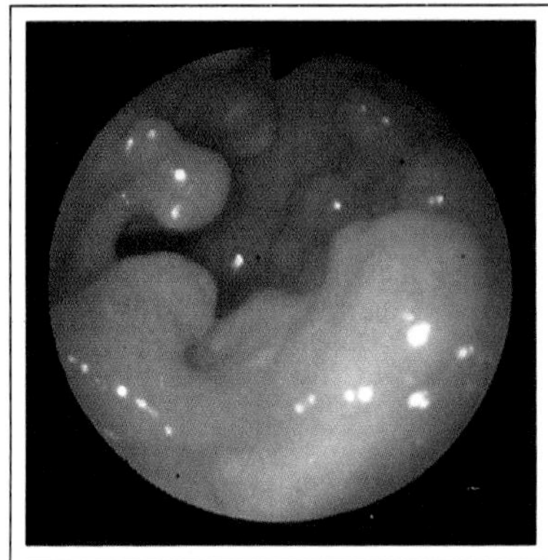
FIG. 30-3d.

FIG. 30-3. Heterotopic gastric mucosa. **a:** Appearing as mucosal nodularity of the duodenal bulb. There is no flat mucosa between individual elevations, ranging in size from 2 to 6 mm. **b:** Appearing as polyps. A cluster was observed in the duodenal bulb with individual lesions ranging in size from 6 to 8 mm. Although having an appearance identical with that of common hyperplastic-inflammatory polyps (Fig. 30-2a), biopsies showed pyloric glands, indicating heterotopic gastric mucosa. **c:** With a larger (1 cm) polyp in addition to the cluster of small lesions [same case as in (b)]. **d:** Appearing as large 1- to 2-cm duodenal polyps confined to the duodenal bulb.

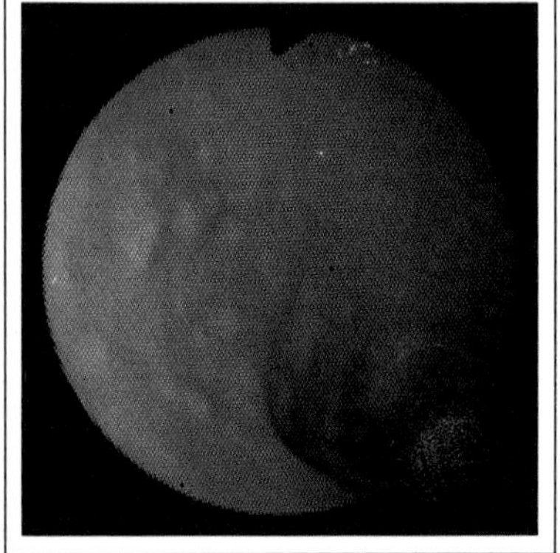
FIG. 30-4a.

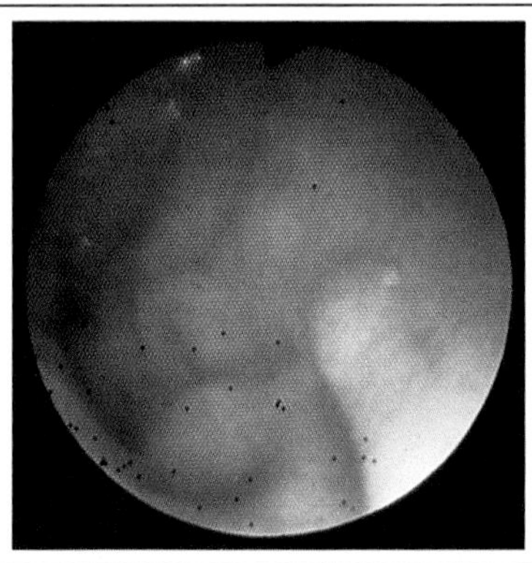
FIG. 30-4b.

FIG. 30-4. Brunner gland hyperplasia. **a:** Appearing as multiple tiny polyps (2 to 4 mm) of the duodenal bulb and descending duodenum. Some intervening flat mucosa between the polyps can be identified. **b:** Seen as larger (5 to 8 mm) polyps observed close together in the duodenal bulb and descending duodenum.

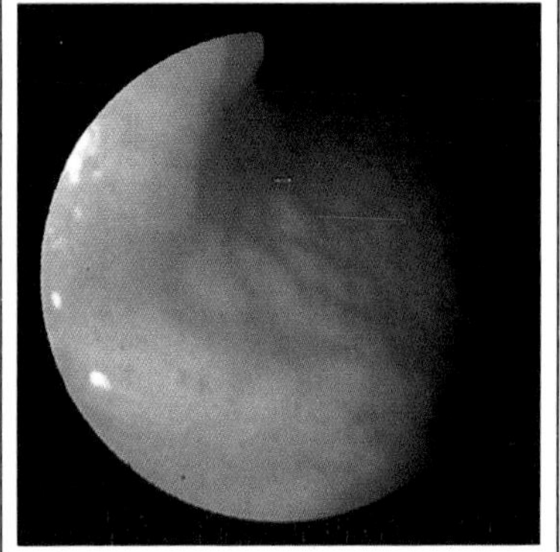
FIG. 30-5a.

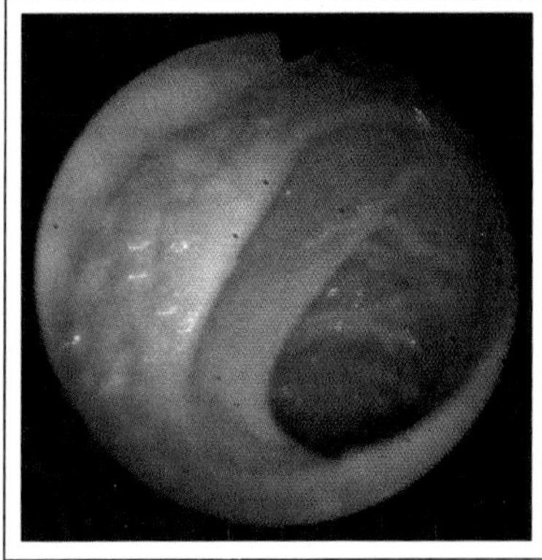
FIG. 30-5b.

FIG. 30-5. a: Lymphoid hyperplasia revealed in biopsies was associated with the finding of multiple tiny (2 to 4 mm) polyps of the duodenal bulb and descending duodenum. The patient had no underlying immunoglobulin deficiency. **b:** Nodular lymphoid hyperplasia of the duodenal bulb and descending duodenum in a patient with hypogammaglobulinemia. A cluster of tiny (2 to 3 mm) polyps was found in the duodenal bulb and descending duodenum which on biopsy was seen to be composed of lymphoid tissue. There is no difference endoscopically between lymphoid hyperplasia which is associated with immunoglobulin deficiency and that which is not.

tend to be more numerous and are located closer together (Fig. 30-4a) than either hyperplastic polyps (Fig. 30-2a) or polyps composed of heterotopic gastric mucosa (Fig. 30-3d).

Lymphoid Hyperplasia

For about 10% of the cases where multiple polyps (Fig. 30-5a) are present, biopsies show lymphoid hyperplasia (Table 30-3), even in the absence of an immunoglobulin deficiency (see Chapter 28). In these cases the appearance at endoscopy is identical to that found with immunoglobulin A (IgA) deficiency, so-called nodular lymphoid hyperplasia (Fig. 30-5b).

Like Brunner gland hyperplasia (Fig. 30-4a), lymphoid hyperplasia tends to be associated with smaller, more closely situated polyps of the descending duodenum (Table 30-4) whereas hyperplastic-inflammatory polyps (Fig. 30-4a) and polyps composed of heterotopic gastric mucosa (Fig. 30-3d) tend to be larger, more widely separated, and confined to the duodenal bulb (Table 30-4).

SINGLE POLYPS

Single polyps represent only one-third of the cases (Table 30-1). They are of three types and are considered in this section separately as: (a) hyperplastic-inflammatory polyps; (b) submucosal polyps, e.g., leiomyomas; and least common (c) adenomatous polyps.

Hyperplastic-Inflammatory Polyps

Single hyperplastic-inflammatory polyps are relatively uncommon, accounting for only 10% of the total cases (Table 30-5). Most range in size between 3 and 6 mm (Fig. 30-6a). A small fraction (two out of seven) are larger than 1 cm (Table 30-5). The size (Fig. 30-6b) as well as the appearance of the mucosa—either eroded (Fig. 30-6c) or granular (Fig. 30-6d)—may cause the endoscopist to suspect an adenoma. Although some have reported that adenomas account for almost 20% of the cases of duodenal polyps,[1] we found only one case among 20 patients who had single duodenal polyps (5%), making it unlikely that any given duodenal polyp is an adenoma. Furthermore, inflammatory-hyperplastic polyps were seven times more common than proved submucosal polyps. Still, one would wish to biopsy any single polyp larger than 5 mm, but especially one with its largest dimension 1 cm or more, that has an eroded or otherwise atypical mucosa (Fig. 30-6d). Most, even those with a seemingly adenomatous appearance, will prove to be nonneoplastic (Table 30-5).

TABLE 30-4. *Distribution of multiple duodenal polyps*

Type	Total no.	Duodenal bulb No.	Duodenal bulb %	Duodenal bulb and descending duodenum No.	Duodenal bulb and descending duodenum %
Hyperplastic-inflammatory	24	19	79	5	21
Brunner gland hyperplasia	9	2	22	7	78
Lymphoid hyperplasia	6	—	—	6	100
Heterotopic gastric mucosa	4	4	100	—	—
Adenomatous polyps[a]	1	—	—	1	100
Total	44	25	57	19	43

[a] Patient with Gardner's syndrome (familial polyposis).

TABLE 30-5. *Single duodenal polyps—20 cases*

Type	No.	% of single polyps	% of total cases
Epithelial			
Hyperplastic	7	35	11.0
<1 cm	5		
≥1 cm	2		
Adenomatous	1	5	1.5
Submucosal			
Leiomyoma	2	10	3.1
Lipoma	1	5	1.5
Carcinoid	3	15	4.6
Benign	2		
Malignant	1		
Brunner gland adenoma	1	5	7.8
Uncertain, possibly submucosal			
Negative forceps biopsy	5	25	1.8
Total	20	100	31.3

Submucosal Polyps

We find single submucosal polyps as commonly as single hyperplastic polyps (Table 30-5). They might even prove to be the most common type of single duodenal polyp if all polyps greater than 1 cm were removed totally and submitted for histologic examination. As most submucosal polyps are incidental findings and their removal is not indicated, we probably will never know the true incidence of this type of polyp, although in all probability they represent less than 15% of the cases.

In this section we consider the four types of submucosal polyp the endoscopist may encounter. These are: (a) leiomyomas; (b) lipomas; (c) carcinoids; and (d) Brunner gland adenomas.

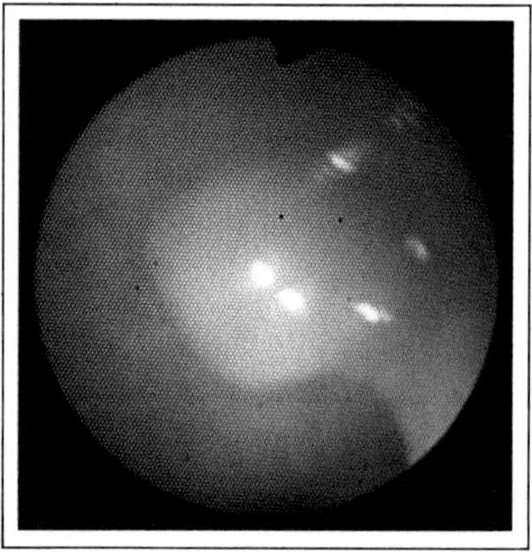

FIG. 30-6a.

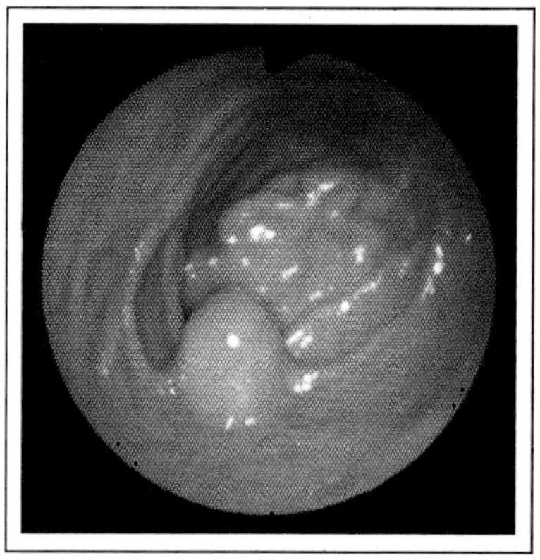

FIG. 30-6b.

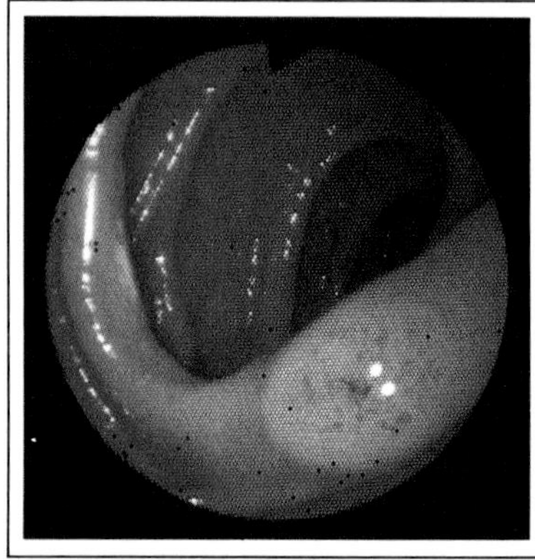

FIG. 30-6c.

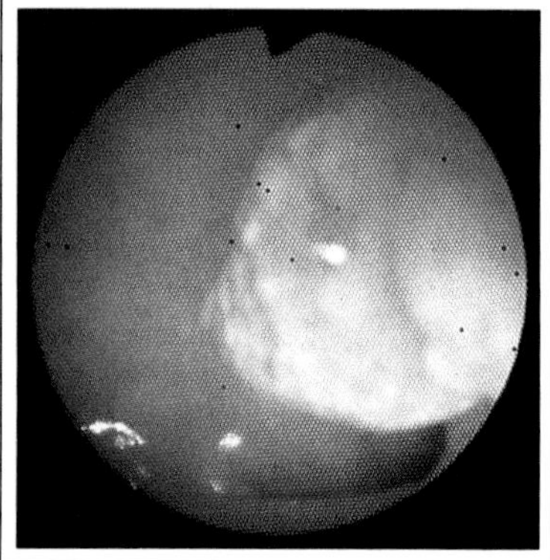

FIG. 30-6d.

FIG. 30-6. a: Hyperplastic-inflammatory polyp. A single 4-mm polyp was found at the apex. Biopsy showed only mild chronic inflammation. **b:** Hyperplastic-inflammatory polyp. An isolated 1-cm polyp of the bulb with intact, smooth surface epithelium. Its appearance caused the endoscopist to suspect a submucosal polyp; however, histologic examination of the completely excised polyp showed it only to be hyperplastic. **c:** A 7-mm hyperplastic-inflammatory polyp with a slightly eroded (superficially ulcerated) surface. **d:** A 1-cm hyperplastic-inflammatory polyp with an eroded surface, which caused it to be mistaken for an adenoma (Fig. 30-12).

Leiomyomas

In surgical series, where the polyps tend to be large (>1 cm), leiomyomas are found either to be the commonest submucosal tumor[2] or to occur no less frequently than lipomas[3]; together these are the commonest duodenal polyps.[2,3] However, in a recent endoscopic series of 45 polyps, although only 12 were excised completely no leiomyomas were found. In such a series, where most polyps are discovered as incidental findings because they are smaller than 1 cm, one would expect that leiomyomas are underrepresented.

When they appear, they are generally larger than 5 mm in maximum dimension and most commonly larger than 1 cm (Fig. 30-7); they have a central ulceration or umbilication, especially when endoscopy was prompted by either acute gastrointestinal (GI) bleeding or an iron deficiency anemia.

The location of leiomyomas is most often the junction of the apex of the bulb and proximal descending duodenum (Fig. 30-7), but they can have more distal locations in the third and fourth portions.[2] Biopsies from the umbilicated or ulcerated portion may reveal spindle cells, pointing toward the nature of the tumor as a leiomyoma.

If the leiomyoma were noted at endoscopy as an incidental finding in a patient with nonspecific symptoms, one would be justified in watching the polyp, especially if biopsies confirmed its nature. In the face of iron deficiency anemia or acute GI bleeding, one would be justified in recommending surgical removal rather than endoscopic electrosurgical treatment; the latter, although feasible, is technically difficult, especially in the locations where the leiomyoma is often found: the apex of the duodenal bulb, the medial wall of the proximal descending duodenum, and the third and fourth portions.

Lipomas

Lipomas occur in some surgical series as commonly as leiomyomas.[2,3] They are more often found in the descending duodenum at its junction with the apex rather than in the bulb itself. Although they represent up to 25% of benign tumors of the duodenum found at surgery, they are an infrequent type of duodenal polyp found at endoscopy, seen in only two of 45 cases reported by Reddy et al.,[1] and in only 1 of 20 single polyps in our series (Table 30-5). They may be overrepresented in surgical series because the more common but smaller hyperplastic-inflammatory polyps are rarely an indication for exploration; however, they are underrepresented in endoscopic reports because their commonest location, the junction of the descending duodenum

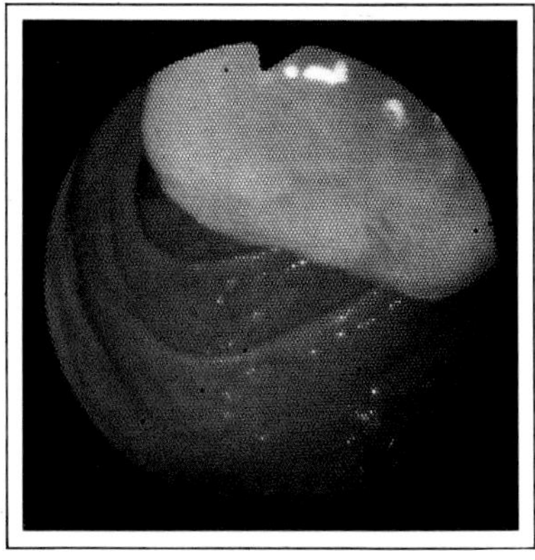

FIG. 30-7.

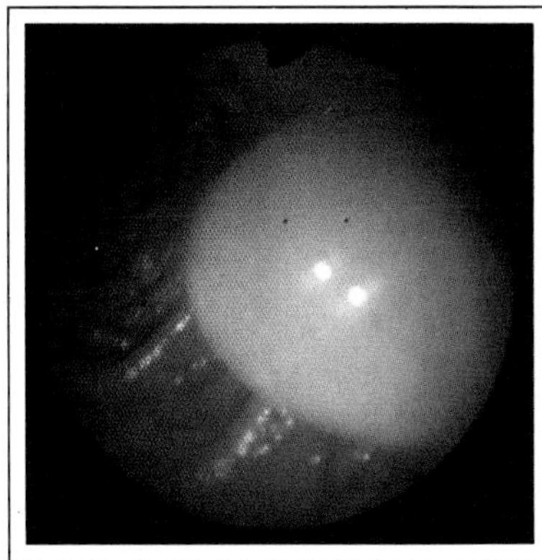

FIG. 30-8.

FIG. 30-7. Duodenal leiomyoma. A 2.5-cm sessile polypoid mass at the apex of the duodenal bulb. The overlying mucosa showed nonspecific erythema. Because of its size and the uncertainty of the diagnosis, the patient was surgically explored, at which time the histology was established.

FIG. 30-8. Duodenal lipoma. A 2-cm sessile polyp with smooth overlying mucosa in a patient with iron deficiency anemia. The diagnosis was established with surgical resection rather than endoscopic removal because of the location of the polyp just below the apex, making polypectomy more hazardous.

at the apex, makes them difficult to remove electrosurgically.

One may suspect a lipoma based on the slightly yellowish coloration and smooth surface of the polyp (Fig. 30-8). Unlike leiomyomas, they are usually not umbilicated or ulcerated. Biopsy—especially if it is of the large-particle, electrosurgical type—may be associated with an ooze of greasy material as in the case of similar biopsies taken from colonic lipomas (see Chapter 41).

Lipomas may present in a variety of ways, including upper GI bleeding and obstruction.[1] Most, however, are incidental findings so that the indication for their removal would be to exclude the polyp's being a carcinoid. Because of the relative rarity of carcinoid tumors of the duodenum, in the absence of GI bleeding, iron deficiency anemia, or an eroded surface, one could legitimately follow the patient rather than attempt electrosurgically to remove the lipoma, which may be situated in a location (Fig. 30-8) to make the procedure hazardous.

Carcinoid Tumors

The likelihood of a submucosal polyp being a carcinoid tumor, to a large extent, depends on the reasons prompting endoscopy. Because the duodenum is the least common site of carcinoid tumors in the small intestine, the likelihood of an asymptomatic submucosal polyp being a carcinoid is low, probably not substantially greater than 10 to 15%, even for polyps which exceed 1 cm in maximum dimension. Reddy et al.[1] found only one carcinoid tumor among 11 cases of either proved submucosal polyps or those strongly suspected of being so based on their size (>1 cm) with a negative biopsy. This was in a patient who presented with nonspecific symptoms and who had an upper GI series showing a 1-cm polyp of the duodenal bulb.[8] In our series of 12 patients with either proved submucosal polyps or those strongly suspected of being so based on their being greater than 1 cm, three carcinoid tumors were found; one presented with pain and weight loss suggestive of a malignancy. Excluding this case, we also noted a low incidence (16.7%—similar to that of Reddy et al.[1]) of carcinoid tumors in largely asymptomatic patients for single 1-cm or larger polyps from which mucosal biopsies were negative.

Both nonmalignant cases of carcinoid in our series presented as GI bleeding. In one case the carcinoid appeared as a smooth, 1.5 × 2 cm sessile lesion. The site of bleeding was presumed to be a mucosal ulceration, but this could not be identified at the time of endoscopy (Fig. 30-9a). In another case, also presenting with upper GI bleeding, the centrally ulcerated portion of a carcinoid of the duodenal bulb was its most prominent feature (Fig. 30-9b). The folds radiating from the ulcer were interpreted as being part of an ulcer scar deformity (Fig. 30-9c). These two nonmalignant cases in which a discrete, smooth, or ulcerated submucosal mass less than 3 cm in maximum dimension was observed contrasts with the case where the carcinoid presented as an extensive malignant neoplasm involving the duodenal bulb and descending duodenum (Fig. 30-10a). In this case an entire mucosal surface was replaced by a raised, nodular, ulcerated tumor mass (Fig. 30-10b).

Because of the low probability of any submucosal mass, even one larger than 1 cm, being a carcinoid, we believe the endoscopist is justified in following such lesions with yearly examinations until the growth pattern of the lesion is ascertained rather than subjecting the patient immediately to either an attempt at electrosurgical removal or laparotomy. We believe that only in cases where the polyp is actually observed to increase in size or a clinical problem such as bleeding or iron deficiency anemia emerges would a more aggressive approach be justified.

Brunner Gland Adenomas

Brunner gland adenomas are widely regarded as being extremely rare.[9,10] A review of the literature in 1973 yielded fewer than 100 reported cases.[9] Nevertheless, Reddy et al.[1] found one case among 11 polyps 1 cm or larger, either proved to be submucosal or strongly suspected because of unrevealing surface mucosal biopsies. Similarly, we found one case among 11 such polyps.

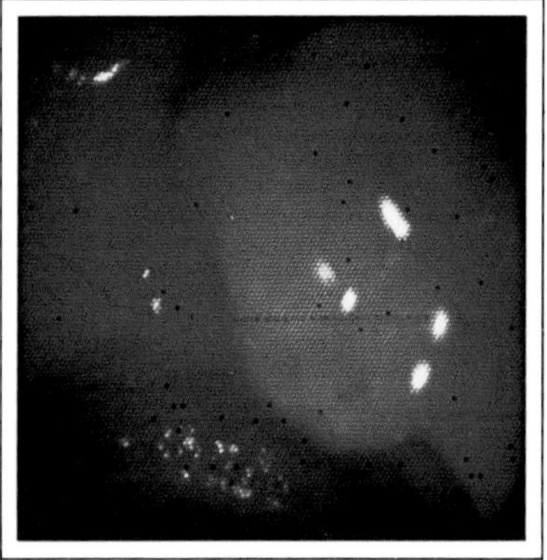

FIG. 30-9a.

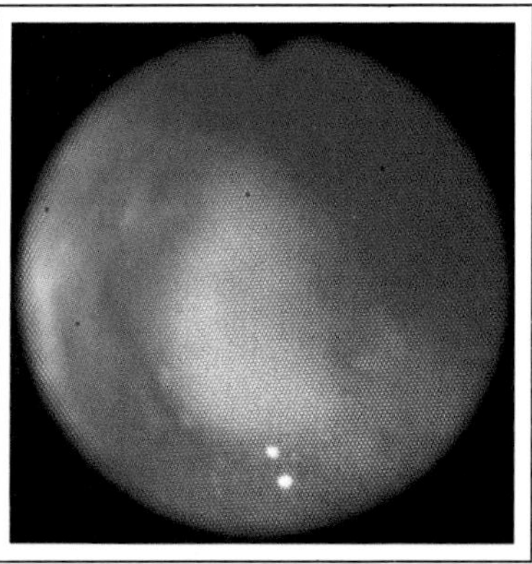

FIG. 30-9b.

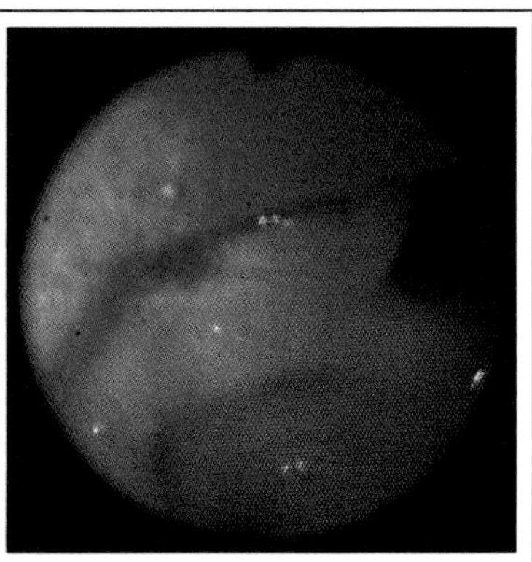

FIG. 30-9c.

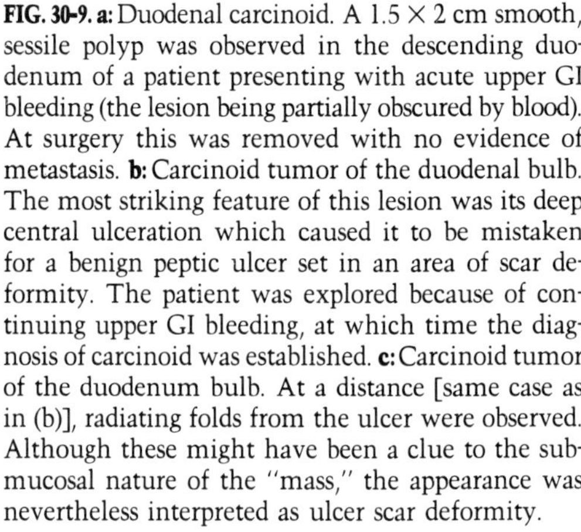

FIG. 30-9. a: Duodenal carcinoid. A 1.5 × 2 cm smooth, sessile polyp was observed in the descending duodenum of a patient presenting with acute upper GI bleeding (the lesion being partially obscured by blood). At surgery this was removed with no evidence of metastasis. **b:** Carcinoid tumor of the duodenal bulb. The most striking feature of this lesion was its deep central ulceration which caused it to be mistaken for a benign peptic ulcer set in an area of scar deformity. The patient was explored because of continuing upper GI bleeding, at which time the diagnosis of carcinoid was established. **c:** Carcinoid tumor of the duodenum bulb. At a distance [same case as in (b)], radiating folds from the ulcer were observed. Although these might have been a clue to the submucosal nature of the "mass," the appearance was nevertheless interpreted as ulcer scar deformity.

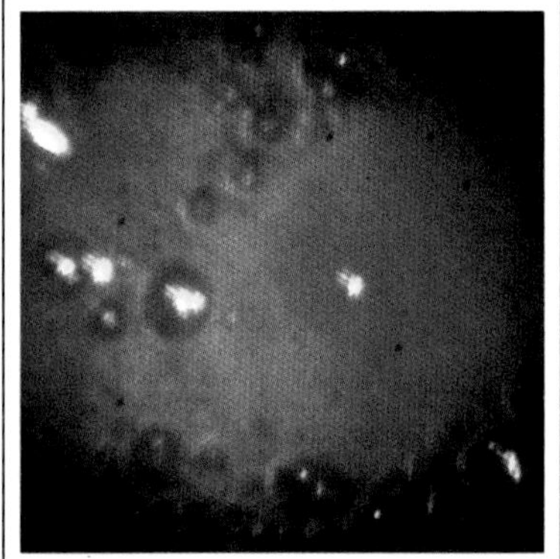

FIG. 30-10a.

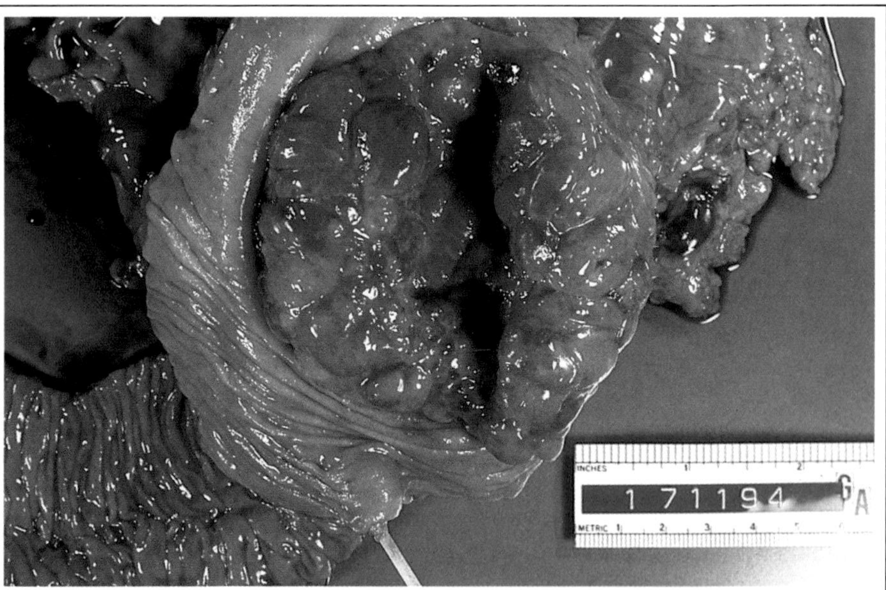

FIG. 30-10b.

FIG. 30-10. Malignant carcinoid of the descending duodenum. **a:** At endoscopy the entire surface of the medial wall was seen to be replaced by an ulcerating mass. **b:** The resected specimen in this case shows fully the large tumor mass, which has replaced the medial wall of the duodenum.

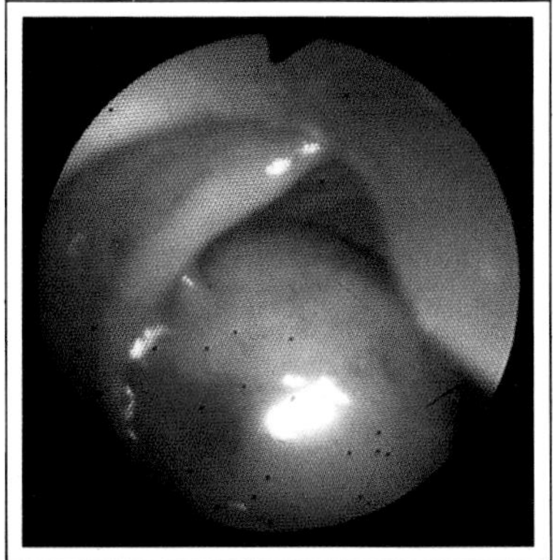

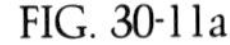

FIG. 30-11a.

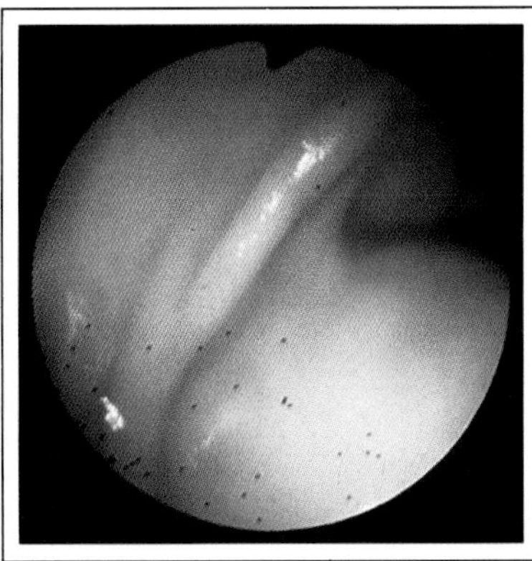

FIG. 30-11b.

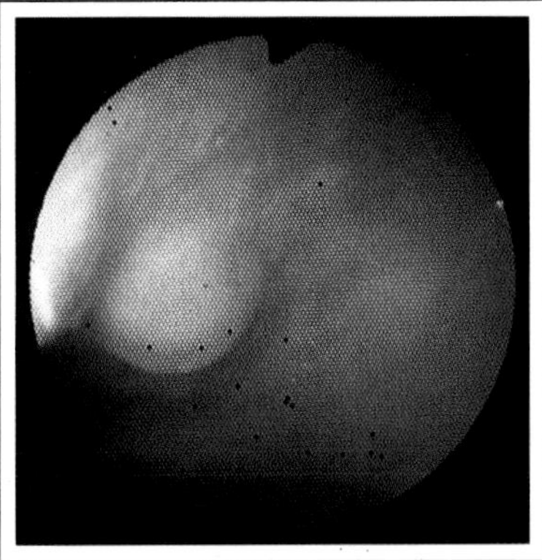

FIG. 30-11c.

FIG. 30-11. a: Brunner gland adenoma. A 2-cm smooth submucosal tumor mass of the descending duodenum was observed in a patient presenting with an upper gastrointestinal bleed from an ulceration of its surface mucosa. Even though the lesion was pedunculated (b), because of its size and location just below the apex the patient underwent surgical excision. **b:** Brunner gland adenoma [same case as in (a)] with pedicle (just off the 12 o'clock position). **c:** Possible Brunner gland cyst. The soft consistency of this polyp made the examiner suspect a (Brunner gland) retention cyst. Biopsy showed only normal mucosa.

The term Brunner gland adenoma is a misnomer because the lesions are in fact not true neoplasms but result from focal enlargement of solitary Brunner glands.[9] Histologically, they have features of hyperplasia with little evidence of cell atypia.[9] Furthermore, in no case has malignant degeneration been reported.[9]

The polyp may be sessile, or when it achieves considerable size it may become pedunculated (Fig. 30-11). These lesions may achieve a maximum dimension of 2 to 4 cm (Fig. 30-11). Smaller Brunner gland adenomas tend to be discovered as incidental findings, whereas the larger polyps may bleed or obstruct.[9,10]

Although endoscopic electrosurgical removal has been advocated, one is justified in simply following those discovered as incidental findings after taking mucosal biopsies to establish their being submucosal rather than epithelial adenomas, which are true neoplasms (see below). For patients who present with GI bleeding or iron deficiency anemia, resection of the Brunner gland adenoma is indicated. Although electrosurgical removal would be attractive and would spare the patient the risks, discomforts, and extra days in the hospital, such an approach is not without hazard. The location of Brunner gland adenomas, being most often apical or just postbulbar, makes the endoscopic approach to them problematic. The endoscopist must therefore critically assess his abilities in terms of the larger lesions of this location. As a rule, the endoscopist may wish to limit the electrosurgical approach for lesions of less than 1.5 cm and advocate laparotomy for larger Brunner gland adenomas in symptomatic patients.

Other Submucosal Polyps of the Duodenum

Benign small bowel tumors, e.g., fibromas, angiomas, lymphangiomas, and myxomas, may be rarely encountered. Although they account for up to 20% of collected surgical series of small bowel tumors,[3] they were not found by Reddy et al.[1]

Adenomatous Polyps

Adenomas, in our experience, are the least common type of duodenal polyps. In our series of 64 cases, out of 15 being 1 cm or larger (Table 30-6), only one (7%) proved to be adenomatous, either by histologic examination of the entire polyp or biopsies of its surface mucosa. Somewhat surprising was the much higher incidence afforded by Reddy et al., where 12 of 23 (52%) polyps larger than 1 cm proved to be adenomatous: in six cases simple adenomas and in the remaining six villous adenomas.[1] To some extent this may represent a selection artifact in that some patients may have had prior endoscopy and were referred for endoscopic polypectomy or surgery. To our knowledge, a similar incidence of adenomatous polyps, representing nearly one-third of all

TABLE 30-6. *Single duodenal polyps (≥1 cm)—15 cases*

Type	Status	No.	%
Hyperplastic-inflammatory	a	2	13
Adenomatous	a	1	7
Leiomyoma	a	2	13
Lipoma	a	1	7
Carcinoid tumor	a	3	20
Brunner gland adenoma	a	1	7
Insufficient tissue for diagnosis	b	5	33
Total		15	100

[a] Completely excised.
[b] Thought to be submucosal, not excised.

duodenal polyps and 50% of those larger than 1 cm, has not been reported by others. In this section we consider adenomatous polyps as (a) simple adenomas and (b) villous adenomas.

Adenomas

The duodenum is an uncommon location for adenomatous polyps occurring in the small bowel, accounting for only 10% of such polyps in one series.[3] Adenomatous polyps accounted for only two of our 64 patients with duodenal polyps, an incidence of 3%. Excluding one case in a patient with known familial polyposis where the incidence of duodenal adenomas is increased (see below), the true incidence of these polyps in other patients might be only 1 to 2%.

Duodenal adenomas may arise from mucosa of the duodenal bulb or descending duodenum, or derive exclusively from the ampulla of Vater. At endoscopy most are found to be 1 cm or larger. The surface mucosa appears finely nodular or superficially ulcerated (Fig. 30-12). Duodenal adenomas may be sessile or pedunculated. Reddy et al.[1] found five of eight to be pedunculated, including one 8-mm and one 2.5 cm polyp. As hyperplastic polyps tend to be sessile, any pedunculated, 1-cm or larger polyp having an irregular surface should be considered a possible adenoma. Biopies taken from the surface of the polyp, even if superficial, would be expected to show the neoplastic epithelium of an adenoma.

Some tubular adenomas arise directly from the ampulla of Vater. Although exceedingly rare in the general population, these are seen in patients with familial polyposis,[11] especially Gardner's syndrome (Fig. 30-13a) where there is a high incidence of periampullary neoplasia.[12] In these patients there may be neoplastic transformation of the mucosa of the ampulla of Vater which appears as faint (Fig. 30-13b) or even gross nodularity of its mucosa in contrast to the normal appearance (Fig. 30-13c). Any nodularity of the ampulla in cases of familial polyposis raises the question of neoplastic change and is a strong indication for biopsy; and if this shows adenomatous tissue, endoscopic polypectomy[12a] or surgical resection of the ampulla is feasible. Because of the high incidence of recurrent adenoma formation within the area of local resection the effects of measures short of radical surgery in reducing the risk of periampullary cancer[12b] are unclear. Like the original appearance, recurrence is indicated by the presence of nodularity or irregular consistency of the surgical scar site (Fig. 30-13d). For that matter, even the appearance of tiny mucosal excrescences of the duodenal bulb, which in others are most likely hyperplastic-inflammatory polyps, in these patients would be regarded as adenomatous until proven otherwise (Fig. 30-14).

Villous Adenoma

Villous adenomas are said to be exceedingly rare[13,14] with fewer than 75 cases having been reported up until recently. However, Reddy et al.[1] encountered six cases among 45 patients with duodenal polyps, suggesting it to be more common than previously thought. Still, we did not find any villous adenomas among our 64 cases.

As noted in all reports,[1,13,14] these polyps are generally large, bulky tumor growths which come to the attention of the endoscopist because of GI bleeding or intermittent obstruction. At endoscopy they appear similar to villous adenomas in the colon (see Chapter 41) as soft, cauliflower-like tumors exceeding 2 cm.[1,13] Although some prefer large-particle electrosurgical biopsies (see Chapter 1) for providing a more representative sample of the tumor, Reddy et al.[1] found that simple forceps biopsy established the diagnosis of villous adenoma in five of six cases.

Therapy for these tumors is surgical excision rather than endoscopic electrosurgery removal because of their tendency to undergo malignant degeneration, especially deep within the tumor, which may not be appreciated with piecemeal endoscopic removal.[13] In cases where at surgery invasive malignancy is demonstrated on frozen section, a Whipple (pancreaticoduodenectomy) procedure has been considered to be the therapy of choice.[13]

Villous Adenomas of the Ampulla of Vater

Even rarer than villous adenomas of the duodenum are those which arise from the ampulla of Vater directly.[4] Still, Reddy et al.[1] observed one case of villous adenoma to be of this type, or one case among 23 polyps larger than 1 cm. We, on the other hand, have yet to observe a case of villous adenoma of either the duodenum or the ampulla of Vater.

Because of their location, they are reported to produce symptoms of intermittent biliary obstruction.[4] In some reported cases they are associated with GI bleeding and duodenal obstruction, as are other duodenal villous adenomas.[1]

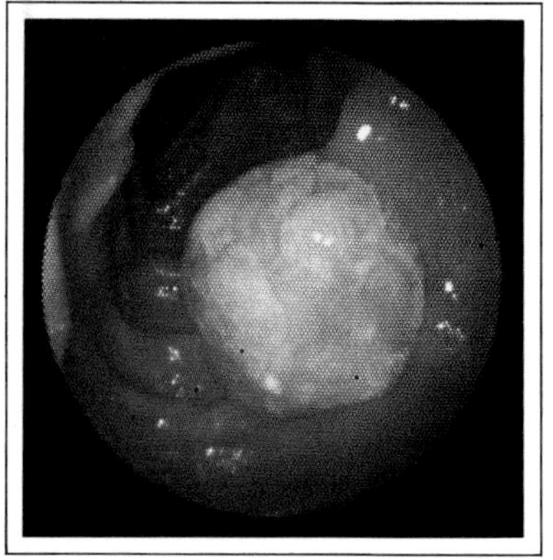

FIG. 30-12a.

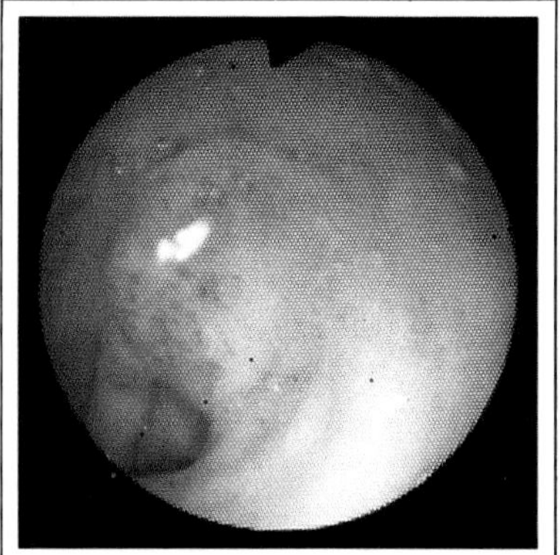

FIG. 30-12b.

FIG. 30-12. a: Duodenal adenoma. A single 1-cm pedunculated polyp of the duodenal bulb was entirely excised electrosurgically. **b:** Small duodenal adenoma. A 5-mm polyp on the apex is indistinguishable from one of the hyperplastic-inflammatory type. Biopsy, however, showed it to be adenomatous.

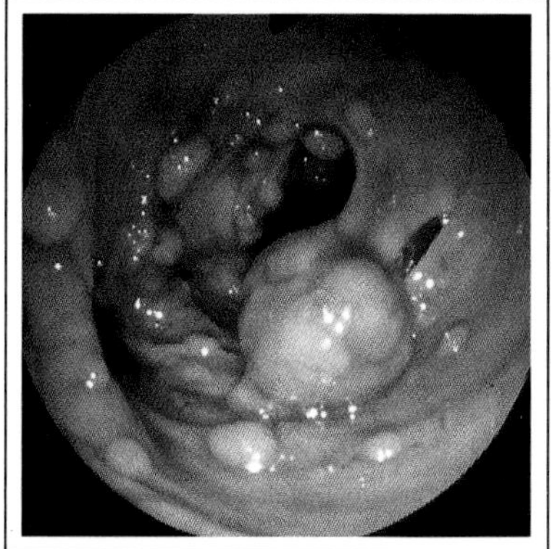

FIG. 30-13a.

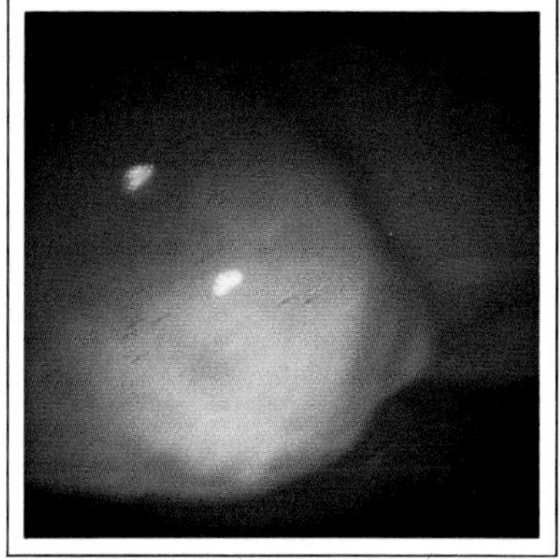

FIG. 30-13b.

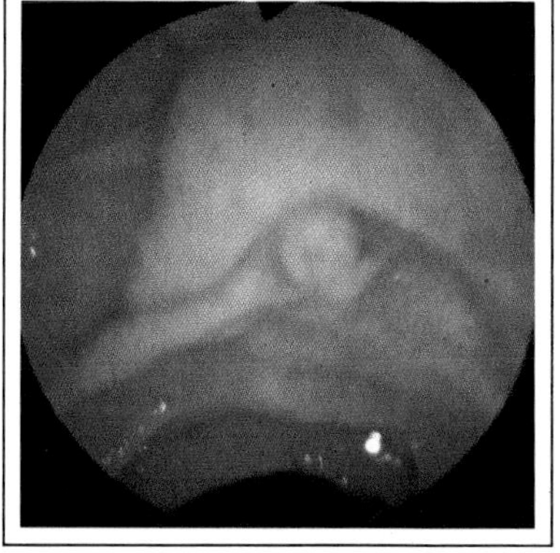

FIG. 30-13c.

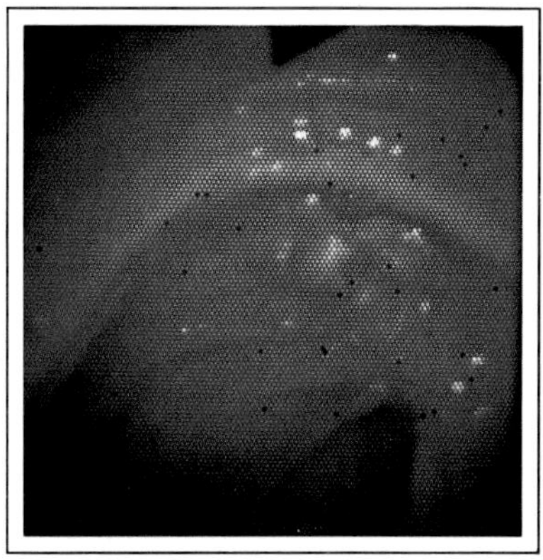

FIG. 30-13d.

FIG. 30-13. a: Colonic involvement with Gardner's syndrome (familial polyposis) of the colon. The colonoscopic view shows multiple adenomatous polyps. **b:** Adenomatous transformation of the duodenal papilla in a patient with Gardner's syndrome (a). Tiny nodular elevations are barely evident in comparison with the normal papilla (c). Biopsies showed these elevations to represent adenomas. **c:** Duodenal papilla, papillary type, normal appearance. **d:** Recurrent adenomas after surgical removal of the duodenal papilla. Multiple elevations appear in the same location where the papilla had been (b) 1 year after surgery.

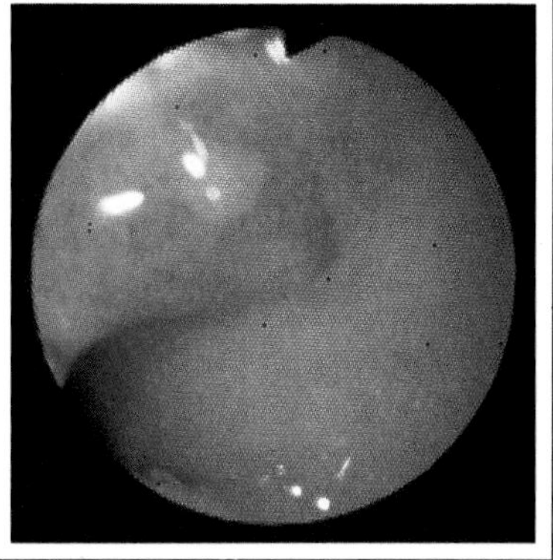

FIG. 30-14.

FIG. 30-14. Multiple tiny adenomas of the apex of the bulb in a patient with Gardner's syndrome (Fig. 30-13a). Innocent mucosal elevations, which in others would most likely be regarded as hyperplastic-inflammatory polyps, were in this patient found to be tiny adenomas.

Like the villous adenomas of the duodenum itself, the diagnosis is considered with any soft, sessile, bulky tumor of the ampulla of Vater. As is true of villous adenomas of the duodenum, surgical therapy is considered because of the high rate of malignant degeneration, where as many as 25% can be expected to show *in situ* or invasive carcinoma at the time of discovery.[4] A finding of invasive carcinoma at surgery on frozen section would necessitate the need for a pancreatoduodenectomy procedure rather than simple excision.

REFERENCES

1. Reddy, R. R., Schuman, B., and Priest, R. J. (1981): Duodenal polyps: diagnosis and management. *J. Clin. Gastroenterol.*, 3:139–145.
2. Kibbey, W. E., Sirinek, K. R., Pose, W. G., and Thomford, N. R. (1976): Primary duodenal tumor: a diagnostic and therapeutic dilemma. *Arch. Surg.*, 111:377–380.
3. Wilson, J. M., Melvin, D. B., Gray, G., and Thorbjarnarson, B. (1975): Benign small bowel tumor. *Ann. Surg.*, 181:247–250.
4. Sobol, S., and Cooperman, A. M. (1978): Villous adenomas of the ampulla of Vater: an unusual cause of biliary colic and obstructive jaundice. *Gastroenterology*, 75:107–109.
5. Fontan, A. N., Rapaport, M., Celener, D., Piskorz, E., Peralta, C. G., and Rubio, H. H. (1978): Chronic nonspecific duodenitis (bulbitis). *Endoscopy*, 10:94–98.
6. Langkemper, R., Hoek, A. C., Dekker, W., and Op den Orth, J. O. (1980): Elevated lesions in the duodenal bulb caused by heterotopic gastric mucosa. *Radiology*, 137:621–624.

6a. Spiller, R. C., Shousha, S., and Barrison, I. G. (1982): Heterotopic gastric tissue in the duodenum. A report of eight cases. *Dig. Dis. Sci.*, 27: 880–883.

7. Maratka, Z., Kocianova, J., Kudrmann, J., Jirko, P., and Pirk, F. (1979): Hyperplasia of Brunner's glands: radiology, endoscopy, and biopsy findings in 11 cases of diffuse, nodular and adenomatous form. *Acta Hepatogastroenterol. (Stuttg.)*, 26:64–69.
8. Godwin, J. D. (1975): Carcinoid tumors: an analysis of 2837 cases. *Cancer*, 36:560–568.
9. Osborne, R., Toffler, R., and Lowman, R. M. (1973): Brunner's gland adenomas of the duodenum. *Am. J. Dig. Dis.*, 18:689–694.
10. Shirazi, S. S., and Deckinga, B. G. (1977): Brunner gland adenoma of the duodenum: resection through the fiberoptic endoscope. *Arch. Surg.*, 112:306–307.
11. Iida, M., Yao, T., Itoh, H., Ohsato, K., and Watanabe, H. (1981): Endoscopic features of adenoma of the duodenal papilla in familial polyposis of the colon. *Gastrointest. Endosc.*, 27:6–8.
12. Naylor, E., and Lebenthal, E. (1980): Gardner's syndrome: recent developments in research and management. *Dig. Dis. Sci.*, 25:945–959.

12a. Sweeny, B. F., and Anderson, D. S. (1982): Endoscopic removal of a duodenal polyp in a patient with Gardner's syndrome. *Dig. Dis. Sci.*, 27:557–560.

12b. Sugihara, K., Muto, T., Kamiya, J., Konishi, F., Sawada, T., and Morioka, Y. (1982): Gardner's syndrome associated with periampullary carcinoma, duodenal and gastric adenomatosis. Report of a case. *Dis. Colon. Rectum*, 25:766–771.

13. Spira, I. A., and Wolff, W. I. (1977): Villous tumors of the duodenum. *Am. J. Gastroenterol.*, 67:63–68.
14. Cooperman, M., Clausen, K., Hecht, C., Lucas, J. G., and Keith, L. M. (1978): Villous adenomas of the duodenum. *Gastroenterology*, 74:1295–1297.

31

UNCOMMON DUODENAL APPEARANCES

We consider in this chapter some structural and mucosal appearances which one may see only once in a career. Still, the endoscopist must be cognizant of their existence so that he may suspect them when confronted with the clinical setting in which they occur. A patient with a duodenal obstruction may have an annular pancreas or other rare cause of duodenal stenosis. An immunosuppressed individual may have developed an opportunistic infection from *Candida, Histoplasma capsulatum,* or cytomegalovirus. In the patient with cavitary pulmonary tuberculosis, the appearance of an ulcerated stenotic lesion of the apex and descending duodenum suggests to the astute endoscopist the possibility of duodenal tuberculosis, an extremely rare lesion but an appropriate consideration in this setting. Finally, an awareness of its characteristic appearance may lead the endoscopist to a diagnosis of *Ascaris Lumbricoides* infestation in a patient with intermittent biliary obstruction or pancreatitis.

STRUCTURAL ABNORMALITIES

In this section we distinguish duodenal narrowing from the better known annular pancreas as well as other rare congenital causes of duodenal stenosis, e.g., diaphragms, bands, and rings.

Annular Pancreas

Annular pancreas, a congenital abnormality, consists of a band or ring of pancreatic tissue which surrounds the second portion of the duodenum. It results from failure of the embryologic ventral anlage to rotate and join with the dorsal limb.[1] Although it usually becomes apparent during infancy, in some cases the condition is encountered for the first time in middle age, with the patient presenting with duodenal obstruction.[1] The late presentation may be a result of pancreatitis, either from the anomaly alone or in combination with chronic changes from longstanding alcohol abuse, causing further encroachment by the annular limb, which ultimately obstructs the duodenum.

Varying degrees of duodenal obstruction occur; however, patients typically present with a fairly high-grade obstruction during the third to fifth decades, often having had several weeks of continuing vomiting and weight loss. In one case we personally observed, profound metabolic alkalosis was present from continued vomiting. In symptomatic patients radiographic studies reveal a stenotic area of the upper midportion of the descending duodenum, generally 1 to 2 cm long (Fig. 31-1a) with extrinsic compression arising from the lateral wall[2,3] proximal to the stenotic area. The duodenal bulb and stomach may be massively dilated (Fig. 31-1b).

Appearance

At endoscopy a stenotic area (Fig. 31-1c) or complete obstruction (Fig. 31-1d) is present, beginning generally within 3 cm of the apex. Just above the stenotic area, extrinsic compression from the lateral wall (Fig. 31-1c) can be observed. In addition, there may be a nonspecific increase in the size of the folds proximal to the stenotic area (Fig. 31-1d).

The duodenal papilla is observed in some but not all cases, its relationship to the stenotic area being variable. In several reported cases, the constricting limb was found to be above the major (Wirsung's) papilla, so that this would not be observed unless the stenotic area itself could be traversed. In one of the two cases we personally observed, the stenosis was above the papilla (Fig. 31-1c), whereas in the other it was below (Fig. 31-1d). In cases where the papilla was above the stenotic area or where it is possible to advance the 10-mm side-viewing duodenoscope through the narrow portion, endoscopic pancreatography has been useful in providing

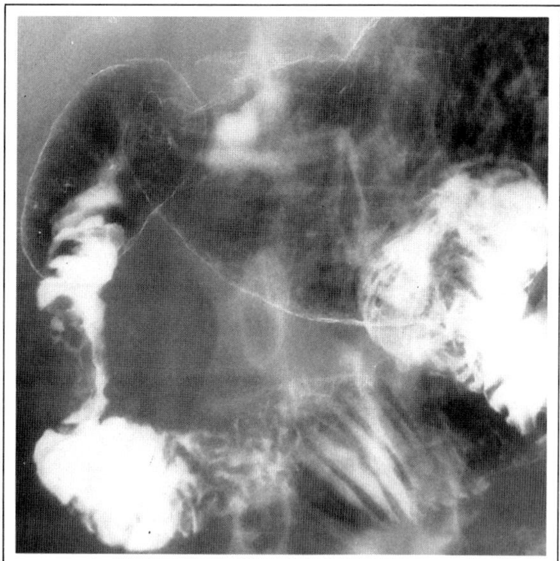

FIG. 31-1a.

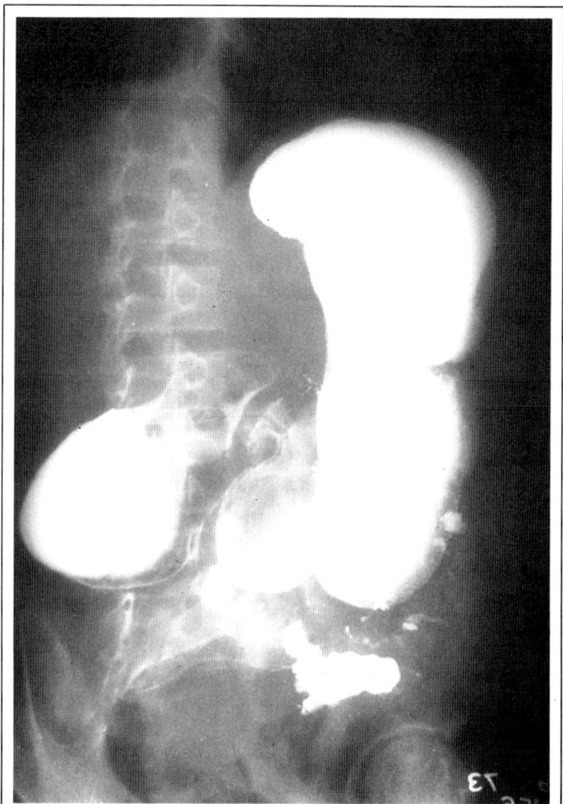

FIG. 31-1b.

FIG. 31-1. Annular pancreas. **a:** Radiographic appearance of the descending duodenum with a long, stenotic area and extrinsic compression from the lateral wall aspect. **b:** Massive gastric and duodenal bulb enlargement in a patient presenting with protracted vomiting and profound metabolic alkalosis. **c:** Narrowing of the lumen corresponding to the stenotic area noted radiographically (a) with extrinsic compression from the lateral (6 o'clock) wall. **d:** With complete obstruction [same patient as in (b)]. Here the lumen narrows abruptly to a pinpoint opening (6 o'clock). The duodenal papilla (at 12 o'clock) was noted 2 cm proximal to the obstruction.

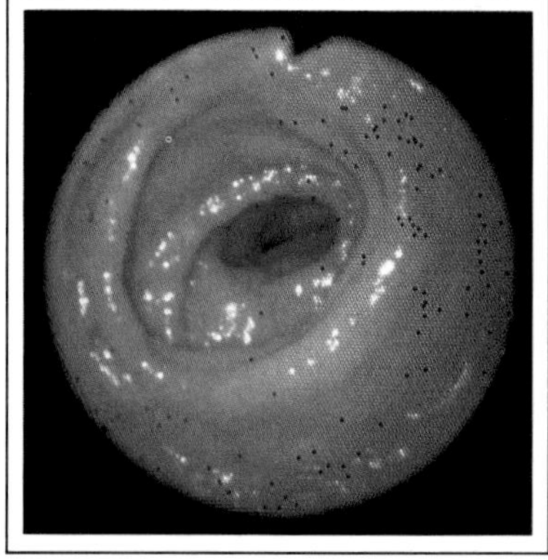

FIG. 31-1c.

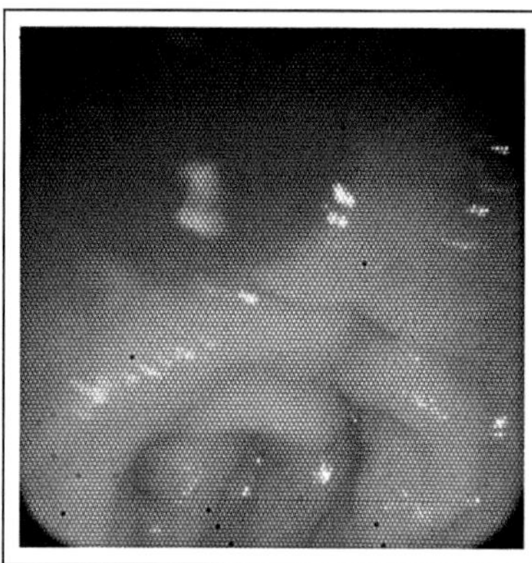

FIG. 31-1d.

radiographic confirmation of the presence of the annular pancreas (Fig. 31-2) prior to surgery.[2-4]

Other Congenital Causes of Duodenal Stenosis

In other cases of duodenal stenosis due to congenital causes, there is a ring-like, focal narrowing 5 to 10 mm in length, rather than the longer 2- to 3-cm narrowing seen with annular pancreas. Like annular pancreas, these are congenital abnormalities which, for unclear reasons, manifest in the adult patient with symptoms of duodenal obstruction. Three types have been observed: (a) duodenal diaphragms; (b) extrinsic bands; and least common (c) congenital stenosis.

Congenital Duodenal Diaphragm

Congenital duodenal diaphragm is rarely seen in adults, only 12 cases having been reported in 1972.[5] When they occur, they present with symptoms of duodenal obstruction, i.e., nausea, vomiting, and weight loss. At endoscopy a characteristic slit-like narrowing or "cervix sign" has been

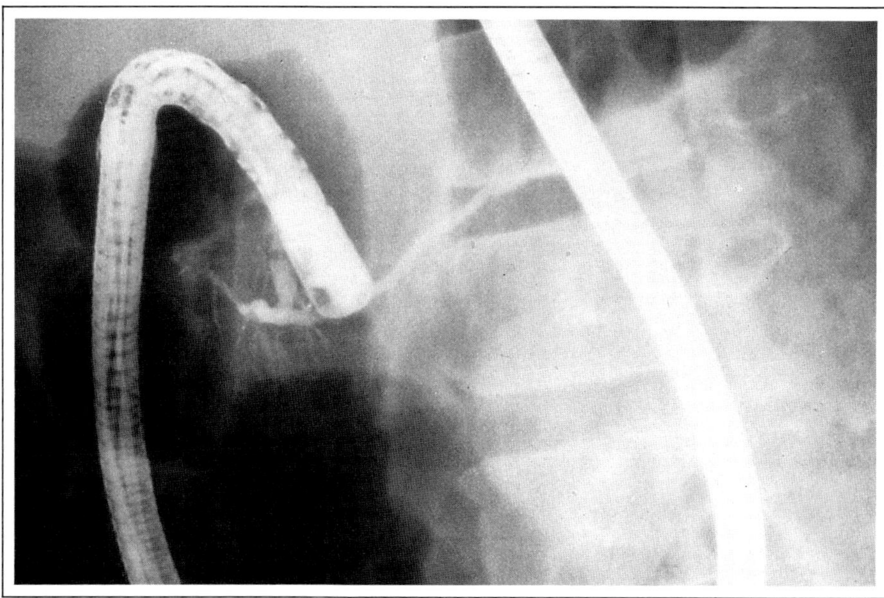

FIG. 31-2. Annular pancreas. An endoscopic retrograde pancreaticogram obtained in a patient with an annular pancreas shows a rightward deviating ductal limb (toward the endoscope shaft) encircling the duodenum and compatible with annular pancreas.

described[6] in the mid-portion of the descending duodenum. In other cases the narrowing is more ring-like. In one reported case, two such diaphragms were found at surgery.[7] In symptomatic patients, surgery is necessary to relieve the obstruction. Endoscopic electrosurgical therapy has been suggested as potentially feasible,[6] but no case of its successful use for this type of obstruction has been reported.

Congenital Duodenal Bands

A patient with an extrinsic fibrous band crossing the duodenum to produce obstruction[8] may present with a relatively brief history or have intermittent symptoms over several years but with recent exacerbation. As in the case of annular pancreas, there may be dilatation radiographically of the proximal duodenum and stomach (Fig. 31-3b). Muscle hypertrophy which occurs in the dilated portion of the proximal duodenum may be responsible for continued emptying despite the obstruction. Ultimately, further dilatation may lead to complete loss of motor function and the onset of obstructive symptoms.

At endoscopy one sees focal narrowing of the lumen of the descending duodenum, down to approximately 5 mm in width and between 5 and 10 mm in length (Fig. 31-3a). This corresponds precisely to the radiographic appearance (Fig. 31-3b). Generally, the obstruction does not allow passage of even the narrow-caliber (9 mm) endoscope. The proximal mucosa as well as that within the stenotic area is intact. The short length of narrowing as well as its ring-like appearance should always suggest this diagnosis even though the condition is rare. The more common causes of duodenal narrowing, e.g., pancreatitis or pancreatic carcinoma (Fig. 31-3c), are not associated with discrete, ring-like folds and narrowing but with extrinsic compression and mucosal changes produced over a longer (>2 cm) portion of the duodenum.

Congenital Duodenal Stenosis

Rarest of all causes of duodenal obstruction is congenital stenosis in which there is failure of the lumen to be reestablished between the proximal and distal embryonic portions of the descending duodenum rather than the overgrowth of epithelial lining which results in the congenital duodenal diaphragm.[9] To date, no cases have been reported in which endoscopy was utilized, so the appearance remains speculative. One would anticipate the finding of a perfect ring-like stenotic area of the mid descending duodenum, in contrast to the slit-like appearance of the congenital diaphragm and the eccentric appearance of the extrinsic band compression.

MUCOSAL ABNORMALITIES

The uncommon conditions considered in this section come to the endoscopist's attention in different ways. In the case of duodenal melanosis, there is an unusually striking endoscopic appearance with a possible but uncertain clinical significance. In eosinophilic gastroenteritis there may be a variety of nonspecific duodenal appearances to prompt endoscopic biopsies which can establish the presence of this condition histologically. In an immunosuppressed patient or one with cavitary tuberculosis, an altered duodenal appearance may be the clue to the presence of duodenal infection which, if confirmed by culture, smear, or biopsy, may lead to crucial therapeutic interventions. Finally, in the case of the intestinal parasite *Ascaris Lumbricoides,*

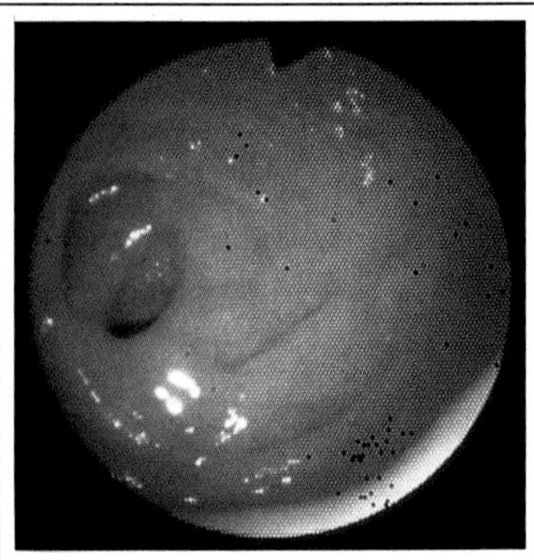

FIG. 31-3a.

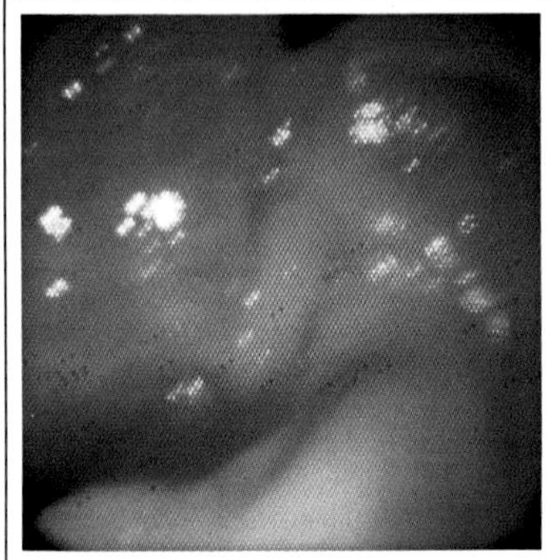

FIG. 31-3c.

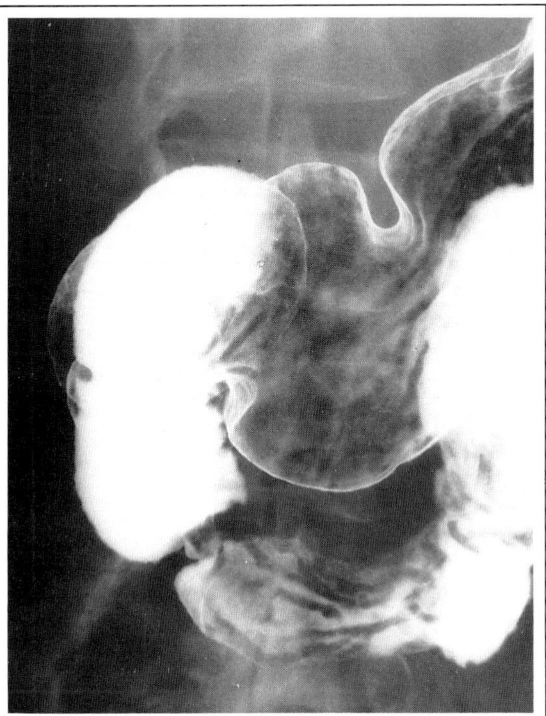

FIG. 31-3b.

FIG. 31-3. a: Congenital extrinsic duodenal band. Extrinsic compression of the lateral wall (6 o'clock) and anterior (3 o'clock) surface of the descending duodenum with narrowing of the lumen for approximately 5 mm. Proximal to this, the duodenum is dilated with a complete absence of Kerckring folds. At surgery a fibrous band (peritoneal reflection) was found between the gallbladder and the ligament of Treitz. **b:** Congenital duodenal band, radiographic appearance. The descending duodenum is obstructed in its mid-portion from the lateral wall by a discrete fibrous band (peritoneal reflection). **c:** Pancreatic cancer, extrinsic compression. In contrast to the discrete (<5 mm) zone of obstruction from the congenital band, there is a much longer portion involved in narrowing from extrinsic compression from either pancreatic cancer or pancreatitis.

observation of the worm itself will lead directly to the diagnosis.

Duodenal Melanosis

In duodenal melanosis brown or black pigmentation is seen scattered throughout the mucosa (Fig. 31-4) as tiny (1 mm) "dots."[10,11] Biopsies show focal deposits of brownish-black pigment in the stroma of villi. In one study careful histologic analysis showed this to most closely resemble the pigment found in melanosis coli rather than true melanin.[10] Unlike melanosis coli, which is the result of chronic exposure to laxatives of the anthracene type (see Chapter 47), no laxative usage has been found to be associated with duodenal melanosis.[10,12] In fact, the etiology of duodenal melanosis remains obscure. In one patient the pigment disappeared with the correction of folate deficiency and healing of a gastric ulcer, suggesting the possible relationship[10]; however, no such association has been noted in other reported cases.[11,12]

Eosinophilic Gastroenteritis

The duodenum itself, although an uncommon site, may nevertheless be involved as a continuation of the disease process from the prepyloric antrum[13] (see Chapter 20). In a patient with prominent, indurated prepyloric antral folds and peripheral eosinophilia, the diagnosis of possible duodenal involvement is considered even if endoscopy showed only nonspecific erythema or nodularity. In these cases biopsy may show the lamina propria to be infiltrated with eosinophils.[13]

Infectious Agents Involving the Duodenum

Candida

Candida may involve the duodenum in an immunosuppressed patient as part of generalized gastrointestinal tract candidiasis,[14] or it may be localized at the base of an ulcer in a similarly compromised patient.[15] Despite the fact that infection of the small bowel with *Candida* species is said to occur in as many as 20% of autopsy cases with a demonstrated gastrointestinal *Candida*,[14] the finding at endoscopy of duodenal plaques similar to those of classic esophageal candidiasis (see Chapter 3) has been reported in only one case, a renal transplant recipient who had esophageal as well as duodenal plaque-like pseudomembranes at endoscopy.[14] In another case, *Candida* was found in the base of an ulcer in a patient with alcoholism and liver disease.[15] We have noted *Candida* at the base of a duodenal ulcer in a patient with longstanding recurrent peptic ulcer

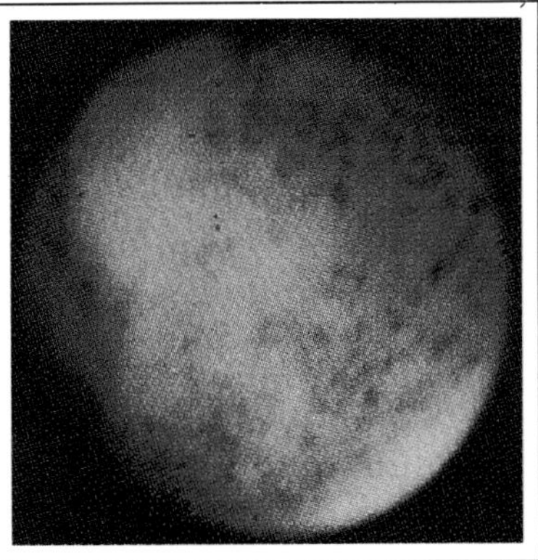

FIG. 31-4.

FIG. 31-4. Duodenal melanosis. Diffusely scattered brown-black dots were apparent within the duodenal bulb and descending duodenum. These have been demonstrated by histochemical techniques to resemble the pseudomelanin of melanosis coli rather than true melanin.[11,12]

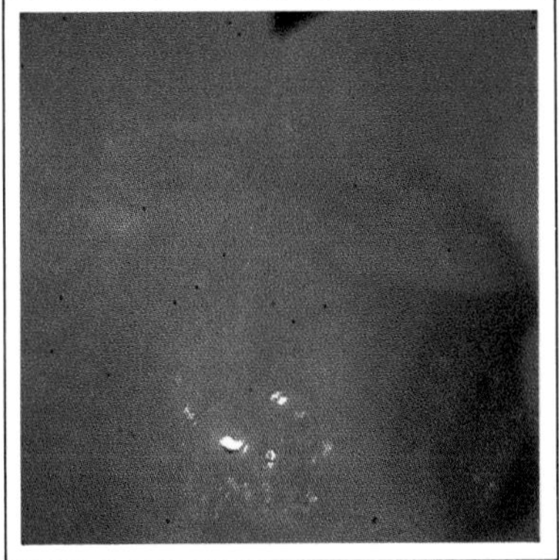

FIG. 31-5a.

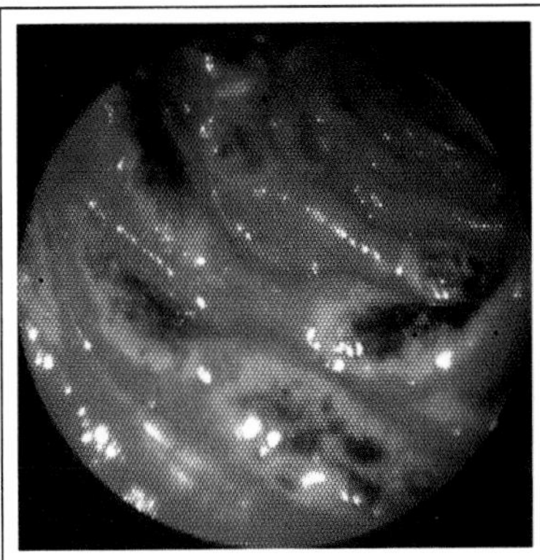

FIG. 31-5b.

FIG. 31-5. Duodenal *Candida.* **a:** A biopsy of the ulcer base (seen just off 3 o'clock) revealed candidal forms in a patient with longstanding peptic ulcer disease who was taking prednisone for chronic hepatitis. **b:** Focal candidal ulcerations with old blood (acid hematin) in their bases were the cause of occult bleeding in this patient with a metastatic hepatoma.

disease who at the time had been receiving prednisone for chronic hepatitis (Fig. 31-5a), as well as in multiple focal 'stress' type ulceration (see Chapter 38) with metastatic hepatoma (Fig. 31-5b). In cases where duodenal *Candida* occurs, a compromised immune state appears to have been responsible for an overgrowth of *Candida* which normally inhabits the duodenum, especially within the base of an ulcer.[15]

Histoplasma Capsulatum

Although the small bowel is the commonest gastrointestinal site for disseminated histoplasmosis in immunosuppressed patients, duodenal involvement is uncommon. In one autopsy series it occurred in only 10% of those cases where the small bowel was involved, and in only 2% of the total. We are not aware of any reports of its having been identified endoscopically; however, as histoplasmosis has been found on blind small intestinal biopsies,[16] endoscopic biopsy of the duodenum would be indicated in any immunosuppressed patient suspected of disseminated histoplasmosis because of diarrhea and malabsorption.[16]

Cytomegalovirus

Cytomegalovirus is found in immunocompromised patients, especially after renal transplant.[17] It has also been noted in patients with immunodeficiency syndromes[18] including homosexuals with the acquired immunodeficiency syndrome (AIDS)[18a] and others with malignancies.[19] A diagnosis of cytomegalovirus should be considered in an immunosuppressed patient with a chronic ulcer in which the virus may inhabit the base, as well as for other appearances, e.g., erosions (Fig. 31-6) or scattered ulcerations.[17,19] Biopsies taken from these lesions may reveal typical cells with prominent intranuclear inclusions.[17,19]

Tuberculosis

Even though extremely rare, the endoscopist should suspect duodenal tuberculosis in a patient with cavitary lesions of the lung with nonspecific abdominal pain, peptic-like symptoms, or gastric outlet obstruction.[20] In these cases the radiologic demonstration of a postbulbar ulcer or constricting lesion of the descending duodenum[20] may be interpreted as peptic ulcer disease, duodenal malignancy, or inflammatory bowel disease.[20,21]

Because the descending duodenum is principally involved at or just beyond the apex of the bulb,[20,21] it may be a problem entering the descending duodenum.[20] In this case, however, it may still be possible to obtain biopsies and especially brushings for smears as well as culture. With the newer, narrower caliber endoscopes, one may more

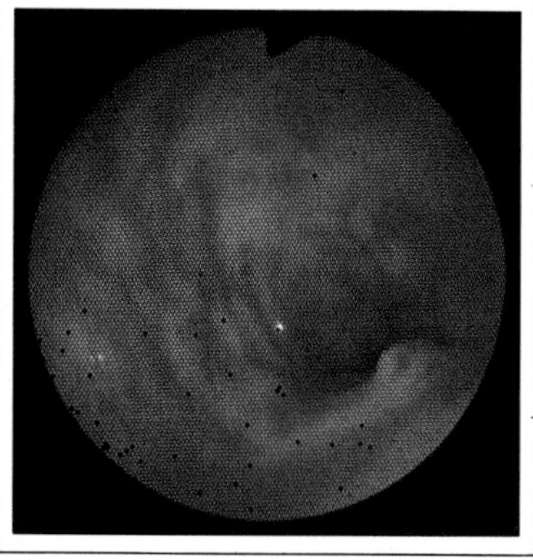

FIG. 31-6.

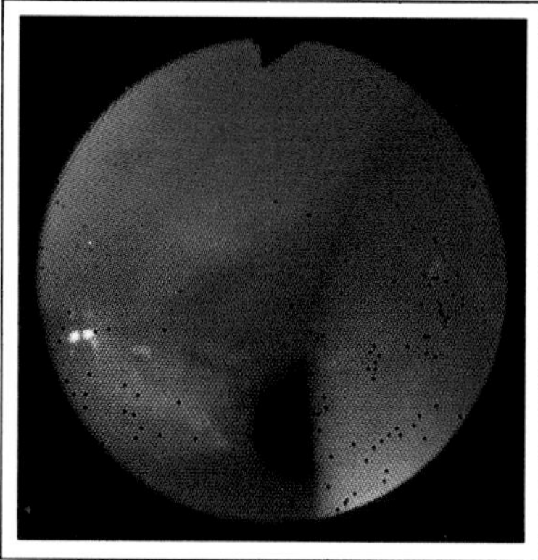

FIG. 31-7.

FIG. 31-6. Duodenal cytomegalovirus. In an immunosuppressed renal transplant recipient, biopsies of nonspecific focal duodenal erythema (erosions) showed cells with prominent intranuclear inclusions typical of the cytomegalovirus.

FIG. 31-7. Duodenal tuberculosis. A stenotic area with enlarged erythematous folds and a deep ulceration beginning at the apex was observed in a patient with ulcer-like symptoms and cavitary tuberculosis. A biopsy from the ulcers showed Langhan's giant cells along with abundant acid-fast bacteria.

readily advance to the proximal descending duodenum and observe the involvement directly (Fig. 31-7). In cases where this has been possible, endoscopy shows deep ulceration, with the surrounding folds markedly enlarged and erythematous (Fig. 31-7). Because the ulcer is irregular and deep, and the surrounding folds are sizable, creating a mass-like deformity, this appearance may be mistaken for carcinoma. Biopsies, however, are diagnostic, revealing clusters of acid-fast bacilli having the typical appearance of *Mycobacterium tuberculosis.*

Parasites Involving the Duodenum

We have already considered *Giardia lamblia* the commonest parasite to involve the duodenum elsewhere (see Chapter 28—Immunoglobulin Deficiency). In this section, we consider two rarely encountered duodenal parasites, *Strongyloides stercoralis,* and *Ascaris lumbricoides.*

Strongyloides

Infection with the intestinal nematode *Strongyloides stercoralis* may be encountered when biopsies are taken from mucosa showing deformity and nonspecific duodenitis in healthy individuals from endemic tropical areas, even when they have lived elsewhere for many years.[22] Biopsies show both adult and larval forms of the organism. Another setting for duodenal involvement is in immunosuppressed individuals undergoing treatment for leukemia lymphoma, as well as in renal transplant recipients. In these patients, a fulminant picture of vomiting, diarrhea, pain, and fever may develop as a result of penetration of large numbers of invasive larvae into the blood. Biopsies of gastroduodenal[23] or colonic ulceration[24] in these cases show the larval form.[24]

Ascaris Lumbricoides

Ascaris lumbricoides, a roundworm is one of the commonest parasites overall, affecting up to one in four of the world's population, particularly in the tropics where its prevalence is as high as 90%.[25] In the United States, it is much less common except in the humid, southeast where rates as high as 40% have been reported.[25] As in one case we personally observed, endoscopy will most often be requested for nonspecific symptoms such as cramping abdominal pain. In rare cases, intermittent biliary obstruction, recurrent pancreatitis or intestinal obstruction will have prompted an endoscopic examination or, in the case of biliary symptoms, ERCP (endoscopic retrograde cholangiopancreatography).[26,27]

In cases where *Ascaris lumbricoides* is present, the examiner finds multiple (5 to 10, or more), cylindrical, motile roundworms, with the width of 1 to 4 mm, ranging in length from 1.5 to more than 10 cm. In cases where biliary obstruction or pancreatitis has occurred, a worm may be seen being extruded from the duodenal papilla,[26] and may be removed by endoscopic means.[26,27]

REFERENCES

1. Kiernan, P. D., ReMine, S. G., Kiernan, P. C., and ReMine, W. H. (1980): Annular pancreas: Mayo Clinic experience from 1957 to 1976 with review of the the literature. *Arch. Surg.,* 115:46–50.
2. Glazer, G. M., and Margulis, A. R. (1979): Annular pancreas: etiology and diagnosis using endoscopic retrograde cholangiopancreatography. *Radiology,* 133:303–306.
3. Clifford, K. M. A. (1980): Annular pancreas diagnosed by endoscopic retrograde-choledochopancreatography (ERCP). *Br. J. Radiol.,* 53:593–595.
4. Dharmsathaphorn, K., Burrell, M., and Dobbins, J. (1979): Diagnosis of annular pancreas with endoscopic retrograde cholangiopancreatography. *Gastroenterology,* 77:1109–1114.
5. Hillson, R. F., den Besten, L., Zike, W. L., and Cohen, W. N. (1972): Congenital duodenal diaphragm in an adult. *Postgrad. Med.,* 51:119–123.
6. Turnbull, A., Kussin, S., and Bains, M. (1980): Radiographic and endoscopic features of a congenital duodenal diaphragm in an adult. *Gastrointest. Endosc.,* 26:46–48.
7. Parker, H., Stewart, E. T., Geenen, J. E., and Hogan, W. J. (1976): Double duodenal diaphragms in an adult: endoscopic, radiographic and operative findings. *Gastroenterology,* 71:663–666.
8. Friedland, G. W., Mason, R., and Poole, G. J. (1970): Ladd's bands in older children, adolescents, and adults. *Radiology,* 95:363–369.
9. Raquel, J. A., Easley, G. W., Watne, A. L., and Mendoza, C. (1972): Congenital duodenal stenosis causing intestinal obstruction in the adult: case report and review of literature. *Am. Surg.,* 38:413–417.

10. Sharp, J. R., Insalaco, S. J., and Johnson, L. F. (1980): "Melanosis" of the duodenum associated with a gastric ulcer and folic acid deficiency. *Gastroenterology,* 78:366–369.
11. Ganju, S., Adomavicius, J., Salgia, K., and Steigmann, F. (1980): The endoscopic picture of melanosis in the duodenum. *Gastrointest. Endosc.,* 26:44–45.
12. Breslaw, L. (1980): Melanosis of the duodenal mucosa. *Gastrointest. Endosc.,* 26:45–46.
13. Caldwell, J. H., Mekhjian, H. S., Hurtubisc, P. H., and Beman, F. M. (1978): Eosinophilic gastroenteritis with obstruction: immunological studies of seven patients. *Gastroenterology,* 74:825–829.
14. Joshi, S. N., Garvin, P. J., and Sunwoo, Y. C. (1981): Candidiasis of the duodenum and jejunum. *Gastroenterology,* 80:829–833.
15. Peters, M., Weiner, J., and Whelan, G. (1980): Fungal infection associated with gastroduodenal ulceration: endoscopic and pathologic appearances. *Gastroenterology,* 78:350–354.
16. Orchard, J. L., Luparello, F., and Brunskill, D. (1979): Malabsorption syndrome occurring in the course of disseminated histoplasmosis: case report and review of gastrointestinal histoplasmosis. *Am. J. Med.,* 66:331–336.
17. Allen, J. J., Silvis, S. E., Sumner, H. W., and McClain, G. J. (1981): Cytomegalic inclusion disease diagnosed endoscopically. *Dig. Dis. Sci.,* 26:133–135.
18. Freeman, H. J., Shnitka, T., Piercey, J. R. A., and Weinstein, W. M. (1977): Cytomegalovirus infection of the gastrointestinal tract in a patient with late onset immunodeficiency syndrome. *Gastroenterology,* 73:1397–1405.
18a. Knapp, A. B., Horst, D. A., Eliopoulos, G., Gramm, H. F., Gaber, L. W., Falchuk, K. R., Falchuk, Z. M., and Trey, C. (1983): Widespread cytomegalovirus gastroenterocolitis in a patient with acquired immunodeficiency syndrome. *Gastroenterology,* 85:1399–1402.
19. Rosen, P., Armstrong, D., and Rice, N. (1973): Gastrointestinal cytomegalovirus infection. *Arch. Intern. Med.,* 132:174–276.
20. Tishler, J. M. (1979): Duodenal tuberculosis. *Radiology,* 130:593–595.
21. Lockwood, C. M., Forster, P. M., Catto, J. V. F., and Stewart, J. S. (1974): A case of duodenal tuberculosis. *Am. J. Dig. Dis.,* 19:575–579.
22. Bone, M. F., Chesner, I. M., Oliver, R., and Asquith, P. (1982): Endoscopic appearances of duodenitis due to strongyloidiasis. *Gastrointest. Endosc.,* 28:190–191.
23. Scowden, E. B., Schaffner, W., and Stone, W. J. (1978): Overwhelming strongyloidiasis. An unappreciated opportunistic infection. *Medicine,* 57:527–544.
24. Drasin, G. F., Moss, J. P., and Cheng, S. H. (1978): *Strongyloides stereoralis* colitis: findings in four cases. *Radiology,* 126:619–621.
25. Denzler, T. B., and Gunning, J.-J. (1976): *Ascaris lumbricoides*—a reminder. *Arch. Intern. Med.,* 136:1044–1045.
26. Dobrilla, G., Valentini, M., and Filippini, M. (1976): A case of common bile duct ascariasis diagnosed by duodenoscopy. *Endoscopy,* 8:211–214.
27. Van der Spuy, S. (1978): Biliary ascariasis—endoscopic aspects. Report of 4 cases. *S. Afr. Med. J.,* 53:1030–1033.

Section 4

UPPER GASTROINTESTINAL BLEEDING

32

ENDOSCOPY AND UPPER GASTROINTESTINAL BLEEDING: AN OVERVIEW

Upper gastrointestinal bleeding requiring hospitalization is a medical emergency with an overall mortality of approximately 10%,[1] increasing to 40% and higher for patients with liver disease or other serious medical illnesses.[2] The physician caring for such patients understandably wishes to know the specific cause of bleeding with the expectation that a treatment plan based on this information offers his patient the best chance for a favorable outcome.

With the introduction during the early 1970s of instruments which allowed a complete examination of the esophagus, stomach, and duodenum to its third portion, fiberoptic endoscopy became widely regarded as the most effective means for providing a precise diagnosis in patients hospitalized for gastrointestinal (GI) bleeding. Supporting this view were three controlled studies[3–5] which showed endoscopy to be superior to conventional single-contrast GI radiology in providing both a correct diagnosis (in the range of 69%[3] to 86%[4]) and a low incidence (under 10%) of erroneous or misleading information.[3–5] Radiology in these studies had a much lower diagnostic yield (a correct answer in less than 50%) along with a higher error rate (erroneous or misleading information in 30%).[3–5] Even in a comparison with the more sensitive double-contrast technique capable of detecting mucosal lesions, the accuracy of endoscopy was still greater (91% versus 76%).[6]

As its increased accuracy began to be perceived, many enthusiastically advocated endoscopy be performed within the first 24 hr ("early" endoscopy) of a hospitalization for any patient with upper GI bleeding in the belief that the increased accuracy would lead to an improved outcome as reflected in a lowering of the overall mortality. More recently, however, this enthusiasm has been tempered with the realization that the mortality for upper GI bleeding remains at 10%,[1] precisely what it was before fiberoptic endoscopy became a widely practiced modality. Indeed, a recent prospective survey of 277 endoscopists (members of the American Society for Gastrointestinal Endoscopy—ASGE) reporting on 2,300 patients hospitalized for uppe GI bleeding (The National ASGE Survey on Upper Gastrointestinal Bleeding) revealed a mortality of 10.8%, even though nearly 70% of these patients underwent endoscopy within the first 24 hr, with 41.5% within the first 12 hr.[1]

The recognition that the overall mortality of upper GI bleeding had not been changed by endoscopy has been the basis of two ongoing controversies: (a) Should endoscopy be performed routinely? (b) If endoscopy is to be performed, should it be "early," within the first 12 hr of admission, or "late," after 24 hr. In the first two sections of this chapter, we examine these questions in some depth, and in the final section we indicate the manner in which we have attempted to answer these questions with a selective approach to endoscopy in patients with upper GI bleeding.

ROUTINE ENDOSCOPY FOR UPPER GI BLEEDING?

When patients with upper GI bleeding are looked at as a group, no clear advantage emerges for patients who have routine endoscopy. As mentioned above, the ASGE survey of 2,300 patients hospitalized for upper GI bleeding and endoscoped, generally within the first 24 hr, showed a mortality of 10.8%,[1] a figure almost identical to what had been noted prior to the introduction of fiberoptic endoscopy.[7] Those who believe endoscopy *should not* be performed routinely focus on the unchanged outcome, as reflected in the fixed mortality rate, whereas those who believe it should cite advantages which are not reflected in this statistic. To do justice to both views, we first present three reasons we believe best explain why the mortality rate is unchanged. This, we believe, provides a better understanding of the viewpoint opposed to routine endoscopy. After this we consider the contrary position, emphasizing the potential advantages of routine endoscopy which are not likely to be reflected in a simple mortality statistic.

Causes of a Fixed Mortality Rate for Upper GI Bleeding

Three reasons for unchanged overall outcome for upper GI bleeding despite precise endoscopic diagnosis are considered under the following headings: (a) the spontaneous cessation of bleeding; (b) the lack of specific, effective medical therapy for those who continue to bleed; and (c) the unchanged surgical mortality from massive bleeding.

Spontaneous Cessation of Bleeding

Depending on the lesion, 40 to 80% of the cases, at endoscopy performed within 24 to 48 hr, have entirely stopped bleeding[8] and do not rebleed.[9] Because bleeding stops and does not recur, for a large percentage of patients with GI bleeding the overall mortality rate tends to remain low because of the favorable outcome. For a patient who spontaneously ceases to bleed, endoscopic diagnosis would be expected to have no influence on outcome because management, which is supportive and largely empiric (i.e., blood replacement, antacids, etc.), would proceed in the same way. Indeed, a recent controlled study, which looked specifically at the influence of endoscopy on the outcome in patients entering the hospital because of upper GI bleeding, but whose bleeding had spontaneously stopped, found no difference for patients who had endoscopy and those who did not.[10] In another study the failure of endoscopic diagnosis to influence management or outcome was apparent when the course of patients who had been endoscoped and the diagnosis transmitted to the responsible physician was contrasted to that of patients for whom the physician was not told the diagnosis.[11]

Lack of Effective Medical Therapy for Patients Who Continue to Bleed

Currently there is no medical therapy for upper GI bleeding of proved effectiveness. There is no convincing evidence that commonly employed ice water lavage,[12] antacids or cimetidine,[13] intravenous vasopressin,[14] or any other general or nonspecific treatment actually works. It is not surprising then that if the treatments are used, even with a precise endoscopic diagnosis, there is no effect on mortality. Furthermore, as the same treatment is likely to be employed with or without an endoscopic diagnosis,[11] the impact specifically of endoscopic diagnosis is negligible. Even when a therapy such as the intraarterial infusion of vasopressin[15] or balloon tamponade follows the specific endoscopic diagnosis of esophageal varix bleeding, as these measures have a doubtful effect on outcome,[16] it is not surprising that mortality is not affected by endoscopic diagnosis in these instances. In the case of endoscopic therapy with electrocoagulation[17] or laser photocoagulation[17a] or sclerotherapy for esophageal varices,[17b] which might follow a precise endoscopic diagnosis, it remains to be seen how these modalities will affect outcome.

Unchanged High Mortality Rate for Patients Requiring Surgery

Although surgical mortality rates have, on the whole, declined over the past 20 years, the decrease has been less marked for patients with upper GI bleeding, particularly from peptic ulcers or esophageal varices, the commonest cases in which surgery would be required.[2] For patients with peptic ulcer bleeding over the age of 60, even with early endoscopy the surgical mortality approaches 30%,[18] similar to what it was before endoscopy became widely available.[19] For esophageal varix bleeding, the surgical mortality may exceed 50%,[20] unchanged from years prior to the use of endoscopy.[20] As a result of the anticipated high surgical mortality in these patients, some surgeons may be unwilling to operate even though a precise endoscopic diagnosis has been established. For those patients who undergo surgery, the mortality rate may still be high, even though the endoscopist provides precise preoperative diagnostic information.

Favorable Effects of Endoscopy on Outcome Not Reflected in the Mortality Rate

By concentrating on mortality rate exclusively, one could ignore four types of potential benefit which routine endoscopy could provide. These are: (a) a definite diagnosis of a surgically remediable lesion in patients who continue to bleed; (b) the indication for close observation in patients with variceal or peptic ulcer bleeding; (c) a sense of security in cases where the bleeding is likely to be self-limited; and (d) effects on long-term management.

Definite Diagnosis of a Surgically Remediable Lesion in Patients Who Continue to Bleed

In patients who are surgical candidates, especially those with peptic ulcer bleeding, establishing a definite diagnosis by endoscopy may mean a shorter preoperative waiting period, which may be translated into fewer preoperative units of blood transfused.[19] For these patients, especially those who receive less than 5 units prior to surgery, a lower operative mortality may be anticipated.[21] As patients undergoing surgery represent less than 20% of those hospitalized because of upper GI bleeding,[1] any improvement on mortality in this group is not likely to be reflected in the overall mortality statistic.

Indication for Close Observation in Patients With Variceal or Peptic Ulcer Bleeding

Although 75%+ of upper GI bleeding ceases on its own, rebleeding may be expected in up to 25%, especially in those with peptic ulcer[9] or esophageal varix bleeding.[22] Endoscopic observation of these lesions, and in particular the "visible vessel" in ulcer bleeding (see Chapters 36 and 38), indicates the need for especially close observation because rebleeding in the hospital, if undetected, is an important cause of death in these patients.[23] Although diagnostic information causing the physician to suspect early rebleeding may be important for the individual case, overall mortality is influenced more by patients who continue to bleed from the time of admission. The effect of endoscopy to prevent undetected rebleeding as a cause of death is therefore unlikely to be reflected in the overall mortality rate.

Sense of Security in Cases Where the Bleeding Is Likely to Be Self-Limited

In cases where acute mucosal injury is found, especially with only a trivial amount of ongoing bleeding, both patient and physician may be relieved by what will most likely be a self-limited bleeding episode. In the ASGE prospective survey, 60% of patients admitted to the hospital for bleeding were found to have inactive lesions (i.e., without any bleeding whatsoever[8]) where 60% of the examinations were performed within the first 48 hr and 80% within the first 72 hr. In a large percentage of the cases where endoscopy is performed, the benefit would not be reflected in the mortality rate but in the alteration of what may be inappropriate management, often in an intensive care setting. For patients who continue to bleed during the first 24 hr of their hospitalization, the finding of acute mucosal injury at endoscopy with its self-limited course could serve to confer a sense of security about continuing medical management even in the face of ongoing bleeding and thereby prevent unnecessary surgery. This is an important effect in the individual case but is unlikely to influence the overall mortality statistic.

Effects on Long-Term Management

Endoscopy in patients with peptic ulcer or esophageal varix bleeding which stops would still have an effect on both in-hospital and long-term management. In the case of peptic ulcer bleeding, the ulcer management which was begun in the hospital would be maintained until complete healing is demonstrated. In such cases we believe that endoscopy must be performed at the time one considers discontinuing the ulcer regimen to ensure that complete healing has occurred. In addition, we question every patient with peptic ulcer bleeding concerning a history of aspirin or other nonsteroidal agent usage (see Chapter 14) which, if continued, could result in disastrous rebleeding. In the case of esophageal varix bleeding which stops, establishing this diagnosis would cause one to consider either one of the newer nonsurgical approaches (i.e., propranolol[24] or endoscopic sclerotherapy[25]) if not surgery itself.

"EARLY" OR "LATE" ENDOSCOPY FOR UPPER GI BLEEDING?

A question related to whether endoscopy should be undertaken routinely is the timing of endoscopy when it is performed. Some continue to advocate that endoscopy be performed early, i.e., within the first 12 hr after admission to the hospital, as an emergency procedure whereas others argue for performing endoscopy late, i.e., after an initial waiting period of 24 hr. In the section which follows, we present the arguments for and against early and late endoscopy.

Early Endoscopy

The Case in Favor

Even though the overall mortality rate is not altered by endoscopy, one might still propose that when endoscopy is performed it be within the first 6 to 12 hr after admission to the hospital on an ***emergent*** (at any time) basis or at least on an ***urgent*** (during the working day) basis. Two reasons for this are: (a) the increased likelihood of observing the suspected lesion actually bleeding; and (b) the benefits of a definitive diagnosis in patients who are likely to continue to bleed.

Observing the suspected lesion bleeding.

Performing endoscopy within the first 12 hr affords one the greatest chance of actually observing the suspected site of bleeding.[26] In the ASGE survey, active bleeding ("oozing" or "pumping") was observed in 41% of those examined within the first 12 hr, in only 30% of those examined between 12 and 36 hr, and in only 20% of those examined after 36 hr. Leinike et al., in fact, found only 20% of lesions to show endoscopic signs of active or recent bleeding after 24 hr.[26] The point in time when one is most likely to observe a lesion bleeding is therefore within the first 12 hr after admission to the hospital. This can be particularly important in a patient who has more than one potential lesion found at endoscopy, e.g., patients with esophageal varix bleeding where other lesions account for 30% or more of the bleeding episodes.[8] In these cases, especially where the management would be vastly different, it is highly desirable to see which of several potential lesions is actually bleeding.

Establishing a diagnosis in patients most likely to continue to bleed.

An important finding of the recent ASGE prospective survey was in support of a long-held concept that those who are actively bleeding at the time of admission and who continue to bleed during the first 12 to 24 hr of hospitalization are at greatest risk of any group of patients with GI bleeding; they have the highest mortality rate, transfusion requirement, incidence of surgical intervention, and complication rate. These patients, in comparison to those who were not bleeding, were shown to have a statistically significant increased mortality (16.1% versus 6.7%), a higher overall complication rate (16.7% versus 8.7%), a transfusion requirement of 5 units of blood or more (37.6% versus 20.1%), and a higher rate of surgical intervention (24.1% versus 11.4%).[8]

By performing endoscopy during the first 12 to 24 hr, one determines a patient's bleeding status and, most importantly, if he belongs to this high-risk group of actively bleeding patients. This would be especially important for patients with bright red blood in the nasogastric aspirate, where active bleeding in the ASGE survey was found at endoscopy in 50%. Even for those patients who had a clear nasogastric aspirate, 16% had active bleeding,[8] making a negative nasogastric aspirate an indication of low likelihood of active bleeding, but not excluding the possibility altogether, especially in the case of duodenal bulb bleeding.

Other clinical indicators in the ASGE survey of an increased likelihood of continued bleeding as evidenced by an excess mortality rate and increased percentage of patients requiring surgery were a hematocrit on admission of under 31, orthostatic (postural) blood pressure changes, and a red (bloody) stool color.[2] Patients with these findings were most likely to have evidence of active bleeding at endoscopy. Because of the increased risk for continued bleeding, patients with these findings would be most deserving of early endoscopy.

The Case Against

The argument against early endoscopy in patients with upper GI bleeding focuses around the following concerns: (a) an increased complication rate for early versus routine endoscopy; (b) an uncertain effect on the outcome of the bleeding episode; and (c) the lack of any definitive changes in management.

Increased complication rate for early endoscopy.

During the first 12 hr of continued upper GI bleeding, within which time early endoscopy would be performed, the patient may not yet have received adequate volume replacement, especially blood, to equal the prehospitalization losses. He may have intermittent or sustained hypotension with acidosis and a compensatory rapid respiratory rate. The premedication required for endoscopy as well as the potentially stressful nature of the procedure itself, especially with a difficult intubation, may further aggravate the hemodynamic instability, be a potential cause of aspiration, cause a perceptible increase in the rate of bleeding, and increase hypotension or be associated with other adverse reactions from the medications given for endoscopy.[27a] Indeed, aspiration, recurrent hemorrhage, hypotension, and medication reaction consituted half of the 21 complications ascribed to endoscopy among the 2,320 examinations performed in the ASGE prospective survey. This complication rate of 0.9% was eight times higher than the 0.13% complication rate found in a previous survey for 211,410 routine procedures.[27] Of the 21 complications in the ASGE survey, 12 were thought to be potentially life-threatening and were considered major. These included five perforations, four instances of aspiration, and three of recurrent hemorrhage. Of these, nine occurred with procedures performed early, i.e., within the first 12 hr. Others have found an even higher complication rate if endoscopy is performed in patients whose hemorrhage is severe enough to require their being placed in an intensive care unit.[28] In one study the complication rate was 8%.[28] It is likely that patients who are unstable hemodynamically and have rapid respiratory rates are the most prone to endoscopic complications from: (a) medications that depress blood pressure and respiration; (b) the procedure itself, resulting in further hypotension from vagovagal responses and arrhythmias; and (c) vomiting or regurgitation of blood during endoscopy, leading to inapparent aspiration along with periods of anoxia. Such patients would be prone to the major complications found in the ASGE survey: aspiration (four patients), medication reactions (three patients), hypotension and arrhythmias (two patients), and an anoxic episode (one patient), accounting for 10 of the 21 complications noted.[8]

In addition to the above, the bleeding patient is also prone to instrumental complications. In the ASGE survey these accounted for 38% (8 of 21) of the complications. Endoscopy was performed as an emergency, rather than elective, procedure in the majority of these patients. Of the instrumental complications, the most obvious is perforation which occurs at two main sites, the cricopharyngeal area, and the pyloroduodenal junction. In the case of the cricopharyngeal type, this occurs especially in elderly patients with cervical spine lordosis which compromises the posterior hypopharynx (see Chapter 1), making it vulnerable to perforation particularly when the intubation is blind. Perforation at the pyloroduodenal junction occurs in patients with deformity of the pylorus or duodenal bulb from ulcer disease. In these cases the endoscopist strives to forcefully intubate areas which he cannot visualize. In yet other cases a bleeding gastric ulcer may be mistaken for the pyloric channel with disastrous consequences.

Less often considered as an instrumental complication is injury to the cardia of the Mallory-Weiss type.[29,30] In these cases endoscopy results in excessive vomiting with forceful prolapse of the cardial mucosa around the endoscope, leading to its being contused or torn.[29,30] In the ASGE survey these accounted for 3 of the 21 complications. Although considered to be "minor" complications, these lesions are potentially a cause for secondary bleeding in patients whose primary lesion has ceased to bleed.

Potentially adverse effect on the outcome of the bleeding episode.

A very difficult matter to determine is if early endoscopy has an adverse effect on outcome, especially in cases of peptic ulcer and esophageal varix bleeding where recurrent hemorrhage occurs in upward of 30%. If endoscopy is capable of inducing vomiting and retching during the intubation and examination itself, might this not have an unfavorable effect on the course of the bleeding? At least one study, that of Sandlow and colleagues, suggested that endoscopy does adversely affect the course of bleeding.[31] In this study the outcome of 150 patients allocated to either an "aggressively managed" or a "conservatively managed" group was compared. Those managed aggressively had endoscopy performed within 24 hr and those managed conservatively had upper GI radiology followed in some but not in all cases by endoscopy. In this study those patients having endoscopy routinely performed within 24 hr had a worse outcome with regard to recurrent bleeding (27% versus 7%) and a greater requirement for emergency surgery (19% versus 7%); there were also a greater number whose hospitalization exceeded 21 days (28% versus 17%). One explanation for this is the effect of endoscopy on hemostasis itself. Vomiting or retching may have been an important factor in dislodging clots which were in the process of forming in the case of the two lesions most likely to rebleed, i.e., peptic ulcers[9] and esophageal varices.[22] Although this is speculative regarding peptic ulcer disease itself, it is noteworthy that in the ASGE study all the patients with recurrent hemorrhage as a complication of endoscopy had esophageal varices. Although the rate of endoscopy-induced bleeding in the ASGE study is small, these were only the cases where the endoscopist was aware of the bleeding recurrence during his examination. It can never be fully known how many cases of recurrent bleeding may have occurred because of endoscopy, as this may not be apparent to either the clinician or the endoscopist.

Management decisions are not altered by early endoscopy.

The risk of early endoscopy as outlined above might seem justified if management decisions were shown to be altered. Three controlled studies[5,11,32] have looked at whether management decisions are affected by endoscopy. In one study, Keller and Logan[5] suggested that endoscopic diagnosis did result in more correct management decisions. Two studies[11,32] have shown the opposite. Indeed, Graham[11] found that even though the initial clinical impression was correct in only 36% of patients in his study, being altered by endoscopy in 64%, management was changed in only 22%, and in only 12% was this considered "important," i.e., to operate or not, to administer vasopressin or not, or to use a Sengstaken-Blackemore tube or not. So long as the management of upper GI bleeding continues to remain largely supportive and empiric, there is little chance that management decisions will be greatly affected by early endoscopy, especially with 70% or more patients who cease to bleed on their own.

Late Endoscopy

The Case in Favor

Because management during the first 24 hr is generally nonspecific,[7] being employed in the same way regardless of the site of bleeding, endoscopy would not be required for therapeutic decisions at this time. Some therefore propose that endoscopy be performed, if at all, only after an initial waiting period of 24 hr, during which time resuscitative efforts may proceed unhindered. Performing endoscopy in patients who continue to bleed beyond 24 hr would mean doing so at a time when precise diagnosis would likely have its greatest impact on management, especially when the need for surgery is indicated in peptic ulcer bleeding or continued medical management is needed in drug-induced mucosal injuries. For patients who stop bleeding during this period, whether endoscopy is performed would be based on clinical considerations; for example, when peptic ulcer disease is suspected and found, medical treatment would be continued beyond the hospitalization along with possibly repeat endoscopy to ensure complete healing prior to its termination.

Although such a policy of late endoscopy (at 24 hr) would somewhat reduce the chances of demonstrating a bleeding lesion, the ASGE survey suggested that this would be only a marginal reduction (41% to 29%)[8] overall, and no reduction at all for patients who continue to bleed.

The Case Against

As attractive as late endoscopy may seem theoretically, there are practical considerations which make the endoscopist reluctant to wait. First, the interpretation of endoscopic findings at 24 hr may be confounded by the presence of numerous artifacts, e.g., the nasogastric tube, antacids, the accumulation of blood itself, or vomiting (see Chapter 3). Because of these, the endoscopist is often unwilling to wait any longer than is absolutely necessary to stabilize the patient. He simply wishes to avoid these interpretive problems by performing endoscopy early. Second, waiting 24 hr or longer in some patients, especially those with previously unexplained bleeding or those with a high likelihood of multiple, potential bleeding sites (e.g., patients with known esophageal varices), may mean a missed opportunity for a specific diagnosis based on the presence of a bleeding lesion. Even though the reduction of actively bleeding lesions seen at 24 hr, compared with 12 hr, was only 12% in the ASGE survey (41% compared with 29%), this represents nearly a 25% loss in the number of lesions actually seen bleeding, another factor which makes the endoscopist unwilling to wait.

Finally, for patients with a high likelihood of rebleeding, e.g., those with peptic ulcer disease or esophageal varices,[31] if endoscopy is not performed at a time within the first 12 hr when bleeding may have slowed or stopped and the stomach is relatively clear the opportunity to actually identify the bleeding lesion may be missed. Waiting 24 hr longer in such patients runs a risk of up to 30% for rebleeding,[8] which would result in an examination being performed during a period of brisk rebleeding at a time when only a general site may be observed, rather than the specific bleeding lesion.

A SELECTIVE APPROACH TO ENDOSCOPY FOR PATIENTS WITH GI BLEEDING

We answer the questions of whether to perform and when to perform endoscopy for upper GI bleeding in a selective fashion. For any given patient, it is our policy to consider endoscopy only after resuscitative measures have been employed, generally for a minimum of 12 hr and often not before 24 hr. In certain patients, however, we consider endoscopy within the first 12 hr because of the high risk of continued or recurrent bleeding. Our highest priority would be for elderly patients, over age 60, with a history of peptic ulcer disease or long-term aspirin consumption who may have surgically remediable peptic ulcer bleeding but who also have the highest risk of fatal outcome if surgery is delayed. In these patients the timing of endoscopy is crucial to the extent that it bears on the timing of surgery. For surgery to be performed with the least mortality in these patients, it must be done early, before an excessive transfusion requirement (>6 units) has accrued.[19,20] A definite diagnosis of peptic ulcer bleeding in these patients, we believe, promotes an earlier decision for surgery.

The second group of patients for whom we especially consider early endoscopy are those with the stigmata of liver disease, particularly those with known esophageal varices who have required in excess of 4 units of blood for stabilization, the presentation suggestive of active variceal bleeding.[33] Variceal bleeding of such magnitude prompts strong consideration for specific medical intervention, e.g., endoscopic sclerotherapy[34] or balloon tamponade,[35] if not emergency shunt surgery.[20] In all of these cases, an endoscopic diagnosis is required before initiation of any of these therapeutic interventions.

A third group of patients we consider for early endoscopy comprises those who present with a history of hematemesis associated with hypotension, orthostatic blood pressure changes in excess of 20 mm Hg, bright red blood in the nasogastric aspirate and/or in the stool, or a transfusion requirement in excess of 4 units during the first 6 hr for hemodynamic stabilization. All indicate an increased likelihood of continued bleeding[8] and an increased mortality[36] that would justify endoscopy as soon as it becomes feasible. In these cases an endoscopic diagnosis allows surgery to be instituted without excessive delay, or if the patient is not a surgical candidate the institution of endoscopy is therefore at a point where survival may still be anticipated.

Finally, with patients who have had undiagnosed upper GI bleeding or who have known varices and in whom several bleeding sites may be present,[8] we advocate endoscopy at the earliest practical time to provide the greatest opportunity for demonstrating an active bleeding lesion.

Although we believe that early endoscopy is desirable in all these patients, we nevertheless view it as being less crucial to the patient's overall chances of survival than the initial resuscitative efforts, which must be well under way before endoscopy can be safely performed.

Results

Our experience over the past 7 years with a selective approach to endoscopy in patients with upper GI bleeding is presented in this section. Here we review our experience with 500 consecutively examined patients. Of these, 15% were performed as emergent examinations, within 6 to 12 hr of the patient's admission to the hospital (Table 32-1). These emergent examinations were largely performed within the medical or surgical intensive care unit, generally within 2 hr of request. An additional 25% of the patients were examined on an urgent basis, generally within 12 to 24 hr of the patient's admission to the hospital. Again these examinations were usually performed in an intensive care unit but at a time convenient for the endoscopist. The majority of these examinations (60%) were performed as routine procedures—whenever the patient could be conveniently scheduled for endoscopy.

A definite diagnosis was made in 87% of the cases. These are presented in Table 32-2. The distribution of these diagnoses is comparable to that found in the ASGE survey[1] with the exception of hemorrhagic-erosive gastritis, which was present in 10.8% of our patients in contrast to 23.4% of the survey patients. This, we believe, is due to the largely referral nature of our hospital, which affects the numbers of admissions of indigent patients who would be more likely to have acute mucosal injury from alcohol (see Chapter 36). Endoscopy failed to reveal the cause of bleeding in

TABLE 32-1. *Timing of 500 consecutive examinations for upper GI bleeding (1974–1980)*

Type of examination	No.	%
Emergency[a]	78	15.6
Urgent[b]	125	25.0
Routine[c]	297	59.4

[a] Whenever requested, within 6 to 12 hr of admission.
[b] Whenever conveniently performed, but within 12 to 24 hr.
[c] Whenever conveniently scheduled, after 24 hr.

TABLE 32-2. *Endoscopic diagnoses for 500 consecutive examinations of patients with upper GI bleeding (1974–1980)*

Diagnosis	No.	%
Esophageal varices	64	12.8
Esophagitis	8	1.6
Mallory-Weiss lesion	22	4.4
Gastric ulcer	121	24.2
Stomal ulcer	5	1.0
Hemorrhagic-erosive gastritis	54	10.8
Gastric cancer	6	1.2
Gastric angiodysplasia (including hereditary hemorrhagic telangiectasia)	5	1.0
Duodenal ulcer	135	27.0
Other lesions	15	3.0
Cause of bleeding not determined	65	13.0
Total	500	100.0

TABLE 32-3. *Patients with undetermined cause of bleeding*

Endoscopic finding	No.	%
Massive amount of blood	38	58
Nonspecific finding	15	24
No finding	12	18
Total	65	100

TABLE 32-4. *Endoscopic complications in 500 patients with upper GI bleeding*

Type	No.	%
Aspiration	4	0.8
Hemorrhage	5	1.0
Perforation	1	0.2
Hypotension	3	0.6
Arrhythmia	1	0.2
Medication reaction	2	0.4
Total	16	3.2

13%. This was comparable to, though somewhat higher than, the 8.1% of failures noted in the ASGE survey.[8] In our patients a massive amount of blood in the stomach was the commonest cause of failure (Table 32-3), representing almost 60% of the cases where endoscopy failed to establish a diagnosis. In 24%, failure resulted from the presence of only nonspecific findings believed insufficient to explain the bleeding, e.g., scattered erosions attributable to the nasogastric tube or nonspecific gastric erythema. Finally, no findings whatsoever were present in 18%. The higher percentage of nondiagnostic examinations in our patients in contrast to those in the ASGE survey may have been due in part to our selective policy. Whereas only 40% of our patients were examined within the first 24 hr, 62.8% of the survey patients were, with the result that, for the additional 20%, transient lesions such as acute gastric mucosal injury may have disappeared by the time the examination was performed.

TABLE 32-5. *Endoscopic complications in relation to the type of examination*

Condition	Type of examination: Emergency	Urgent	Routine
Aspiration	2	1	1
Hemorrhage	2	2	1
Perforation	1	—	—
Hypotension	2	1	—
Arrhythmia	1	—	1
Medication reaction	1	—	—
Total complications	9	4	3
Total examinations	78	125	297
Percent	11.5	3.2	1.0

TABLE 32-6. *Mortality attributable to complications*

Complication	No. with complication	No. dying with complication	Mortality attributable to complication (%)
Aspiration	4	1	25
Hemorrhage	5	2	40
Hypotension	3	1	33
Other complications	4	—	—
Total complications	16	4	25
Total examinations	500	4	0.8

Even with a selective policy, our complication rate was high at 3.2% (Table 32-4), almost 3.5 times higher than the 0.9% reported in the ASGE survey, although the complications were similar (Table 32-4), with aspiration and hemorrhage predominating in both series. As noted by others,[28] the complication rate from endoscopy was increased for patients examined emergently in an intensive care unit setting. In our emergent cases, with the endoscopic procedure being almost always performed in an intensive care unit, the complication rate was 11.5%; it was considerably less (3.2%) for those performed later as urgent procedures and was least of all (1.1%) for patients in whom endoscopy could be performed on a routine basis (Table 32-5).

The mortality directly relating to endoscopy in these patients is low (Table 32-6), being only 0.8%; however, it was 25% in patients having an endoscopic complication. This is comparable though somewhat higher than the 14% mortality rate associated with endoscopic complications in the ASGE survey.[8] Not surprisingly, mortality from endoscopy was highest in the emergent group, which also had the highest complication rate (Table 32-7). In this group the mortality from endoscopy was 2.5% in contrast to the 0.8% for the urgent group, 0.34% for the routine group, and 0.8% overall.

TABLE 32-7. *Mortality from complications related to type of examination*

Type of examination	No.	Deaths from endoscopic complications (No.)	Mortality from endoscopy (%)
Emergency	78	2	2.56
Urgent	125	1	0.80
Routine	297	1	0.34
Total	500	4	0.80

REFERENCES

1. Silverstein, F. E., Gilbert, D. A., Tedesco, F. J., Buenger, N. K., Persing, J., and 277 members of the ASGE (1981): The national ASGE survey on upper gastrointestinal bleeding. I. Study and baseline data. *Gastrointest. Endosc.*, 27:73–79.
2. Silverstein, F. E., Gilbert, D. A., Tedesco, F. J., Buenger, N. K., Persing, J., and 277 members of the ASGE (1981): The national ASGE survey on upper gastrointestinal bleeding. II. Clinical prognostic factors. *Gastrointest. Endosc.*, 27:80–93.
3. Morris, D. W., Levine, G. M., Soloway, R. D., Miller, W. T., Marin, G. A., and the Gastrointestinal Section of the University of Pennsylvania (1975): Prospective randomized study of diagnosis and outcome in acute upper gastrointestinal bleeding: endoscopy versus conventional radiography. *Am. J. Dig. Dis.*, 20:1103–1109.
4. McGinn, F. P., Guyer, P. B., Wilken, B. J., and Steer, H. W. (1975): A prospective comparative trial between early endoscopy and radiology in acute upper gastrointestinal hemorrhage. *Gut,* 16:707–713.
5. Keller, R. T., and Logan, G. M. (1976): Comparison of emergent endoscopy and upper gastrointestinal series radiography in acute gastrointestinal hemorrhage. *Gut,* 17:180–184.
6. Thoeni, R. F., and Cello, J. P. (1980): A critical look at accuracy of endoscopy and double-contrast radiography of the upper gastrointestinal (UGI) tract in patients with substantial UGI hemorrhage. *Radiology,* 135:305–308.
7. Winans, C. S. (1977): Emergency upper gastrointestinal endoscopy: does haste make waste? *Am. J. Dig. Dis.*, 22:536–540.
8. Gilbert, D. A., Silverstein, F. E., Tedesco, F. J., Buenger, N. K., Persing, J., and 277 members of the ASGE (1981): The national ASGE survey on upper gastrointestinal bleeding. III. Endoscopy in upper GI bleeding. *Gastrointest. Endosc.*, 27:94–102.
9. Morgan, A. G., McAdam, W. A. F., Walmsley, G. L., Jessop, A., Horrocks, J. C., and DeDombal, F. T. (1977): Clinical findings, early endoscopy and multivariate analysis in patients bleeding from the upper gastrointestinal tract. *Br. Med. J.*, 2:237–260.
10. Peterson, W. L., Barnett, C. C., Smith, H. J., Allen, M. H., and Corbett, D. B. (1981): Routine early endoscopy in upper gastrointestinal tract bleeding: a randomized, controlled trial. *N. Engl. J. Med.*, 304:925–929.
11. Graham, D. Y. (1980): Limited value of early endoscopy in the management of acute upper gastrointestinal bleeding: prospective controlled trial. *Am. J. Surg.*, 140:284–290.
12. Silverstein, F. E., Feld, A. D., and Gilbert, D. A. (1981): Upper gastrointestinal tract bleeding: predisposing factors, diagnosis and therapy. *Arch. Intern. Med.*, 141:322–327.
13. La Brooy, S. G., Misiewicz, J. J., Edwards, J., Smith, P. M., Haggie, S. J., Libman, L., Sarner, M., Wyllie, J. H., Croker, J., and Cotton, P. (1979): Controlled trial of cimetidine in upper gastrointestinal haemorrhage. *Gut,* 20:892–895.
14. Fogel, M. R., Knauer, C. M., Andres, L. L., Mahal, A. S., Stein, D. E. T., Kemeny, M. J., Rinki, M. M., Walker, J. E., Siegmund, D., and Gregory, P. B. (1982): Continuous intravenous vasopressin in active upper gastrointestinal bleeding: a placebo-controlled trial. *Ann. Intern. Med.*, 96:565–569.
15. Conn, H. O., Ramsby, G. R., Storer, E. H., Mutchnick, M. G., Joshi, P. H., Phillips, M. M., Cohen, G. A., Fields, G. N., and Petroski, D. (1975): Intraarterial vasopressin in the treatment of upper gastrointestinal hemorrhage: a prospective, controlled clinical trial. *Gastroenterology,* 68:211–221.
16. Chojkier, M., and Conn, H. O. (1980): Esophageal tamponade in the treatment of bleeding varices. *Dig. Dis. Sci.*, 25:267–272.
17. Papp, J. P. (1982): Endoscopic electrocoagulation in the management of upper gastrointestinal tract bleeding. *Surg. Clin. N. Am.*, 62:797–806.

17a. Vallon, A. G., Cotton, P. B., Laurence, B. H., Armengol Miro, J. R., and Salord Oses, J. C. (1981): Randomized trial of endoscopic argon laser photocoagulation in bleeding peptic ulcers. *Gut,* 22:228–233.

17b. Allison, J. G. (1983): The role of injection sclerotherapy in emergency and definitive management of bleeding esophageal varices. *J.A.M.A.*, 249:1484–1487.

18. Kim, U., Rudick, J., and Aufses, A. H. (1978): Surgical management of acute upper gastrointestinal bleeding: value of early diagnosis and prompt surgical intervention. *Arch. Surg.*, 113:1444–1447.
19. Brooks, J. R., and Eraklis, A. (1964): Factors affecting the mortality from peptic ulcer: the bleeding ulcer and ulcer in the aged. *N. Engl. J. Med.*, 271:803–809.
20. Prandi, D., Rueff, B., Roche-Sicot, J., Sicot, C., Maillard, J. N., Benhamou, J. P., and Fauvert, R. (1976): Life-threatening hemorrhage of the digestive tract in cirrhotic patients: an assessment of the postoperative mortality after emergency portacaval shunt. *Am. J. Surg.*, 131:204–209.
21. Hunt, P. S., Hansky, J., and Korman, M. G. (1979): Mortality in patients with haematemesis and melaena: a prospective study. *Br. Med. J.*, 1:1238–1240.
22. Graham, D. Y., and Smith, J. L. (1981): The course of patients after variceal hemorrhage. *Gastroenterology,* 80:800–809.
23. Devitt, J. E. (1969): Upper gastrointestinal bleeding with special reference to peptic ulcer. *Gastroenterology,* 57:89–94.
24. Lebrec, D., Poynard, T., Hillon, P., and Benhamou, J.-P. (1981): Propranolol for prevention of recurrent gastrointestinal bleeding in patients with cirrhosis. *N. Engl. J. Med.*, 305:1371–1374.
25. Clark, A. W., Macdougall, B. R. D., Westaby, D., Mitchell, K. J., Silk, D. B. A., Strunin, L., Dawson, J. L., and Williams, R. (1980): Prospective controlled trial of injection sclerotherapy in patients with cirrhosis and recent variceal haemorrhage. *Lancet,* 2:552–554.
26. Leinike, J. A., Schaffer, R. D., Hogan, W. J., and Geenen, J. E. (1976): Does timing affect the significance of diagnostic yield? *Gastrointest. Endosc.*, 22:228.
27. Silvis, S., Nebel, O., Rogers, G., Sugawa, C., and Mandelstam, P. (1976): Endoscopic complications: results of the 1974 American Society for Gastrointestinal Endoscopy survey. *JAMA,* 235:928–930.

27a. Katon, R. M. (1981): Complications of upper gastrointestinal endoscopy in the gastrointestinal bleeder. *Dig. Dis. Sci.*, 26(July Suppl):47S–54S.

28. Paul, F., and Huchzermeyer, H. (1980): Results and complications of emergency endoscopy for acute gastrointestinal bleeding in patients on intensive care units. In: *Abstracts of the IV European Congress of Gastrointestinal Endoscopy,* p. 103. George Thieme Verlag, Stuttgart.
29. Watts, H. D. (1976): Mallory-Weiss syndrome occurring as a complication of endoscopy. *Gastrointest. Endosc.*, 22:171–172.
30. Baker, R. W., Spiro, A. H., and Trnka, Y. (1982): Mallory-Weiss tear complicating upper endoscopy: case reports and review of the literature. *Gastroenterology,* 82:140–142.
31. Sandlow, L. J., Becker, G. H., Spellberg, M. A., Allen, H. A., Berg, M., Berry, L. H., and Newman, E. A. (1974): A prospective randomized study of the management of upper gastrointestinal hemorrhage. *Am. J. Gastroenterol.*, 61:282–289.
32. Dronfield, M. W., McIlmurray, M. B., Ferguson, R., Atkinson, M., and Langman, M. J. S. (1977): A prospective randomized study of endoscopy and radiology in acute upper-gastrointestinal-tract bleeding. *Lancet,* 1:1167–1169.
33. Morris, S. J., Greenwald, R. A., and Tedesco, F. J. (1978): Characteristics of variceal versus nonvariceal hemorrhage in cirrhosis with varices. *Gastroenterology,* 74:1070.
34. Hughes, R. W., Larson, D. E., Vigiano, T. R., Adson, M. A., Van Heerden, J. A., and Reeves, C. B. (1982): Endoscopic variceal sclerosis: a one year experience. *Gastrointest. Endosc.*, 28:62–67.
35. Hunt, P. S., Korman, M. G., Hansky, J., and Parkin, W. G. (1982): An 8-year prospective experience with balloon tamponade in emergency control of bleeding varices. *Dig. Dis. Sci.*, 27:413–416.
36. Fleischer, D. (1981): Incidence and etiology of severe UGI bleeding which is not self-limited. *Gastroenterology,* 80:1148.

33

ENDOSCOPIC TECHNIQUE AND ACCOMPANYING INTERPRETIVE PROBLEMS

ENDOSCOPIC TECHNIQUE

Performing endoscopy in patients with active upper gastrointestinal (GI) bleeding challenges the skill of the most experienced examiner. Here the visual field may be partially or almost completely obscured by either blood (Fig. 33-1a), clots (Fig. 33-1b), or antacid (Fig. 33-1c), alone and in combination (Fig. 33-1d). In order to cope, especially in cases where the usual visual clues (esophageal columns, rugal folds, gastric angulus, superior duodenal angle, etc.) are not always apparent, the endoscopist must rely on his knowledge of endoscopic anatomy and orientation of the esophagus, stomach, and duodenum to guide his movements (see Chapters 1, 11, and 24). Because of the forced circumstances of a critically ill patient who has received either little or no sedation, the examination must be completed within the shortest period of time with the least number of false moves. Because of the visual constraints as well as the

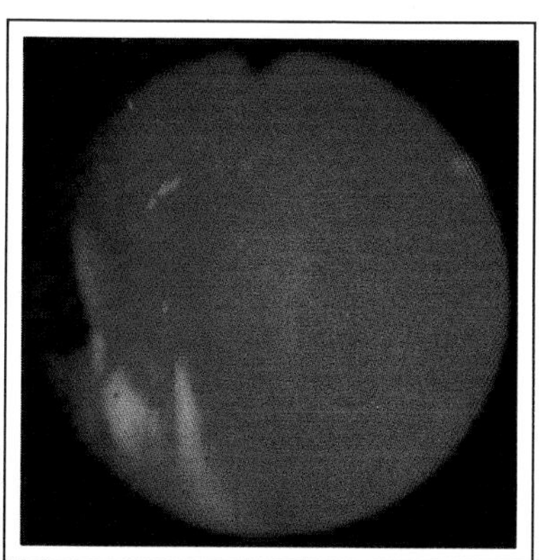

FIG. 33-1a.

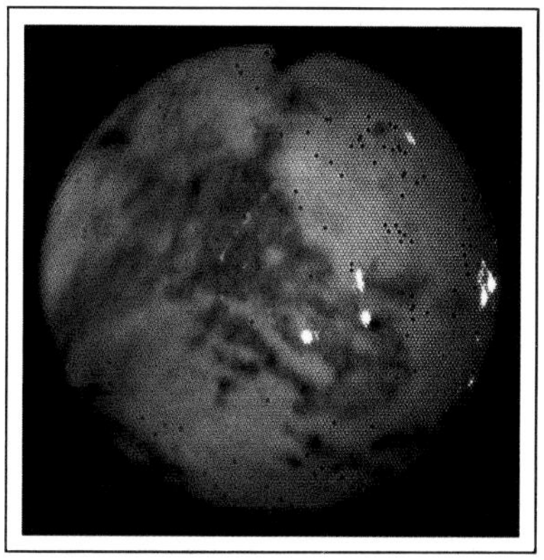

FIG. 33-1b.

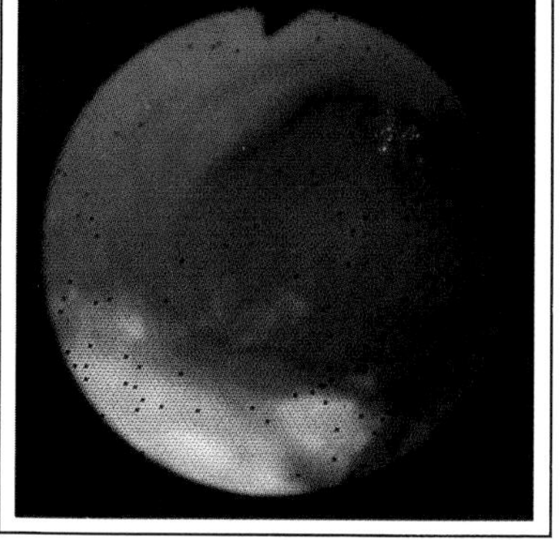

FIG. 33-1c.

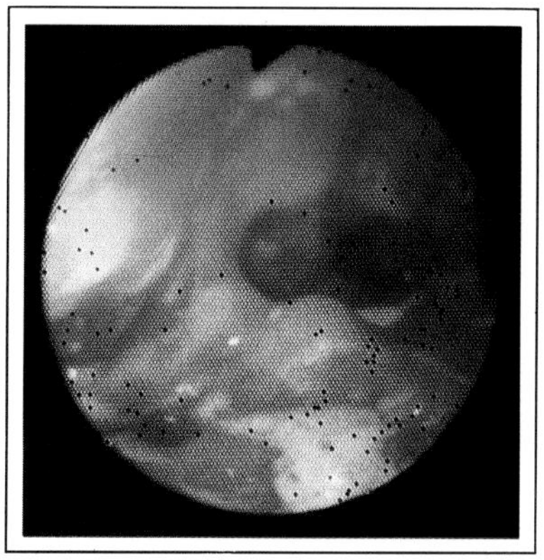

FIG. 33-1d.

FIG. 33-1. a: Active gastric bleeding. Bright red blood completely obscures the bleeding site, a prepyloric antral ulcer. **b:** Antral clots. Although the bleeding has stopped, the clots obscure the mucosa and may potentially hide the bleeding site or erroneously suggest acute gastric mucosal injury (see Chapter 36). **c:** Pool of antacid simulating a large gastric ulcer. The antacid which collects within the recesses between rugal folds may simulate an ulcer appearance. **d:** Blood and antacid taken together may be mistaken for the base of a large bleeding ulcer.

rapidity with which the examination must be performed, many, the author included, find examination of the actively bleeding patient to be among the most difficult of any the endoscopist is called on to perform, certainly from the interpretive standpoint.

In this section we discuss the technique for performing endoscopy in patients with upper GI bleeding. Specifically, we consider the following: (a) the role of preliminary nasogastric lavage and aspiration; (b) premedication; (c) the choice of instruments; and (d) our method of examination. After presenting the endoscopic technique, we consider in a separate section the types of interpretive problems inherent in the endoscopic examination of bleeding patients.

Preliminary Nasogastric Lavage and Aspiration

Experienced endoscopists are generally divided over the question of a preliminary nasogastric lavage and suction for 30 min to 1 hr prior to the examination. Some advocate a preliminary lavage with iced saline in all cases, hoping to remove clots and accumulated blood as well as to temporarily halt the rate of bleeding.[1,2] Morrissey recommends lavage only in cases where a large amount of blood is suspected which the patient could aspirate.[3] Rather than iced saline,[4] he employs tepid water.[3] If lavage is to be employed, most[1-3] find the use of conventional nasogastric tubes with a diameter of 16 to 18 Fr to be inadequate in the face of sizable (>500 to 700 cc) accumulations of blood and clots. Even the Ewald tube with a diameter of 30 Fr may be insufficient for massive amounts of bleeding. What has been advocated is the use of even larger-bore rubber tubes of the "garden hose" type having diameters of 40 to 50 Fr and passed in the manner of an endoscope.[1-3] More recently, a Silastic "overtube" has been used which can be passed over the endoscope and introduced along with it so that when large amounts of blood and/or clots are encountered the endoscope can be withdrawn and these accumulations removed with suction.

Although these tubes are helpful in some cases, truly massive accumulations are rarely removed to a degree which allows all surfaces of the stomach to be examined with ease. Some accumulation generally remains; moreover, the tubes themselves and the suctioning of blood and clots through them may be responsible for producing mucosal trauma (nasogastric tube artifacts) which would detract from the value of the procedure. The risk of artifacts has led us to abandon the use of routine nasogastric lavage, employing it only where an initial aspirate from the stomach reveals large quantities of blood and clots which may both preclude a satisfactory examination from being performed and predispose the patient to aspirate during the procedure.[3]

Premedication

The role of premedication is unsettled. A recently published prospective survey of 277 endoscopists, members of the American Society for Gastrointestinal Endoscopy (the National ASGE Survey on Upper Gastrointestinal Bleeding), reporting on some 2,300 examinations,[5] indicated that some premedication was used in 85.4%; Valium was the most commonly used. Among the survey patients, 70.2% received Valium with a mean dose of 10 ± 6.9 mg. In contrast, Demerol was used in only 39.2%, with a mean dose of 50 ± 22.0 mg. Whether a complete examination was performed, however, was not influenced by whether the patient received premedication, with a success rate of 85% in either case.[5]

We find that a highly satisfactory examination can be performed in a cooperative patient with only topical pharyngeal anesthesia as premedication. Often complete cooperation can be achieved simply with a brief yet full explanation of the procedure prior to intubation, particularly if the patient is forewarned about the major discomforts he will experience. For the anxious patient who does not respond simply to reassurance, light to moderate sedation can be achieved through intravenous Valium. We find this helps relax the patient and thus speeds the examination as well as enhances its accuracy in that the endoscopist can concentrate on the examination rather than on the patient. In some patients, however, especially alcoholics, the use of Valium particularly in amounts greater than 20 mg frequently leads to increasing confusion with "paradoxical hyperagitation" resulting. If this is not recognized and even larger amounts of Valium are administered, prolonged stupor and even coma may result, especially in patients with underlying cirrhosis.[6]

Our approach to premedication is to individualize as much as possible. We attempt to perform the procedure without sedation, relying only on simple verbal reassurance. Should this fail, we administer 10 to 20 mg Valium before intubation is tried again. If the patient remains resistant, further attempts at intubation are abandoned.

We neither sedate nor perform endoscopic procedures in patients who are hypotensive or who have a respiratory rate in excess of 30 breaths per minute unless absolutely mandated by the clinical situation. In these patients we advise continued efforts at resuscitation with intensive blood replacement, endoscopy being deferred for at least 4 to 12 hr until these resuscitative efforts are completed. Ill-timed endoscopy during this critical phase of resuscitation, especially if premedication with Valium is used, is very likely to result in endoscopic complications, e.g., aspiration or hypotension, which in the ASGE survey carried a 15 to 25% mortality[5] (see Chapter 32).

Choice of Instrument

There are three factors to consider when choosing an instrument for diagnostic purposes, quite apart from any consideration of therapeutic procedures, e.g., electrocoagulation, which might be performed at the same time. These factors are: (a) ease of intubation; (b) illumination; and (c) suction capability.

Intubation

A very important consideration in the choice of an instrument lies in whether it offers the greatest likelihood of a complete examination of the esophagus, stomach, and duodenum (to its third portion). Large-caliber (11 to 13 mm) single-channel instruments or even larger two-channel endoscopes may be desired because of their greater irrigation and suction capacities[7]; however, they have the disadvantage of a more difficult intubation, especially in elderly patients where the posterior hypopharynx might be compromised due to cervical spine lordosis or osteoarthritis with osteophyte formation.[8] Moreover, these instruments might not readily pass across a scarred pyloroduodenal junction into an even more scarred duodenal bulb; nor would they be ideal for examining a scarred bulb. Whether a complete examination can be performed is often determined by the choice of instrument. In the ASGE survey, 11.3% of the examinations were incomplete. Poor patient cooperation and other "technical difficulties" accounted for 40% of these failures.[5] In our experience, three groups of patients are likely to prove poor technical failures if a large-caliber (11 to 13 mm) instrument is used: (a) patients who cannot or will not swallow on command; (b) elderly patients; and (c) patients with a history suggestive of peptic ulcer disease in whom there may be significant pyloroduodenal junction scarring. The choice of a narrow-caliber (9 mm) pediatric-type endoscope is especially appropriate for these patients as the smaller endoscope easily passes through a "tight" posterior hypopharynx by direct intubation with only modest patient cooperation. Furthermore, they can usually be passed through even a considerably deformed pyloric channel and contracted duodenal bulb with a modicum of effort. In one series a high diagnostic yield was achieved using an 8.8-mm pediatric-type endoscope (Olympus GIF-P2), with a complete examination achieved in 97% (67/69), especially in elderly and marginally cooperative patients.[9]

Illumination

A major reason for an unsuccessful examination in a bleeding patient is inadequate illumination due to the capacity of a large amount of blood "absorbing" much of the light the endoscope transmits. In the past, adequate illumination was provided by only the largest-caliber (≥13 mm) instruments when used with the most powerful cold (xenon) light sources (outputs of 300 to 500 watts). The newer generation of medium-caliber (11 mm) endoscopes now seem to have better illumination than that provided by the older instruments.

The medium-caliber endoscopes capable of delivering bright illumination are especially important for patients with active bleeding. An indication of the patient's bleeding status was found in the ASGE survey to be the nasogastric aspirate, with a finding of red blood an indication of 50% likelihood of active bleeding being encountered at endoscopy.[5] For this group of patients, maximum illumination is highly desirable, and one would use a medium-caliber, rather than a narrow-caliber, instrument provided the patient is not elderly or uncooperative, or has a history of duodenal ulcer disease. For the latter, the pediatric instrument with its somewhat diminished illumination potential is still the instrument of choice. This is especially true if the nasogastric tube return suggested that the bleeding had either slowed (initially bright red, turning pink) or stopped altogether (initially bright red, turning to coffee-ground color or completely clear).

Another group of patients for whom illumination is critical are those in whom acute gastric mucosal injuries are suspected. In these patients the most powerful illumination is required because blood, by absorbing much of the light and then reflecting only the red end of the spectrum, causes normal gastric mucosa to appear reddened and thus creates an erroneous impression of diffuse gastritis (Fig. 33-2).

Removal of Blood and Clots

Some advocate the use of a two-channel operating, large-caliber (15 mm) gastroscope for the examination of actively bleeding patients. If the patient can be intubated, this would allow for lavage through one of the channels and aspiration of blood and clots through the other.[3,7] It has been proposed that these instruments are highly effective for removing clots and provide intense illumination because of their size.[3] It is not known if this advantage is offset by difficulties in intubating the cricopharyngeus in elderly patients and the duodenal bulb in 20 to 30% of patients who have bleeding duodenal ulcers. Most workers at present prefer the ease of examination provided by the smaller instruments even though they are largely ineffective in the removal of blood and clots. Even so, it is still possible to provide crucial diagnostic information (e.g., the demonstration of bleeding varices, diffuse gastric mucosal injury, bleeding duodenal ulcers), even though the stomach contains a considerable amount of blood and clots. Controlled trials are necessary to determine if there is a benefit from using the larger, more cumbersome double-channel instrument.

Method of Examination

The endoscopic examination of a patient who is bleeding proceeds in a fashion similar to that in a nonbleeding patient (see Chapters 1, 11, 21, and 24). However, certain areas in the bleeding patient take on an even greater significance as potential sites of bleeding and must be observed if the examination is to be successful, in both finding the actual cause and excluding other lesions. These areas are: (a) the cardioesophageal junction; (b) the fundus and upper body of the stomach; (c) the gastric angle and adjacent lesser curve; (d) the posterior wall of the duodenal bulb; and (e)

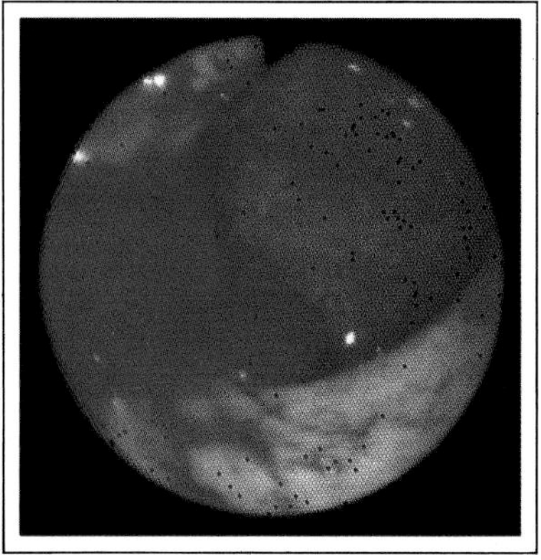

FIG. 33-2

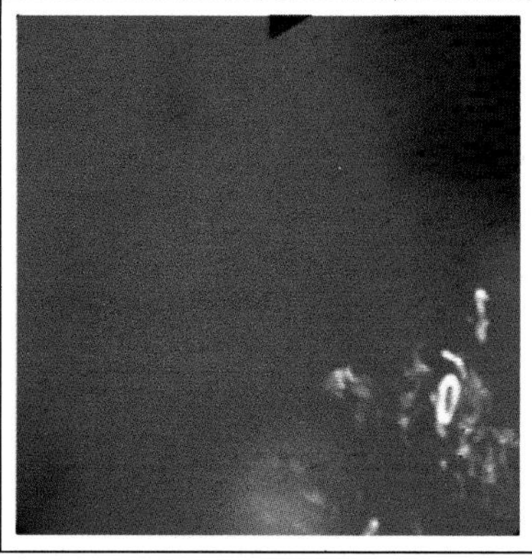

FIG. 33-3.

FIG. 33-2. Gastric mucosal appearance in the presence of bright red blood. The blood itself covers a large area of mucosal surface. The diminished illumination, as well as the blood itself, gives any mucosa that is relatively free of blood (at 6 o'clock) a reddish cast which could erroneously suggest acute mucosal injury. Further confusion is caused by blood which clots between mucosal folds, giving the appearance of erosions.

FIG. 33-3. Bright red blood in the gastric lake completely obscures the upper body and fundus.

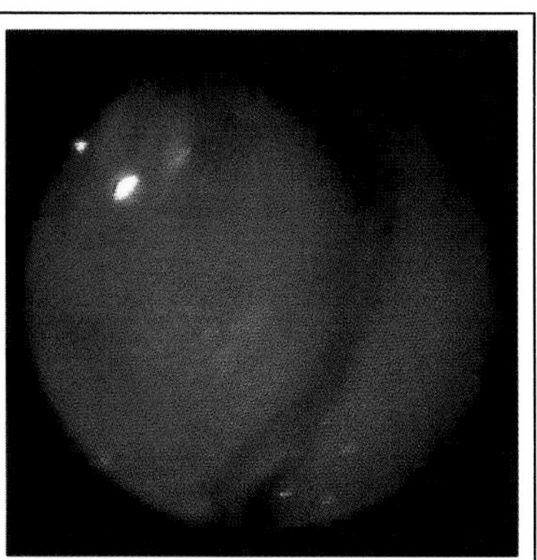

FIG. 33-4.

FIG. 33-4. Blood clot in the third portion of the duodenum. In this case, with the stomach free of blood, a distal duodenal bleeding site was suspected, and examination of the third portion revealed an ulcerating mass, eventually proved to be lymphoma.

the inferior duodenal angle and, if possible, the third portion of the duodenum.

Logistics

The examination may be performed at the bedside or in a standard endoscopy suite. For unstable patients with hypotension (systolic pressure < 90 mm Hg), rapid pulse (>100 beats per min), or respiratory rate (>24 per min), the examination should be performed in an intensive care unit where the patient could be immediately resuscitated should a cardiac or respiratory arrest occur during or immediately after the procedure. The endoscopist should be assisted by at least one other individual who monitors the patient's pulse and respiration and who clears the oropharynx of secretions through constant suctioning so as to minimize the chances of aspiration.

Procedure

The patient is initially placed in a left lateral recumbent position. The intubation of the cricopharyngeus and esophagus proceeds as previously described (see Chapter 1). Beginning in the mid-esophagus, the examiner observes the mucosa carefully for the appearance of varices (see Chapters 7 and 34). As he proceeds into the distal esophagus, he searches carefully for erosions and/or a pseudomembrane, which would suggest peptic esophagitis (see Chapters 3 and 34). The gastroesophageal (GE) junction is located and the cardia inspected, especially in its right-posterior (3 to 6 o'clock) aspect for a Mallory-Weiss lesion (see Chapter 35). The stomach is entered, but the blood and clots within the gastric lake (Fig. 33-3) are avoided by an immediate 90° to 120° clockwise torquing maneuver, and upward deflection bringing the tip in line with the lesser curve (see Chapter 11). The lesser curve of the body is briefly examined as the instrument is advanced into the antrum, at which point the angle is quickly observed for any evidence of gross ulceration. The antrum is intubated rapidly as is the pyloric channel (Chapter 21), and the instrument is thereupon advanced across the pyloric channel into the duodenal bulb (see Chapter 24). It is desirable to continue the examination into the descending duodenum; this is usually possible by using either the direct or indirect intubation technique (see Chapter 24). Should this prove difficult or the patient's toleration for the procedure begin to wane, attempts at further intubation should be abandoned and a careful examination of the duodenal bulb begun. If the descending duodenum can be entered, it is desirable to carry the examination down to the inferior duodenal angle and, if possible, view the third portion, especially if bright red blood is present in the descending duodenum but not in the duodenal bulb or stomach (Fig. 33-4). The instrument is thereupon withdrawn slowly and the medial wall of the

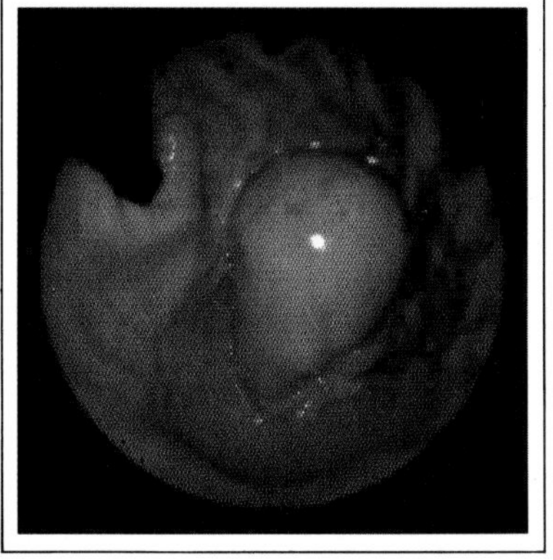

FIG. 33-5a.

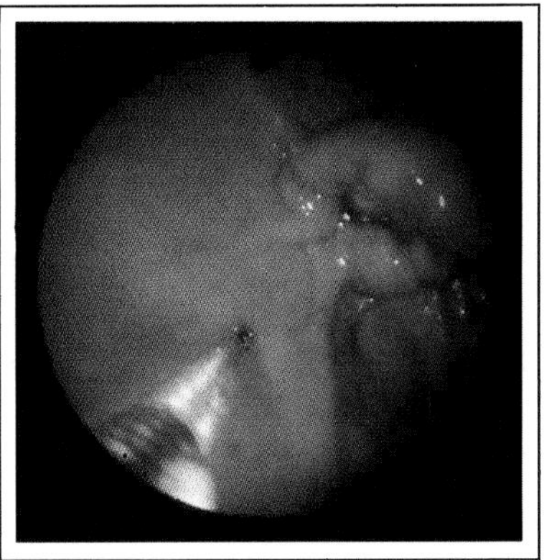

FIG. 33-5b.

FIG. 33-5. Bleeding leiomyoma of the fundus. **a:** Because of its location, this lesion can be seen only with retroflexion, which must be attempted in all cases. **b:** A close-up view of the leiomyoma reveals a central ulcer from which there is active bleeding.

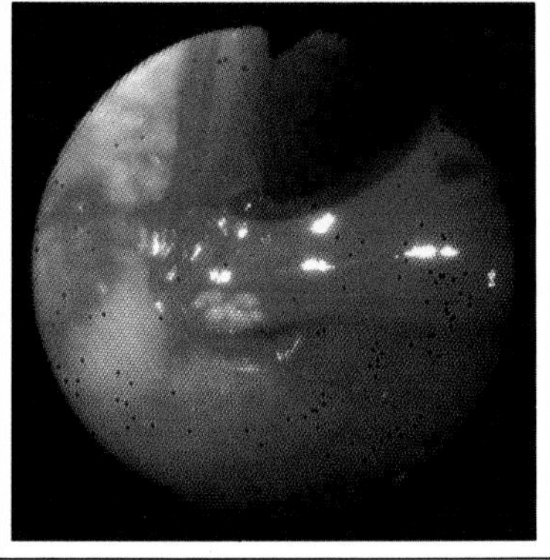

FIG. 33-6.

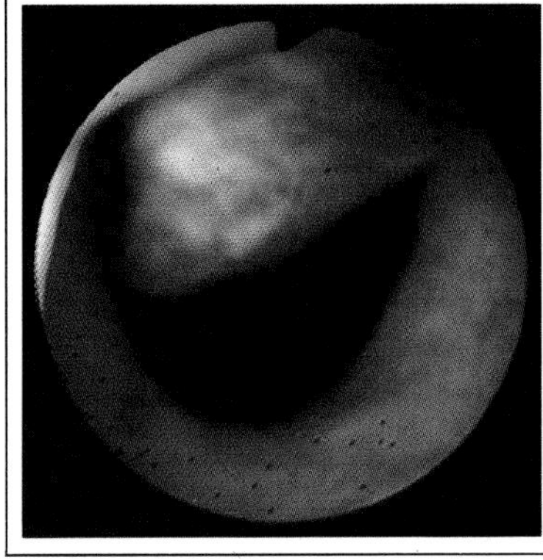

FIG. 33-7.

FIG. 33-6. Bleeding Mallory-Weiss lesion. A retroflexed view of the cardia reveals a discrete clot present (at 9 o'clock) from which blood can be seen dripping down.

FIG. 33-7. Mallory-Weiss lesion with an overlying clot seen on slow withdrawal from the cardia. The clot (at 12 o'clock) covering the Mallory-Weiss tear was not seen when the stomach was first entered.

descending duodenum carefully examined, especially in the mid-portion, for evidence of hemobilia or a bleeding diverticulum (see Chapter 38).

Once back in the duodenal bulb, it is critical that the posterior wall (see Chapter 24) be carefully examined, as it is a common site of ulcer disease as well as a location from which massive bleeding may occur as an ulcer erodes into the gastroduodenal artery (see Chapter 38). After examination of the bulb, the instrument is withdrawn into the antrum, where the prepyloric area as well as the posterior wall and lesser curve adjacent to the angle receive careful attention—all common locations of gastric ulcers (see Chapter 15).

The examination continues in the body where special attention is given to the lesser curve and posterior wall, particularly the proximal lesser curve (within 15 cm of the cardia), an especially common site of gastric ulcers in elderly patients (see Chapter 15). Should the examination have been unrevealing at this point, especially with copious amounts of blood and clots in the gastric lake, this may be shifted from the anterior to the posterior wall by simply changing the position of the patient. To view the posterior wall of the body, the patient lies anteriorly in a prone position; conversely, to view the anterior wall, blood may be shifted onto the posterior wall by rotating the patient into the supine position or onto the right side to examine the greater curve by shifting blood toward the lesser curve aspect.[10] With any of these positional changes, careful attention must be given to the patient's mouth and throat, not allowing them to become supine, which would increase the likelihood of aspiration. Another maneuver to shift the position of clots is to tilt the head of the bed or examining table up or down to relocate them in either the proximal or distal stomach.

The final phase of the stomach examination consists of a U-turn maneuver (see Chapter 11), which is performed in all patients to view the cardia and the fundus. While in the U position, the endoscope is further advanced so that there is yet another opportunity for viewing the proximal lesser curve (see Chapter 11). We have found such a maneuver to be occasionally the best single means of finding a bleeding gastric ulcer of the proximal lesser curve, common in elderly patients (see Chapter 36). After this, the fundus is carefully examined for the presence of a leiomyoma (Fig. 33-5) or gastric varices (see Chapter 37), and the cardia inspected for a Mallory-Weiss lesion (see Chapter 35) which may appear as blood dripping down from the cardia (Fig. 33-6). After the U maneuver, the body is again inspected for evidence of diffuse mucosal hemorrhage and erosions characteristic of hemorrhagic erosive gastritis (see Chapter 36). Finally, as the endoscope is withdrawn back through the cardia into the esophagus, this area is again examined for evidence of varices, esophagitis, or a Mallory-Weiss tear (Fig. 33-7), all of which can be missed if the endoscope had been originally advanced rapidly through the esophagus and into the stomach.

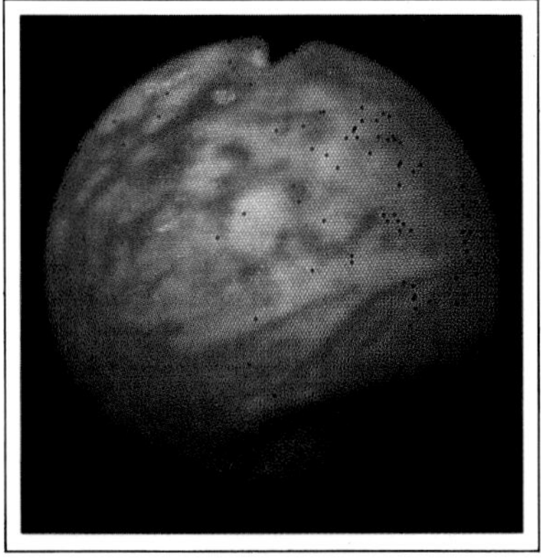

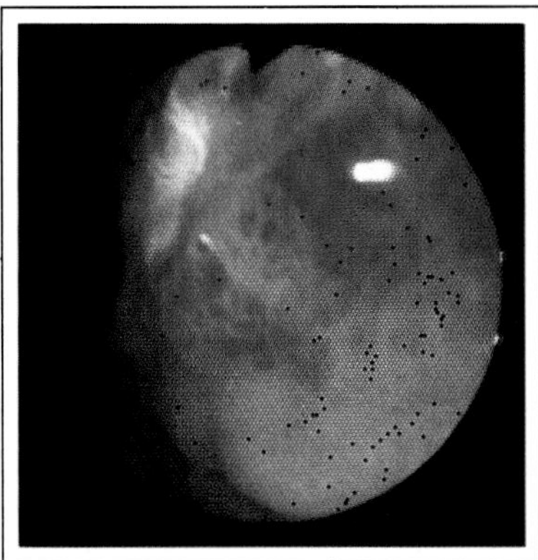

FIG. 33-8. a: Bright red blood from a bleeding duodenal ulcer simulating gastric erosions. The blood collects in recesses between the folds, giving the appearance of linear erosions. The decreased illumination and the blood itself create a reddish background, further suggesting diffuse mucosal injury. The absence of erosions on the elevated portion of the folds is an important clue to the appearance being simply an artifact of blood. **b:** Gastric erosions in aspirin-induced acute mucosal injury. The lesions seen representing areas of intramucosal hemorrhage occur both within recesses and on elevated portions of folds.

FIG. 33-8a.

FIG. 33-8b.

INTERPRETIVE PROBLEMS IN PATIENTS WITH UPPER GI BLEEDING

Although the goal of a complete, rapid, and safe examination in the actively bleeding patient is an enormous challenge, an even greater one is correct interpretation of the visual appearances encountered. In subsequent chapters we address specific interpretive problems pertaining to the various bleeding sites. In what follows here, we discuss in more general terms the problems which confound the interpretation of endoscopic findings in patients with upper GI bleeding. The problems presented are: (a) active bleeding; (b) the presence of antacids; (c) multiple potential bleeding sites; (d) distal bleeding sites; and finally (e) nasogastric suction artifacts.

Active Bleeding

Of all the potential causes of interpretive error, blood itself is the most difficult to cope with in a satisfactory way. In cases where there has been massive bleeding, blood covers and adheres to wide areas of mucosa, especially in the most dependent portions of the stomach, e.g., the fundus and greater curve (Fig. 33-3). Because blood in massive amounts from an actively bleeding lesion is only partially removed, much of it remains, absorbing light and decreasing the total amount of illumination available for examining areas free of blood; in addition, the blood may intermittently coat the lens and result in a further decrease in illumination. The result of decreased illumination is to give the mucosa a reddish cast erroneously interpreted as acute mucosal injury (Fig. 33-2). In cases where this problem is recognized, the examiner concentrates primarily on examining mucosa less likely to accumulate blood. In these areas any blood present is more easily washed away, thus exposing mucosa which is likely to be representative of neighboring areas covered with blood.

In some cases, despite vigorous washing, the blood remains absorbed to mucosal surfaces (Fig. 33-2). Generally, the blood is found in the recesses between rugal folds (Fig. 33-8a). This stands in contrast to the mucosal ridges and erosions of hemorrhagic gastritis, which form discrete red areas covering the mucosa of folds (Fig. 33-8b).

Antacids

As a rule, the endoscopist requests the physician caring for the bleeding patient to withhold antacids for at least 8 hr prior to the procedure. Often this is ignored, however, and antacids are administered right up to the time of endoscopy. In the stomach these are combined with blood and clots and together are adsorbed onto the mucosa, which can simulate the appearance of a bleeding ulcer (Fig. 33-9a). Most of the time, however, there is a sufficient amount of free-floating antacid to make the endoscopist suspicious of such an appearance (Fig. 33-9b). Often the examiner can remove the congealed blood and antacids with a spray of water from a polyethylene cannula and thus assure himself that an ulcer is not present. If this cannot be done, however, and uncertainty remains, the examiner is justified in gently probing the clot with the polyethylene cannula to expose either a normal undersurface or the base of an ulcer, a manuever which he would not attempt if any part of an ulcer base was seen with certainty (Fig. 33-9c).

Multiple Potential Bleeding Sites

Multiple endoscopic findings were observed in one-third of the cases in the ASGE prospective survey.[5] In almost half of these, or in a total of 15% of all cases, it was impossible to determine which site was actually the cause of bleeding. In cases where multiple bleeding sites are present, the endoscopist hopes to find evidence of active bleeding from one of the potential sources to indicate which is the cause. However, one must expect that in many of these cases this is impossible.

The problem of multiple bleeding sites is illustrated with the example of esophageal varices, the commonest case in which multiple potential bleeding sites are found (Fig. 33-10a). In the ASGE prospective study, bleeding was attributed

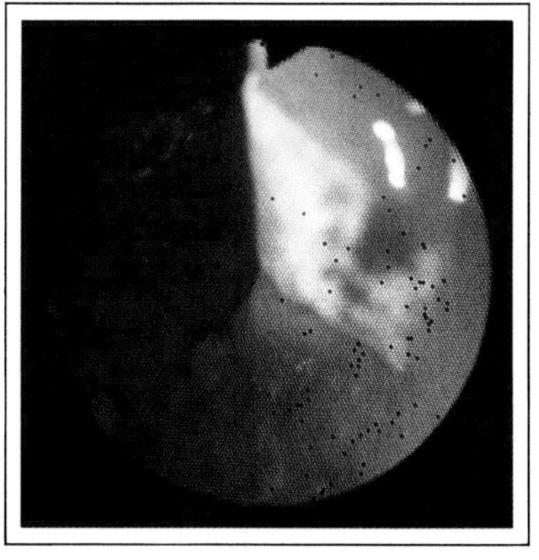

FIG. 33-9a.

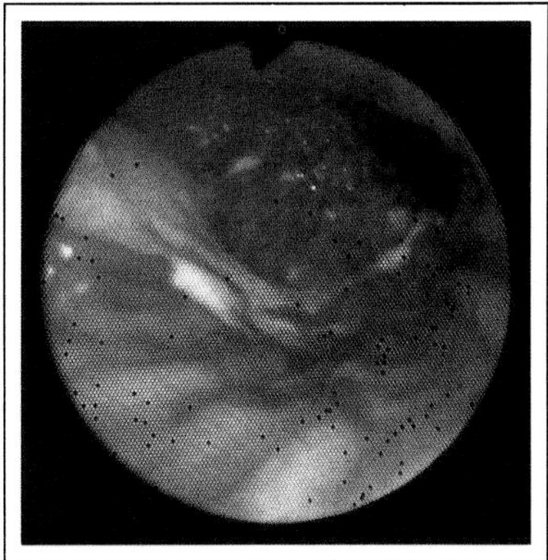

FIG. 33-9b.

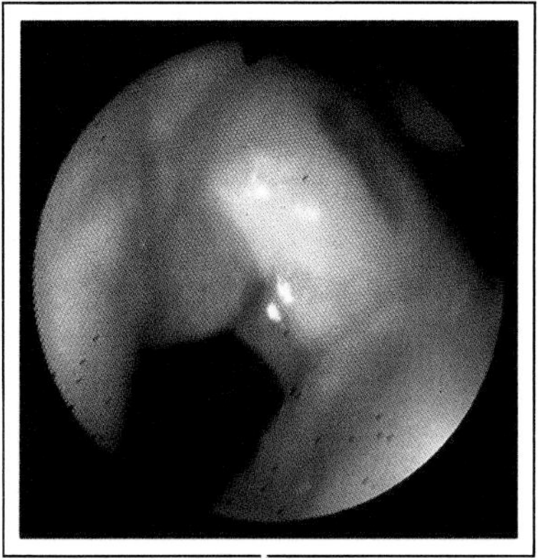

FIG. 33-9c.

FIG. 33-9. a: Antacid residue with blood clot simulating an ulcer base with an active bleeding site. The absence of an excavation was an important clue to it being an artifactual appearance, which was easily removed with a water spray. **b:** Antacid simulating a giant gastric ulcer. The pool of antacid might be mistaken for an ulcer base except for its being raised above the level of the rugal folds. **c:** Gastric ulcer base with clots. The base with clot at 2 o'clock has a depressed position in relation to the surrounding folds.

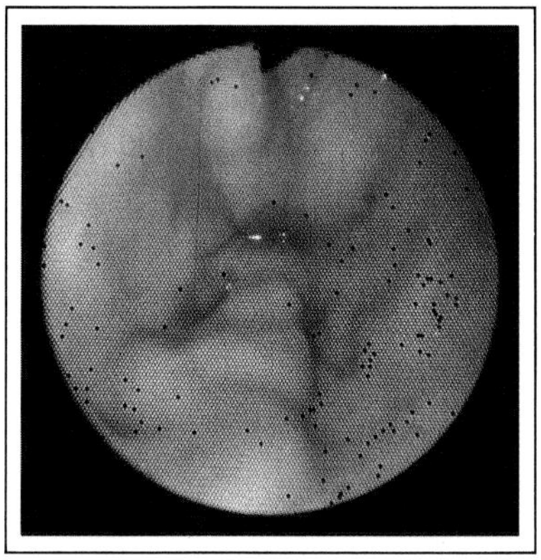

FIG. 33-10a.

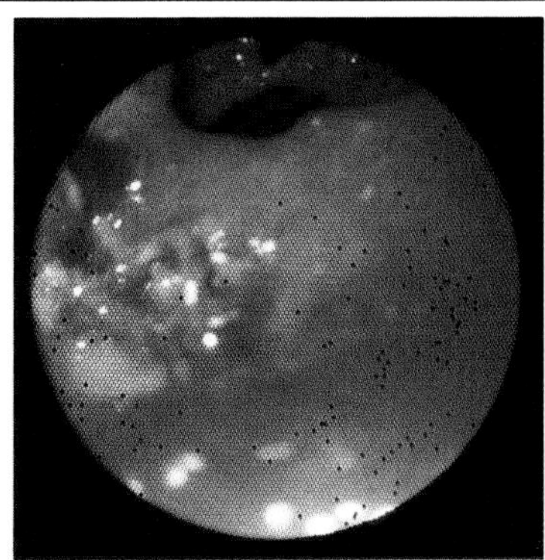

FIG. 33-10b.

FIG. 33-10. a: Esophageal varices that are not the site of bleeding. These lack any sign of recent bleeding. **b:** Duodenal bulb ulcer as a site of bleeding in a patient with esophageal varices (a). The blood clot within the base indicates this to be the true bleeding site.

to other sites (Fig. 33-10b) in one-third of the cases where esophageal varices were present.[5] In other series the prevalence of other bleeding lesions in patients with esophageal varices has been as high as 60%.[11] In these cases and others with multiple potential bleeding sites, the interpretive problems result from the following: (a) the ubiquitousness of blood; (b) the ease with which esophageal varices are demonstrated; and (c) the potential for artifactual "other" sites of bleeding.

Ubiquitousness of Blood

Blood is not stationary in the face of active bleeding from a gastric or duodenal site but may be refluxed back into the esophagus (Fig. 33-11a). In the presence of esophageal varices (Fig. 33-11b), this may simulate variceal bleeding. To avoid interpretive problems, one must patiently observe the region just above the cardia for the moment when blood may be cleared from the esophagus (Fig. 33-11b) and for the opportunity to arise for direct observation in order to determine if there is a continued ooze of blood from the varices themselves. In cases where blood seems to clear from the lower esophagus, the endoscopist re-enters the stomach (Fig. 33-11c) and carefully examines the lesser curve, gastric angle, and duodenal bulb for the actual bleeding site.

Ease With Which Varices Are Identified

Also serving to confuse, along with the ubiquitousness of blood, is the ease with which varices, especially if sizable (grade IV—see Chapter 8), are readily found and identified (Fig. 33-11b). With the reflux of blood into the esophagus from a gastric lesion (Fig. 33-11a), the endoscopic diagnosis of variceal bleeding may seem inescapable. Still, one must attempt to observe the distal esophagus after some of the accumulated blood has cleared (Fig. 33-11b) so as to derive a sense of whether the varices (Fig. 33-12b) or another site (Fig. 33-12a) are the likely cause of bleeding.

Questionable "Other Sites" of Bleeding

Although the finding of "other sites" of bleeding in patients with esophageal varices, e.g., peptic ulcers (Fig. 33-12a), is a positive benefit of endoscopy, some of these are questionable, in that they cannot be separated visually, or even conceptually, from variceal bleeding. Whether, for example, one can separate variceal bleeding from a contig-

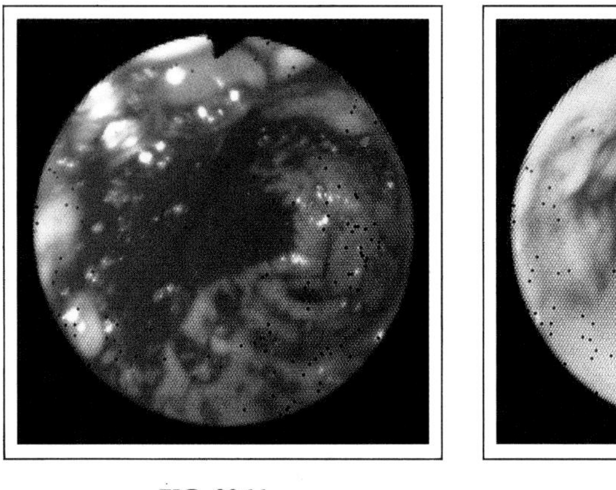

FIG. 33-11a.

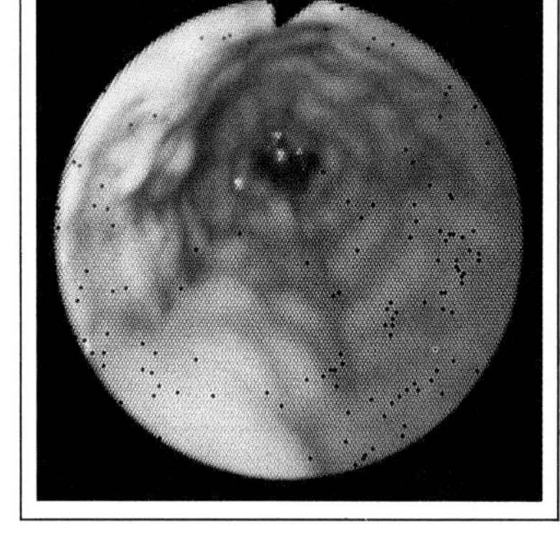

FIG. 33-11b.

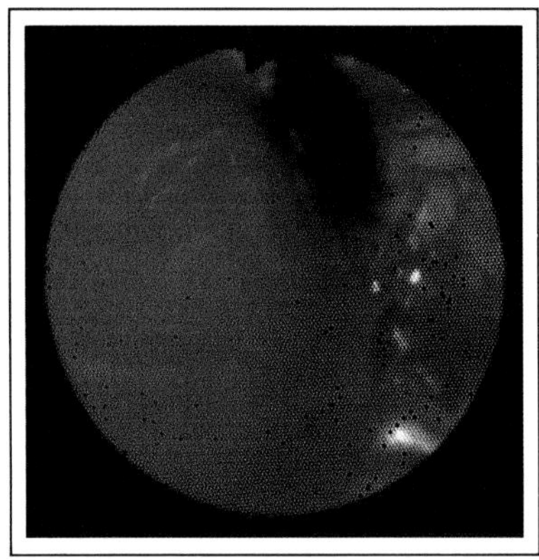

FIG. 33-11c.

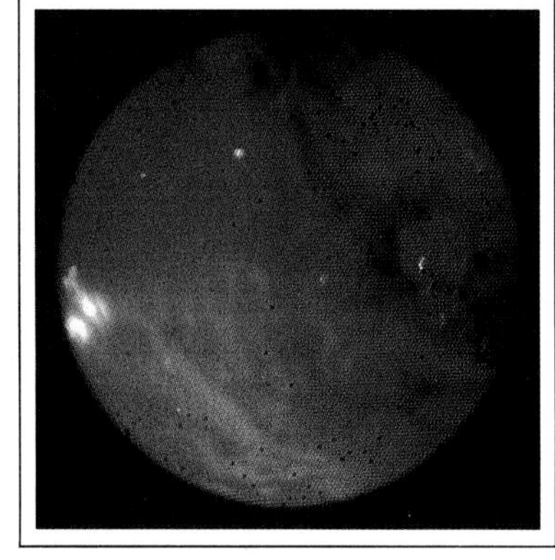

FIG. 33-11d.

FIG. 33-11. Esophageal varices. **a:** With a massively bleeding pyloric channel ulcer. The reflux of blood into the esophagus makes the esophagogastric junction seem to be the bleeding site. **b:** With an actively bleeding pyloric channel ulcer. With continued observation, the esophagogastric junction is now seen to be free of blood, suggesting that it is not the bleeding site. **c:** With an actively bleeding pyloric channel ulcer. On entry into the stomach, a massive amount of bright red blood is present with no apparent bleeding site. **d:** With an actively bleeding pyloric channel ulcer. Advancing the endoscope into the prepyloric region reveals an actively "pumping" bleeding site from which blood could be seen to be entering the stomach.

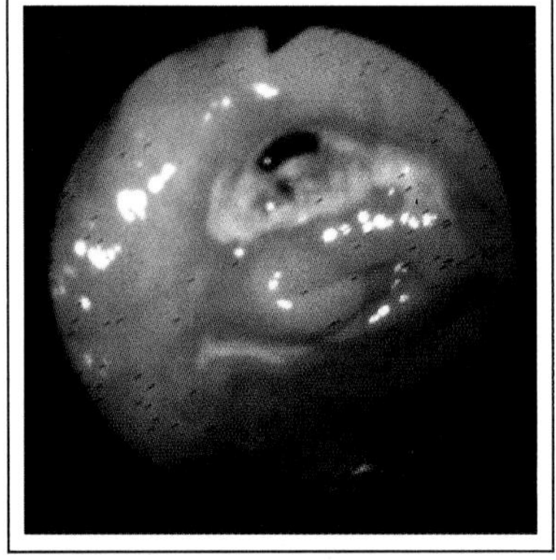

FIG. 33-12a.

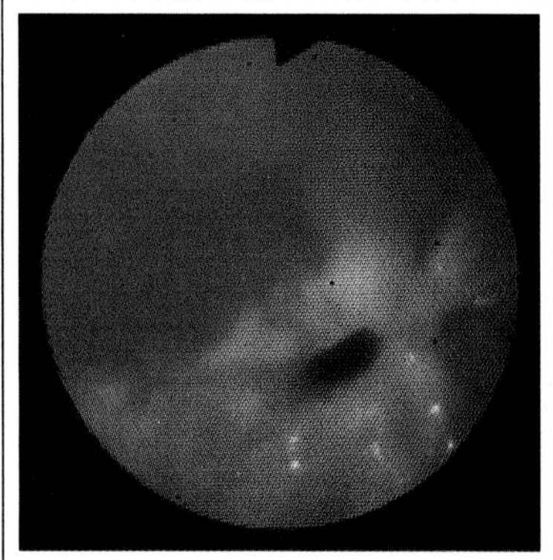

FIG. 33-12b.

FIG. 33-12. a: Gastric ulcer with evidence of recent bleeding in a patient with esophageal varices. The coffee-ground (acid hematin) material in the base marks this as a site of recent bleeding (see Chapter 36). **b:** Esophageal varix bleeding. Bright red blood wells up in the distal esophagus and completely obscures the varices.

uous Mallory-Weiss lesion or esophagitis is doubtful (Fig. 33-13), at least as far as this author is concerned. Moreover, it is uncertain whether such a distinction as bleeding from a Mallory-Weiss lesion adjacent to, but separate from, esophageal varices is useful, particularly when the outcome of such bleeding in our experience is more often like that of variceal bleeding (see Chapter 34) than the self-limited Mallory-Weiss tear (see Chapter 35). One would believe just the contrary, that the genesis of variceal bleeding and Mallory-Weiss tears are both the same—a sudden increase in intra-abdominal pressure with prolapse and dilatation of the esophagogastric junction[12]—making a Mallory-Weiss type mucosal tear which is contiguous to varices a most likely point for their rupture.

Another type of problematic case is that of gastric erosions taken as the site of bleeding in patients with esophageal varices. In the ASGE survey these accounted for half of the "other sites" of bleeding in patients with esophageal varices and approximately 20% of the final diagnoses of bleeding for all patients with esophageal varices.[5] In some of these cases, bleeding is undoubtedly from acute mucosal injury from alcohol or aspirin (see Chapter 36), but in others the erosions may have been artifacts from the placement of a nasogastric tube (see below) or from the endoscopic

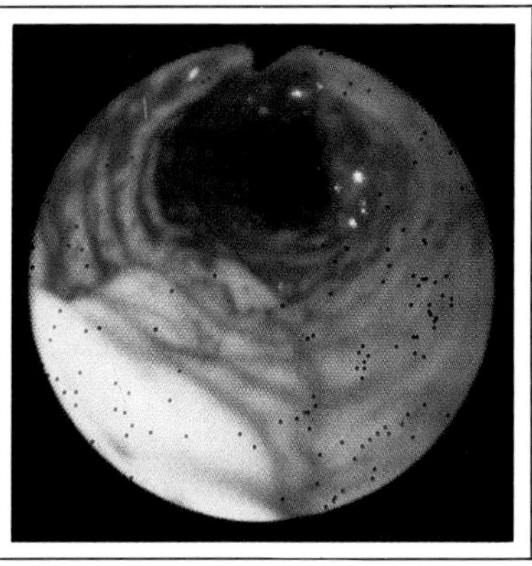

FIG. 33-13.

FIG. 33-13. Cardial bleeding thought to be from a Mallory-Weiss lesion in a patient with large esophageal varices. Cardial varices were not apparent. Because of the separation between the esophageal varices and the bleeding site and a history of vomiting just prior to the bleeding episode, a Mallory-Weiss lesion was suspected. At autopsy this was found to overlie a large submucosal varix.

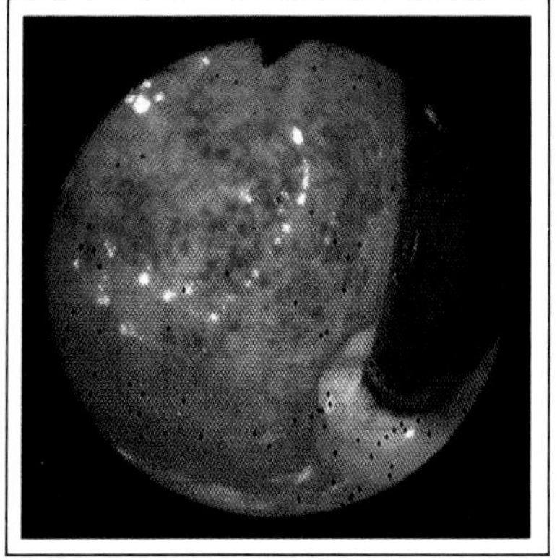

FIG. 33-14a.

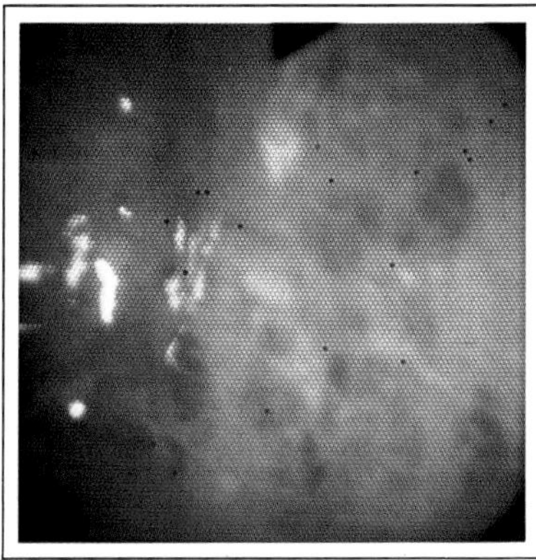

FIG. 33-14b.

FIG. 33-14. a: Endoscope-induced intramucosal hemorrhage simulating acute mucosal injury. Multiple petechiae were seen on U-type retroflexion in a patient with atrophic gastritis. The prominent mucosal capillaries in this condition are subject to instrument-induced trauma with resulting injury and mucosal bleeding. The uniform size of the petechiae serves to differentiate the appearance from that of acute mucosal injury (b). **b:** Acute mucosal injury secondary to alcohol. The petechiae are similar to those found in instrument-induced injury (a). The variation in size and shape, however, serves to differentiate them from those found with endoscope-induced trauma.

examination itself (Fig. 33-14a). Because both types of artifacts are identical in appearance—the erosions of acute mucosal injury—an erroneous impression of a bleeding site other than a varix would be created (Fig. 33-14b). In such a case, especially where a nasogastric tube has been previously placed, we regard the cause of the bleeding as indeterminate, with varices not excluded as a cause.

Distal Bleeding Sites

Bleeding which originates from the distal duodenum or even the jejunum can reflux back into the stomach, particularly if the bleeding lesion is obstructive, as in the case of a leiomyoma, a malignancy, or Crohn's disease (Fig. 33-15a). The blood in the stomach itself may create the picture of hemorrhagic gastritis (see above), and an erroneous interpretation would result if the duodenum itself were not carefully examined. One must suspect a distal bleeding site with the appearance of blood welling up in the descending duodenum (Fig. 33-15a), especially if it is disproportionate to the amount of blood in the stomach (Fig. 33-15b) or duodenal bulb.

Another finding we have encountered in patients with a distal duodenal bleeding site is the presence of blood mixed with bile in the gastric lake, giving it a dark brown (muddy) appearance (Fig. 33-15c), with no obvious bleeding site in either the stomach or the duodenal bulb.

In cases where a distal bleeding site is suspected, the examiner attempts to advance either a standard-length forward-viewing panendoscope at least into the third if not the fourth portion (Fig. 33-15d). In some cases the additional length provided by the side-viewing duodenoscope facilitates examination of the distal duodenum in order to find bleeding sites in cases which would otherwise have been left undiagnosed or with an erroneous interpretation of hemorrhagic gastritis.

Although blood welling up into the descending duodenum is an indication for careful examination of the third and fourth portions, the examiner must not neglect the commonest site of massive duodenal bleeding, which is the posterior wall of the duodenal bulb. Careful examination of this surface is mandatory in such cases so as to avoid the misinterpretation of a distal site in a patient with a bleeding posterior wall duodenal bulb ulcer (Fig. 33-16).

Nasogastric Suction Artifacts

Continuous or intermittent suction applied to the gastric mucosa through the side holes of a nasogastric tube can promote mucosal hemorrhage and erosions, which may: (a) simulate the picture of drug-induced (see Chapter 36) or emetogenic (see Chapter 35) mucosal injury; and (b) be itself a factor in perpetuating the bleeding episode. Although

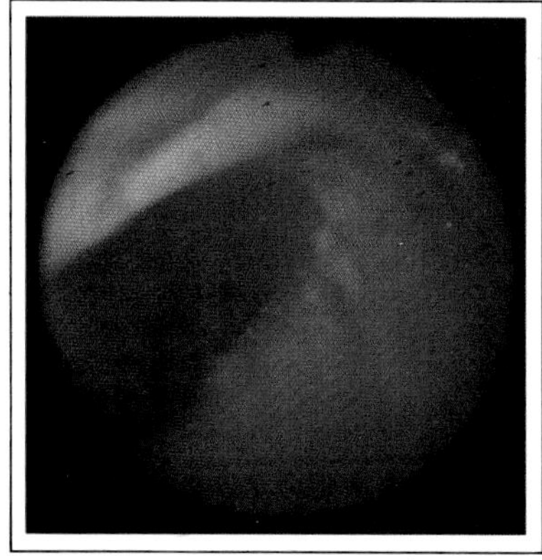

FIG. 33-15a.

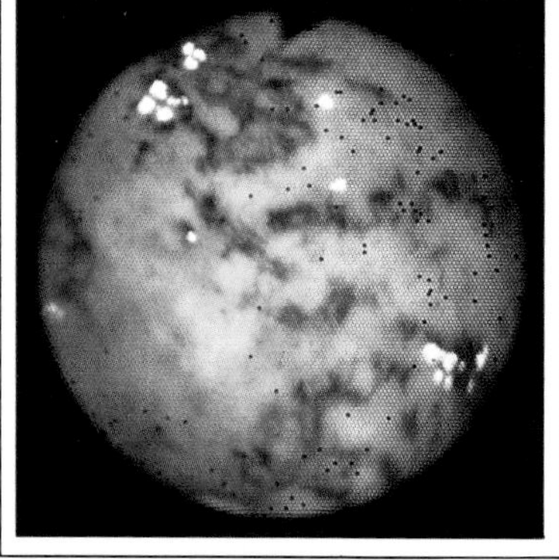

FIG. 33-15b.

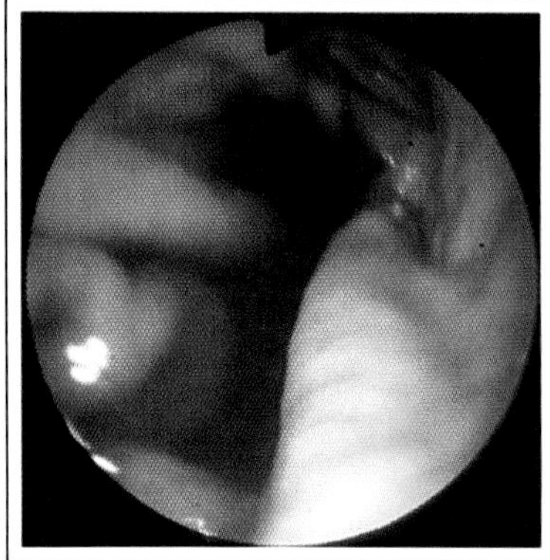

FIG. 33-15c.

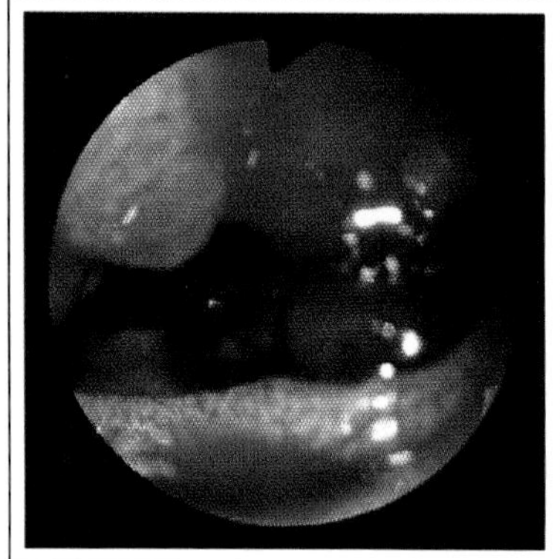

FIG. 33-15d.

FIG. 33-15. Distal (duodenal) bleeding site. **a:** Blood was observed to well up in the distal second portion. A distal bleeding site was suspected with only coffee-ground material (b) in the stomach and no proximal duodenal site found. **b:** Only scattered clots and coffee-ground (acid hematin) material were present in the stomach. **c:** Rather than clots (b), dark blood (acid hematin) mixed with bile, causing the gastric lake to appear muddy, may be the finding that suggests a distal bleeding site. **d:** An actively bleeding duodenal lymphoma was found on examination of the third portion. A clue to the presence of this was a muddy gastric lake (acid hematin material mixed with bile).

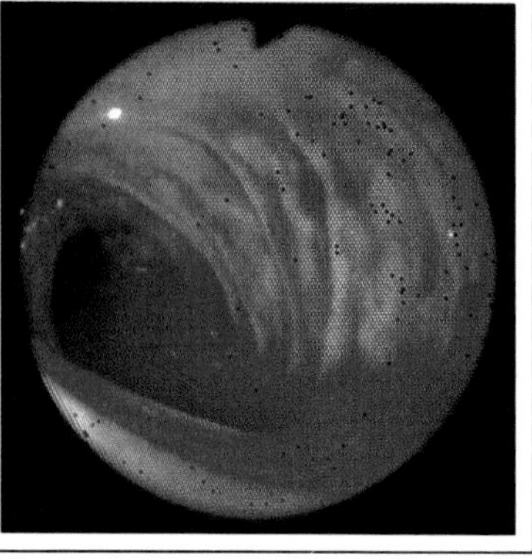

FIG. 33-16.

FIG. 33-16. Massive duodenal bulb ulcer bleeding (surgically proved) simulating a distal bleeding site. Blood seems to be welling up from the junction of the second and third portions. However, the presence of blood proximally (at 6 o'clock) should always make one suspect the bulb, the commonest site of duodenal bleeding.

scarcely mentioned in the literature,[3] these lesions deserve recognition because of their similarity to other sites of bleeding, which could potentially be both a source of interpretive error as to the cause of bleeding as well as a factor in the delay of treatment, i.e., removal of the nasogastric tube.

Incidence

The true incidence of these lesions is unknown. What is certain is that the nasogastric tube is commonly inserted in patients with GI bleeding to decompress the stomach, prevent further vomiting and hematemesis, serve as a means for administering antacids in a stuperous or uncooperative patient, and serve as a monitor for continued bleeding.

In the ASGE prospective survey, the nasogastric tube had been placed prior to endoscopy in 71% (1,498 of 2,097) of patients. At endoscopy, gastric erosions were found in 620 of the 2,097, which in 152 cases were not believed to be the cause of bleeding. However, there was no mention in the survey as to how often the examiner thought the erosions were attributable to the nasogastric tube. If one were to assume that in many of these cases the erosions may have been nasogastric-tube-induced, then the incidence of

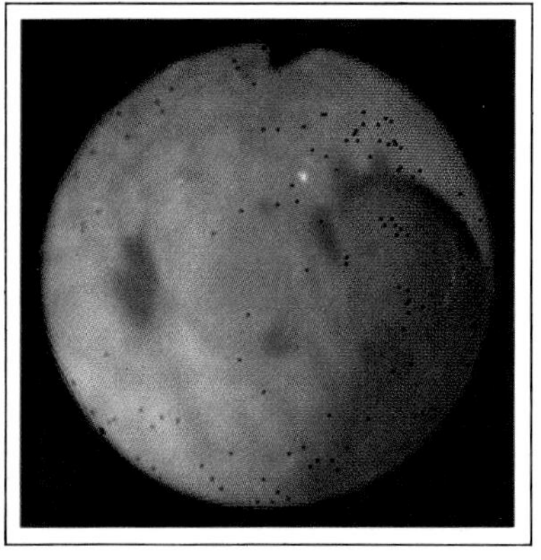

FIG. 33-17a.

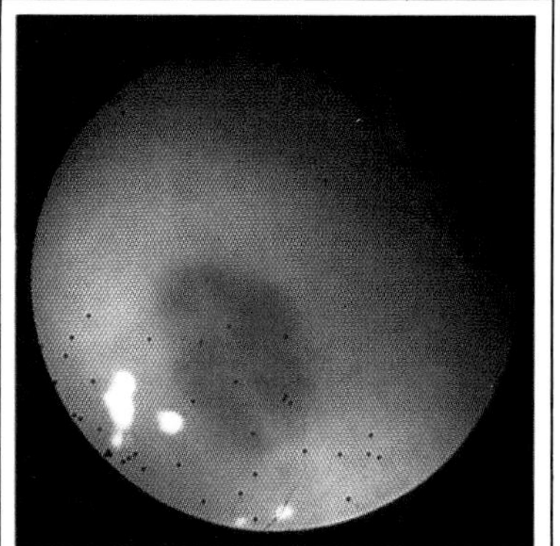

FIG. 33-17b.

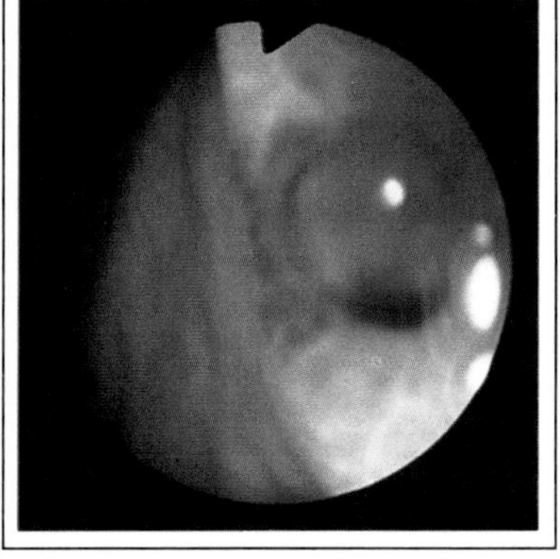

FIG. 33-17c.

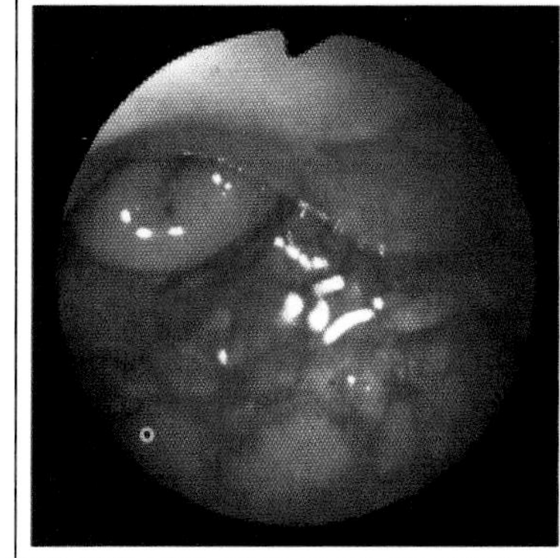

FIG. 33-17d.

FIG. 33-17. Nasogastric suction artifacts. **a:** Early lesions. Endoscopy was performed because of coffee-ground returns in a patient with intestinal obstruction who had had a nasogastric tube in place for 12 hr. Multiple, focal 3- to 5-mm areas of intramucosal hemorrhage were found, some (not pictured) having adherent clots (erosions). In this case continuous suction (wall type) had been used, being set at the maximum pressures (>100 mm Hg). **b:** Early lesion. A close-up view shows this to consist of small foci of intramucosal hemorrhage. **c:** Early lesion. A clot is seen within the center of the lesion indicating that a break in the mucosa has occurred, i.e., the presence of an erosion. A peripheral zone of intramucosal hemorrhage having a diameter of more than 1 cm is also seen. **d:** Actively bleeding. Bright red blood can be seen to ooze from a large early lesion [similar to that in (c)]. The indication for nasogastric suction in this case was intestinal obstruction.

nasogastric tube artifacts could approach up to 10% of the cases where the nasogastric tube had been placed prior to endoscopy.

Clinical Setting

We find that virtually all patients who have had continuous nasogastric suction for more than 24 hr for reasons other than bleeding and who subsequently have endoscopy, particularly those in whom continuous (wall-type) suction with pressures in excess of 100 mm Hg was employed, show discrete areas of gastric intramucosal hemorrhage and erosions with focal bleeding. With the use of intermittent suction at this pressure, the incidence of bleeding is reduced but acute injury effects are still present in at least 50% at 24 hr and in a higher percentage (≥80%) if the suction was continued at this pressure for more than 48 hr. In cases where continuous suction is employed at lower pressures (35 to 75 mm Hg), the incidence of nasogastric suction artifacts is somewhat reduced; however, these artifacts are found in a percentage comparable to that associated with the use of higher intermittent suction pressures when sustained for more than 48 hr. These lesions are usually not seen with low intermittent suction (bedside-Gomco type) with pressure settings of less than 35 mm Hg.

Appearance

Multiple acute mucosal lesions in a patient who has had nasogastric aspiration at high continuous or intermittent pressures would make the examiner consider suction artifacts, especially in the absence of a history suggestive of drug-induced mucosal injury. Like the lesions associated with alcohol- or aspirin-induced mucosal injury (see Chapter 36), suction artifacts have a typical early and late appearance.

Early lesions.

Early lesions are found as multiple (generally 5 to 10) sites of intramucosal hemorrhage running along a line on the greater curve. The lesions themselves appear as discrete bright or dark circular areas, 4 to 8 mm in diameter (Fig. 33-17a). They are probably formed because of suction trauma to the mucosa with rupture of capillaries and resultant intramucosal hemorrhage. On close examination these appear as multiple focal, minute reddened areas (Fig. 33-17b). In some cases the injury appears along with bleeding from the mucosal surface and so justifies the term erosion. Here, we find the evidence of bleeding in the form of adherent clots (Fig. 33-17c). Although most of these erosions are similar in size to that of intramucosal hemorrhages, 4 to

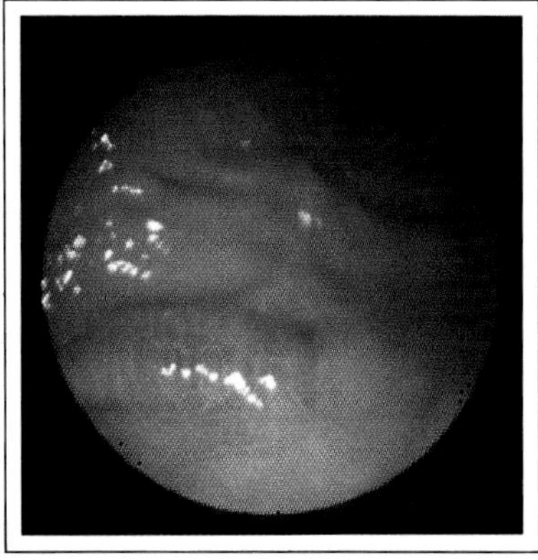

FIG. 33-18a.

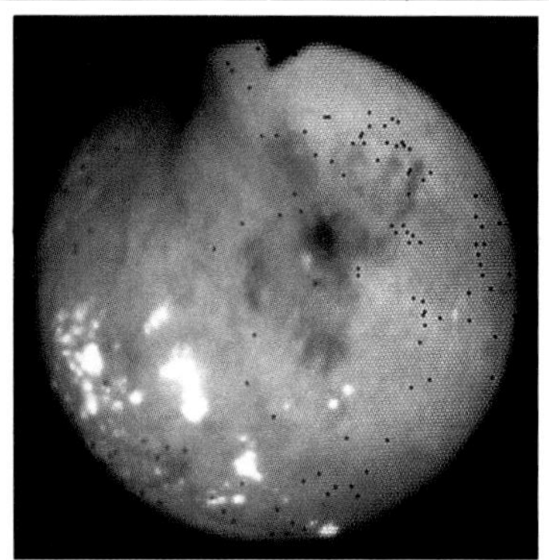

FIG. 33-18b.

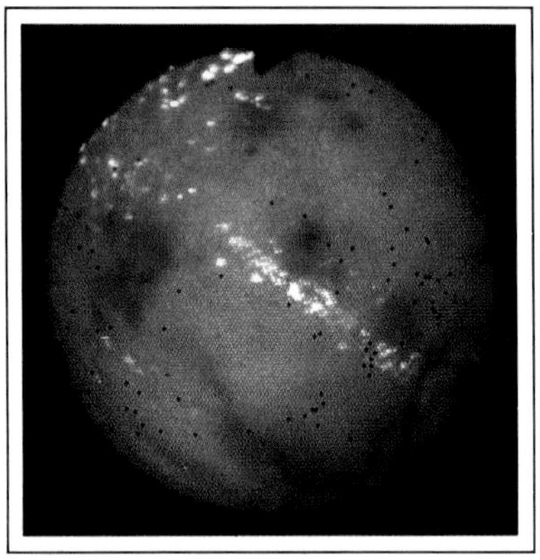

FIG. 33-18c.

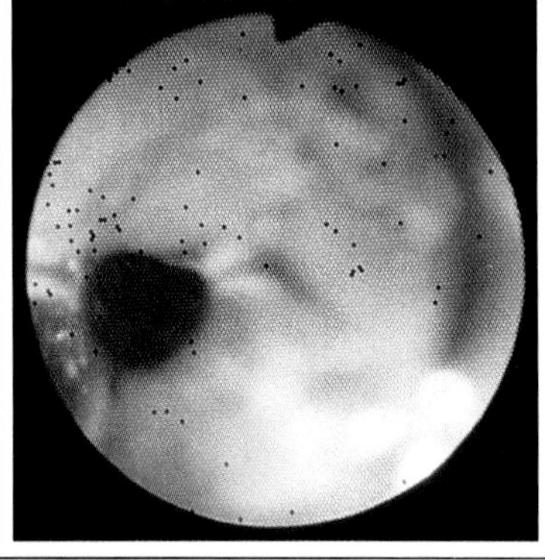

FIG. 33-18d.

FIG. 33-18. Nasogastric suction artifact. **a:** Late lesion. A patient in whom a nasogastric tube had been placed after surgery was examined because of coffee-ground returns. The procedure was performed 24 hr after the nasogastric tube had been withdrawn. The 1.5-cm area of focal erythema seen at 7 o'clock probably represents a suction artifact that had the appearance seen in Fig. 33-17c, but which at the time it was examined was fading. **b:** Late lesion. Some peripheral fading has probably occurred where there was only intramucosal hemorrhage. The central clot remains, marking the point of maximum mucosal injury. **c:** Multiple early lesions. In this case, where the nasogastric tube had remained for 5 days, multiple areas of focal intramusocal hemorrhage and erosions cause the inherent linear pattern of these artifacts (Fig. 33-17a) to be lost. The focal nature of these lesions, however, still serves to differentiate them from acute drug-induced mucosal injury (Fig. 33-14b). **d:** Late lesions, in a patient who had had prolonged nasogastric suction. There is an extensive exudative lesion around the cardia with signs of recent bleeding (acid hematin material). The location of this lesion in the cardia, as well as the use of continuous ("wall-type") suction exceeding 100 mm Hg, is compatible with the diagnosis of a nasogastric suction artifact.

8 mm in diameter, some are larger, exceeding 1.5 cm (Fig. 33-17c). In these cases where larger erosions are present, active bleeding may be observed in the form of oozing (Fig. 33-17d).

Late lesions.

If the nasogastric tube has already been removed at 24 hr, smaller areas of intramucosal hemorrhage may have already begun to fade (Fig. 33-18a). Some of the larger erosions still show the central clot but with peripheral fading (Fig. 33-18b). Continuation of nasogastric suction may cause multiple lines of erosions to form, so that the linear distribution of the nasogastric suction artifacts may be obscured, causing them to further resemble acute drug-induced mucosal injury (Fig. 33-18b). The larger lesions, especially those in which overlying clots appear, develop acute inflammatory exudate in association with a clot as it begins to organize. As in the case of late hemorrhagic erosive gastritis (see Chapter 36), the exudate may become more apparent after the clot has fallen off (Fig. 33-18c). At 24 hr of continuous 100 mm Hg suction, 50 to 75% of the lesions are of the exudative type (Fig. 33-18d). Some of the blood clot is present within the exudate, and blood may be seen to ooze from the lesion into the surrounding mucosa.

Treatment

The obvious therapeutic maneuver in these cases is removal of the nasogastric tube even in the presence of some ongoing bleeding, which generally stops if the cause of the continued injury is eliminated. To use antacids or other agents (e.g., cimetidine) for these lesions and not remove the cause, we believe, places the patient in jeopardy of continued bleeding, which is occasionally substantial.

Prevention

As these lesions rarely form with intermittent suction employed at pressures of less than 35 mm Hg, the endoscopist should attempt to educate all concerned in the care of patients with upper GI bleeding about the dangers of intermittent suction at high pressure and continuous suction at any pressure, especially that exceeding 50 mm Hg. The use of a suction apparatus which routinely achieves pressures in excess of 100 mm Hg (wall suction) should be discouraged.

REFERENCES

1. Palmer, E. D. (1969): The vigorous diagnostic approach to upper gastrointestinal tract hemorrhage. *JAMA*, 207:1477–1480.

2. Dagradi, A. E., and Stempien, S. J. (1969): Esophagogastroscopy during active upper gastrointestinal bleeding. *Am. J. Gastroenterol.*, 51:498–505.
3. Morrissey, J. F. (1981): Clinical approach to diagnostic endoscopy in patients with upper gastrointestinal bleeding. *Dig. Dis. Sci. (Suppl.)*, 26:65–115.
4. Waterman, N. G., and Walker, J. L. (1973): The effect of gastric cooling on hemostasis. *Surg. Gynecol. Obstet.*, 137:80–82.
5. Gilbert, D. A., Silverstein, F. E., Tedesco, F. J., Buenger, N. K., Persing, J., and 277 members of the ASGE (1981): The national ASGE survey on upper gastrointestinal bleeding. III. Endoscopy in upper gastrointestinal bleeding. *Gastrointest. Endosc.*, 27:94–102.
6. Greenblatt, D. J., and Koch-Weser, J. (1973): Adverse reactions to intravenous diazepam. *Am. J. Med. Sci.*, 266:261–266.
7. Wissler, D. W., and Morrissey, J. F. (1980): Use of an external suction-irrigation device in endoscopy. *Gastrointest. Endosc.*, 26:11–12.
8. Wright, R. A. (1980): Upper-esophageal perforation with a flexible endoscope secondary to cervical osteophytes. *Dig. Dis. Sci.*, 25:66–68.
9. Mogan, G. R., Gottfried, E. B., and Waye, J. D. (1980): A technique of emergency upper gastrointestinal endoscopy in adults using a small caliber endoscope (GIF-P2). *Gastrointest. Endosc.*, 26:126–127.
10. Gaisford, W. D. (1979): Endoscopic electrohemostasis of active upper gastrointestinal bleeding. *Am. J. Surg.*, 137:47–53.
11. Pitcher, J. L. (1977): Variceal hemorrhage among patients with varices and upper gastrointestinal hemorrhage. *South. Med. J.*, 70:1183–1185.
12. Liebowitz, H. R. (1961): Pathogenesis of esophageal varix rupture. *JAMA*, 175:874–879.

34

ESOPHAGEAL BLEEDING

Esophageal bleeding may be from a variety of sites; however, as was true in the ASGE prospective survey, the predominant cause is esophageal varix bleeding.[1] Varices (apart from exceptional cases of "downhill" varices—see Chapter 8) do not originate in the esophagus but are derived from short gastric veins and may have an esophagogastric junction component. Nevertheless, we regard them as a cause of esophageal bleeding because they are principally recognized as esophageal structures both in the nonbleeding patient (see Chapter 8) and in the course of a bleeding episode. The finding of varices in the body of the esophagus is the decisive visual clue.

In this chapter our major concern is with bleeding esophageal varices. Our approach is to briefly describe the clinical presentation and pathogenesis of the bleeding, the rationale for endoscopy, the endoscopic appearance, and particular types of interpretive problems for this type of bleeding. In a subsequent section we similarly discuss esophagitis, an important although less frequent cause of esophageal bleeding, and in a concluding section we briefly present a variety of uncommon causes of esophageal bleeding, including carcinoma and other tumors, achalasia, and vascular lesions, all of which account for less than 1% of cases of esophageal bleeding.

ESOPHAGEAL VARICES

As esophageal varix bleeding occurs for the most part as sequela of alcoholic cirrhosis,[2] the frequency with which the individual endoscopist encounters this type of bleeding depends to a large extent on the prevalence of alcoholism and alcoholic liver disease in the hospital population served. As summarized by Graham and Davis,[3] the largest proportion of cases of variceal bleeding in endoscopic series reported for 1969 through 1976 (15 to 20% of the total) was found in those from municipal or military (including Veterans Administration) centers where the prevalence of alcoholism may approach 50%.[4,5] Endoscopic series reporting the lowest proportion of variceal bleeding (less than 5%) have been largely from community and private university hospitals where the incidence of alcoholism is generally less than 20%.[6] In the ASGE prospective survey[1] varices were considered to be the cause of bleeding for 10.3%, midway between the higher percentage reported from centers with a high prevalence (50%) of alcoholism and those where it is lower (less than 20%). Similar to the ASGE survey, among our patients (see Table 32-2) variceal bleeding accounted for 12.8% of the total.

The typical patient is one with known or strongly suspected advanced alcoholic liver disease.[2] The stigmata of liver disease, particularly ascites, are present in many but not all cases. The patient with variceal bleeding characteristically presents at endoscopy having had a substantial or massive bleeding episode evident by vomiting or by a nasogastric tube return of bright red blood and with transfusion requirements in excess of 4 units of blood within the first 24 hr.[7,7a,8] Other causes of bleeding may be found in 30 to 60% of patients with esophageal varices, but usually such patients present with less bleeding.[7,7a]

Pathogenesis

There is no general agreement as to what determines the degree to which varices bleed or if they bleed at all. It is our view that variceal bleeding is best thought of as a "blowout" of a varix.[9] This has been likened by Conn to the eruption of a volcano.[10] The likelihood of a blowout has been related to the size of a varix, with patients who have the largest varices (most prominently projecting into the lumen) but not necessarily the highest portal pressures standing the greatest chance of bleeding.[11] What predisposes such varices to bleed, we believe, is that the mucosa which overlies them is already stretched to the breaking point. Any further stretching of the mucosa, as might occur with vomiting, retching, heavy lifting, or coughing,[9] could exert enough of a shearing force to split it. It seems likely that a combination of the sudden application of a shearing force to the mucosa overlying the varix and an abrupt increase in portal pressure would be capable of producing a blowout at the point where the mucosa is split. Larger tears might be expected over larger varices, which in our experience are associated with the most massive bleeding.

Rationale for Endoscopy

Variceal bleeding is a serious, highly lethal condition that carries the highest mortality rate (30%+) of any of the major causes of gastrointestinal (GI) bleeding. In the ASGE prospective survey, the mortality rate for variceal bleeding was 30.1%,[12] in contrast to a 10.8% mortality rate for the entire study population.[1] Because of the serious loss during variceal bleeding, as reflected in the associated mortality rate,[6] endoscopy is requested whenever the diagnosis is suspected both in cases with continued bleeding and where the bleeding appears to stop. The thoughtful endoscopist wonders just when endoscopy for variceal bleeding is likely to be the most beneficial.

Continued Bleeding

We believe endoscopy is indicated in a patient with known or suspected esophageal varices whose bleeding has been continuous for 12 hr because of the high probability that a specific intervention such as endoscopic sclerotherapy,[12a] placement of Sengstaken-Blakemore tube,[12b] or emergency shunt or surgery[12c] will be considered necessary. Before any specific therapeutic intervention occurs, endoscopy would almost certainly be sought to establish a definite diagnosis of variceal bleeding.

Bleeding Which Appears to Have Stopped

Sixty percent of variceal bleeding spontaneously stops within the first 24 hr; however, up to one-third of these cases may be expected to rebleed.[8] Such bleeding places the patient at the same high risk as those in whom bleeding has continued; it also increases the likelihood that a specific therapeutic intervention will be required. The decision to examine a patient whose bleeding has stopped is made somewhat more difficult by the fact that there is a small but definite risk of rebleeding as a result of endoscopy itself. In the ASGE prospective survey, 215 patients with variceal bleeding were endoscoped at the time the bleeding had stopped; of these the bleeding resumed in three (1.4%) after endoscopy.[12] In one of these cases, the bleeding resulted in the death of the patient, who exsanguinated during the procedure. If one considered the risk for patients to rebleed spontaneously to be on the order of 20% (one-third of 60% who spontaneously stop bleeding), and if the risk of a rebleed with endoscopy were itself only on the order of 1 to 2%, then endoscopy would be justified, especially if benefit results from a precise diagnosis obtained at a time the patient is not bleeding. One would expect this to be more likely to occur in a patient who would be a candidate for a therapeutic intervention, e.g., endoscopic sclerosis[12a] or surgery.[12c] A critically ill patient with advanced liver disease, early encephalopathy, or other major medical problems, however, would not be a candidate for endoscopy especially if a specific therapeutic intervention, such as sclerotherapy, was not to follow.

Appearance of Variceal Bleeding

The endoscopist may expect three types of appearance at endoscopy in patients with an episode of variceal bleeding: (a) torrential bleeding; (b) slow bleeding; and (c) no bleeding.

Torrential Bleeding

It is often said that massive, continuous hemorrhage is found in up to one-third of the cases of variceal bleeding[7]; however, the endoscopist probably encounters this type of torrential bleeding less often—in more like 5 to 10% of the cases. In the ASGE prospective survey, only 7.5% of the cases of variceal bleeding were found at endoscopy to be "pumping" and so would likely have received the designation torrential—but not the 25.3% observed to be "oozing" and certainly not the remainder who had either no blood (55.9%) or only a clot (11.2%).[13] The lower percentage of torrential bleeding observed by endoscopists may be the result of a bias against examining patients with the most active bleeding. Rather than performing endoscopy during this phase, many recommend arteriography to define the varices and to allow vasopressin administration, which could lead to the bleeding either slowing down or stopping in up to one-third of the cases.[14] One might expect that the more aggressive the endoscopist is about studying such patients with massive variceal bleeding early the higher the percentage of torrential bleeding he might encounter. In our experience, the incidence of torrential bleeding lies somewhere between the ASGE figure of 7.5% and that from reported series (20 to 30%).[7] Of 64 patients with variceal bleeding studied in our Unit, the bleeding was considered to be massive or torrential in nine (15%).

In patients with torrential bleeding, the examiner finds bright red blood welling up in the distal 3 to 5 cm of the esophagus (Fig. 34-1a), the site of most variceal bleeding.[14a] The varices themselves are first seen only above this pool of blood in the mid or mid-distal portion (Fig. 34-1b).

The varices seen in the presence of torrential bleeding are often not the largest (grade IV—see Chapter 8), even though recent studies suggest that these are the varices most likely to bleed.[10,11] Several reasons may be given for this. First, the endoscopist may be viewing the varices at a considerable distance from the gastroesophageal (GE) junction, where they are expected to be at their maximum size. Second, the bleeding itself may have resulted in a decrease of variceal size, associated with a reduction in portal pressure

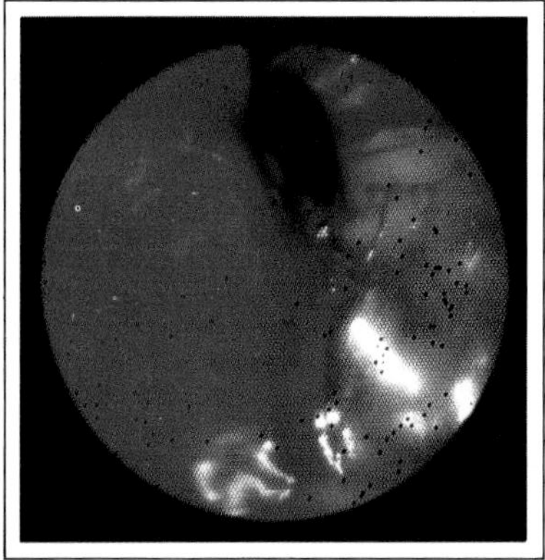

FIG. 34-1a.

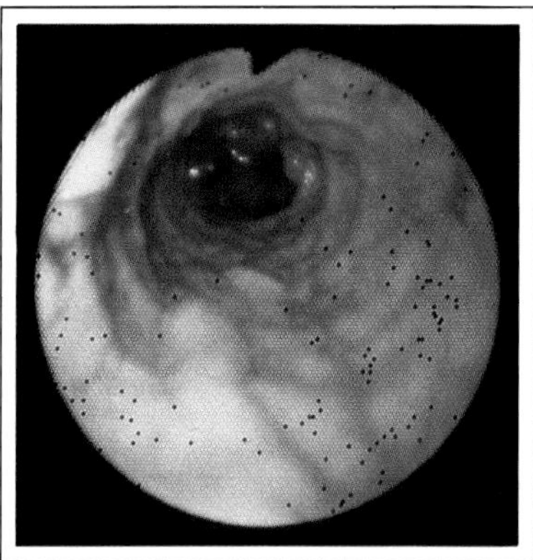

FIG. 34-1b.

FIG. 34-1. Bleeding esophageal varices. **a:** Blood wells up in the distal esophagus, obscuring the varices present. **b:** The varices themselves are identified in the mid-distal portion above the site of active bleeding, which is most commonly in the distal 2 to 3 cm. Because of the location (mid-esophagus, as well as the bleeding itself), the varices appear small (grade II).

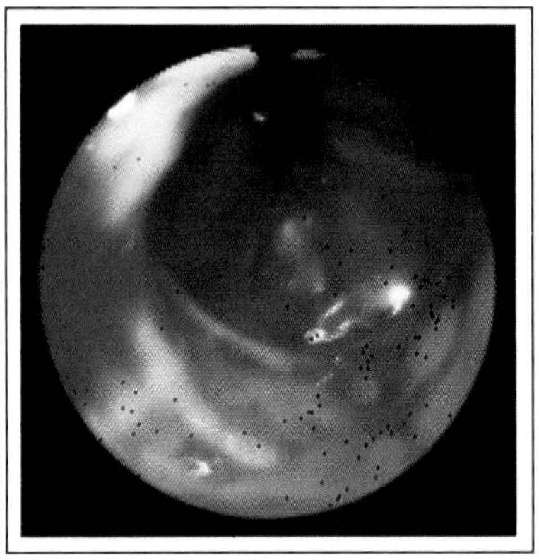

FIG. 34-2a.

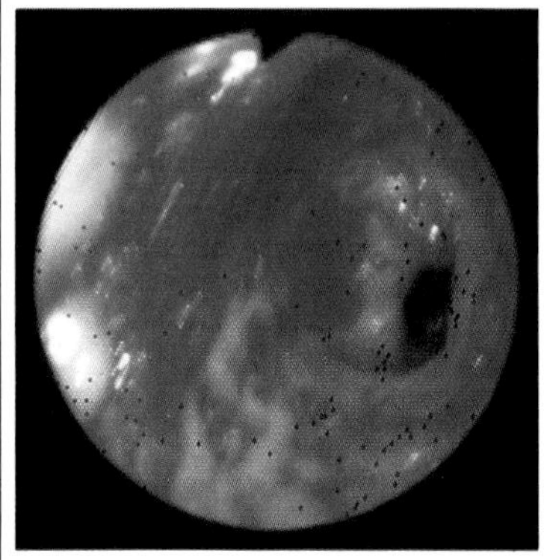

FIG. 34-2b.

FIG. 34-2. Esophageal varices in the distal esophagus with slow ooze. **a:** A small pool of blood obscures the varices. With the patient on his left side, the ongoing ooze produces a collection of bright red blood on the left (9 o'clock) wall. **b:** Clearing of the pool of blood which had obscured the distal esophagus (a) allows the varices to be seen as small, gray-blue elevations (9 o'clock). From within the center of this field, bright red blood emanates, indicating a variceal bleed. The varices themselves are most likely collapsed (grade II) from the magnitude of the bleed.

from the bleeding itself, especially when it is torrential (Fig. 34-1b).

Because the actual bleeding or blowout site generally lies within the pool of blood where the magnitude of bleeding would be regarded as massive or torrential, the endoscopist does not fruitlessly search for the specific point. Rather, he proceeds to examine as best as he can the stomach, especially the lesser curve, 2 cm on either side of the gastric angle, the prepyloric antrum, and the posterior wall of the duodenal bulb to exclude a bleeding ulcer which could mimic a massive reflux of blood (see Chapter 33).

Slow Bleeding

In the majority of cases the endoscopist sees variceal bleeding which appears as a slow ooze from the varices themselves, generally in association with clot formation (Fig. 34-2a). These clots tend to adhere to the mucosa overlying the actual rupture of the varix in the distal 2 cm of the esophagus. In the ASGE survey, an ooze or clot was found in 36.5% of the cases overall and 51% (117 of 229) of the cases with the final diagnosis of variceal bleeding. In these patients this appearance was five times more common than a pumping varix (51% versus 10.5%), giving rise to torrential bleeding.

The varices themselves (Fig. 34-3a) are generally of the large, grade IV type (see Chapter 8) unless there has been prior massive bleeding for which the patient has not received adequate volume replacement (Fig. 34-2b). In fact, if the patient has had only a modest bleed with adequate volume replacement, the appearance of small varices is an indication for a careful search of the stomach and duodenum to exclude other sites of bleeding.

No Bleeding

In many cases the endoscopist concludes that the varices were the cause of bleeding in the absence of other potential sites. In 40% of the cases where variceal bleeding was the final diagnosis in the ASGE survey, the endoscopist observed only varices, without either bleeding (as pumping or oozing) or clot. In these cases the endoscopist saw no other sites of bleeding, either potential or actual.[13]

As in the case of slow bleeding, the endoscopist expects to find large, grade IV varices, especially in patients whose blood volume has been adequately restored (Fig. 34-3b). In a small percentage there are adherent clots marking the site of bleeding even though no blood is observed. We have occasionally noted the appearance of a discrete, elevated red point (Fig. 34-3c) which may represent the site of blowout after disruption of the clot. As the site of a recent variceal blowout, it may be that this finding indicates an increased risk for rebleeding over and above the 30% rebleeding rate overall.[8]

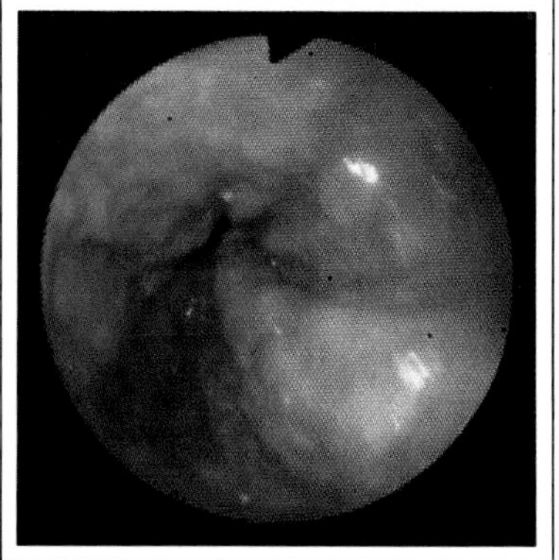

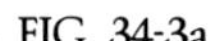
FIG. 34-3a.

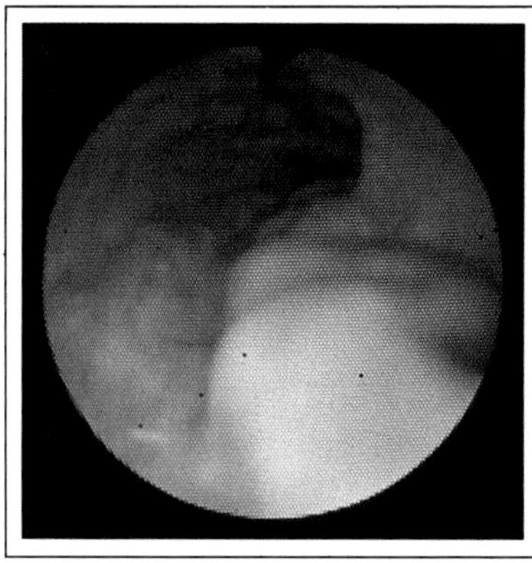

FIG. 34-3b.

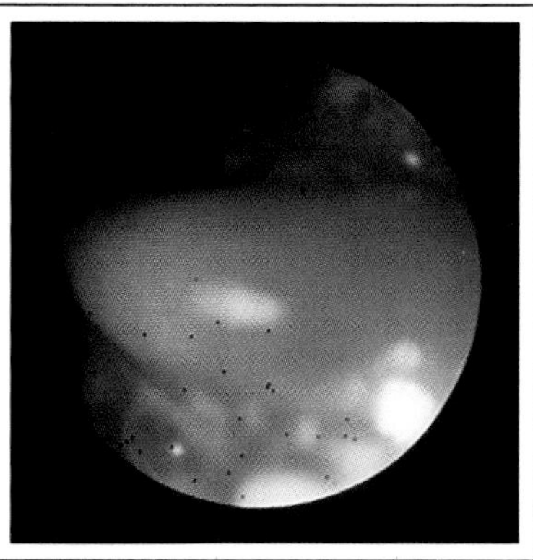

FIG. 34-3c.

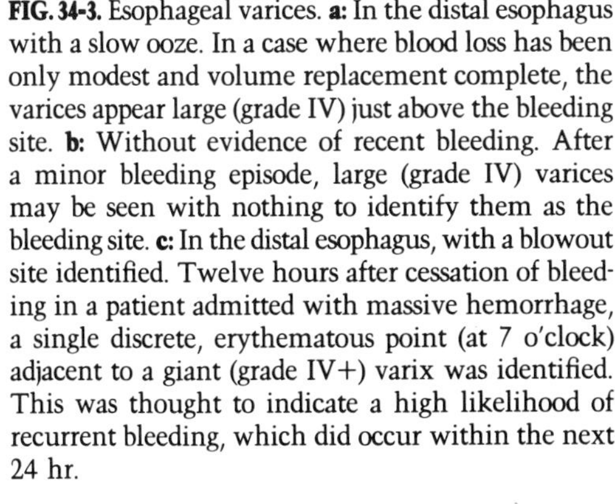
FIG. 34-3. Esophageal varices. **a:** In the distal esophagus with a slow ooze. In a case where blood loss has been only modest and volume replacement complete, the varices appear large (grade IV) just above the bleeding site. **b:** Without evidence of recent bleeding. After a minor bleeding episode, large (grade IV) varices may be seen with nothing to identify them as the bleeding site. **c:** In the distal esophagus, with a blowout site identified. Twelve hours after cessation of bleeding in a patient admitted with massive hemorrhage, a single discrete, erythematous point (at 7 o'clock) adjacent to a giant (grade IV+) varix was identified. This was thought to indicate a high likelihood of recurrent bleeding, which did occur within the next 24 hr.

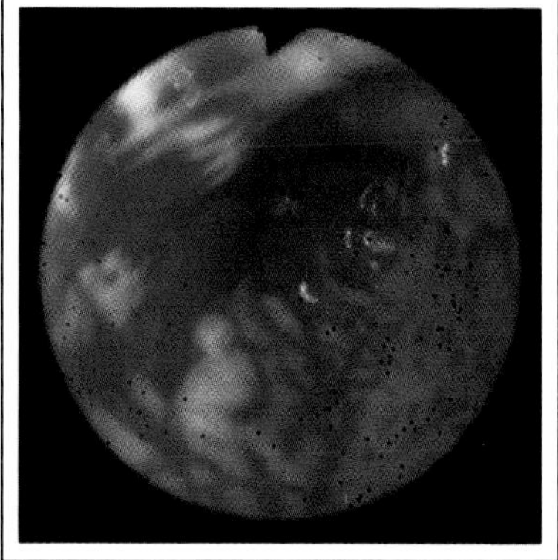

FIG. 34-4a.

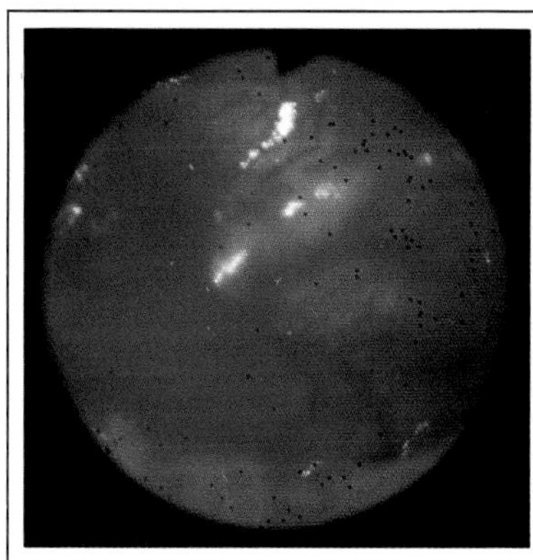

FIG. 34-4b.

FIG. 34-4. a: Esophageal varices covered by blood from a nonvariceal bleeding site. Blood has refluxed into the distal esophagus and covers varices so as to appear as a variceal bleed. In this case massive bleeding had occurred from the pyloroduodenal junction (b). **b:** Pyloroduodenal ulcer bleed in a patient with esophageal varices. In this patient the bleeding site is the pyloroduodenal junction. With massive bleeding, there is reflux into the esophagus, which gives an erroneous impression of variceal bleeding (a).

Interpretive Problems

The correct identification of the source of bleeding in patients with esophageal varices is often considered a difficult judgment by many endoscopists. As one might expect, correct diagnosis means avoiding two kinds of error: (a) attributing bleeding from other causes to varices; (b) confusing true variceal bleeding with that from other sites.

Other Causes of Bleeding Which May Be Called Variceal

As was considered in our general discussion of interpretive problems confronting the endoscopist in the bleeding patient (see Chapter 33), blood present in the stomach in massive amounts may freely reflux into the esophagus (Fig. 33-4a). Although much of the blood is eventually cleared from the esophagus, clots may be left behind which adhere to the esophageal mucosa. The blood from a massively bleeding gastric site may be bright red or maroon, which along with the clots creates a picture that in the presence of sizable varices may be indistinguishable from that of actual variceal bleeding (Fig. 34-4a). Were the endoscopist reluctant to enter the stomach because of a massive amount of blood in the distal esophagus, on the basis of that appearance alone he would erroneously conclude the bleeding to be variceal.

This problem will be obviated to the extent that the stomach can be examined adequately. Despite the amount

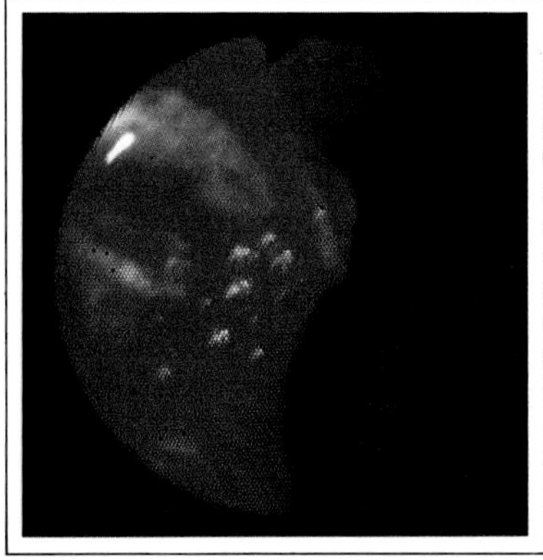

FIG. 34-5a.

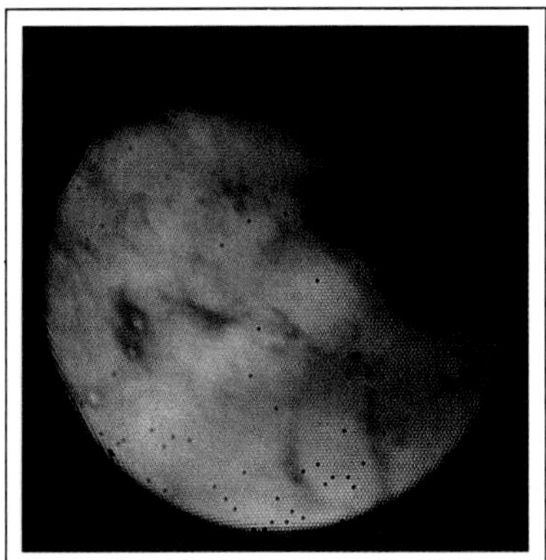

FIG. 34-5b.

FIG. 34-5. a: Variceal bleeding, raising the possibility of a separate Mallory-Weiss lesion. Because of the cardial location of the bleeding point, as well as its puckered appearance, a Mallory-Weiss tear (see Chapter 35) was considered; however, the clinical course favored the diagnosis of variceal bleeding. **b:** Nonspecific acute gastric mucosal injury in a patient with variceal bleeding which has stopped (Fig. 34-3a). Nonspecific acute focal intramucosal hemorrhage—which in this case could well have been from nasogastric suction—might be mistaken for a true bleeding site.

of blood in the distal esophagus, it is generally possible to enter the stomach, even if largely by a blind "slide-by" maneuver, i.e., torquing the tip while still in the esophagus in a counterclockwise (anterior) direction, an up deflection, and advancing into the upper body (see Chapter 11). Once the stomach is entered, the endoscopist attempts to examine three critical areas; this may be accomplished even if the stomach is full of blood. These are: (a) the lesser curvature of the body; (b) the gastric angle; and (c) the duodenal bulb. By carefully examining these surfaces, he may find an actively bleeding ulcer (Fig. 34-4b) which could mimic variceal bleeding clinically[7] and endoscopically.

True Variceal Bleeding Interpreted as Bleeding from Other Sites

Because it is now well known that varices coexist with other causes of bleeding in at least 30% of the patients,[12] the endoscopist, even in the face of obvious variceal bleeding (Fig. 34-5a) may wonder about nonspecific appearances, e.g., scattered gastric erosions (Fig. 33-5b), as possibly being indicative of acute mucosal injury (hemorrhagic-erosive gastritis) bleeding from alcohol (see Chapter 36). Some endoscopists consider other appearances of the mucosa overlying or contiguous with varices—e.g., multiple erosions or single cleft-like defects (Fig. 34-5a) suggestive of Mallory-Weiss lesions—as indicative of an alternative cause of bleeding (see Chapter 33). In the ASGE survey, 25% of the "other" sites of bleeding in patients with esophageal varices were either Mallory-Weiss lesions (14.6%) or esophagitis (11%). We believe such appearances do not constitute strong evidence of an alternate cause, especially if the bleeding has been massive, which is the characteristic clinical picture of variceal bleeding.[7,7a] Indeed, any Mallory-Weiss lesion of the cardia could well represent the blowout point of a submucosal varix in that area. An appearance such as that of gastric erosions located at some distance from the varices does warrant consideration as a potential alternate bleeding site. However, these lesions should be generalized rather than focal and should in all other ways be truly representative of bleeding from acute mucosal injury (see Chapter 36). Even with a more diffuse mucosal effect, if the bleeding is truly massive with a sizable transfusion requirement and peptic ulcer disease is not present, the diagnosis of variceal bleeding is still favored. This is so because of the predisposition of varices rather than gastric erosions to produce massive bleeding[7] with the latter appearance possibly caused by shock or other "stress" factors (see Chapter 37).

ESOPHAGITIS

Esophagitis as a cause of upper GI bleeding is encountered in occasional patients. We found it to account for only 1.6% of our cases over a 7-year period (see Table 32-2). This accords with an incidence of 2%, similar to that reportea from at least four centers.[3] Somewhat surprising was the relatively large number of patients (8%) in the ASGE prospective survey who had esophagitis (6.3%) or closely related esophageal ulcer bleeding (1.7%) as a final diagnosis. Among these patients, the incidence of esophagitis bleeding was similar to that from esophageal varices (10.3%). The commonest types of esophagitis associated with bleeding are the peptic and drug-induced (largely aspirin) forms. These are considered in the next section along with the other less common varieties of esophagitis which are associated with bleeding from time to time.

Peptic Esophagitis

Bleeding in patients with peptic esophagitis is not uncommon. In a 20-year prospective study, Palmer found that 26.6% of patients in whom this diagnosis had been established had at least one bleeding episode.[15] This is similar to the reported cumulative incidence of bleeding in patients with peptic ulcer disease[16] even though frank ulceration or its equivalent adherent inflammatory exudate (pseudomembrane) is found at endoscopy in only one-third of the patients with symptomatic esophageal reflux.[17] In most cases symptoms of peptic esophagitis are well established prior to the bleed, often with a history of an increase in symptoms or superimposed vomiting prior to hematemesis.[18] Another setting is in the patient with nasogastric-tube-induced esophagitis where the tube has been in place for several weeks (see Chapter 3).

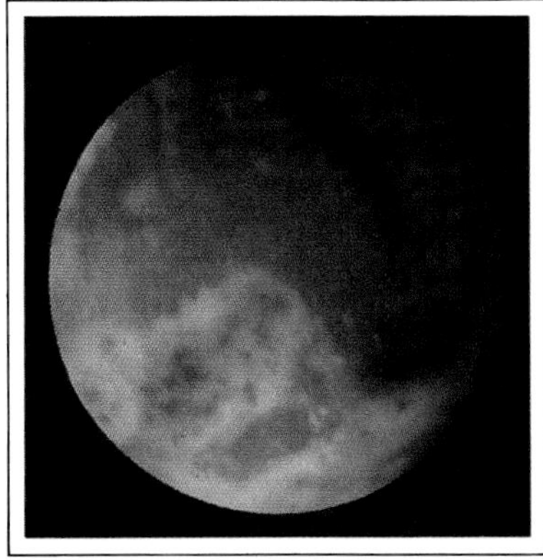

FIG. 34-6a.

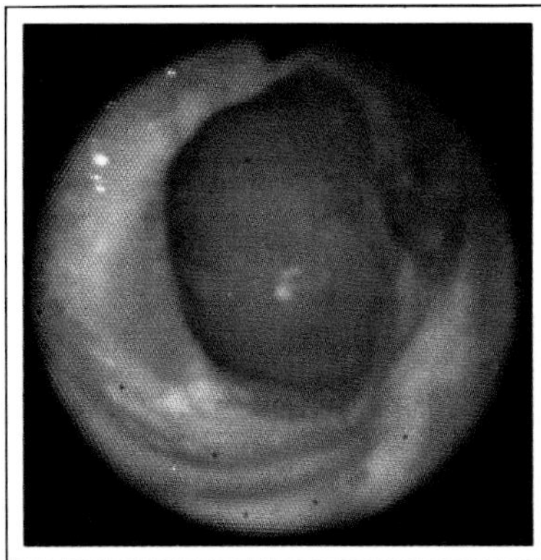

FIG. 34-6b.

FIG. 34-6. Peptic esophagitis after recent bleeding. **a:** The old blood (acid hematin) embedded in the pseudomembrane is a marker for bleeding in a patient with longstanding reflux symptoms and recent hematemesis. **b:** An erythematous elevated area (at 2 o'clock) was identified within the pseudomembrane. Because of its coloration and focal nature, it was thought possibly to represent a neoplastic lesion; it was biopsied, resulting in torrential bleeding. In all likelihood the erythematous lesion represented an organizing blood clot surrounding a small or medium-sized artery and should have been regarded as a "visible vessel" or equivalent.

Despite a mortality rate of 15% reported in older series,[18] a lower rate of only 8.5% was found in the ASGE survey for bleeding associated with esophagitis.[12] In addition, a significantly lower transfusion requirement and lower rate of surgical intervention were found in these patients, reflecting the general self-limiting nature of esophagitis bleeding. Further indicative of this was the fact that nearly 70% of patients had no evidence of bleeding at the time of endoscopy.[12] An additional 5.6% had a clot adherent to the involved mucosa but without active bleeding, whereas in only 22.5% was there evidence of bleeding as oozing. In less than 1% (0.5%) was there more active bleeding, as pumping.[12]

Appearance

Typically, in patients with peptic esophagitis-associated bleeding, one notes ulceration or its equivalent—pseudomembrane formation (see Chapter 3)—confined to the distal 4 to 6 cm of the esophagus (Fig. 34-6a). Within this area, old blood (acid hematin pigment) may be seen embedded within the ulcer base or pseudomembrane. In cases where the bleeding is recent, adherent clot and a small amount of oozing from within are noted. Rarely, as in the case of gastric or duodenal or ulcer bleeding (see Chapters 36 and 38) a "visible vessel" is noted within the pseudomembrane or ulcer base as a small, discrete, pink, granular mound. If it is not bleeding, it may be, as in one case observed by us, mistaken for a small polyp and biopsied with the disastrous result of massive bleeding (Fig. 34-6b).

Aspirin-Related Esophagitis

Bleeding from acute esophageal erosions is occasionally encountered in patients with recent heavy (eight or more pills) per day aspirin ingestion. In some cases, there are associated conditions which predispose to an increased contact time of the aspirin with esophageal mucosa resulting in acute mucosal injury.[19] We believe conditions such as a Schatzki ring, esophageal stricture, achalasia (see below), or an acute angulation of the distal esophagus in elderly patients associated with vascular compression (see Chapter 10) predispose to aspirin injury. Patients with preexisting esophagitis may be at even greater risk because of prior mucosal injury. Like bleeding associated with peptic esophagitis, that found with aspirin is generally of a self-limited nature in our experience.

Appearance

Focal, acute erosions (intermucosal hemorrhage with adherent clot) in the distal esophagus in a patient with recent heavy aspirin ingestion suggest a diagnosis of aspirin-related esophagitis (Fig. 34-7). Often the underlying anatomic predisposition, e.g., a Schatzki ring, is found as well. The finding of ulceration or its equivalent pseudomembrane argues for an aspirin-precipitated bleeding episode in a patient with preexisting peptic esophagitis.

Esophagitis Associated with Cancer Chemotherapy

In patients with cancer, especially those receiving cytotoxic agents for hematologic and other malignancies, esophagitis may account for up to 10% of the cases of upper GI bleeding.[20] The cause of the esophagitis is varied (see Chapter 3). In many cases it is related to opportunistic infections, e.g., *Candida* or herpes simplex. In other cases acute emetogenic mucosal injury (see Chapter 35) may play a role. In at least one-third of the cases we encounter there is no obvious cause for the esophagitis, which we attribute to a combination of factors including the inhibition of esophageal basal cell proliferation by the cytotoxic agent as well as a possible increase in the susceptibility of the mucosa to bacterial injury in the presence of granulocytopenia, which commonly occurs in these patients. In those with bleeding from these lesions, additional effects of cytotoxic agents on platelets may also play a role.

Appearance

There is often an extensive adherent exudate composed of necrotic tissue and debris in these patients (Fig. 34-8). These areas are extremely friable and bleed if only gently

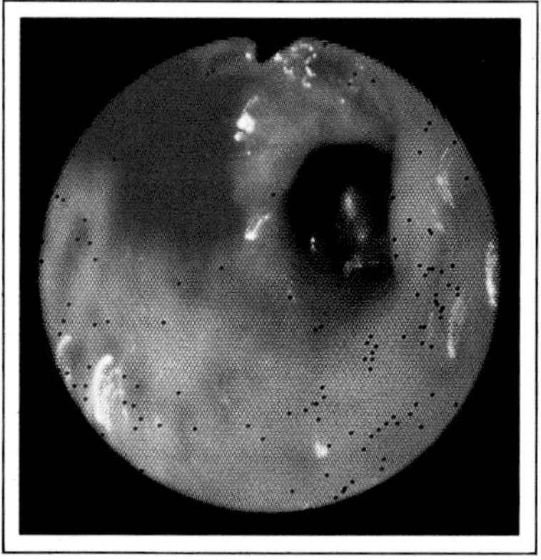

FIG. 34-7.

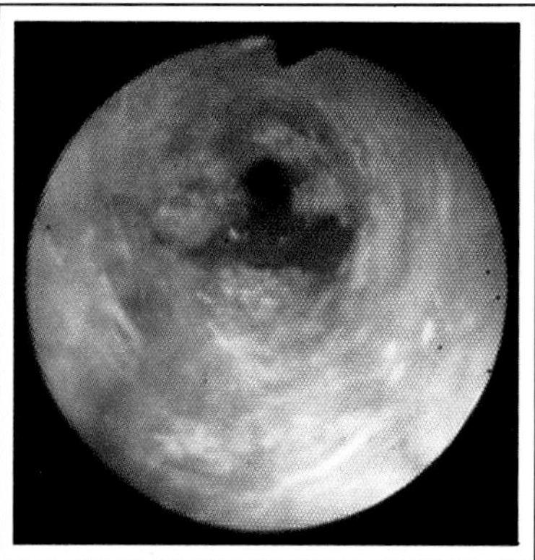

FIG. 34-8.

FIG. 34-7. Aspirin-related acute esophagitis. Multiple focal bleeding points, especially along the anterior (12 o'clock) wall, were found in the distal esophagus in a patient with recent heavy aspirin ingestion; no other potential site was identified.

FIG. 34-8. Chemotherapy-associated esophagitic bleeding. A dense pseudomembrane was found in a patient with bleeding 1 week after chemotherapy for acute leukemia. In the absence of opportunistic infection, the severe injury with resulting bleeding was probably multifactorial, related to vomiting, possibly the direct effects of the chemotherapy on mucosal integrity, and thrombocytopenia (see text).

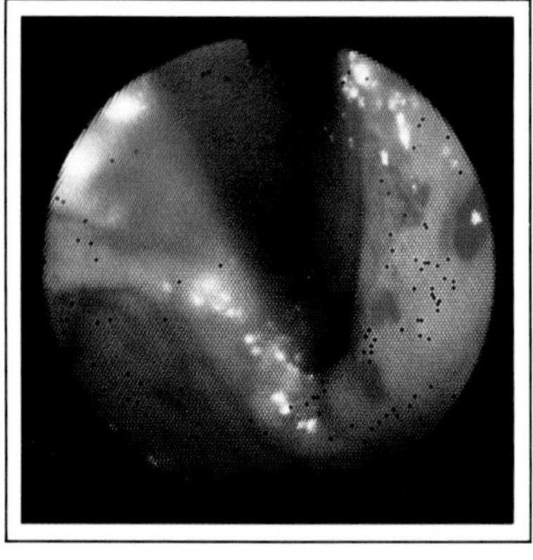

FIG. 34-9a.

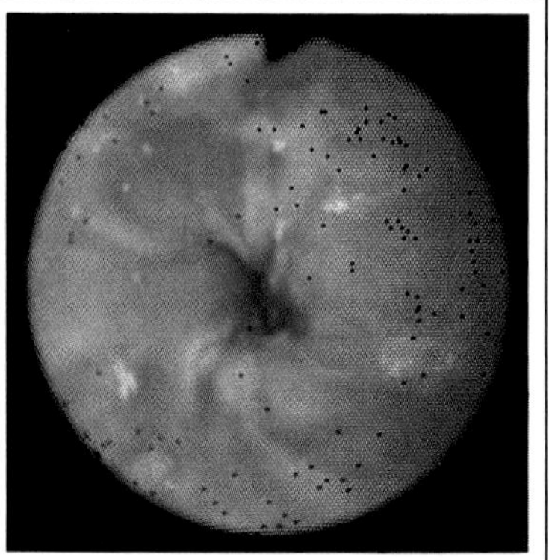

FIG. 34-9b.

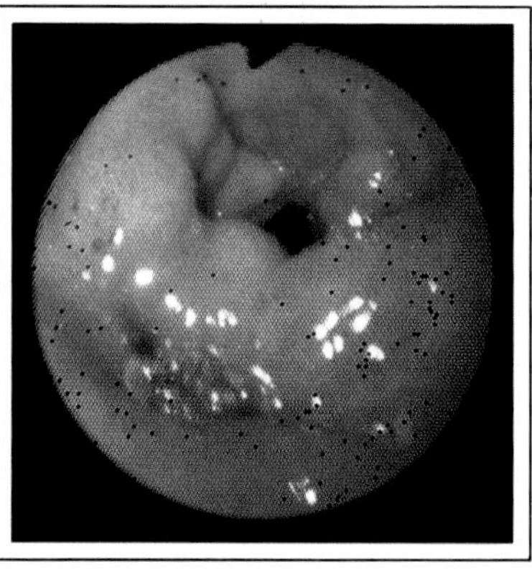

FIG. 34-9c.

FIG. 34-9. a: Nasogastric tube injury of the cardia. In this case, bleeding had occurred 24 hr after nasogastric tube placement for intestinal obstruction. The acute mucosal injury was confined to the cardia and lower esophagus, suggesting that injury was related to improper positioning of the nasogastric tube. These nasogastric suction artifacts have an appearance similar to that of drug-induced acute mucosal injury confined to the esophagogastric junction (see Chapter 35). **b:** Nasogastric tube injury after prolonged intubation. With the tube in place for more than 72 hr, peptic injury to the distal esophagus may occur, as in this patient with postoperative ileus. The pseudomembrane in this case is identical to that which would be found in peptic esophagitis bleeding. **c:** Duodenal ulcer bleeding in a patient with severe distal esophagitis [similar to that in (b)]. In contrast to the esophagitis, old blood (acid hematin) was embedded in the ulcer base, indicating this to be the bleeding site.

touched by the endoscope tip. Most often, the injury involves the middle and distal esophagus, beginning as high as 24 to 26 cm and continuing down to the GE junction. We find that if protracted vomiting has preceded the bleeding, or if a nasogastric tube has been in place for a protracted length of time (>1 week), one may see even more extensive injury that involves nearly the entire length of the esophagus.

Interpretive Problems

The finding of a focal distal esophageal injury, even if severe with adherent pseudomembrane, may still be nonspecific, relating to events following the initiation of the bleed and its treatment rather than being indicative of the cause of bleeding. In an ASGE survey,[12] esophagitis with or without an esophageal ulcer was noted in 15% of the cases but considered the cause of bleeding in only 8%, or roughly half the patients in whom it was present. Even in those cases in which the esophageal ulcer itself was found, it was considered the cause of bleeding in only 71.7%, whereas esophagitis itself had the lowest specificity for bleeding of any endoscopic finding, being considered the cause of bleeding in only 48.3%. The low specificity of esophagitis in patients with upper GI bleeding can be accounted for by any one of the following, which pose interpretive problems for the endoscopist. These are: (a) na-

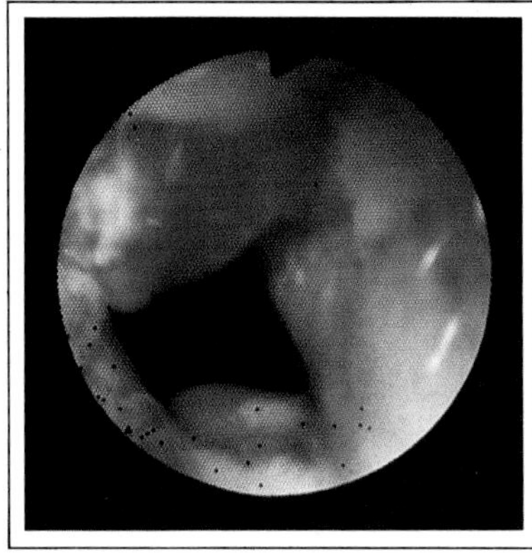

FIG. 34-10a.

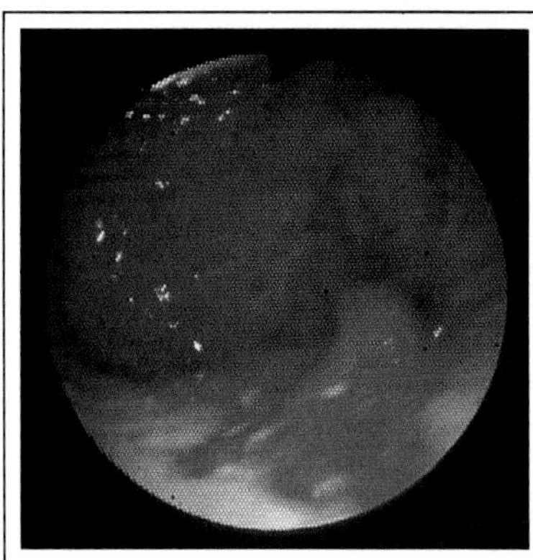

FIG. 34-10b.

FIG. 34-10. a: Distal esophageal erosions in a patient with massive hematemesis from an actively bleeding gastric ulcer. No nasogastric tube had been used prior to endoscopy. The erosions in the distal esophagus are possibly the result of emetogenic injury from repeated bouts of hematemesis prior to endoscopy. But for a careful examination of the stomach, the bleeding might have been ascribed to this site as a localized (esophagogastric) form of hemorrhagic gastritis (see Chapter 35). **b:** Actively bleeding gastric ulcer associated with hematemesis and possible emetogenic injury to the cardioesophageal junction (a). A careful examination of the stomach revealed this elevated blood clot with active bleeding. At surgery this was confirmed to be a bleeding gastric ulcer.

sogastric suction (tube) induced injury to the esophagus; (b) emetogenic injury secondary to recurrent hematemesis; (c) preexisting but nonbleeding peptic esophagitis as part of an ulcer diathesis; and (d) blood and foreign material simulating peptic esophagitis.

Nasogastric-Tube-Induced Injury

Nasogastric tube placement is often a routine procedure in patients with upper GI bleeding. In the ASGE survey, 70% had had it placed prior to endoscopy.[12] A nasogastric tube may be associated with esophageal injury in a variety of ways. In some patients, the tip may be located in the cardial (Fig. 34-9) or distal esophagus rather than more distally, predisposing the mucosa of the cardioesophageal junction to focal suction-type injury (see Chapter 33). These erosions can be easily confused with appearances which suggest esophagitis as a cause of bleeding, as in the case of aspirin-induced injury (Fig. 34-7). In other cases, especially where the bleeding has stopped, the nasogastric tube itself, placed because of bleeding, may be a precipitant of severe peptic injury to the distal esophagus (see Chapter 3) within a short period of time. In susceptible patients this can occur within 24 hr of its placement (Fig. 34-9b), so that in a patient examined 24 to 48 hr after admission to the hospital and who has had a nasogastric tube in place from the time of admission the endoscopist may observe acute inflammatory exudate with erosions leading him to conclude that esophagitis was the cause of bleeding, especially where a careful examination of the stomach and duodenum is not performed to exclude other sites (Fig. 34-9c).

Emetogenic Esophagitis Related to Hematemesis

Recurrent vomiting from any cause may produce acute injury to the distal esophagus (see Chapter 35) that appears as focal areas of acute intramucosal injury with adherent clot, i.e., acute erosions. When found in the distal esophagus (Fig. 34-10a), especially in the presence of adherent clots, it may be interpreted as the bleeding site if a careful examination is not performed of the stomach and duodenum to reveal the true bleeding site (Fig. 34-10b).

Peptic Esophagitis as Part of a Generalized Peptic Ulcer Diathesis

Even in patients with an appearance suggestive of true peptic esophagitis (Fig. 34-9b) because peptic ulcer disease may predispose to peptic esophagitis a careful search of the usual ulcer-bearing surfaces of the stomach and duodenum is necessary to exclude coexisting ulcers, which in some cases are the actual cause of bleeding.

Blood and Foreign Material Simulating Peptic Esophagitis

Blood, as already noted (see Chapter 33), can be found in the distal esophagus. This, in association with clots which adhere to the mucosa, gives the appearance of erosions. Similarly, bleeding ulcerations may be found which are in fact adherent clot and antacid (Fig. 34-11). Washing the distal esophagus may help remove some of the adherent material; however, in many cases this proves to be only partially successful. Rather than continue at this attempt, the endoscopist would more profitably turn his attention to the important surfaces of the stomach and duodenal bulb to find the actual site of bleeding. In some cases the passage of the endoscope through the distal esophagus helps remove such accumulated foreign material so that when the mucosa is examined on the return to the esophagus the previously noted erosions and/or ulcerations have disappeared.

OTHER INFREQUENT CAUSES OF ESOPHAGEAL BLEEDING

Esophageal Carcinoma

Although squamous carcinomas of the esophagus are often bulky, extremely friable tumors, bleeding easily after only a light touch (see Chapter 5), only rarely does one encounter carcinoma of the esophagus presenting as an upper GI bleed. We have encountered one case among the 500 consecutive bleeding patients examined over a 7-year

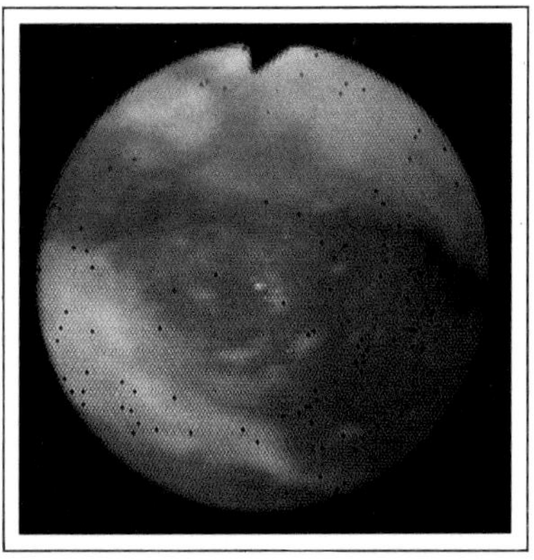

FIG. 34-11.

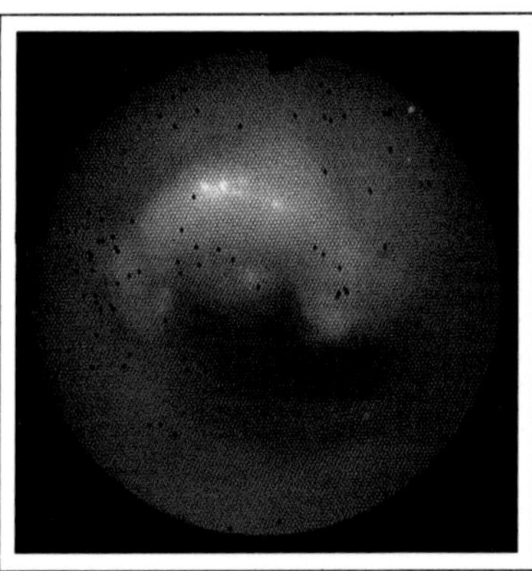

FIG. 34-12.

FIG. 34-11. Antacids and some blood in the distal esophagus which could be mistaken for peptic esophagitis bleeding.

FIG. 34-12. Esophageal cancer presenting with upper GI bleeding. The ulcerated mass probably eroded into the vascular bed of the esophagus.

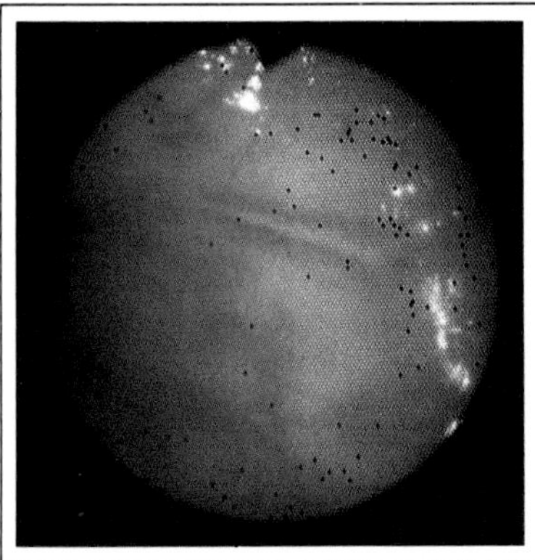

FIG. 34-13.

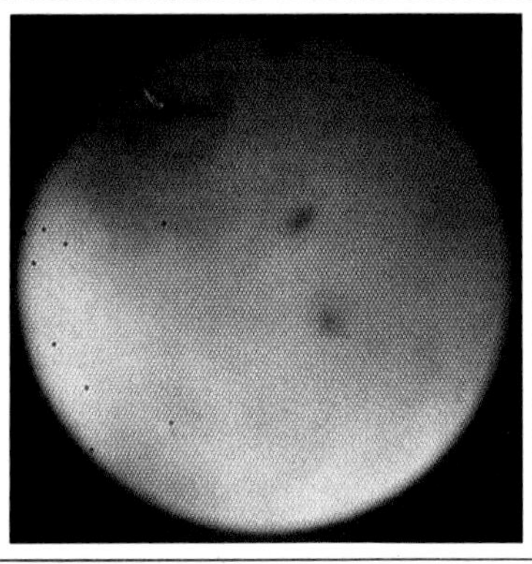

FIG. 34-14.

FIG. 34-13. Achalasia with bleeding. Recent heavy aspirin usage in a patient with known achalasia was probably responsible for the linear esophageal exudate from which hematemesis was thought to occur.

FIG. 34-14. Hereditary hemorrhagic telangiectasia involving the esophagus in a patient with recurrent occult GI bleeding, though not necessarily from the esophagus.

period. In this case (Fig. 34-12) there was a large mass with central ulcerations where the tumor had eroded into the vascular bed of the esophagus.

Submucosal Esophageal Tumors

Even rarer than esophageal malignancy as a cause of bleeding are submucosal tumors, e.g., leiomyomas or lipomas. We did not encounter a single case of these over a 7-year period. As with submucosal tumors elsewhere, bleeding occurs when the lesion develops a deep central ulceration.

Achalasia

Esophageal bleeding is rarely a manifestation of achalasia, occurring in probably only 1 to 2% of the cases. Of 95 patients with achalasia studied in our Unit over a 7-year period, bleeding was the indication for endoscopy in only one. In this patient the bleeding was from erosions in ulcerations just above the lower esophageal high-pressure zone. In this patient, who had consumed up to 12 aspirin tablets per day during the preceding 2 weeks, the postulated mechanism was that of acute mucosal injury from the tablets becoming lodged at the high-pressure zone rather than passing into the stomach (Fig. 34-13).

Also reported in achalasia as a cause of bleeding is the phenomenon of "downhill" varices[21] in which the sac-like dilatation of the mid and upper esophagus causes a redirection of blood from the azygos system across the submucosal veins of the esophagus into the portal venous system via a coronary (left gastric) vein. These varices are found to be largest in the upper and mid-esophagus and get smaller as the distal esophagus is traversed. Whereas "downhill" varices immediately come to mind as a cause of esophageal bleeding in achalasia, we suspect that bleeding from a topical injury from aspirin or other drug capable of causing mucosal injury (see Chapter 3) is the commonest cause of esophageal bleeding in achalasia.

Vascular Lesions

Hereditary Hemorrhagic Telangiectasia

Although not widely reported,[22] esophageal involvement may occur as part of hereditary hemorrhagic telangiectasia (Fig. 34-14). With esophageal involvement there is usually gastric (see Chapter 37) as well as duodenal lesions. In cases with esophageal involvement we have noted only small

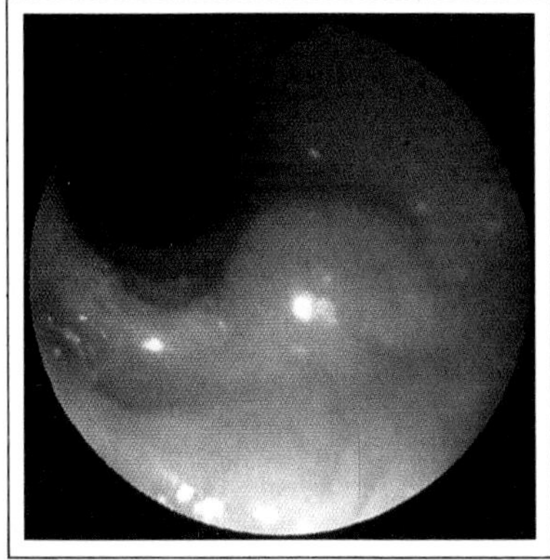

FIG. 34-15a.

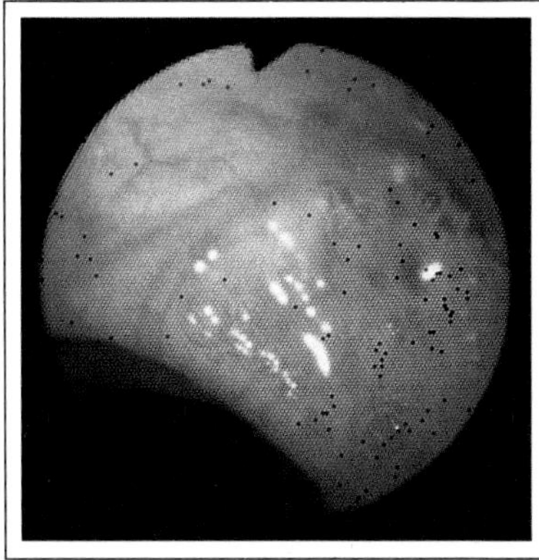

FIG. 34-15b.

FIG. 34-15. Possible esophageal hemangioma. **a:** A 2-cm raised lesion with bluish discoloration at 4 o'clock in a patient without a history of bleeding was nonetheless—because of its size and coloration—thought to represent a small hemangioma. In view of its asymptomatic nature, no further treatment was considered. **b:** Multiple, small (2 to 4 mm), blue, rounded and distinct elevations were thought to be consistent with the appearance of a hemangioma. As the patient was asymptomatic, with the examination being performed because of occult blood in the stool, surgery was not advised.

(<5 mm) lesions in contrast to the larger lesions found in the stomach and duodenum.

Hemangiomas of the Esophagus

Esophageal hemangiomas are rare vascular tumors that have been reported as an occasional cause of esophageal bleeding.[23] They characteristically appear as a smooth submucosal mass, generally having a bluish color (Fig. 34-15a), which allows them visually to be differentiated from other submucosal lesions of the esophagus, e.g., lipomas or leiomyomas. Another type of hemangioma appearance we have encountered is that of small, multiple blue elevations (Fig. 34-15b). Surgery is advised in cases where bleeding has occurred.[23]

REFERENCES

1. Silverstein, F. E., Gilbert, D. A., Tedesco, F. J., Buenger, N. K., Persing, J., and 277 members of the ASGE (1981): The national ASGE survey on upper gastrointestinal bleeding. I. Study design and baseline data. *Gastrointest. Endosc.*, 27:73–79.
2. Baggenstoss, A. H., and Stauffer, M. H. (1952): Posthepatitic and alcoholic cirrhosis: clinicopathologic study of 43 cases each. *Gastroenterology*, 22:157–180.
3. Graham, D. Y., and Davis, R. E. (1978): Acute upper-gastrointestinal hemorrhage: new observations on an old problem. *Am. J. Dig. Dis.*, 23:76–83.
4. McCusker, J., Cherubin, C. E., and Zimberg, S. (1971): Prevalence of alcoholism in a general municipal hospital population. *N.Y. State J. Med.*, 71:731–754.
5. Maletsky, B. M., and Klotter, J. (1975): The prevalence of alcoholism in a military hospital. *Milit. Med.*, 140:273–275.
6. Nolan, J. P. (1965): Alcohol as a factor in the illness of university service patients. *Am. J. Med. Sci.*, 37:135–142.
7. Fleischer D. (1983): Etiology and prevalence of severe persistent upper gastrointestinal bleeding. *Gastroenterology*, 84:538–543.

7a. Morris, S. J., Greenwald, R. A., and Tedesco, F. J. (1978): Characteristics of variceal versus non-variceal hemorrhage in cirrhotics with varices. *Gastroenterology*, 74:1070.

8. Graham, D. Y., and Smith, J. L. (1981): The course of patients after variceal hemorrhage. *Gastroenterology*, 80:800–809.
9. Liebowitz, H. R. (1961): Pathogenesis of esophageal varix rupture. *JAMA*, 175:874–879.
10. Conn, H. O. (1980): The varix volcano connection. *Gastroenterology*, 79:1333–1337.
11. Lebrec, D., De Fleury, P., Rueff, B., Nahum, H., and Benhamou, J.-P. (1980): Portal hypertension, size of esophageal varices and risk of gastrointestinal bleeding in alcoholic cirrhosis. *Gastroenterology*, 79:1139–1144.
12. Silverstein, F. E., Gilbert, D. A., Tedesco, F. J., Buenger, N. K., Persing, J., and 277 members of the ASGE (1981): The national ASGE survey on upper gastrointestinal bleeding. II. Clinical prognostic factors. *Gastrointest. Endosc.*, 27:80–93.

12a. Allison, J. G. (1983): The role of injection sclerotherapy in the emergency and definitive management of bleeding esophageal varices. *JAMA*, 249:1484–1487.

12b. Hunt, P. S., Korman, M. G., Hansky, J., and Parkin, W. G. (1982): An 8-year prospective experience with balloon tamponade in emergency control of bleeding varices. *Dig. Dis. Sci.*, 27:413–416.

12c. Orloff, M. J., Bell, R. H., Hyde, P. V., and Skivolocki, W. P. (1980): Long-term results of emergency portalaval shunt for bleeding esophageal varices in unselected patients with alcoholic cirrhosis. *Ann. Surg.*, 192:325–340.

13. Gilbert, D. A., Silverstein, F. E., Tedesco, F. J., Buenger, N. K., Persing, J., and 277 members of the ASGE (1981): The national ASGE survey on upper gastrointestinal bleeding. III. Endoscopy in upper gastrointestinal bleeding. *Gastrointest. Endosc.*, 27:94–102.
14. Conn, H. O., Ramsby, G. R., Storer, E. H., Mutchnick, M. G., Joshi, P., Phillips, M. M., Cohen, G. A., Fields, G. N., and Petroski, D. (1975): Intraarterial vasopressin in the treatment of upper gastrointestinal hemorrhage: a prospective controlled clinical trial. *Gastroenterology*, 68:211–221.

14a. Orloff, M. J., and Thomas, H. S. (1963): Pathogenesis of esophageal varix rupture. *Arch. Surg.*, 87:131–137.

15. Palmer, E. D. (1968): The hiatus hernia-esophagitis-esophageal stricture complex: twenty year prospective study. *Am. J. Med.*, 44:566–579.
16. Walker, C. O. (1978): Complications of peptic ulcer disease and indications for surgery. In: *Gastrointestinal Disease: Pathophysiology, Diagnosis, Management*, edited by M. H. Sleisenger and J. S. Fordtran, p. 914. Saunders, Philadelphia.
17. Kobayashi, S., and Kasugai, T. (1974): Endoscopic and biopsy criteria for diagnosis of esophagitis with a fiberoptic esophagoscope. *Am. J. Dig. Dis.*, 19:345–352.
18. Safaie-Shirazi, S., and Hardy, B. M. (1976): Treatment of reflux esophagitis resulting in massive esophageal bleeding. *Arch. Surg.*, 111:365–367.
19. Smith, V. M. (1978): Association of aspirin ingestion with symptomatic esophageal hiatus hernia. *South. Med. J. (Suppl. 1)*, 71:45–47.
20. Lightdale, C. J., Kurtz, R. C., Sherlock, P., and Winawer, S. J. (1974): Aggressive endoscopy in critically ill patients with upper gastrointestinal bleeding in cancer. *Gastrointest. Endosc.*, 20:152–153.
21. Kraft, A. R., Frank, H. A., and Glotzer, D. J. (1973): Achalasia of the esophagus complicated by varices and massive hemorrhage. *N. Engl. J. Med.*, 288:405–406.
22. Mayer, I. E., and Hersh, T. (1981): Endoscopic diagnosis of hereditary hemorrhagic telangiectasia. *J. Clin. Gastroenterol.*, 3:361–365.
23. Hanel, K., Taley, N. A., and Hunt, D. R. (1981): Hemangioma of the esophagus: an unusual cause of upper gastrointestinal bleeding. *Dig. Dis. Sci.*, 26:257–263.

35

CARDIOESOPHAGEAL BLEEDING

Bleeding sites within 5 cm of the gastroesophageal (GE) junction are being increasingly recognized. In a series reported by Katz and colleagues, the cardioesophageal junction represented the site of bleeding in over 35% of the cases.[1] Even excluding esophageal varices, as we would (see Chapter 34), cardioesophageal sites constituted nearly 20% of their cases.[1] It is noteworthy that this series with its high prevalence of cardioesophageal bleeding was reported from Metropolitan Hospital in New York City, a municipal hospital that serves an inner city population with a high incidence of alcoholism, which would predispose to the commonest cause of cardioesophageal bleeding, the Mallory-Weiss lesion. Among our patients (see Table 32-2), a mixture of referral and inner city individuals, cardioesophageal bleeding (largely as Mallory-Weiss lesions) constituted approximately 5% of the cases.

Cardioesophageal bleeding is most commonly the result of injury to previous normal mucosa, the injury being either from vomiting alone or seen in association with mucosal injuries from alcohol or aspirin. Less commonly, cardioesophageal bleeding occurs from cardial varices or other lesions of the cardia.

In this chapter we consider in some detail the commonest cause of cardioesophageal bleeding—acute emetogenic injury—considering separately the better appreciated discrete Mallory-Weiss type of injury and a less well known, more diffuse type of emetogenic injury to the cardioesophageal junction. Finally, we briefly touch on several uncommon causes of cardioesophageal bleeding, e.g., cardial varices and tumors.

ACUTE EMETOGENIC INJURY

Vomiting may be associated with two types of injury appearance: (a) a discrete mucosal lesion, the Mallory-Weiss tear; and (b) a more diffuse injury consisting of multiple areas of hemorrhage and erosion of the distal esophagus, cardia, and upper body. Although these are not mutually exclusive and can occur in the same patient, because of their different endoscopic features we treat them separately, recognizing that they are likely to be different manifestations of the same injury phenomena.

Mallory-Weiss Tear

The Mallory-Weiss tear is the most commonly recognized type of acute emetogenic injury. In one series it accounted for almost 15% of the cases, with only peptic ulcer bleeding being more common.[2] In the ASGE survey,[3] a final diagnosis of Mallory-Weiss tear was made in 7.2% of the cases, a figure which accords with our own experience (see Table 32-2), where it was encountered in almost 5%. Others have reported a lower incidence, on the order of 1 to 2%.[2] Although Mallory-Weiss tears may be seen in any clinical setting, its association with alcoholism seems inescapable. Not surprisingly, its highest incidence has been found in patients from military (including Veterans Administration) and city hospitals where the incidence of heavy alcohol intake approaches 50 to 60% of the patient population.[4]

The classic setting for the Mallory-Weiss tear is in the longstanding alcoholic patient with a history of recent binge drinking and protracted vomiting followed by hematemesis. The percentage of patients reporting this history varies with individual series. Bubrick et al.[5] found this history in more than half their patients, whereas Graham and Schwartz[6] reported it in only 29%. The presence of a hiatus hernia also seems to predispose to a Mallory-Weiss-type injury, being present in 75% or more of the cases.[6] According to Watts, the pathogenesis is directly related to the presence of the hiatus hernia.[7] With vomiting, there is a sudden forcible dilatation of the herniated cardia just above the diaphragm as gastric contents are ejected upward through the esophagus. A shearing force results which is greatest at the point of maximum dilatation, resulting in a typical

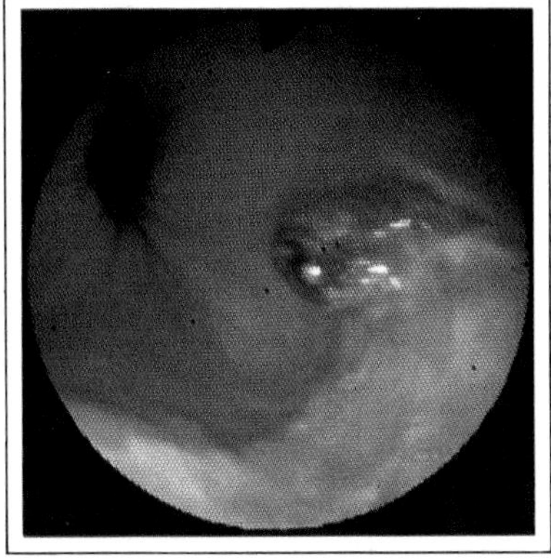

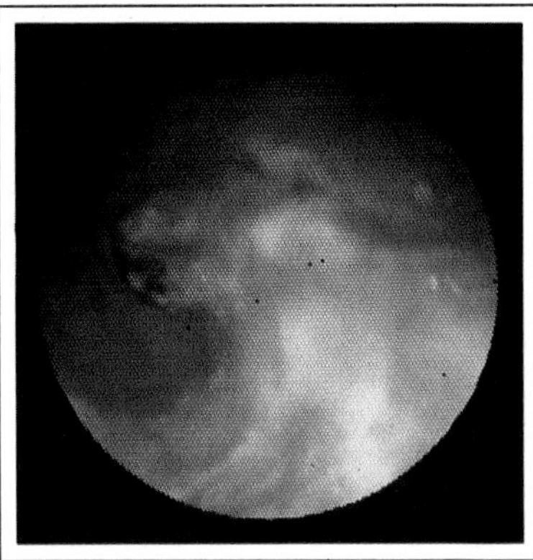

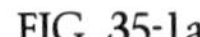

FIG. 35-1a. FIG. 35-1b.

FIG. 35-1. Mallory-Weiss tear. **a:** A characteristic longitudinal cleft was observed in the typical location on the right (3 o'clock) wall of the GE junction. At the termination of the cleft is an adherent clot marking this as the site of bleeding. **b:** A close-up view of (a) better demonstrates the cleft-like nature of the tear with its characteristic overhanging, gaping margins.

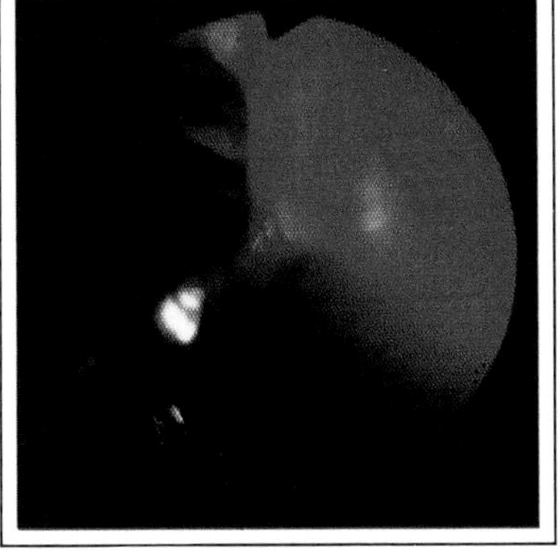

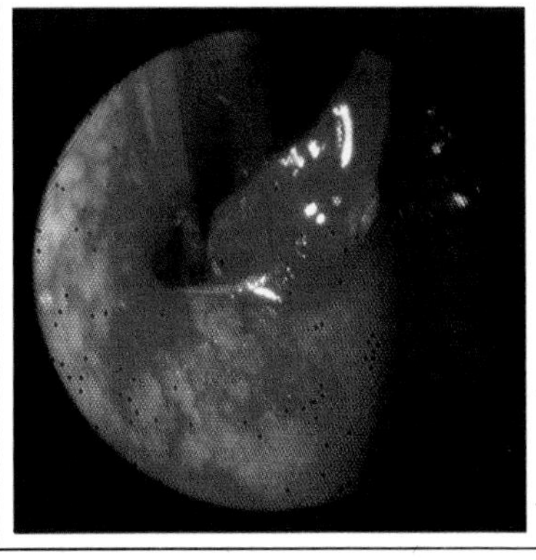

FIG. 35-2. FIG. 35-3.

FIG. 35-2. Mallory-Weiss tear and arterial bleeding point with pumping were found on the posterior wall of a hiatus hernia at the level of the diaphragmatic impression.

FIG. 35-3. Mallory-Weiss tear. A blood clot and bright red blood are seen dripping down from the cardia on U-type retroflexion. This was not apparent on direct examination of the cardia.

linear Mallory-Weiss tear. The position of the tear is related to the amount of stomach herniated. In cases where there is only a small hiatus hernia or none at all, maximum dilatation occurs at or just below the GE junction.[6] With large hiatal hernias, the injury point occurs more distally as a greater amount of stomach is herniated, with the point of maximum dilatation being at a more distal point relative to the GE junction. Most Mallory-Weiss tears, however, are either at the GE junction or within 2 cm of it within the cardia.[6]

Rationale for Endoscopy

The natural history of bleeding associated with the Mallory-Weiss tear is for it to cease spontaneously with conservative management,[5–8] which explains its low overall mortality. In the ASGE survey the mortality rate associated with Mallory-Weiss tears was 4.4%, contrasted with the 10.8% mortality for all patients.[9] Another indication of the self-limited nature of the bleeding was the low proportion (8.8%) of cases which required surgery, in contrast to 16.1% for the survey patients overall.[9]

Because most patients with Mallory-Weiss tears stop bleeding on their own without recurrence, endoscopy has a limited impact on these patients overall. However, patients in the ASGE survey with Mallory-Weiss tears who continued to bleed over the first 24 hr and at endoscopy had oozing (39.4%) or pumping (3%) had a higher mortality than those whose bleeding had stopped (8.6% versus 2.1%); a higher percentage of them received in excess of 5 units of blood transfusions (28.6% versus 14.7%) as well, and more required surgery (18.6% versus 3.2%). It therefore is the patient with a history suggestive of a Mallory-Weiss tear and clinical evidence of continued bleeding at 24 hr on whom endoscopy has its greatest impact.

Appearance

The endoscopic finding most suggestive of a Mallory-Weiss tear is a 1- to 2-cm, linear, cleft-like mucosal defect running longitudinally on the right posterior aspect of the GE junction (Fig. 35-1a) toward the cardia. For reasons not well understood, tears usually occur on the right (lesser curve) posterior aspect of the cardia (between 2 and 6 o'clock). Knauer, in fact, found 70% of tears in this location (Fig. 35-1b), with only 7% being anterior (between 11 and 1 o'clock) and 23% on the left (greater curve) aspect of the cardia (between 8 and 11 o'clock).[8] In the presence of a large hiatus hernia, the expected position of the tear is on the lesser curve posterior (3 o'clock) aspect of the hernia just above the diaphragmatic impression (Fig. 35-2).

If endoscopy is performed during the first 12 to 24 hr, active bleeding (Fig. 35-3) or an adherent clot (Fig. 35-4) is observed rather than the tear itself. If endoscopy is performed

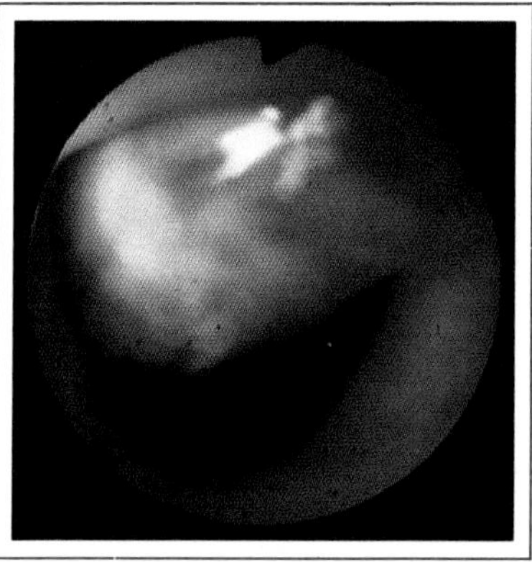

FIG. 35-4.

FIG. 35-4. Mallory-Weiss tear. A large organizing clot (with exudate) is apparent on the anterior (12 o'clock) wall of the cardia just below the GE junction, marking the presumptive site of a Mallory-Weiss tear. No further bleeding occurred, and on repeat examination 3 weeks later the cardia was entirely normal.

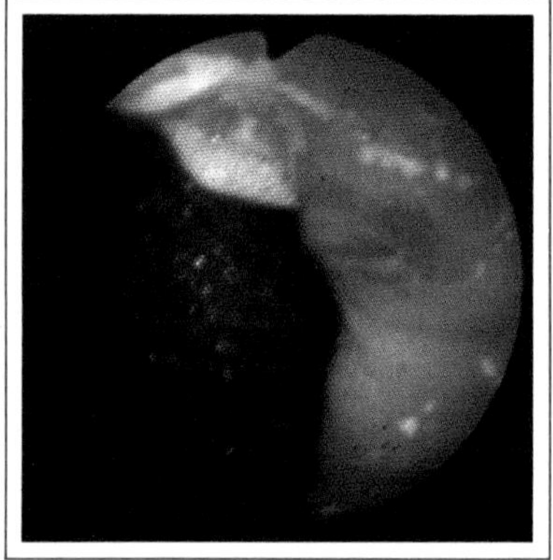

FIG. 35-5a.

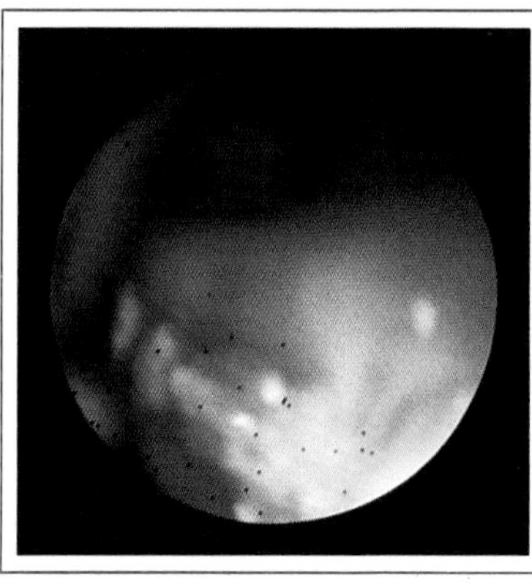

FIG. 35-5b.

FIG. 35-5. a: Esophageal erosion simulating a Mallory-Weiss tear. This linear erosion observed in a patient with protracted retching finally becoming hematemesis could be mistaken for a resolving Mallory-Weiss tear. In this case, although the pathogenesis may be similar there is no visual evidence of a tear. **b:** Mallory-Weiss tear adjacent to an esophageal varix. A longitudinal cleft with a puckered appearance of the mucosa (at 6 o'clock) suggests a Mallory-Weiss tear. The proximity of this to a varix was interpreted as indicative of a blowout point. At 24 hr after endoscopy, the patient rebled massively. At autopsy a bleeding point from a cardial varix was definitely identified.

later, with the bleeding having subsided and the clot fallen off, the puckered or erythematous margin of the longitudinally running tear (Fig. 35-1a) with its linear defect of granulation tissue is observed. In the majority of patients a single tear is seen, but occasionally two, three, or four such lesions may be observed.[6]

Interpretive Problems

In cases where the Mallory-Weiss lesion is considered, two interpretive problems arise. These are: (a) cardial erosions which simulate a true Mallory-Weiss tear; and (b) other potential bleeding sites.

Cardial erosions simulating a Mallory-Weiss tear.

If a nasogastric tube has been in place for 12 to 24 hr, the possibility of a suction artifact should be considered especially if the Mallory-Weiss tear consisted of only a single linear erosion set in a recess between prominent cardial folds (Fig. 35-5a). The finding of other such tears around the cardia strongly suggests nasogastric tube artifacts due to improper placement of the tip and the use of high suction pressures (> 50 mm Hg).

Other potential bleeding sites.

Mallory-Weiss tears have been reported to be frequently associated with other potential bleeding sites. In the series reported by Knauer,[8] 83% were associated with other lesions, principally esophageal varices, esophagitis, and hemorrhagic gastritis. Graham and Schwartz[6] found a lower but substantial proportion, 35% (32 of 93 patients), who had other lesions; 5 of the 32 had varices and 13 had peptic ulcer disease. In cases where the other lesion is located some distance from the Mallory-Weiss tear, proper attribution of the bleeding to one or the other is straightforward based on the evidence of recent or active bleeding from the presumed site. In most cases, if endoscopy is performed within the first 24 hr, it is possible to observe the Mallory-Weiss tear either bleeding or with evidence of recent bleeding (clot formation). In the ASGE survey, where the majority of examinations were performed within 24 hr, 78.8% of the Mallory-Weiss tears showed evidence of bleeding and were considered to be the actual bleeding sites in 89.3% of the cases where they were observed. The high percentage can be contrasted with that found in the ASGE survey for a lesion such as peptic esophagitis, where no bleeding was found in 71.1% and where the bleeding was attributed to only 48.3% of the cases where it was initially seen at endoscopy. Seeing blood in some form in association with a Mallory-Weiss tear is the crucial factor in determining whether one can ascribe bleeding to the lesion.

More difficult is the attribution of bleeding in cases where the Mallory-Weiss tear is associated with varices (see Chapter 34). We find it impossible in such cases to determine if the Mallory-Weiss tear is separate (Fig. 35-5b), although

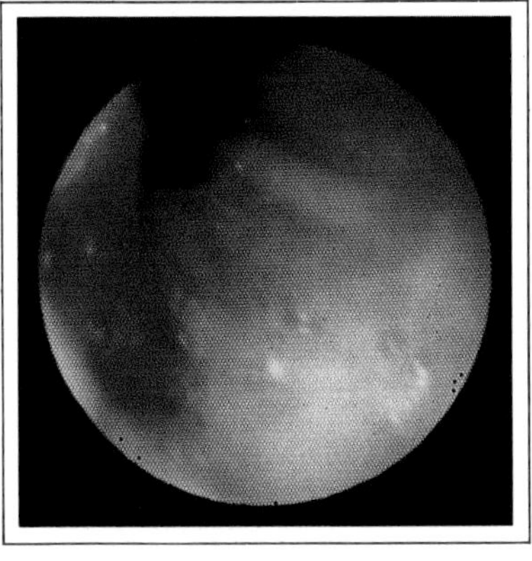

FIG. 35-6.

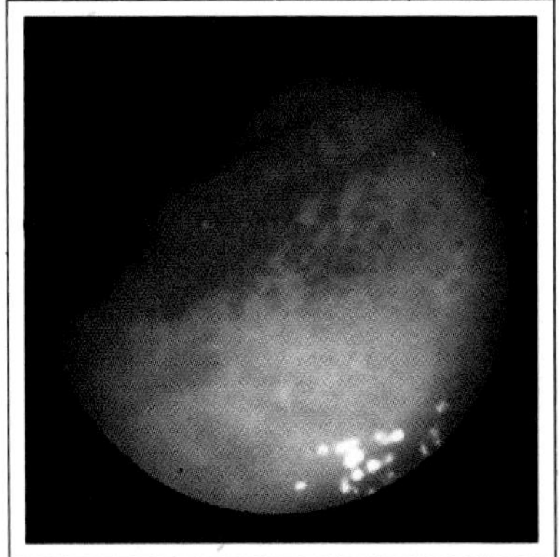

FIG. 35-7a.

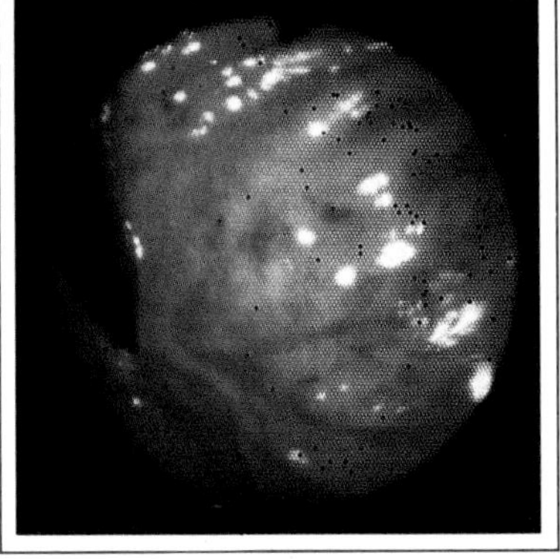

FIG. 35-7b.

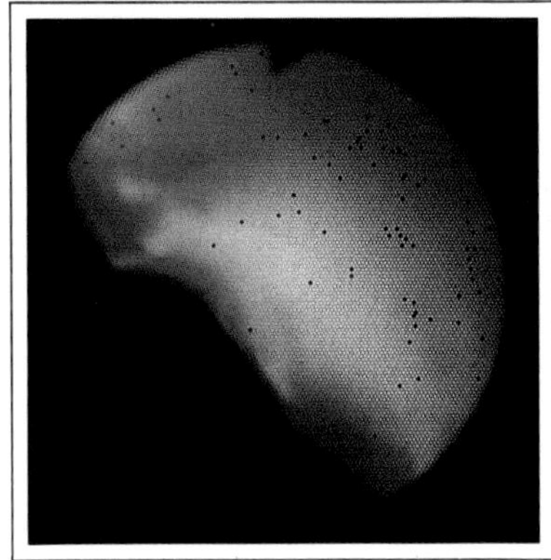

FIG. 35-7c.

FIG. 35-6. Emetogenic esophagogastritis. Forceful prolapse of cardial mucosa into the esophagus may result in intermucosal hemorrhage seen on the anterior (9 o'clock) wall of the cardia.

FIG. 35-7. Emetogenic esophagogastritis. **a:** Forceful prolapse of the mucosa could be responsible for this discrete red injury site seen on the posterior (3 o'clock) body of the stomach. **b:** In this case forceful prolapse resulted in the appearance of diffuse petechiae and intermucosal hemorrhage surrounding the cardial portion of a large hiatus hernia. **c:** An extensive area of acute ulceration on the posterior wall of the cardia was seen in a patient with bleeding after prolonged vomiting. In this case the acute mucosal injury was extensive and severe, resulting in mucosal slough and ulceration.

Knauer states that it was possible in 20% of his cases of Mallory-Weiss bleeding to differentiate this as a site of bleeding from varices present.[8] Similarly, in the ASGE survey of 109 patients with varices at endoscopy which were not the cause of bleeding, 14.6% were thought to have bleeding Mallory-Weiss tears.[10] Although some Mallory-Weiss tears are located at a distance from the varices, enabling one to ascribe bleeding directly to them, most are located close to the varices, making it impossible to exclude variceal bleeding. It is therefore our policy to consider the bleeding as variceal if the Mallory-Weiss tear is located within 3 cm of the esophagogastric junction (Fig. 35-5b) so as to alert the clinician to the potential seriousness of the bleeding as well as the increased likelihood of recurrence, which is expected from esophageal varices but not from a Mallory-Weiss tear, where bleeding is self-limited in 90% or more of the cases.[6]

Emetogenic Esophagogastritis

In some cases bleeding associated with vomiting does not result in a discrete Mallory-Weiss type of linear lesion but in a larger though circumscribed area of acute mucosal injury of the cardia or upper body.[11] The mechanism for this type of injury appears to be forceful prolapse of cardial mucosa into the esophagus, where it forms a plug which stops the stream of vomitus; this in turn has a traumatic effect on the mucosa of the entrapped cardia.[11] In cases where a larger zone of gastric mucosa has prolapsed, a ring-like area of injury involving the cardia and upper body may be seen.[12] In cases where only one portion of the upper body (typically the lesser curve) is prolapsed, a smaller area of injury is produced.

Another mechanism postulated by LaForet[12] is that of incarceration of the prolapsed mucosa during vomiting with obstruction of its venous outflow tract and progressive engorgement, edema, and finally intramucosal bleeding at the apex of the incarcerated mass of cardial mucosa. Still another injury route could be simply forceful prolapse and the formation of a submucosal hematoma.[13]

Appearance

In acute emetogenic esophagogastritis, the specific finding is that of a zone of hemorrhagic mucosa at or just below the GE junction, especially in the presence of hiatus hernia with prolapsing cardial mucosa (Fig. 35-6). In other cases, ring-like areas of intense erythema are apparent, especially on a retroflexed examination of the cardia and upper body, although this can be identified on direct examination of the upper body as focal, linear intramucosal hemorrhage (Fig. 35-7a).[11,12]

In addition to these findings, we have noted pleomorphic areas of intermucosal hemorrhage, 1.5 to 2 cm or more in maximum dimension (Fig. 35-7b). These are especially prevalent in patients with a history of profound vomiting.

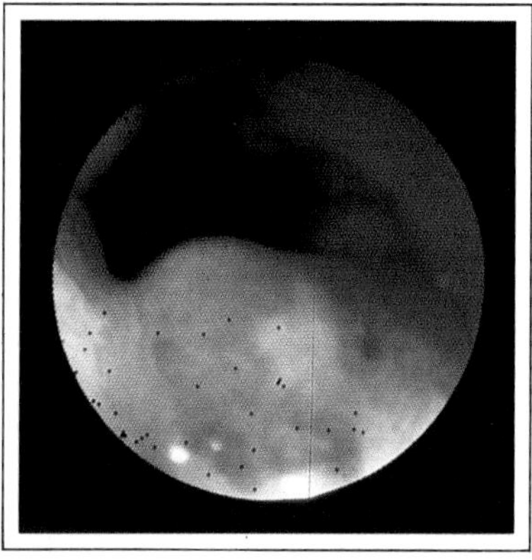

FIG. 35-8a.

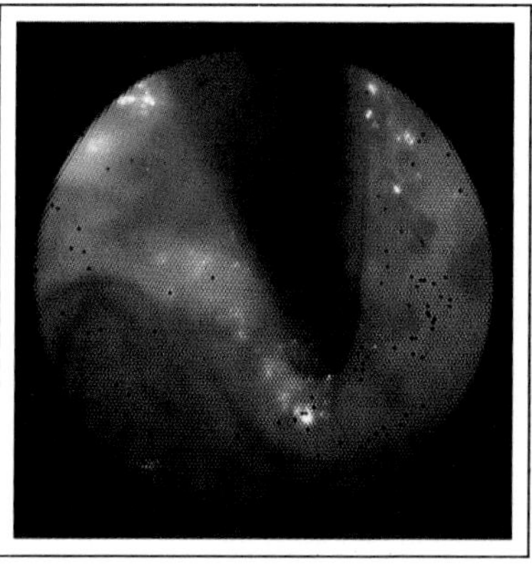

FIG. 35-8b.

FIG. 35-8. a: Hemorrhagic-erosive gastritis in a patient with a history of recent heavy alcohol ingestion. The appearance of the cardia in patients with hemorrhagic (erosive) esophagitis may in part be related to emetogenic injury. The acute inflammatory exudate and ulceration in this case were similar in appearance to that seen with severe emetogenic injury (Fig. 35-7c). **b:** Cardial erosion secondary to improper nasogastric tube placement. Multiple areas of intramucosal hemorrhage are seen in a patient with bleeding after nasogastric intubation. This appearance is similar to that found in emetogenic injury (Fig. 35-7a).

In some cases a slow ooze of blood is observed from these lesions, which in the absence of other definable causes we believe is attributable to vomiting. In some, the intramucosal hemorrhage (without clot) and erosions (intramucosal hemorrhage with adhering clot) involve the distal esophagus as well as the cardia and upper body. We have noted that the evolution of these lesions over 24 to 48 hr is similar to that of hemorrhagic-erosive gastritis (see Chapter 36) with the lesion either fading or associated with an organizing clot (clot mixed with exudate) or with lesions devoid of clot in the presence of yellow-white exudate alone (Fig. 35-7c). The latter appearances are generally found in cases where the bleeding is associated with protracted vomiting.

Interpretive Problems

Emetogenic esophagogastritis needs to be differentiated from drug-induced acute mucosal injury confined to the esophagogastric junction (Fig. 35-8a; see also Chapter 36) and nasogastric suction-induced injury (Fig. 35-8b; see also Chapter 33).

Differentiation from drug-induced acute mucosal injury.

The difficulty of differentiation from drug-induced injury lies in the fact that in up to one-third of the cases hemorrhagic-erosive gastritis may be confined to the cardia and upper body within 5 cm of the GE junction, precisely the same location for emetogenic esophagogastritis.[1] The appearance may be virtually identical, so that a diagnosis of emetogenic esophagogastritis rests on a history of profound vomiting alone in the absence of aspirin or alcohol ingestion. In cases where the latter have been used and hemorrhagic-erosive gastritis is likely, it may well be that some of the injury, especially when confined to an area within 5 cm of the GE junction, is related to vomiting itself.

Differentiation from nasogastric suction injury.

Nasogastric suction injury is another condition which produces an appearance similar to that of emetogenic esophagogastritis. It occurs in cases where the tip of the nasogastric tube has become lodged in the cardia (Fig. 35-8b), especially when high (100 mm Hg) continuous (wall type) suction has been used (see Chapter 33). In any case, when a nasogastric tube has been placed for the treatment of protracted vomiting and an appearance suggestive of emetogenic esophagogastritis is observed, there should always be concern about the suction pressures employed which may have contributed to this injury appearance.

OTHER CAUSES OF CARDIOESOPHAGEAL BLEEDING

Cardial Varices

Commonly, esophageal varices disappear in the cardia when they assume a deep submucosal or subserosal location (Fig. 35-9a). In 20 to 30% of the cases, however, they remain in a superficial submucosal location (Fig. 35-9b) and become potential sites for a blowout, similar to the more usual location in the distal 2 to 3 cm of the esophagus (see Chapter 34).

Another setting of cardial varices is as part of a system of gastric varices from splenic vein obstruction (see Chapter 37). A clue to this condition is the absence of esophageal varices or their being small in comparison to the size of the cardial varices.

Appearance

The presence of prominent mucosal folds of cardia in a patient with esophageal varices suggests the diagnosis. Some bluish discoloration may be apparent (Fig. 35-9b), but because of the submucosal location their coloration may be simply that of the surrounding mucosa. Bleeding from cardial varices may be appreciated only on examination of the cardia by retroflexion, where one observes a dripping down from the varices themselves (Fig. 35-9c). On withdrawal back into the cardia the bleeding site is again identified. The tendency of these sites to be on the lesser curve-posterior aspect of the cardia (2 to 6 o'clock) in precisely the same location as one most commonly finds a Mallory-Weiss tear

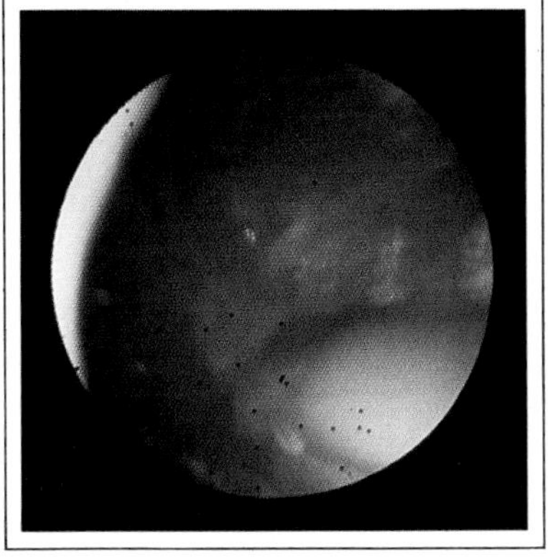

FIG. 35-9a.

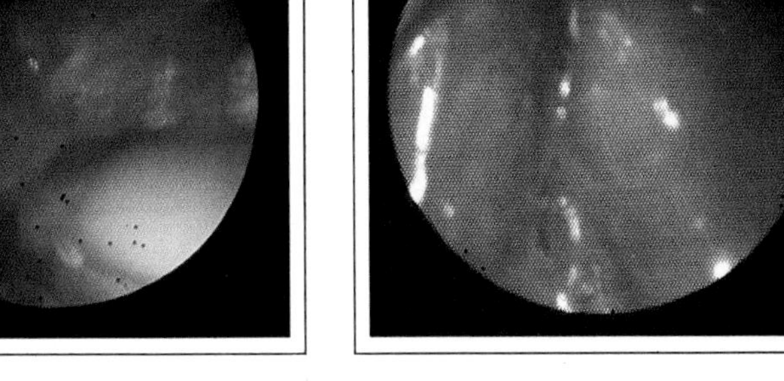

FIG. 35-9b.

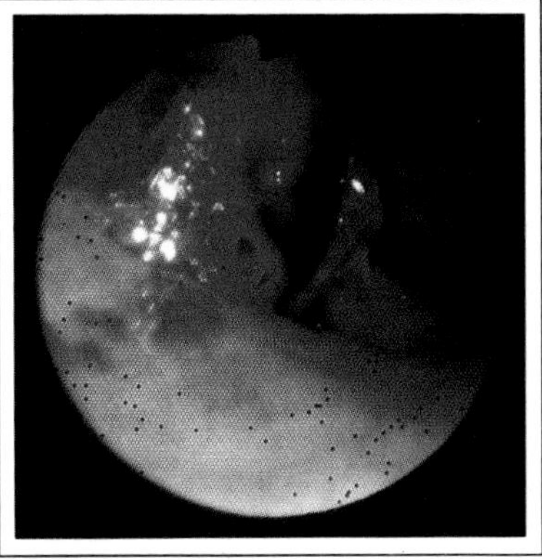

FIG. 35-9c

FIG. 35-9. a: Esophageal varices. These usually appear to terminate at the GE junction (at 6 o'clock), assuming a deeper location within the wall of the cardia (toward 9 o'clock) and fundus. **b:** Cardial varices. In some cases the varices maintain a more superficial location than can be observed across the cardia. **c:** Bleeding cardial varices. This was noted only on U-type retroflexion where the cardia was completely observed. The location of the bleeding point on the posterior (3 o'clock) wall was confirmed on direct examination of the cardia. Because vomiting preceded the variceal bleeding, and with the bleeding site being typically that of a Mallory-Weiss tear, it is believed that a mucosal tear overlying the varix could have contributed to the blowout of the varix, causing it to bleed.

may lead to the speculation that the pathogenesis of cardial varix bleeding is the production of a Mallory-Weiss tear of the mucosa overlying the varix (Fig. 35-9c).

Uncommon Types of Cardioesophageal Bleeding

A variety of cardial lesions, including malignancy, benign epithelial or submucosal polyps, and peptic ulcer disease involving the cardia, may cause bleeding from this area. In the series reported by Katz et al., these causes accounted for 6% of bleeding from this area and 2.1% of cases of upper GI bleeding overall.[1]

The endoscopist may visualize these lesions on direct examination of the GE junction and cardia, but in many cases lesions of the cardia are present only on U-type retroflexion where the entire cardia as well as a contiguous upper body and fundus can be thoroughly examined.

REFERENCES

1. Katz, D., Pitchumoni, C. S., Thomas, E., and Antonelle, M. (1978): Bleeding at the gastroesophageal junction. *South. Med. J. (Suppl. 1)*, 71:29–30.
2. Graham, D. Y., and Davis, R. E. (1978): Acute upper-gastrointestinal hemorrhage: new observations on an old problem. *Am. J. Dig. Dis.*, 23:76–83.
3. Silverstein, F. E., Gilbert, D. A., Tedesco, F. J., Buenger, N. K., Persing, J., and 277 members of the ASGE (1981): The national ASGE survey on upper gastrointestinal bleeding. I. Study design and baseline data. *Gastrointest. Endosc.*, 27:73–79.
4. McCusker, J., Cherubin, C. E., and Zimberg, S. (1971): Prevalence of alcoholism in a general municipal hospital population. *N.Y. State J. Med.*, 71:751–754.
5. Bubrick, M., Lundeen, J. W., Onstad, G. R., and Hitchcock, C. R. (1980): Mallory-Weiss syndrome: analysis of fifty-nine cases. *Surgery*, 88:400–405.
6. Graham, D. Y., and Schwartz, J. T. (1977): The spectrum of the Mallory-Weiss tear. *Medicine*, 57:307–318.
7. Watts, H. D. (1976): Lesions brought on by vomiting: the effect of hiatus hernia on the site of injury. *Gastroenterology*, 71:683–688.
8. Knauer, C. M. (1976): Characterization of 75 Mallory-Weiss lacerations in 528 patients with upper gastrointestinal hemorrhage. *Gastroenterology*, 71:5–8.
9. Silverstein, F. E., Gilbert, D. A., Tedesco, F. J., Buenger, N. K., Persing, T., and 277 members of the ASGE (1981): The national ASGE survey on upper gastrointestinal hemorrhage. II. Clinical prognostic factors. *Gastrointest. Endosc.*, 27:80–93.
10. Gilbert, D. A., Silverstein, F. E., Tedesco, F. J., Buenger, N. K., Persing, J., and the 277 members of the ASGE (1981): The national ASGE survey on upper gastrointestinal bleeding. III. Endoscopy in upper gastrointestinal bleeding. *Gastrointest. Endosc.*, 27:94–102.
11. Axon, A. T. R., and Clark, A. (1975): Haematemesis: a new syndrome. *Br. Med. J.*, 1:491–492.
12. LaForet, E. G. (1976): Acute hemorrhagic incarceration of prolapsed gastric mucosa. *Gastroenterology*, 70:589–591.
13. Watts, H. D. (1976): Postemetic hematomas: a variant of the Mallory-Weiss syndrome. *Am. J. Surg.*, 132:320–326.

36

GASTRIC BLEEDING—MAJOR CAUSES: HEMORRHAGIC-EROSIVE GASTRITIS AND GASTRIC ULCERS

Between 25 and 50% of upper gastrointestinal (GI) bleeding originates from gastric sources. Two causes predominate: (a) acute (drug-induced) hemorrhagic-erosive gastritis; and (b) peptic ulcer disease, including postsurgical (stomal) ulcers. In the ASGE prospective survey (see Chapter 32) these causes accounted for 46.5% of the 2,225 patients included in the study.[1]

These two important causes of upper GI bleeding are considered in detail in this chapter. As elsewhere in this section on upper GI bleeding, various clinical and pathogenetic aspects are considered as a basis for understanding the endoscopy of each condition. This is followed by the rationale for endoscopy and then by the expected endoscopic findings and associated interpretive problems.

HEMORRHAGIC-EROSIVE GASTRITIS

Hemorrhagic-erosive gastritis has been found to be the commonest cause of gastric bleeding in several recent endoscopic series reported from municipal hospitals or others with a high prevalence of alcoholism.[2] Some authors, however, find it to be an uncommon cause of upper GI bleeding, accounting for under 10% of the total cases, and in some series 5% or less.[2]

In the ASGE survey, the incidence of gastric erosions as a final diagnosis (which one assumes to have been for the most part cases of hemorrhagic-erosive gastritis) was 23.4%.[1] This figure stands half-way between the lower percentage reported for hemorrhagic-erosive gastritis in endoscopic series since 1969 (2 to 8.7%[2]) and the highest percentages (33%[3] and 42%[4]) reported from municipal hospitals serving an inner city population with an expected incidence of alcoholism that exceeds 50%.[5]

For 500 patients consecutively endoscoped for upper GI bleeding in our Unit over a 7-year period (see Table 32-2), hemorrhagic-erosive gastritis accounted for only 10.8%, reflecting both the largely private referral center type patients served by our institution as well as the timing of endoscopy, with most of our patients being studied late (after 24 hr) at a time when a diagnosis of hemorrhagic-erosive gastritis may not have been readily made. Still, of 11 endoscopic series reported between 1969 and 1976, summarized by Graham and Davis, our incidence of erosive-hemorrhagic gastritis exceeded those of five.[2]

Pathogenesis of Hemorrhagic-Erosive Gastritis

Alcohol

Alcohol is the commonest drug-implicated cause of hemorrhagic-erosive gastritis. A history of recent "binge drinking" was obtained by Dagradi and colleagues in 44% of 117 patients with this lesion at endoscopy.[6] In these patients alcohol was consumed in close proximity to the onset of bleeding, with an acute effect of the high concentration of alcohol postulated by these authors as the cause of the acute mucosal injury found at endoscopy. Support for this concept is derived from animal experiments, where an ultrastructural injury effect can be demonstrated after exposure of gastric mucosa to concentrations of alcohol in excess of 12% by volume, as well as an alteration in the gastric mucosal barrier allowing for entry (back-diffusion) of hydrogen ions into the mucosa.[7,8] The latter effect is postulated to lead to a local release of histamine, capillary dilatation, and intramucosal hemorrhage, ultimately resulting in cellular destruction that produces macroscopic areas of mucosal breakdown (erosions) which bleed.[8]

Supporting this sequence of events in humans was a study of seven male alcoholic volunteers who ingested a 40% solution (approximately 80 proof) of alcohol and then had endoscopy performed within an hour of ingestion.[9] Moderate to severe antral erythema and friability was found in all of these volunteers, with two of the seven having erosions and hemorrhage. Biopsies showed evidence of mucosal hemorrhage in four of the seven.

The fact that all alcoholic patients do not bleed after heavy alcohol ingestion has led some to consider the effects of prior alcohol injury.[10,11] In one study, fecal blood loss in alcoholic patients, measured by ^{51}Cr-tagged red blood cells, was significantly greater in patients with atrophic gastritis than where the mucosa was normal or showed only superficial gastritis.[10] Another study was conducted in army personnel who had a history and endoscopic examination compatible with alcoholic hemorrhagic gastritis; of those biopsied 3 months after the bleeding episode, a higher percentage had atrophic gastritis than did patients with comparable alcohol ingestion but without a history of bleeding[11] Thus thinning of the mucosa with atrophic gastritis may bring the capillary bed closer to the surface and predispose such patients to bleed if the mucosa is subjected to a high, potentially toxic concentration of alcohol.

Aspirin

Like alcohol, aspirin is capable of producing bleeding via acute mucosal injury. A history of recent heavy aspirin ingestion was obtained by Dagradi et al. in 22% of 117 patients with endoscopically proved hemorrhagic-erosive gastritis.[6] In an additional 25% there was a history of combined alcohol and aspirin usage. Aspirin was therefore implicated in almost half (47%) of the patients presenting with hemorrhagic-erosive gastritis. Typically, the aspirin had been ingested for short periods of time (3 days or less) prior to the onset of bleeding.

Of 54 patients with hemorrhagic-erosive gastritis found by us over a 7-year period, 16 (32%) gave a history of recent ingestion of aspirin (6 to 12+ tablets per day) in close proximity to the bleeding episode that prompted admission. In roughly one-third of these, there was also a history of chronic alcohol usage, similar to the finding of Dagradi et al.[6]

Two mechanisms have been proposed for aspirin-related gastric mucosal injury: (a) effects on the gastric mucosal barrier; and (b) a decrease in gastric mucus production with attendant loss of its cytoprotective effects.

Effects on the gastric mucosal barrier.

A well-known injury effect of aspirin relates to the tight junctions of surface cell membranes.[12] Aspirin in high enough concentrations, like other detergents such as bile acids, break down these tight junctions. This effect depends on the physical state of aspirin, which at the usual gastric pH is almost entirely non-ionized and readily penetrates the cell membrane, effectively destroying the tight junctions. This allows for back-diffusion of detergent ions into the mucosa which, as in the case of alcohol, has been postulated to lead to histamine release, capillary dilatation, and intramucosal hemorrhage.[8] In addition, some aspirin enters the cell itself and at intercellular pH is converted to its ionized form, leading to further cell injury.[12]

Effects on mucus production.

A second mechanism for aspirin injury appears to be the result of a decrease in gastric mucus production through the inhibition of mucosal prostaglandin synthesis.[13] Gastric mucus production has been proposed as one of the principal mechanisms by which prostaglandins exert their cytoprotection against the potentially deleterious effects of luminal constituents, e.g., gastric acid or bile salts.[13] Along with decreased production of mucus, aspirin seems to reduce the associated secretion of bicarbonate by surface epithelial cells as well as intracellular bicarbonate, which potentially makes the cells more vulnerable to luminal acids.[14] Finally, in addition to decreasing mucus production and its bicarbonate buffering capacity, aspirin seems to alter the viscosity of the mucus as well, making it less resistant to proteolysis.[14]

The amount of aspirin required to produce enough mucosal injury to cause bleeding is unknown. Evidence of mucosal injury has been found for as little as 600 mg (two 5-grain tablets) when administered with 10 mEq hydrochloric acid.[15] The administration of 2.4 g aspirin per day uniformly produces antral erythema and erosions (see below) in all subjects[16] and occult bleeding in some but not all.[14] Although a potential injury effect for aspirin was demonstrated in all subjects, in none of these studies did gross hemorrhage occur. Furthermore, the injury effects noted in these studies were in the distal body and antrum rather than the upper body and fundus, where at least 50% of the lesions of aspirin-induced hemorrhagic-erosive gastritis occur.[17]

Alcohol Combined with Aspirin

Although alcohol and aspirin alone are capable of inducing gastric mucosal injury, the combination is synergistic.[17a] In experimental animals, Robert et al. found that for amounts of aspirin that produced no mucosal injury, the addition of alcohol resulted in significant numbers of lesions, despite the aspirin alone being harmless in the concentration and amount used.[17a] Dagradi et al.[6] noted the combination of aspirin and alcohol as common a cause of hemorrhagic-erosive gastritis as aspirin alone. Needham and colleagues found in their patients a significant association of gastrointestinal hemorrhage with the combination of aspirin and alcohol, as well as with aspirin alone, but not with alcohol alone.[17b] It may be that the potentiating effect of aspirin to promote alcohol induced mucosal injury acts to reduce levels of mucosal prostaglandins[13] and to decrease cytoprotection against alcohol injury.[17c]

Other Drugs

In addition to aspirin, other anti-inflammatory agents, e.g., phenylbutazone, corticosteroids, and nonsteroidal analgesic agents, have been suggested as possible causes of hemorrhagic-erosive gastritis. Of these, nonsteroidal analgesic agents, e.g., indomethacin and naproxen, have the clearest association with upper GI bleeding,[18] although not exclusively as a result of acute mucosal injury. Several endoscopic studies performed on normal volunteers who ingested either aspirin or other nonsteroidal analgesics have found acute effects indistinguishable from aspirin effects: intramucosal hemorrhage, erosions, inflammatory exudate, and superficial ulceration.[19,20]

Among 54 patients with hemorrhagic-erosive gastritis examined by us over a 7-year period, four (8%) had used a nonsteroidal analgesic other than aspirin immediately prior to their episode of bleeding. In these patients there was a history of either alcohol or aspirin usage.

Rationale for Endoscopy

Because hemorrhagic gastritis represents a self-limited acute injury effect in 90% of patients—in whom bleeding spontaneously ceases with only supportive measures and surgery is not required[6]—endoscopy seems unnecessary for most of these patients. There are, however, two clinical considerations which, for us, prompt endoscopy in any patient suspected of having hemorrhagic-erosive gastritis. These are: (a) signs of liver disease; and (b) continued or recurrent bleeding.

Signs of Liver Disease

Patients with alcohol-induced hemorrhagic-erosive gastritis often have underlying liver disease and esophageal varices. Dagradi et al.[6] found evidence of liver disease in nearly 50% of patients whose hemorrhagic-erosive gastritis was caused by either alcohol or alcohol combined with aspirin. Of those with liver disease, varices were present in 80% (or 40% of the total). Sugawa and colleagues[17] found varices in a smaller number of patients with hemorrhagic-erosive gastritis, 8 of 75 (almost 10%). Still, for many patients with hemorrhagic-erosive gastritis, the possibility of bleeding esophageal varices is a major diagnostic consideration. For such patients, a secure endoscopic diagnosis of hemorrhagic-erosive gastritis serves both to confirm the correctness of medical management and to remove any consideration for therapy, medical or surgical, directed at the varices.

Continued or Recurrent Bleeding

The large majority of patients (90%) with hemorrhagic-erosive gastritis stop bleeding within 24 to 48 hr; however, one-third (30%) rebleed, with approximately 10% of these showing continuous bleeding with high transfusion requirements as well as an increased mortality rate, which in the face of liver disease and the need for surgical intervention may approach 50%.[6] Endoscopy is desirable in patients with suspected hemorrhagic-erosive gastritis who have had continuous bleeding for 24 to 36 hr or who have stopped within the first 24 hr but who have re-bled. Endoscopic confirmation of the clinical diagnosis of hemorrhagic-erosive gastritis is critical, especially if surgery with its attendant high mortality is being considered.

Appearance

A variety of appearances await the endoscopist in patients with hemorrhagic-erosive gastritis relating to the acute mucosal injury itself which we consider in this section, as well as others, e.g., the presence of blood, superimposed mucosal lesions, and other potential sites of bleeding, which we discuss in the next section. The reader must appreciate this separation as artificial because one rarely encounters hemorrhagic-erosive gastritis in a clear-cut fashion, completely free of interpretive problems. Our hope in presenting hemorrhagic-erosive gastritis in this way is that the interpretive problems may be better understood and recognized once the endoscopist becomes familiar with the appearance of the "pure" lesion.

Site

One thinks of hemorrhagic gastritis primarily as a proximal lesion involving principally the body but this is variable. Dagradi et al.[6] found antral involvement in over half of their cases (46 of 91),[6] and Sugawa et al.[17] noted antral involvement in 54% of their cases of alcohol-associated and 37% of aspirin-associated hemorrhagic-erosive gastritis. Yet others have found the lesions to be almost exclusively proximal, with a high proportion of alcohol-associated hemorrhagic-erosive gastritis (one-third of their cases) confined to the esophagogastric junction, with no involvement of the antrum or remainder of the body.[21]

Among the 54 patients with hemorrhagic-erosive gastritis observed by our group, antral involvement was infrequent, occurring in only four patients (7.5%); and in only one case (1.9%) was the principal area of involvement the cardia and upper body. Unlike the results of Sugawa et al.,[17] there appeared to be no difference between the distribution of lesions in patients who had alcohol or aspirin as the cause.

Intramucosal Hemorrhage

Because the principal mechanism for both alcohol- and aspirin-induced acute mucosal injury is the breakdown of the gastric mucosal barrier (see above), with back-diffusion of hydrogen ions, histamine release, capillary engorgement, and breakdown,[8] it is not surprising that intramucosal hemorrhage is a characteristic endoscopic feature (Fig. 36-1a). The endoscopist is already familiar with intramucosal hemorrhage, which he sees as an artifact of the endoscopic examination where the endoscope may come into forceful

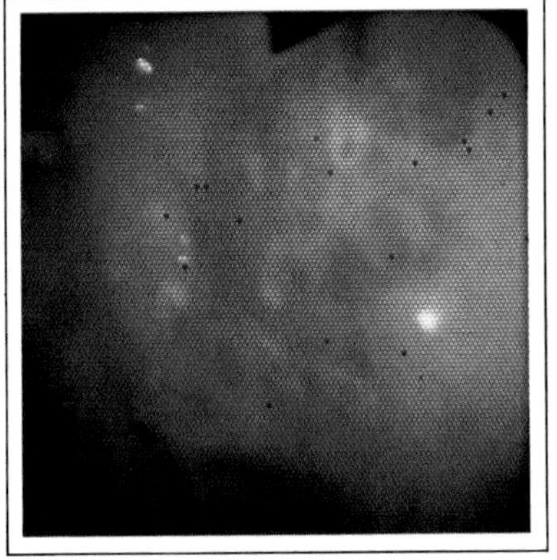

FIG. 36-1a.

FIG. 36-1b.

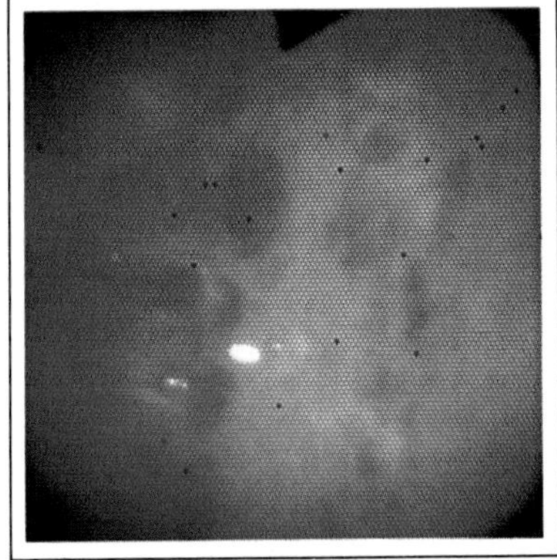

FIG. 36-1c.

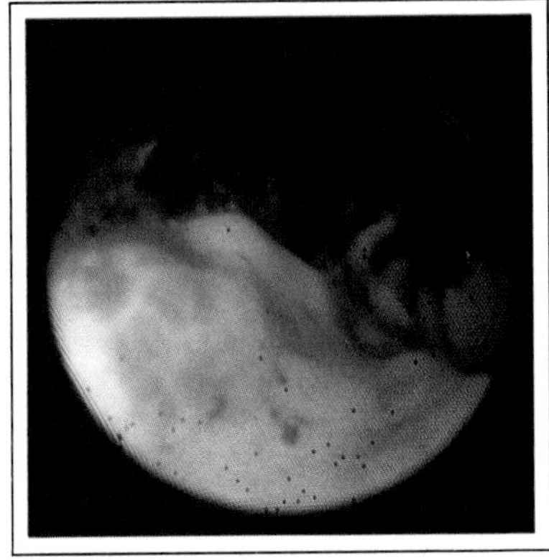

FIG. 36-1d.

FIG. 36-1. a: Hemorrhagic-erosive gastritis. Scattered areas of intramucosal hemorrhage (serpiginous reddened areas) are present on an erythematous background. These were seen in conjunction with adherent clot (7 o'clock), suggesting the presence of a break in the mucosa or an erosion. The focal whitish exudate (toward 12 o'clock) further suggests a mucosal response to the acute injury, implying that the erosions are late (see text). **b:** Endoscopy (instrument) induced intramucosal hemorrhage and erosions in a patient with atrophic gastritis. The relatively uniform size of the petechiae and the linear distribution of the larger ecchymoses and bleeding erosions on a pale rather than an erythematous background all suggest instrument trauma. This appearance must always be differentiated from that of hemorrhagic-erosive gastritis (a). **c:** Hemorrhagic-erosive gastritis. The zones of intramucosal hemorrhage are pleomorphic, ranging in size from the petechiae at 7 o'clock to the larger (5 to 10 mm) ecchymoses at 9 o'clock. **d:** Hemorrhagic-erosive gastritis. Several small intramucosal hemorrhages (at 9 o'clock) are seen together with larger (15 to 30 mm) areas of intramucosal hemorrhage running along the rugal folds at 9 o'clock.

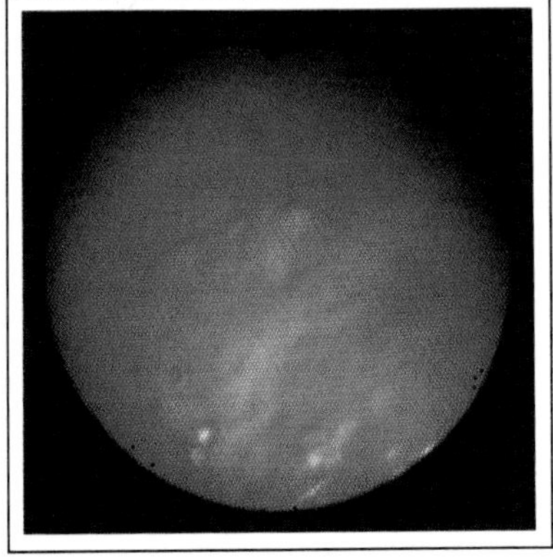

FIG. 36-2.

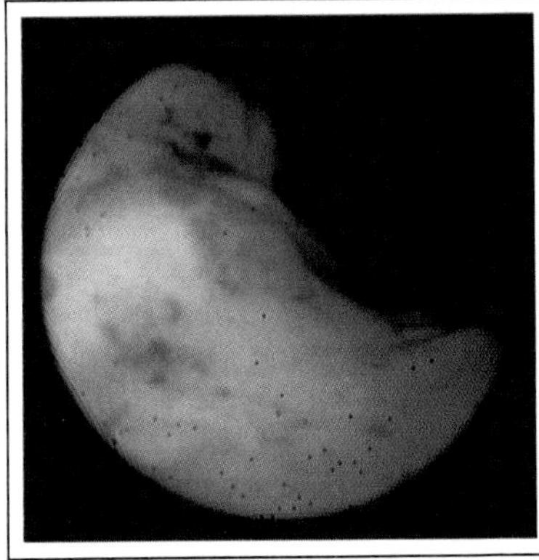

FIG. 36-3.

FIG. 36-2. Hemorrhagic-erosive gastritis. The diffuse erythema tends to obscure individual areas of intramucosal hemorrhage into a single erythematous background in a patient with a history of recent heavy alcohol consumption (binge drinking) and hematemesis.

FIG. 36-3. Hemorrhagic-erosive gastritis. In this case there is a relative paucity of lesions confined to the upper body despite massive bleeding.

contact with the mucosa as part of blind advancement or as a result of suctioning (Fig. 36-1b). Here the endoscopist sees small (3 to 5 mm), discrete, intensely reddened areas of mucosa.

Similar areas are observed in hemorrhagic-erosive gastritis and were classically described by Dagradi et al.[22] as "brilliant or dusky red" ranging from petechial (1 to 2 mm) to macular (5 to 10 mm) type lesions (Fig. 36-1c) or even ecchymotic (15 to 30 mm) areas (Fig. 36-1d). These areas of injury are pleomorphic, being either circular, ovoid, linear, or irregularly angulated (Fig. 36-1c). They appear on a mucosal background which is either entirely unremarkable (Fig. 36-1c) or, because of the presence of larger areas of intramucosal hemorrhage, diffusely erythematous, so that individual areas of mucosal injury may not be easily identified (Fig. 36-2). The areas of intramucosal hemorrhage are generally present for up to 72 hr or even longer, although they begin to fade after 24 hr. They are said to be characteristically numerous[22]; however, we find this to be usually not the case, especially if the patients are examined after 24 hr. At this time, one may see relatively few intramucosal hemorrhages (Fig. 36-3), rather than the scores or even hundreds of such lesions suggested by Dagradi et al.[22] to be the characteristic appearance.

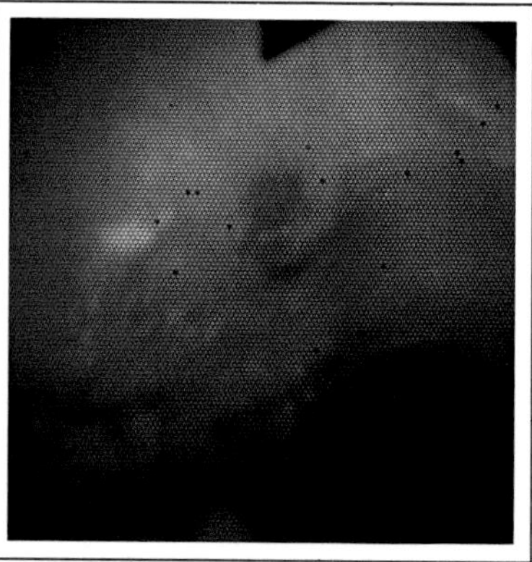

FIG. 36-4.

FIG. 36-4. Hemorrhagic-erosive gastritis erosions. The adherent clot over an area of intramucosal hemorrhage suggests mucosal breakdown from which point bleeding has occurred.

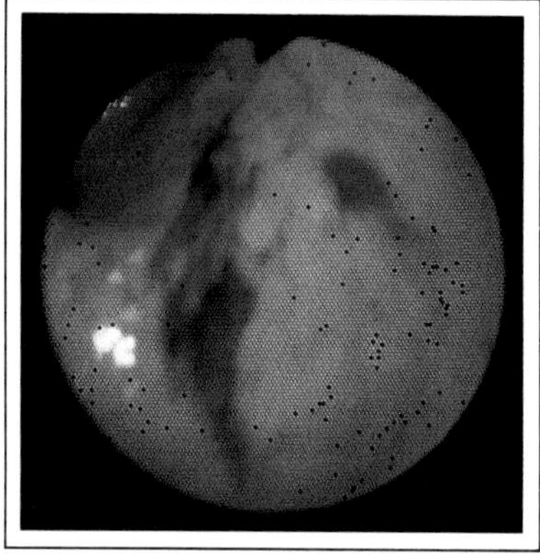

FIG. 36-5a.

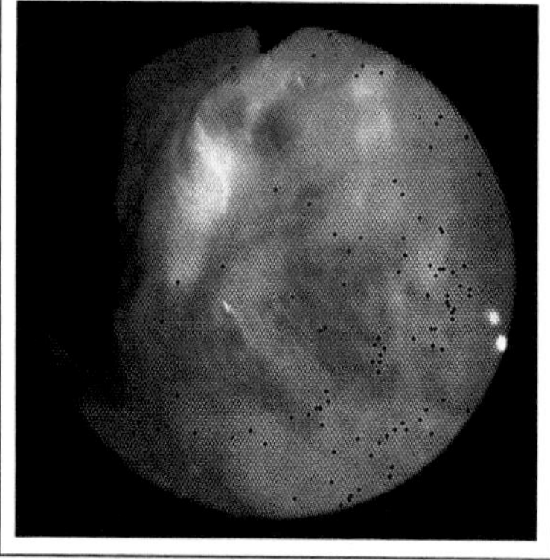

FIG. 36-5b.

FIG. 36-5. Hemorrhagic-erosive gastritis. **a:** Early erosions. Adhering clots overlie areas of intramucosal hemorrhage without, at this point, evidence of a tissue reaction (an inflammatory exudate). **b:** Late erosions. In this case the whitish exudate (at 10 o'clock) was biopsied and found to be a pure, acute inflammatory exudate indicating a later stage of injury (see text).

Mucosal Erosions

The term erosion implies a break in the mucosal surface. Visual evidence of this must be more than simply the presence of intramucosal hemorrhage, i.e., discrete reddened areas of mucosa. To qualify as an erosion, there must be either evidence of bleeding in association with the reddened area (active bleeding or adherent clot) or an inflammatory exudate or ulceration (Fig. 36-4) to indicate a break having occurred in the mucosal surface. One may consider erosions as "early" if they show active bleeding or an adherent clot and "late" if they show evidence of tissue reaction (organization) around a clot or inflammatory exudate/superficial ulceration in the absence of a clot.[22]

Whether one sees early or late erosion depends on both the timing of endoscopy and if there is continuing acute mucosal injury, which occurs in a minority of patients even after 72 hr.[22] In these cases one sees both early and late erosions as well as others in various stages of evolution.

Early erosions.

Early erosions are seen most often if endoscopy is performed within the first 24 hr of the hospitalization. Here blood is observed either to ooze in areas of intramucosal hemorrhage or, in cases where bleeding has stopped, as an intramucosal hemorrhage with adherent overlying clots (Fig. 36-5a). In these cases only a rim of intense erythema serves as evidence of the underlying intramucosal hemorrhage.

Late erosions.

An acute inflammatory response at the site of an erosion may be expected after 24 hr. In cases where a clot is still present, it is seen in association with a yellow-white inflammatory exudate (pseudomembrane) which surrounds and actually becomes part of the clot (Fig. 36-4). In cases where the clot no longer adheres, acute inflammatory exudate is seen at the site of the erosion (Fig. 36-5b). This may be observed as a sharply marginated thin pseudomembrane, often with a rim of intense erythema remaining. In contrast to the intensely erythematous appearance of intramucosal hemorrhage, the erythema at this later stage appears as regenerative mucosa with distinct areae and lineae gastricae, an appearance identical to that of regenerating mucosa surrounding a healing gastric ulcer (see Chapter 15). This regenerative epithelium replaces the inflammatory exudate, finally evolving into completely normal-appearing mucosa.

Although the acute injury effect giving rise to hemorrhagic-erosive gastritis may persist beyond 72 hr, one can nevertheless consider other possibilities for late lesions, especially in the face of continued bleeding after 72 hr. These include: (a) nasogastric suction artifacts (see Chapter

33); (b) superimposed emetogenic injury from continued bleeding and vomiting (see Chapter 35); or (c) concomitant stress lesions (see Chapter 37), especially in the setting of sustained hypotension or fulminant hepatic failure. Unfortunately, because the mucosal appearance found in association with these other conditions is indistinguishable from that of late erosions, the endoscopist can only suggest these other conditions and cannot conclude with certainty that any are actually the cause of continued bleeding.

Interpretive Problems

Hemorrhagic-erosive gastritis is frequently reported as a major cause of upper GI bleeding in many series,[2] but its appearance presents endoscopists with a variety of difficult interpretive problems. To what extent these affect the overall accuracy of endoscopy is unknown. One suspects that at centers where the prevalence of alcoholism and therefore hemorrhagic gastritis is truly high the accuracy is least affected both because of the endoscopists' familiarity with the condition as well as the increased statistical likelihood of a diagnosis of hemorrhagic-erosive gastritis being correct. At centers where the true prevalence of hemorrhagic-erosive gastritis is low, the accuracy may suffer overall because of the increased likelihood that a diagnosis of hemorrhagic-erosive gastritis is incorrect. Still, even in the setting of a low prevalence of hemorrhagic-erosive gastritis, one may be able to avoid interpretive errors, especially if the potential for them is kept in mind and a diagnosis of hemorrhagic-erosive gastritis made only on the basis of classic endoscopic features. To do this, one may be forced in 10% of the cases or more to state that no diagnosis can be made. In their series of 107 patients, Kim et al.[23] found an incidence of hemorrhagic-erosive gastritis (surgery or autopsy proved) in only 5.3%. Their error rate for the entire series was also low, only 3.7%; one suspects that this was so because they were unwilling to make a diagnosis in 12%, offering only an impression as to the level of bleeding. One imagines that interpretive problems such as the ones we present below may have made the endoscopist unwilling to make a specific diagnosis, especially a potentially erroneous one of hemorrhagic-erosive gastritis.

The interpretive problems associated with hemorrhagic-erosive gastritis may be considered as: (a) those leading to erroneous diagnosis because of the presence of blood and/or superimposed mucosal lesions; and (b) those resulting from the failure to recognize hemorrhagic-erosive gastritis.

Erroneous Diagnosis of Hemorrhagic-Erosive Gastritis

The percentage of incorrect diagnoses of hemorrhagic-erosive gastritis made at endoscopy is unknown, but some indication of the frequency with which the appearance of gastric erosions would be found in patients with another final diagnosis to account for their bleeding episode can be derived from the ASGE prospective survey. Of 2,097 patients in whom a final diagnosis was reported,[24] gastric erosions were noted at endoscopy in 620; however, in only 458 of the 620 (75.5%) was this the final diagnosis. In the remaining 152 (24.6%) another diagnosis was made. Therefore in any case where gastric erosions occurred, there was a one in four chance that these would not be the cause of the bleeding episode. Our own experience has been precisely this in patients with an endoscopic diagnosis of hemorrhagic-erosive gastritis where a tissue diagnosis was obtained. Of 54 patients with this diagnosis encountered over a 7-year period, 12 had either surgical (eight) or autopsy (four) examinations of the stomach. The diagnosis of hemorrhagic-erosive gastritis was confirmed in nine patients (75%), but in three (25%) another lesion was found to be the cause of bleeding; two of these had gastric ulcers, and the third had a large fundic leiomyoma which was not observed by the endoscopist.

The cause of misinterpretation leading to an erroneous diagnosis of hemorrhagic-erosive gastritis can, we believe, be accounted for by the two commonest artifacts associated with significant upper GI bleeding: (a) the presence of blood itself; and (b) superimposed acute mucosal lesions.

Blood.

The accumulation of blood and clots (Fig. 36-6a) in the dependent portions of the stomach is, in our experience, the major source of error. The blood itself effectively diminishes illumination, giving mucosa a reddish cast, which misleads the endoscopist in the direction of hemorrhagic-erosive gastritis. Coupled with this background are blood and clots which adhere to the mucosa (Fig. 36-6a). Often these can be washed off (Fig. 36-6b) so that the true nature of the "lesions"—blood—is revealed. Not uncommonly, however, the mucosa resists washing, especially in the presence of massive bleeding (Fig. 36-6c) so that at no time is the mucosa free of blood. Although the careful endoscopist learns to disregard clots which are not adherent to areas of intramucosal hemorrhage or associated with acute inflammatory exudate (see above), the presence of numerous clots with essentially poor illumination may cause even the most experienced to err.

Superimposed mucosal lesions.

Acute mucosal lesions may result from traumatic nasogastric suction (see Chapter 33), emetogenic injury (see Chapter 35), and stress conditions (see Chapter 37) relating to the bleeding episode itself (hypotension or associated fulminant hepatic failure). These superimposed acute mucosal lesions appear as intramucosal hemorrhage (Fig. 36-7a) or erosions (Fig. 36-7b) and are indistinguishable from the findings of hemorrhagic-erosive gastritis (Fig. 36-7c). In

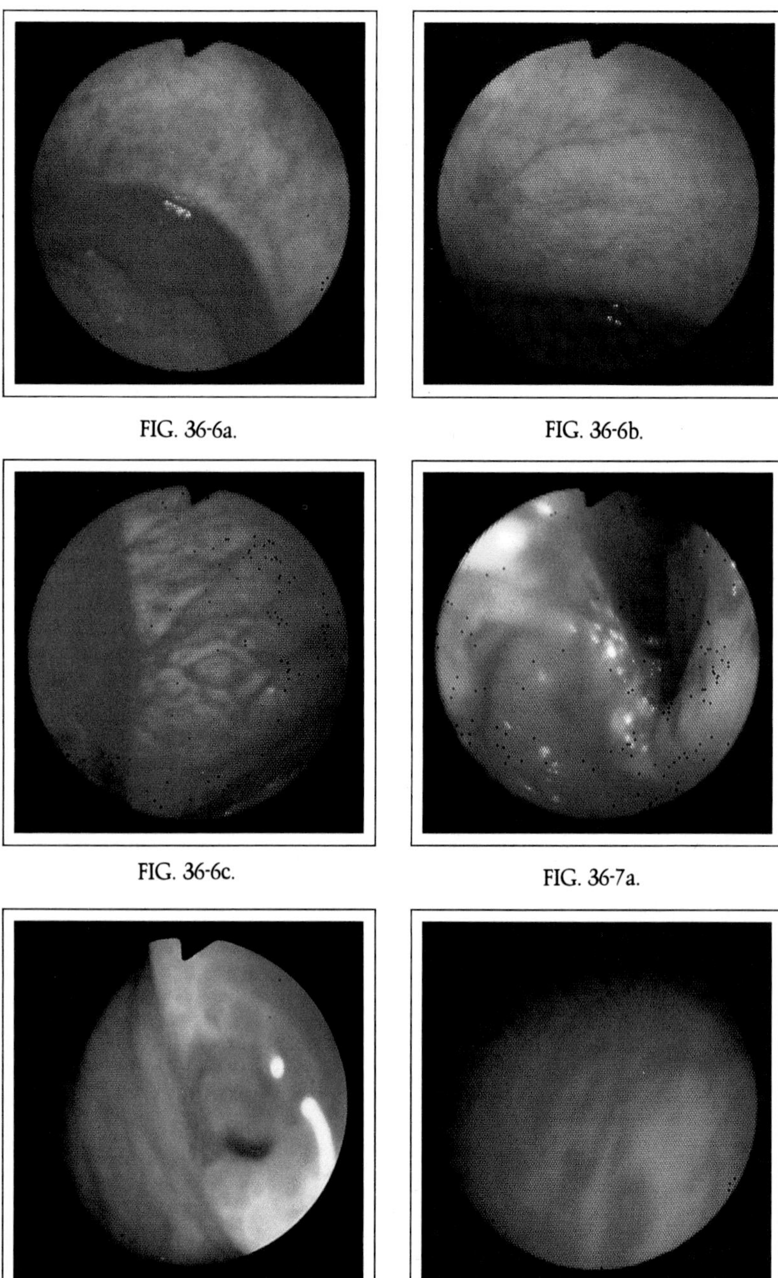

FIG. 36-6a. FIG. 36-6b. FIG. 36-6c. FIG. 36-7a. FIG. 36-7b. FIG. 36-7c.

FIG. 36-6. Blood simulating hemorrhagic-erosive gastritis. **a:** The presence of large amounts of blood and clots gives the mucosa of the lesser curve (between 9 and 4 o'clock) a reddish cast. In addition, blood adheres to the mucosa and simulates the appearance of intramucosal hemorrhage (at 2 o'clock). **b:** The blood which was adherent to the mucosa of the lesser curve (a) could be washed away, revealing the underlying mucosa that is essentially normal. This observation led to the endoscopist finding the true source of bleeding, an ulcer of the pyloroduodenal junction. **c:** Because of the presence of a massive amount of blood, attempts at washing the mucosa proved fruitless. Still, the site of bleeding could be localized to the pyloroduodenal junction.

FIG. 36-7. a: Acute mucosal injury to the cardia, a nasogastric suction artifact. Multiple irregular areas of intramucosal hemorrhage in a patient on prolonged nasogastric suction (see Chapter 33) examined because of coffee ground returns. The appearance of intramucosal hemorrhage is indistinguishable from those of hemorrhagic-erosive gastritis (Fig. 36-1a). **b:** Acute mucosal injury to the cardia, a nasogastric suction artifact. A large erosion (intramucosal hemorrhage with clots) is similar to the erosions of hemorrhagic-erosive gastritis (Fig. 36-4). **c:** Hemorrhagic-erosive gastritis confined to the esophagogastric junction. Large intramucosal hemorrhages are seen in this area and not elsewhere. This appearance may be indistinguishable from that found as part of nasogastric suction artifacts or stress gastritis (see Chapter 37).

one of our three cases in which a diagnosis of hemorrhagic-erosive gastritis was proved to be in error, nasogastric suction artifacts were interpreted as hemorrhagic-erosive gastritis and a fundic leiomyoma was overlooked. In another case a diagnosis of hemorrhagic-erosive gastritis caused by aspirin was made in a patient who had been hypotensive for 2 days prior to surgery from what was, in fact, a giant gastric ulcer with a large exposed artery in its base. We find that to avoid such interpretive errors one must always view a diagnosis of hemorrhagic-erosive gastritis as one of exclusion. Even with a history of binge drinking or heavy aspirin usage prior to the bleeding episode, a careful examination of the duodenal bulb, the gastric angle, and lesser curve, especially in the proximal 10 to 15 cm, must always be performed as well as inspection of the cardiofundic area by retroflexion (see Chapter 33). If a careful examination is precluded by the amount of bleeding, the endoscopist must always interpret the appearance of acute mucosal lesions cautiously as only "compatible with" hemorrhagic-erosive gastritis, one which does not exlude another diagnosis.

Failure to Recognize Hemorrhagic Gastritis

Just as there are no secure data concerning the percentage of false-positive diagnoses, the frequency with which the

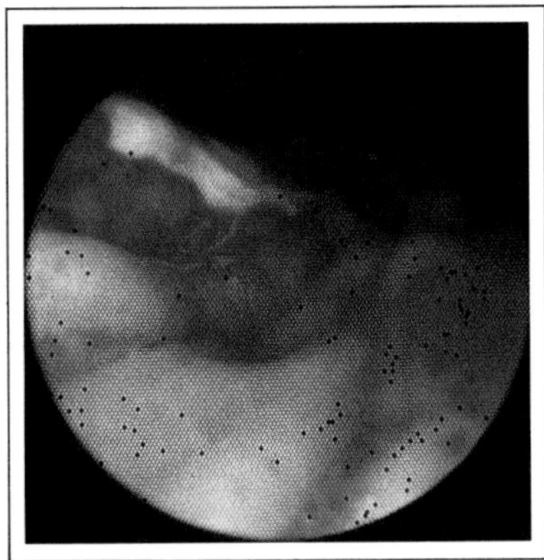

FIG. 36-8.

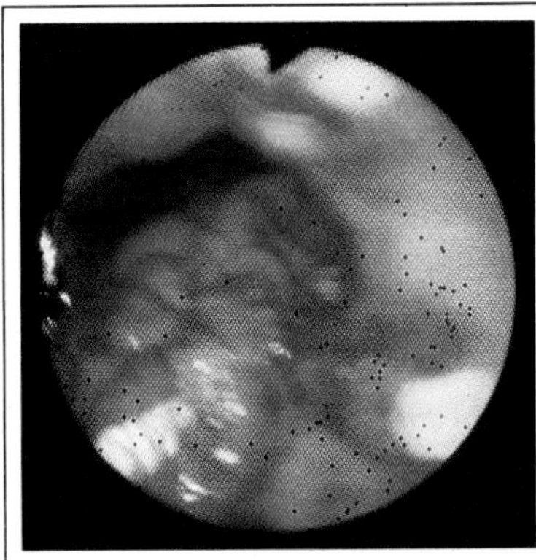

FIG. 36-9.

FIG. 36-8. Hemorrhagic-erosive gastritis. Several large ecchymoses are present which could be confused with nasogastric suction artifacts (Fig. 36-9). These were found on histologic examination of a surgically resected specimen to represent discrete areas of intramucosal injury.

FIG. 36-9. Nasogastric suction artifacts in a patient with relatively discrete zones of intramucosal hemorrhage.

endoscopist fails to make a correct diagnosis of hemorrhagic-erosive gastritis is unknown. Because the lesion is both transient and subtle, one suspects that in some of the cases where an endoscopic diagnosis is not made (8% in the ASGE prospective survey[24] and up to 20% in other series[2]) the diagnosis of hemorrhagic-erosive gastritis may have been missed. This would be especially true for patients in whom endoscopy was performed after the first 48 hr where, in contrast to the first 12 hr,[25] clear-cut evidence of bleeding from hemorrhagic-erosive gastritis may be absent.

For those patients with hemorrhagic-erosive gastritis in whom endoscopy is performed at the time the lesion is still present, the diagnosis may nevertheless prove illusive because of: (a) the absence of discrete lesions; (b) the small number of lesions present; and (c) the similarity of the lesions of hemorrhagic gastritis, especially in terms of their location relative to other acute mucosal lesions.

Absence of discrete lesions.

With identifiable intramucosal hemorrhage (Fig. 36-1a) or erosions (Fig. 36-2) the injury may be so extensive it causes the entire mucosal surface to bleed; in these cases one sees only blood and diffuse gastric erythema (Fig. 36-4). Moreover, the erythema is variable, not necessarily intense but sometimes simply disproportionate to the expected mucosal coloration, i.e., a pale yellow-gray color, observed when uninvolved mucosal surfaces are encountered in the face of significant bleeding (with a hematocrit of less than 30). Fortunately, cases where the finding of erythema is the predominant appearance are infrequent. In our series it occurred in only one of nine patients (11%) in whom the endoscopic diagnosis was confirmed histologically (surgical resection or autopsy).

Small number of lesions present.

Although one would expect that the injury phenomenon in hemorrhagic-erosive gastritis would be wide and easily identified, the number of discrete areas of intramucosal hemorrhage and/or erosions may not be great (Fig. 36-8) even in the resected or autopsy specimen. There may be only a few erosions in cases even where the bleeding was profound. Nevertheless, the endoscopist may be unwilling to ascribe the bleeding to an appearance which shows so little in the way of actual bleeding points. Yet in our experience, the expected appearance of numerous lesions is not found in as many as 30% of the cases where hemorrhagic-erosive gastritis is either the most probable or proved cause of bleeding.

Similarity of lesions of hemorrhagic gastritis, especially their location with regard to other acute mucosal lesions.

In up to 40% of cases with hemorrhagic gastritis in the series reported by Katz et al., the lesions were confined to the esophagogastric junction.[21] With a circumscribed rather than a diffuse distribution of lesions, the endoscopic picture may not be thought compatible with hemorrhagic-erosive gastritis (Fig. 36-8). Rather, the appearance may be interpreted as nasogastric suction artifacts, which they closely resemble (Fig. 36-9), if there had been a nasogastric tube in place, or as lesions of emetogenic injury (see Chapter 35), especially if there has been severe or protracted vomiting. In these cases one cannot arrive at a firm conclusion from the endoscopic appearance itself; indeed, to some extent the lesions present may be derived from several sources in addition to the drug-induced injury. Nevertheless, in the face of a strong clinical history for hemorrhagic-erosive gastritis, this diagnosis should be suspected even in cases where the injury effects are not "diffuse."

GASTRIC ULCER BLEEDING

Gastric ulcers are a common cause of gastric bleeding in virtually all recent endoscopic series. Of the 11 series reported between 1969 and 1976 and summarized by Graham and Davis,[2] ulcers were the commonest cause of gastric bleeding in three, with an incidence equal to (or within four percentage points of) hemorrhagic-erosive gastritis in an additional five. In only three series was the percentage of patients having hemorrhagic-erosive gastritis substantially higher, and these were in series from municipal hospitals

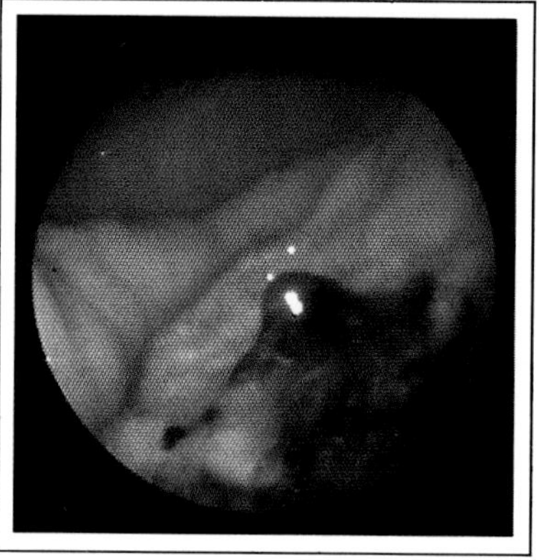

FIG. 36-10.

FIG. 36-10. Gastric ulcer bleeding, with a visible vessel in the ulcer base. At the time of endoscopy the protruding, conical blood clot suggested the presence of a large visible vessel (see text); bleeding had stopped at this point, but it recurred 24 hr later. A large exposed artery was found within the ulcer base in the surgically resected specimen.

in two cases and a naval base hospital in a third—known settings for a high prevalence of alcohol-induced hemorrhagic-erosive gastritis.

In the ASGE prospective survey, the percentage of cases of gastric ulcer bleeding was 21.3%, being equivalent to that for hemorrhagic-erosive gastritis (listed as gastric erosions), which was 23.4%.[1] This parallel incidence may reflect the balanced makeup of the study population in that there was not a predominance of either alcoholic inner city or military-Veterans Administration (VA) reporting centers versus private community or university referral hospitals.

In our patients, gastric ulcer bleeding predominated over hemorrhagic-erosive gastritis (see Table 32-2), being twice as frequent (24.2% versus 10.8%), which we attribute to the largely referral makeup of our patient population with only 30% derived from the inner city neighborhood, partially served by our hospital.

Patients with gastric ulcer bleeding may have had typical ulcer symptoms prior to the hemorrhage; however, for some, especially elderly patients over age 60 who are consuming aspirin or other nonsteroidal analgesic agents, bleeding is the initial presentation of the ulcer.

Pathogenesis of Gastric Ulcer Bleeding

Prospective studies indicate that for patients with gastric ulcers the cumulative incidence of bleeding is 10 to 15% if patients are followed for a 20- to 25-year period.[26] The factors which determine if a given ulcer will bleed are uncertain, but two kinds may be considered: (a) vascular factors; and (b) the effects of drugs, e.g., aspirin.

Vascular Determinants of Gastric Ulcer Bleeding

Although any gastric ulcer may bleed from the blood vessels of the margin or base which become exposed to the surface, only a minority of ulcers (<15%) actually do bleed. What appear to protect these vessels are reactive, inflammatory changes that occur especially in the intimal layer of a vessel, causing occlusion of its lumen.[27] These changes result in a mucinous infiltration of the intima which thickens it and makes it resistant to bleeding.[27] If these intimal changes keep pace with the rate of ulcer formation, bleeding does not occur. Conversely, bleeding would be expected if the ulcer were to progress at a rate which either does not allow for intimal changes to occur, causes the exposed part of the vessel where the changes have occurred to be digested away, or exposes deeper vessels where the reactive changes are absent.[27] In cases where intimal changes have not occurred, especially where larger vessels are exposed to the surface, one finds massive bleeding.[27] Even vessels that have undergone intimal changes may nevertheless become prone to bleed if they protrude from the surface of an ulcer base. Such vessels may be observed endoscopically and are currently designated "visible vessels." Because of their reactive intimal changes, they appear rigid and often "stand up" from the ulcer base (Fig. 36-10). They are associated with both continuous protracted bleeding as well as rebleeding, seemingly because of the vulnerability of the exposed portion of the vessel.[28]

Another potential reason for the protracted and/or recurrent bleeding from such ulcers is the rigidity of the vessel wall in cases where intimal changes have occurred.[27] Because of the reactive intimal changes (but not arteriosclerosis)[27] those vessels do not contract in response to bleeding; this causes defective clot formation and ultimately makes the vessel more likely to rebleed.[28]

Aspirin-Related Causes of Bleeding

To date, the single best studied drug predisposing to gastric ulcer bleeding is aspirin, although other nonsteroidal analgesic agents may have a similar effect. Aspirin, when taken more than 4 days per week for periods of 12 weeks or more, is associated with an increased likelihood that the patient will be admitted to the hospital for gastric ulcer bleeding compared to patients who do not take aspirin.[29] Curiously, however, there is not an increased likelihood of duodenal ulcer bleeding for these patients. The reason for this selective effect on gastric ulcers may relate to the fact that aspirin exerts its toxic effect principally on gastric mucosa.[16] For patients on aspirin, bleeding seems to be promoted by a combination of: (a) the effects of aspirin on the ulcer diathesis; and (b) coagulation effects.

Effects of aspirin on the ulcer diathesis.

Evidence exists for an association between aspirin ingestion and deep ulcers which present as gastric perforations. That a history of "heavy" aspirin usage (4 days or more per week) is obtained in a higher percentage of patients with recent gastric ulcer perforation[30] than in the general population suggests that aspirin usage may aggravate an ulcer diathesis in two ways which may cause it to be associated with bleeding. First, it may accelerate the ulcer process to a rate which does not allow for intimal changes to occur that protect the vessel from bleeding. Second, the larger and deeper ulcers[30,31] found in association with aspirin usage (see Chapter 15) predispose to more sizable vessels being brought to the surface of the ulcer base as visible vessels, an effect which places them at an increased risk to bleed.[28]

Coagulation effects of aspirin.

Because of its well-known alteration of platelet function, aspirin increases the likelihood of any lesion capable of bleeding to actually bleed.[32] It also promotes gross bleeding in those in whom the bleeding may have been occult and so would predispose a patient to present with an actively bleeding gastric ulcer.[29]

Corticosteroids and Nonsteroidal Analgesic Agents

The evidence that corticosteroids and nonsteroidal analgesics are associated with gastric ulcer bleeding is less certain than that for aspirin and is largely from anecdotal reports and retrospective series.[33] The precise role these agents play in causing gastric ulcer bleeding is unclear. As a group they cause gastric ulceration less predictably than aspirin or not at all; therefore their important effect with regard to whether bleeding occurs may be seen in the patient who already has an ulcer diathesis. Such drugs may shift the balance toward more rapid ulceration with diminished healing.[33] Any such effect would predispose to the formation of deep ulcers, potentially exposing larger vessels to the surface where they are more likely to bleed.[28]

Rationale for Endoscopy

Patients with bleeding gastric ulcers tend to be older, with a mean age approaching 60 years.[34] For such patients an increased mortality rate can be expected from any cause of bleeding, particularly in those who require surgery after receiving 6 units (3,000 cc) or more of blood; with the rate approaching 50% among patients in whom more than 10 units have been transfused.[35]

Endoscopy helps in the management of patients with bleeding gastric ulcers by identifying those with signs (stigmata) of ongoing or recent bleeding who stand the greatest likelihood of continued or recurrent bleeding. In one study, stigmata such as fresh bleeding, fresh or altered blood adherent to or within the base, or a visible vessel (see below) were associated with a 45% rate of surgical intervention for gastric ulcer bleeding, in contrast to no requirement for surgery for patients without such stigmata.[36] In the ASGE survey[24] the observation of active gastric ulcer bleeding (blood oozing or pumping) was associated with a requirement for 6 units or more of blood transfusion, nearly twice that found of patients in whom there is no active bleeding (38.2% versus 21.3%), along with a similar twofold increase in the rate of surgical intervention (24.5% versus 12.2%). A higher mortality rate was also seen in the "active" group (11.8% versus 6.8%) although it did not differ from the overall mortality rate for the entire survey group (10.8%).[24] However, the mortality rate specifically for elderly patients (over age 60) was not determined, a group which has been identified in other studies as having an overall unfavorable prognosis associated with GI bleeding.[35,37] Endoscopy therefore plays an especially important role in elderly patients with suspected gastric ulcer bleeding; that is, it identifies those with stigmata of recent or continued bleeding who are at the greatest risk without early definitive therapy. Until recently this has meant surgical intervention,[38] but in the future a subgroup may be defined that benefits from endoscopic coagulation (photocoagulation[39] or electrocoagulation[40]) of the ulcer base.

Finally, whether actively bleeding or not, the identification of a blood vessel in the ulcer base, i.e., the visible vessel phenomenon (Fig. 36-10), carries with it a high likelihood of persisting or recurrent hemorrhage, placing the patient who does not undergo surgery or definitive endoscopic therapy (photo- or electrocoagulation) at greatest risk. In one series such vessels were recognized in 9% of ulcer patients observed without vigorous washing of the base[28] and in 48% in another series[41] where the base was washed prior to photocoagulation.[39] In both series[28,41] there was continued or recurrent bleeding in a high percentage (50[41] and 80+[28]). Recognition of a visible vessel therefore affects management dramatically, allowing the patient to have either early surgery or, if feasible, endoscopic therapy[39,40] without which the mortality rate may be in excess of 80%.[28]

Location

The location of bleeding gastric ulcers, like others presenting for endoscopy, can be related to three variables: (a) age; (b) coexisting duodenal ulcer disease; and (c) aspirin usage prior to the bleeding episode (see Chapter 15). Of these, the age of the patient seems to be the most important, with advancing age (60+ years) favoring location in the

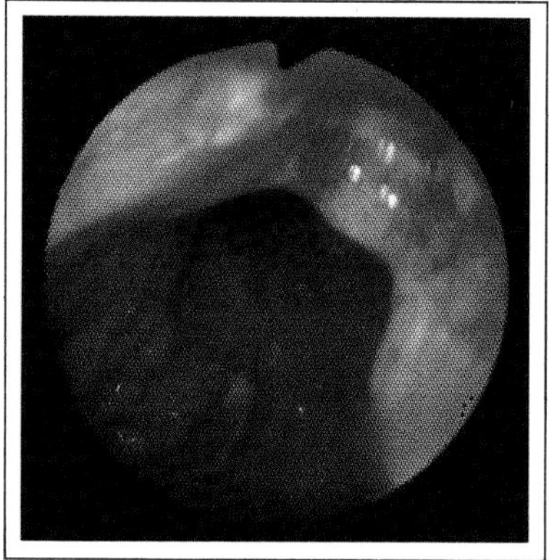

FIG. 36-11a.

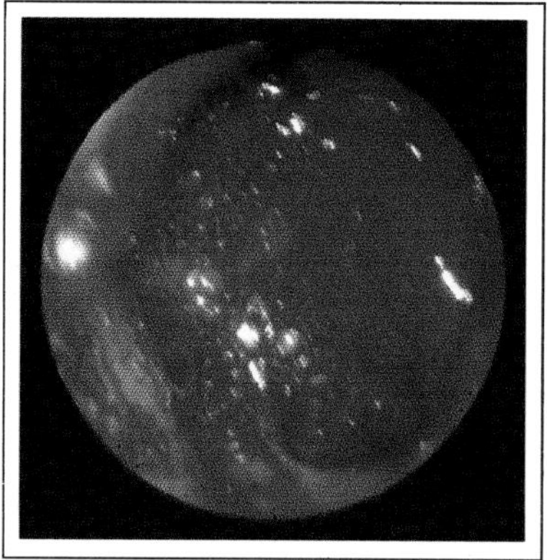

FIG. 36-11b.

FIG. 36-11. Gastric ulcer bleeding. **a:** Oozing. This can be seen from an ulcer of the gastric angle. Even though the base is obscured by the bleeding, an angular (V-type) deformity pointed the endoscopist to the bleeding site. **b:** Pumping. The blood itself obscures the ulcer base. In this case the diagnosis is suspected largely on the basis of scar deformity of the pyloroduodenal junction.

mid and upper body.[34] Coexisting peptic ulcer disease of the duodenal bulb, found in 15 to 20% of patients with gastric ulcers, favors a prepyloric antral or angular location (see Chapter 26). Finally, aspirin usage, especially if heavy (4 days or more per week for 12 weeks), also favors an angular or prepyloric antral location (see Chapter 15).

Gastric Body and Angle

The lesser curve of the gastric body, including the angle, is the commonest location for bleeding gastric ulcers. Of 121 patients with bleeding gastric ulcers endoscoped by us over a 7-year period, 79 (65%) of the ulcers were found in the gastric body including the angle. In nearly half (35) of these 79 patients, the ulcer was located within 10 to 15 cm of the cardia. The predisposition for gastric ulcers to be located high on the lesser curve, within 10 to 15 cm of the cardia, has been noted by others.[34] In one study, 52% of gastric ulcers in patients between the ages of 60 and 69 were found at this location, the figure rising to 66% in patients aged 70 to 79.[34] The cause of this upward shift in the location of gastric ulcers in the elderly has been attributed to the ascent of pyloric mucosa along the lesser curve, resulting in an upward shift of the junctional zone between pyloric and parietal mucosa, an area which may be particularly predisposed to ulcerate (see Chapter 15).

Gastric Antrum

Less common as a site of bleeding gastric ulcers, in our experience, is the gastric antrum. Of 121 patients in our series with bleeding gastric ulcers, only 42 of the ulcers were in this location. Within the antrum, the commonest site is the pyloroduodenal junction area, including a 2- to 3-cm zone of prepyloric antrum. The pyloroduodenal junction is an especially important site of bleeding in patients with marked duodenal bulb deformity from previous peptic ulcer disease and scarring (see Chapter 26), as well as in those with a history of heavy aspirin use (see Chapter 15).

Appearance

The findings in patients with gastric ulcers whose examination is performed because of bleeding depend on the ulcer's bleeding status at the time of endoscopy. As was found in the ASGE survey, there is active bleeding (pumping or oozing) in only a minority of the cases (22.5%). In about one-third of patients (32.8% in the ASGE survey), the bleeding has ceased by the time endoscopy is performed but a clot is seen within the ulcer base signifying recent bleeding. In almost half the patients with gastric ulcer bleeding (44.7% in the ASGE survey) there is no evidence of bleeding, with only the ulcer itself seen as a potential site. We may therefore consider the appearance of gastric ulcers in patients examined because of bleeding under three categories: (a) those actively bleeding; (b) those whose bleeding has stopped but who have signs, or stigmata, of recent bleeding; and (c) those without such stigmata.

Active Bleeding

In 20 to 30% of the cases active bleeding is present as either a visible ooze of blood from the base of a well-defined ulcer (Fig. 36-11a) or more vigorous bleeding seen as blood either pumping or spurting, which tends to obscure the ulcer, making it possible only to establish the site of bleeding with certainty. In these cases, however, the presence of some type of ulcer deformity, i.e., converging folds, suggests the source of bleeding to be a gastric ulcer.

Another active bleeding appearance is that of oozing from a blood clot overlying the base of an ulcer (Fig. 36-12). In these cases it may be possible to identify only a small portion of the ulcer base as a clue to the nature of the bleeding.

Visible Vessel—An Active Bleeding Equivalent

If the bleeding temporarily ceases, especially if the endoscopist washes away clots adhering to the ulcer base,[41]

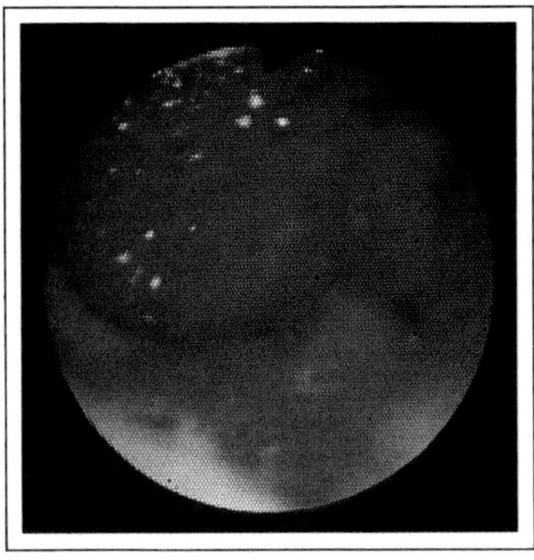

FIG. 36-12.

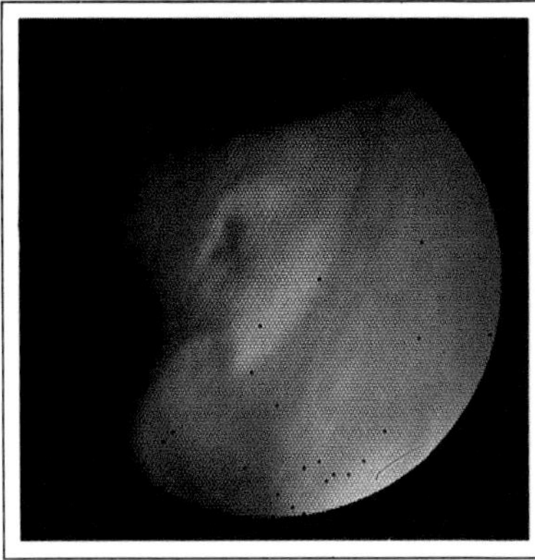

FIG. 36-13.

FIG. 36-12. Gastric ulcer bleeding from a visible vessel. Blood in this case can be seen to spurt from a small, raised conical point on the posterior wall of the upper body. The ulcer base is entirely obscured by the bleeding. A bleeding ulcer was found at surgery and within its base was a large pumping artery.

FIG. 36-13. Gastric ulcer with a possible visible vessel equivalent. A discrete red spot is present within an ulcer base of the patient examined because of bleeding. The bleeding had completely ceased at the time of examination; however, it recurred, and surgery was ultimately required. In the resected specimen, several arterioles were found at the surface of the ulcer base.

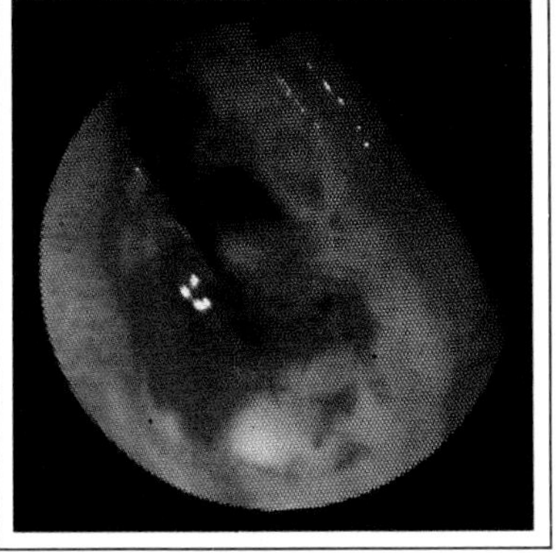

FIG. 36-14a.

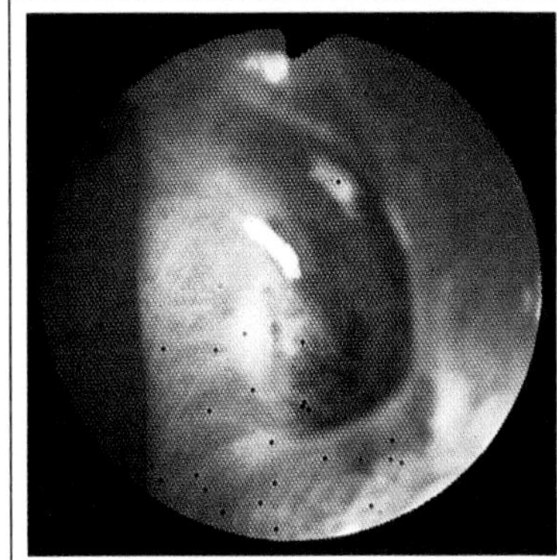

FIG. 36-14b.

FIG. 36-14. Gastric ulcer. **a:** With a fresh clot. This marks the ulcer as the site of a recent bleeding episode and indicates a greater likelihood of rebleeding in contrast to a clot which is embedded in the ulcer base (b). **b:** With old blood (acid hematin) embedded in its base. This indicates an ulcer less likely to rebleed than one with a fresh clot (Fig. 36-15a) or a visible vessel (Fig. 36-10).

he may observe a visible vessel (Fig. 36-10). This has been described typically as a focal, red-pink elevation within the ulcer base which represents a large or medium-sized artery (Fig. 36-10). We have also seen a visible vessel simply as several punctate (1 to 3 mm) intensely red areas with an ulcer base (Fig. 36-13) in a patient in whom subsequent bleeding necessitated surgery and where the resected specimen showed two arterioles at the surface of the ulcer base from which bleeding had occurred. An, vascular-like structure observed in an ulcer base, especially if raised, should be suspected as representing a visible vessel. As already mentioned (see "Rationale for Endoscopy," this chapter), a visible vessel implies the high likelihood of continuous or recurrent bleeding.

Stigmata of Recent Bleeding

In 20 to 30% of the cases, there is no active bleeding observed at endoscopy, but evidence of recent bleeding is found as either a clot overlying the ulcer base, appearing fresh (Fig. 36-14a) or bulky. As some of these clots cover what would otherwise be a visible vessel,[41] we are not surprised to find for this appearance a risk of rebleeding that approaches 20 to 30%. This stands in contrast to the finding of old blood (acid hematin) embedded in the base, which is characteristic of the appearance after 48 hr (Fig. 36-14b) with a likelihood of rebleeding of less than 10%.[41] In these cases, the base and margin of the ulcer can be clearly demonstrated and the size accurately determined, unlike the case of an actively bleeding ulcer where the endoscopist can observe only a small portion of the ulcer that may be free of blood.

No Stigmata of Recent Bleeding

The incidence of patients whose gastric ulcers are thought to be the cause of bleeding but who have no stigmata varies between 20 and 40%. In some cases whether the endoscopist sees stigmata depends on whether the entire ulcer base (Fig. 36-15a) is examined or only partially observed (Fig. 36-15b). Another factor is the timing of endoscopy with the lowest incidence of true stigmata-less ulcers probably found in series where endoscopy is routinely performed within the first 24 hr, although stigmata associated with gastric ulcers tend to persist even after 48 hr. Even so, the percentage of stigmata-less ulcers may comprise one-third or more of the cases where bleeding is ultimately ascribed to a gastric ulcer. In the ASGE survey, even though 62.8% had endoscopy within the first 24 hr the incidence of stigmata-less ulcers was 44.7%. Of these, however, only a small fraction (15%)

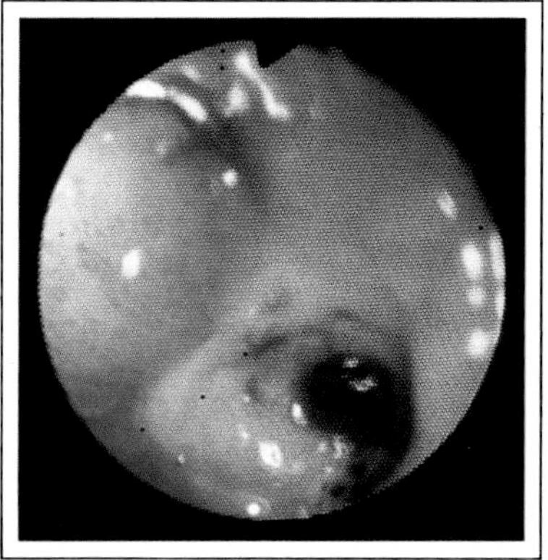

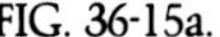
FIG. 36-15a.

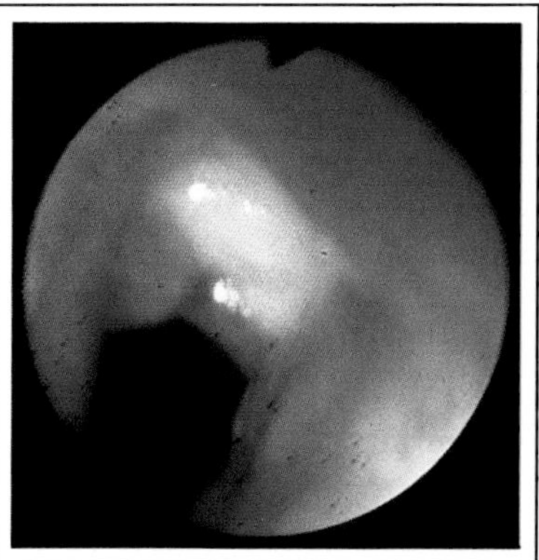

FIG. 36-15b.

FIG. 36-15. Gastric ulcer. **a:** With an adherent blood clot. Unless carefully looked for, stigmata such as this, indicating both recent bleeding and an increased predisposition to rebleed, can be missed. **b:** Recent bleeding with no obvious stigmata. Careful examination of the ulcer base revealed an adherent clot (a) not yet embedded in the ulcer base and thereby indicating the need for continued, close observation because of an increased risk of rebleeding, which may occur in 20 to 30% of cases. As it was, massive rebleeding occurred 1 week later, requiring surgery.

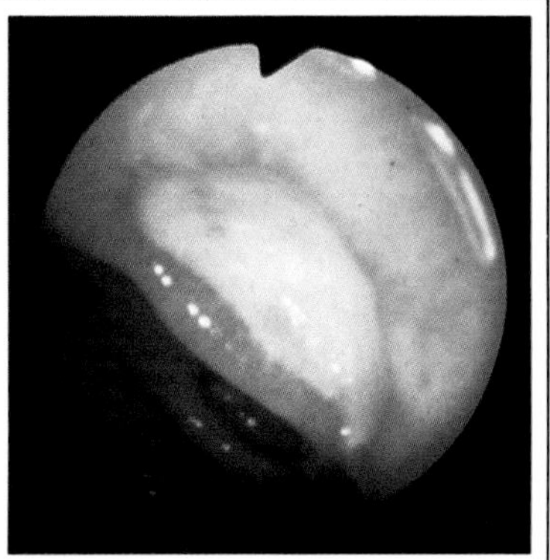

FIG. 36-16a.

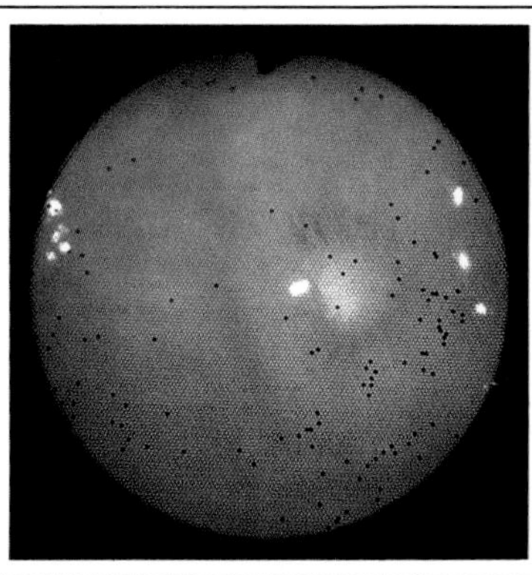

FIG. 36-16b.

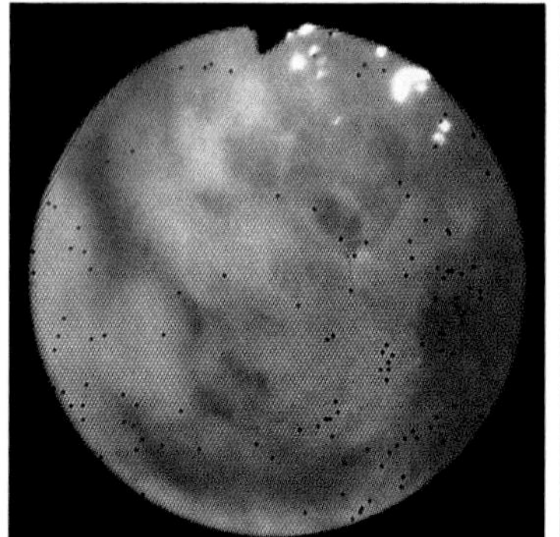

FIG. 36-16c.

FIG. 36-16. a: Gastric ulcer with a recent bleeding episode but no stigmata. The ulcer is of the size (7 × 10 mm) which suggests it could have been responsible for a small bleed (2 to 4 transfusion units). **b:** Gastric ulcer bleeding. This small (3 mm) ulcer with no stigmata is unlikely to be the source of bleeding. **c:** Gastric ulcer bleeding. A large (2 cm) ulcer was found with evidence of continued bleeding in a patient with a second small ulcer (b).

were found in association with other lesions which were considered to be a more likely source of bleeding than the ulcer. In 85% of the cases where stigmata-less ulcers were found, they were nonetheless considered the site of bleeding.[24] In cases where bleeding had been substantial, one would expect stigmata-less ulcers to be sizable (at least 5 mm if not over 1 cm) and deep (Fig. 36-16a) as well as being associated with some evidence of chronicity, i.e., scar deformity (see Chapter 18). The presence of a small (<5 mm), shallow ulceration prompts the endoscopist to look for a more likely bleeding site (Fig. 36-16c).

Interpretive Problems

The commonest causes of interpretive error in patients with bleeding gastric ulcers are: (a) large amounts of blood and clots; (b) nasogastric suction artifacts; and (c) an incomplete endoscopic examination.

Large Amounts of Blood and Clots

In the face of active bleeding or that which has been massive, the presence of copious amounts of blood and clots

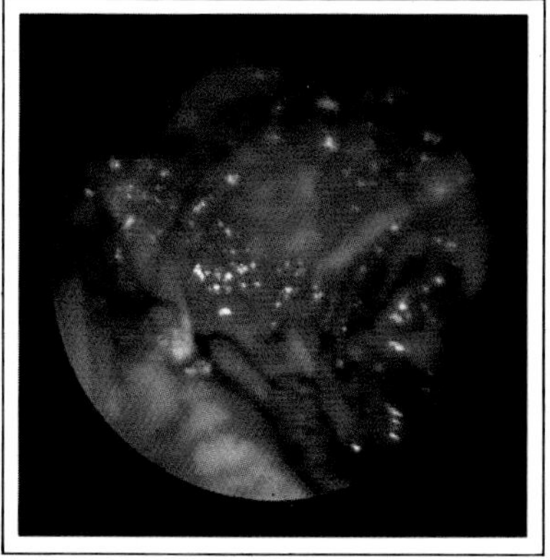

FIG. 36-17a.

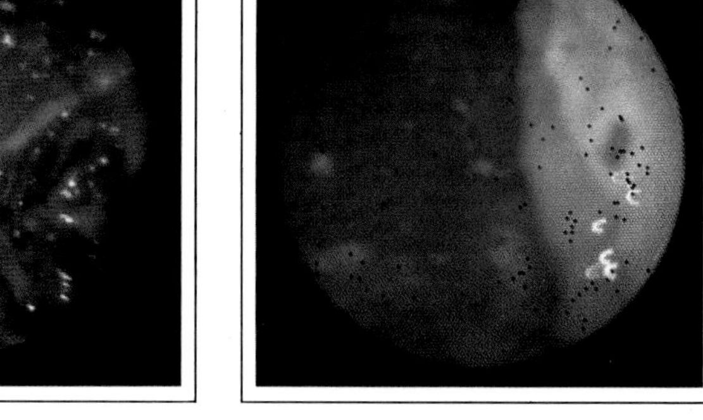

FIG. 36-17b.

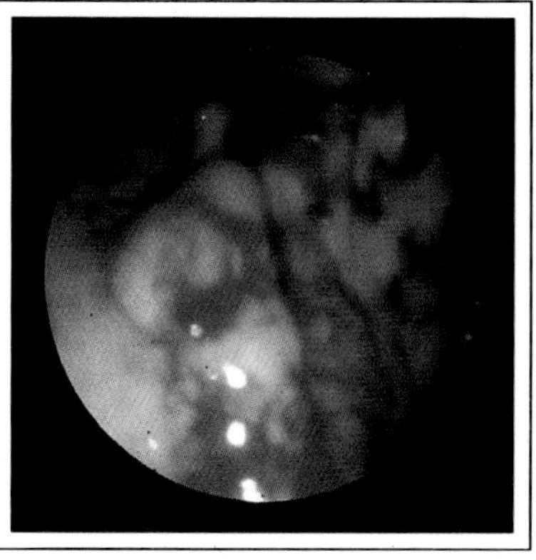

FIG. 36-17c.

FIG. 36-17. a: Gastric ulcer bleeding. Because of the bright red blood which adheres to the mucosa (at 9 o'clock), this appearance was initially thought to represent the intramucosal hemorrhages of hemorrhagic-erosive gastritis. Careful observation, however, reveals scar deformity and an ulcer base on the gastric angle (at 9 o'clock). **b:** Gastric ulcer bleeding, gastric angle. Viewing an ulcer (a) at close range revealed several blood clots embedded in its base as stigmata of recent bleeding. **c:** Two gastric suction artifacts in gastric ulcer bleeding. These acute mucosal hemorrhages and erosions are so striking they mislead the examiner into making a diagnosis of hemorrhagic-erosive gastritis, missing the bleeding gastric ulcer (b).

may seem an insurmountable problem (Fig. 36-17a) as this obscures the area which needs to be observed in the mid and upper body. Moreover, blood may adhere to the mucosa and simulate acute mucosal hemorrhages and erosions, leading the endoscopist to an erroneous diagnosis of hemorrhagic-erosive gastritis (Fig. 36-17a). Fortunately, most of the blood and clots tends to accumulate on the greater curve aspect. The fact that most bleeding ulcers, like gastric ulcers in general, are located on the lesser curve[34] means that the endoscopist may still demonstrate ulcers even with sizable accumulations of blood in the gastric lake and along the dependent greater curve (Fig. 36-17b). In cases where active bleeding precludes an adequate examination of the lesser curve or where neither an ulcer nor another site can be diagnosed, the endoscopist recommends arteriography to determine whether the bleeding site is diffuse (as in hemorrhagic-erosive gastritis) or localized (suggestive of an ulcer).

Nasogastric Suction Artifacts

With prolonged nasogastric suction, especially if continuous and at pressures exceeding 50 mm Hg (see Chapter 33), acute mucosal injury effects in the upper body may be so striking as to cause the endoscopist to diagnose hemorrhagic-erosive gastritis, especially if any history of alcohol or aspirin ingestion is elicited. Even if the injury is confined to the upper body and cardia, the endoscopist may still conclude it is part of a circumscribed rather than a diffuse presentation of hemorrhagic-erosive gastritis.[21] Despite an appearance suggesting hemorrhagic-erosive gastritis, the careful endoscopist nevertheless thoroughly examines the lesser curve as best as he can, looking for a specific area of bleeding associated with scar deformity (Fig. 36-11a) which would strongly suggest a diagnosis of gastric ulcer bleeding.

Inadequate Examination

A complete examination of the stomach may be impossible to perform in the presence of large amounts of blood. This may lead the endoscopist to "give up" on an examination of the stomach, especially the lesser curve. However, we often find the entire lesser curve, especially the supra-angular 10 cm, to be surprisingly amenable to visualization even when there is a considerable amount of blood elsewhere (Fig. 36-6b). Still, it is the proximal lesser curve—which can be the site of up to 30% of gastric ulcers overall and up to 60% in patients over age 60[34]—which is the most crucial for the endoscopist to examine. For him not to do this would place the patient with gastric ulcer bleeding at a serious disadvantage, potentially causing a delay in definitive management for the bleeding which could result in an increased likelihood of an adverse outcome, in terms of both postsurgical complications and mortality.[35,37,38]

Data concerning the frequency with which failure to examine the proximal lesser curve leads to an erroneous diagnosis are difficult to obtain. A suggestion of this, however, is found in a recent series reported by Forrest and colleagues[42] in which the endoscopic diagnosis was compared with that obtained from surgery and autopsy in 104 patients. In this series endoscopy missed 4 of 24 (17%) gastric ulcers. As excess blood was believed to have precluded adequate examination in only 3% of the cases overall, one might legitimately conclude that failure to examine the lesser curve adequately was an important contributing factor to the error rate for gastric ulcers, which may have caused the endoscopist(s) in that study to interpret nonspecific intramucosal hemorrhage and erosions as the site of bleeding.

To avoid this type of error, our approach is to attempt to examine the lesser curve with sweeping arc-like movements on both entry to the stomach and withdrawal (see Chapter 11). On withdrawal, we attempt to visualize the proximal lesser curve first by means of J-type retroflexion; wherever possible, we also utilize U-type retroflexion to examine the proximal lesser curve (see Chapter 11). In this way we believe that we can minimize the "miss rate" for gastric ulcers of the proximal lesser curve.

ULCER BLEEDING AFTER GASTRIC SURGERY

Bleeding from ulcers in patients who have had prior gastric surgery, usually for peptic ulcer disease, is relatively uncommon, but it still constitutes 2 to 6% of the cases of upper GI bleeding.[2] In the ASGE survey, postsurgical (stomal) ulcers were found to be the cause of 1.8% of the cases, similar to our own 1% (see Table 32-2). One could actually expect this type of ulcer bleeding to decrease in frequency during the coming years as the use of potent antisecretory agents (e.g., cimetidine) decreases the number of ulcer operations performed[43] and thereby lowers the absolute number of patients who ultimately present with postsurgical (stomal) ulcer bleeding. For those patients having gastric surgery, especially for duodenal ulcer disease, recurrent ulcers may be expected overall in approximately 5% of the patients.[44] For patients with postsurgical ulcers, bleeding is the presenting symptom in 50%[45] to 60%,[46] appearing as painless melena or episodes of massive GI bleeding and causing the patient to be admitted to the hospital.[46,47] The patients with postsurgical ulcer bleeding tend to be middle-aged, with the ulcer occurring within 1 to 3 years of the surgery, although some investigators have found recurrence in up to 36% of patients documented by endoscopy after 10 years or more.[46]

Pathogenesis of Postsurgical (Stomal) Ulcer Bleeding

It has not been clearly established what factors predispose to postsurgical ulcer bleeding. The original indication for ulcer surgery—bleeding or intractability—seems not to be a factor.[46] As bleeding is a common presentation of postsurgical ulcers, it may be that if an ulcer develops in surgically created junctional mucosa, its natural history is to proceed to the point where larger vessels located deep within the wall become exposed to the ulcer process (see p. 354, "Pathogenesis of Gastric Ulcer Bleeding") and are thus predisposed to bleed. Also involved, but in an as yet unclear fashion, in the pathogenesis of bleeding undoubtedly are factors which predispose to the formation of stomal ulcers in the first place: (a) increased preoperative gastric acid secretion which is (b) inadequately corrected by the surgery; and (c) the presence of a gastrojejunal anastomosis.

Increased Preoperative Gastric Acid Secretion

Increased gastric secretion preoperatively (basal acid output $>$ 5 mEq/hr) in one series was associated with an ulcer rate of 9.5%. For patients with a basal acid output of 7 mEq/hr, this rose to 18%, whereas in those who had a basal secretion of 2 to 5 mEq/hr the recurrence rate was 4.4%; when it was less than 2 mEq/hr the recurrence rate was 1.4%.[44] The reason for this relationship may be the relatively fixed reduction in gastric acid secretion which may be expected from standard ulcer operations (see below); thus the higher the preoperative acid secretion, the higher is the postoperative secretory rate.[44] Patients with a postoperative secretory rate in these higher ranges seem to be predisposed to recurrent ulceration given the usual types of ulcer operations performed (see below).

Inadequate Operative Reduction of Gastric Secretion

Other factors relating to the surgery itself may be responsible for the failure of adequate control of acid secretion, thus predisposing to the formation of recurrent ulcers and bleeding. These are: (a) an incomplete vagotomy; (b) an antral sparing operation, i.e., vagotomy and pyloroplasty, in the presence of (c) an underlying hypersecretory state. Of these, the commonest appears to be the presence of an incomplete vagotomy.[43] Whereas an effective vagotomy may reduce acid secretion by up to 60%, this reduction is not achieved if the vagotomy is technically inadequate. Even with a complete vagotomy, patients with initially high rates of gastric secretion may still have an inadequate operation if an antrectomy (with its major reduction in gastrin) was performed, decreasing secretion a further 30%.[44]

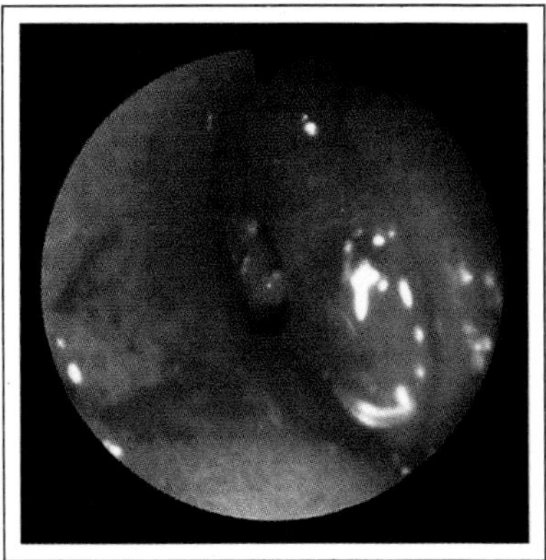

FIG. 36-18. Postsurgical (stomal) ulcer bleeding. A deep ulcer with oozing appears within the efferent limb of a gastrojejunostomy stoma created at the time of a resection for pancreatic cancer 1 year before.

FIG. 36-18.

Gastrojejunal Anastomosis

The jejunum tends to be more vulnerable to the effects of acid and allied ulcerogenic substances than the duodenum so that the recurrence rate of a gastrojejunostomy, even with a complete vagotomy, approaches 10%, whereas the recurrence rate for vagotomy and pyloroplasty is only 5%.[44] For a gastrojejunostomy performed without a vagotomy (as is the case when it is fashioned as part of a cancer operation), postsurgical ulcers may occur in at least 10% if not more, as is the case where a gastrojejunostomy (without vagotomy) is performed at an ulcer operation with a recurrence rate of 30%.[44]

It is our impression that elderly patients who have a gastrojejunal anastomosis with a postsurgical ulcer on the jejunal side are at greatest risk for massive bleeding because of the decreased resistance of the jejunum to peptic injury, as well as possibly other vascular factors which may alter rates of healing for the perianastomotic mucosal surface. As recurrence with a gastrojejunal anastomosis is said to occur later than those at a gastroduodenal junction site,[43] one might imagine that vascular factors related to chronic changes around the stoma itself from longstanding stomatitis scarring might predispose to the accelerated type of ulceration which exposes large blood vessels to the surface where they can bleed massively.[27] In this regard, like gastric ulcer bleeding, the potentiating role of aspirin or other anti-inflammatory agents should always be considered and a history of recent ingestion sought.

Rationale for Endoscopy

Patients with stomal ulcer bleeding, like patients with gastric ulcer hemorrhage in general, are at risk to die if the bleeding is continuous or recurs in the hospital.[37] Although the overall mortality for postsurgical (stomal) ulcer bleeding in the ASGE survey was only 9.8%, not differing from the mortality overall, this was higher than for bleeding gastric or duodenal ulcers (7.8% and 6.7%, respectively). The mortality rate for those ulcers observed at endoscopy to be bleeding, however, was double the overall mortality for this type of bleeding (18.8% versus 10%).[24] In addition, patients with active bleeding had a three times greater rate of transfusion, exceeding 5 units of blood (37% versus 10%), and seven times higher rate of surgical intervention (31.3% versus 4.4%).[24] As in the case of gastric ulcer bleeding itself, the higher transfusion requirement, the rate of surgical intervention, and the mortality rate for patients actively bleeding make one anxious to perform endoscopy early, within the first 6 to 12 hr on patients with previous gastric surgery, where the incidence of active bleeding found at endoscopy is high, in the range of 30 to 50%.[24] Such patients would be those with a hematocrit of less than 30, orthostatic hypotension, or pulse changes, as well as a nasogastric aspirate showing either bright red blood or coffee-ground material. The role of endoscopy in these patients is to confirm the presence of a bleeding postsurgical (stomal) ulcer so that surgery, at present the only uniformly effective therapy, is not delayed for lack of a definite diagnosis.

Location of Bleeding Postsurgical (Stomal) Ulcers

A generally held view is that most ulcers occurring in patients with previous gastric surgery are at the anastomotic junction and that the commonest site is intestinal, especially jejunal, within 2 cm of the actual anastomotic line (Fig. 36-18) because of a supposedly increased disposition of jejunal mucosa to ulcerate (see above).

Questioning this view is a recent series reported by Sharaiha et al.[46] in which 60% of recurrent ulcers were located proximal to the anastomosis; only 27% were on the intestinal side and only 10% at the anastomotic margin, with the remaining 3% being esophageal. The site of recurrence bore no relationship to the original type of ulcer disease, the indication for surgery, or the presentation of the recurrence, particularly whether there was bleeding. This contrasts with the traditional view and our own experience where the recurrent ulcer tends to be anastomotic (Fig. 36-18), with

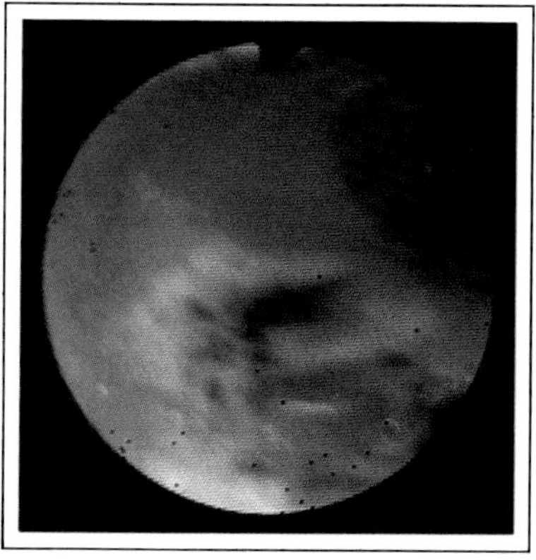

FIG. 36-19.

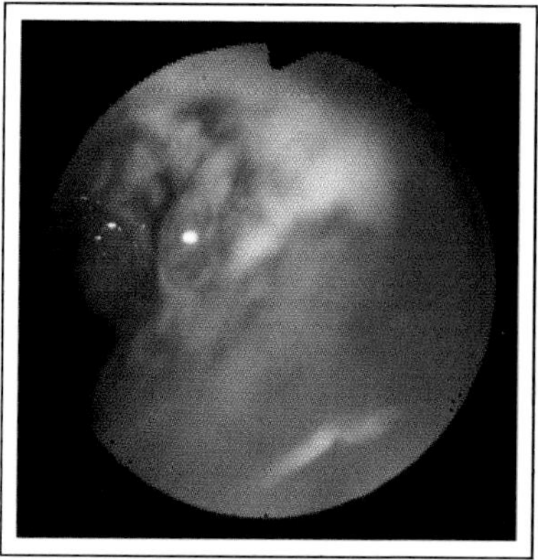

FIG. 36-20.

FIG. 36-19. Postsurgical (stomal) ulcer bleeding. Old blood is embedded within the base of an ulcer located on the bridging fold between the afferent and efferent limbs (the efferent limb is running off toward 3 o'clock). The previous surgery (vagotomy and antrectomy) had been performed 3 years earlier because of intractable ulcer symptoms, with the bleeding episode being the presentation of ulcer recurrence.

FIG. 36-20. A postsurgical ulcer located high on the lesser curve of the gastric remnant. Blood clots embedded within its base are stigmata of its being the site of a recent bleeding episode.

those that bleed involving the intestinal mucosa. Of the five patients with recurrent ulcer bleeding in our series, all of the ulcers were within 2 cm of the anastomotic line, on either the gastric side (one) or the intestinal side (two duodenal, two jejunal).

Nevertheless, the implication from this study is clear. Endoscopists must expect recurrent ulcers, especially those which bleed, not to be confined solely to a small area on either side of the anastomotic line but with a variable percentage sometimes to be found elsewhere (possibly up to 60%).[46]

Appearance

In patients with postsurgical (stomal) ulcers who are examined because of recent hemorrhage, the ulcer is commonly observed to be actively bleeding. Of 39 postsurgical (stomal) ulcers reported in the ASGE survey, 33.3% showed oozing and an additional 7.7% were pumping as evidence of more massive bleeding. Only esophageal varices had a comparable percentage (7.5%) of the massive bleeding.[24] The majority of postsurgical (stomal) ulcers in the ASGE survey, as for gastric ulcers in general, had ceased to bleed (59%) by the time endoscopy was performed, with 12.8% showing a clot overlying the base (Fig. 36-19) and 46.2% no stigmata or recent bleeding. Nevertheless, because the stomal ulcer was generally the sole lesion in the 92.3% of the cases where it was found it was taken to be the site of bleeding.

In our experience, the typical finding for a postsurgical (stomal) ulcer examined because of recent bleeding is an ulcer generally within 2 cm of the anastomotic line on the jejunal side of the gastrojejunostomy stoma (Fig. 36-19). A common location for the ulcer is on the bridging fold between the afferent and efferent loops or just proximal to it (Fig. 36-19). The ulcer is deep and appears punched-out and well marginated (Fig. 36-18). In cases where endoscopy is performed after the bleeding has clinically stopped, the ulcer base is generally free of stigmata of recent bleeding; conversely, in those patients who clinically appear to be continuing to bleed, active bleeding from the ulcer is expected. In the case of active bleeding, the ulcer itself may not be seen because of the blood which tends to well up in the compartment between the stoma and marginal folds. The presence of bright red blood at this site, however, would make the endoscopist very suspicious of a stomal ulcer bleed.

In some patients, although not the majority in our experience, the ulcer is located on the gastric side of the stoma but still within 2 cm of the anastomotic line. Only rarely do we find, in contrast to others,[46] that the ulcer is located a considerable distance from the stoma (Fig. 36-20). Deformity of the stoma, with radiating folds to it or to another area within the remaining stomach, can be a clue that causes the endoscopist to suspect a postsurgical (stomal) ulcer as the cause of the bleeding episode.

Interpretive Problems

There are three major sources of interpretive error in patients with postsurgical (stomal) ulcer bleeding. These are derived from: (a) the blood itself; (b) appearances within the gastric remnant; and (c) the appearance of the stoma.

Active Bleeding Simulating Hemorrhagic-Erosive Gastritis

Active bleeding is found in slightly less than half the cases according to the ASGE survey; however, when it occurs it may be massive in 7%[24] to 10%.[47] Copious accumulations of blood in a relatively small gastric remnant quickly lead to the interpretive problems associated with large amounts of blood in the stomach (see Chapter 33). Fresh blood in the stomach in amounts associated with massive hemorrhage may simply, by its adherence to mucosal surfaces, create an appearance which simulates that of hemorrhagic-erosive gastritis, leading the endoscopist to an erroneous diagnosis. Such an interpretation could result in the death of the patient if surgery were withheld despite

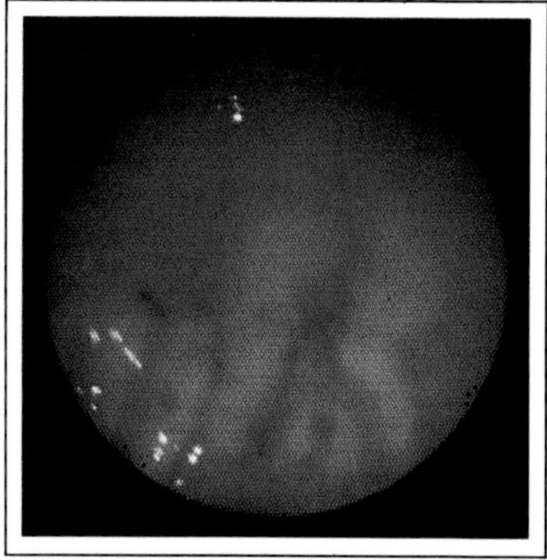

FIG. 36-21.

FIG. 36-21. Hemorrhagic-erosive gastritis in the gastric remnant of a patient with a Billroth II resection. Diffuse intramucosal hemorrhage and erosions were found within the mucosa of a patient with a history of recently having ingested large amounts of aspirin. Blood in and around the stoma, however, made the endoscopic diagnosis a stomal ulcer bleed. Examination of the surgically resected specimens revealed only hemorrhagic-erosive gastritis.

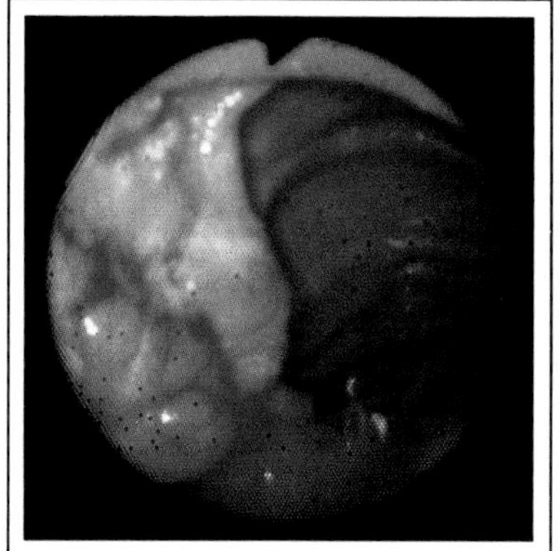

FIG. 36-22a.

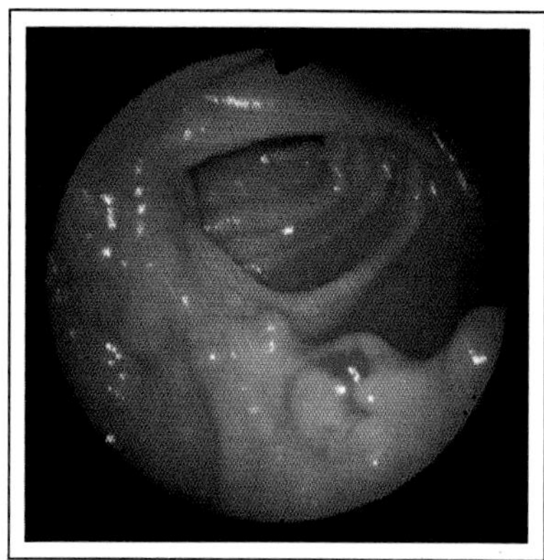

FIG. 36-22b.

FIG. 36-22. a: Stomatitis in a patient with hematemesis and a recent bleeding episode. Erythema and friability of the stoma suggest it to be a possible bleeding site but only by exclusion of other causes. In a questionable case, arteriography would be indicated to exclude a proximal small bowel site, e.g., a leiomyoma (see text). **b:** Hyperplastic polyps in a patient with prior gastric resection (Billroth II) as a cause of bleeding. Multiple hyperplastic polyps with friable surfaces pose the risk of recurrent bleeding such as occurred in this patient until a total gastrectomy was performed.

high transfusion requirements because of the generally high surgical mortality found in patients operated on for hemorrhagic-erosive gastritis.[6] Had a correct diagnosis been made, simple ligation of the bleeding vessel may have been possible with an acceptable surgical mortality (<10%).[35] In cases where massive bleeding precludes adequate examination of the stoma and gastric remnant, the endoscopist should not attempt to make a diagnosis but should recommend that arteriography be attempted to determine whether the bleeding site is diffuse or localized to a site which suggests a postsurgical (stomal) ulcer as the source.

Bleeding from Hemorrhagic-Erosive Gastritis

The presence of previous gastric surgery does not exclude hemorrhagic-erosive gastritis in an appropriate clinical setting (Fig. 36-21). Nevertheless, because the blood tends to well up at the stoma, the endoscopist may find the diagnosis of stomal ulcer bleeding irresistible. In typical clinical setting, one looks for intramucosal hemorrhage and erosions alone (see "Hemorrhagic-Erosive Gastritis," p. 346) occurring diffusely throughout the mucosa of the remnant. Finding this, especially in the setting of only modest bleeding, the endoscopist may suggest that hemorrhagic-erosive gastritis is the likely source with recurrent (stomal) ulcer bleeding unlikely, although not excluded, especially if old or fresh blood compromises the examination of the stomal area.

Appearance of the Stoma

The endoscopist may encounter a stoma with marked erythema, edema, and friability but no ulcer (Fig. 36-22a) and may conclude that this is the site of bleeding if a careful examination of the esophagus and other portions of the remaining stomach and adjacent small bowel reveals no other potential source. Under these circumstances, he may tentatively regard stomatitis as a possible ulcer-equivalent, although at the same time cautioning all concerned that another bleeding site in the proximal small bowel, e.g., a leiomyoma,[48] or arteriovenous malformation[48a] is not excluded. In cases where the indication of the original surgery was bleeding, and the pathologic findings were not that of a definite ulcer, angiography is mandatory with an endoscopic finding of only stomatitis.

Another potentially confusing appearance which involves the stoma is that of hyperplastic polyps (Fig. 36-22b). Although these are seen in the absence of bleeding, they may also be a source.[48] As in the case of stomatitis bleeding, careful search for other bleeding sites must be carried out. If none is found, one may conclude that the stomal hyperplastic polyps[49] are a likely source but by no means does this exclude another site.

REFERENCES

1. Silverstein, F. E., Gilbert, D. A., Tedesco, F. J., Buenger, N. K., Persing, J., and 277 members of the ASGE (1981): The national ASGE survey on upper gastrointestinal bleeding. I. Study design and baseline data. *Gastrointest. Endosc.,* 27:73–79.
2. Graham, D. Y., and Davis, R. E. (1978): Acute upper-gastrointestinal hemorrhage: new observations on an old problem. *Am. J. Dig. Dis.,* 23:76–84.
3. Katz, D., Pitchumoni, C. S., Thomas, E., and Antonelle, M. (1976): The endoscopic diagnosis of upper-gastrointestinal hemorrhage: changing concepts of etiology and management. *Am. J. Dig. Dis.,* 21:182–187.
4. Sugawa, C., Werner, M. H., Hayes, D. F., Lucas, C. E., and Walt, A. J. (1973): Early endoscopy: a guide to therapy for acute hemorrhage in the upper gastrointestinal tract. *Arch. Surg.,* 107:133–137.
5. McCusker, J., Cherubin, C. E., and Zimberg, S. (1971): Prevalence of alcoholism in a general municipal hospital population. *N.Y. State J. Med.,* 71:751–754.
6. Dagradi, A., Lee, E. R., Bosco, D. L., and Stempien, S. J. (1973): The clinical spectrum of hemorrhagic erosive gastritis. *Am. J. Gastroenterol.,* 60:30–46.
7. Dinoso, V., Ming, S.-C., and McNiff, J. (1976): Ultrastructural changes of the canine gastric mucosa after topical application of graded concentrations of ethanol. *Am. J. Dig. Dis.,* 21:626–632.
8. Davenport, H. W. (1969): Gastric mucosal hemorrhage in dogs—effects of acid, aspirin and alcohol. *Gastroenterology,* 56:439–449.
9. Gottfried, E. B., Korsten, M. A., and Lieber, C. S. (1978): Alcohol-induced gastric and duodenal lesions in man. *Am. J. Gastroenterol.,* 70:587–592.
10. Dinoso, V. P., Meshkinpour, H., and Lorber, S. H. (1973): Gastric mucosal morphology and faecal blood loss during ethanol ingestion. *Gut,* 14:289–292.
11. Winawer, S. J., Bejar, J., McCray, R. S., and Zamcheck, N. (1971): Hemorrhagic gastritis: importance of associated chronic gastritis. *Arch. Intern. Med.,* 127:129–131.
12. Fromm, D. (1978): Gastric mucosal defense mechanisms: effects of salicylate and histamine. *Am. J. Surg.,* 135:379–383.
13. Konturek, S. J., Piastucki, I., Brozozowski, T., Radecki, T., Dembinska-Kiec, A., Zmuda, A., and Gryglewski, R. (1981): Role of prostaglandins in the formation of aspirin-induced gastric ulcers. *Gastroenterology,* 80:4–9.
14. Rees, W. D. W., and Turnberg, L. A. (1980): Reappraisal of the effects of aspirin on the stomach. *Lancet,* 2:410–413.
15. Baskin, W. N., Ivey, K. J., Krause, W. J., Jeffrey, G. E., and Gemmell, R. T. (1976): Aspirin-induced ultrastructural changes in human gastric mucosa: correlation with potential difference. *Ann. Intern. Med.,* 85:299–303.
16. Hoftiezer, J. W., Silvoso, G. R., Burks, M., and Ivey, K. (1980): Comparison of the effects of regular and enteric-coated aspirin on gastroduodenal mucosa of man. *Lancet,* 2:609–612.
17. Sugawa, C., Lucas, C. E., Rosenberg, B. F., Riddle, J. M., and Walt, A. J. (1973): Differential topography of acute erosive gastritis due to trauma or sepsis, ethanol and aspirin. *Gastrointest. Endosc.,* 19:127–130.

17a. Robert, A., Nezamis, J. E., Hanchar, A. J., and Lancaster, C. (1980): Aspirin combined with alcohol is ulcerogenic. *Gastroenterology,* 80:1245.

17b. Needham, C. D., Kyle, J., Jones, P. F., Johnston, S. J., and Kerridge, D. F. (1971): Aspirin and alcohol in gastrointestinal haemorrhage. *Gut,* 12:819–821.

17c. Miller, T. A., Gum, E. T., Guinn, E. J., and Henagan, J. M. (1982): Prostaglandin prevents alteration in DNA, RNA, and protein in damaged gastric mucosa. *Dig. Dis. Sci.,* 27:776–781.

18. Hart, F. D. (1974): Naproxen and gastrointestinal hemorrhage. *Br. Med. J.,* 2:51–52.
19. Lanza, F. L., Royer, G. L., Nelson, R. S., Chen, T. T., Seckman, C. E., and Rack, M. F. (1979): The effects of ibuprofen, indomethacin, aspirin, naproxen, and placebo on the gastric mucosa of normal volunteers: a gastroscopic and photographic study. *Dig. Dis. Sci.,* 24:823–828.
20. Caruso, I., and Bianchi Porro, G. (1980): Gastroscopic evaluation of anti-inflammatory agents. *Br. Med. J.,* 1:75–78.
21. Katz, D., Pitchumoni, C. S., Thomas, E., and Antonelle, M. (1978): Bleeding at the gastro-esophageal junction. *South. Med. J. (Suppl. 1),* 71:29–30.
22. Dagradi, A. E., Stempien, S. J., Lee, E. R., and Juler, G. (1968): Hemorrhagic-erosive gastritis. *Gastrointest. Endosc.,* 14:147–150.
23. Kim, U., Rudick, J., and Aufses, A. H. (1978): Surgical management of acute upper gastrointestinal bleeding. *Arch. Surg.,* 113:1444–1447.
24. Gilbert, D. A., Silverstein, F. E., Tedesco, F. J., Buenger, N. K., Persing, J., and 277 members of the ASGE (1981): The national ASGE survey on upper gastrointestinal bleeding. III. Endoscopy in upper gastrointestinal bleeding. *Gastrointest. Endosc.,* 27:94–102.
25. Leinicke, J. A., Shaffer, R. D., Hogan, W. J., and Geenen, J. E. (1976): Emergency endoscopy in acute upper GI bleeding: does timing affect the significance of the diagnostic yield? *Gastrointest. Endosc.,* 22:228.
26. Walker, C. O. (1978): Complications of peptic ulcer disease. In: *Gastrointestinal Disease,* edited by M. H. Sleisenger and J. S. Fordtran, p. 916. Saunders, Philadelphia.
27. Osborn, G. R. (1954): The pathology of gastric ulcers, with special reference to fatal haemorrhage from peptic ulcer. *Br. J. Surg.,* 41:585–594.
28. Griffiths, W. J., Neumann, D. A., and Welsh, J. D. (1979): The visible vessel as an indicator of uncontrolled or recurrent gastrointestinal hemorrhage. *N. Engl. J. Med.,* 300:1411–1413.
29. Levy, M. (1974): Aspirin use in patients with major upper gastrointestinal bleeding and peptic ulcer disease. *N. Engl. J. Med.,* 290:1158–1162.
30. Muggan, M. (1972): Aspirin ingestion and perforated peptic ulcer. *Gut,* 13:631–633.
31. Hamilton, S. R., and Yardley, J. H. (1980): Endoscopic biopsy diagnosis of aspirin-associated chronic gastric ulcers. *Gastroenterology,* 78:1178.
32. Bick, L. L., Admas, T., and Schmalhorst, W. R. (1976): Bleeding times, platelet adhesion, and aspirin. *Am. J. Clin. Pathol.,* 65:69–72.
33. Emmanuel, J. H., and Montgomery, R. D. (1981): Gastric ulcer and the anti-arthritic drugs. *Postgrad. Med. J.,* 47:227–232.
34. Sheppard, M. C., Holmes, G. K. T., and Cockel, R. (1977): Clinical picture of peptic ulceration diagnosed endoscopically. *Gut,* 18:524–530.
35. Himal, H. S., Watson, W. W., Jones, C. W., Miller, L., and MacClean, L. D. (1974): The management of upper gastrointestinal hemorrhage: a multi-parametric computer analysis. *Ann. Surg.,* 179:489–493.
36. Forster, D. N., Miloszewski, K. J. A., and Losowsky, M. S. (1978): Stigmata of recent haemorrhage in diagnosis and prognosis of upper gastrointestinal hemorrhage. *Br. Med. J.,* 1:1173–1177.
37. Morgan, A. G., MacAdam, W. A. F., Walmsley, G. L., Jessop, A., Horrocks, J. C., and de Dombal, F. T. (1977): Clinical findings, early endoscopy, and multivariate analysis in patients bleeding from the upper gastrointestinal tract. *Br. Med. J.,* 2:237–240.
38. Hunt, P. S., Hansky, J., and Korman, M. G. (1979): Mortality in patients with haematemesis and melaena: a prospective study. *Br. Med. J.,* 1:1238–1240.
39. Swain, C. P., Bown, S. G., Storey, D. W., Kirckham, J. S., Northfield, T. C., and Salmon, P. R. (1981): Controlled trial of argon laser photocoagulation in bleeding peptic ulcers. *Lancet,* 2:1313–1316.
40. Papp, J. P. (1981): Electrocoagulation in upper gastrointestinal bleeding. *Dig. Dis. Sci. (Suppl.)* 26:41–43.
41. Storey, D. W., Bown, S. G., Swain, C. P., Salmon, P. R., Kirhan, J. S., and Northfield, T. C. (1981): Endoscopic prediction of recurrent bleeding in peptic ulcers. *N. Engl. J. Med.,* 305:915–916.
42. Forrest, J. A. H., Finlayson, N. D. C., and Shearman, D. J. C. (1974): Endoscopy in gastrointestinal bleeding. *Lancet,* 2:394–397.
43. Wylie, J. H., Clark, C. G., Alexander-Williams, J., Bell, P. R. F., Kennedy, T. L., Kirk, R. M., and MacKay, C. (1981): Effect of cimetidine for surgery for duodenal ulcer. *Lancet,* 1:1307–1309.

44. Stabile, B. E., and Passaro, E. (1976): Recurrent peptic ulcer. *Gastroenterology*, 70:124–135.

45. Lindenauer, S. M., and Dent, T. L. (1975): Management of the recurrent ulcer. *Arch. Surg.*, 110:531–536.

46. Sharaiha, Z., Graham, D. Y., Smith, J. L., Schwartz, J. T., and Cain, G. D. (1981): Location and presentation of recurrent ulcer after peptic ulcer surgery: a modern reassessment. *Gastroenterology*, 80:1281.

47. Neustein, C. L., Buskin, F. L., Weinshelbaum, E. I., and Woodward, E. R. (1977): Reoperation for postsurgical peptic ulcer recurrence: appraisal of ten years' experience. *Ann. Surg.*, 185:169–174.

48. Stothert, J. C., Riaz, A., Joyce, P. F., and Kaminski, D. L. (1978): Preoperative angiographic diagnosis of small bowel leiomyomas. *Arch. Surg.*, 113:643–645.

48a. Case records of the Massachusetts General Hospital (case 30-1981) (1981): *N. Engl. J. Med.*, 305:211–216.

49. Joffee, N., Goldman, H., and Antonioli, D. A. (1978): Recurring hyperplastic gastric polyps following subtotal gastrectomy. *Am. J. Roentgenol.*, 130:301–305.

37

GASTRIC BLEEDING—VASCULAR AND OTHER UNCOMMON CAUSES

The conditions we consider in this chapter are rarely observed. Taken together, they account for less than 5% of the cases of upper gastrointestinal (GI) bleeding.[1] Still, an awareness that there are vascular and other uncommon causes of gastric bleeding is necessary, especially in the particular setting of GI hemorrhage where they are most likely to be found. Given an elderly patient with recurrent, unexplained GI bleeding, the endoscopist searches the stomach and duodenum for areas of angiodysplasia[2] which he might otherwise have overlooked or dismissed as erosions were he not actively considering this condition.

In a patient with known chronic pancreatitis, the thoughtful endoscopist, on seeing unusually prominent or otherwise atypical cardiofundic folds, suspects gastric varices, knowing that chronic pancreatitis is the setting where he is most likely to encounter them.[3] Although bleeding from neoplasms accounts for only 2 to 4% of cases of gastric bleeding,[1] it is always a consideration in older patients with a history of weight loss. In patients with known malignancy, the endoscopist looks for evidence of the major causes of gastric bleeding elsewhere (see Chapter 36), searching especially for hemorrhagic-erosive gastritis from aspirin or alcohol usage and for acute mucosal injury from stress conditions, e.g., superinfection.[4] The endoscopist is mindful as well that in a minority of these patients, especially those with breast or lung cancer or melanoma,[5] the stomach may be the site of metastasis presenting gastric bleeding. Finally, in other patients with acute mucosal "stress" conditions, e.g., burns, sustained hypotension, renal failure, or fulminant hepatic failure, acute mucosal lesions are encountered as a cause of bleeding.[6]

The purpose then of this chapter is to present a brief discussion of each of these significant but infrequently encountered conditions.

VASCULAR CAUSES OF GASTRIC BLEEDING

Vascular Malformations

Vascular abnormalities of gastric mucosa that occur as part of a generalized disorder (hereditary hemorrhagic telangiectasia) with mucocutaneous and intestinal lesions or which are confined to the stomach (with duodenal sites in some cases) account for less than 1% of patients with GI bleeding.[7] In most of these, the bleeding is chronic, with endoscopy being performed selectively, rather than necessarily, within the first 24 to 48 hr after the patient's admission to the hospital. These are therefore rare findings among patients examined urgently for upper GI bleeding. Because they are uncommon and easily overlooked or misinterpreted as artifacts or focal erosions if the examiner is unaware of their appearance, they may escape detection. In the case of gastric angiodysplasia this is regrettable, as definitive therapy is available either in the form of surgery or endoscopic therapy in cases where the lesions are amenable to electrocoagulation.[2]

In this section, we consider first vascular abnormalities occurring as part of generalized hereditary hemorrhagic telangiectasia (Osler-Weber-Rendu disease) followed by a discussion of localized vascular abnormalities, e.g., gastric angiodysplasia.

Hereditary Hemorrhagic Telangiectasia

Hereditary hemorrhagic telangiectasia (HHT) is infrequently encountered in patients who have endoscopy for upper GI bleeding. Of the 2,225 cases in the ASGE prospective survey with a final diagnosis of the cause of bleeding, HHT was the cause in only 11 (0.5%).[7] In our own

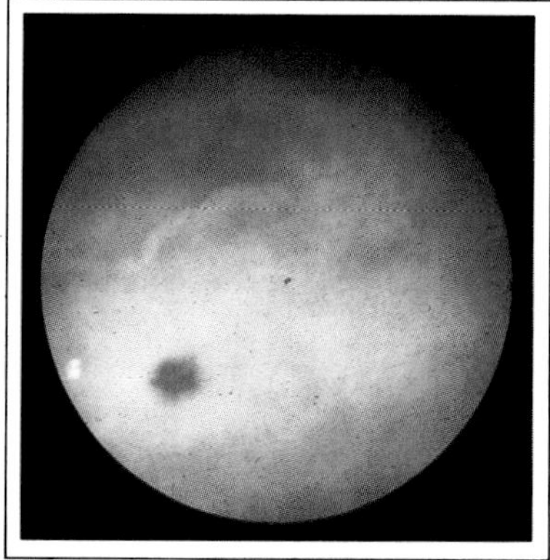

FIG. 37-1a.

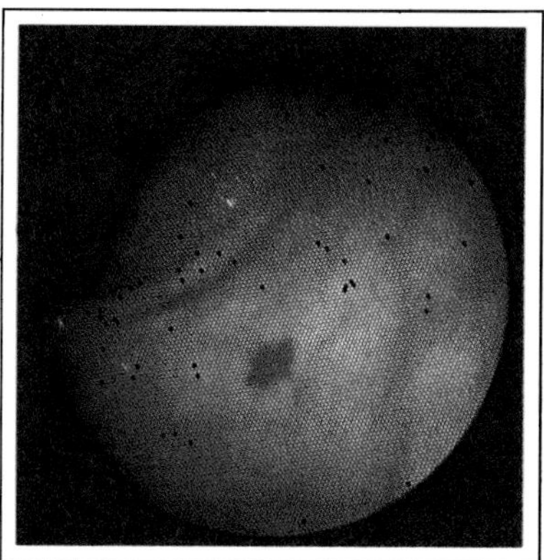

FIG. 37-1b.

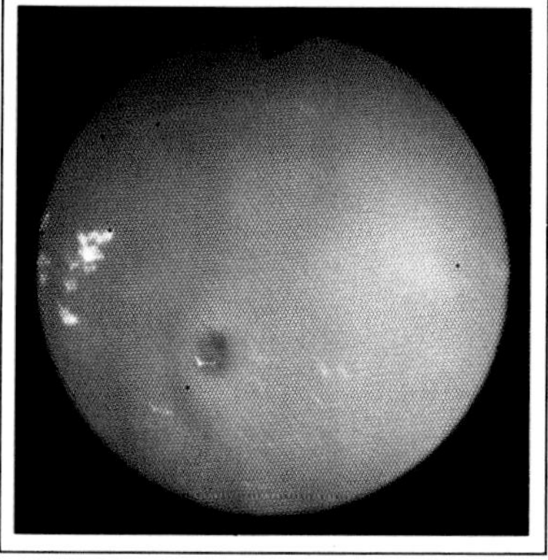

FIG. 37-1c.

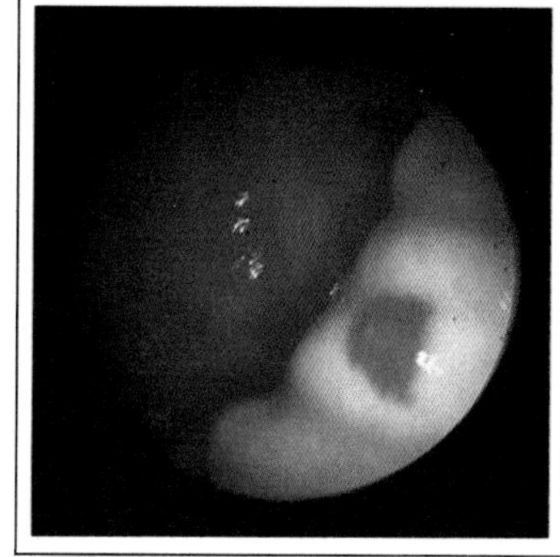

FIG. 37-1d.

FIG. 37-1. a: Hereditary hemorrhagic telangiectasia. One of several (five) 2-mm cherry-red spots in the stomach of a patient with a long history of nose bleeds and recent hematemesis. **b:** Hereditary hemorrhagic telangiectasia. At closer range the margin appears irregular from projections to neighboring capillaries. **c:** A suction artifact simulating a telangiectatic lesion. This lesion was noted in a patient with no history of bleeding after entry into the stomach during which suction had been applied. Its perfectly rounded margin is a clue to its being an artifact. **d:** Hereditary hemorrhagic telangiectasia, large (6 mm) lesion.

series of 500 consecutively studied patients (see Chapter 32), only two cases of HHT were observed (0.4%). In one, the bleeding was chronic, the patient having been admitted to the hospital for transfusion; the other had had an acute bleeding episode. Similar to the experience of others,[8] in both of our cases the diagnosis had been considered prior to endoscopy with a typical history of long-standing epistaxis, the GI bleeding, generally occult and chronic, beginning in adulthood. In both of our patients, the skin and mucous membranes of the nose and mouth showed typical 1- to 3-mm telangiectatic lesions. Endoscopy in these cases was generally requested to determine specifically the presence of esophageal, gastric, or duodenal involvement and to exclude the presence of other essentially treatable causes of bleeding, e.g., peptic ulcer disease. In the one case presenting as an acute upper GI bleed, hematemesis, and orthostatic blood pressure changes, a diagnosis of acute hemorrhagic-erosive gastritis from aspirin usage was made, and was confirmed on subsequent endoscopy with the clearing of multiple intramucosal hemorrhages and erosions. This is consistent with results from the ASGE survey, where two of the 10 patients who had had HHT as the initial diagnosis had a different final diagnosis.[9]

Apart from determining whether other treatable conditions are present, endoscopy is requested in patients with HHT for possible electrocoagulation of gastric lesions, which in at least one report seems to be associated with a temporary remission from continued GI bleeding.[10]

Appearance.

Typically, these lesions are seen as cherry-red spots, similar to their appearance in nasal or buccal mucosa. They range in size between 2 and 4 mm (Fig. 37-1a) but are occasionally larger. At a distance their margins appear irregular, and on close inspection they are noted to be irregular with filamentous projections, representing the communication of the telangiectasia with neighboring capillaries (Fig. 37-1b). This irregular marginal appearance is important because it allows the endoscopist to differentiate a vascular lesion from acute mucosal injury or trauma (Fig. 37-1c). In these cases the margins tend to be regular, especially with suction artifacts, where there may be a rim of edema seen around the cherry-red spot.

Although vascular lesions of HHT are less than 5 mm as a rule, occasionally the telangiectasias are larger, being on the order of 5 to 10 mm (Fig. 37-1d). A rare appearance which has been reported is that of an antral mass, which when resected proved to be composed of a proliferation of blood vessels.[11]

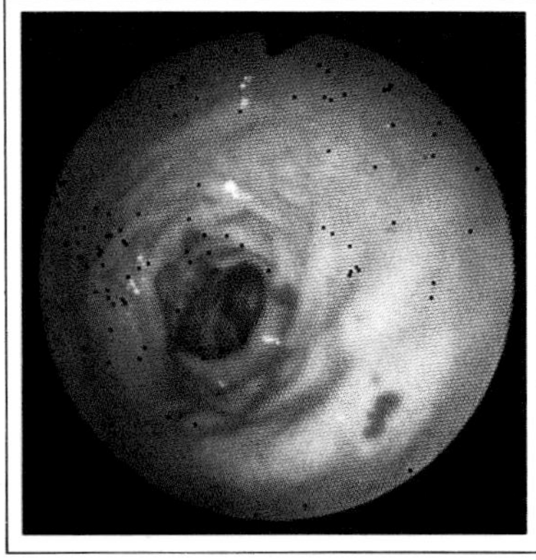

FIG. 37-2a.

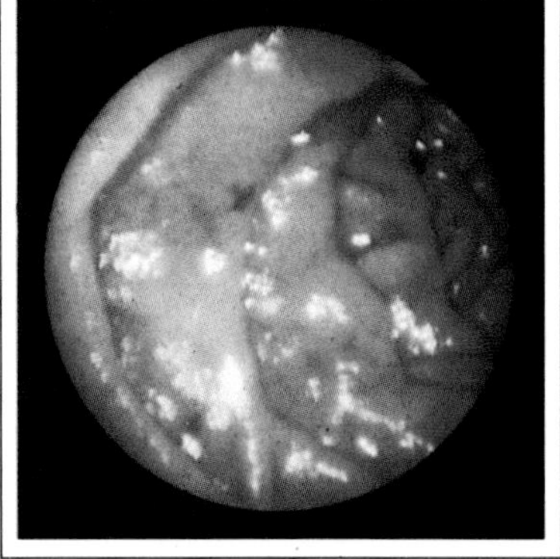

FIG. 37-2b.

FIG. 37-2. a: Hereditary hemorrhagic telangiectasia in the duodenum. Several 2- to 4-mm cherry-red spots were found in the duodenal bulb of a patient with similar lesions in the stomach and recurrent bleeding. **b:** Hereditary hemorrhagic telangiectasia in the colon. Several cherry-red spots were found in the right colon of a patient with gastric and duodenal telangiectasia as evidence of diffuse GI involvement.

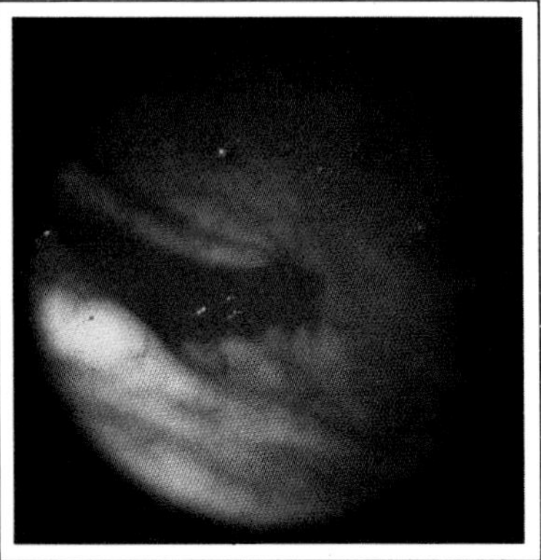

FIG. 37-3a.

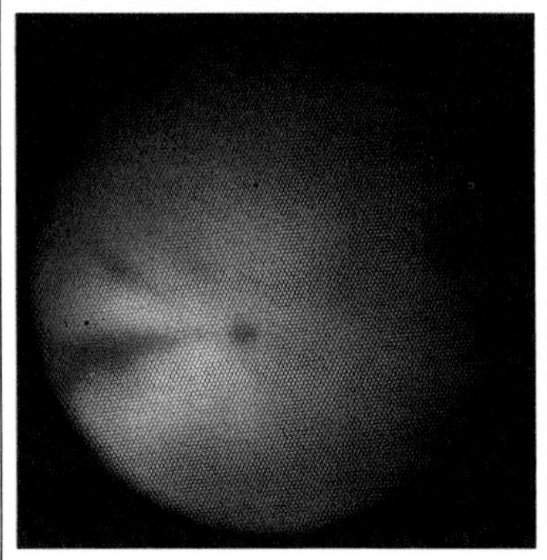

FIG. 37-3b.

FIG. 37-3. Gastric angiodysplasia, bleeding. **a:** Active bleeding appeared to emanate from a solitary point. After washing, this was actually seen to be from an angiodysplasia lesion (b). **b:** The blood can be seen to ooze from a 2-mm cherry-red spot. This was one of several lesions found and then treated electrosurgically.

In addition to gastric lesions, esophageal and duodenal (Fig. 37-2a) sites may be identified along with colonic sites (Fig. 37-2b) in patients subjected to colonoscopy.

Gastric Angiodysplasia

The term angiodysplasia is currently used by endoscopists to indicate the presence of vascular abnormalities. Although histologically these may be quite variable, including even true vascular neoplasms, i.e., hemangiomas, most angiodysplasia lesions are similar to the vascular ectasias (telangiectasias) of HHT (see above). A variable but probably high percentage of these cases are found in association with aortic valvular disease.[2] Other cases where the vascular ectasias have been referred to as abnormal blood vessels (of the gastric antrum) have been reported in association with liver disease.[12] Vascular ectasias with an endoscopic appearance identical to that of lesions associated with aortic valvular disease have been found with histologic evidence of cholesterol emboli to gastric vessels[13]; in the absence of associated conditions, oversized arterial branches in the submucosa, termed "caliber-persistence" lesions, have been described[14] in which the endoscopic appearance is similar to that of other angiodysplasias.[14] These are thought to be rarely occurring congenital vascular malformations.[14] More recently, gastric angiodysplasia has been reported in patients with chronic renal failure, particularly those on long term (4 years or more) hemodialysis.[14a]

Endoscopy is requested in patients with both acute and chronic GI bleeding. Even combining the two, gastric angiodysplasia probably accounts for, at most, only about 1% of patients having upper GI endoscopy because of bleeding. In a Norwegian series of 650 patients endoscoped for GI bleeding over a 4-year period, only nine cases of angiodysplasia (called telangiopathy) were found, constituting 1.4% of the cases.[15] Of these, only a small percentage were examined at the time the angiodysplasia lesion was actually bleeding (Fig. 37-3). Among our 500 consecutively studied patients (see Table 32-2), only three (0.6%) had gastric angiodysplasia.

Unlike patients with HHT in whom the diagnosis is generally suspected prior to endoscopy, the possibility of gastric angiodysplasia is less commonly considered. The association of aortic stenosis and gastric angiodysplasia[2] should prompt one to suspect it when confronted with patients with this type of valvular heart disease who have unexplained GI bleeding. Another presentation is that of multiple, unexplained upper GI bleeding episodes in which prior endoscopy showed "areas of nonspecific capillary dilatation," "focal erosions," or other questionable findings.[2]

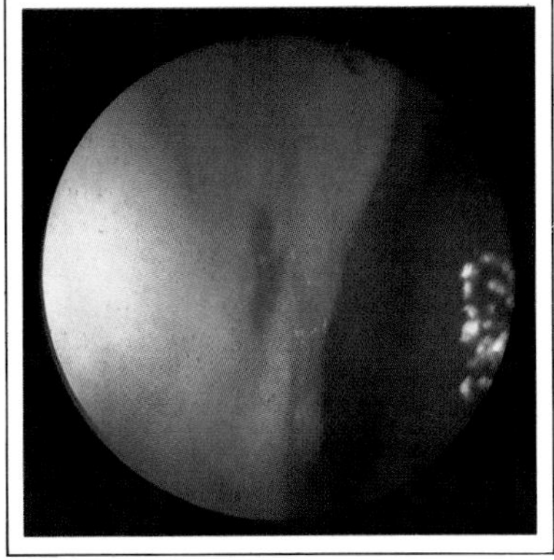

FIG. 37-4a.

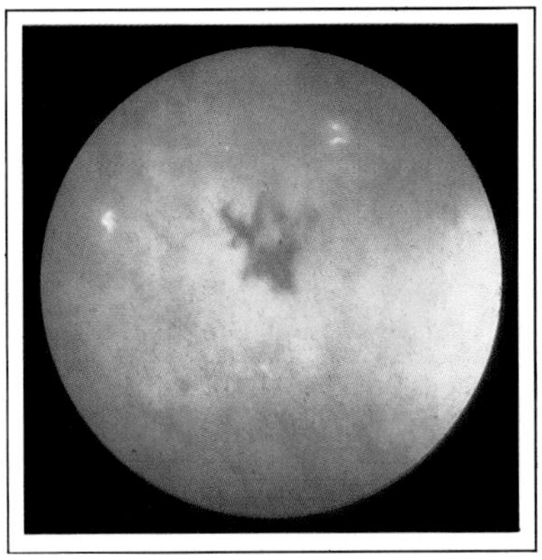

FIG. 37-4b.

FIG. 37-4. a: Gastric angiodysplasia. A 3-mm cherry-red spot was noted on the lesser curve of the lower body; a second lesion (b) was found in the antrum. **b:** A close-up view of the lesion revealed a markedly irregular border with filamentous projections to the neighboring capillaries. An area of central clearing can also be seen which may have resulted from previous bleeding with some destruction of the lesion with healing.

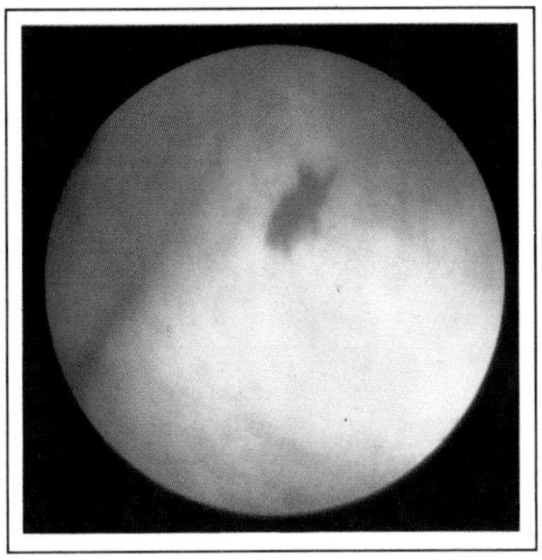

FIG. 37-5a.

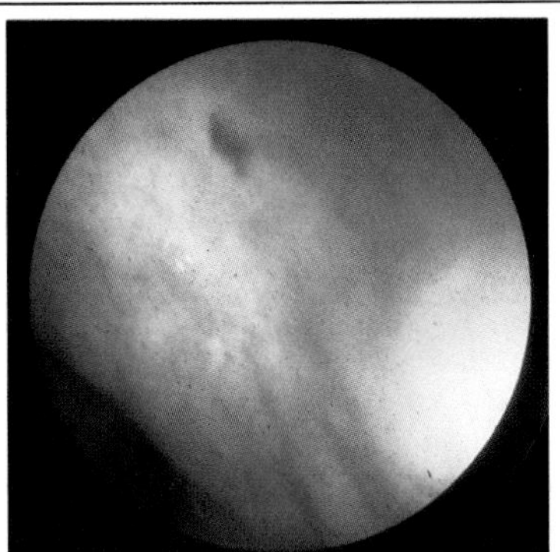

FIG. 37-5b.

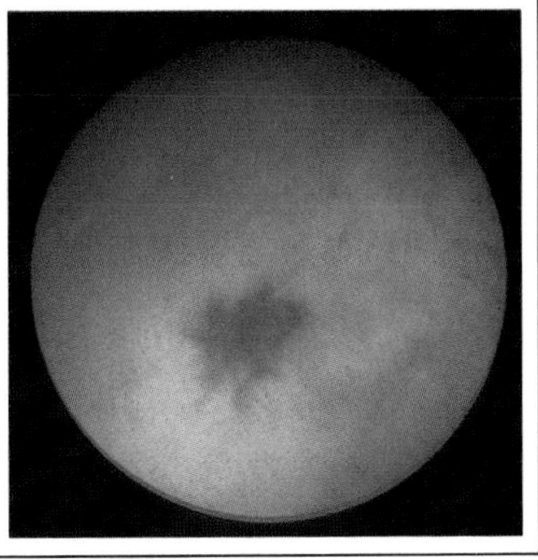

FIG. 37-5c.

FIG. 37-5. a: Gastric angiodysplasia. The typical cherry-red spot of angiodysplasia is indistinguishable from that of hereditary hemorrhagic telangiectasia (b). **b:** Hereditary hemorrhagic telangiectasia. The cherry-red spots of these lesions, though tending to be smaller than gastric angiodysplasia and more widely distributed, are in themselves indistinguishable. **c:** Gastric angiodysplasia, a 7.5-mm lesion. A close-up view of a somewhat large angiodysplasia lesion shows the typical filamentous communications to neighboring capillaries.

In cases where the angiodysplasia lesions are focal (≤1.5 cm), they may be treated with electrocoagulation[2,15] with no additional bleeding episodes.

Appearances.

Four distinctive types of endoscopic findings may be expected in patients with gastric angiodysplasia: (a) small angiodysplasias (<5 mm); (b) large angiodysplasias (>5 mm, occasionally >1 cm); (c) mixed type (large and small lesions); and (d) antral lesions (as discrete or confluent areas of vascular abnormality).

1. *Small angiodysplasias:* The commonest appearance we find is that of single, small lesions (Fig. 37-4a) confined to the body alone or seen in conjunction with antral lesions (Fig. 37-4b). The lesions themselves (Fig. 37-5a) are indistinguishable from the cherry-red spots of hereditary hemorrhagic telangiectasia (Fig. 37-5b). We and others[3] have found esophageal or duodenal angiodysplasia in cases where gastric lesions are of the small type. It has been suggested that when esophageal or duodenal lesions are present the cases might be considered an incomplete form of hereditary telangiectasia.[16] As is true of the lesions in that condition,

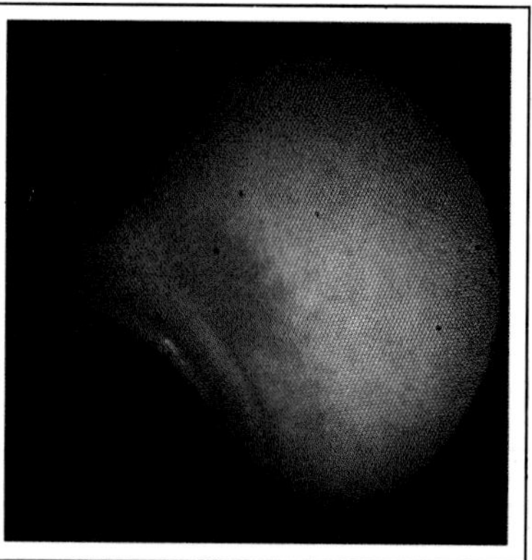

FIG. 37-6.

FIG. 37-6. Gastric angiodysplasia. This 1-cm lesion of the lower body was located just above the gastric angle in a patient with recurrent bleeding. On one occasion the patient was endoscoped and a diagnosis of "atypical erosive gastritis" made. Bleeding was finally controlled electrosurgically.

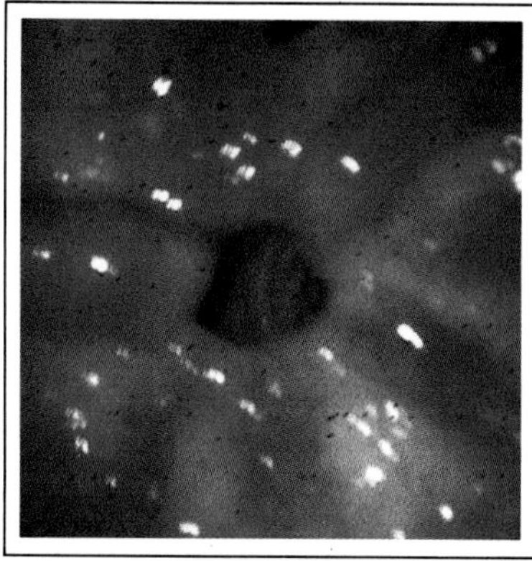

FIG. 37-7a.

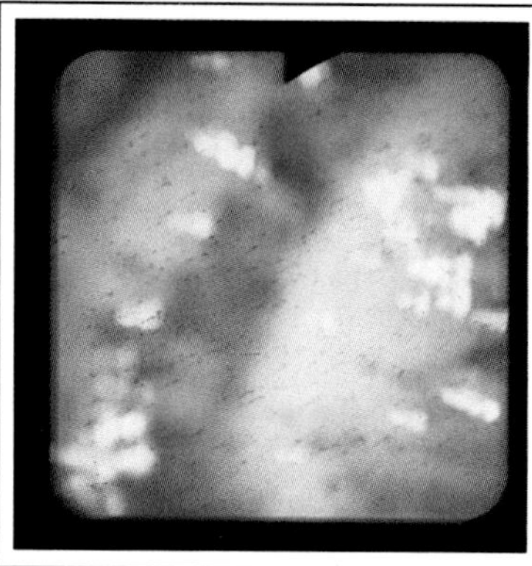

FIG. 37-7b.

FIG. 37-7. a: Gastric angiodysplasia, antral type. Intensely erythematous folds, called angioid streaks (see text), radiate to the pyloric channel in a patient with recurrent gastric bleeding which ultimately required antrectomy. Histologic examination of the resected specimen revealed dilated capillaries similar to what has been called "abnormal blood vessels of the gastric antrum."[17] **b:** Antral angiodysplasia, with angioid streaks. In this case, these appear as a continuous linear area of interconnected petechial lesions running along the mucosal folds of the gastric antrum. Recurrent bleeding in this patient could only be controlled with antrectomy.

the margins of gastric angiodysplasia are irregular with apparent filamentous projections to the neighboring capillary beds (Fig. 37-5c). Also, as in hereditary hemorrhagic telangiectasia, the lesions may evolve so that on serial examinations they may disappear from one area of the stomach and reappear in another or evolve from a red to a brown appearance, which indicates breakdown of the telangiectatic vessel and the beginning of resorption of intramucosal blood.[2]

2. *Large angiodysplasias:* Less common in our experience and that of others[2] is the finding of one or two large lesions (Fig. 37-6) below the body and the antrum. In some cases these exceed 1 cm and have a characteristically irregular, fern-like margin of interconnections with the neighboring capillaries. Large lesions seem more likely to bleed significantly over time and prove to be the most important type of lesion to consider for endoscopic therapy in that most large lesions persist and continue to bleed intermittently.[2]

3. *Mixed type:* Large and small angiodysplasias may coexist in the body and antrum. Generally the large lesions are responsible for the bleeding.

4. *Antral type:* A distinctive type of gastric angiodysplasia is that in which the lesion is confined entirely to the antrum. This may be seen as a discrete small, large, or mixed type of angiodysplasia as discussed above. Distinct from these lesions are confluent areas of vascular abnormality, appearing as erythematous linear zones (angioid streaks)[17,18] running along the ridges of antral folds toward the pyloric channel (Fig. 37-7a). These vascular abnormalities have been referred to as abnormal blood vessels in the gastric antrum[17] or as antral vascular lesions.[18] In patients where abnormal blood vessels of the prepyloric antrum have been described in association with liver disease, the angioid streaks seem to be made up of multiple petechial-type lesions (Fig. 37-7b).[12]

Relation of gastric to colonic angiodysplasia.

The pathogenesis of both gastric and colonic angiodysplasia is uncertain, but both may be a consequence of age-related degenerative changes involving the submucosal vascular bed. In some cases there may be the additional factor of diminished cardiac output related to aortic valve stenosis.[12] In an as yet uncertain but possibly significant percent of patients with gastric angiodysplasia, one or more colonic lesions may be expected, particularly on the right side. Weaver et al. performed colonoscopy in 4 of 10 patients with gastric angiodysplasia (but without cutaneous or other manifestations of HHT) and found colonic angiodysplasia in two cases (50%).[12] One might, therefore, consider performing colonoscopy in patients with gastric angiodysplasia, particularly those with some suggestion of lower GI bleeding such as the passage of maroon-colored stool or bright red blood.

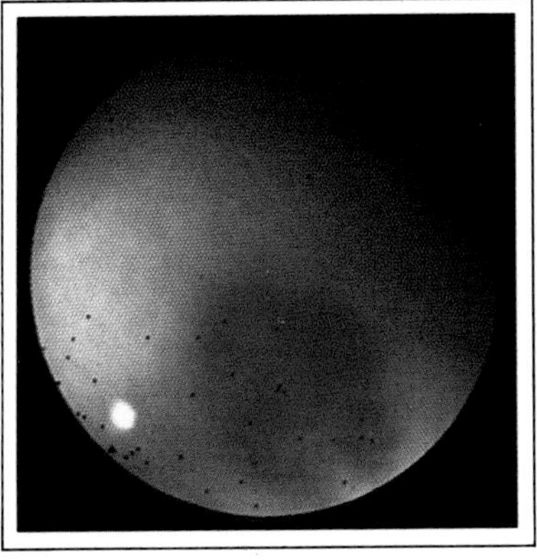

FIG. 37-8.

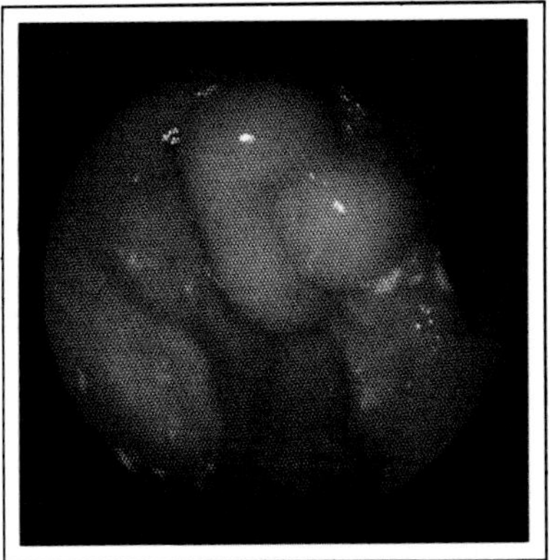

FIG. 37-9a.

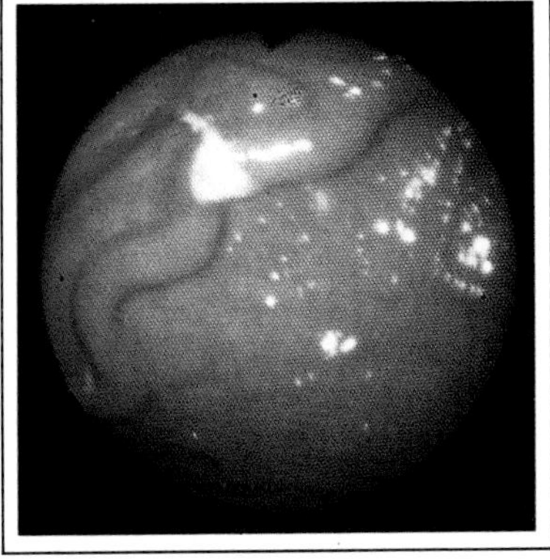

FIG. 37-9b.

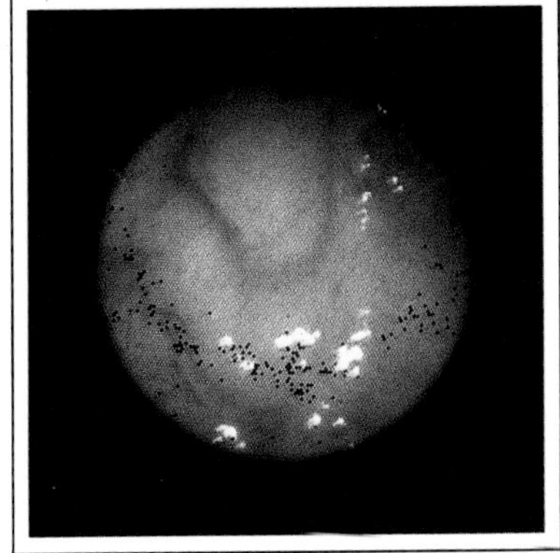

FIG. 37-9c.

FIG. 37-8. Suction artifact appearing as gastric angiodysplasia: one of multiple nasogastric suction artifacts in a patient with prolonged intubation. A clue to its being an artifact lies in its essentially regular margin despite some inhomogeneity within.

FIG. 37-9. a: Gastric varices appearing as a cardiofundic mass. Large serpiginous folds of the cardiofundic area create the impression of a fundic mass. In a patient with chronic pancreatitis, this appearance immediately suggests a diagnosis of gastric varices. **b:** Gastric varices, serpiginous folds. Undulating folds of the upper body, especially with interconnections at right angles with other folds (c), always suggest a diagnosis of gastric varices. **c:** Gastric varices, appearing as interconnected (intercalated) folds. The interconnections between the straight coursing rugal folds and gastric varices of the upper body create the impression of a latticework.

Interpretive problems.

The commonest type of interpretive problem in gastric angiodysplasia is distinguishing the discrete, small angiodysplastic lesions of the body or antrum from the intramucosal hemorrhage that is associated with mucosal trauma caused by either placement of the nasogastric tube or the endoscopic procedure itself. In both types of mucosal trauma, discrete intensely red areas 1 to 3 mm in size are found (Fig. 37-8). The absence of an irregular margin (lacking filamentous extensions) is a clue to the presence of an artifact; however, the lesions of mucosal trauma, especially suction artifacts, may also display some marginal irregularities (Fig. 37-8) although not usually to the same extent as the angiodysplasias.

Gastric Varices

Unlike esophageal varices, which are common and have a distinctive appearance (see Chapter 8), gastric varices, when present alone, are both subtle in their appearance and relatively uncommon. Although precise data concerning their incidence are not available, our experience is probably representative, with gastric varices accounting for only two of 500 cases consecutively examined over a 7-year period.

Gastric varices result from splenic vein obstruction, which forces splenic blood flow to be rerouted across the short gastric vein into the fundus and cardia, and finally to empty into the portal system via the left gastric (coronary) vein.[2] One of the most commonly recognized causes of splenic vein obstruction leading to gastric varices is chronic pancreatitis, often seen in association with pseudocyst formation.[2] In chronic pancreatitis, abnormalities of the splenic vein can be found in half the cases examined by splenoportography and, as a result, places such patients at risk of developing obstruction secondary to splenic vein thrombosis.[19] Patients with pancreatic malignancies also frequently have splenic vein thromboses, which occur as a result of spontaneous intravascular clotting or direct tumor extension to occlude the splenic vein.

Clinically, the endoscopist suspects gastric varices when called on to examine the patient with pancreatic disease who presents with acute GI hemorrhage, especially in whom a mass of the cardiofundic area has been demonstrated on an upper GI series.

Appearance.

The endoscopic findings may be: (a) a cardiofundic mass; (b) interconnected (intercalated) fundic folds; or (c) giant gastric folds.

1. *Cardiofundic mass:* In these cases gastric varices, as they course across the fundus and around the cardia, take

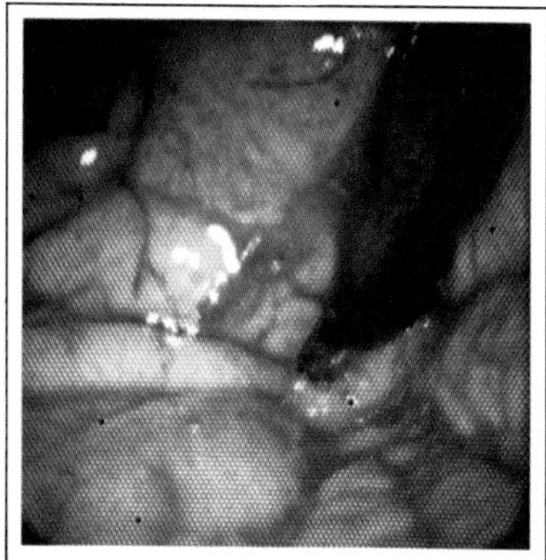

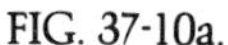

FIG. 37-10a.

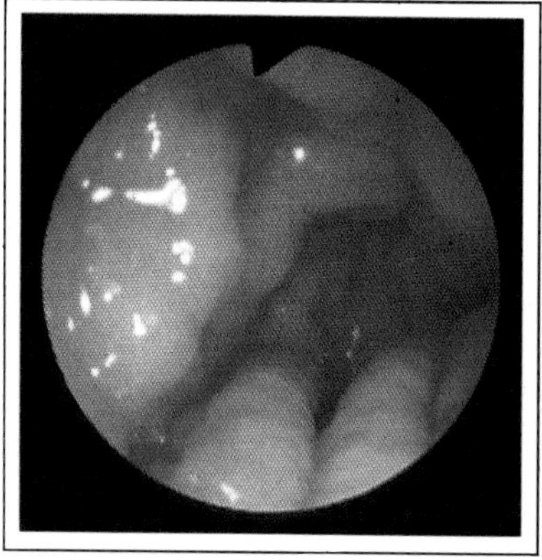

FIG. 37-10b.

FIG. 37-10. a: Gastric varices as giant gastric folds. In this case, their appearance is giant folds (>1.5 cm in height and width) and could be confused with that of an infiltrating malignancy. However, their extreme compressibility (with a closed biopsy forceps) helps to distinguish them (Fig. 37-11). **b:** Giant gastric fold of an infiltrating malignancy. The hard, rubbery character of the folds, which can be determined with a closed biopsy forceps, serves to differentiate these gastric varices (a).

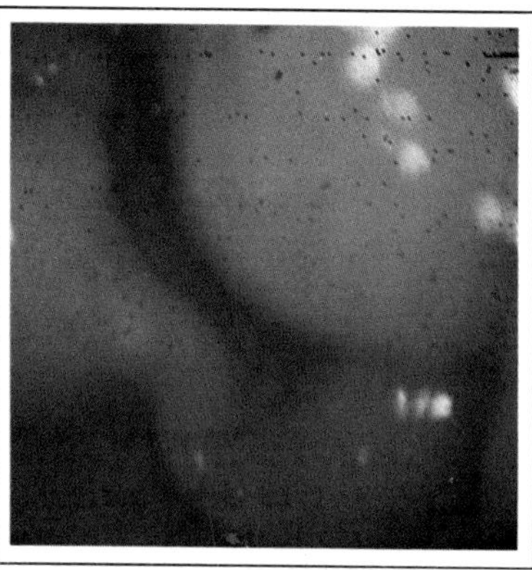

FIG. 37-11.

FIG. 37-11. Gastric varices, antral location. In this patient with known end-stage cirrhosis, these giant antral folds were suspected of being varices because they were easily compressed with a closed biopsy forceps. The diagnosis was subsequently proved angiographically.

on the appearance of a mass (Fig. 37-9a). The projection of this mass into the lumen becomes the most striking feature. Although the undulating or serpiginous arrangement of these folds can still be made out (Fig. 37-9a), because of the mass-like configuration and the impression of nodularity which the folds themselves create in the clinical context of weight loss or pain the endoscopist may be tempted to interpret this appearance as suggesting infiltrating carcinoma. This erroneous conclusion is avoided if the folds are simply touched with a closed biopsy forceps. Here the endoscopist finds that rather than their being indurated they are soft and quite easily compressed. Furthermore, on close inspection the "mass" and "nodules" may show a faint, bluish discoloration from the venous blood within, although this feature is not required for diagnosis.[19]

2. *Interconnected (intercalated) fundic folds:* A more subtle appearance for gastric varices is that of interconnected (intercalated) folds of the fundus and upper body. Because of the deep submucosal position of the varices as well as their size (>5 mm to 1.5+ cm), they may appear simply as prominent rugal folds although having a somewhat more tortuous appearance (Fig. 37-9b). It is their tendency, however, to course perpendicular to the rugal folds themselves, creating a latticework appearance (Fig. 37-9c), which gives them a characteristic intercalated appearance.

3. *Giant gastric folds:* In rare cases (we have seen only one) the varices, because of their size (>1.5 cm in diameter) and location principally in the body, appear as giant gastric folds (Fig. 37-10a). Interconnections between the folds are not apparent. Although their size may cause the endoscopist to consider the possibility of an infiltrating malignancy (Fig. 37-10b), their pliancy and compressibility (which can be tested using a closed biopsy forceps) leads the endoscopist to suspect gastric varices. In such a case, rather than risking biopsy, which could prove castastrophic, the endoscopist recommends that arteriography first be performed.

Another appearance of gastric varices of the giant fold type is one where the folds are found exclusively in the antrum (Fig. 37-11).

Interpretive problems.

The commonest interpretive problem we find is the differentiation of gastric varices from prominent fundic veins (see Chapter 12), which are seen especially in elderly patients with atrophic gastritis. Generally, fundic veins are less than 5 mm, usually less than 3 mm. They are straight, superficial, and often intensely purple-blue. By contrast, fundic varices are almost always greater than 5 mm in diameter, often exceeding 1 cm or more (Fig. 37-9a), and are distinct from fundic veins, running at right angles with typical rugal folds of the body to create the characteristic interconnected (intercalated) appearance.

OTHER UNCOMMON CAUSES OF GASTRIC BLEEDING

Gastric Tumors

Gastric neoplasms are an infrequent cause of GI bleeding, with the commonest of these, carcinoma, accounting for 1 to 2% of the cases.[1] In some series they have accounted for a higher percentage (4% and 8%),[1] approaching the incidence of esophageal varices or Mallory-Weiss lesions.

A variety of tumors in addition to carcinoma, both epithelial and submucosal (mesenchymal) in origin, may cause GI bleeding. Most investigators, however, including ourselves, find all gastric tumors, even when taken together, an unusual source of bleeding. In this section, we touch briefly on these tumors and their associated interpretive problems.

Gastric Epithelial Tumors

Gastric carcinoma.

Gastric carcinoma is the commonest reported tumor that causes upper GI bleeding. Hematemesis and/or melana is a presenting symptom in at least 10% of patients with gastric carcinoma.[20] Most of these patients have a history of weight loss, loss of appetite, or other symptoms suggestive of malignancy at the time of their presentation with GI bleeding[20]; however, in others the bleeding itself is the initial clinical manifestation.

In our series of 500 patients consecutively examined because of upper GI bleeding (see Table 32-2), gastric cancer was the final diagnosis in six (1.2%). The appearance of these lesions varied, the commonest being an ulcerated mass (Fig. 37-12a). Bleeding was either from friable tumor nodules or, as in one case (Fig. 37-12b), massive bleeding from involvement of a large artery in the central portion of the tumor.

Of the six gastric cancers, four were located in the body, one in the antrum, and one in the cardiofundic area. One of the six cases arose in the remaining portion of the stomach 25 years after a Billroth II hemigastrectomy (see Chapter 19). In this case the bleeding episode was the first clinical manifestation of malignancy.

Other gastric malignancies.

Gastric lymphoma or metastases to the stomach from distant primaries may also be a rare cause of GI bleeding. In the case of metastases from the breast, lung, or kidney, or from a melanoma (Fig. 37-12c), bleeding may be the first manifestation of gastric involvement.[5]

Nonmalignant polyps.

When sizable (>2 cm), nonmalignant polyps may be associated with acute bleeding although chronic blood loss and iron deficiency anemia is more usually the case. We have observed two such cases. In one, a giant hyperplastic polyp was the cause of bleeding in a patient who required hospitalization because of the melanoma and orthostatic blood pressure changes (Fig. 37-12d). In another case a giant villous adenoma was responsible. Others have reported massive bleeding from similar polyps.[21]

Submucosal Tumors

Leiomyomas.

Of the many types of gastric submucosal tumors, the leiomyoma is both the commonest[22] (see Chapter 17) and the most frequent cause of submucosal tumor bleeding. Among our 500 patients, three (0.6%) had bleeding leiomyomas at endoscopy. Generally the lesions which bleed are greater than 2 cm in diameter (Fig. 37-13) and have a characteristic central ulceration from which a clot may be observed (Fig. 37-13) or blood is oozing (Fig. 37-14b).

Carcinoids.

Like leiomyomas, large carcinoids (>1.5 cm) bleed from ulcerations of the overlying mucosa.[23] Because they are uncommon in the stomach,[23] they are an exceedingly rare cause of gastric bleeding, with none being observed among our 500 consecutively studied cases.

Other submucosal tumors.

Pancreatic rests, although not neoplasms, appear as polypoid lesions and may be endoscopically indistinguishable from leiomyomas.[24] Occasionally they attain a size where they may be associated with mucosal ulcerations and bleeding.[25] Another type of nonneoplastic tumor we have encountered in association with bleeding has been an area of eosinophilic gastritis confined to the fundus which appeared indistinguishable from a leiomyoma, with only peripheral eosinophilia as a clue to the nature of the fundic tumor.[26]

Interpretive Problems

There are two major sources of diagnostic error in patients with gastric tumor bleeding: (a) blood which obscures the tumor or otherwise causes the examination to be inadequate; and (b) a blood clot simulating a tumor.

Blood which obscures the tumor.

Gastric tumors tend to be found along the greater curve of the body or antrum and, in the case of leiomyoma, in the fundus. This location makes them potentially inaccessible if bleeding is substantial and fills these areas with blood. Even after meticulous lavage, the area in question may be obscured (Fig. 37-14a).

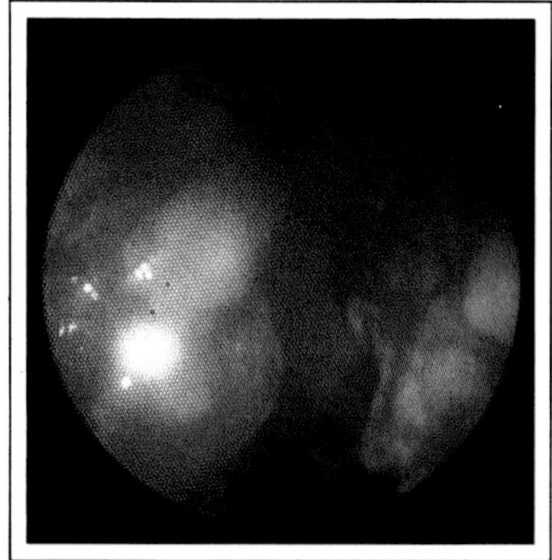

FIG. 37-12a.

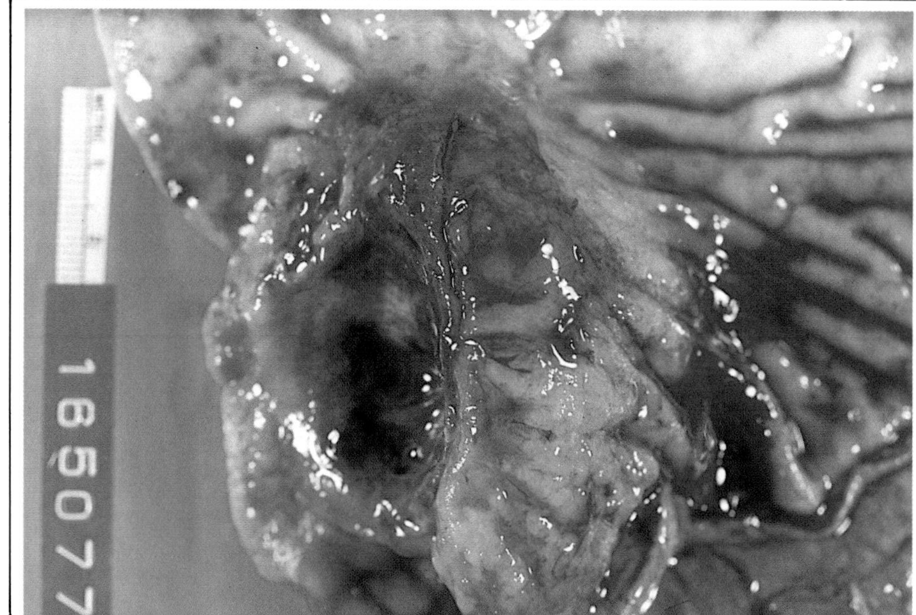

FIG. 37-12b.

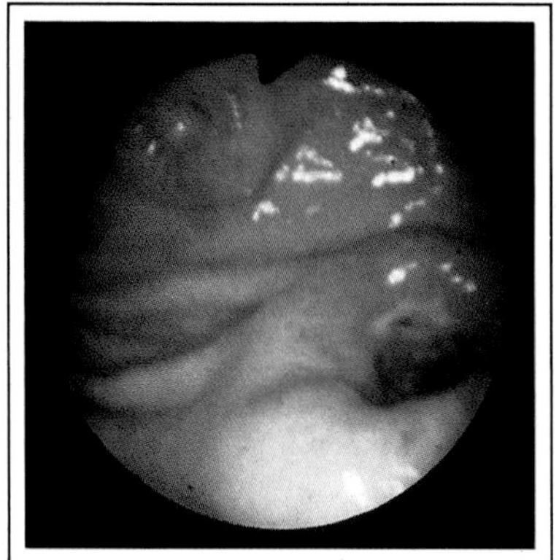

FIG. 37-12c.

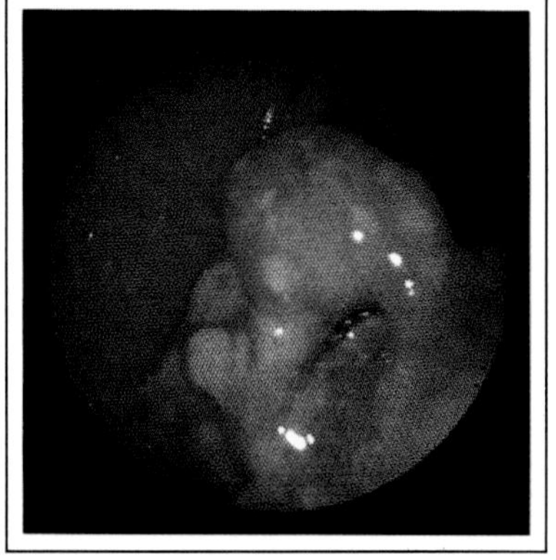

FIG. 37-12d.

FIG. 37-12. a: Gastric cancer, bleeding. Despite the lesion being largely obscured by blood, the raised nodular margin of this ulcer caused the endoscopist to suspect carcinoma. **b:** Gastric cancer, bleeding, resected specimen (a). Within the centrally ulcerated portion of this lesion there is a clot which was adherent to a large exposed artery. **c:** Melanoma, metastatic to the stomach, presenting as gastric bleeding. This appeared as multiple submucosal masses (5 and 11 o'clock) which contained within their central ulcerations melanotic material that was actually a combination of old blood (melena) and the melanoma implant. **d:** Giant hyperplastic polyp, bleeding. Some adherent clot is seen within the ulcerated portion of this giant (10 cm) polypoid mass. Because of its size, surgery was required for its removal.

The best defense against missing gastric tumor bleeding is to suspect this diagnosis, especially in patients lacking the more common sites of bleeding, e.g., esophageal varices, hemorrhagic-erosive gastritis, or peptic ulcer disease. In such instances one attempts to reposition the patient so as to afford the greatest opportunity for examining both the anterior wall (with the patient in the supine position) and the greater curve aspects (with the patient in the right lateral recumbent position). Most importantly, in all patients in whom no obvious bleeding site has been found, the endoscopist must make a special effort to examine the proximal portion of the upper body and cardiofundic areas (Fig. 37-14b). Failing to do this may mean missing the opportunity to make a diagnosis of a surgically treatable tumor at a time when an operation might be performed with acceptable mortality and morbidity rates.

Blood clots simulating tumor.

The blood clot itself, lying relatively fixed on the greater curve, may simulate the appearance of a gastric tumor (Fig. 37-14c). If found in association with a large gastric ulcer that has an irregular margin, the temptation to view this as a neoplasm, especially a carcinoma, can be great (Fig. 37-14d). In the presence of much blood and clot, the en-

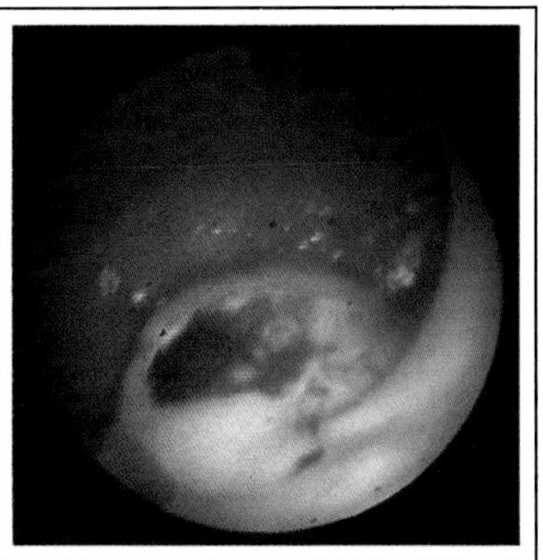

FIG. 37-13.

FIG. 37-13. Leiomyoma, bleeding. A submucosal mass is seen at the junction of the body and fundus with a central ulceration containing adherent clot and old blood (acid hematin) embedded in the base, as evidence of recent bleeding.

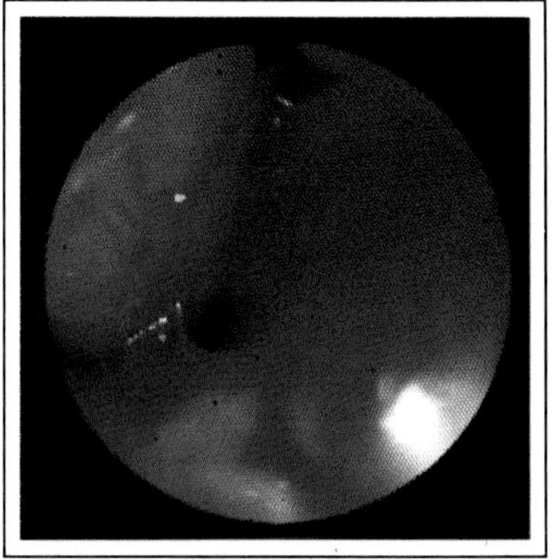

FIG. 37-14a.

FIG. 37-14b.

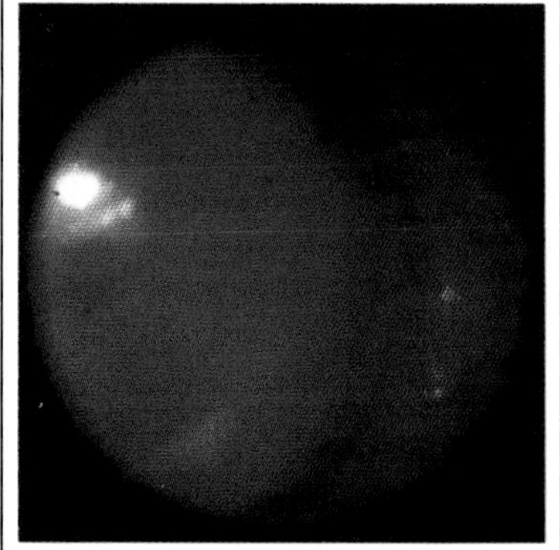

FIG. 37-14c.

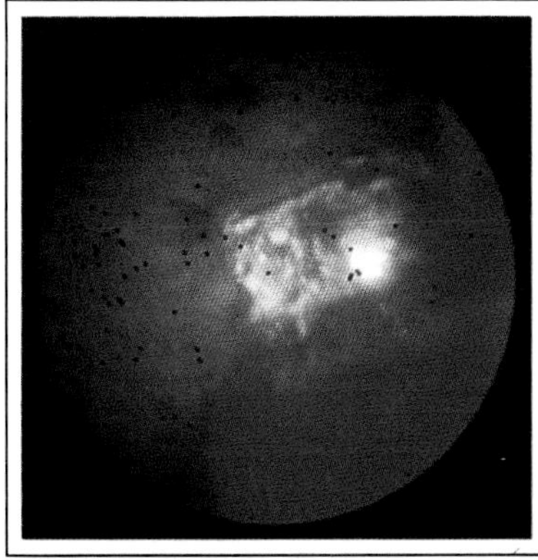

FIG. 37-14d.

FIG. 37-14. a: Gastric cancer, bleeding. The blood largely obscures the lesion. However, the asymmetrical, nodular appearance of the folds causes the endoscopist to suspect a malignant lesion. **b:** Leiomyoma, bleeding. Unless retroflexion was performed (a U-type maneuver in this case), the leiomyoma with bleeding from its central ulceration would not have been detected. **c:** A large clot in the fundus simulating tumor. The clot itself has a mass-like appearance which is a reflection only of its size. **d:** Gastric ulcer bleeding simulating malignancy. The size of this ulcer (2 cm), the irregularity of its base and margin, and the mass-like appearance created by the blood create the impression of a malignant lesion. Unless features are present which strongly suggest malignancy, e.g., an elevated nodular margin, the ulcer should be called indeterminate; re-examination is advised once bleeding ceases.

doscopist wisely remains cautious in his interpretation of the ulcer unless he can identify a raised nodular margin (Fig. 37-14a) or other feature which would be highly suspicious for malignancy.

Nontumor Gastric Bleeding in Patients With Malignancy

Patients with known hematologic or solid-type malignancies and nontumor-related gastric bleeding represent a small but appreciable percentage of those endoscoped because of GI hemorrhage. In the ASGE survey, 152 of 2,223 patients (7%) had a history of either a hematologic (25) or solid-type (127) malignancy, although the number with active malignancies (i.e., undergoing treatment) versus those in remission was not stated.[27] Our own experience is comparable to that of the ASGE survey in that of 500 patients consecutively endoscoped for GI bleeding over a 7-year period 23 (4.6%) were patients with known malignancy undergoing treatment (irradiation or chemotherapy) or who had had treatment within the previous 6 months.

The causes of gastric bleeding in patients with malignancy are varied. For the large majority, the bleeding derives not from the tumor itself but from nonmalignant sources.[4,28]

Of these, the commonest is acute mucosal injury, accounting for up to 40% of the cases. Because of its importance, we consider this cause in some detail below. Two other nonmalignant causes of bleeding which we have discussed elsewhere account for an additional 40%: Peptic ulcer disease (see Chapters 36 and 38) accounts for 30%, and esophagitis (see Chapter 34) accounts for the remaining 10%. Only 20% of bleeding episodes are caused by the tumor.[28]

Bleeding from Acute Mucosal Injury

The commonest single cause of GI bleeding in patients with malignancy is acute mucosal injury. This accounts for nearly half the cases in most series[4,28] and is related to either stress-type mucosal injury or gastric irritants.

Stress-related mucosal injury.

In up to 65% of cases the mucosal injury is best accounted for by stress-related conditions (see "Stress Lesion Bleeding," this chapter). In a study reported from the Memorial-Sloan Kettering Hospital in New York, sepsis was the commonest of these stress factors, being found in 63%; other factors, e.g., recent surgery (37%), debility from advanced cancer (35%), jaundice (19%), uremia (16%), respiratory failure (12%), and shock (10%), were found less often.[29]

Mucosal injury from gastric irritants.

As in patients without malignancy, the commonest of the gastric irritants that cause mucosal injury are alcohol and aspirin. In one series of 26 patients with acute mucosal injury attributable to this cause, aspirin had been taken by 25 of 26 such patients.[29] Only four (13%) had received cytotoxic agents, e.g., 5-fluorouracil, cyclophosphamide, or bleomycin. Therefore aspirin, rather than cytotoxic agents, seems to be the drug which is most often incriminated in these patients, especially as the potential of cytotoxic agents for gastric injury is uncertain (see Chapter 14).

Rationale for endoscopy.

The outcome for patients with acute mucosal injury bleeding and malignancy is much like that of patients without malignancy. The natural history of acute mucosal bleeding related to irritants is one of cessation of bleeding, generally within 48 to 72 hr. The mortality in such patients is low, being less than 10% on the whole. In one series of gastric bleeding associated with malignancy, the mortality for the episode was nil.[29] However, patients with stress-related bleeding do poorly, with a mortality rate which may exceed 50%.[29]

Because of differing sites of mucosal injury relating to gastric irritants or stress factors (see below), endoscopy potentially may serve to suggest a patient's having acute mucosal injury associated with a low mortality from an irritant (e.g., aspirin) or an excessive mortality if from stress-related injury. In addition, endoscopy identifies still other high risk patients, those with a bleeding peptic ulcer, where a mortality rate of up to 30% is found.[30] Under certain circumstances (i.e., malignancy in remission) these patients might still be operable with acceptable morbidity and mortality if surgery is performed early. Other patients may be candidates for endoscopic therapy. In any event, endoscopy indicates to those caring for the patient the prognosis of a bleed based on the type of lesion as well as whether bleeding was observed to be ongoing or have stopped.

Location of the acute mucosal injury.

An important determining factor for the location of the lesion seems to be the etiology of the acute mucosal injury—whether it is related to gastric irritants or to stress-related causes. Chait et al. found that 60%[29] of acute mucosal lesions occurred in the body and fundus in patients in whom a stress condition could be defined; this was twice the incidence of lesions found in this location in patients whose injury was believed to be caused by gastric irritants. In the latter only one-third of the lesions were found in the body or fundus. Conversely, the incidence of a primarily antral location was found in only 13% with stress-related lesions but in 54% where they were related to gastric irritants. In addition, the incidence of a generalized distribution (body and antrum) was twice as great for stress-associated lesions (27%) compared with those associated with gastric irritants (13%).

In cancer patients, therefore, the finding of acute mucosal lesions primarily in the upper body and fundus points toward an underlying stress condition with a poor prognosis, whereas usually a distal location points toward a gastric irritant, e.g., aspirin, with a favorable outcome.[29]

Appearance.

Both superficial acute mucosal erosions (Fig. 37-15), such as those described for drug-induced acute mucosal injury (see Chapter 36), and deeper acute mucosal ulcerative stress-type lesions (see below) are described for patients with gastric bleeding related to malignancy. Although overlap exists, erosions tend to be more characteristic of gastric irritant type bleeding, whereas deep ulcerations were more typical of patients with an underlying stress condition.[29]

Thrombocytopenia as a determinant of appearance.

A diminished platelet count is not uncommon in patients with malignancies, especially those undergoing chemotherapy. We have previously described (see Chapter 14) a distinct endoscopic appearance of thrombocytopenia, especially with platelet counts below 30,000/cu mm. Increased

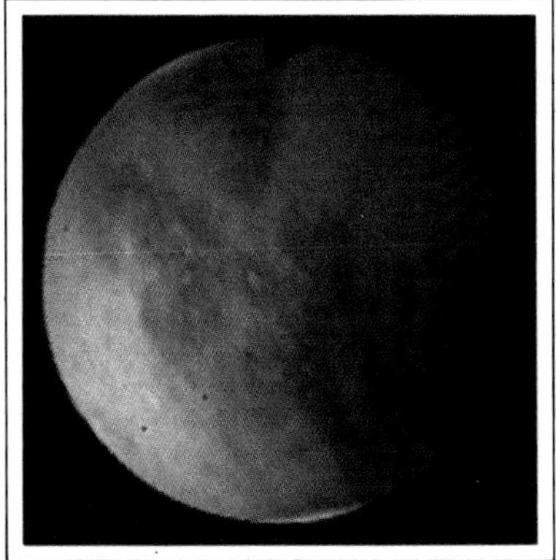

FIG. 37-15a.

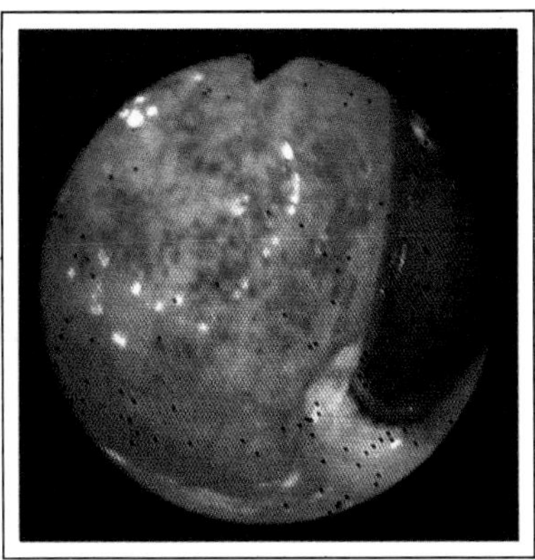

FIG. 37-15b.

FIG. 37-15. Bleeding from acute mucosal injury. **a:** In a patient with lung cancer. Multiple erosions were seen after ingestion of large amounts of aspirin. **b:** In a cancer patient with chemotherapy-induced thrombocytopenia. The multiple petechiae were seen throughout the upper body as a clue to the underlying thrombocytopenia.

capillary fragility associated with thrombocytopenia tends to produce a picture of diffuse intramucosal hemorrhage simulating the petechial type of intramucosal hemorrhage of acute mucosal injury (Fig. 37-15). In one series a pattern of multiple or diffuse injury was rarely seen in patients with a platelet count above 40,000/cu mm, whereas its incidence in patients with counts below 40,000/cu mm was 11%.[31] Although an uncommon appearance, to be sure, a diffuse petechial type of intramucosal hemorrhage should always prompt the endoscopist to suspect the patient of having thrombocytopenia, rather than simply attributing this appearance to gastric irritants or stress-related causes.

Interpretive Problems

As the commonest cause of gastric bleeding in patients with underlying malignancy is acute mucosal injury, having a range of appearance similar to that of hemorrhagic-erosive gastritis, the interpretive problems for that condition (see Chapter 36) apply here. The presence of blood itself, superimposed mucosal lesions, vomiting, or nasogastric suction artifacts, as well as the subtlety and often the paucity of lesions themselves, all create interpretive problems for the endoscopist who may erroneously be expecting to find gastric involvement by tumor as a common cause of bleeding. With this expectation in mind, the endoscopist may erroneously regard such nonspecific features as thickening of the rugal folds as evidence of malignancy. The best protection for such error would be to properly regard patients with malignancy and GI bleeding as a group of individuals always predisposed to acute gastric mucosal injury, with this the commonest type of bleeding, and the malignancy itself an infrequent cause.

Stress Lesion Bleeding

Critically ill patients are particularly prone to bleed from areas of acute mucosal injury (erosions and/or deeper ulcerations) called stress lesions. The conditions most often associated with bleeding are: (a) extensive burns; (b) head injuries; (c) sepsis; (d) prolonged hypotension; (e) the post-surgical state in critically ill patients or those with multiple, recent operations; and (f) fulminant hepatic failure.[32,33] Overall significant bleeding may occur in 20% of these cases.[33]

Critically ill patients with GI bleeding may constitute up to 5% of those for whom endoscopy is requested. In the ASGE survey, a history suggesting a critically ill patient potentially having stress lesion bleeding was obtained for 107 (4.8%) of the 2,223 constituting the study group.[27] Unfortunately, no information was provided as to how many patients actually did have stress lesion bleeding and how many were bleeding from other causes. Where endoscopy has been performed in patients with stress conditions and bleeding, virtually all have had acute mucosal lesions; about 10% of these appear as deep ulcerations but lack any type of ulcer scarring to suggest they would have preceded the stress condition.[34]

Pathogenesis

The mechanism by which acute mucosal injury occurs in stress conditions is uncertain. Some gastric acid seems to be required in virtually all experimental models[32]; moreover, the prevention of acute mucosal injury related to stress can be affected if gastric pH is held above 4.0.[33] Just how the presence of acid results in mucosal injury is not clear. A sequence of events where stress would cause disruption of the gastric mucosal barrier to acid, resulting in injury similar to that which occurs with aspirin or alcohol (see Chapter 36), is not supported by experimental studies.[32] An alternate explanation has centered around the role of altered mucosal blood flow[32] and a related decrease in mucosal energy stores[35] leading to a low energy state where the mucosa, particularly that of the body, becomes more vulnerable to its luminal environment, especially to bile salts, which are known to promote stress-related injury.[35] Despite numerous studies, however, the precise mechanism by which stress affects mucosal integrity remains to be elucidated.

Rationale for Endoscopy

Patients with stress conditions and GI bleeding are gravely ill with a mortality rate which is substantially higher than that seen in other conditions. In the ASGE survey, the mortality in these patients was three to four times higher than the overall mortality of 10.8%, with that for sepsis being 45.7%, acute liver failure 27%, trauma and shock 33%, and burns 33%.[27] The high mortality of the bleeding episode is attributable to both the severity of the underlying stress condition and the nature of the bleeding, which tends to be heavy, continuous, and in those with temporary cessation, recurrent. A sense of this is derived from the fact that in the ASGE survey 50% of patients with sepsis or trauma with shock required 6 units of blood transfusion for a given episode compared with 25.1% of patients with other causes of bleeding.[27]

For patients with stress lesion bleeding, the value of endoscopy may be seriously questioned, with medical management largely supportive and of limited efficacy and surgery infrequently resorted to because of the high overall mortality. Still, endoscopy can be important in such patients for two reasons. First, a precise diagnosis of the bleeding site may offer consideration of a specific pharmacologic approach, e.g., the use of growth hormone[36] or prostaglandins,[37] which can produce a favorable outcome in some patients with this type of bleeding. Surgery itself may become more of a consideration if the lesion actually is found to be circumscribed, which suggests a limited operative procedure, rather than if the lesion were generalized to involve the stomach and duodenum (see below).

Apart from considerations of management is the prognostic information which endoscopy provides. A patient who is observed to be actively bleeding from a stress lesion after 24 or 48 hr of medical therapy will have a mortality in excess of 50% unless the underlying stress is eliminated. This information is especially important to the physician who cares directly for the patient and the patient's family. On the other hand, if endoscopy shows that bleeding has stopped and the underlying stress condition is resolving, a more favorable outcome may be anticipated.

Appearance

The endoscopic features of stress lesions have been best studied in burn patients in whom serial observations of the lesions have been made over time.[34] This has resulted in a concept of two types of stress lesion related to time: (a) acute mucosal erosions (early lesions); and (b) ulcerations (late lesions).

Acute mucosal erosions (early lesions).

Early lesions occur within the first 24 hr and appear as discrete areas of erythema, commonly along with intramucosal hemorrhage and erosions, with the latter evidenced by focal bleeding (Fig. 37-16a). In some cases, rather than intramucosal hemorrhage there is a central area of pallor within a zone of erythema. Acute mucosal erosions occurred in more than 75% of patients with extensive burns (>30% total body surface area) studied by Czaja et al.,[34] having a distribution which was equally divided between proximal (fundus and body) and distal (antrum) areas. Sugawa et al. found stress-related bleeding from trauma or sepsis mostly in proximal locations, with 87% located in the fundus and upper body and only 5% in the antrum.[6]

Acute mucosal ulcerations (late lesions).

At 96 hr and afterward, Czaja et al. found acute ulcerations in 22% of the burn patients studied.[34] Bleeding had occurred in nearly half of these (9% of the total), in contrast to only 4% of patients with acute mucosal erosions. Acute mucosal erosions (early lesions) were present in all patients with ulcerations. The ulcers themselves appear as discrete, punched-out lesions (Fig. 37-16b), generally 1 cm or less in size. Some old blood may be observed within the base as evidence of recent bleeding (Fig. 37-16b). Czaja et al.[37] found ulcerations to be typically located within areas of intense, acute mucosal injury, although we have noted these in stress ulcers to be set in mucosa which appears endoscopically normal (Fig. 37-16c).

Associated duodenal lesions.

Similar appearances of acute mucosal injury (intramucosal hemorrhage, erosions, and ulcerations) were found by Czaja et al. in 82% of patients studied within 72 hr, although not necessarily at 24 hr, suggesting that the duodenum may be involved somewhat later than the stomach. Evidence of gastric mucosal injury was present in the majority of these patients (21 of 23). Acute duodenal ulcerations were present in almost 40% (9 of 23), with bleeding occurring in one-third of these (three of nine), in contrast to no bleeding in 14 cases having only erythema and erosions.

Interpretive Problems

The interpretive problems confronting the endoscopist examining patients with stress conditions are similar to those already discussed for hemorrhagic-erosive gastritis (see Chapter 36), resulting mainly from the presence of blood itself and superimposed nasogastric tube trauma. The differentiation of acute mucosal injury related to stress conditions and nasogastric suction artifacts may be particularly difficult if the nasogastric tube has been left in place for a considerable length of time (see Chapter 33), as is often the case in critically ill patients. In these cases nasogastric injury phenomena can be multiple, pleomorphic, and diffuse (see Chapter 33). In general, one expects to find nasogastric suction artifacts as mucosal erosions rather than discrete punched-out ulcerations (Fig. 37-16b). The finding of such

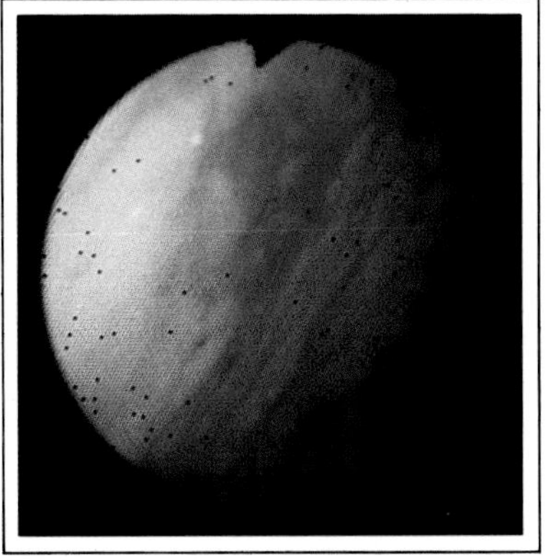

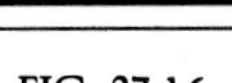

FIG. 37-16a.

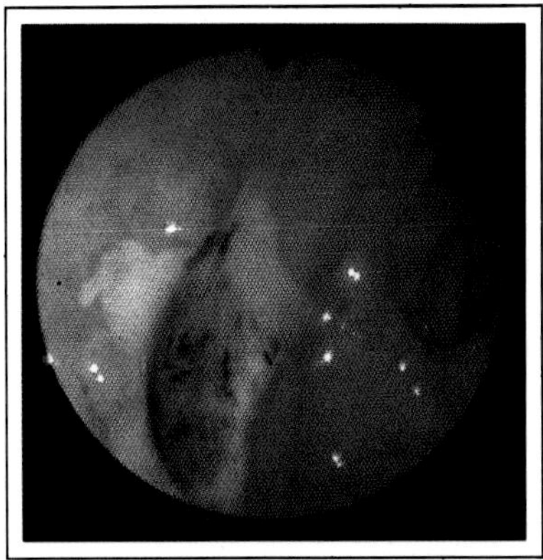

FIG. 37-16b.

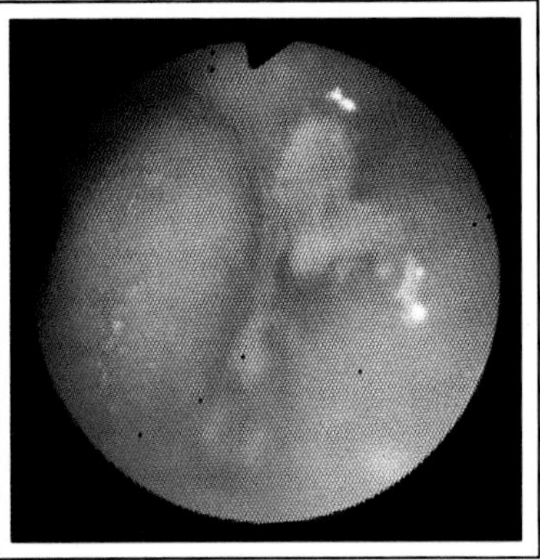

FIG. 37-16c.

FIG. 37-16. a: Stress-type acute mucosal injury; bleeding in a patient with respiratory failure. Discrete areas of intramucosal hemorrhage and erosions were identified. In this patient bleeding was of an insignificant amount. **b:** Stress-type acute mucosal ulceration. One of several discrete 1-cm ulcerations found in a patient recovering from sepsis which had been complicated by significant bleeding. The mucosa surrounding the ulcer was diffusely erythematous. **c:** Stress-type acute mucosal ulceration and erosion. These are set in otherwise almost normal mucosa. They were found on examination of a patient with bleeding after a decompressive laminectomy for a spinal abscess complicated by sepsis.

lesions as well as a distal distribution of other acute mucosal injury effects favors, in the appropriate clinical setting, a diagnosis of stress lesion bleeding.

Gastric Bleeding Associated With Renal Failure

Patients with gastric bleeding and renal failure are infrequently encountered except at centers where there is an active hemodialysis and/or renal transplant program. In the ASGE survey, patients with renal failure constituted only 4.5% of the total sample.[27] Bleeding in these patients such as that in those with stress conditions is a serious medical emergency with a high mortality, 31.5% for those with chronic renal failure and 63.6% for those with acute renal failure.[27]

Patients with renal failure are a diverse group and may be expected to have many potential sources of bleeding.[38,39] The commonest of these are the conditions which account for most cases of upper GI bleeding (i.e., acute mucosal injury secondary to aspirin or alcohol and peptic ulcer bleeding), although the specific instances vary in different series, with either acute mucosal injury (gastritis)[38] or peptic ulcer disease[39] being the single commonest cause, accounting for 30 to 40% of the cases. Interestingly, although peptic ulcer disease accounts for up to 30% of the cases of bleeding in renal failure,[39] it was not found at all in one series of patients who underwent endoscopy for reasons other than bleeding.[40] This suggests that the ulcers themselves, when they occur, may be more acute and stress-like with a greater predisposition to bleed than peptic ulcers in general. Our own experience bears out this notion in that ulcers seen in association with renal failure bleeding tend to be of the acute type (Fig. 37-16b), actually indistinguishable from ulcers found in stress conditions.

In addition to the general type of patient with chronic renal failure and bleeding are two special cases which require consideration. These are patients with marked renal insufficiency who may have uremic gastritis and patients with bleeding after renal transplant.

Uremic Gastritis

For many patients found at endoscopy to have acute mucosal injury as a cause of bleeding in chronic renal failure, the use of gastrotoxins, e.g., aspirin or alcohol, is not found. In our experience, this is particularly the case in patients bleeding in association with a blood urea nitrogen (BUN) of greater than 100 mg/dl, a condition referred to as uremic gastritis. The cause of this condition is unknown but may be related to the injurious effect of high concentrations of urea either in the mucosa or as part of the luminal contents. In this regard, urea is capable of diminishing the functional integrity of the gastric mucosal barrier.[41] The well-known disturbances of coagulation, espe-

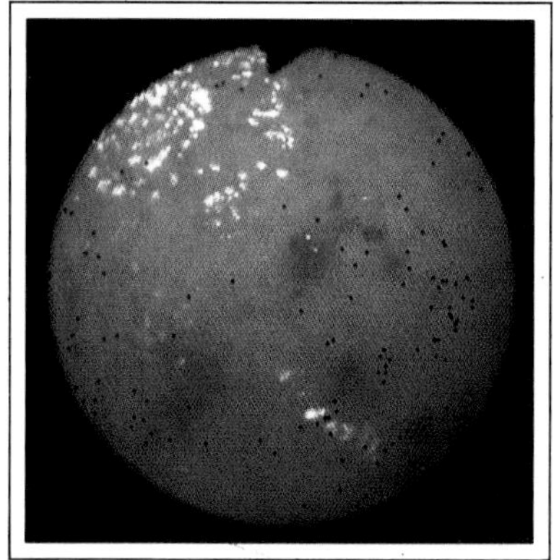

FIG. 37-17a.

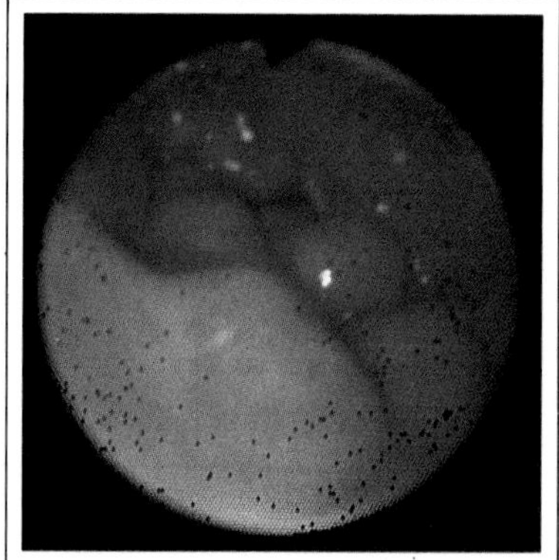

FIG. 37-17b.

FIG. 37-17. a: Uremic gastritis. Acute focal injury with focal erosions in a patient with worsening chronic renal failure (BUN > 150 mg/dl). **b:** Nonspecific gastric erythema of the body and antrum in a patient with chronic renal failure and bleeding. The erythema itself is not evidence of uremic gastritis.

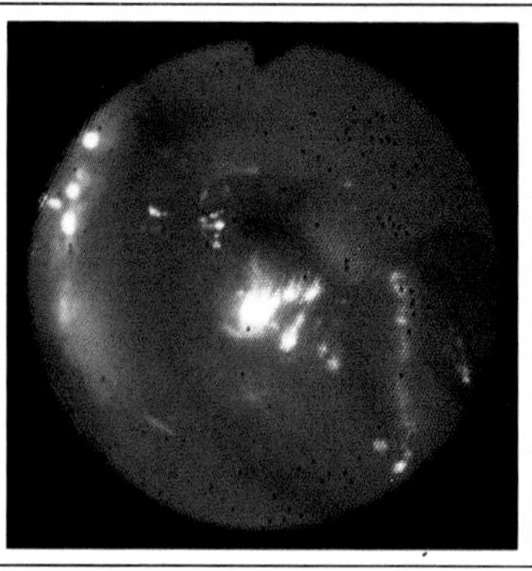

FIG. 37-18.

FIG. 37-18. Pyloric channel ulcer bleeding 2 months after renal transplant. The marked scar deformity suggests that an ulcer diathesis preceded the renal transplant, with activation of this possibly by the immunosuppressive agents (especially the corticosteroids) administered to prevent rejection.

cially in patients with a BUN greater than 100 mg/dl, also may promote bleeding.

We have also encountered patients with bleeding from uremic gastritis with a lower BUN (<100 mg/dl), with this occurring immediately after hemodialysis. In these cases, apart from the effects of heparin which patients receive during hemodialysis, continued loss of the functional integrity of the gastric mucosal barrier coupled with a high rate of gastric secretion has been suggested as a precipitant of bleeding.[42]

Appearance.

The appearance is characteristically a diffuse mucosal lesion involving the body and fundus (Fig. 37-17a), primarily with multiple 4- to 8-mm areas of intramucosal hemorrhage and erosions in various stages of evolution, either with clot alone or in association with acute inflammatory exudate.

Interpretive problems.

Added to the difficulties encountered in differentiating acute mucosal lesions from blood and nasogastric suction artifacts (see Chapter 36) is the problem in patients with renal failure of enlarged, often erythematous mucosal folds.[40] Although these could be a site of bleeding, especially in the presence of an altered coagulation status and diminished functional integrity of the gastric mucosal barrier, actual bleeding from them is uncommon in our experience. Moreover, we do not regard this as evidence of uremic gastritis, a term we reserve for cases in which there is evidence of acute mucosal injury. The finding of enlarged, erythematous rugal or antral folds (Fig. 37-17b) prompts us to examine the proximal stomach for evidence of acute mucosal lesions as well as the duodenal bulb for the presence of an acute ulcer.

Bleeding in Patients with Renal Transplants

As in patients with chronic renal failure, the causes of bleeding in those with renal transplants are varied; however, they must be regarded in terms of the timing of the bleed relative to when the transplant was performed, as well as the status of the transplant. Patients who bleed early after transplantation or in association with rejection may have a stress-type acute mucosal injury (see "Stress Lesion Bleeding," this chapter); this is most often a large acute ulcer.[43] In bleeds associated with rejection, the bleeding from these ulcers is protracted and associated with mortality.[43]

For bleeding that occurs after 30 days, especially in the absence of rejection, peptic ulcers (Fig. 37-18) of the duodenal bulb or pyloroduodenal junction are most often incriminated. In addition to the chronic ulcer (associated with scar deformity) are acute stress ulcers of the upper body, generally occurring multiply (three or more). Chronic ulcers are thought to have been present at the time of transplantation;

they then enlarge and deepen over the next several months possibly in relation to the high dose of corticosteroids used to prevent rejection. In other patients, acute ulcers observed in the upper body may be the result of this or other stress factors related to the initial posttransplantation period. In both cases the bleeding is massive with a high mortality (in excess of 40%).[43]

REFERENCES

1. Graham, D. Y., and Davis, R. E. (1978): Acute upper-gastrointestinal hemorrhage: new observations on an old problem. *Am. J. Dig. Dis.*, 23:76–84.
2. Weaver, G. A., Alpern, H. D., Davis, J. S., Ramsey, W. H., and Reichelderfer, M. (1979): Gastrointestinal angiodysplasia with aortic valve disease: part of a spectrum of angiodysplasia of the gut. *Gastroenterology*, 77:1–11.
3. Little, A. G., and Moossa, A. R. (1981): Gastrointestinal hemorrhage from left-sided portal hypertension: an unappreciated complication of pancreatitis. *Am. J. Surg.*, 141:153–158.
4. Lightdale, C. J., Kurtz, R. C., Sherlock, P., and Winawer, S. J. (1974): Aggressive endoscopy in critically ill patients with upper gastrointestinal bleeding and cancer. *Gastrointest. Endosc.*, 20:152–153.
5. Menuck, L. S., and Amberg, J. R. (1975): Metastatic disease involving the stomach. *Am. J. Dig. Dis.*, 20:903–913.
6. Sugawa, C., Lucas, C. E., Rosenberg, B. F., Riddle, J. M., and Walt, A. J. (1975): Differential topography of acute erosive gastritis due to trauma or sepsis, ethanol or aspirin. *Gastrointest. Endosc.*, 19:127–130.
7. Silverstein, F. E., Gilbert, D. A., Tedesco, F. J., Buenger, N. K., Persing, J., and 277 members of the ASGE (1981): The national ASGE survey on upper gastrointestinal bleeding. I. Study design and baseline data. *Gastrointest. Endosc.*, 27:73–79.
8. Mayer, I. E., and Hersh, T. (1981): Endoscopic diagnosis of hereditary hemorrhagic telangiectasia. *J. Clin. Gastroenterol.*, 3:361–365.
9. Gilbert, D. A., Silverstein, F. E., Tedesco, F. J., Buenger, N. K., Persing, J., and 277 members of the ASGE (1981): The national ASGE survey on upper gastrointestinal bleeding. III. Endoscopy in upper gastrointestinal bleeding. *Gastrointest. Endosc.*, 27:94–102.
10. Weaver, G. A., Wilk, H. E., and Olson, J. E. (1981): Successful endoscopic electrocoagulation of gastric lesions of hereditary hemorrhagic telangiectasia responsible for repeated hemorrhages. *Gastrointest. Endosc.*, 27:181–183.
11. Tedesco, F. J., Hosty, T. A., and Sumner, H. W. (1975): Hereditary hemorrhagic telangiectasia: presenting as an unusual gastric lesion. *Gastroenterology*, 68:384–386.
12. Van Vliet, A. C. M., ten Kate, F. J. W., Dees, J., and van Blankenstein, M. (1978): Abnormal blood vessels of the prepyloric antrum in cirrhosis of the liver as a cause of chronic gastrointestinal bleeding. *Endoscopy*, 10:89–94.
13. Bourdages, R., Prentice, R. S. A., Beck, I. T., Da Costa, L. R., and Paloschi, G. B. (1976): Atheromatous embolization to the stomach: an unusual cause of gastrointestinal bleeding. *Am. J. Dig. Dis.*, 21: 889–894.
14. Domjan, L., Biliczki, F., Lorand, P., Cserenyi, L., and Bordas, F. (1975): Endoscopic diagnosis of "calibre-persistence," a rare cause of massive gastric hemorrhage. *Endoscopy*, 7:169–173.

14a. Cunningham, J. T. (1981): Gastric telangiectasias in chronic hemodialysis patients: A report of six cases. *Gastroenterology*, 81:1131–1133.

15. Farup, P. G., Rosseland, A. R., Stray, N., Pytte, R., Valnes, K., and Rand, A. A. (1981): Localized telangiopathy of the stomach and duodenum diagnosed and treated endoscopically: case reports and review. *Endoscopy*, 13:1–6.
16. Bongiovi, J. H., and Duffy, J. L. (1967): Gastric hemangioma associated with upper gastrointestinal bleeding. *Arch. Surg.*, 95:93–98.
17. Wheeler, M. H., Smith, P. M., Cotton, P. B., Evans, D. M. D., and Lawrie, B. W. (1979): Abnormal blood vessels in the gastric antrum: a cause of upper-gastrointestinal bleeding. *Dig. Dis. Sci.*, 24:155–158.
18. Calam, J., and Walker, R. J. (1980): Antral vascular lesion, achlorhydria, and chronic gastrointestinal blood loss: response to steroids. *Dig. Dis. Sci.*, 25:236–240.
19. Marshall, J. P., Smith, P. D., and Hoyumpa, A. M. (1977): Gastric varices: preliminary diagnosis. *Am. J. Dig. Dis.*, 22:947–955.
20. Cassell, P., and Robinson, J. O. (1976): Cancer of the stomach: a review of 854 patients. *Br. J. Surg.*, 63:603–607.
21. Brand, B., and Bernstein, L. H. (1973): Emergency gastroscopic polypectomy for control of hemorrhage. *Gastroenterology*, 65:956–958.
22. Brandborg, L. L. (1978): Polyps, tumors, and cancer of the stomach. In: *Gastrointestinal Disease*, edited by M. H. Sleisenger and J. S. Fordtran, p. 772. Saunders, Philadelphia.
23. Pao-Huei, Ch., Chuan-Pau, S., Kuang-Yang, L., Gonq-Chin, Jean-Dean, L., Hsian-Chong, K., and Ting-Yao, Ch. (1980): Carcinoids of the gastrointestinal tract. *Endoscopy*, 12:299–305.
24. Perillo, R. P., Zuckerman, G. R., and Shatz, B. A. (1977): Aberrent pancreas and leiomyoma of the stomach: indistinguishable radiologic and endoscopic features. *Gastrointest. Endosc.*, 23:162–163.
25. Clark, R. E., and Teplick, S. K. (1975): Ectopic pancreas causing massive upper gastrointestinal hemorrhage. *Gastroenterology*, 69:1331–1333.
26. Eschar, J., Kimerling, J. J., and Gilboa, Y. (1973): Eosinophilic granuloma of the stomach simulating leiomyoma. *Gastrointest. Endosc.*, 20:72.
27. Silverstein, F. E., Gilbert, D. A., Tedesco, F. J., Buenger, N. K., Persing, J., and 277 members of the ASGE (1981): The national ASGE survey on upper gastrointestinal bleeding. II. Clinical prognostic factors. *Gastrointest. Endosc.*, 27:80–93.
28. Padmanabhan, A., Douglass, H. O., and Nava, H. R. (1980): Role of endoscopy in upper gastrointestinal bleeding in patients with malignancy. *Endoscopy*, 12:10–104.
29. Chait, M. M., Turnbull, A. D., and Winawer, S. J. (1978): The anatomic distribution of gastric erosions from stress and gastric irritants in patients with cancer. *Gastrointest. Endosc.*, 24:233–235.
30. Chait, M. M., Turnbull, A. D., and Winawer, S. J. (1979): Risk factors and mortality in patients with cancer and hemorrhage from stress ulcer. *Am. J. Gastroenterol.*, 72:227–233.
31. Shivshanker, K., Stroehlein, J. R., and Nelson, R. S. (1981): Acute major gastrointestinal bleeding in the cancer patient: effect of myelosuppression and safety of endoscopy. *Gastroenterology*, 80:1284.
32. Moody, F. G., Cheung, L. Y., Simons, M. A., and Zalewsky, C. (1976): Stress and the acute gastric mucosal lesion. *Am. J. Dig. Dis.*, 21:148–154.
33. Hastings, P. R., Skillman, J. J., Bushnell, L. S., and Silen, W. (1978): Antacid titration in the prevention of acute gastrointestinal bleeding: a controlled, randomized trial in 100 critically ill patients. *N. Engl. J. Med.*, 298:1041–1045.
34. Czaja, A., McAlhany, J. C., and Pruitt, B. A. (1974): Acute gastroduodenal disease after thermal injury: an endoscopic evaluation of incidence and natural history. *N. Engl. J. Med.*, 291:925–929.
35. Menguy, R., and Masters, Y. F. (1976): Mechanism of stress ulcer: influence of sodium taurocholate on gastric mucosal energy metabolism during hemorrhagic shock, and on mitochondrial respiration and ATPase in gastric mucosa. *Am. J. Dig. Dis.*, 21:1001–1007.
36. Winawer, S. J., Sherlock, P., Sonenberg, M., and Vanamee, P. (1975): Beneficial effects of human growth hormone on stress ulcers. *Arch. Intern. Med.*, 135:569–572.
37. Weiss, J. B., Peskin, G. W., and Isenberg, J. I. (1982): Treatment of hemorrhagic gastritis with 15(R)-15 methyl prostaglandin E_2: report of a case. *Gastroenterology*, 82:558–560.
38. Posner, G., Huded, F. V., Fink, S. M., Dunn, I., Calderone, P., and Joglekar, S. (1982): Endoscopic findings in chronic hemodialysis patients with upper gastrointestinal bleeding. *Gastrointest. Endosc.*, 28:142.
39. Johnston, B., and Boyle, J. M. (1981): Non-variceal upper gastrointestinal hemorrhage in patients with chronic renal insufficiency. *Am. J. Gastroenterol.*, 76:181.
40. Margolis, D. M., Saylor, J. L., Geisse, G., DeSchryver-Kecskemeti, K., Harter, H. R., and Zuckerman, G. R. (1978): Upper gastrointestinal disease in chronic renal failure: a prospective evaluation. *Arch. Intern. Med.*, 138:1214–1217.
41. Davenport, H. W. (1968): Destruction of the gastric mucosal barrier by detergents and urea. *Gastroenterology*, 54:175–186.
42. McConnell, J. B., Stewart, W. K., Thjodleifsson, B., and Wormseley, K. G. (1975): Gastric function in chronic renal failure: effects of maintenance haemodialysis. *Lancet*, 2:1121–1123.
43. Stuart, F. P., Reckard, C. R., Schulak, J. A., and Ketel, B. L. (1981): Gastroduodenal complications in kidney transplant recipients. *Ann. Surg.*, 194:339–344.

38

DUODENAL BLEEDING

The duodenum is a frequent site of upper gastrointestinal (GI) bleeding, accounting in recent endoscopic series for 20 to 30% of the cases.[1] In the ASGE survey conducted in 1978, cases of duodenal bleeding (peptic ulcer and erosive duodenitis) accounted for 30.1%,[2] which was an even higher percentage than was found in all but two of 11 endoscopic series reported between 1969 and 1976, summarized by Graham and Davis.[1] That duodenal bleeding sites were recognized in this high percentage may in some part be due to the ease with which the duodenum can be entered using currently available narrow-caliber endoscopes, which also allow for a more complete examination of the duodenal bulb than did earlier instruments, especially a bulb contracted and scarred by peptic ulcer disease (see Chapter 24).

Of the causes of duodenal bleeding, peptic ulcer disease stands as the commonest, being one of the leading causes of upper GI bleeding, especially in elderly patients (over age 60), where it accounts for up to 40% of all bleeding episodes.[3]

In young patients, especially those who present to municipal, county, or Veterans Administration (VA) hospitals with a history of heavy alcohol consumption, erosive duodenitis, the duodenal equivalent of hemorrhagic-erosive gastritis, has accounted for up to 9% of the cases.[1] Also seen by the endoscopist from time to time are a variety of less common causes of duodenal bleeding, including tumors, diverticula, Crohn's disease of the duodenum, aortoenteric fistulas, and other vascular causes.

In this chapter we consider the endoscopic features of duodenal causes of bleeding, starting with the commonest cause, peptic ulcer disease, continuing with erosive duodenitis, and concluding with briefer discussions of the rarely encountered causes.

DUODENAL ULCER BLEEDING

Duodenal ulcers are generally found at endoscopy in 20 to 35% of cases examined because of upper GI bleeding.[1] In the ASGE survey, it was the final diagnosis in 24.3%,[2] according with our own experience of 27% (see Table 32-2). The percentage of duodenal ulcer bleeding has been lowest (in the range of 11 to 16%)[1] in reports from municipal hospitals, presumably because of the disproportionate number of patients who are admitted because of bleeding from alcoholic hemorrhagic-erosive gastritis[1] (see Chapter 36).

Patients with duodenal ulcers commonly present for endoscopy because of bleeding. Sheppard et al. noted bleeding as the presentation for endoscopy of 31% of patients with duodenal ulcers.[4] This was especially true for elderly patients with duodenal ulcers in whom bleeding prompted endoscopy in 44% of patients aged 60 to 69, and in 60% of patients between the ages of 70 and 79. In up to 25% of the cases[3] bleeding is the first presentation of peptic ulcer disease so the diagnosis may not always be suspected clinically. This is particularly true of patients who present with melena alone, where because of a negative nasogastric aspirate the patient may be first considered to have a lower GI bleeding site. In our experience about 20% of patients with a duodenal site of bleeding found at endoscopy (Fig. 38-1a) have a nasogastric aspirate negative for blood (Fig. 38-1b).[5]

The treacherousness of a nasogastric aspirate for excluding an upper GI bleeding site was confirmed by the ASGE survey, where 15.9% patients who had a clear nasogastric aspirate had active bleeding sites at endoscopy.[6] Contrary to the view of some authors,[7] a negative nasogastric aspirate should never be regarded as an indication not to perform endoscopy, particularly in elderly patients in whom bleeding in the form of melena is not an uncommon presentation of a duodenal ulcer.

GI bleeding may be expected in up to 20% of patients with well-established peptic ulcer disease if the patients are followed over a 15- to 25-year period.[8] A history of a duodenal ulcer is significant in predicting the cause of a subsequent bleed. In the ASGE survey the finding of duodenal ulcer bleeding was three times more prevalent among those with a history of duodenal ulcers (43.6%) than in those without such history (16.6%).[6]

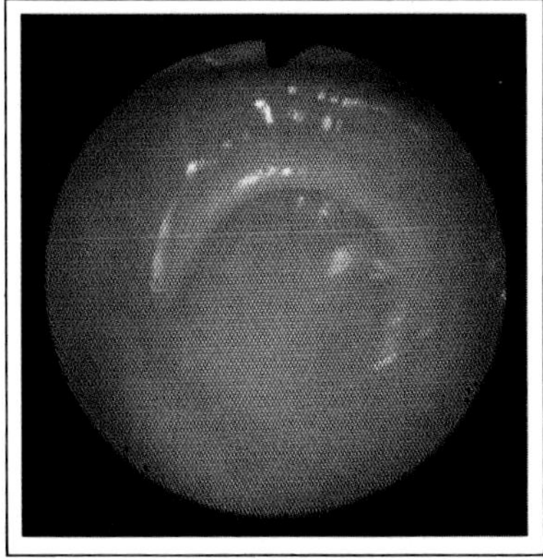

FIG. 38-1a.

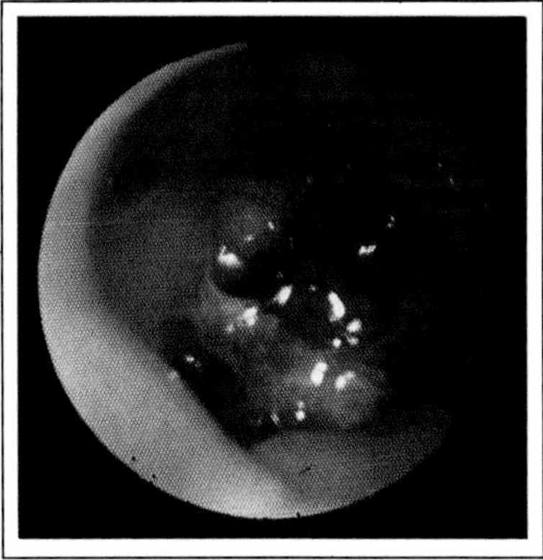

FIG. 38-1b.

FIG. 38-1. a: Clear gastric antrum in a patient with a bleeding duodenal ulcer (b). A nasogastric aspirate was negative for blood, despite a four-unit transfusion requirement. **b:** Duodenal ulcer, bleeding. A large clot partially obscures a 2-cm ulcer base in a patient presenting with melena but without a history of peptic ulcer disease. In such cases endoscopy is indicated to examine the duodenal bulb, irrespective of the status of the nasogastric aspirate.[5]

Pathogenesis of Duodenal Ulcer Bleeding

Like that of gastric ulcer bleeding (see Chapter 36), the pathogenesis of duodenal ulcers is uncertain. As is true for gastric ulcers, one supposes that when the rate of ulceration outstrips the occurrence of protective changes in blood vessels within the base (e.g., reactive thickening of the intimal layer), exposed vessels lacking these changes are more prone to bleed as are others where the portion of the vessel that has undergone reactive changes is destroyed, as in a case where an ulcer is rapidly enlarging and/or deepening. Surprisingly, in contrast to gastric ulcers, prior heavy aspirin usage has not been found to increase the likelihood of a patient presenting to the hospital because of duodenal bleeding, suggesting that aspirin does not change a duodenal ulcer diathesis in some fundamental way to predispose it to bleed.[9]

Rationale for Endoscopy

Although the overall mortality for duodenal ulcer bleeding is low—in fact it is significantly lower than for all other causes of bleeding considered together (a mortality of 6.7% in the ASGE survey for duodenal ulcer bleeding compared with 12.2% overall for other conditions)[10]—there is still an excess mortality for this common cause of GI bleeding in patients over age 60 whose bleeding continues or recurs in hospital.[3] Endoscopy provides a means of determining the likelihood of continuing or recurrent bleeding by identifying the stigmata of recent bleeding, including actively bleeding ulcers, those with adherent clots, or the appearance of a visible vessel within the ulcer base. Foster et al.[11] found that 50% of patients with duodenal ulcers who had these stigmata at endoscopy performed within the first 24 hr of admission to the hospital had both further hemorrhage and emergency surgery, in contrast to 5% of patients without stigmata. In the ASGE survey, a similar difference was noted in the transfusion requirement (as an indication of continued or recurrent bleeding) and the rate of surgical intervention for patients observed at endoscopy to be actively bleeding and those who were not, with 43.7% having a 6+ unit transfusion requirement and 41.6% surgical intervention for those observed with active bleeding (pumping or oozing from the ulcer site), in contrast to 21.3% and 12.9%, respectively, for those whose bleeding was inactive (clots alone or no blood).[6] In addition, the mortality rate for patients with actively bleeding ulcers was 10.6%, in contrast to a 3% rate for ulcers not bleeding. Moreover, there was a complication rate (largely surgical complications) of 18.3% for actively bleeding ulcers contrasted to 7.2% for those where bleeding has stopped.[6]

The role of endoscopy therefore is to identify patients with stigmata of recent bleeding, including active bleeding itself, who require very close observation over the first 48 hr following endoscopy for evidence of continued or recurrent bleeding[12] and consideration for endoscopic therapy (electrocoagulation[12a] or laser photocoagulation[12b]) or, if this fails[12a,12b] or is unavailable, early surgery.[12] This is especially important for patients over the age of 60[13] with massive bleeding who require more than six units in the first 24 hr and are not amenable to endoscopic therapy.[12a,12b] In cases that finally come to surgery after having received six units of blood or more, the mortality rate approaches 30%, in contrast to a rate of under 15% for patients who receive five units or less.[12]

Location

Bleeding duodenal ulcers are found in the usual locations (see Chapter 26). As the anterior wall tends to be the commonest site of duodenal ulcers in general, not surprisingly this was found in one series to be the commonest site of bleeding ulcers.[4] However, massively bleeding duodenal ulcers tend, in our experience, to be located on the posterior wall where the ulcer has eroded into the gastroduodenal artery. A review of our experience with 135 bleeding ulcers seen over a 7-year period disclosed 20 that required emergency surgical intervention (15%). Of these, 14 (60%) were located on the posterior wall, in contrast to only 35% of ulcers found in this location at endoscopy performed in nonbleeding patients (see Chapter 26).

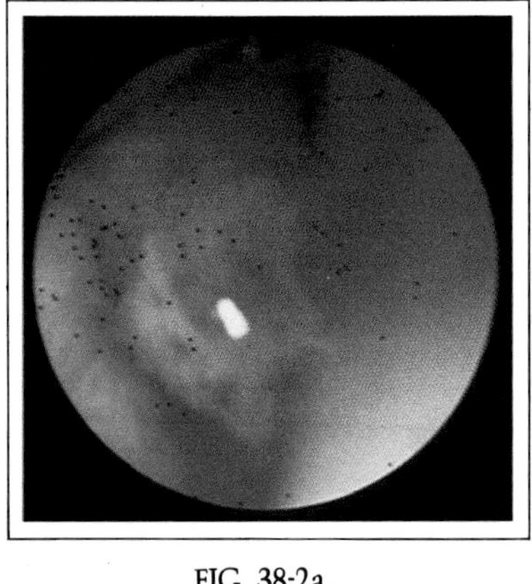

FIG. 38-2a.

FIG. 38-2b.

FIG. 38-2c.

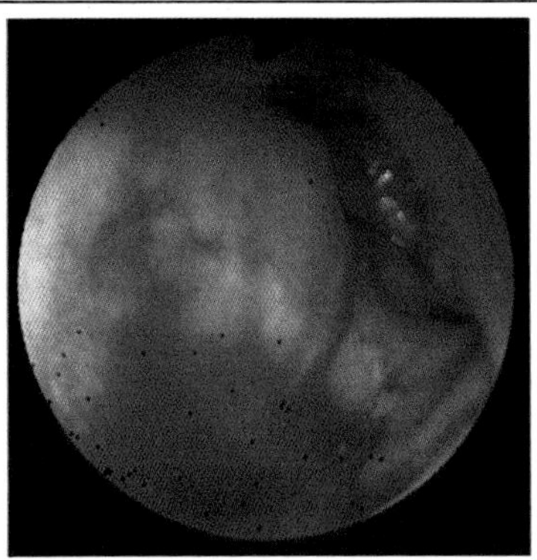

FIG. 38-2d.

FIG. 38-2. a: Duodenal ulcer bleeding, slow ooze. Blood can be seen to trickle down from the ulcer margin. **b:** Duodenal ulcer bleeding, slow ooze. Blood emerges from around a clot, which largely obscures the base. **c:** Duodenal ulcer bleeding with fresh clot and continued oozing. Despite the large adherent clot, the base of the ulcer can still be seen at 9 o'clock with oozing at 3 o'clock. **d:** Duodenal ulcer bleeding with a small amount of residual oozing. Little is seen of the ulcer base. The deep depression on the anterior wall in which the blood collects is evidence of ulcer scar deformity and a high likelihood of ulcer bleeding.

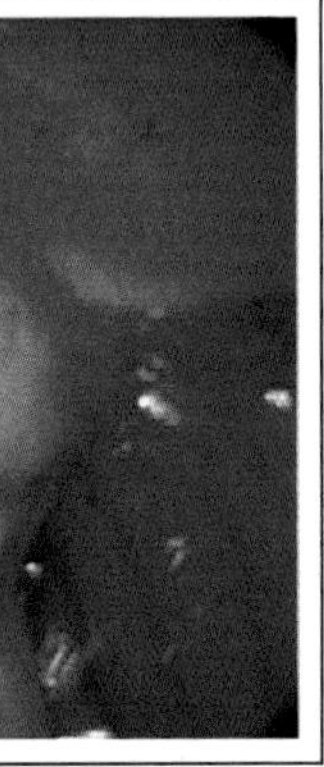

FIG. 38-3a.

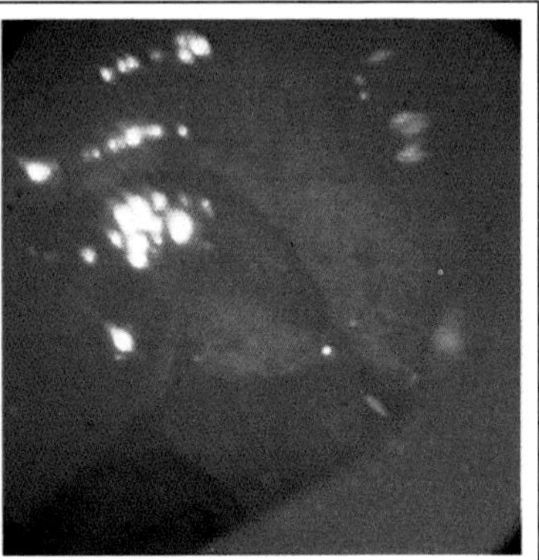

FIG. 38-3b.

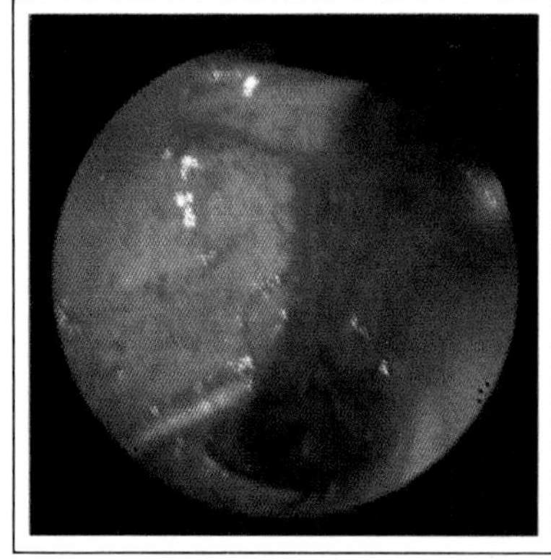

FIG. 38-3c.

FIG. 38-3. Duodenal bleeding, pumping. **a:** A large amount of blood covers the posterior wall of the bulb and descending duodenum. The welling up of blood on the posterior wall as well as the large amount of blood suggested that the ulcer had eroded into the gastroduodenal artery. This was confirmed by arteriography. **b:** The mucosal surfaces of the descending duodenum and bulb are almost completely covered by blood. **c:** With gastric reflux. The large amount of blood in the bulb streams back into the stomach from the pyloric channel at 6 o'clock.

Appearance

The endoscopist encounters ulcer bleeding as: (a) an actively bleeding ulcer; (b) an ulcer with stigmata of recent bleeding, including visible vessel; and (c) an ulcer with no stigmata.

Actively Bleeding Ulcer

The endoscopist may see active bleeding in about one-third of the cases. Here the blood is seen to either trickle from the ulcer, referred to as oozing (Fig. 38-2a), or spurt from the ulcer base (Fig. 38-3a) called pumping. In the ASGE survey, active bleeding was seen in 29.9%, with most of this the oozing variety (24.2%); pumping occurred in a smaller number (5.57%).[8] The ulcer which is oozing is often denoted by an adherent clot around which the blood is seen to ooze (Fig. 38-2b). The ulcer base may be quite indistinct because of the bleeding, with only a part of it, at best, being seen adjacent to the clot (Fig. 38-2c). Often the correct diagnosis of duodenal ulcer bleeding is suspected by the blood and clot being set in an area of scar deformity with the ulcer base entirely obscured (Fig. 38-2d).

Pumping of blood (Fig. 38-3a) is seen in 5 to 10% of the cases (5.7% in the ASGE survey).[8] In this case the blood seems to spurt from a point generally along the posterior

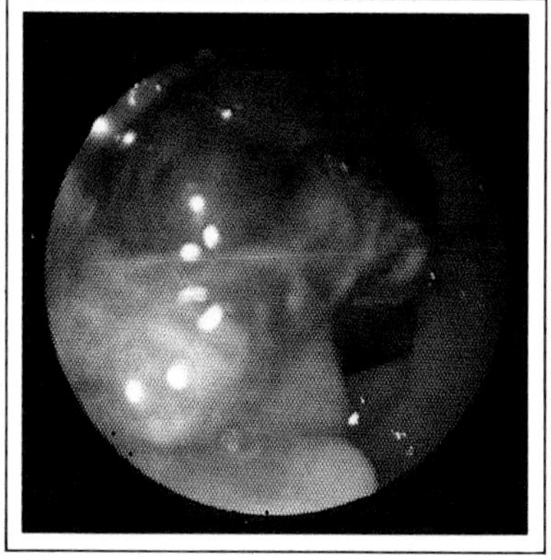

FIG. 38-4a.

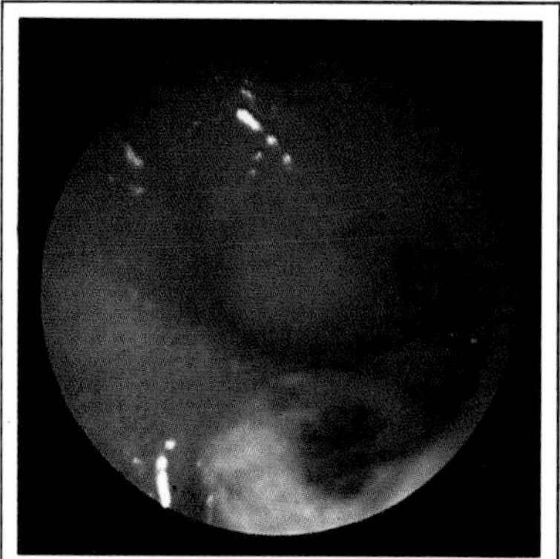

FIG. 38-4b.

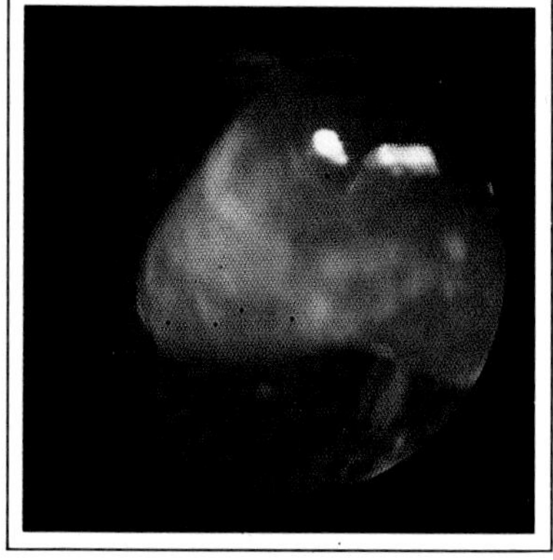

FIG. 38-4c.

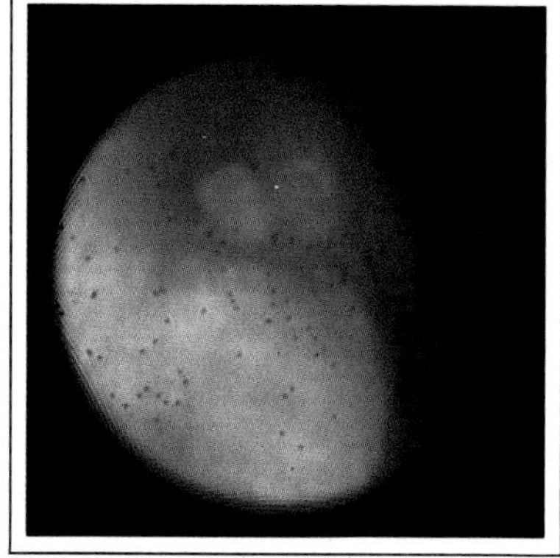

FIG. 38-4d.

FIG. 38-4. a: Duodenal ulcer with a large bulky clot, indicating recent bleeding. We find that ulcers with bulky clots are prone to rebleed in about 30% of cases (see text). **b:** Duodenal ulcer with old blood in its base as an indicator of recent bleeding. The likelihood of recurrent bleeding in these cases is less than 10% (see text). **c:** Duodenal ulcer with a visible vessel within its base. A 5-mm cylindrical vascular-appearing structure was seen protruding from the base of a deep ulcer on the posterior wall. By arteriography this was shown to be the gastroduodenal artery. The finding of a visible vessel carries a 50% or greater likelihood of recurrent bleeding and therefore requires close observation and definitive therapy, either surgical or endoscopic (photocoagulation[17] or electrocoagulation[16]). **d:** Duodenal ulcer with no stigmata of recent bleeding. The patient was examined 48 hr after admission to the hospital. At this time there were no stigmata of recent bleeding. With this appearance, the likelihood of bleeding is less than 5%.

wall. Frequently the blood is so copious it completely obscures an entire surface of the bulb, usually the posterior wall (Fig. 38-3b)—the site, in our experience, most often associated with pumping (Fig. 38-3a)—where the ulcer has eroded into the gastroduodenal artery. In these cases only bright red blood is seen with no part of the ulcer visible (Fig. 38-3a). A not uncommon special case of pumping is that where the pyloroduodenal junction is deformed from previous ulcer scarring such that the duodenal bulb cannot be entered. The endoscopist nevertheless may see bright red blood emanating from the pyloric channel (Fig. 38-3c). In this instance he would be justified in suspecting that the most likely source of bleeding is a posterior wall ulcer eroding into the gastroduodenal artery and in offering this interpretation rather than simply stating the level of bleeding without a diagnosis.

Stigmata of Recent Bleeding, Including the Visible Vessel

In about 20% of the cases active bleeding is not seen, with only stigmata indicating that recent bleeding occurred. The commonest of these stigmata is a clot which is seen to cover the ulcer base (Fig. 38-4a), either partially or entirely, with only a small area of the ulcer projecting from the clot. Early on, the clot may be mound-like, projecting out into the lumen (Fig. 38-4a). Such clots are generally seen within the first 36 hr of the patient's admission to the hospital. Later, only a residual of this may be observed as a small amount of old blood (acid hematin) embedded in the base of the ulcer, denoting a previous bleeding site (Fig. 38-4b). We find that the presence of a fresh clot, especially with mound-like appearance, indicates an increased likelihood of recurrent hemorrhage. Although we do not know the precise risk, because many such clots cover what would otherwise be a visible vessel (see below), we believe it to be on the order of 30% of cases, a figure somewhere between that associated with the risk of recurrent bleeding with the finding of a visible vessel (50% or more)[14] and that associated with finding a clot embedded in the ulcer base, where the risk is 10% or less.[14]

Visible Vessel

The finding of a blood vessel projecting from the ulcer base (Fig. 38-4c) is of great prognostic significance, being associated with recurrent or continuous bleeding in more than 50% of patients in whom it is observed.[14,15] In one study a visible vessel was found in 13.7% (11 of 80) of bleeding duodenal ulcers.[15] If overlying clots are washed away,[14,16] as in other studies, the percentage is found to equal this[16] or be even higher.[14] We, however, have only rarely seen a duodenal ulcer visible vessel, possibly because it is not our policy to routinely attempt to wash a clot

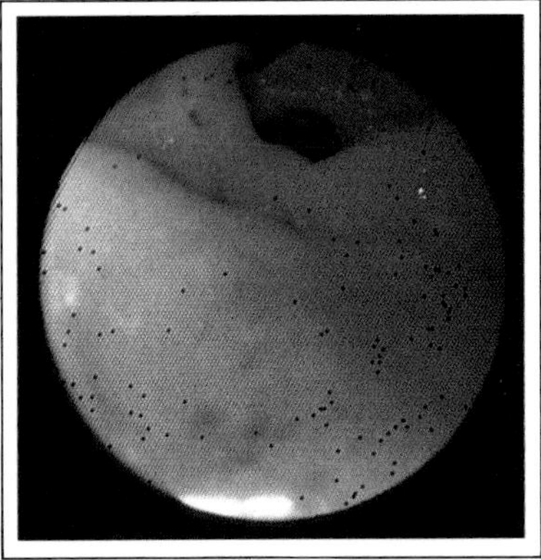

FIG. 38-5a.

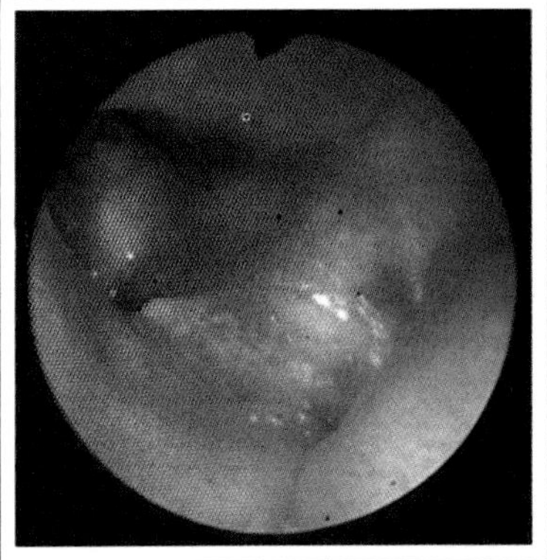

FIG. 38-5b.

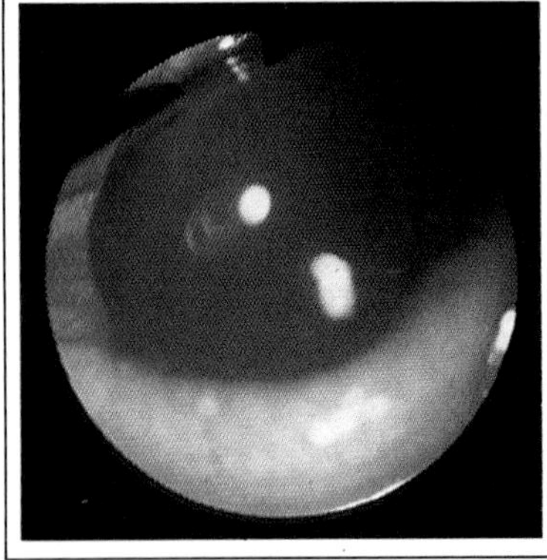

FIG. 38-5c.

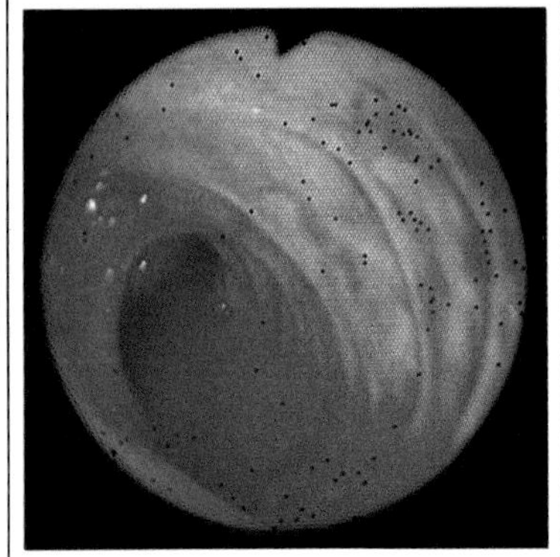

FIG. 38-5d.

FIG. 38-5. a: Duodenal ulcer bleeding with marked scar deformity. If the bleeding ulcer is set within a depression just proximal to the apical V-shaped deformity, careful examination of this recess area is required to demonstrate the ulcer. **b:** Duodenal ulcer after a recent bleeding episode, appearing tumor-like. The irregular outline as well as the mass-like character of the clot gives the ulcer a tumor-like appearance. Because of the rarity of such tumors in the duodenal bulb, any such appearance should still be regarded as probably that of a peptic ulcer. **c:** Duodenal ulcer bleeding with large clots simulating a duodenal polyp (e.g., that in Fig. 38-9). Closer examination, however, reveals it to be only a large clot, which in the duodenal bulb is almost always caused by peptic ulcer disease. **d:** Duodenal ulcer bleed simulating a distal bleeding site. The large amount of bright red blood and especially the clot found at the junction of the second and third portions caused the endoscopist to believe this was from a distal site (as in Fig. 38-10d). The fact that blood was also seen in the proximal descending duodenum and duodenal bulb should have made him suspect a duodenal bulb origin.

away and therefore risk an exacerbation of bleeding. In a series where visible vessels were encountered in 15% of patients endoscoped because of bleeding, any clot present was routinely washed away with the expectation that if a visible vessel was demonstrated it would be electrocoagulated[16] because in the absence of such treatment bleeding uniformly recurred. It seems likely that a policy of aggressive washing to discover an appreciable percentage of ulcers with visible vessels may predispose patients to an adverse outcome, i.e., rebleeding, especially if endoscopic therapy (electro- or photocoagulation) is not immediately forthcoming.[17] In a controlled study of laser photocoagulation of 24 cases where a visible vessel was identified but not treated, 13 (54%) rebled with a mortality of 21% (5 of 24).[17]

Ulcer with No Stigmata

No stigmata of bleeding were found in association with the ulcer in 30 to 40% of patients with the final diagnosis of duodenal ulcer bleeding (Fig. 38-4d). In the ASGE survey, duodenal ulcers lacking stigmata were present in 41.9% of the cases where duodenal ulcer was listed as the final diagnosis for the bleeding episode. In practice, if an ulcer is observed without stigmata it is generally seen as the only potential site. Although the endoscopist cannot be certain that such an ulcer was, in fact, the cause of the patient's bleeding, he may nonetheless be quite confident that bleeding will not recur from the ulcer at least during the course of hospitalization. The risk of bleeding from a stigmataless ulcer found at endoscopy seems to be on the order of 5% or less.[11,14]

Interpretive Problems

Four interpretive problems are found in patients with duodenal ulcers. These are: (a) the finding of duodenal bulb deformity/duodenitis but with no ulcers seen; (b) the ulcer and clot simulating the appearance of a tumor mass; (c) blood in the descending duodenum suggesting a distal bleeding site; and (d) a duodenal ulcer which is not the bleeding site.

Duodenal Bulb Deformity and Duodenitis Without a Definite Ulcer Seen

Most duodenal ulcers can be seen with the currently employed narrow-caliber instruments. Still, in our experience, even in the absence of bleeding 3 to 5% of duodenal ulcers which are ultimately proved at surgery or autopsy may not be observed endoscopically, being for the most part obscured by the scar deformity (Fig. 38-5a). Confronted with the appearance of scar deformity alone or with focal erythema that suggests duodenitis, the endoscopist may reject the finding as indicative of the cause of bleeding and state categorically that no convincing bleeding site has been identified. We believe that it is unwise to do this, especially if the character of the bleeding suggests duodenal ulcers or melena in a patient with a history of a duodenal ulcer.[6] In such a case, one suggests that while a definite ulcer has not been observed there is a high probability that the bleeding was from this site. One then recommends that the patient be managed as if a definite ulcer had been observed, with the provision that with any suggestion of recurrent bleeding endoscopy be immediately performed with a hope of demonstrating blood in the duodenum. Should blood in this instance not be found, an evaluation from a more distal bleeding site (small intestinal or colonic) would be appropriate.

Ulcer and Clot With Features Suggestive of a Tumor Mass

The margin of the bleeding ulcer may be quite irregular (Fig. 38-5b). This, taken with the presence of a large overlying clot with a "mass-like" appearance (Fig. 38-5c), may cause the endoscopist to conclude erroneously that he is observing a carcinoma or a duodenal neoplasm. Statistically, however, the commonest cause of duodenal bulb bleeding is peptic ulcer disease. As such, only in a case where a duodenal bulb lesion with suspicious features is well demonstrated and entirely free of blood might one wish to suggest the possibility of a neoplasm, though never dismissing the diagnosis of peptic ulcer disease.

Blood in the Descending Duodenum Suggesting a Site Distal to the Bulb

For patients in the midst of a massive bleeding episode from the duodenal bulb, the descending duodenum as well as the third portion may be full of blood, leading to the erroneous impression of a distal bleeding site (Fig. 38-5d). Even in the face of copious amounts of blood, however, it is still possible to observe the presence of bright red blood on the posterior wall of the duodenal bulb. Although it is possible that blood from a distal site in the duodenum could reflux back into the bulb or even the stomach, statistically it is much more probable that bright red blood found in both the descending duodenum and the duodenal bulb is from the duodenal bulb. In such cases the careful endoscopist suggests both possibilities, i.e., a duodenal bulb or descending origin, but with duodenal ulcer bleeding being the most probable. He further suggests that to determine which is actually the case, especially in the face of massive bleeding, arteriography is the next indicated step.

Duodenal Ulcer Which Is Not the Site of Bleeding

The finding of a duodenal ulcer with or without stigmata of recent bleeding is in most cases accepted as the bleeding site. In the ASGE survey, duodenal ulcer bleeding was the final diagnosis in 94.3% of the cases in which a duodenal ulcer was found at endoscopy.[8] Still, in 5% of the cases the endoscopist rejected this finding in favor of another, although the other sites to which the bleeding was ultimately attributed were not defined. As a rule, one tends to reject stigmata-less ulcers of less than 5 mm as likely sites of bleeding. Finding this type of ulcer in the bulb (Fig. 38-6a) prompts the endoscopist to examine the prepyloric antrum (Fig. 38-6b) and gastric angle as likely sites of peptic ulcer disease which would be associated with a duodenal bulb ulcer. Even finding a larger ulcer with apparent stigmata (Fig. 38-6c) does not eliminate the need to carefully examine the distal esophagus and fundus for another lesion which could also account for the bleeding episode (Fig. 38-6d).

EROSIVE DUODENITIS

In many but not all recent endoscopic series, the finding of mucosal erosions of the duodenal bulb—erosive duodenitis—accounts for 1 to 5% of cases of upper GI bleeding.[1] In the ASGE survey erosive duodenitis was the final diagnosis in 5.8%, approaching the frequency of esophagitis (6.3%) and Mallory-Weiss tears (7.2%) as the final diagnosis.

The commonest presentation reported has been hematemesis after heavy alcohol consumption[18]; however, it has also been described as a "stress" lesion associated with a recent myocardial infarction or extensive surgery.[19]

Pathogenesis

Alcohol-Related Erosive Duodenitis

Alcohol-induced erosive duodenitis seems to result from a direct toxic mucosal effect of alcohol at a critical concentration. Gottfried et al. performed endoscopy in seven alcoholic subjects who had had prior normal examinations of their duodenal bulb, followed by oral administration of alcohol (1 g/kg body weight) in a 35 g/100 ml solution (approximately 80 proof).[20] At endoscopy the duodenal bulb was abnormal in five of the seven cases, with erythema and friability in three and hemorrhage or petechiae in two. In four of the five, evidence of subepithelial hemorrhage was found on biopsy. These observations suggested that alcohol, when ingested in an amount of 1 g/kg and at a concentration of 35% is capable of producing an acute injury reaction in some but not all patients. However, the factors which predispose individuals to develop these lesions with associated bleeding are unknown.

Stress-Related Duodenitis

Erosive duodenitis as a cause of significant bleeding in the absence of gastric lesions has been reported in patients

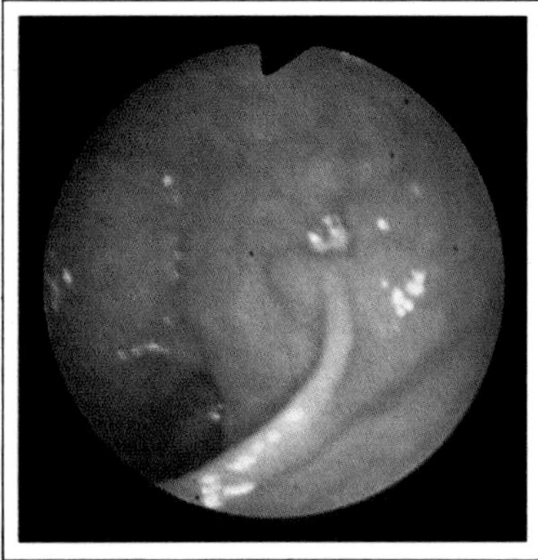

FIG. 38-6a.

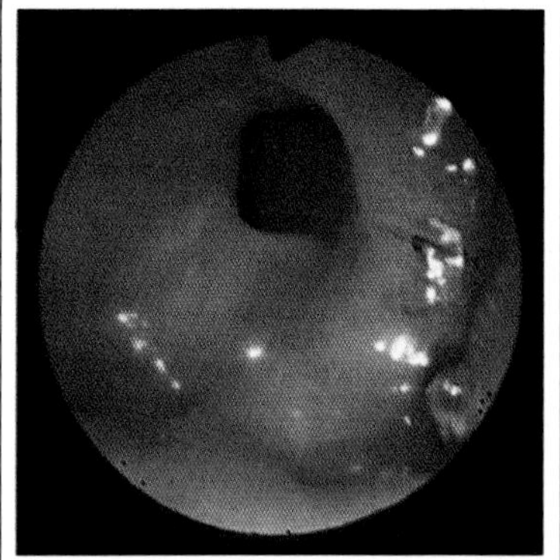

FIG. 38-6b.

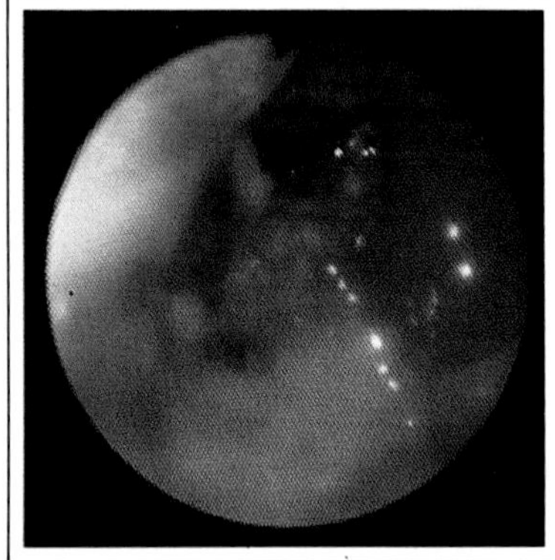

FIG. 38-6c.

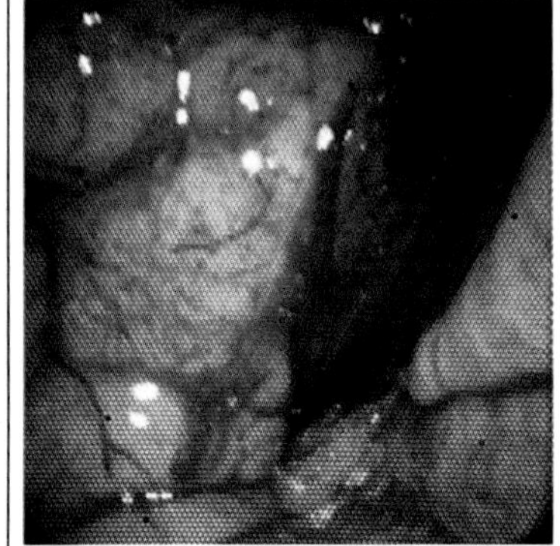

FIG. 38-6d.

FIG. 38-6. a: Small duodenal ulcer, unlikely to be a bleeding site. The size (<5 mm) as well as the absence of stigmata or recent bleeding suggested another bleeding site (d). **b:** Prepyloric ulcer with stigmata of recent bleeding (clot embedded in base). This was initially overlooked upon entry into the duodenal bulb; the finding of a small ulcer (a) caused the endoscopist to carefully examine the prepyloric antrum on his return into the stomach. **c:** Large duodenal ulcer with apparent stigmata of recent bleeding, as old blood (acid hematin) within the base (where the bright red blood was thought to represent endoscope-induced trauma). Somewhat unsettling was the fact that most of the old blood could be washed off with similar material free-floating in the stomach, in a patient having bled in the past from gastric varices (d). **d:** Gastric varices, covered with old blood in a patient with a large duodenal ulcer (c). These, not the ulcer, proved to be the bleeding site.

after myocardial infarction or extensive surgery.[19] Although stress lesions of the duodenum, i.e., intramucosal hemorrhage, erosions, and superficial ulcerations, are found in up to 30% of patients with stress lesion bleeding (see Chapter 37), their presence as an isolated finding is somewhat surprising, especially in view of the probable role of altered blood flow in the etiology of stress lesions (see Chapter 37). In this regard, with the blood supply of the duodenal bulb richer than that to proximal stomach, it is surprising that isolated duodenal lesions occur. That they are a rare manifestation of stress effects on gastroduodenal mucosa is probably a reflection of this. The particular circulatory alterations which might predispose to their occurring in an isolated fashion to involve only the duodenal bulb have not been determined.

Rationale for Endoscopy

Bleeding associated with erosive duodenitis is on the whole self-limited, with a low mortality rate and a low incidence of protracted bleeding that requires surgery. In the ASGE survey, it had the lowest mortality rate (2.3%) in contrast to the 11.4% for other conditions, the second lowest number requiring 6 units or more of blood transfusion (11.7% versus 27.3% for other conditions), and the lowest rate of surgical interventions (1.6% versus 16.4% for other conditions).[6] In view of the self-limited nature of this condition, the role of endoscopy if any is to suggest a self-limited bleeding episode based on the natural history of erosive duodenitis bleeding. Such informtion would affect decisions concerning the patient's discharge from an intensive care unit or, more importantly, alter a decision for early surgical intervention based on the erroneous clinical diagnosis of duodenal ulcer bleeding.

Appearance

The characteristic endoscopic finding[18] for erosive duodenitis is that of focal areas of erythema, friability, with intramucosal hemorrhage and acute erosions (Fig. 38-7a), much like the appearance of hemorrhagic-erosive gastritis (see Chapter 36). Erosions have several shapes and vary in size from millimeters to several centimeters. The Kerckring folds, when seen, are prominent and erythematous (Fig. 38-7b). With active bleeding, which occurs in approximately 25%, on entering the bulb one sees blood oozing around clots adherent to the mucosal erosions.

Intramucosal hemorrhage and erosions tend to be confined to the bulb. Within the descending duodenum there may be nonspecific erythema along with enlarged folds. Intense erythema, especially in and around the duodenal

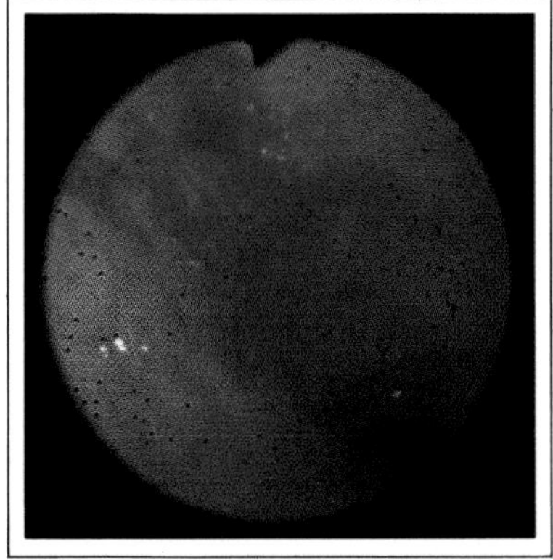

FIG. 38-7a.

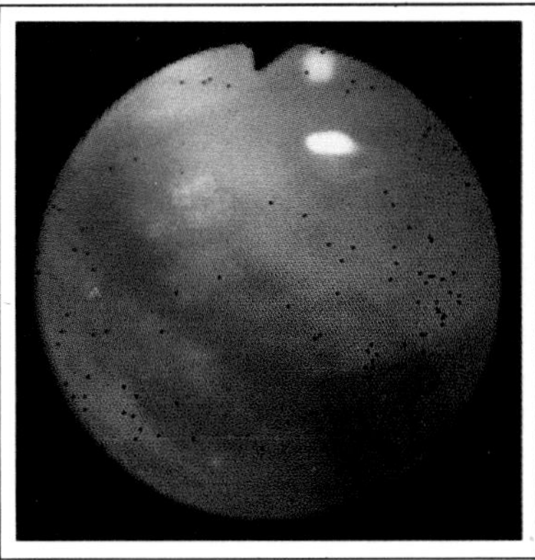

FIG. 38-7b.

FIG. 38-7. Erosive duodenitis. **a:** In a patient with recent heavy alcohol intake, intramucosal hemorrhage with some areas of adherent clot and oozing suggested this to be the bleeding site. At the time of examination there was no evidence of acute gastric mucosal injury. **b:** The acute alcohol injury phenomenon continues into the descending duodenum as enlargement (edema) of the Kerckring folds. A focal area of bleeding is noted at 9 o'clock.

papilla suggests the presence of coexisting pancreatitis (see Chapter 28).

Interpretive Problems

The difficulties confronting the endoscopist who is considering a diagnosis of erosive duodenitis as a cause of bleeding are: (a) blood simulating acute mucosal injury; (b) duodenitis coexisting with an inapparent ulcer; and (c) the presence of nonspecific acute duodenitis as a longstanding mucosal change.

Blood Simulating Acute Mucosal Injury

The presence of blood in the duodenal bulb can be extremely misleading. Blood here, as in the stomach, tends to accumulate on the dependent surfaces, adhering to the mucosa in such a way as to simulate the appearance of an intramucosal hemorrhage or erosions with clots. The bleeding, if substantial, tends to obscure an ulcer, with the blood itself simulating the appearance of erosive duodenitis (Fig. 38-8a). In the face of substantial bleeding which continues or is recurrent (which is not the pattern of erosive duodenitis bleeding), the endoscopist is well advised to suspect peptic ulcer bleeding, especially in the face of duodenal bulb deformity or a history of prior ulcer disease.[6]

Duodenitis from a Coexisting but Inapparent Ulcer

For 20 to 40% of duodenal ulcers, endoscopic changes of duodenitis are present within a circumferential area having a width of 5 mm or more (Fig. 38-8b). In cases where the acute duodenitis is extensive, and where scar deformity obscures the ulcer, only duodenitis may be seen. Some authors, e.g., Katz et al.,[21] suggest that one may diagnose erosive duodenitis as the cause of bleeding even if a duodenal ulcer base is seen. However, as ulcers may bleed from the margins as well as their base (in which case the actual bleeding site may be confusing), we believe it is unwise to postulate bleeding from duodenitis in the face of a frank ulcer, especially if the bleeding is brisk and protracted, features which are clearly more characteristic of peptic ulcer bleeding.[6]

Longstanding Acute Duodenitis

We find endoscopic abnormalities in the duodenal bulb suggestive of nonspecific duodenitis in up to 5% of patients undergoing endoscopy for reasons other than duodenal bleeding (see Chapter 25). Erosions are present in one-third of these (Fig. 38-8c) along with friability, which continues to be present at subsequent endoscopies. Because of the erythema and friability associated with acute nonspecific duodenitis, entry into the bulb may be associated with some bleeding. Bleeding sometimes occurs also as a result of traumatic entry in patients with preexisting acute nonspecific duodenitis (Fig. 38-8d). Indeed, in the ASGE survey there was a significant discrepancy between the endoscopic finding of duodenitis and the final diagnosis. In only 65% was the initial endoscopic diagnosis of duodenitis believed to be the actual cause of bleeding.[6] For this reason, endoscopists and clinicians alike are well advised to view any diagnosis of erosive duodenitis with great suspicion. The endoscopist might prudently suggest a repeat endoscopy within a month of the bleeding episode to evaluate the status of the duodenal mucosa. A diagnosis of erosive duodenitis for a bleeding episode is accepted only if at that time no lesion is found. If nonspecific acute duodenitis is still present, the endoscopist advises that the cause of the prior bleeding episode be considered undetermined.

TUMOR-RELATED BLEEDING

In our experience, tumors of the duodenum account for about 1% of upper GI bleeding. In our series of 500 consecutive cases examined over a 7-year period, six (1.3%) were the result of duodenal tumor bleeding. Of these, two were benign and four were malignant. In five of the six cases, bleeding was brisk, producing syncope or orthostatic changes in addition to melena. The nasogastric aspirate was positive in only one, being negative in four, and trace-positive in the remaining case, again pointing up the treach-

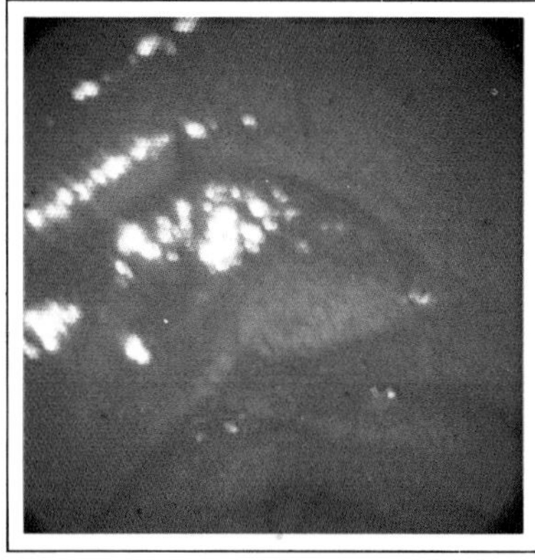

FIG. 38-8a.

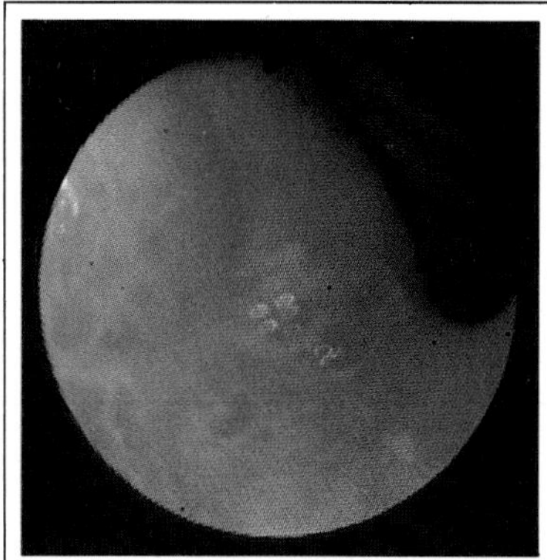

FIG. 38-8b.

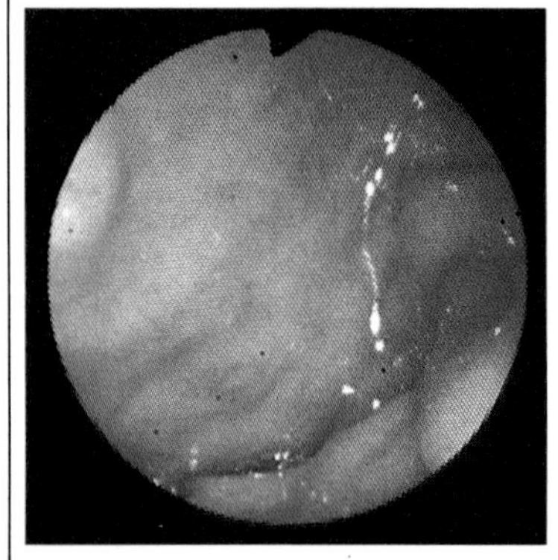

FIG. 38-8c.

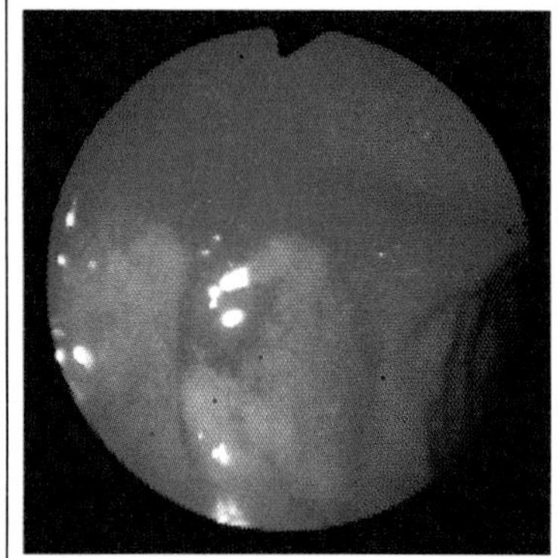

FIG. 38-8d.

FIG. 38-8. a: Bleeding duodenal ulcer, coating the mucosal surface with blood to simulate erosive duodenitis. **b:** Duodenitis surrounding a peptic ulcer which may be confused with acute erosive duodenitis. In this case the clot within the base (rather than the duodenitis) indicates the ulcer to be the bleeding site. **c:** Nonspecific acute duodenitis in a patient with bleeding 1 month before. The continued presence of duodenitis would make one suspect that the previous bleeding episode may have had another origin. **d:** Traumatized acute duodenitis in a nonbleeding patient examined because of atypical ulcer pain. Entry into a deformed bulb with duodenitis produced the appearance of hemorrhage. Were this to have occurred in a bleeding patient, the appearance could have been mistaken for bleeding erosive duodenitis.

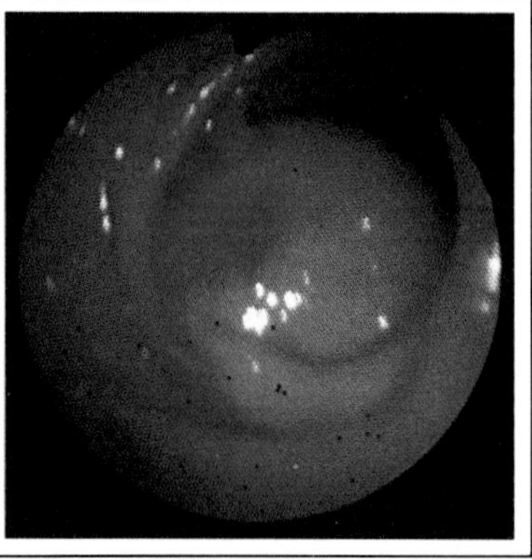

FIG. 38-9.

FIG. 38-9. Brunner gland adenoma, bleeding. A large 2-cm adenoma with an active bleeding site was removed surgically.

erousness of a negative nasogastric aspirate in excluding an upper GI site of bleeding.[5]

In these cases the commonest clinical diagnosis prior to endoscopy was duodenal ulcer bleeding. In three of the four patients' malignant tumors, two had known cancer elsewhere, suggesting the duodenum might also be involved (see below), and in the remaining patient with a metastatic carcinoid, substantial weight loss had occurred prior to the bleeding episode.

Benign Tumors

The two commonest benign tumors which are associated with bleeding are leiomyomas and adenomatous polyps.[23] Less commonly, lipomas or Brunner gland adenomas are associated with bleeding if they grow large enough (>2 cm) to cause mucosal (central) ulceration (see Chapter 30). The commonest location for these tumors is the descending duodenum, except for Brunner gland adenomas and lipomas, which are most often found at the apex of the duodenal bulb or just beyond (Fig. 38-9).[22]

Malignant Tumors

Gastrointestinal bleeding may be associated with primary duodenal carcinoma, malignancies of mesenchymal origin

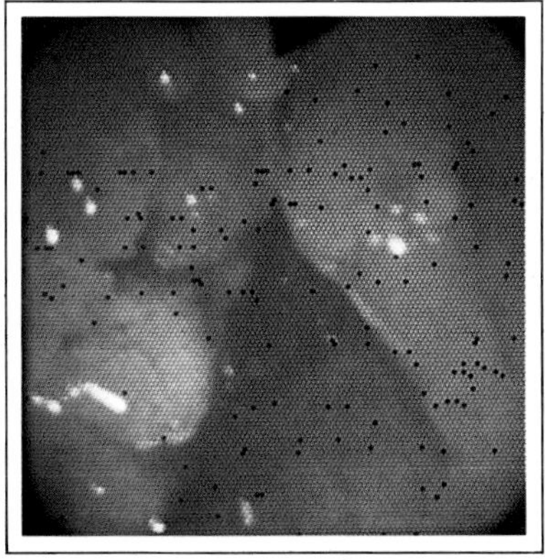

FIG. 38-10a.

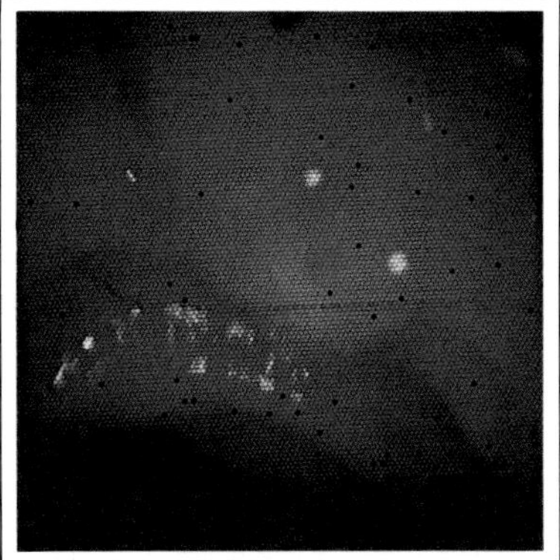

FIG. 38-10b.

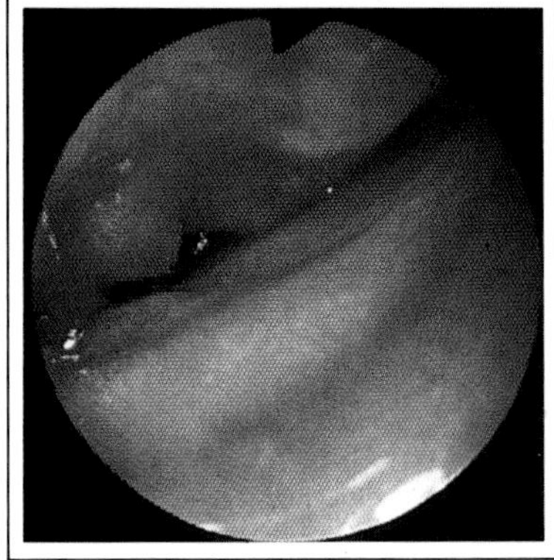

FIG. 38-10c.

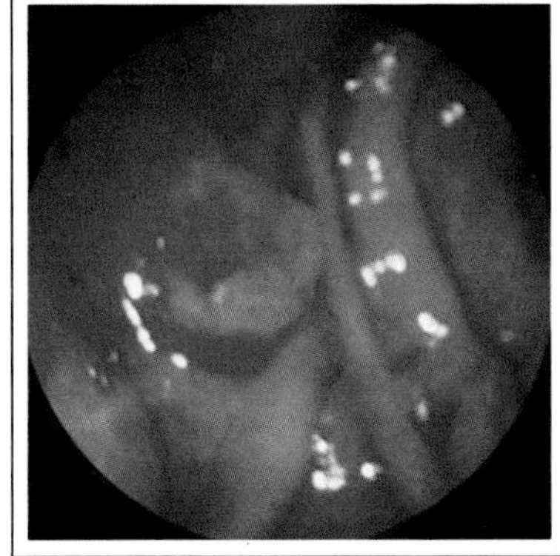

FIG. 38-10d.

FIG. 38-10. a: Primary carcinoma of the duodenum presenting with upper GI bleeding. In this case examination of the third portion of the duodenum revealed an excavated tumor mass to be the bleeding site marked by the clot (at 9 o'clock). **b:** Metastatic carcinoid tumors of the descending duodenum, actively bleeding. An ulcerated mass lesion on the lateral wall required emergency surgery for control of the bleeding. At surgery multiple peritoneal implants were found. **c:** Abdominal histiocytic lymphoma involving the third portion of the duodenum presenting with duodenal bleeding. An ulcerated tumor mass of the duodenum was responsible for the bleeding episode. **d:** Metastatic renal carcinoma to the duodenum. Recurrent GI bleeding in this patient with known metastatic renal carcinoma was finally traced to this large (2.5 × 3 cm) tumor mass in the fourth portion of the duodenum.

(leiomyosarcoma, metastatic carcinoma, etc.), or those metastatic to the duodenum from distant primaries. Bleeding was the presentation in 4 of 25 malignant tumors of the duodenum encountered over a 7-year period (see Chapter 29). One case was a primary duodenal carcinoma, another a large metastatic carcinoid mass involving the duodenal bulb of the descending duodenum; in two cases the duodenum was involved with metastatic spread of tumor, in one case from a neighboring retroperitoneal lymphoma and in the other from a distant (skin) primary (metastatic melanoma).

Primary Carcinoma of the Duodenum

Massive GI bleeding as a presentation for primary carcinoma of the duodenum is not unknown. In one series it was the presentation of 2 of 12 duodenal carcinomas.[24] Generally, the tumors which bleed are large (>3 cm) and ulcerated (Fig. 38-10a), similar to bleeding gastric carcinomas (see Chapter 37).

Other Primary Malignancies of the Duodenum

Carcinoid tumors[25] (Fig. 38-10b) and leiomyosarcoma[26] are the other primary malignancies of the duodenum which are found to be causes of bleeding. These are large submucosal tumors that may have extensive areas of ulceration into the tumor itself which may involve larger vessels and be associated with massive bleeding.

Of the carcinoids we have seen, the commonest location is the distal duodenal bulb in conjunction with the descending duodenum (Fig. 38-10b). The size of the tumor, its location, and the nodularity and irregularity of the ulcerated portion are clues to its malignant nature. In some sense, bleeding from these tumors may exert a favorable influence on outcome as it leads to their being detected.

Metastatic Tumors to the Duodenum

Although the commonest cancer to involve the duodenum is pancreatic, we did not observe any such lesion associated with bleeding over a 7-year period, in contrast to Sharon et al.,[23] who found pancreatic carcinoma accounting for nearly half their cases (four of nine) of duodenal malignancies presenting as GI hemorrhage.

Among our patients, lymphoma involving the duodenum by direct extension accounted for two of three cases of metastatic-tumor-associated bleeding. These were both non-Hodgkin's, histiocytic-type lesions, where duodenal involvement may occur in 5% of the cases.[27] Here the involvement may be associated with bulky ulcerated masses (Fig. 38-10c) which bleed.

The remaining type of metastatic tumor to the duodenum is that from distant primaries, e.g., from the breast or skin (melanoma), bronchogenic carcinoma, and hypernephroma (Fig. 38-10d).[28] As with lymphomas involving the duodenum, a metastatic lesion from a distant primary appears as a bulky, friable ulcerated tumor (Fig. 38-10d). These masses are extremely friable and bleed copiously on biopsy or even after slight trauma. Their tendency to bleed is not surprising; it is especially true of melanoma, which is bulky, and hypernephroma because of its neovascularity.[28]

RARE CAUSES OF DUODENAL BLEEDING

Hemobilia

Although the term hemobilia was originally used to denote hemorrhage into the biliary system,[29] it now encompasses any bleeding which passes through the ampulla of Vater, from both the liver and bile ducts[29] as well as the pancreas.[30] The rarity of this condition is reflected in the fact that over a 7-year period we encountered only two cases among 500 patients consecutively examined because of upper GI bleeding (0.4%).

Hepatic Hemobilia

In most series almost half the cases result from blunt trauma to the liver sustained during automobile accidents, as well as liver lacerations from gunshot wounds, liver biopsy, or percutaneous transhepatic cholangiography.[29] The injury results in the formation of a communication between the hepatic arterial system and the bile ducts. In these cases the onset of symptoms may be immediate in the case of liver biopsy, or it may be delayed up to several weeks in the case of trauma or even many months after liver laceration from gunshot wounds associated with the formation of hepatic artery aneurysms (see below).

Vascular lesions are the second commonest cause, accounting for 10% of the cases. These are mainly hepatic artery aneurysms which form direct communications with the biliary system.[31] In most of these cases this is the right hepatic artery, which communicates directly with the common bile duct or right hepatic duct. Commonly in these cases there is a history of either hepatic trauma or prior cholecystectomy within the preceding 1 to 2 years, but especially within 3 months of the onset of hemobilia.[31]

Other rare causes include acute cholecystitis associated with hemorrhage from the wall of the gallbladder, erosion of a gallstone into the wall of the cystic duct with injury of the cystic artery, or metastatic liver disease.[29]

The clinical triad which suggests hepatic hemobilia prior to endoscopy is: (a) intermittent right upper quadrant pain; (b) fluctuating jaundice; and (c) melena.[29]

With a diagnosis of hepatic hemobilia suspected, especially by suggestive endoscopic findings (see below), the site of communication of the hepatic arterial and biliary system is best demonstrated by arteriography.[31] Recently arteriographic means have been developed to control bleeding from hemobilia, either with selective embolization of small amounts of gelatin (Gelfoam) sponge[32] or metallic coils into the right hepatic artery.[31] This has obviated the need for surgery, which in the past, as the only specific treatment, carried a high mortality rate and incidence of rebleeding.[32]

Pancreatic Hemobilia

Pancreatitis may be associated with a small number of cases of hemobilia, probably no more than 5% of the total. In these, there is commonly a pseudocyst which erodes into the splenic artery leading to bleeding into the pseudocyst. In cases where the pseudocyst communicates with the main pancreatic duct, blood finds an egress by way of the main pancreatic duct and duodenal papilla.[30,33,34] In these cases there is often recurrent, unexplained GI bleeding in the setting of chronic pancreatitis, but without other findings. Unfortunately, a diagnosis of pancreatic hemobilia may not be considered in the absence of the clinical triad observed in hepatic hemobilia (see above). As in the case of hepatic hemobilia, once the diagnosis is suspected, arteriography can be definitive by showing a direct communication between the splenic artery and the pancreatic ductal system.[34]

If the diagnosis is suspected prior to endoscopy, a side-viewing instrument is chosen for optimal visualization of the duodenal papilla from which blood is seen to ooze or clots are extruded.[35] In cases where the diagnosis is not suspected, the finding of bright red blood (Fig. 38-11a) in the second portion of the duodenum but not in the duodenal bulb or stomach, in the appropriate clinical setting (see above), causes the endoscopist to consider this diagnosis (Fig. 38-11b). He then exchanges the forward-viewing instrument for a side-viewing endoscope (Fig. 38-11c).

Appearance

1. *Hepatic hemobilia:* In cases of hepatic hemobilia fresh blood or a clot may be observed.[35] We have found the clot itself to have a distinctive filiform appearance, shaped by the bile duct as well as its passage through the duodenal papilla (Fig. 38-11c). We have noted this filiform appearance only in association with hepatic hemobilia, where the blood itself may remain for longer periods within the biliary system, allowing a clot to form, compared with the shorter clearance time expected for the pancreatic duct.

2. *Pancreatic hemobilia:* In cases of pancreatic hemobilia, blood (Fig. 38-11d) rather than clot seems to ooze from the duodenal papilla. We observed at least one case where accumulation into the duodenum was considerable but clot formation was still not observed. This may be the result of rapid transit through the pancreatic duct as well as an

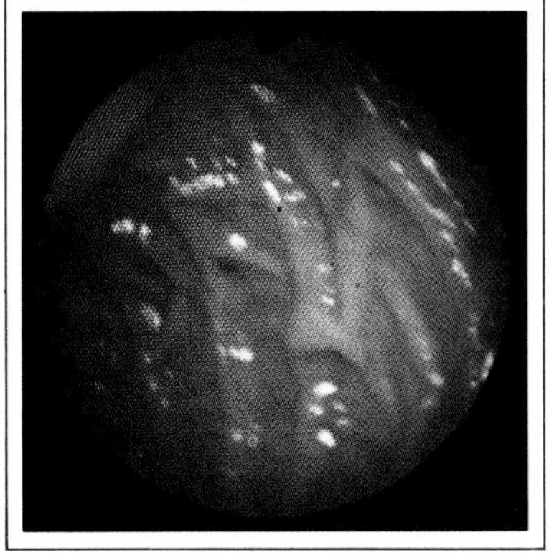

FIG. 38-11a.

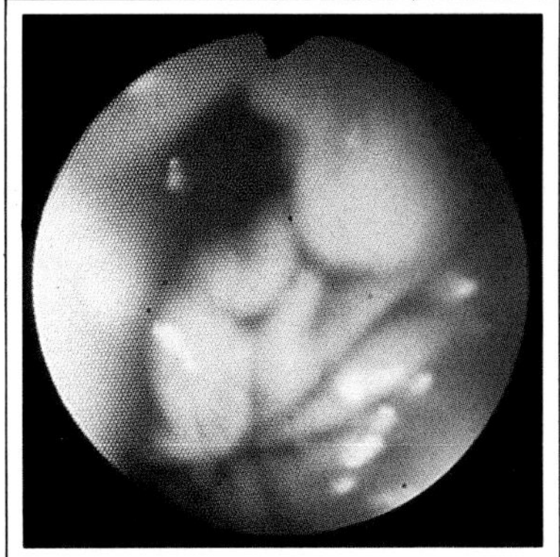

FIG. 38-11b.

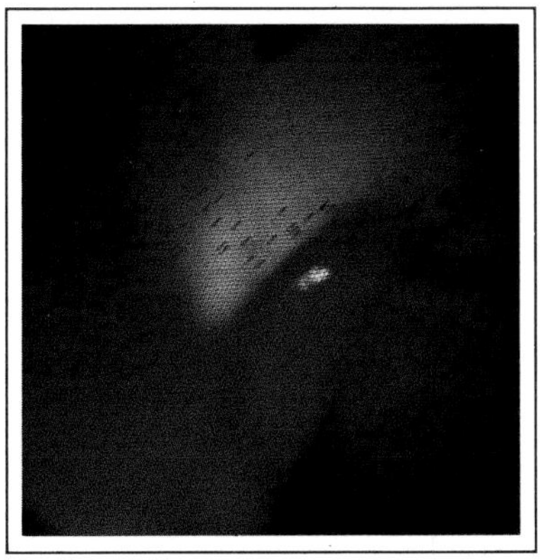

FIG. 38-11c.

FIG. 38-11d.

FIG. 38-11. a: Hepatic hemobilia. A focal area of bright red blood is just barely seen in the region of the duodenal papilla at 11 o'clock. The patient had a history of traumatic injury to the liver 3 months before. **b:** Hepatic hemobilia. Better positioning (counterclockwise torquing) and upward deflection to bring the papilla into view. A cylindrical "toothpaste"-like clot is beginning to be extruded from the papilla at 10 o'clock. **c:** Hepatic hemobilia. Better demonstration of the extrusion of the clot from the duodenal papilla is afforded by the use of a side-viewing duodenoscope. **d:** Pancreatic hemobilia. Active bleeding from the papilla was observed in a patient with known chronic pancreatitis and a pseudocyst who had had a recent history of multiple, unexplained bleeding episodes. An arteriogram showed a pseudoaneurysm of the splenic artery communicating with the pseudocyst.

effect of pancreatic enzymes, especially trypsin, which in the presence of blood within the pancreatic duct may become an active fibrinolytic agent.

Duodenal Diverticula

Although duodenal diverticula may be encountered in 1 to 5% of radiologic studies of the duodenum,[36] they are uncommon at endoscopy, at least in our experience, where over a 7-year period only 10 cases were noted out of 500 patients examined (0.2%). The incidence of GI bleeding from duodenal diverticula has been reported to be as high as 16%[36]; however, because of their relative rarity at endoscopy, diverticula are not found to be a cause of bleeding in many large endoscopy series, including our own.

Duodenal diverticular bleeding has been attributed to ulceration within the diverticulum eroding into the gastroduodenal artery. In addition, in cases where the diverticulum was found in association with pancreatitis, reactive changes with the diverticulum were associated with peridiverticular fat necrosis leading to mucosal ulceration and bleeding.[36]

The expected endoscopic finding for diverticular bleeding is bright red blood oozing from the medial wall where there is an abrupt termination of the Kerckring folds. The latter finding—the hallmark of duodenal diverticula (see Chapter 27)—in association with bleeding causes the endoscopist to suspect a duodenal diverticular site. As in the case of hemobilia, the appearance of bright red blood in the descending duodenum and not in the duodenal bulb or stomach suggests a duodenal bleeding site even though the diverticulum itself may not be visualized. In such cases the endoscopist advises arteriography to determine the precise location of bleeding as well as its likely origin.[36]

Crohn's Disease of the Duodenum or Upper Small Intestine

Massive GI bleeding in Crohn's disease is uncommon, occurring at most in only 10% of patients and in these being almost entirely from the distal small bowel or a colonic site.[37] Less than 10% of the cases (and therefore less than 1% of the total) are from proximal small intestinal or duodenal sites. The rarity of this is also suggested by our own experience, where only two cases were seen out of a total 500 patients examined for upper GI bleeding over a 7-year period. In both cases, the site of the bleeding (later confirmed at surgery in one and suspected in the other) was the upper jejunum. In these cases, obstruction from the Crohn's disease resulted in significant retrograde return of blood into the duodenum.

In addition to small intestinal sites, the bleeding may occur from duodenal involvement.[38] In the cases observed by us, the bleeding site was in the proximal small bowel

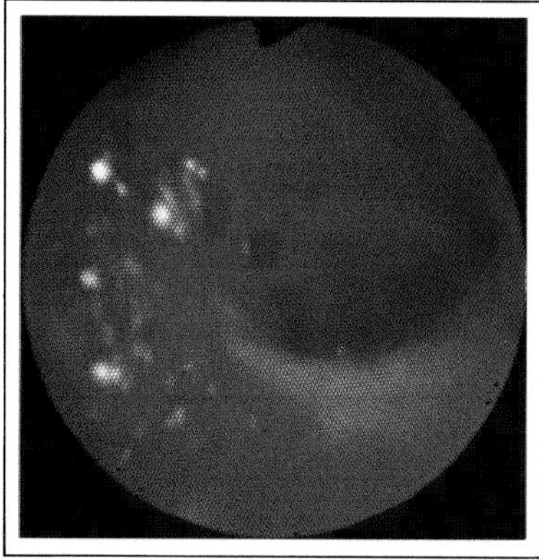

FIG. 38-12.

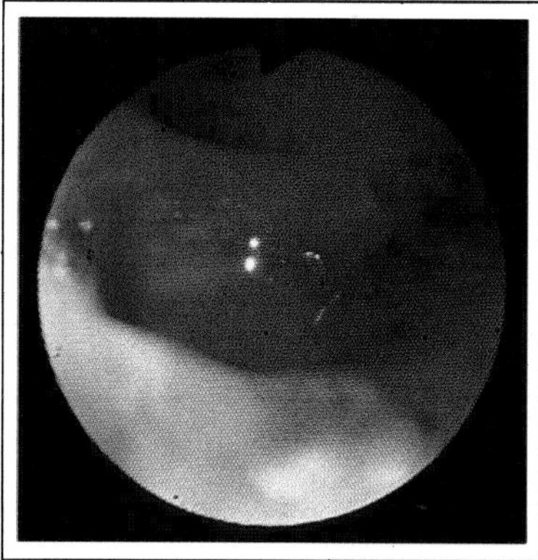

FIG. 38-13.

FIG. 38-12. Active bleeding from Crohn's disease of the proximal jejunum. Because of obstruction, there is significant retrograde flow of bright red blood into the proximal duodenum.

FIG. 38-13. Bleeding aortoduodenal fistula 9 months after placement of an aortic graft. A depression on the superior-posterior wall (6 to 9 o'clock) of the third portion would immediately raise the question of an aortoduodenal fistula (confirmed in this case arteriographically). Because of the bleeding, the graft itself is not seen.

in the absence of gastroduodenal involvement. The site of bleeding was suspected because of the appearance of fresh blood in the descending duodenum and the third portion (Fig. 38-12), with no blood in the stomach or duodenal bulb. A history of small bowel involvement in Crohn's disease in both cases caused the endoscopist to suspect a proximal small bowel site with Crohn's disease causing the bleeding.

Bleeding may occur in other patients with well-established duodenal Crohn's disease,[38] so that at endoscopy one would expect to find blood and clots in the duodenal bulb and stomach with stricture formation and especially deep ulceration within the duodenal bulb (see Chapter 28).

Aortoduodenal Fistula

Gastrointestinal bleeding in patients who have had prior placement of an aortic graft should always make one suspect the presence of an aortoduodenal fistula. Such fistulas have been reported as complications of aortic graft placement in up to 2%.[39] Usually this has been with the placement of a Dacron graft just below the renal arteries; however, aortoduodenal fistulas have also been reported after placement of renal[40] and femoral artery bypass grafts. Less commonly, aortoduodenal fistulas arise as a primary condition from large aortic aneurysms.[41]

Aortoduodenal fistulas are of two types. The commonest is that which forms at the proximal margin of the graft and aorta, with this junction eroding into the duodenum. In other cases, the prosthesis itself replaces the posterior wall of the duodenum as a paraprosthetic-enteric fistula.[42]

Pathogenesis

Why aortoduodenal fistulas occur is uncertain. Several mechanisms have been proposed, especially to account for their commonest location, the third portion of the duodenum where the posterior wall lies in direct apposition with the aorta, just distal to the origin of the renal artery.[39] Here, the wall often has part of the aneurysm sac, so often inflammatory changes may occur which could impair the blood supply to this portion of the duodenum after surgery.[34] Inapparent injury to the wall may also occur at the time of surgery which does not heal either because of prior circulatory changes or superimposed bacterial contamination.[39]

Presentation

The patient with aortoduodenal fistula bleeding presents months or even years after aortic graft surgery with a history generally of anemia and intermittent GI bleeding, usually with melena. Generally, the bleeding pattern remains intermittent with only one or two episodes of massive bleeding which are life-threatening, often exsanguinating. The intermittent bleeding pattern is thought to be the result of clotting within the fistula, providing a tamponade effect.

The evaluation of patients in whom a diagnosis of aortoduodenal fistula is suspected may include barium contrast studies, abdominal ultrasound, and arteriography, as well as endoscopy. In cases where other studies, even arteriography, are equivocal or nondiagnostic, endoscopy may be decisive if the third portion of the duodenum can be reached.

Appearance

The endoscopic finding which has most often been reported is that of the a bile-stained graft which has eroded through the inferior-posterior wall of the third portion of the duodenum.[42] If the descending duodenum has been intubated in such a way that the 12 o'clock lens position comes to view the medial wall (see Chapter 24), the location of the fistula will be most probably seen in the 6 to 9 o'clock position, just beyond the junction of the descending duodenum and third portion (Fig. 38-13). In cases where the fistula involves the suture line (aortoduodenal fistula), some blood present may prevent visualization of the bile-stained graft. In other cases (paraprosthetic-enteric fistulas), the bile-stained graft may be completely visualized.[42]

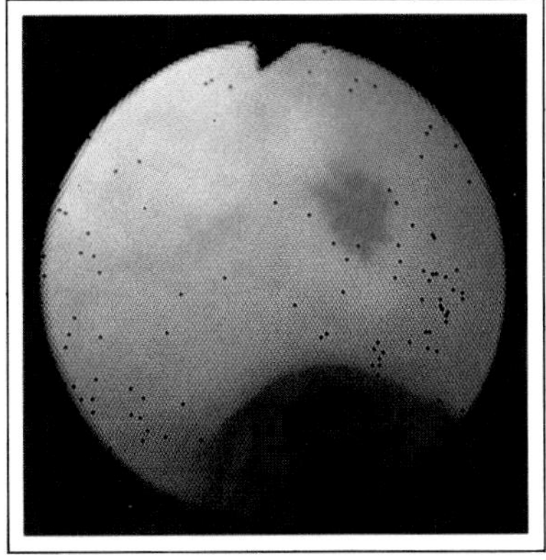

FIG. 38-14a.

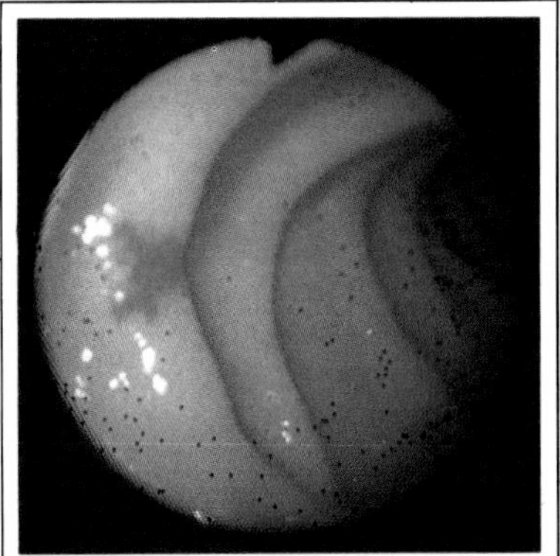

FIG. 38-14b.

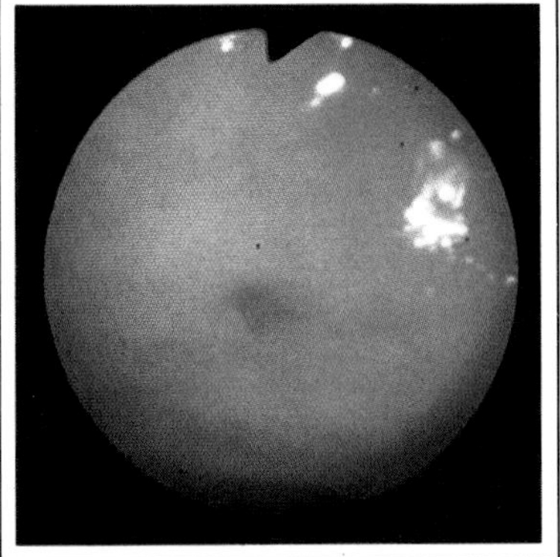

FIG. 38-14c.

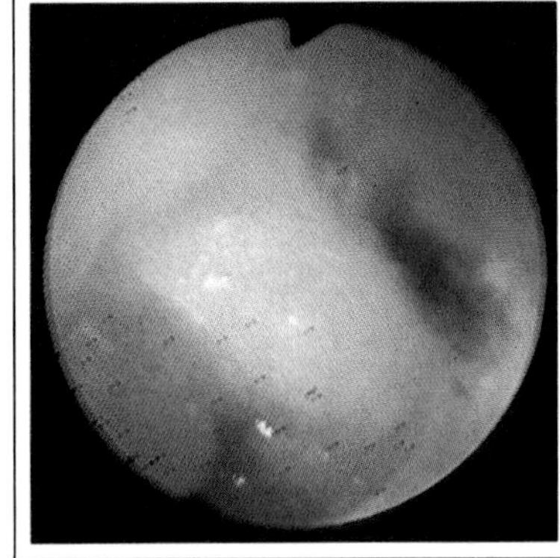

FIG. 38-14d.

FIG. 38-14. a: Duodenal angiodysplasia. A single 3-mm cherry-red spot is seen in the duodenal bulb. **b:** Multiple duodenal angiodysplasias of the duodenal bulb and descending duodenum. One of many 2- to 4-mm cherry-red spots. The margin is made irregular by filamentous or pseudopod-like projections. **c:** Duodenal angiodysplasia, not the site of bleeding. The finding of this 4-mm cherry-red spot initially made the endoscopist suspect that it caused the bleeding; however, careful examination of the stomach revealed the true bleeding site. **d:** Gastric ulcer base with stigmata of recent bleeding at an adherent clot.

Two less common appearances have been reported in association with aortoduodenal fistulas where an aneurysm forms at the junction of the aorta and graft. In these cases, ulceration is seen either in the center of the the mass-like deformity which simulates a leiomyoma[44] or as simply a large ulceration with prominent, heaped-up margins at a location where one would expect to encounter the fistula.[43] In these cases there is a mass effect from the aneurysm pushing up against the posterior wall of the duodenum.

Other Vascular Causes

Duodenal Angiodysplasia

Between 8%[45] and 33%[46] of upper GI angiodysplasias identified at endoscopy may be found exclusively in the duodenum. In this location they tend to be single (Fig. 38-14a) but can be multiple (Fig. 38-14b). Most are found in the duodenal bulb (Fig. 38-14a) or in the second portion (Fig. 38-14b), although the third and fourth portions are occasionally the sites of these lesions.[46] Colonic angiodysplasia was present in at least one case,[45] although it is not seen in most patients in whom colonoscopy has been performed.[46] Similarly, the association of these lesions with aortic stenosis[45] appears to be inconstant.[46]

As in the case of gastric angiodysplasia, most duodenal angiodysplasia lesions range in size between 2 and 4 mm (Fig. 38-14a). The margins are distorted by projections, either filamentous or pseudopod-like, to the neighboring capillaries.

Although duodenal angiodysplasia lesions are in fact the source of bleeding in most instances where they are found, we have seen at least one case where apparent duodenal angiodysplasia (Fig. 38-14c) was found in a case where bleeding had occurred from a gastric ulcer (Fig. 38-14d) with an adherent clot in its base, indicating it to have been the bleeding site. The presence of a single angiodysplasia lesion still warrants a careful search for other potential sites of bleeding.

As in the case of gastric angiodysplasia, bleeding from duodenal angiodysplasia may be controlled endoscopically with electrosurgical destruction of the lesion.[46,47]

Duodenal Varices

The duodenum is an unusual site for varices associated with cirrhosis or extrahepatic portal hypertension.[47] In cases where they occur, the patient presents with hematemesis and melena or melena alone. The esophageal varices present are generally small and thought to be insignificant. During the bleeding episode the blood and clots found within the duodenal bulb obscure the varices. Endoscopy performed

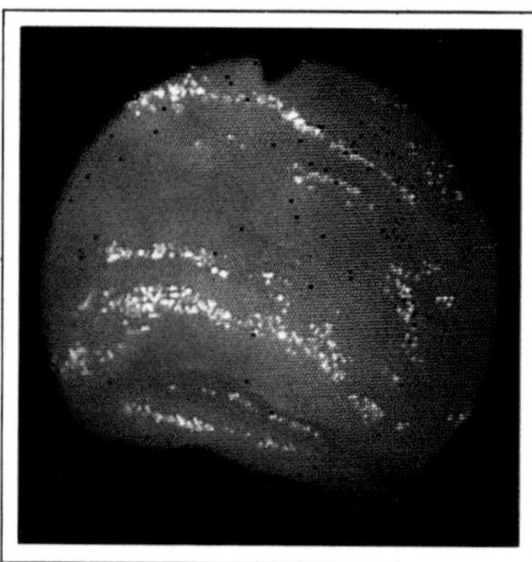

FIG. 38-15.

FIG. 38-15. Duodenal varix, nonbleeding. A 5-mm, slightly raised, somewhat serpiginous vascular structure between two Kerckring folds. Because of its proximity to the surface, it displays a gray-blue coloration. This was found in a patient with cirrhosis and several recent unexplained bleeding episodes.

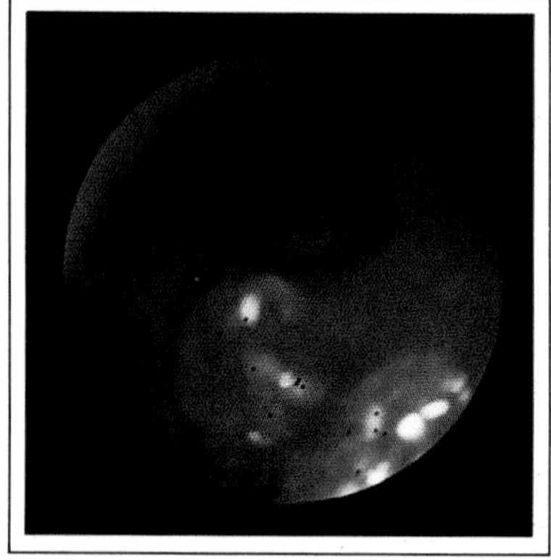

FIG. 38-16a.

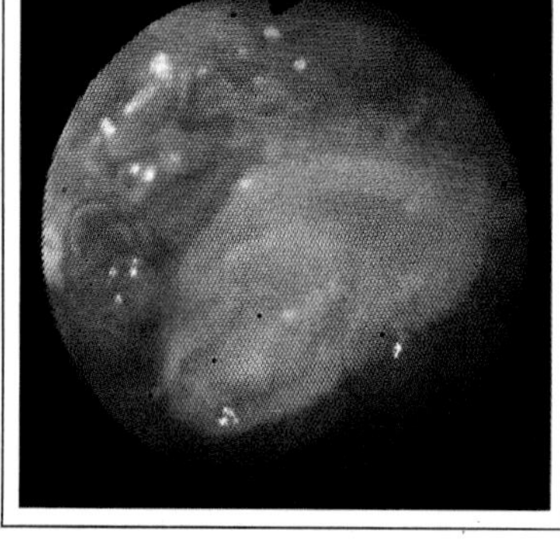

FIG. 38-16b.

FIG. 38-16. a: Bleeding posterior wall duodenal ulcer associated with a hepatic artery catheter. This patient presented with massive bleeding 3 weeks into chemotherapy for a hepatoma. A large visible vessel was identified at endoscopy; however, despite electrocoagulation of its base, bleeding continued. At surgery a tumor was found to have eroded into the posterior wall of the duodenum, with the base of the ulcer being tumor. **b:** A large (2 cm) posterior superior wall duodenal ulcer in a patient with a recently implanted hepatic artery catheter. Rather than bleeding, this patient presented with refractory ulcer symptoms.

after bleeding has stopped shows large, serpiginous submucosal vessels running between Kerckring folds (Fig. 38-15) or focally enlarging these folds, particularly on the posterior wall of the apex.[47a] Because of their location close to the mucosal surface, they may have a gray-blue coloration, or like gastric varices have the same color as the surrounding mucosa.[47a] Bleeding from duodenal varices has been treated with endoscopic sclerosis.[47a]

Chemotherapy Infusion Catheter Associated Bleeding

Selective hepatic artery catheterization for infusion of chemotherapeutic agents is an established technique for the treatment of primary and metastatic carcinoma of the liver.[48] A rare complication of these catheters is duodenal bleeding from mucosal erosions[48] or ulcers.[49] These are apparently common in patients with infusion catheters, found in one recent series in over 40%.[50] As the placement of these catheters may involve ligation of the right gastric and gastroduodenal arteries to ensure selective infusion of the liver, some mucosal injury may result from a decrease in duodenal blood flow after catheter placement.[49] Other mechanisms suggested by Crowley[49] for the pathogenesis of these ulcers include mucosal injury from the chemotherapeutic agents, injury from concurrent irradiation, and pressure necrosis of the wall of the duodenum from the catheter residing in the gastroduodenal artery. Possibly worsening the injury effects of any of these is erosion into the wall of the duodenum by the tumor itself.

We have observed two ulcers associated with infusion catheters. In one case where erosion of tumor into the posterior wall of the duodenum was found at surgery, bleeding occurred from a large (2 cm) posterior wall ulcer with a visible vessel (Fig. 38-16a). In the other, rather than for bleeding, the patient was examined because of refractory symptoms (Fig. 38-16b).

Bleeding in Hemophilia

Bleeding in hemophilia, while it may occur anywhere in the GI tract, is most often found to be from duodenal ulcers.[51,52] Prior to the availability of factor VIII concentrate for emergency replacement, GI bleeding accounted for up to one third of all disease-related deaths in hemophiliacs,[53,54] but since it began to be widely used, this has been reduced to 5%. However, factor VIII replacement does not stop bleeding in all cases; where bleeding continues it becomes of paramount importance to know whether it is from a duodenal ulcer, gastroduodenal hematoma, or from some other distal site. Endoscopy should be the diagnostic modality first employed, because it is the most accurate means of determining whether an ulcer is present,[55] and, if one were identified, it allows endoscopic therapy (electrocoagulation[12a] or laser photocoagulation[12b]) to be utilized. Nevertheless, some physicians may be reluctant to subject bleeding hemophilic patients to the risk of hematoma formation, especially retropharyngeal which could occur with a difficult intubation. As traumatic hematomas have not been reported with the current generation of narrow caliber instruments (8–9 mm), we believe the risk to be exceedingly small, especially if sufficient factor VIII concentrate has been given beforehand to raise the activity level to 30% or more.[56]

The endoscopic appearance of duodenal ulcers in hemophiliacs presenting because of GI bleeding will not differ from that in other patients (see above), including both those actively bleeding and those with only stigmata of recent bleeding. In other patients without ulcers, but with gastroduodenal bleeding, one would expect to find single or multiple intramucosal hematomata, consisting of masses of variable size associated with a purplish discoloration of the mucosa.

REFERENCES

1. Graham, D. Y., and Davis, R. E. (1978): Acute upper-gastrointestinal hemorrhage: new observations on an old problem. *Am. J. Dig. Dis.*, 23:76–84.
2. Silverstein, F. E., Gilbert, D. A., Tedesco, F. J., Buenger, N. K., Persing, J., and 277 members of the ASGE (1981): The national ASGE survey on upper gastrointestinal bleeding. I. Study design and baseline data. *Gastrointest. Endosc.*, 27:73–79.
3. Devitt, J. E. (1969): Upper gastrointestinal bleeding with special reference to peptic ulcer. *Gastroenterology*, 57:89–93.
4. Sheppard, M. C., Holmes, G. K. T., and Cockel, R. (1977): Clinical picture of peptic ulceration diagnosed endoscopically. *Gut*, 18:524–530.
5. Blackstone, M. O. (1979): Establishing the site of gastrointestinal bleeding (editorial). *JAMA*, 241:599.
6. Gilbert, D. A., Silverstein, F. E., Tedesco, F. J., Buenger, N. K., Persing, J., and 277 members of the ASGE (1981): The national ASGE survey on upper gastrointestinal bleeding. III. Endoscopy in upper gastrointestinal bleeding. *Gastrointest. Endosc.*, 27:94–102.
7. Luk, G., Bynum, T. E., and Hendrix, T. R. (1979): Gastric aspiration in localization of gastrointestinal hemorrhage. *JAMA*, 241:576–578.
8. Walker, C. O. (1978): Complications of peptic ulcer disease. In: *Gastrointestinal Disease*, edited by M. H. Sleisenger and J. S. Fordtran, p. 916. Saunders, Philadelphia.
9. Levy, M. (1974): Aspirin use in patients with major upper gastrointestinal bleeding of peptic ulcer disease. *N. Engl. J. Med.*, 290:1158–1162.
10. Silverstein, F. E., Gilbert, D. A., Tedesco, F. J., Buenger, N. K., Persing, J., and 277 members of the ASGE (1981): The national ASGE survey on upper gastrointestinal bleeding. II. Clinical prognostic factors. *Gastrointest. Endosc.*, 27:80–93.
11. Foster, D. N., Miloszewski, K. J. A., and Losowsky, M. S. (1978): Stigmata of recent haemorrhage in diagnosis and prognosis of upper gastrointestinal bleeding. *Br. Med. J.*, 1:1173–1177.
12. Himal, H. S., Watson, W. W., Jones, C. W., Miller, L., and Maclean, L. D. (1974): The management of upper gastrointestinal hemorrhage: a multiparametric computer analysis. *Ann. Surg.*, 179: 489–493.

12a. Wara, P., Hojsgaard, A., and Amdrup, E. (1980): Endoscopic electrocoagulation. An alternative to operative hemostasis in active gastroduodenal bleeding? *Endoscopy*, 12:237–240.

12b. Rutgeerts, P., Vantrappen, G., Broeckaert, L., Janssens, J., Coremans, G., Geboes, K., and Schurmans, P. (1982): Controlled trial of YAG laser treatment of upper digestive hemorrhage. *Gastroenterology*, 83:410–416.

13. Hunt, P. S., Hansky, J., and Korman, M. G. (1979): Mortality in patients with haematemesis and melaena: a prospective study. *Br. Med. J.*, 1:1238–1240.
14. Storey, D. W., Brown, S. G., Swain, C. P., Salmon, P. R., Kirkham, J. S., and Northfield, T. C. (1981): Endoscopic prediction of recurrent bleeding in peptic ulcers. *N. Engl. J. Med.*, 305:915–916.
15. Griffiths, W. J., Neumann, D. A., and Welsh, J. D. (1979): The visible vessel as an indicator of uncontrolled or recurrent gastrointestinal hemorrhage. *N. Engl. J. Med.*, 300:1411–1413.
16. Papp, J. P. (1979): Endoscopic electrocoagulation of the nonbleeding visible ulcer vessel. *Gastrointest. Endosc.*, 25:45–46.
17. Swain, C. P., Bown, S. G., Storey, D. W., Kirkham, J. S., Northfield, T. C., and Salmon, P. R. (1981): Controlled trial of argon laser photocoagulation in bleeding peptic ulcers. *Lancet*, 2:1313–1316.
18. Gelzayd, E. A., and Gelfand, D. W. (1973): Hemorrhagic duodenitis as a significant cause of gastrointestinal bleeding. *Gastrointest. Endosc.*, 20:59–60.
19. Katz, A. M. (1959): Hemorrhagic duodenitis in myocardial infarction. *Ann. Intern. Med.*, 51:212–215.
20. Gottfried, E. B., Korsten, M. A., and Lieber, C. S. (1973): Alcohol-induced gastric and duodenal lesions in man. *Am. J. Gastroenterol.*, 70:587–592.
21. Katz, D., Pitchumoni, C. S., Thomas, E., and Antonelle, M. (1976): The endoscopic diagnosis of upper-gastrointestinal hemorrhage: changing concepts of etiology and management. *Am. J. Dig. Dis.*, 21:182–188.
22. Reddy, R. R., Schuman, B. M., and Priest, R. J. (1981): Duodenal polyps: diagnosis and management. *J. Clin. Gastroenterol.*, 3:139–145.
23. Sharon, P., Stalnikowicz, R., and Rachmilewitz, D. (1982): Endoscopic analysis of duodenal neoplasms causing upper gastrointestinal bleeding. *J. Clin. Gastroenterol.*, 4:35–38.
24. Kerremans, R. P., Larut, J., and Penninckx, F. M. (1979): Primary malignant duodenal tumors. *Ann. Surg.*, 190:179–182.
25. Zakariai, Y. M., Quan, S. H., and Hajdu, S. I. (1975): Carcinoid tumors of the gastrointestinal tract. *Cancer*, 35:588–591.
26. Yassinger, S., Imperato, T. J., Midgley, R., Machas, C., and Bolt, R. J. (1977): Leiomyosarcoma of the duodenum. *Gastrointest. Endosc.*, 24:38–40.
27. Burgener, F. A., and Hamlin, D. J. (1981): Histiocytic lymphoma of the abdomen: radiographic spectrum. *Am. J. Roentgenol.*, 137:337–342.
28. Theodors, A., Sivak, M. V., and Carey, W. D. (1980): Hypernephroma with metastasis to the duodenum: endoscopic features. *Gastrointest. Endosc.*, 26:48–51.
29. Bismuth, H. (1973): Hemobilia. *N. Engl. J. Med.*, 288:617–619.
30. Brintnall, B. B., Laidlaw, W., and Papp, J. (1974): Hemobilia: pancreatic pseudocyst hemorrhage demonstrated by endoscopy and arteriography. *Am. J. Dig. Dis.*, 14:186–188.
31. Harlaftis, N. N., and Akin, J. T. (1977): Hemobilia from ruptured hepatic aneurysm: report of a case and review of the literature. *Am. J. Surg.*, 133:229–232.
32. Fagan, E. A., Allison, D. J., Chadwick, V. S., and Hodgson, H. J. F. (1980): Treatment of haemobilia by selective embolisation. *Gut*, 21:541–544.
33. Starling, J. R., and Crummey, A. B. (1979): Hemosuccus pancreaticus secondary to ruptured splenic artery aneurysm. *Dig. Dis. Sci.*, 24:726–729.
34. Ambos, M., Redmond, P., and De Grazin, J. (1980): Hemoductal pancreatitis. *Gastrointest. Radiol.*, 5:349–351.
35. Lehman, G. A., and Bash, D. (1979): Endoscopic observations of hemobilia. *Gastrointest. Endosc.*, 25:110–112.
36. Ghahremani, G. G., and Hietala, S.-O. (1977): Arteriography of a bleeding duodenal diverticulum. *Dig. Dis. Sci.*, 22:445–448.
37. Rubin, M., Herrington, L., and Schneider, R. (1980): Regional enteritis with major gastrointestinal hemorrhage as the initial manifestation. *Arch. Intern. Med.*, 140:217–219.
38. Nugent, F. W., Richmond, M., and Park, S. K. (1977): Crohn's disease of the duodenum. *Gut*, 18:115–120.
39. Champion, M. C., Sullivan, S. N., Coles, J. C., Goldbach, M., and Watson, W. C. (1982): Aortoenteric fistula. *Ann. Surg.*, 195:314–317.
40. Keeffe, E. B., Krippaehne, W. W., Rosch, J., and Melnyk, C. (1974):

Aortoduodenal fistula: complication of renal artery bypass graft. *Gastroenterology,* 67:1240–1244.

41. Reiner, M. A., Brau, S. A., and Schanzer, H. (1978): Primary aortoduodenal fistula: case presentation and review of the literature. *Am. J. Gastroenterol.,* 70:292–296.
42. Skibba, R. M., Greenberger, N. J., and Hardin, C. A. (1975): Paraprosthetic-enteric fistula: role of preoperative endoscopy. *Am. J. Dig. Dis.,* 20:1081–1086.
43. Puppala, A. R., Munaswamy, M., Doshi, A., and Steinheber, F. U. (1980): Endoscopic diagnosis of aortoduodenal fistula: complication of aortic by-pass grafts. *Am. J. Gastroenterol.,* 73:414–417.
44. Ott, D. J., Kerr, R. M., and Gelfand, D. W. (1978): Aortoduodenal fistula: an unusual endoscopic and radiographic appearance simulating leiomyoma. *Gastrointest. Endosc.,* 24:246–298.
45. Weaver, G. A., Alpern, H. D., Davis, J. S., Ramsey, W. H., and Reichelderfer, M. (1979): Gastrointestinal angiodysplasia with aortic valve disease: part of a spectrum of angiodysplasia of the gut. *Gastroenterology,* 77:1–11.
46. Farup, P. G., Rosseland, A. R., Stray, N., Pytte, R., Valnes, K., and Rand, A. A. (1981): Localized telangiopathy of the stomach and duodenum diagnosed and treated endoscopically. *Endoscopy,* 13:1–6.
47. Rapazzo, J. A., Kozarek, R. A., and Altman, M. (1981): Duodenal varices: Endoscopic diagnosis of an unusual source of upper gastrointestinal hemorrhage. *Gastrointest. Endosc.,* 27:227–288.

47a. Sauerbruch, T., Weinzierl, M., Dietrich, H. P., Antes, G., Eisenburg, J., and Paumgartner, G. (1982): Sclerotherapy of a bleeding duodenal varix. *Endoscopy,* 14:187–189.

48. Ansfield, F. J., Ramierez, G., and Davis, H. L. (1975): Further clinical studies with intrahepatic arterial infusion with 5-fluorouracil. *Cancer,* 36:2413–2417.
49. Crowley, M. L. (1982): Penetrating duodenal ulcer associated with an operatively implanted arterial chemotherapy infusion catheter. *Gastroenterology,* 83:118–120.
50. Gillin, J. S., Kemeny, N., Daly, J. M., Balis, M. B., Kurtz, R. C., and Shike, M. (1983): Severe gastroduodenal ulcerations complicating hepatic artery infusion chemotherapy for metastatic colon cancer *Gastroenterology,* 84:1166.
51. Carron, D. B., Boon, T. H., and Walker, F. C. (1965): Peptic ulcer in the haemophiliac and its relation to gastrointestinal bleeding. *Lancet,* 2:1036–1039.
52. Forbes, C. D., Barr, R. D., Prentice, C. R. M., and Douglas, A. S. (1973): Gastrointestinal bleeding in haemophilia. *Quart. J. Med.,* 42:503–511.
53. Wilkinson, J. F., Nour-Eldin, F., Israels, M. C. G., and Barrett, K. E. (1961): Haemophilia syndromes: A survey of 267 patients. *Lancet,* 2:947–950.
54. Kerr, C. B. (1964): Operative surgery in haemophilia. *Aust. N.Z. J. Surg.,* 33:241–249.
55. McGinn, F. P., Guyer, P. B., Wilken, B. J., and Steer, H. W. (1975): A prospective comparative trial between early endoscopy and radiology in acute upper gastrointestinal haemorrhage. *Gut,* 16:707–713.
56. Boggs, R. (1977): Haemophilia treatment in the United Kingdom from 1969 to 1974. *Brit. J. Haematol.,* 35:487–504.

Section 5

THE COLON AND TERMINAL ILEUM

39

THE COLON—ENDOSCOPIC ORIENTATION, TECHNIQUE OF EXAMINATION, AND NORMAL APPEARANCE

ENDOSCOPIC ORIENTATION

The colon, because of its length, mobility, and complex course, is the most difficult portion of the gastrointestinal (GI) tract for the endoscopist to examine. The technical challenge of a complete examination of this 4- to 6-foot length of bowel that is capable of assuming a variety of shapes and configurations is enormous. In the course of performing the examination, the endoscopist utilizes a variety of visual cues to determine his present position and that of the segment he is about to enter. Although it is possible to describe the visual cues in relation to both the lens optical system and specific anatomic landmarks, much the same as we do for upper GI endoscopy (see Chapters 1, 11, and 24), the utility of this for the endoscopist is diminished because of the greater mobility of the colon and tendency of the colonoscope tip to twist as it is advanced rather than to maintain a constant position. The result is that the image seen by the examiner bears a far less precise relationship to its actual anatomic position than elsewhere in the GI tract. Still, it remains for the endoscopist himself to decide how useful it is to think about these relationships, especially when they help him recognize and overcome colonic configurations which impede the progress of the examination.

Image Positions of the Lens in Relation to Those of the Eyepiece

The optical system of a colonoscope is similar to that of instruments used for upper GI endoscopy in that the positions of the visual image in the eyepiece are based on corresponding positions in the lens which relate to the upturn point of the bending portion (see Fig. 1-1). With the bending portion of the colonoscope deflected upward, as is the case on entry into the rectum (Fig. 39-1a), the lens position closest to the point transmits that part of the visual image which is seen in the 12 o'clock position of the eyepiece; the point of the lens just opposite transmits the 6 o'clock position, that to the left of the upturn point the 9 o'clock position, and that to the right of this point the 3 o'clock position. To the extent that the endoscope tip is twisted, these positions are not well maintained, resulting in an altered relationship between that which the tip "sees" and that which the endoscopist observes in the eyepiece. Because much twisting occurs during intubation, the endoscopist must expect an altered relationship to be present during much of this part of the procedure; however, on withdrawal, the expected relationships can often be re-established, particularly if the endoscopist aligns the tip with a fixed landmark, e.g., the rectosigmoid angulus so that it occupies its expected position (Fig. 39-1b).

Segments of the Colon

The orientation for each of the colonic segments differs, and these are considered separately in this section.

Rectum

With the patient lying in left lateral recumbency, the usual starting position, if the colonoscope is passed across the anus into the rectum, as is our practice (see below, "Technique of Colonoscopy"), in the direction of the rectal vault (Fig. 39-1a), the lens image as just defined (see above) has the following relation to anatomic structures: the 12 o'clock position (closest to the upturn point) views the posterior wall; the 9 o'clock position inspects the left wall; the 3 o'clock position surveys the right wall; and the 6 o'clock position visualizes the anterior wall.

Were the endoscopist to continue to intubate the rectum in this orientation (Fig. 39-2a), the retroflexed view of the distal rectum showing the colonoscope entering from

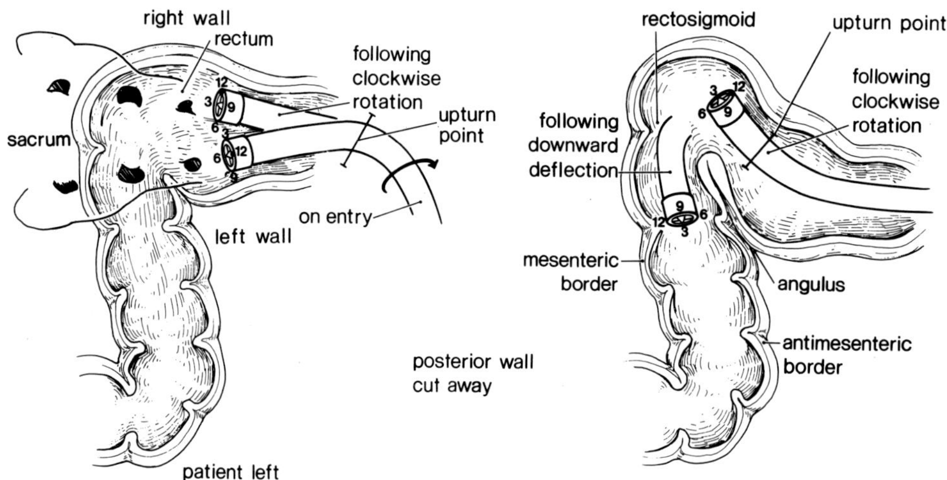

FIG. 39-1. a: Lens image position on entry into the rectum. Here the tip is deflected toward the sacrum. Clockwise rotation causes the tip to deflect up toward the right wall. **b:** Lens image position at the angulus of the rectosigmoid junction after downward deflection into the sigmoid.

the anus would be obtained (Fig. 39-2b). Although this is an important view, it is not the one the endoscopist wishes at this point in the examination. In order to advance the colonoscope through the rectum to the rectosigmoid junction, which is an extension of the right anterior wall (Fig. 39-1), the tip must be rotated in a clockwise fashion by 90° to 120° so that the 12 o'clock position now comes to view the right wall, the 6 o'clock position the left wall, the 9 o'clock position the posterior wall, and the 3 o'clock position the anterior wall (Fig. 39-1a). In this position (Fig. 39-2c), forward advancement of the colonoscope leads to identification of the angulus of the rectosigmoid junction in its expected 6 o'clock position (Fig. 39-2d).

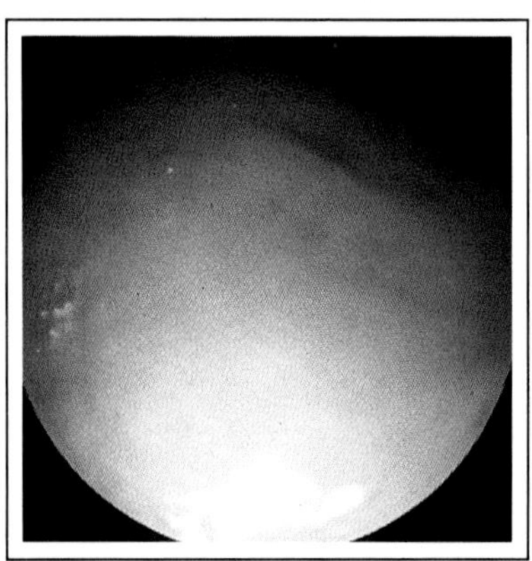

FIG. 39-2a.

FIG. 39-2b.

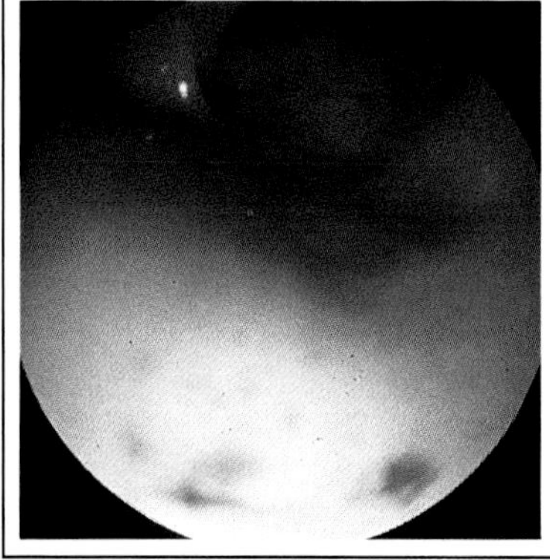

FIG. 39-2c.

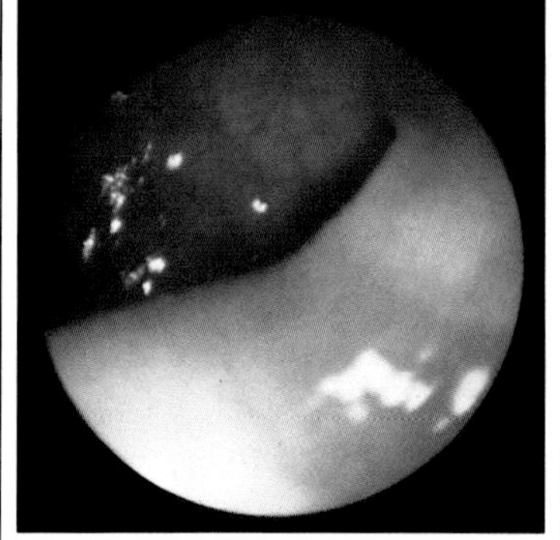

FIG. 39-2d.

FIG. 39-2. a: Rectum on entry. Here the tip is turned up slightly and points toward the sacrum. The lumen is seen in the right anterior direction (3 to 6 o'clock). **b:** Retroflexed view of the endoscope coming through the anus. **c:** Rectum after initial clockwise rotation. The lumen and rectosigmoid are now in the 12 o'clock position in the direction of the right wall (see Fig. 39-1a). **d:** Rectosigmoid junction. With continued advancement after clockwise rotation, the rectosigmoid appears with its angulus in the 6 o'clock position. Downward deflection (Fig. 39-1b) allows entry into the sigmoid.

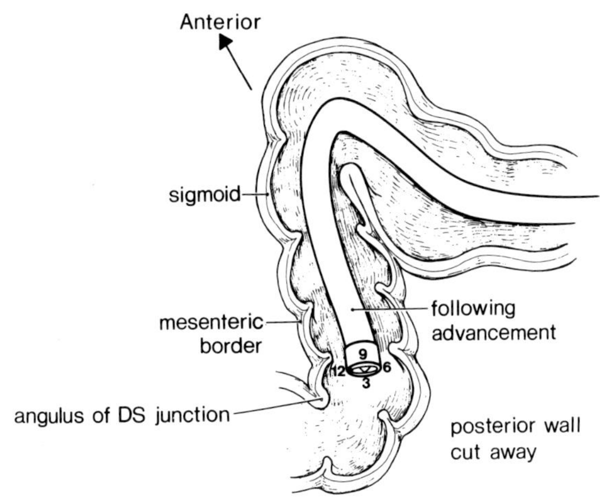

FIG. 39-3. Lens positions after intubation of the sigmoid.

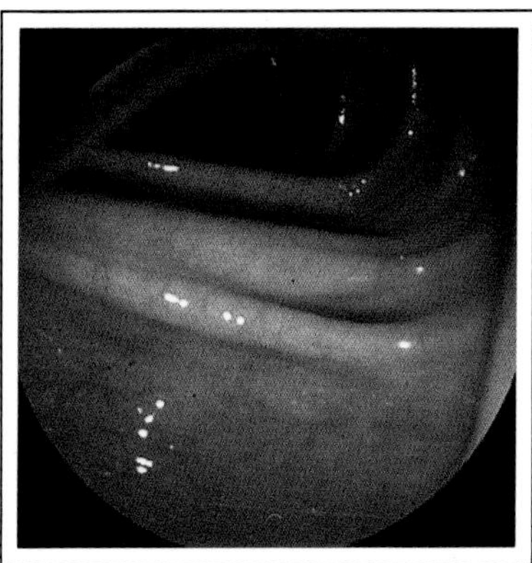

FIG. 39-4.

FIG. 39-4. Sigmoid colon after advancement to its midpoint. The lumen continues in an anterior (3 o'clock) direction. With the tip down, rightward deflection as well as counterclockwise rotation (torquing) of the instrument shaft would cause better alignment of the tip in the anterior direction and allow for easier intubation of the proximal sigmoid.

Rectosigmoid Junction

The rectosigmoid junction may be considered a continuation of the proximal rectum with a similar orientation. In most cases the angulus of the rectosigmoid is formed by a downturn of the left wall of the rectum to become the antimesenteric border of the sigmoid (Fig. 39-1b). As a continuation of the left wall of the rectum, the angulus is expected in the 6 o'clock position (Fig. 39-1b), assuming that a clockwise torquing maneuver has been performed (see above). As the sigmoid is entered, its mesenteric wall, being the direct extension of the right wall of the rectum, is expected in the 12 o'clock position with the posterior wall observed in the 9 o'clock position and the anterior wall at 3 o'clock.

In most cases, with the sigmoid running leftward, the rectosigmoid angulus is found in the 6 o'clock position. In 20 to 30% of the cases, there is redundancy, with initial rightward deviation of the sigmoid. In this case there is first an angulus in the 12 o'clock position, reflecting the initial right-hand course followed by one at 6 o'clock as the sigmoid finally deviates to the left.

Sigmoid

After entry into the sigmoid, the lens-wall relationship remains as it was in the rectosigmoid junction where the mesenteric wall is found in the 12 o'clock position, the posterior wall at 9 o'clock, the anterior wall at 3 o'clock, and antimesenteric wall at 6 o'clock (Fig. 39-3). These relationships may be expected to hold throughout the sigmoid to the descending colon-sigmoid junction (see below) so long as the intubation is reasonably direct (Fig. 39-4).

Descending Colon-Sigmoid Junction

If the sigmoid has been intubated with full view of the lumen, with a minimum of both blind intubation and twisting of the tip, the orientation at the descending colon-sigmoid (DS) junction remains as it was in the sigmoid so that the angulus of the DS junction (Fig. 39-3), which is made by the juncture of the mesenteric wall of the sigmoid and descending colon, is seen in the 12 o'clock position (Fig. 39-5), with the antimesenteric wall observed at 6 o'clock. The posterior wall is again seen at 9 o'clock (Fig. 39-3), and the anterior wall is in the 3 o'clock position (Fig. 39-5). The angulus at 12 o'clock (Fig. 39-5) defines for the endoscopist the upward direction the tip must pursue (Fig. 39-6a) in order to enter the descending colon (Fig. 39-6b).

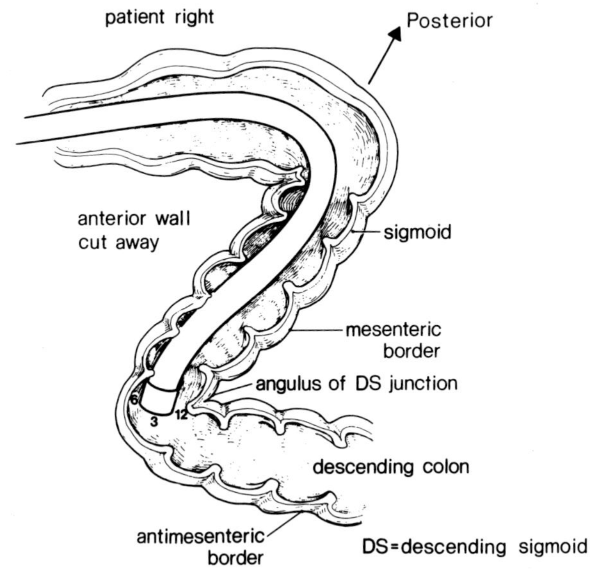

FIG. 39-5. After intubation of the sigmoid to the DS junction, with ideal alignment the angulus of the DS junction would appear in the 12 o'clock image position.

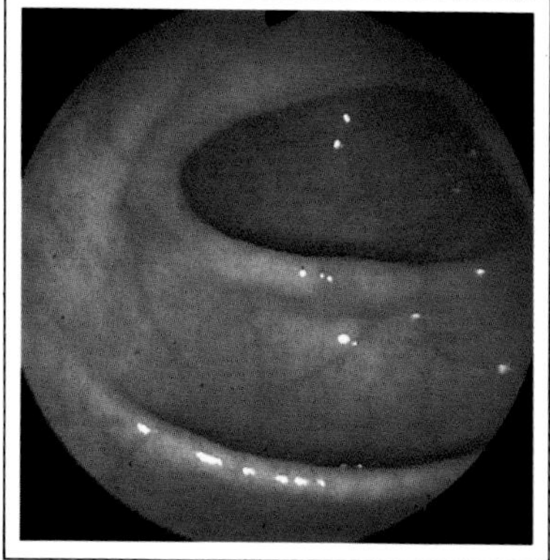

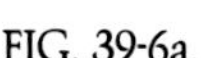

FIG. 39-6a.

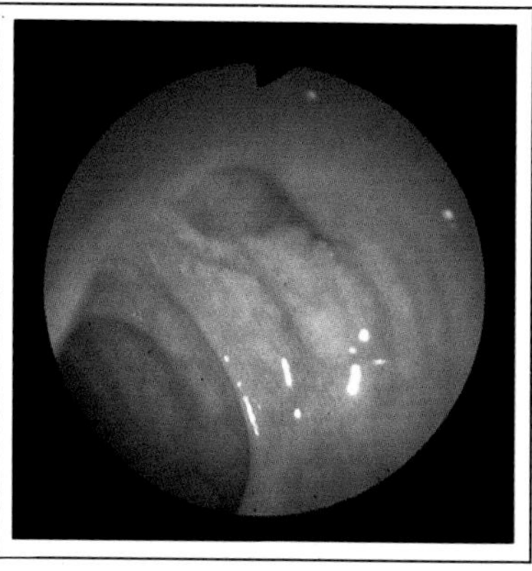

FIG. 39-6b.

FIG. 39-6. a: Angulus of the DS junction. This is seen in the 12 o'clock lens image position, indicating ideal alignment just prior to upward deflection and entry into the descending colon (b). **b:** Descending colon after entry. The mesenteric wall is located just off the 12 o'clock position with the anterior wall at 3 o'clock (Fig. 39-9).

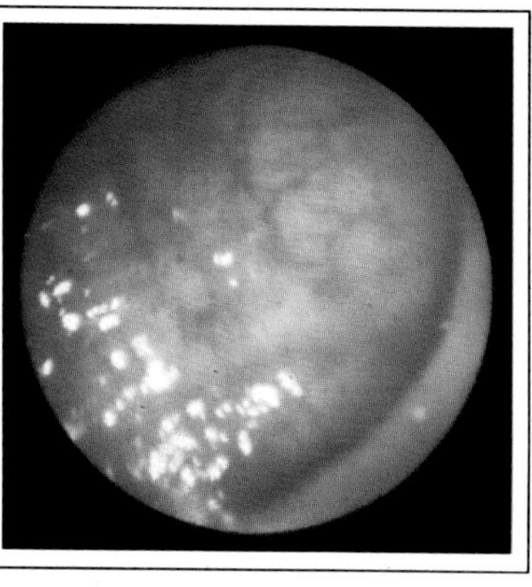

FIG. 39-7.

FIG. 39-7. Sigmoid gamma loop configuration (Fig. 39-8) is recognized endoscopically by the location of the angulus of the DS junction in the 6 o'clock (rather than the 12 o'clock) lens position.

This angulus is utilized in the hooking maneuver which is most often applied when intubating the descending colon (see "Technique of Colonoscopy," this chapter). Should the DS junction be seen in the 6 o'clock position, with further advancement into the descending colon possible (Fig. 39-7), the endoscopist correctly suspects that in the course of sigmoid intubation a gamma loop formed (Fig. 39-8), which generally precludes entry into the descending colon. At this point the endoscopist withdraws the instrument into the distal sigmoid and repeats the intubation.

Descending Colon

If the descending colon has been entered in the usual manner with an upward hooking maneuver (see "Technique of Colonoscopy," this chapter), with the patient remaining in the left lateral recumbent position, the orientation continues to be as it was in the sigmoid (Fig. 39-9). The 12 o'clock lens position views the mesenteric border; the 6 o'clock position finds the antimesenteric border; and the 9 o'clock and 3 o'clock positions view the posterior and anterior walls, respectively (Fig. 39-9). That the mesenteric border is in the 12 o'clock position (Fig. 39-10a) can be confirmed fluoroscopically as the tip is deflected upward toward it.

As the descending colon is intubated, the 12 o'clock lens position may come to lie adjacent to the anterior wall (Fig. 39-9). This occurs for two reasons. First, the anterior wall may be the path of least resistance so that the tip naturally deflects toward it, as if it had been rotated clockwise (Fig. 39-9). Second, the patient's position may be changed from left lateral recumbency to supine, which in effect rotates

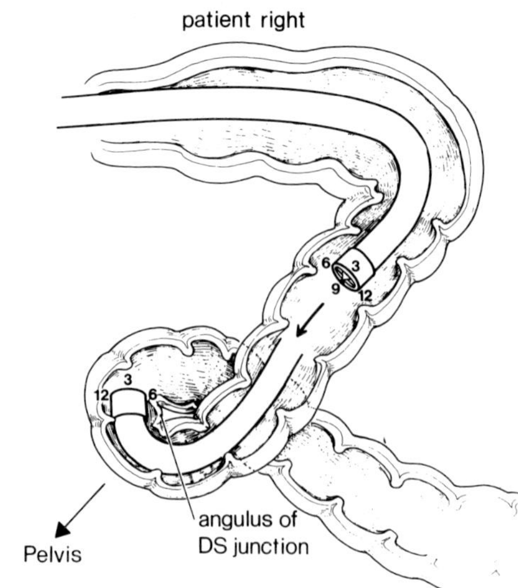

FIG. 39-8. Lens image positions for gamma configuration of the sigmoid. The DS junction is found in relation to the 6 o'clock rather than the 12 o'clock lens position (Fig. 39-5) because of formation of the gamma loop. Passage of the colonoscope beyond this point is generally impossible.

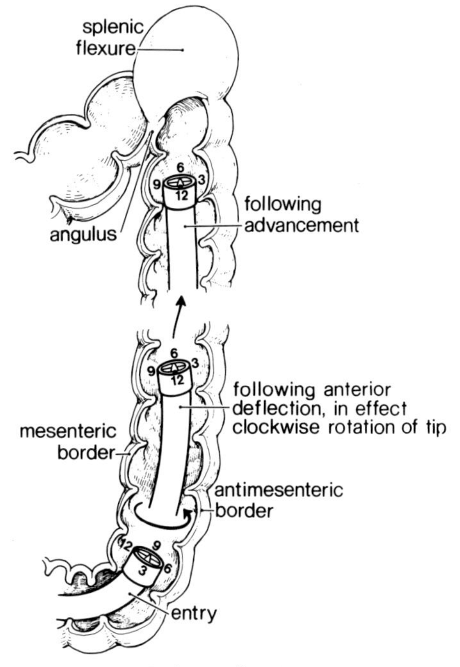

FIG. 39-9. Lens image positions for intubation of the descending colon. On entry the positions are as they were at the DS junction (Fig. 39-5). With continued intubation there is tip rotation toward the anterior wall, as if the instrument had been turned clockwise. When the patient is placed in the supine position (from left lateral recumbency), because the endoscope tip is relatively fixed, the tip in effect also rotates in the clockwise direction so that the 9 o'clock position comes to be aligned with the mesenteric (medial) border.

the colon counterclockwise with the tip position relatively fixed. This counterclockwise rotation of the colon would have the effect of a clockwise rotation of the tip, bringing the 12 o'clock position into alignment with the anterior wall (Fig. 39-9). In this case the 6 o'clock position is the posterior wall, the 9 o'clock position now looks at the mesenteric border, and the 3 o'clock position views the antimesenteric border (Fig. 39-10b).

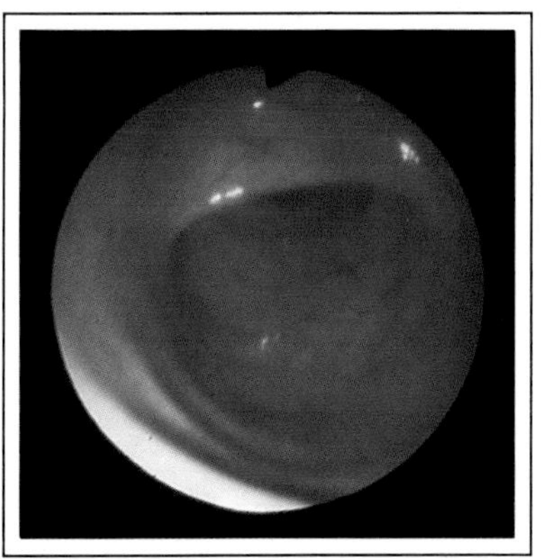

FIG. 39-10a.

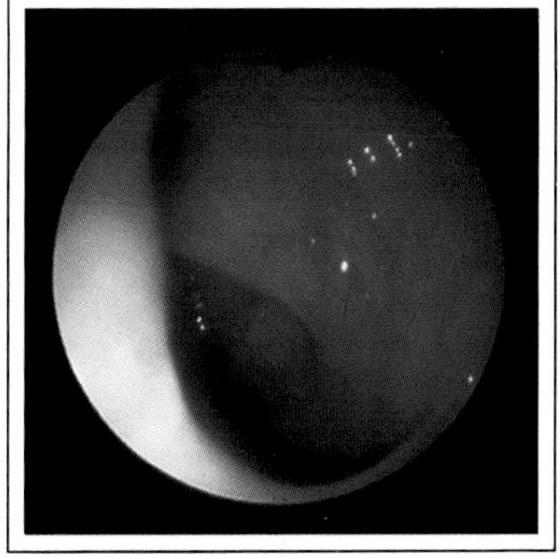

FIG. 39-10b.

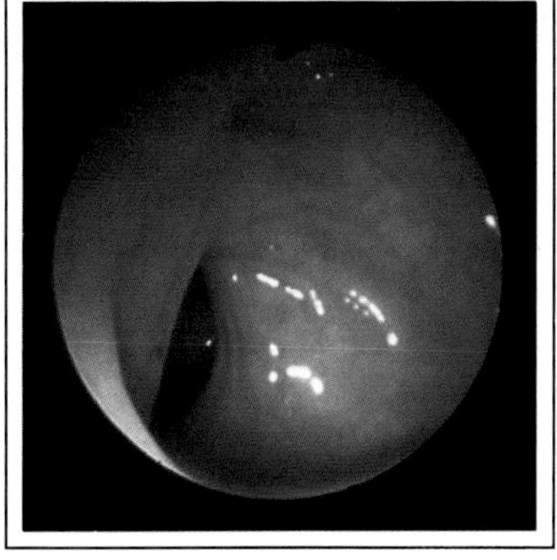

FIG. 39-10c.

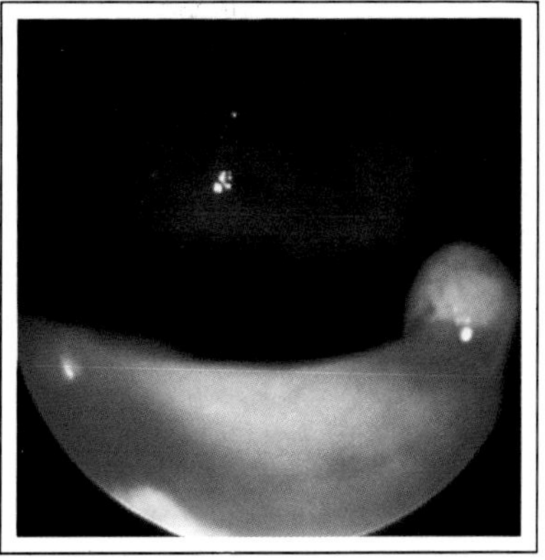

FIG. 39-10d.

FIG. 39-10. a: Descending colon on entry. An angulus of the mesenteric border is noted at 12 o'clock precisely in the same orientation (Fig. 39-9) as the angulus of the DS junction seen in the sigmoid (Fig. 39-6a). **b:** Proximal descending colon after intubation. At this location fluoroscopy confirms the wall observed in the 9 o'clock position as the mesenteric (medial) border. **c:** Splenic flexure prior to additional clockwise rotation. The angulus of the splenic flexure, a landmark for the mesenteric border, is seen at 9 o'clock. **d:** Splenic flexure angulus. After further clockwise rotation (Fig. 39-12) the angulus is now seen in the 6 o'clock position. Downward deflection at the tip of this point facilitates advancement into the transverse colon (Fig. 39-11).

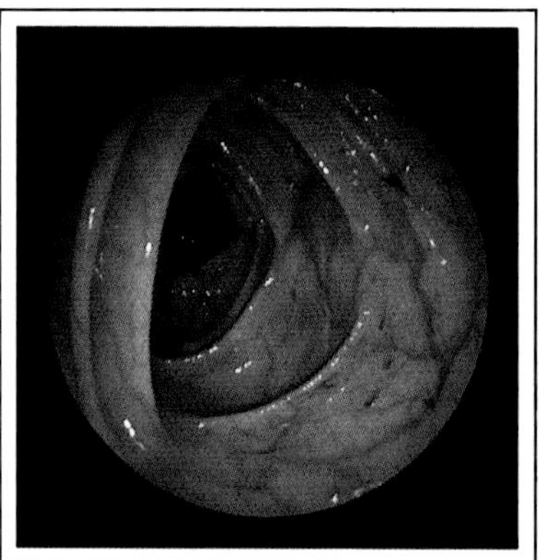

FIG. 39-11.

FIG. 39-11. Transverse colon on entry. After downward deflection just beyond the angulus of the splenic flexure at 6 o'clock, the transverse colon is entered, which is marked by its characteristic triangular interhaustral folds. With the angulus of the splenic flexure, a mesenteric border landmark at 6 o'clock, the antimesenteric border is observed in the 12 o'clock position with the anterior and posterior walls seen in the 9 and 3 o'clock positions, respectively (Fig. 39-12).

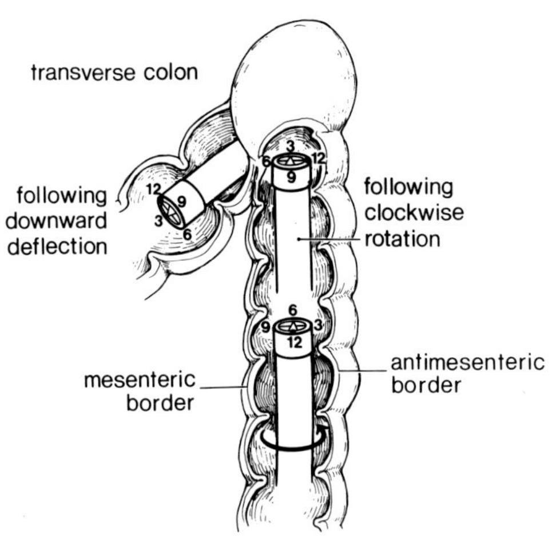

FIG. 39-12. Lens image positions of the splenic flexure before and after entry into the transverse colon. The additional clockwise rotation of the tip aligns the 6 o'clock position with the angulus, which facilitates entry into the transverse colon with downward deflection.

Splenic Flexure

The acute angulation the mesenteric wall of the transverse colon makes with its descending colon counterpart forms the angulus of the splenic flexure. Because of the anterior (and clockwise) tip rotation which occurs as the descending colon is intubated (see above), the angulus of the splenic flexure is expected in the 9 o'clock position (Fig. 39-10c) rather than the 12 o'clock position where the angulus of the DS junction had appeared (Fig. 39-9). Additional clockwise rotation of the tip would bring the angulus of the splenic flexure into a more natural position at 6 o'clock (Fig. 39-10d) for downward deflection into the transverse colon (Fig. 39-11). With the angulus of the splenic flexure in the 6 o'clock lens position, the antimesenteric wall is expected in the 12 o'clock position, with the anterior and posterior walls in the 9 o'clock and 3 o'clock positions, respectively (Fig. 39-12).

Transverse Colon

Because of the extreme mobility of the transverse colon, the orientation which had been established at the splenic flexure can easily be lost. However, to the extent that intubation is direct, the orientation established upon entry will be maintained, especially with identification of the mid-transverse colon (antimesenteric border) angulus (Fig. 39-13), which forms during intubation as a result of the descent of the transverse colon into the lower abdomen and pelvic area leading to an acute angulation of its antimesenteric wall (Fig. 39-14). If the splenic flexure angulus formed by the corresponding mesenteric borders of the transverse and descending colon was observed in the 6 o'clock position, and if the transverse colon has been entered by means of downward deflection, the mid-transverse colon (antimesenteric) angulus is expected in the 12 o'clock position. With this orientation, the anterior and posterior walls are seen in the 9 o'clock and 3 o'clock positions, respectively, and the mesenteric border is found in the 6 o'clock position (Fig. 39-13).

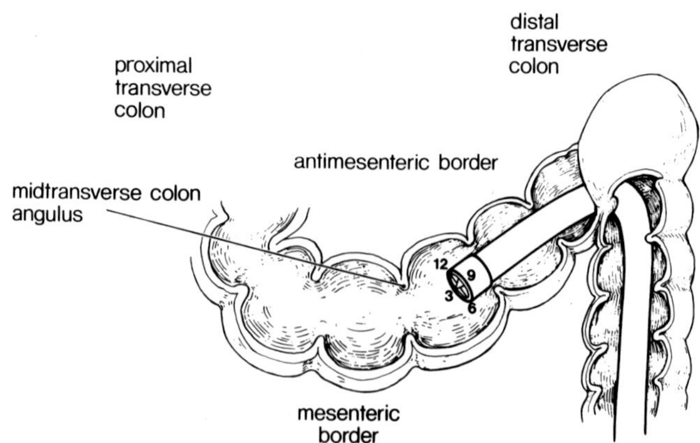

FIG. 39-13. Lens image positions after intubation of the mid-transverse colon. An angulus is formed, which is seen in the 12 o'clock position (Fig. 39-14), from bowing of the transverse colon toward the pelvis.

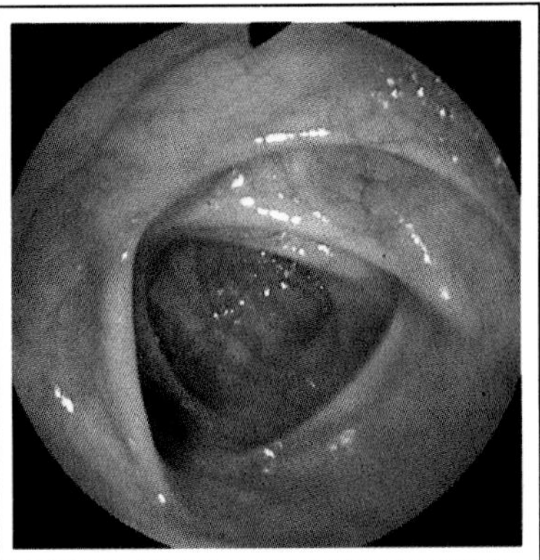

FIG. 39-14.

FIG. 39-14. Mid-transverse colon angulus. This formed as a result of transverse colon bowing on the antimesenteric border (Fig. 39-13).

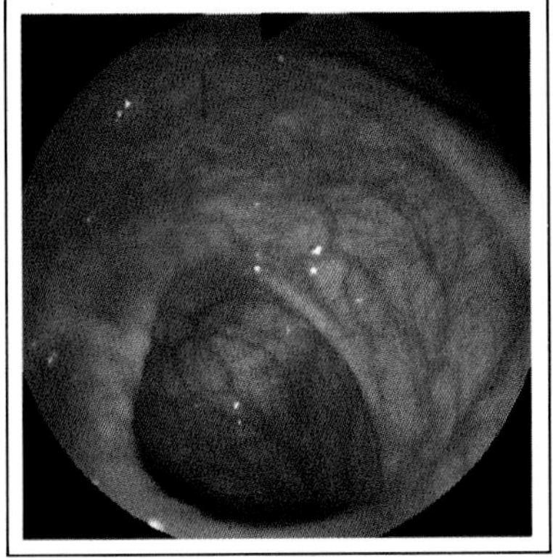

FIG. 39-15a.

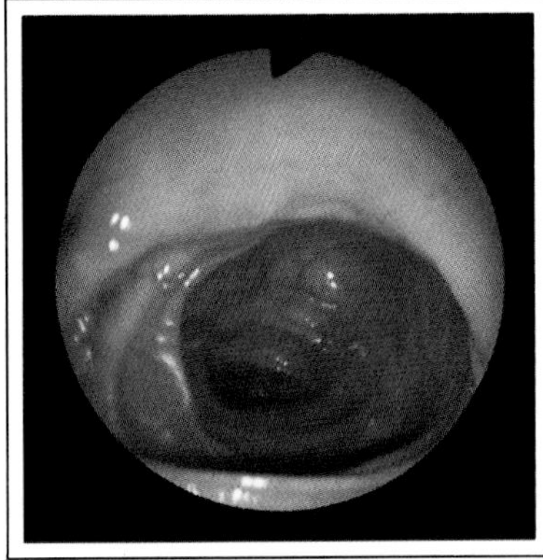

FIG. 39-15b.

FIG. 39-15. a: Proximal transverse colon and hepatic flexure just beyond the mid-transverse colon angulus (Fig. 39-14). The proximal transverse colon and hepatic flexure in the distance as seen with the angulus of the hepatic flexure in the 6 o'clock position. **b:** Ascending colon on entry. With identification of the hepatic flexure angulus at 6 o'clock, downward deflection causes the tip to enter the ascending colon with the antimesenteric border in the 12 o'clock lens position (Fig. 39-16).

Hepatic Flexure

The sharp angulation made by the mesenteric borders of the transverse and ascending colon forms the angulus of the hepatic flexure (Fig. 39-15a). If the angulus of the mid-transverse colon is observed in the 12 o'clock position, then, as was true of the splenic flexure, the hepatic flexure angulus is observed in the 6 o'clock position (Fig. 39-16). Finding the hepatic flexure angulus in this position facilitates entry into the ascending colon by downward deflection (see "Technique of Colonoscopy," this chapter). With the hepatic flexure angulus in this position, the opposite (antimesenteric) border of the hepatic flexure is observed in the 12 o'clock position, with the anterior and posterior walls in the 9 and 3 o'clock positions (Fig. 39-16). If the ascending colon is not entered, but forward advancement continues in the hepatic flexure toward the antimesenteric wall at 12 o'clock, a retroflexed position within the hepatic flexure results (Fig. 39-16), indicated by the appearance of the endoscope itself in the visual field. To correct this so that advancement continues, the tip is withdrawn into the proximal transverse colon before the entry point of the hepatic flexure; intubation then proceeds with the tip deflected downward toward the mesenteric (6 o'clock) wall to anticipate the location of the hepatic flexure angulus (Fig. 39-15b).

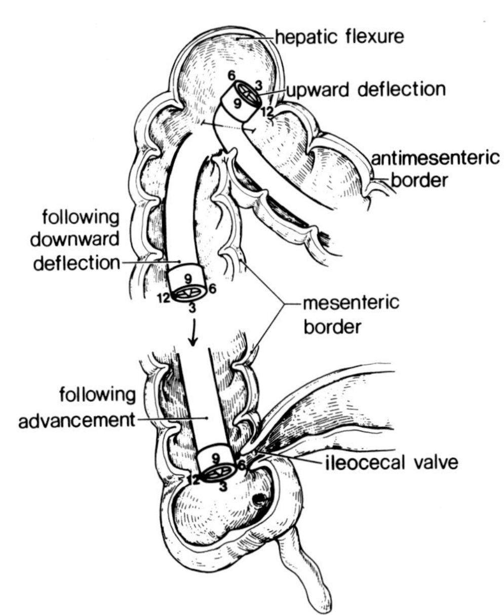

FIG. 39-16. Lens image position of the hepatic flexure, ascending colon, and cecum. The right colon has been entered directly with downward deflection at the hepatic angulus.

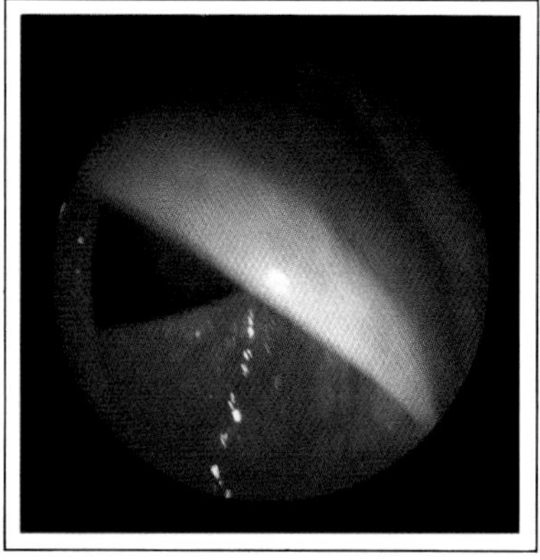

FIG. 39-17a.

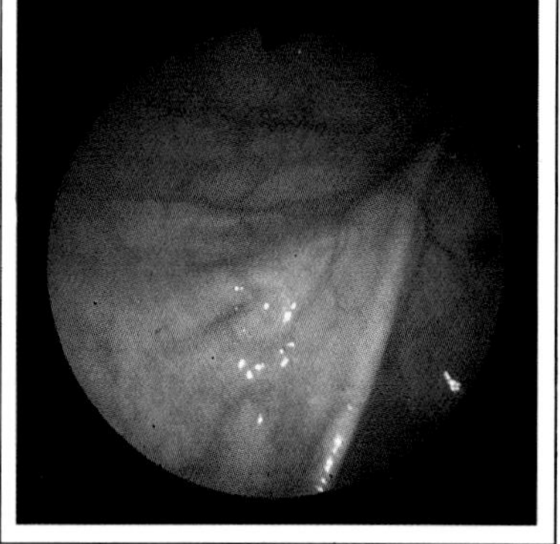

FIG. 39-17b.

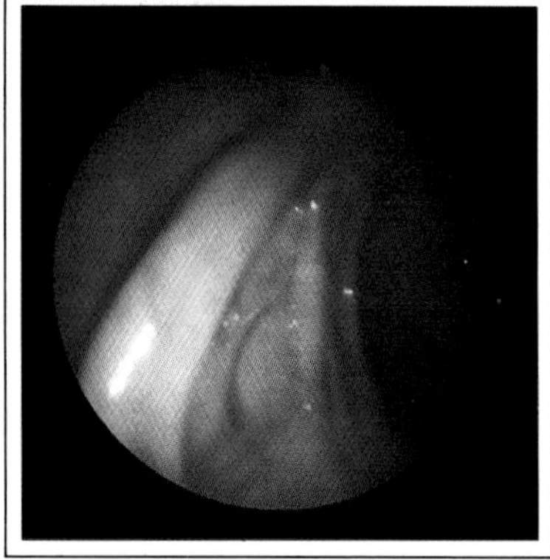

FIG. 39-17c.

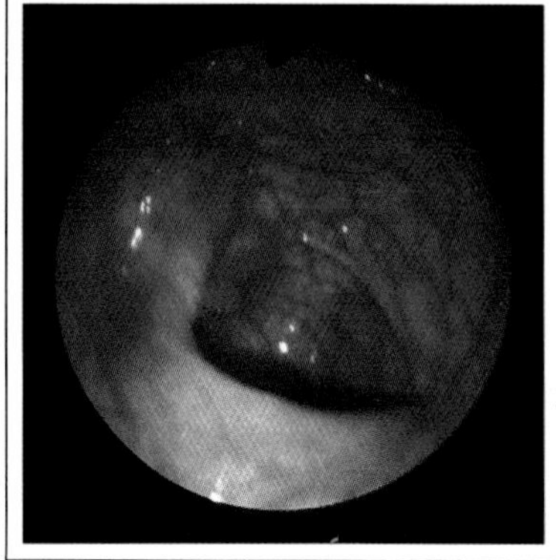

FIG. 39-17d.

FIG. 39-17. a: Ascending colon after downward deflection and advancement. That the antimesenteric border was aligned with the 12 o'clock position was confirmed fluoroscopically. **b:** Cecum, entered directly from the ascending colon. Downward deflection along the angulus of the hepatic flexure and 6 o'clock lens position and further intubation caused it to enter the cecum directly. In this orientation, the 12 o'clock image position is aligned with the antimesenteric border, whereas the 6 o'clock position observes the mesenteric (medial) border. The anterior walls are observed in the 9 and 3 o'clock positions, respectively, with the appendiceal orifice, posterior and medial, being observed in the 3 to 6 o'clock quadrant. **c:** Appendiceal orifice. In this case, where the cecum was entered directly (Fig. 39-16), the orifice was seen in the 4 o'clock position. **d:** Ileocecal valve. With direct entry into the cecum (Fig. 39-16), the ileocecal valve is observed off the mesenteric wall in the 6 o'clock position (Fig. 39-16).

Ascending Colon and Cecum

With the ascending colon entered by downward deflection toward its mesenteric (medial) border, observed in the 6 o'clock position, the antimesenteric (lateral) border is expected in the 12 o'clock position, and the anterior and posterior walls are found in the 9 and 3 o'clock positions, respectively (Fig. 39-16). As in the case of the descending colon, the location of the tip can be checked fluoroscopically from the orientation of the mesenteric border (Fig. 39-17a).

Further direct intubation within the ascending colon brings into view the strut-like folds of the cecum (Fig. 39-17b). If the cecum has been reached by a relatively direct intubation of the ascending colon, the orientation within it remains as it was in the ascending colon, with its antimesenteric (lateral) border viewed in the 12 o'clock position, its mesenteric (medial) in the 6 o'clock position, and its anterior and posterior walls in the 9 and 3 o'clock positions, respectively. Careful inspection of the cecum often reveals the mouth of the appendix or appendiceal stump if an appendectomy has been performed. As the appendix tends to be located posteriorly (Fig. 39-16), if this orientation has been maintained the appendix is found between the 3 and 6 o'clock positions (Fig. 39-17c).

In many cases the orientation on entry is not maintained, as the ascending colon is intubated. Most often there is clockwise rotation of the tip (Fig. 39-18), possibly because the right colon, when entered, is posterior to the transverse colon, causing a counterclockwise torque to be exerted at the hepatic flexure, which in turn rotates the downwardly deflected tip clockwise. In any event, this clockwise rotation causes the posterior appendix to be seen in the 6 to 9 o'clock

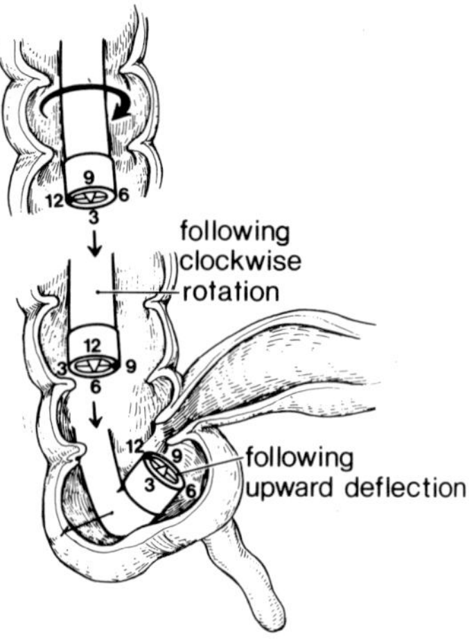

FIG. 39-18. Lens image position of the cecum and ileocecal valve after an initial clockwise rotation. This is performed to bring the mesenteric wall into alignment with the 12 o'clock position. With upward deflection and retroflexion within the cecum, the ileocecal valve is best visualized (in the 12 o'clock lens position).

quadrant (Fig. 39-19a) rather than in the 3 to 6 o'clock quadrant (Fig. 39-17c).

Ileocecal Valve

As the ileocecal valve is located on the mesenteric (medial) aspect of the cecum, some difficulty is often encountered in locating it when intubation of the cecum has proceeded with the orientation of the antimesenteric (lateral) border (Fig. 39-17d) in the 12 o'clock lens position. The problem occurs because the optical system of many instruments has a wider depth of field for the 12 o'clock lens position than the 6 o'clock position. One could correct for this by advancing the endoscope into the cecum with persistent downward deflection of the tip, causing it to assume a retroflexed position, with the ileocecal valve now being observed in the 6 o'clock position and the opposite (antimesenteric) wall in the 12 o'clock position. It is easier, however, to take advantage of the clockwise tip rotation which occurs as the right colon is being intubated (Fig. 34-18). As this rotation may paradoxically result from a counterclockwise torque exerted on the shaft in the anterior transverse colon as the tip is advanced through the more posterior right colon, the examiner continues to rotate the shaft in this direction in order to bring the mesenteric border and ileocecal valve in alignment with the 12 o'clock position (Fig. 39-19b). In this orientation (Fig. 39-18) the lens positions are reversed so that the 9 o'clock position now views the posterior wall and the 3 o'clock position views the anterior wall (Fig. 39-18). This new orientation results in the medial (mesenteric) border being observed more easily, especially on upward deflection (Fig. 39-19c), and the ileocecal valve (Fig. 39-19d) being entered with less difficulty than in the original orientation (see Chapter 48).

TECHNIQUE OF EXAMINATION

The goal of colonoscopy is both a general examination of the colon and, as often as possible, of a portion of the terminal ileum, as well as any specific areas because of radiologic findings. Realizing this goal obviously depends on the ability of the examiner to execute the required techniques for reaching the cecum and terminal ileum. To some extent, however, the successful execution of these techniques also depends on the examiner's choice of instrument as well as the preparation of both the colon and the patient for the examination. If these areas are neglected, the examination may fail to achieve its goal despite the technical expertise of the endoscopist.

In this section, we consider the four components of the colonoscopic examination: (a) preparation of the colon; (b) preparation of the patient, including premedication; (c) choice of instrument; and (d) method of examination.

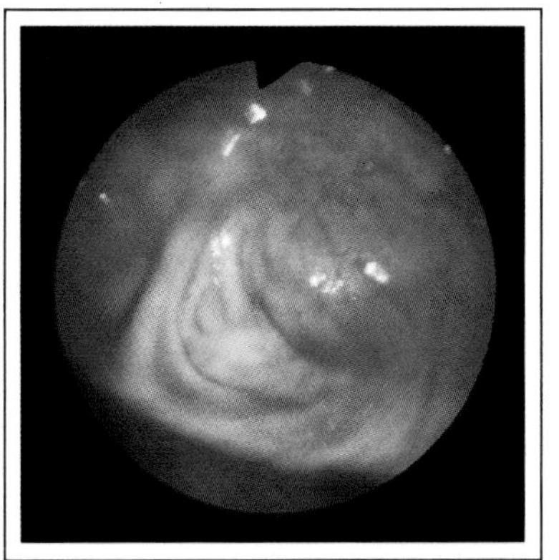

FIG. 39-19a.

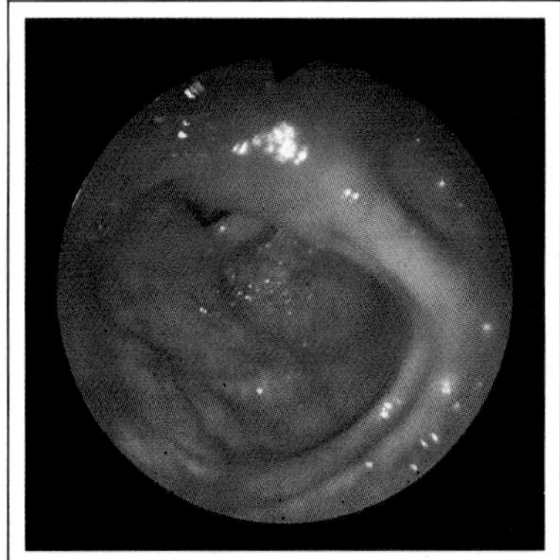

FIG. 39-19b.

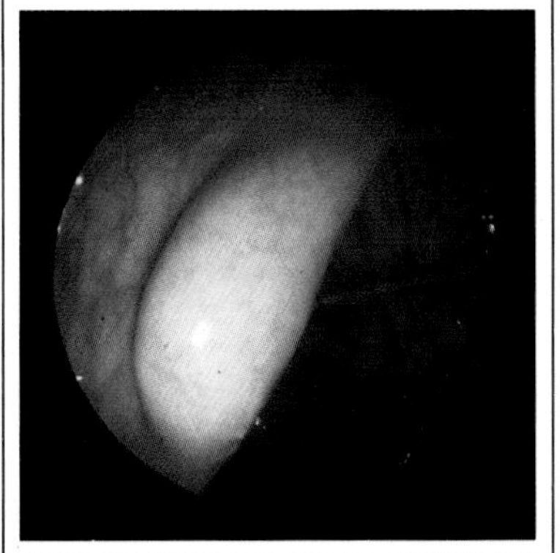

FIG. 39-19c.

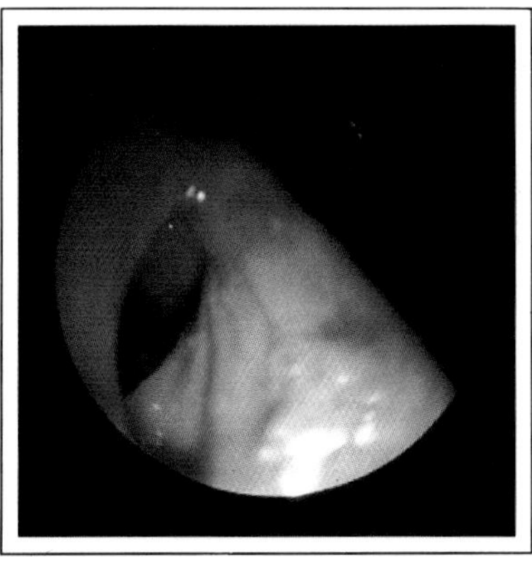

FIG. 39-19d.

FIG. 39-19. a: Appendiceal orifice. With clockwise rotation of the tip (Fig. 39-18), this is now observed at 9 o'clock. **b:** Ileocecal valve observed in the 12 o'clock lens position after clockwise rotation of the tip. **c:** Ileocecal valve, "labial" type, after clockwise rotation and upward deflection. These maneuvers allow better visualization of the ileocecal valve. **d:** Ileocecal valve opening just prior to entry. Better visualization after clockwise rotation allows the examiner to see the slit-like opening, which facilitates entry.

Preparation of the Colon

A well-prepared colon is crucial to the success of the colonoscopic examination.[1] No amount of effort from the colonoscopist succeeds in removing an excessive amount of fecal material; therefore even if the cecum can be reached in these cases, any significant pathology which may lie under fecal material will likely remain hidden. Currently, there are a variety of liquid regimens for cleansing the colon prior to the examination. Some examiners utilize commercially available kits,[2] whereas others use a combination of laxatives and cleansing enemas which are readily obtained by the patient.

Any successful preparation[1] essentially relies on three components: (a) a liquid diet (clear or full liquids, including nutritional supplements) for at least 2 days prior to the examination to minimize stool formation; (b) vigorous laxation with two kinds of laxative, an osmotic type (e.g., magnesium citrate) taken with large amounts of water and another principally with peristaltic effect (e.g., Dulcolax); and (c) vigorous use of enemas (2 to 3 liters) during 3 to 4 hr just prior to colonoscopy to clear the distal colon where residual stool may accumulate. Recently the use of whole gut irrigation with electrolyte solutions has been shown to be effective for colonoscopy as well. This may be an improvement over the older combination when combined with a 48-hr liquid diet, magnesium citrate the night before, and tap water enemas 2 to 4 hr before the procedure.[3]

When considering the preparation of the colon, the examiner must always take into account the underlying condition. For example, in the case of active ulcerative colitis, a reduced (by half) amount of laxative is used or none at all.[1]

Preparation of the Patient

Like a well-prepared colon, a fully cooperative patient is essential to the success of the examination.[1] A full, prior explanation of the procedure with its benefits and risks is extremely helpful. The patient wants to know the kind of discomfort he will experience during the examination. We find that if the patient understands this and why the procedure is necessary, he allows the examination to proceed even though from time to time he is experiencing great discomfort, bordering on intense physical pain.

The actual analgesia used is, of necessity, modest because the vigorous laxative preparation and the prior liquid diet often result in a mildly dehydrated patient; in these cases substantial doses of narcotics and sedation carry a real risk of hypotension and/or respiratory depression, especially if the patient is elderly. We use meperidine (Demerol) generally in no larger dose than 0.75 mg/kg, combined with 20 to 50 mg of promethazine (Phenergan) administered 30 min prior to the procedure and 5 to 20 mg of intravenous diazepam (Valium) administered at the time of the procedure. In most patients, especially if polypectomy is contemplated, we start an intravenous infusion of dextrose in water just before the premedication is administered. Some use atropine (0.4 mg) or glucagon (1.0 mg) as part of the premedication regimen; however, the added efficacy of these medications is questionable.

Choice of a Colonoscope

At present, with four manufacturers of colonoscopes (Olympus Corporation of America, New Hyde Park, New York; American Cystoscope Makers, Inc.—ACMI, Stamford, Connecticut; Fujinon Optical, Inc. of America, Scarsdale, New York; and Pentax Corporation, Norwood, New Jersey) providing a variety of different instruments, the choice of an instrument is ultimately a personal one. Some endoscopists are strongly influenced by the optics, preferring the sharper resolution provided by Olympus and Fujinon instruments. Others simply choose the instrument with which they first performed colonoscopy. The decision is an important one because much depends on the examiner's ability in relation to a particular instrument. The following factors should therefore be taken into account in the choice of an instrument: (a) the length of the instrument required for full insertion into the cecum; (b) the flexibility of the colonoscope; and (c) the nature of the tip control.

Length of Instrument

The goal of most examinations is to reach the cecum. With a technique that heavily depends on telescoping (see "Technique of Colonoscopy," this chapter), this can be reached with a medium (105 to 140 cm) length instrument. However, the technique employed by most examiners does not heavily rely on telescoping, with the result that considerable loop formation and bowing occur, so that a full-length (165 to 180 cm) colonoscope is mandatory. For those who perform the examination utilizing telescoping technique, however, the medium-length instrument, because it is stiffer and resists bow formation, allows the experienced examiner to rapidly intubate the cecum in a large percentage of the cases, whereas others must employ a full-length instrument. In addition, because they are shorter, the medium-length instruments allow better tip control for reduction of loops and greater tip deflection for passage of the instrument across sharply angulated segments.

Flexibility

Although the newer generation of colonoscopes being offered by the principal manufacturers are stiffer than the older instruments, which frequently required stiffening external sheaths (overtubes) or stiffening wires placed within their biopsy channels (internal stiffeners), excessive flexibility is still a problem, especially with full-length (180

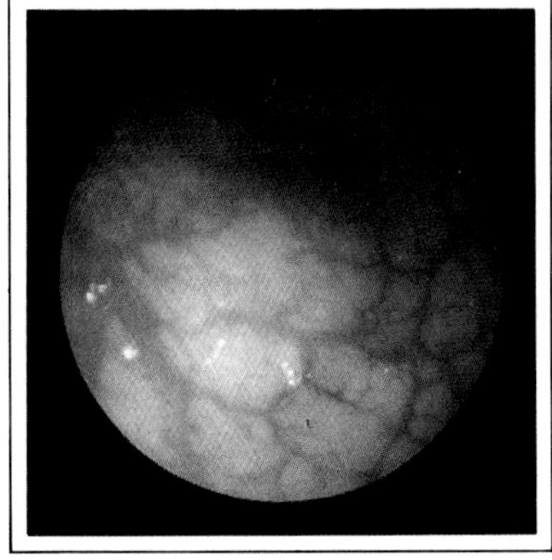

FIG. 39-20a.

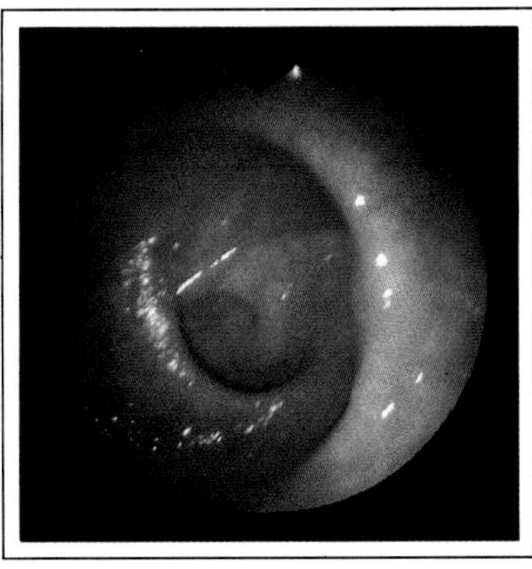

FIG. 39-20b.

FIG. 39-20. a: Rectum on entry. The tip is deflected toward the posterior wall (sacral vault) viewed in the 12 o'clock lens position. The lumen is seen to run in the direction of the right wall in the 3 o'clock position. **b:** Rectum, Houston valve, after initial clockwise rotation (see Fig. 39-1a). A characteristic mucosal fold at 6 o'clock marks the left wall.

cm), single-channel instruments. The use of such instruments is often associated with an excessive amount of bowing, especially of the sigmoid and transverse colon, which may be difficult or impossible to reduce. Some instrument flexibility is necessary as evidenced by the unsuitability of larger-caliber double-channel instruments for general use because their stiffness precludes certain basic techniques, e.g., the alpha loop maneuver (see "Technique of Colonoscopy," this chapter), as well as passage across areas where adhesions have formed from previous surgery. Therefore when choosing an instrument, the colonoscopist must weigh carefully the amount of flexibility or stiffness which he personally requires in an instrument if he is to use it successfully.

One- or Two-Handed Tip Controls

Those examiners who had their initial experience with instruments whose tip controls are not easily operated by one hand (the other hand executing intubation) have become accustomed to a two-man colonoscopy technique. Most instruments now, however, are designed so that their tip controls may be operated by one hand alone but not necessarily with the same ease. For those examiners who wish to perform colonoscopy as a one-man procedure, it is of utmost importance that the tip control be easily operated by one hand. We find Olympus, Fijinon, and Pentax colonoscopes better designed for the one-man technique, whereas ACMI instruments are best suited for individuals performing colonoscopy as a two-man procedure.

Technique of Colonoscopy

For some, performing colonoscopy remains a series of trial and error maneuvers, performed with the hope that one will somehow advance the tip of the instrument at least to the segment of the colon in question, if not to the cecum. We believe, however, that there is a rationale behind colonoscopy and that it can be integrated with the concepts already presented in the orientation section of this chapter. An understanding of the rationale behind colonoscopy, we believe, provides the reader with a better understanding of the technique he employs, as well as forms a basis for him to pursue more comprehensive descriptions of the technique elsewhere.[4-6]

Introduction, Rectum, and Rectosigmoid Junction

The usual starting position for the patient is in left lateral recumbency.[4-6] With the patient in this position, lubricating jelly is applied to the anus; then, with the tip itself well lubricated and in the "up" position, the colonoscope is inserted into the anus and advanced blindly in the direction of the rectal ampulla (presacral rectal vault). Once the tip is securely in the rectal vault, one proceeds to insufflate so that the direction of the lumen can be ascertained. With the 12 o'clock position of the lumen lens facing the posterior wall, as would be expected after insertion (Fig. 39-1), one expects the lumen seen in the direction of the right wall (Fig. 39-20a) to be found in the 3 o'clock position (Fig. 39-1a). With insufflation, Houston valves may be seen coming off the left and right walls in the 9 and 3 o'clock positions, respectively (Fig. 39-20b). In order to align the tip in the direction of the rectosigmoid, which comes off the right wall (Fig. 39-1a), the colonoscope itself must be turned (torqued) 90° to 100° in the clockwise direction so that the 12 o'clock lens position now views the right wall (Fig. 39-20b) so that further intubation causes the tip to advance in the direction of the rectosigmoid junction. In this orientation, one expects to see the rectosigmoid junction as an opening with a ridge-like angulus at 6 o'clock (Fig. 39-21a), with the angulus being the junction of the left wall of the rectum and the antimesenteric border the sigmoid (Fig. 39-1b). The endoscope tip is introduced into the rectosigmoid junction and deflected downward. The direction of the sigmoid is both to the left (6 o'clock) side as well as anterior (toward 3 o'clock) to the posteriorly situated rectum, joining the even more anteriorly located descending colon. As a result, intubation is facilitated by a combination of downward and rightward tip deflection, as well as coun-

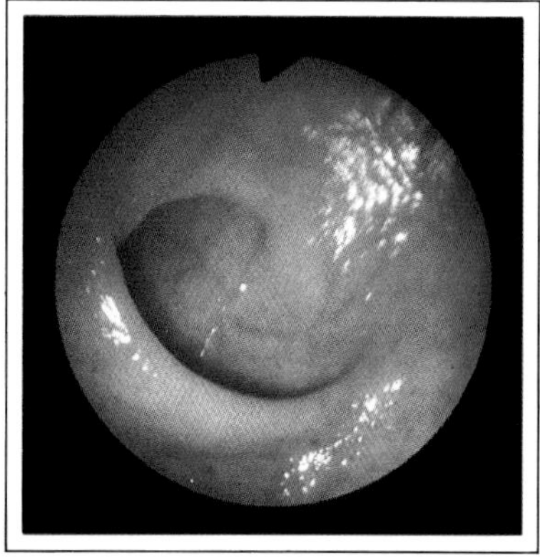

FIG. 39-21a.

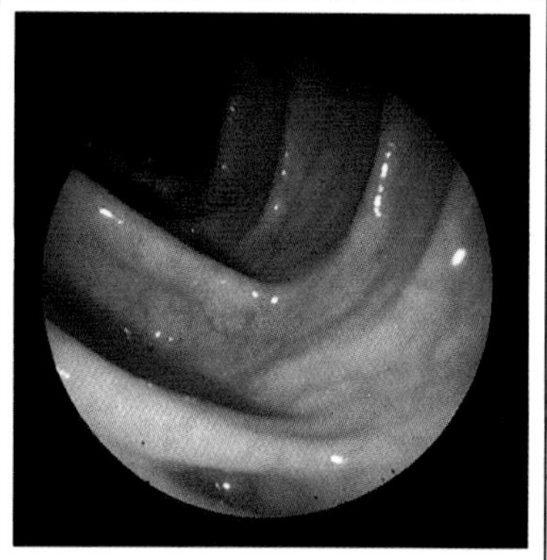

FIG. 39-21b.

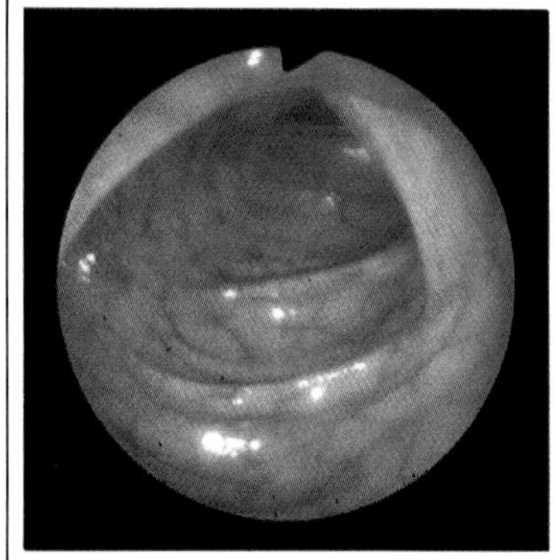

FIG. 39-21c.

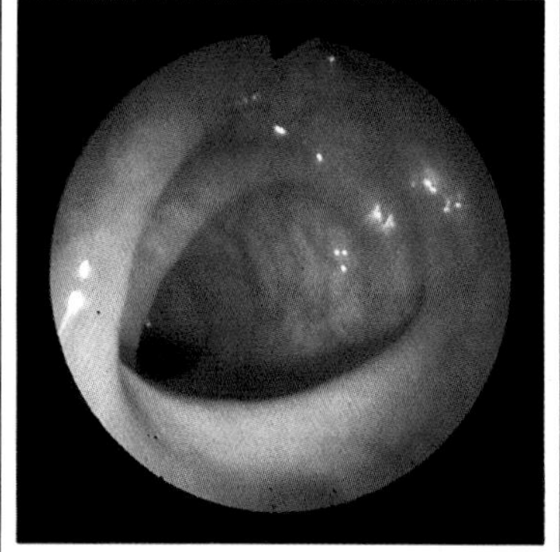

FIG. 39-21d.

FIG. 39-21. a: Rectosigmoid junction after clockwise rotation and intubation into the proximal rectum. Downward deflection across the angulus at 6 o'clock facilitates entry into the sigmoid. **b:** Sigmoid. After downward deflection and intubation, the lumen becomes obscured by an angulus. As a sigmoid bow enlarges, the technique of sigmoid straightening (Fig. 39-22) allows reduction for this bow and facilitates passage across the DS junction. **c:** DS junction. This is seen as a crescent-shaped angulus running down from the mesenteric border located in the 12 o'clock position. Just beyond this angulus, the descending colon is reached (d) by upward deflection. **d:** Descending colon. After advancement and upward deflection, the mesenteric wall is seen in the 9 to 12 o'clock position, similar to its location in the sigmoid.

terclockwise instrument rotation (which with the tip in the "down" position accentuates rightward tip deflection), which keeps the endoscope running in the general anterior direction of the lumen of the sigmoid (Fig. 39-21b).

Intubation of the Sigmoid and Passage Across the DS Junction

Once in the sigmoid, which is recognized by its prominent circular valvulae (Fig. 39-21b), ideally the tip is advanced only with the lumen in view; when this is lost, the tip is immediately withdrawn in upward deflection until the lumen is seen again. Intubation of the sigmoid colon using this technique of "sigmoid straightening" prevents excessive bow formation as well as helps to telescope the sigmoid, i.e., to cause it to contract onto the colonoscope (Fig. 39-22). This has the effect of reducing the angulation found at the DS junction. In practice, sigmoid straightening is assisted by additional twisting or jiggling of the insertion tube as the instrument is advanced.[5] Although less desirable than sigmoid straightening where the lumen is kept in view, some blind intubation (called "slide by") appears to be inevitable. This may be performed for short distances provided the mucosa does not appear excessively whitened, which suggests that a dangerous amount of stretching (to the point of perforation) has occurred. However, even though it may be performed safely, it is more often than not associated with the formation of such configurations as the gamma loop (see below), which does not allow further advancement.

As intubation of the sigmoid proceeds, the examiner becomes aware of the natural tendency of the colonoscope tip to deflect downward rather than stay in a neutral position or in one of upward deflection. However, even though the intubation seems to be going well, the examiner is well advised to resist this natural inclination, as it is almost certainly causing the tip to be directed downward into the pelvis. This increases both the acuteness of the DS junction angulation as well as the size of the sigmoid bow, which results in the formation of a configuration that makes further advancement impossible, e.g., a gamma loop (Fig. 39-8). This the examiner recognizes by seeing the DS junction angulus at 6 o'clock rather than at the expected 12 o'clock position (Fig. 39-7).

If the sigmoid has been kept reasonably straight, the DS junction can be easily traversed by direct intubation (Fig. 39-21c) and the descending colon easily entered (Fig. 39-21d). The DS junction is recognized by its crescent-shaped angulus descending from the 12 o'clock position (Fig. 39-21c). Deflecting the endoscope tip upward so that it goes just beyond this point allows one to glimpse the descending colon, which can then be entered directly. If the sigmoid is relatively straight or the bowing which has occurred not

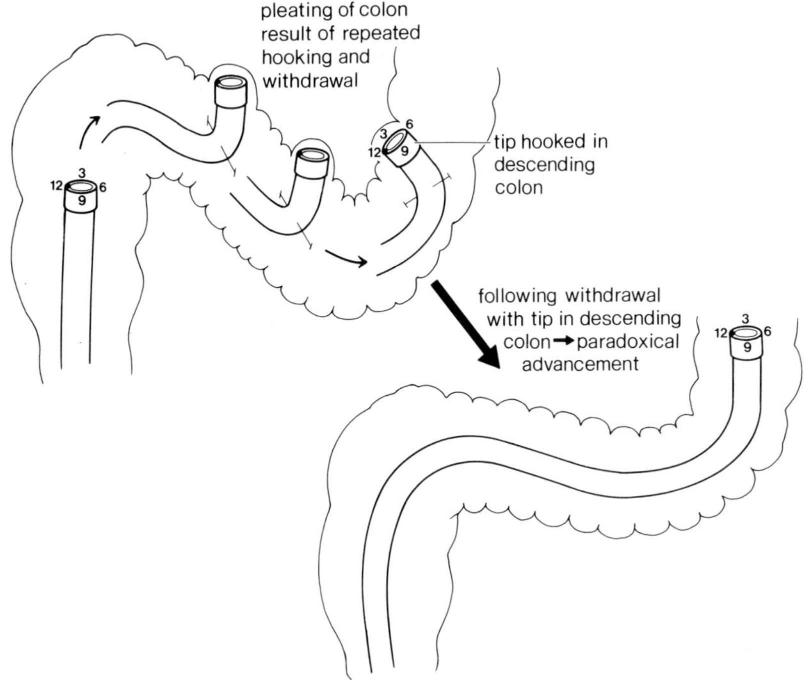

FIG. 39-22. Technique of sigmoid straightening. With repeat upward deflection of the sigmoid into the mesenteric border and advancement with a twisting or a jiggling movement,[5] the tip is advanced with the result that the sigmoid becomes "pleated" onto the colonoscope. This ultimately allows the instrument to be withdrawn and the angle of the DS junction to be reduced, thereby avoiding the formation of a gamma loop (Fig. 39-8).

excessive, it is still possible to hook into the descending colon and, with the tip position fixed in upward deflection, for the instrument to be slowly withdrawn. This results in further advancement of the tip, as any sigmoid bowing which has occurred is reduced and the force which had been forming it directly transmitted to the endoscope tip resulting in so-called paradoxical advancement (Fig. 39-22).

Additional Techniques for Sigmoid Intubation and Passage Across the DS Junction

In the event that a hooking maneuver across the DS junction into the descending colon cannot be performed, two additional maneuvers may be employed: (a) external compression; and (b) the alpha maneuver.

External compression.

With external compression, excessive bow formation is prevented by placing the patient in the supine position and pressing down in the midline or just to the left of it to prevent the sigmoid from bowing up beyond this point and forming an impossible configuration. As the bow forms, to some extent because of posterior tip deflection, counter to the direction of the sigmoid toward the descending colon, the application of a counterclockwise torque to the insertion tube to correct for this is performed along with the application of pressure.

Alpha maneuver.

In a case where there is an excessively redundant sigmoid leading to massive bowing when direct intubation is performed, the DS junction may nevertheless be crossed after application of the alpha maneuver. The idea of this is to fix the redundant portion of the sigmoid by diverting it first to the right side and then straightening the DS junction, allowing it to be easily traversed (Fig. 39-23). To perform this maneuver, the patient is initially placed in the supine or right lateral recumbent position, with the tip advanced so that it is just within the distal sigmoid; a 180° counterclockwise rotation is then performed so that the tip turns the entire sigmoid over to the right. After this, the lumen is identified and the tip quickly advanced to the DS junction beyond. Once in the descending colon, with the alpha loop configuration maintained by constant application of counterclockwise torque, the tip is further advanced into the splenic flexure and finally hooked into the distal transverse colon (Fig. 39-23). At this point, the alpha loop may be reduced by a 90° to 130° clockwise rotation so that it does not interfere with further advancement.

Descending Colon, Splenic Flexure, and Entry into the Transverse Colon

Once the descending colon has been entered, it is possible, with the patient in either the prone or left lateral recumbent position, to advance the tip directly to the splenic flexure by following the lumen (Fig. 39-24a). Should a sigmoid bow form and impede further advancement, this may be overcome by placing the patient in the supine position, applying pressure at a point midway between the umbilicus and the pubis, just to the left of the midline, as was done for intubation of the sigmoid.

The splenic flexure is recognized by the large cavernous area (Fig. 39-24a) with an angulus located usually just off

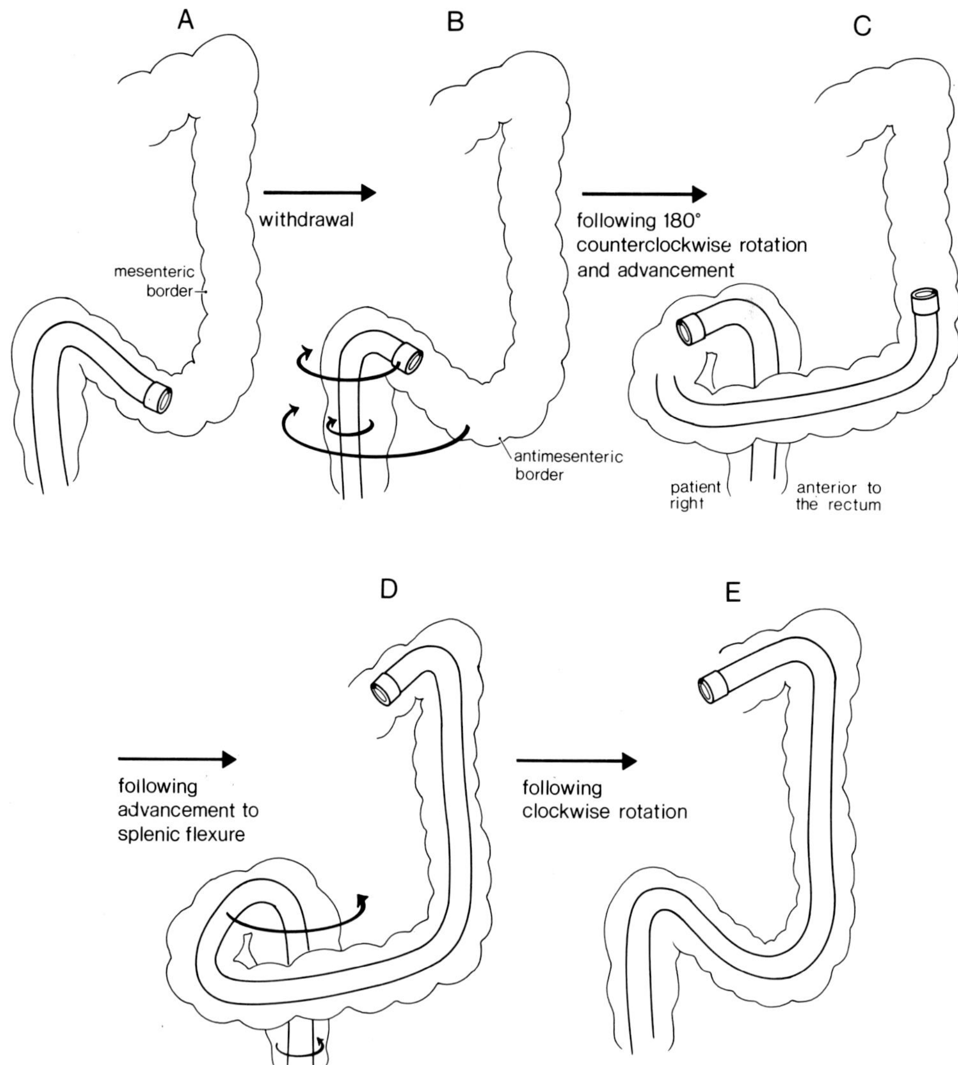

FIG. 39-23. Technique for the alpha maneuver. A redundant sigmoid initially resists the standard technique of sigmoid straightening (*frame A*). This is overcome by an initial 180° counterclockwise rotation (*frame B*), causing the sigmoid to become located to the right and anterior to the rectum (*frame C*). This facilitates intubation of the sigmoid (*frame C*) as well as the descending colon (*frame D*). Once the colonoscope has been advanced into the transverse colon (*frame D*), the alpha loop may be reduced (*frame D*) with clockwise rotation (*frame E*).

the 9 o'clock position (Fig. 24b). As was discussed previously (see "Endoscopic Orientation, Splenic Flexure," this chapter), the tip rotation in a clockwise direction just off the mesenteric border toward the anterior wall and antimesenteric border accounts for this location (Fig. 39-9). Entry into the transverse colon is facilitated by continuing this clockwise rotation so that the angulus of the splenic flexure is seen in the 6 o'clock position (Fig. 39-24c). Downward deflection of the tip allows entry into the distal transverse colon, recognized by its characteristically triangular interhaustral folds (Fig. 39-24d). If the lumen of the transverse colon is not immediately apparent after downward deflection, changing the patient's position from left lateral recumbent to supine or from supine to right lateral recumbent often causes the lumen to come into view.

Transverse Colon, Hepatic Flexure, and Entry into the Ascending Colon

The transverse colon is entered by downward deflection toward its mesenteric wall so that the antimesenteric border is seen in the 12 o'clock position (Fig. 39-24d). Downward deflection toward the mesenteric wall, which is the natural inclination of the tip as the transverse colon is intubated, often causes the mid-transverse colon to descend downward toward the lower abdomen and pelvis resulting in the formation of a large bow, which must be overcome if further advancement is to occur. If orientation on entry into the transverse colon is maintained, the angulation (Fig. 39-25a) of this bow (formed by the antimesenteric border of the proximal-mid and mid-distal transverse colon) actually

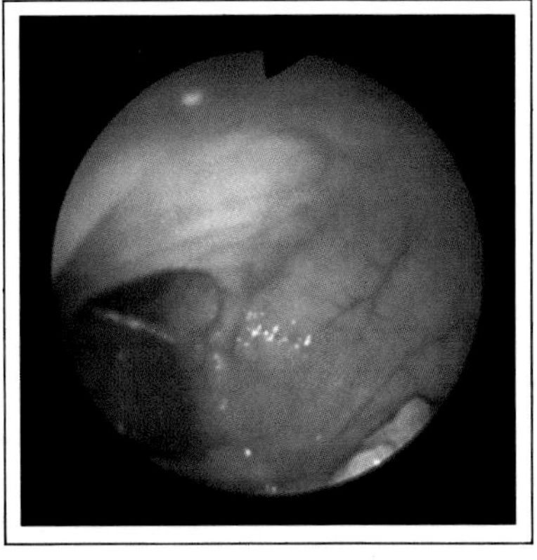

FIG. 39-24a.

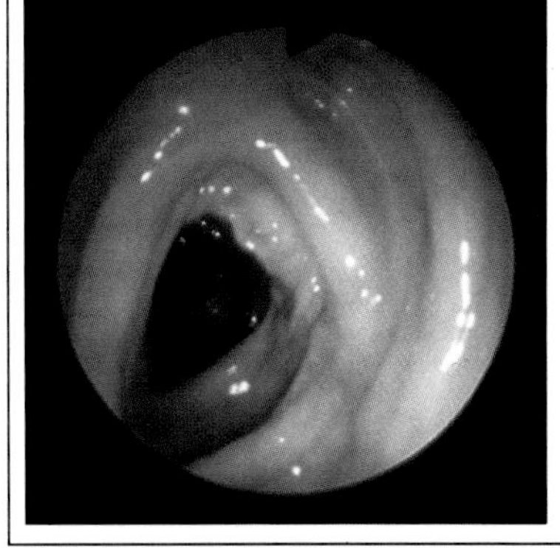

FIG. 39-24b.

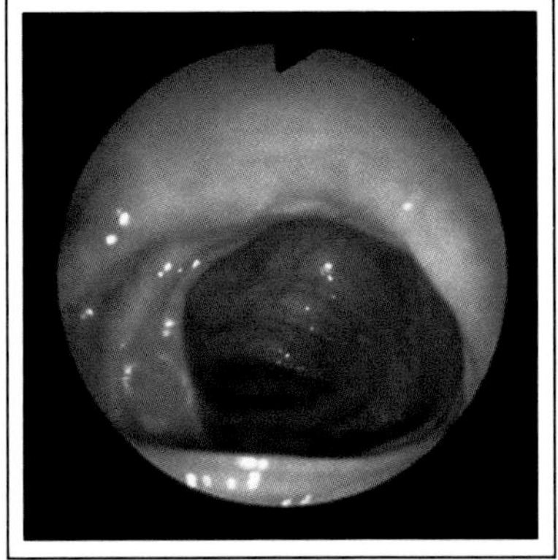

FIG. 39-24c.

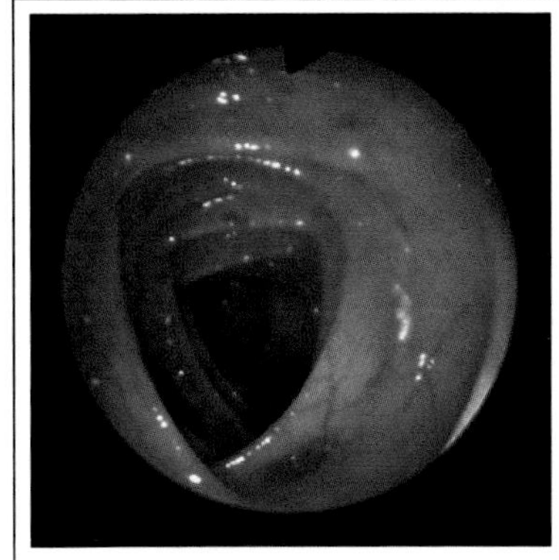

FIG. 39-24d.

FIG. 39-24. a: Proximal descending colon just distal to the splenic flexure. **b:** Angulus of the splenic flexure. Here this is aligned with the 9 o'clock lens position rather than the 12 o'clock position, the result of anterior (clockwise) rotation of the tip during advancement as well as changing the patient from left lateral recumbency to the supine position (Fig. 39-9). **c:** Angulus of the splenic flexure aligned with the 6 o'clock lens position just prior to entry into the transverse colon. **d:** Transverse colon on entry from the splenic flexure. This has been reached by downward deflection on the splenic flexure angulus and further intubation. In this orientation the antimesenteric border is seen in the 12 o'clock lens position, the mesenteric wall in the 6 o'clock position, and the anterior posterior walls in the 9 and 3 o'clock positions, respectively (Fig. 39-13).

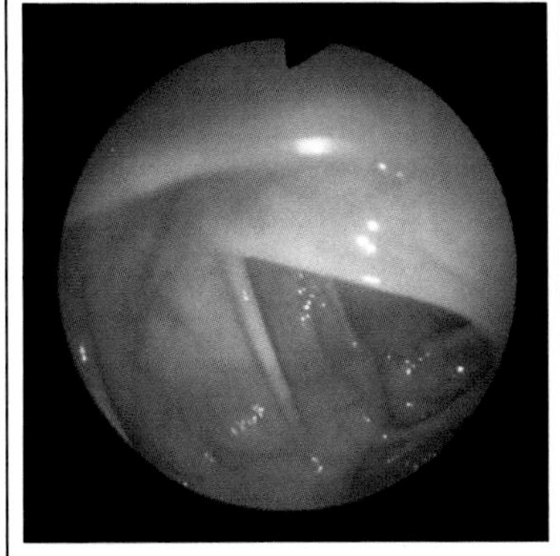

FIG. 39-25a.

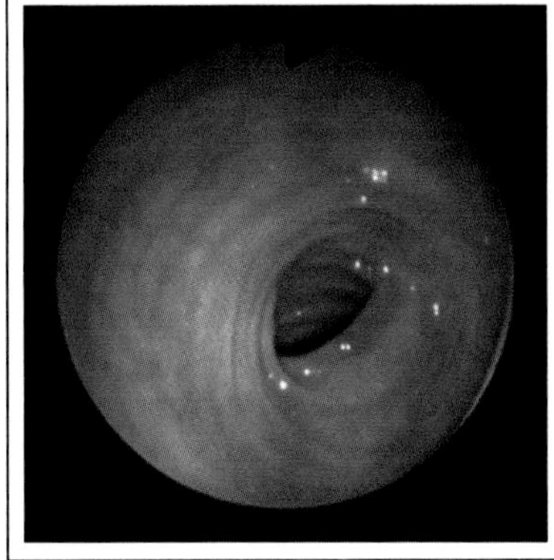

FIG. 39-25b.

FIG. 39-25. a: Transverse colon angulus. This formed on the antimesenteric wall (in the 12 o'clock lens position) as a result of bowing of the transverse colon during intubation toward the pelvis (Fig. 39-13). **b:** Proximal transverse colon and hepatic flexure after the lift and hook maneuver (Fig. 39-26). The hepatic flexure is seen in the distance devoid of interhaustral folds.

forms two compartments (proximal and distal) for the transverse colon (Fig. 39-13). To enter the proximal compartment from the distal colon, the angulus of the bow must be traversed (Fig. 39-13). To do this, the tip is deflected up and held in a fixed position while the instrument is withdrawn (Fig. 39-26). This "hooking-lifting-telescoping" maneuver is necessary to raise the tip so that it is in position to be advanced into the proximal transverse colon (Fig. 39-25b) and hepatic flexure (Fig. 39-25b) rather than bowing excessively in the pelvis. To prevent the latter from occurring, pressure must be applied to the epigastrium just to the right of the midline as the tip is advanced.

The hepatic flexure (Fig. 39-25b), like the splenic flexure, is recognized as a cavernous space, generally devoid of the typical angular intrahaustral folds of the transverse colon. Within the hepatic flexure, the liver impression may be seen (Fig. 39-27a). If the orientation on entry into the transverse colon is maintained, this is just anterior to the mesenteric border (between 9 and 12 o'clock) with the angulus of the hepatic flexure expected in the 6 o'clock position. If the angulus of the hepatic flexure, the entry point into the ascending colon, is not immediately apparent, further advancement of the tip may lead to its becoming retroflexed, resulting in a view of the shaft entering the hepatic flexure

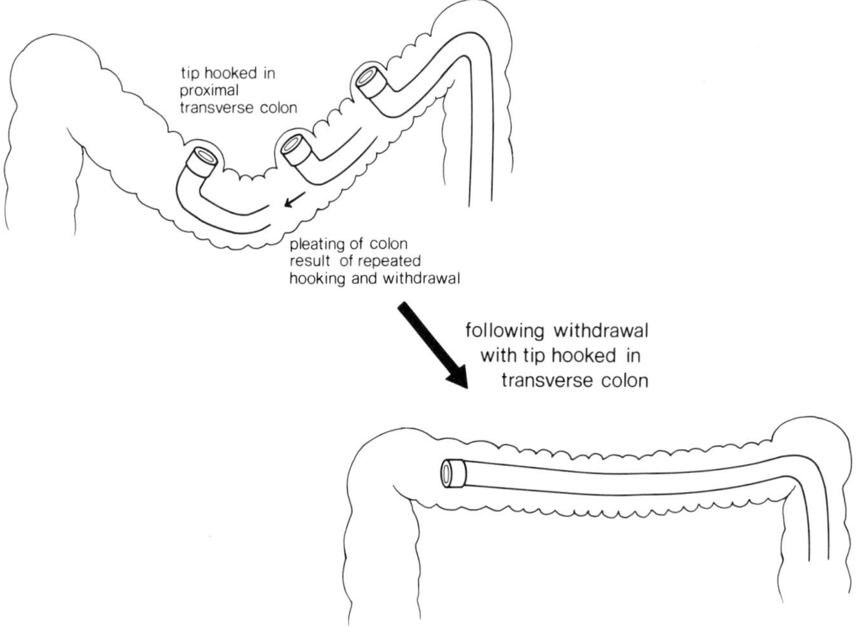

FIG. 39-26. Technique for lift and hook maneuver to reduce bowing of the transverse colon. As in the case of the technique for sigmoid straightening (Fig. 39-22), the distal transverse colon is pleated onto the colonoscope by a series of upward deflections and withdrawals which prevents bowing and facilitates entry into the proximal transverse colon.

from the proximal transverse colon (Fig. 39-16). To prevent this, once the examiner determines that he is in the hepatic flexure, the direction of the tip must be changed to become downward. In this direction the angulus between the mesenteric walls of the proximal transverse colon of the ascending colon is seen at 6 o'clock (Fig. 39-16). The tip is advanced across this view in this position (Fig. 39-27a) until the lumen of the ascending colon (Fig. 39-27b) with its widely spaced, prominent interhaustral folds is seen. In some cases the tip does not cross into the ascending colon

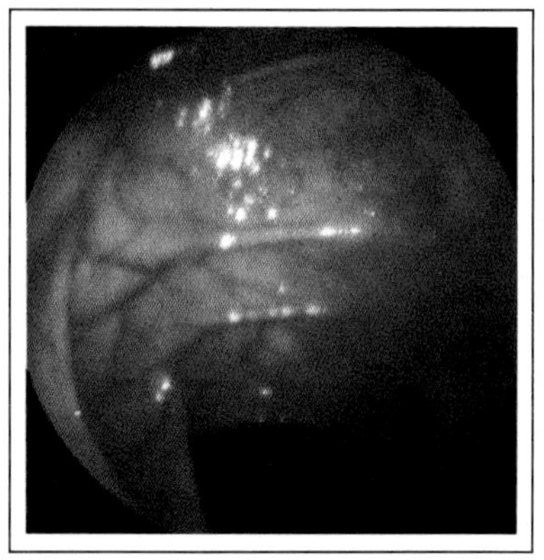

FIG. 39-27a.

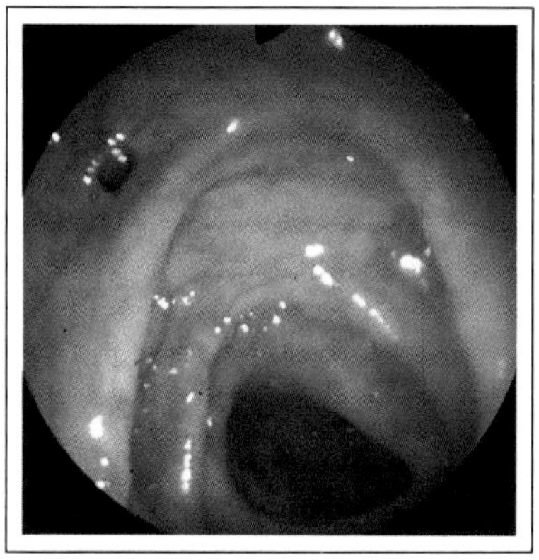

FIG. 39-27b.

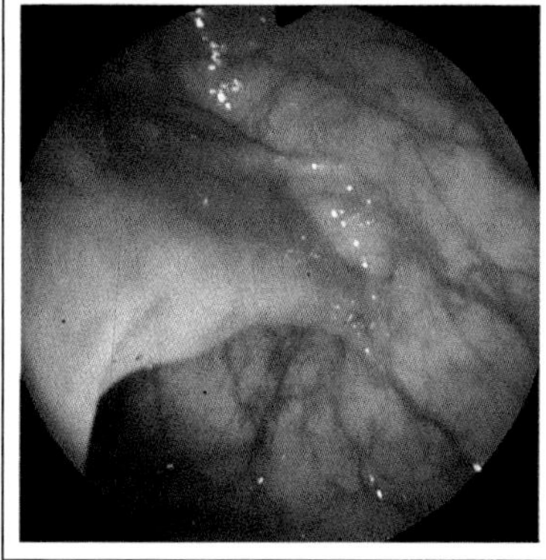

FIG. 39-27c.

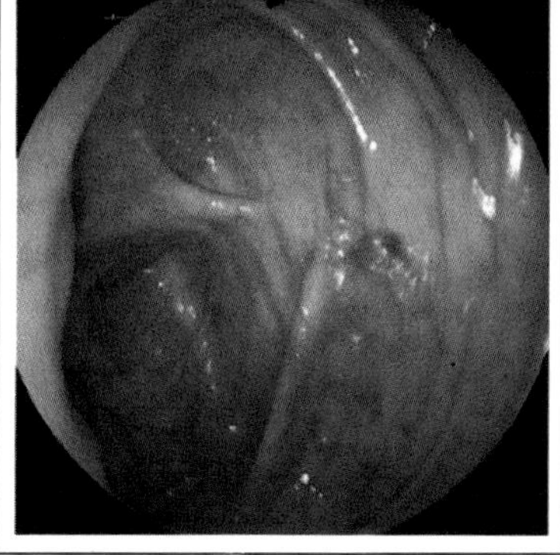

FIG. 39-27d.

FIG. 39-27. a: Hepatic flexure. The liver impression is seen as a gray-blue zone on the anterior aspect of the antimesenteric border (in the 11 to 1 o'clock lens position). **b:** Ascending colon on entry from the hepatic flexure. **c:** Ascending colon with prominent widely spaced interhaustral folds. **d:** Cecum with its characteristic strut-like folds.

unless external compression is applied to the right upper quadrant, which forces it from the hepatic flexure into the more posteriorly lying ascending colon. Additional compression may be required in the more medial right upper quadrant to prevent reformation of the transverse colon bow, another factor which would prevent further advancement.

Ascending Colon and Cecum

Once the ascending colon has been entered (Fig. 39-27c), further advancement usually leads to cecal intubation. This may be facilitated by applying pressure to the upper mid-abdomen to prevent a transverse colon bow from either forming or expanding and thus dissipating the force of advancement before it reaches the tip. The cecum is recognized by its own distinctive, strut-like fold pattern (Fig. 39-27d). This may be confirmed fluoroscopically as well as by seeing light transmitted through the abdominal wall in the right lower quadrant.

If the ascending colon has been entered by a downward deflection to advance across the hepatic flexure angulus in the 6 o'clock position, the antimesenteric border of the cecum may remain in the 12 o'clock position. This means that the ileocecal valve is expected in the 6 o'clock position 2 cm proximal to the base of the cecum (Fig. 39-17d). However, it may not be seen until the tip is rotated so that the 12 o'clock lens position, often having the greatest depth of field, is now aligned with the mesenteric (medial) border (Fig. 39-19b). As already noted (see "Endoscopic Orientation, Ileocecal Valve," this chapter), there is a natural tendency for the tip to rotate clockwise, paradoxically from a counterclockwise torque exerted at the hepatic flexure, causing the downward deflected tip to enter the more posterior right colon. Once entered, to align the 12 o'clock position with the mesenteric border one continues to apply a counterclockwise torque to the shaft, so that further advancement of the endoscope tip with upward deflection brings the ileocecal valve into ideal view for both observation and intubation (Fig. 39-19c) (see Chapter 48).

Examination of the Colon upon Withdrawal

Intubation of the colon may leave the examiner as well as the patient exhausted. Psychologically both may feel that the examination is over once the cecum has been reached. In fact, it has just begun. The critical part of any colonoscopic examination is withdrawal. The tremendous effort which may have been expended in reaching the cecum is wasted if a large polyp or polypoid carcinoma is missed simply because the withdrawal phase has occurred too rapidly. Each examiner has his own system for surveying the various segments of the colon. As in the examination of the stomach (see Chapter 11), we recommend that the examiner establish in his own mind a set of survey arcs he wishes to make at 5- to 10-cm intervals (as in the stomach—see Chapter 11). At least 5 min should be provided in each of the segments above the rectum with an additional 5 to 10 min for the flexures so that the withdrawal phase should take at least 20 min, especially if the indication for colonoscopy was rectal bleeding or a positive fecal occult blood test. Any area where based on an X-ray study there is a suspicion of a polyp, especially one greater than 1 cm in diameter, deserves particular attention, and we recommend that the patient be examined in both left and right lateral recumbency as well as the prone and supine positions. Once the tip is withdrawn back into the rectum, one may, prior to concluding the examination, perform a retroflexed maneuver (deflecting up in the same orientation as on entering the rectum—see above) to examine the distal rectum which is not seen on entry (Fig. 39-2b).

NORMAL ENDOSCOPIC APPEARANCE OF THE COLON

In this section we first consider the distinctive endoscopic features of the various sections of the colon and then discuss the normal colonic mucosal appearance.

Segmental Endoscopic Anatomy

Rectum

The semilunar valves of Houston are the characteristic feature of the rectum. These are found in the mid-distal portion (Fig. 39-20b). They are best appreciated on withdrawal as semilunar mucosal projections of variable shape and thickness alternating from the anterior and posterior walls (Fig. 39-20b). Proximal to these, the rectum is generally devoid of folds until the angulus of the rectosigmoid junction is reached (Fig. 39-28a).

Sigmoid

The sigmoid is a striking contrast to the featureless character of the proximal rectum (Fig. 39-28a). The typical appearance of the sigmoid is that of concentric ring-like (Fig. 39-28b) valvulae (interhaustral folds). These have a variable thickness but are generally 5 mm or less. They may be especially prominent where their width approaches 1 cm (Fig. 39-28c), which is generally thought to be the result of hypertrophy of the circular as well as the longitudinal muscle bands. In cases where they are especially prominent, the valvulae appear triangular resulting from hypertrophy and contraction of the longitudinal muscle of the wall of the sigmoid. When the valvulae are triangular (Fig. 39-28c), their similarity to the interhaustral folds of the transverse colon (Fig. 39-29a) may cause the examiner to believe he has intubated farther than the sigmoid, especially when as much as 80 cm or more of the instrument

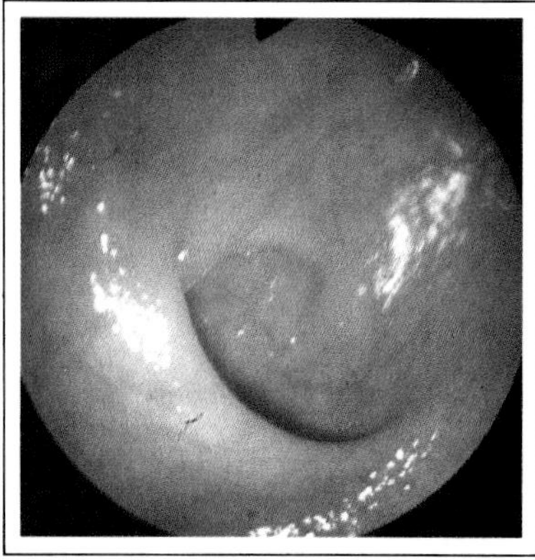

FIG. 39-28a.

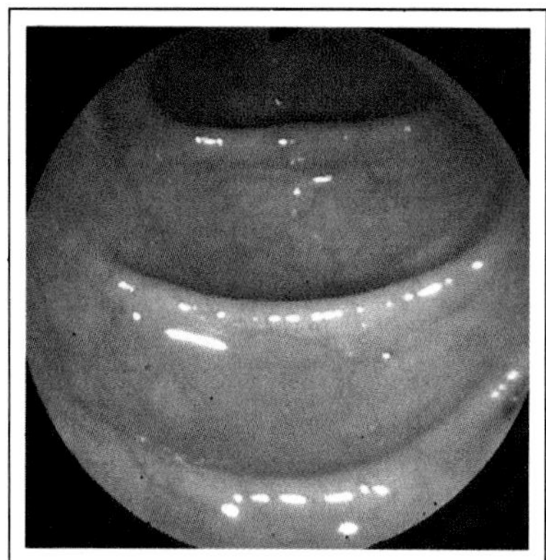

FIG. 39-28b.

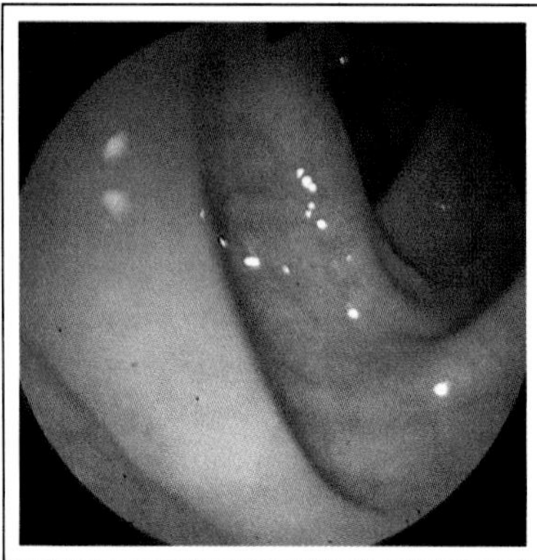

FIG. 39-28c.

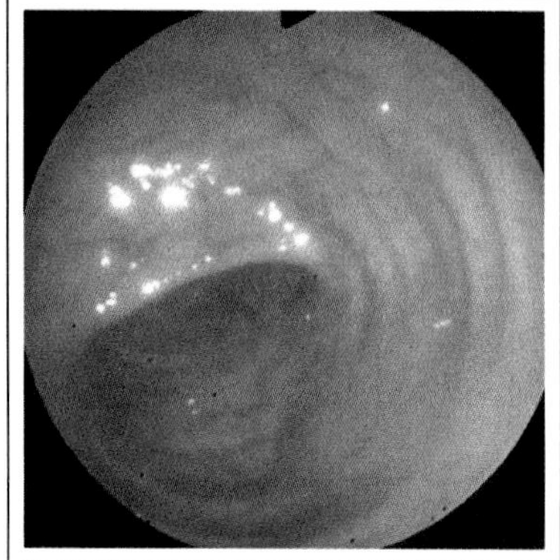

FIG. 39-28d.

FIG. 39-28. a: Rectum. Just above the Houston valves one can see the characteristic featureless appearance of a prominent mucosal vascular pattern. **b:** Sigmoid with thin valvulae (interhaustral folds). **c:** Sigmoid with prominent valvulae thought to be the result of circular muscle hypertrophy (see Chapter 46). **d:** Descending colon. In this case the descending colon was largely devoid of folds.

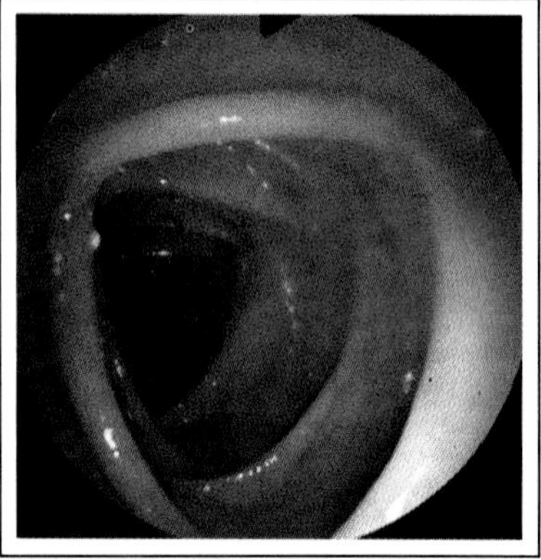

FIG. 39-29a.

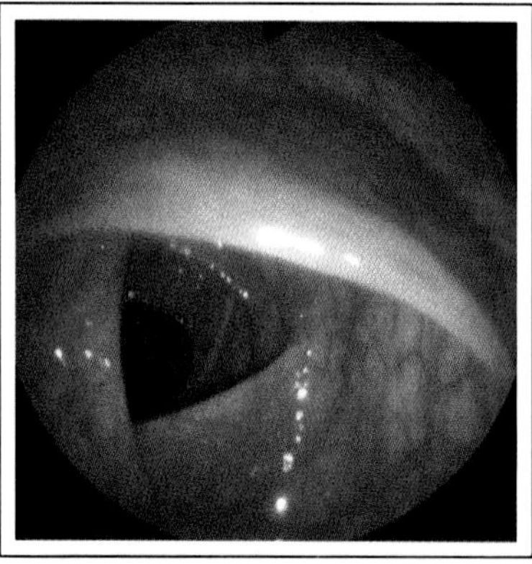

FIG. 39-29b.

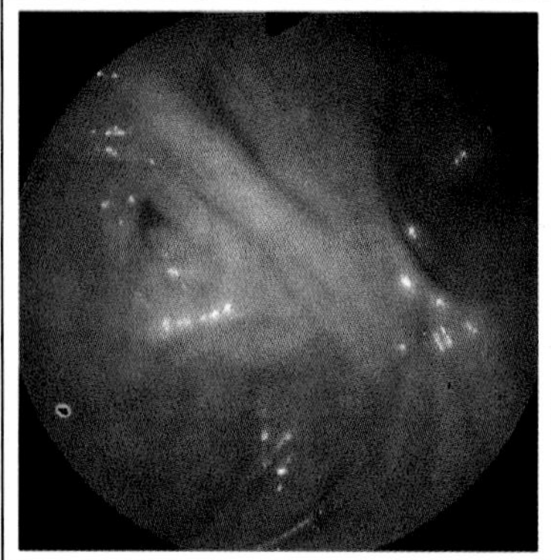

FIG. 39-29c.

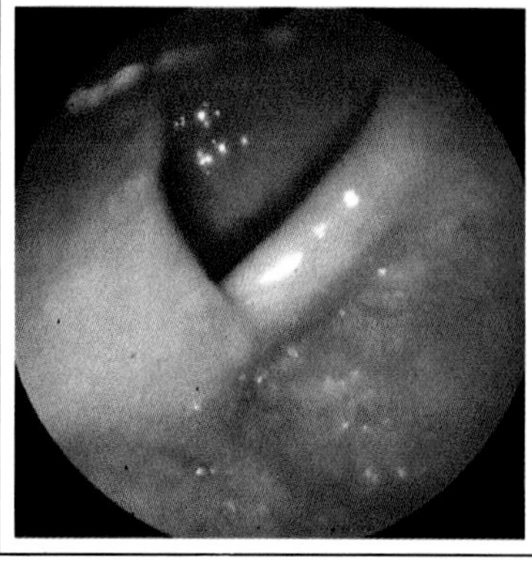

FIG. 39-29d.

FIG. 39-29. a: Transverse colon. The triangular interhaustral folds are a typical feature; these are tall but thin with a width at their peaks of less than 3 mm. **b:** Ascending colon. The width of this segment exceeds 10 cm with tall, widely spaced interhaustral folds. **c:** Cecum. The characteristic strut-like folds on the base of the cecum. Clockwise rotation of the tip on intubation of the right colon causes 3-mm dimple-like orifices to appear at 9 o'clock (Fig. 39-19). **d:** Ileocecal valve. This was identified 2 cm above the cecum as a focally prominent fold in the 6 o'clock position, indicating that the orientation on entry into the ascending colon (with the mesenteric wall in the 6 o'clock position) has been maintained.

has been inserted in the process of forming a giant sigmoid bow.

Descending Colon

In contrast to the relatively narrow sigmoid colon, the lumen of the descending colon is considerably more expansive (Fig. 39-28d). The valvulae tend to be more widely spaced in the descending colon than in the sigmoid. We find that in roughly one-third of the cases, in the absence of any histologic abnormality, the valvulae are entirely absent, giving the descending colon a completely featureless appearance.

Transverse Colon

The striking appearance of the transverse colon, indeed one of the most characteristic endoscopic features of any segment of the colon, are the large triangular folds (Fig. 39-29a). These folds are created by contraction of the three longitudinal bands of muscle, the taeniae coli. These generally occur at 1.5- to 2-cm intervals with sac-like segments, the haustrae located between. The triangular folds are tall, up to 1.5 cm, and sharp, with the width at their peaks being 4 mm or less (Fig. 39-29a).

Ascending Colon

The ascending colon and the cecum are the widest segments of the colon. When fully distended, their lumens may exceed 10 to 15 cm in width (Fig. 39-29b). In contrast to the transverse colon, the interhaustral folds are irregular and can be widely spaced. In addition, they are taller than those of the transverse colon, with some being more than 2 cm in height although still sharp, typically 4 mm or less in width at their peaks. The haustrae between the folds are large, with spaces of 2 to 3 cm not unusual (Fig. 39-29b).

Cecum

Advancing the tip beyond the ascending colon reveals the cecum. It is often cavernous so that with air insufflation it is not unusual to distend it beyond 15 cm in width (Fig. 39-29c). The interhaustral folds have a characteristic strut-like appearance as they run toward a central point in the base of the cecum. These folds are 3 to 5 cm long and may be 5 to 10 mm high, but they still appear sharp, with the width at their peaks being less than 5 mm (Fig. 39-29c). Rather than having one typical pattern, the folds of the cecum show great variation so that any type of fold is not unexpected. The appendiceal opening may be found within the cecum in up to 20% of the cases. If the orientation on entry into the right colon with the angulus of the hepatic flexure at 6 o'clock has been maintained down to the cecum, the appendiceal opening is expected in the 3 to 6 o'clock lens position, in which the posterior aspect of the mesenteric wall is expected (Fig. 39-16). To the extent that either clockwise (or counterclockwise) rotation has occurred, with the 12 o'clock position now viewing the mesenteric (medial) border (Fig. 39-18), the opening to the appendix is expected in the 9 to 12 o'clock quadrant of the visual field (Fig. 39-29c). The characteristic appearance of the appendiceal opening is a dimple-like depression about 5 mm in diameter. When there has been previous surgery, the mouth of the appendix may be eroded, giving the appendiceal stump a polypoid appearance.

Ileocecal Valve

The ileocecal valve is found approximately 3 cm above the terminal portion of the cecum (Fig. 39-29d) and denotes the junction between the cecum and the ascending colon. It is best seen if the tip has been rotated off the antimesenteric (lateral) border so that the mesenteric border (Fig. 39-30a) and ileocecal valve appear toward the 12 o'clock position (Fig. 39-18), a position which can be confirmed fluoroscopically. Further intubation and upward deflection facilitate identification of its opening and entry (see Chapter 48).

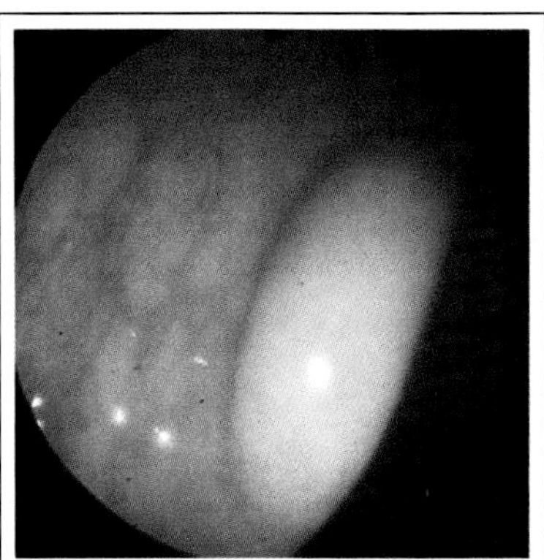

FIG. 39-30a.

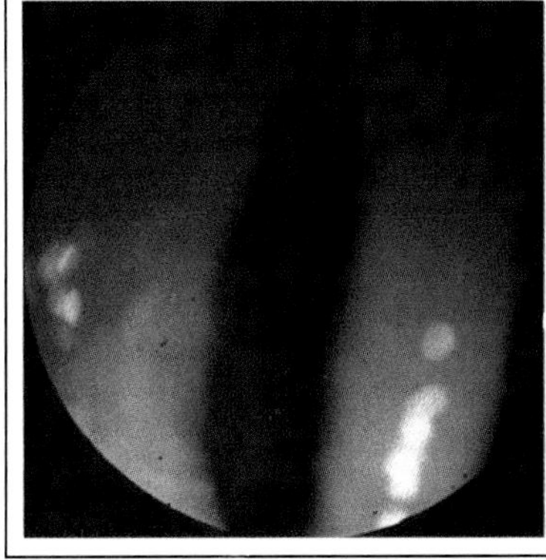

FIG. 39-30b.

FIG. 39-30. Ileocecal valve, labial type. **a:** Identification and entry into the ileocecal valve is facilitated by clockwise rotation to align the 12 o'clock lens position with the mesenteric border (Fig. 39-19). **b:** After clockwise rotation (a) and retroflexion within the cecum. These maneuvers facilitate the identification of its opening between its upper and lower limbs.

Three types of ileocecal valve have been described[7]: (a) the labial type (Fig. 39-30a), a slightly raised fold in which the mouth of the ileocecal valve is set between an upper and lower part; (b) the papillary type with a dome-like protrusion and the mouth at its apex; and (c) an intermediate-type appearance with features of both the labial and papillary types.[6] In any given ileocecal valve, one may observe any of these three shapes, with the appearance dependent on the content of the terminal ileum.[6] For the labial type, the terminal ileum is empty and motionless; for the papillary type, the ileum is full and about to discharge its contents; and for the intermediate type, the ileum has some content, although it is not full.[7]

Normal Mucosal Appearance

The visual characteristics of normal mucosa depend, as is true elsewhere in the GI tract, on a variety of factors which we may call intrinsic or extrinsic. Intrinsic factors relate to actual mucosal characteristics, and those which are extrinsic relate to conditions under which the examination is performed, e.g.: (a) the amount and quality of the illumination provided in relation to the width and length of the segment to be examined; (b) the presence of stool or fluid; and (c) the sharpness of resolution provided by the endoscopic optical system. These extrinsic factors need to be considered when assessing, for example, a somewhat reddened appearance of the mucosa in a segment of poorly prepared colon where there is either extraneous fecal material or fluid to absorb much of the light. Another example is when the segment to be examined is so large it diffuses the light (Fig. 39-29a) so that what is reflected is of low intensity and therefore red (Fig. 39-31a). We consider these extrinsic factors in more detail in Chapter 40. What follows is a consideration of the normal mucosa appearance which would be expected under conditions of perfect illumination and preparation.

Color

The color is typically gray-pink with yellow highlighting (Fig. 39-31b). With more intense illumination, as can be provided by some light sources, the highlighting appears yellow-white (Fig. 39-31c). Conversely, when the illumination is less bright, the mucosa appears a deeper pink or even red (Fig. 39-31a).

Character

As observed with currently used instruments, the mucosa is essentially smooth. Mucus secretion provides the mucosa

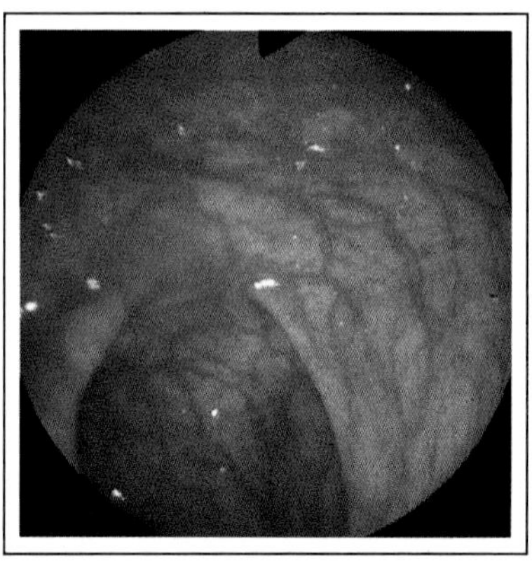

FIG. 39-31a.

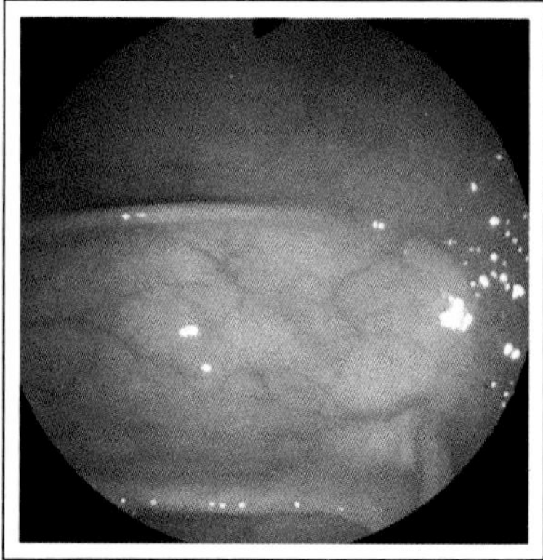

FIG. 39-31b.

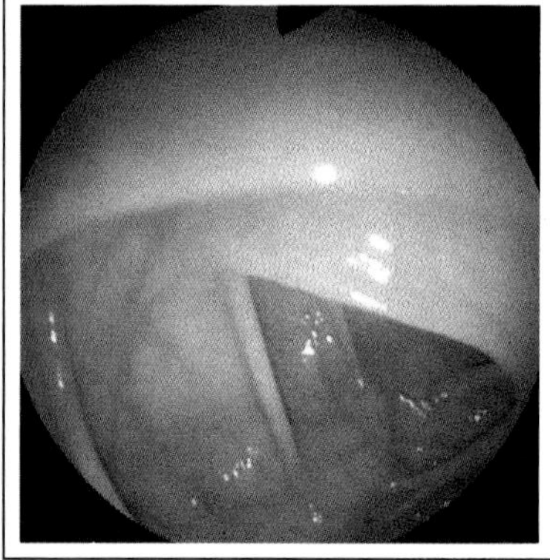

FIG. 39-31c.

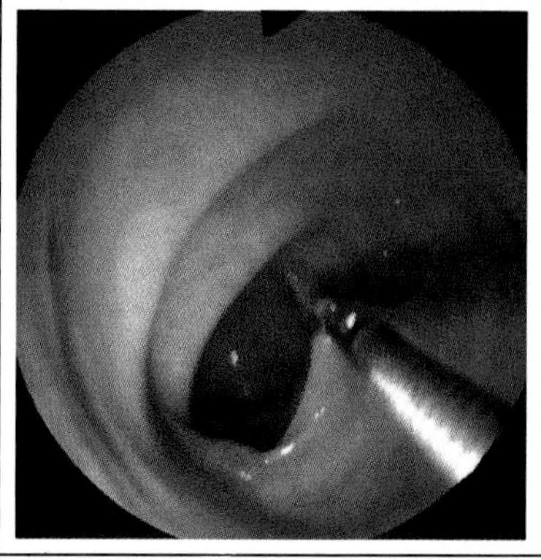

FIG. 39-31d.

FIG. 39-31. a: Normal colonic mucosa (ascending colon). Because of the width of the segment, the mucosa is poorly illuminated and appears reddened. Biopsies, however, were entirely normal. **b:** Normal colonic mucosa (sigmoid). With adequate illumination the mucosa appears gray-pink with yellow highlights. The vascular pattern, although somewhat diminished, is appropriate for the sigmoid. Overall the mucosa has a glistening surface quality. **c:** Normal colonic mucosa (transverse colon). With intense illumination, the mucosa appears yellow-white with little pink. **d:** Tenting of a sigmoid valvular fold. Even though prominent, the fold tents freely, being pulled up for a considerable distance with a biopsy forceps.

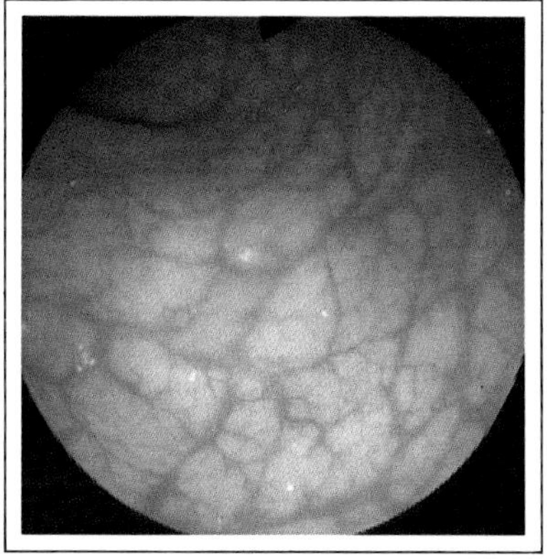

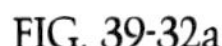

FIG. 39-32a.

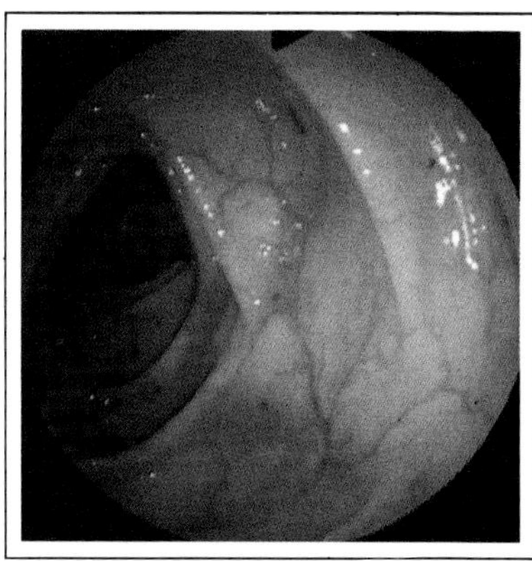

FIG. 39-32b.

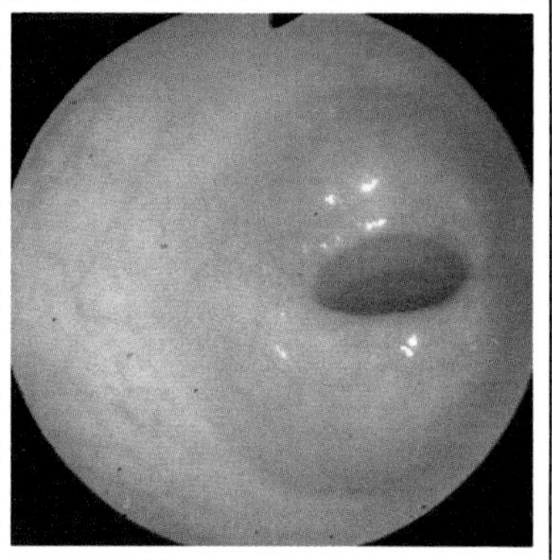

FIG. 39-32c.

FIG. 39-32. a: Normal mucosal vascular pattern in the rectum. At close range, several orders of fine branching can be identified, similar to the branching of a tree. **b:** Normal mucosal vascular pattern, transverse colon. The large mucosal vessels are found in the transverse colon. **c:** Normally absent vascular pattern, descending colon. Just distal to the splenic flexure it is not unusual to find vascular pattern absent. Biopsies were entirely normal.

with a film, giving it its characteristic moist, glistening appearance (Fig. 39-31b).

Mucosal Folds

The most characteristic feature of colonic mucosa is its arrangement into interhaustral folds (or valvulae). These vary tremendously as to height and intervening distance throughout the colon. They may be separated by only millimeters as in the sigmoid (Fig. 39-31b) or by several centimeters as in the ascending colon (Fig. 39-29b). They may be short as in the descending colon or sigmoid (less than 5 mm tall) (Fig. 39-31b) or greater than 1.5 cm as in the transverse colon (Fig. 39-29a). Regardless of their other characteristics, they generally have sharp terminations with a maximum width at their peaks of less than 5 mm (Fig. 39-29d). In addition, they are exceedingly pliant, being freely movable for a considerable distance when tented with a biopsy forceps (Fig. 39-31d).

Mucosal Vascular Pattern

A striking feature of colonic mucosa is its vascular pattern. This consists of submucosal vessels which are readily observed through the normally transparent mucosa. They are typically reddish blue, 1 to 2 mm in diameter, and can be observed to branch for at least one if not several divisions into extremely fine capillaries (Fig. 39-32a). The particular mucosal vascular pattern depends on the location, with the most prominent vessels being seen in the rectum (Fig. 39-32a) and transverse colon (Fig. 39-32b) with a less apparent to absent vascular pattern in the sigmoid or descending colon (Fig. 39-32c).

REFERENCES

1. Nagy, G. S. (1981): Preparing the patient. In: *Colonoscopy*, edited by R. H. Hunt and J. D. Waye, pp. 19–26. Chapman and Hall, London.
2. DeLuca, V. A. (1980): Preparation of the colon for flexible sigmoidoscopy and colonoscopy. *Gastrointest. Endosc. (Suppl.)*, 26:7S–9S.
3. Thomas, G., Brozinsky, S., and Isenberg, J. I. (1982): Patient acceptance and effectiveness of a balanced lavage solution (Golytely) versus the standard preparation of colonoscopy. *Gastroenterology*, 82:435–437.
4. Hunt, R. H. (1981): Colonoscopy intubation techniques with fluoroscopy. In: *Colonoscopy*, edited by R. H. Hunt and J. D. Waye, pp. 109–146. Chapman and Hall, London.
5. Waye, J. D. (1981): Colonoscopy intubation techniques without fluoroscopy. In: *Colonoscopy*, edited by R. H. Hunt and J. D. Waye, pp. 147–178. Chapman and Hall, London.
6. Shinya, H. (1982): *Colonoscopy: Diagnosis and Treatment of Colonic Diseases.* Igaku-Shoin Medical Publishers, New York.
7. Nagasako, K., and Takemoto, T. (1973): Endoscopy of the ileocecal area. *Gastroenterology*, 65:403–411.

40

THE COLON—VARIATIONS FROM THE NORMAL APPEARANCE

As in the case of other parts of the gastrointestinal (GI) tract, during the examination of the colon the endoscopist may encounter structural and mucosal appearances which have an uncertain meaning. Some of these relate to the shape of the lumen, as in the case where it seems to terminate abruptly, giving the examiner the impression of either fixation, angulation, or spasm—singly or in combination. Other structural findings of uncertain significance relate to the appearance of an unusually prominent interhaustral fold or ileocecal valve. Finally, the mucosal appearances themselves, e.g., erythema or erosions, may come to be regarded as suggestive of inflammation unless their entirely nonspecific nature is appreciated.

STRUCTURAL APPEARANCES

Shape of the Lumen

The shape of the lumen most often comes into question in cases where the colon can not be examined in its entirety. Although it is often stated that with experience an examiner can expect to reach the cecum 90% of the time or more, some report a different result, especially when the endoscopist has performed fewer than 50 examinations. In one such series the cecum was reached in only 36% of cases.[1] Even experienced examiners may fail to reach the cecum more than 10% of the time.[2] The commonest reason for an incomplete examination is generally the examiner's inability to overcome "difficult colonic anatomy" with the commonest site of termination the transverse colon.[1] We find, along with the transverse colon and the descending colon, that the sigmoid function is a frequent terminating point for the examination, especially if there is a gamma loop (see Chapter 39) or other unreducible type of sigmoid bow. In these instances the endoscopist wonders if an anatomic reason may account for his failure, e.g., fixation of a loop by adhesions from previous surgery, mesenteric fibrosis, or even occult carcinoma. In some cases there may be adhesions from pelvic surgery[2] or other anatomic causes of a configuration of the sigmoid or transverse colon that makes further advancement impossible. However, we find that in most cases it is the particular colonic anatomy itself, i.e., redundant sigmoid or transverse colon, which causes the examination to fail. In these cases no technique suffices. Still, there are some appearances which cause the examiner to consider the failure the result of pathologic obstruction rather than inadequate technique. These are: (a) fixation; (b) angulation; (c) an atypical location of the lumen; and (d) spasm.

Fixation

The point at which the examiner is forced to terminate the procedure short of the cecum may give the subjective impression that failure was due to the colon's being fixed; that is, the tip is prevented from further advancement because of something external to the segment of the colon which has been reached (Fig. 40-1a). This impression, however, is based solely on the fact that the tip does not move. In fact, for many such cases no fixation of the colon is found at surgery. Therefore for the endoscopist to suggest either adhesions, mesenteric fibrosis, or occult carcinoma based on his subjective impression of fixation is unjustified. All one can legitimately state from failure to advance beyond some point is simply that the examination could proceed no farther. No other conclusion is warranted unless there were other findings, e.g., a mass, a narrowing associated with the loss of the mucosal fold pattern, or extrinsic compression to suggest mechanical obstruction (see Chapter 45). Another "proof" of fixation sometimes suggested is the failure to reduce or straighten a sigmoid or transverse colon bow using standard techniques because of the instability of the tip. However, straightening is dependent on

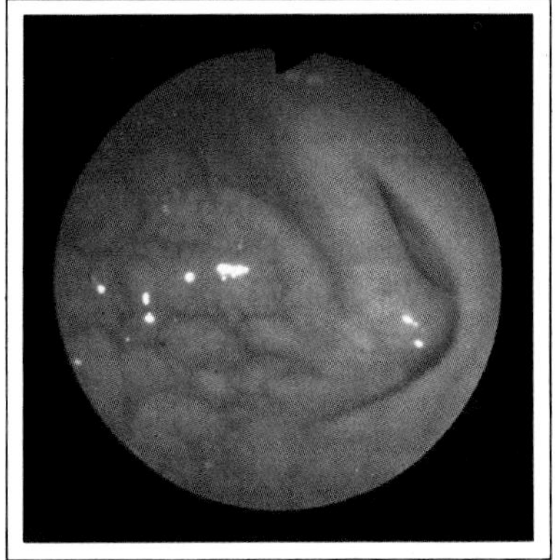

FIG. 40-1a.

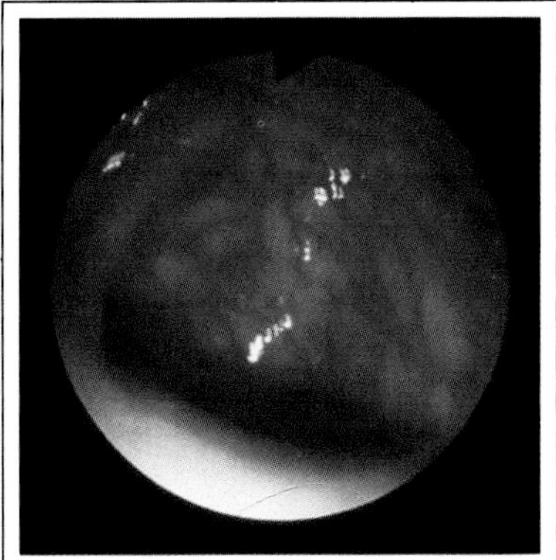

FIG. 40-1b.

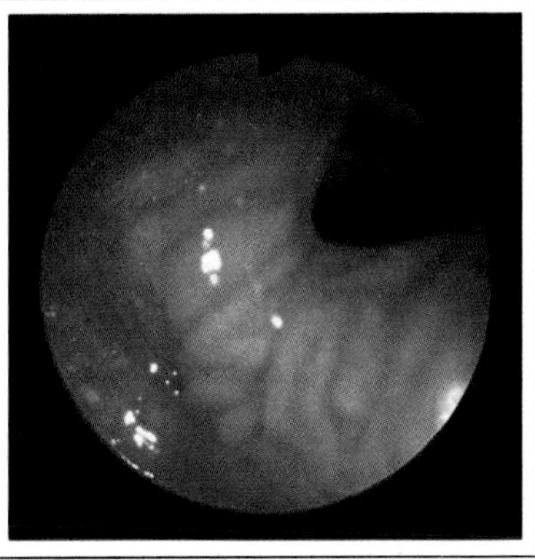

FIG. 40-1c.

FIG. 40-1. a: Splenic flexure, with fixation. The examination, performed because of a suspected carcinoma of the transverse colon, could not proceed beyond this point. The direction of the lumen (confirmed fluoroscopically) toward the left side of the patient rather than to the right could not be changed despite a variety of maneuvers, suggesting fixation of this segment. At subsequent surgery, however, neither fixation nor any other explanation was forthcoming for this appearance. **b:** Descending colon-sigmoid (DS) junction, angulation. The DS junction could not be traversed. The location of its angulus in the 6 o'clock lens position suggests that in the course of sigmoid intubation a gamma loop was formed (see Chapter 39). The colonoscopist's inability to continue the examination past this point was attributed to fixation and sharp angulation of the DS junction, but at subsequent surgery neither fixation nor any other anatomic explanation was forthcoming to explain the examiner's inability to pass into the descending colon. **c:** Sigmoid colon, spasm. The examiner had to terminate in the proximal sigmoid. Although some relaxation of the valvulae was noted after the administration of glucagon (seen as an increase in luminal diameter), it was insufficient to allow further intubation of the cecum. A change in luminal diameter after glucagon suggested spasm of enlarged valvulae; whether this is of any clinical significance is unknown.

the success of the hooking maneuver (see Chapter 39), which itself is highly variable. Failure to maintain the tip position says only that the technique itself was unsuccessful, not that the segment was fixed.

Angulation

Closely related to the idea of fixation is the concept that failure to hook into an adjacent loop implies a sharply angulated junction (Fig. 40-1b) and therefore some underlying pathology. The ability to perform the hooking maneuver is a matter of technique which can be accomplished routinely by some examiners and only occasionally by others. The sharply angulated junction may be more in the mind of the examiner who fails to hook successfully into an adjacent segment. Generally, failure to advance is associated with the formation of a bow in the loop where the tip is positioned. This may cause stretching of the mucosa around the tip and make it appear narrow or otherwise deformed, giving the examiner the impression of a pathologic stricture. However, the intactness and pliancy of the mucosal folds at the point where the tip is lodged should suggest an alternate and usually correct explanation to the examiner that the angulation is simply the result of technical failure rather than underlying pathology.

Atypical Location of the Lumen

As already mentioned, the formation of a bow may distort the appearance of the termination point, causing it to appear deformed with an eccentric appearance of one of its walls (Fig. 40-1a). In the case of a transverse colon bow, this is the result of the descent of the transverse colon into the lower abdomen or pelvis with a sharp angulation point created on its antimesenteric border. It is not uncommon to see this as an eccentrically appearing angulus, which could lead one to suspect extrinsic compression. However, the careful examiner considers the position of the endoscope as well as the presence of a bow when judging the significance of any alteration in the shape of the lumen.

Spasm

If the valvulae of the sigmoid are especially prominent and initial attempts at passing these prove fruitless, the endoscopist may view this as evidence of spasm (Fig. 40-1c). This is especially true if after the administration of 1 to 2 mg of glucagon these valvulae relax, so that the tip can be negotiated beyond this point. If this sequence is witnessed, some endoscopists conclude that they have observed the colonoscopic equivalent of the irritable digestive tract syndrome. The significance of relaxation of the val-

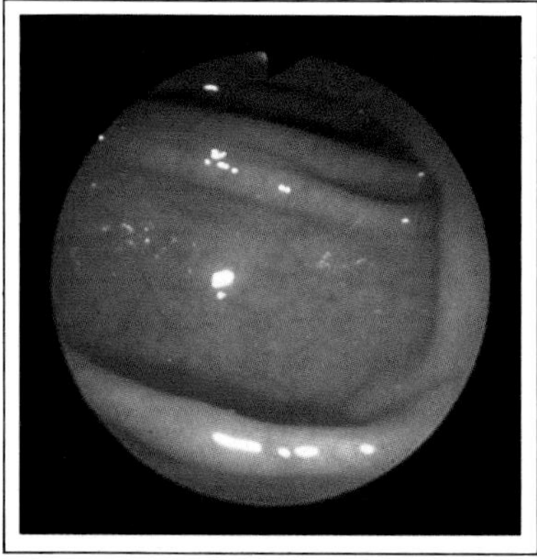

FIG. 40-2a.

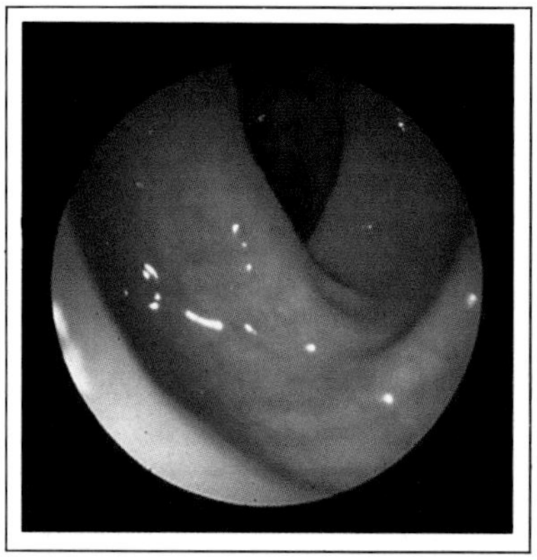

FIG. 40-2b.

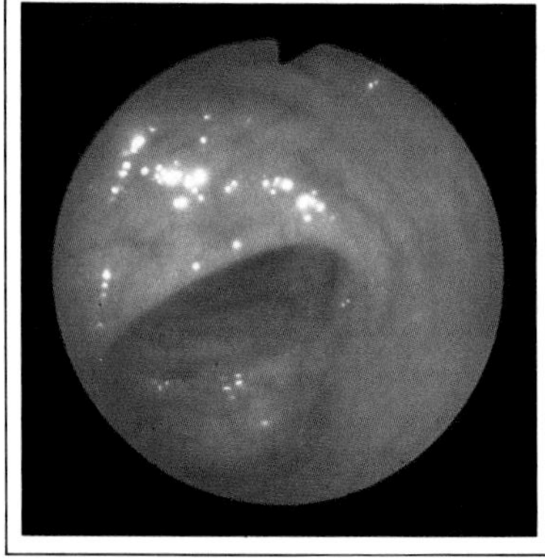

FIG. 40-2c.

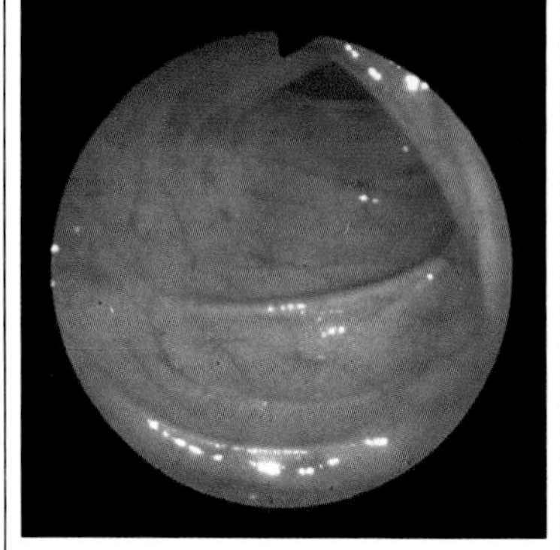

FIG. 40-2d.

FIG. 40-2. a: Sigmoid colon valvulae. The individual valvulae, 5 mm in height and 3 mm in width, are well within the expected range. **b:** Sigmoid colon, enlarged valvulae. In this case the height of the valvulae ranges between 5 and 10 mm and the width in excess of 5 mm. This enlargement may be from circular muscle hypertrophy; however, the clinical significance of this finding, particularly in relation to the irritable bowel syndrome,[3] is unsettled. **c:** Descending colon, valvulae. Just distal to the splenic flexure the valvulae are decreased to absent as a normal finding, even with a diminished or an absent mucosal vascular pattern (d). **d:** Descending colon, decreased vascular pattern. The diminutive valvulae as well as the markedly decreased vascular pattern were interpreted as "possible quiescent ulcerative colitis." Biopsies in this case, however, revealed normal histology.

vulae in response to glucagon is uncertain, however. In cases where the spasm occurs in conjunction with prominent, thickened valvulae, it may be reasonable to conclude that the symptoms which prompted colonoscopy may be related to this finding. This is especially true if the symptoms are characteristic of the irritable digestive tract syndrome, i.e., pain after meals relieved by defecation or pain associated with chronic constipation.[3] However, as the colonoscopist should be quick to point out, the finding of prominent sigmoid valvulae which relax in response to glucagon is by no means proof that this condition is present.

Appearance of the Mucosal Folds (Valvulae)

The endoscopist who expects to find uniformity in the appearance of the mucosal folds of the colon, especially of the sigmoid or descending colon, will be disappointed by the extreme variability in these areas.[4] This variability has not been systematically studied, nor have appearances such as enlarged valvulae of the sigmoid been correlated with symptoms. It is therefore a finding which must be regarded as of unknown significance. In this section we consider briefly two appearances of the valvulae which may impress the endoscopist as being atypical or abnormal: (a) enlarged valvulae, especially those of the sigmoid; and (b) its opposite, the absence of valvulae.

Enlarged Valvulae of the Sigmoid

The variation in the size of the valvulae of the sigmoid is striking, ranging from a height and width of just several millimeters (Fig. 40-2a) to greater than 5 mm in both dimensions. Such valvulae frequently come to one's attention because they are difficult to negotiate and may be associated with spasm (Fig. 40-2b). As already mentioned, the significance of enlarged valvulae in relation to symptoms suggestive of the irritable digestive tract syndrome remains speculative.[3]

Absent Valvulae

In contrast to the closely set valvulae of the sigmoid, those of the descending colon are spaced more widely apart and in some cases are absent altogether (Fig. 40-2c). Here the descending colon appears as a hollow tube and resembles the featureless appearance of quiescent ulcerative colitis (see Chapter 43), especially if the mucosal vascular pattern is absent, as not uncommonly occurs in the descending colon (Fig. 40-2d) with a completely normal histologic appearance (see below). We find that absent valvulae occur in as many as 15% of the descending colons we examine, and this in itself or even a colon with an altered vascular pattern should not make one conclude that inflammatory bowel disease is present.

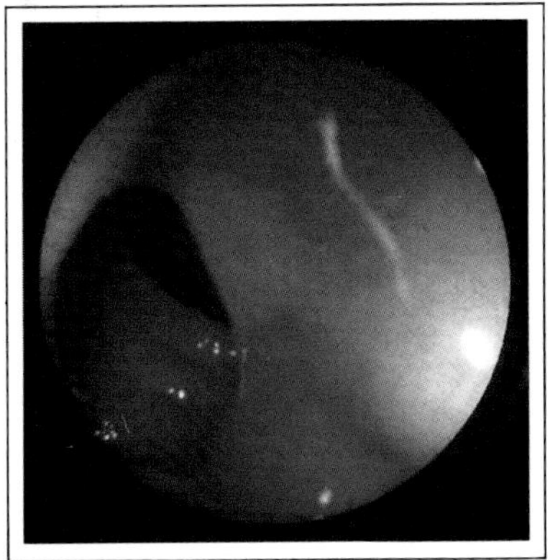

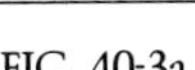

FIG. 40-3a.

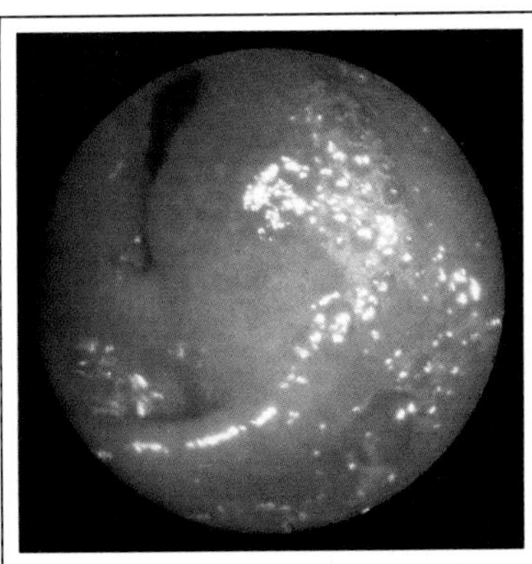

FIG. 40-3b.

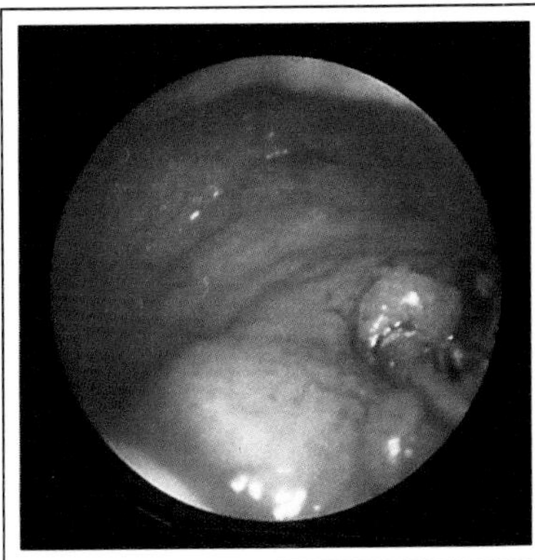

FIG. 40-3c.

FIG. 40-3. a: Prominent (cecal) valvulae simulating a mass. The shape of this mass changed as the mucosa was tented. This along with a biopsy showing normal mucosa suggested that the mass was just a prominent fold. **b:** Mass-like ileocecal valve. The prominent ileocecal valve in this case, especially when viewed eccentrically, gives the appearance of a mass. Tenting suggested that the mass was, in reality, redundant mucosa. Even if the enlargement were believed to be smooth muscle hypertrophy, its clinical significance would still be questionable.[6] **c:** Ileocecal valve lipomatosis. The mass-like ileocecal valve had a somewhat yellow coloration, suggesting the possibility of fatty infiltration (lipomatosis). At the biopsy site a greasy exudate is seen (at 4 o'clock) which was confirmed histologically as fat. Like other mass-like appearances of the ileocecal valve, the clinical significance of lipomatosis is unclear.

Mass-Like Appearances

Three mass-like appearances require special consideration. These are: (a) mass-like mucosal folds (valvulae); (b) mass-like appearances of the ileocecal valve; and (c) the everted appendiceal stump.

Mass-Like Folds

Prominent valvulae, especially if redundant, may appear mass-like and simulate lesions (Fig. 40-3a), especially submucosal polyps (see Chapter 41). In these cases the mucosa of the mass appears perfectly intact, and when tented (see Chapter 12) proves to be extremely pliant. Moreover, the shape of the mass may change dramatically on tenting, additional evidence that the mass is simply a fold. This should make one extremely cautious about proceeding with snare biopsy or polypectomy (Fig. 40-3b).

Mass-Like Appearance of the Ileocecal Valve

The papillary-type appearance of the ileocecal valve (see Chapter 39), especially if prominent, may suggest a polypoid mass.[5] Some suggest that this appearance is the result of hypertrophy of the ileocecal valve.[6] There is no general agreement as to the significance, if any, of this finding. In some cases enlargement of the ileocecal valve (Fig. 40-3c) results from fatty infiltration (lipomatosis).[7] Ulceration and bleeding of the ileocecal valve have been described in association with lipomatosis but, like ileocecal hypertrophy, this finding for the most part lacks any clinical significance, being found in many asymptomatic patients.[7] Finally, yet another cause of a mass-like appearance of the ileocecal valve is prolapse.[8] As with the other causes of this appearance, its principal significance is in the potential confusion of this appearance with that of polyps or even cancer.

To determine the type of ileocecal valve appearance, the endoscopist may first wish to administer a peristaltic agent, e.g., metoclopramide 10 mg intramuscularly, to contract the terminal ileum and thus cause it to deposit its contents in the cecum. This serves to both localize the os and potentially change the configuration of the valve once the terminal ileum is empty (see Chapter 39). This maneuver in itself may resolve the issue of the mass-like appearance in that the mass may disappear completely or a significant change may take place in its shape, suggesting its origin to be a prolapse.[8] Some consider the persistence of the mass-like appearance an indication for snare biopsy, although in the absence of ulceration or other feature to suggest carcinoma (see Chapter 42) the utility of determining the histologic origin of the mass-like appearance must be weighed against the potential for injury of the ileocecal valve and possible obstruction if the biopsy is too large or deep.

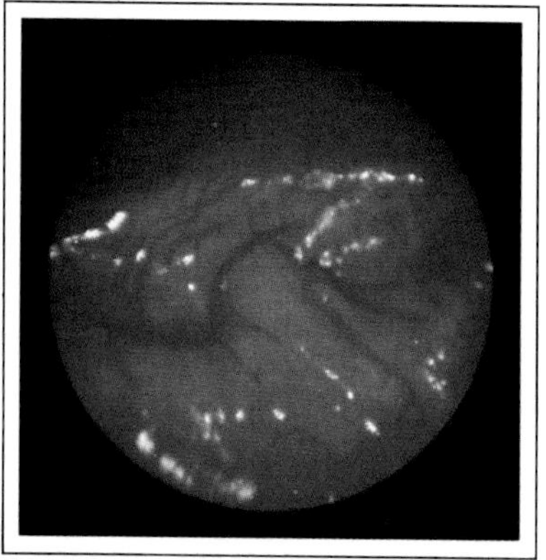

FIG. 40-4a.

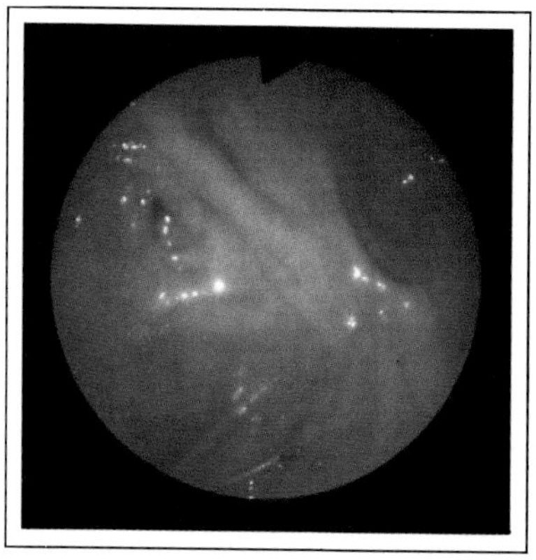

FIG. 40-4b.

FIG. 40-4. a: Everted appendiceal stump. A prominent mucosal fold appears in the cecum in a location where the appendix is expected. This finding in a patient with a previous appendectomy suggests an everted appendiceal stump. **b:** The expected appearance of the appendiceal orifice (at 9 o'clock) is that of a dimple-like depression.

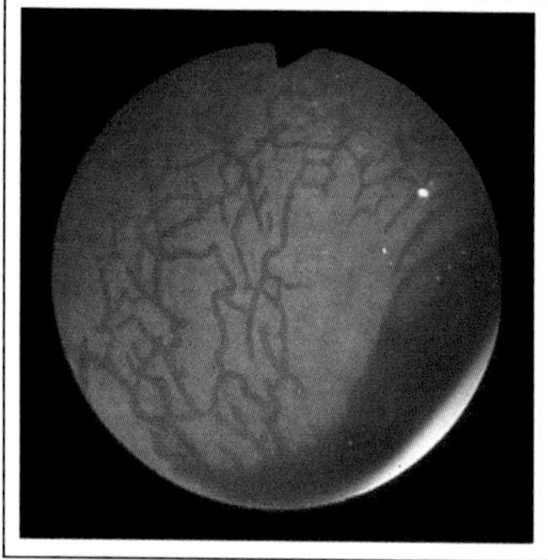

FIG. 40-5a.

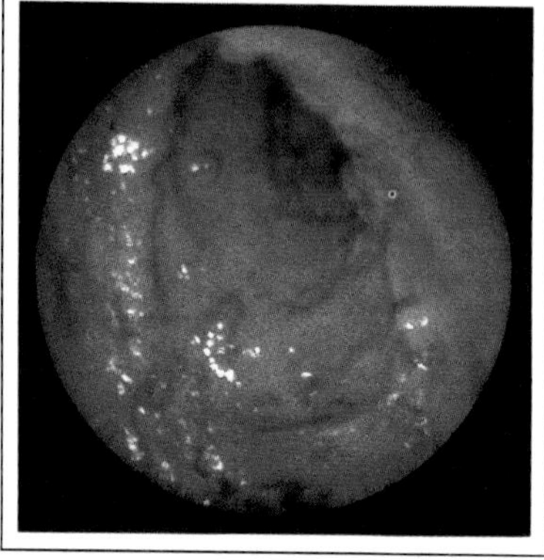

FIG. 40-5b.

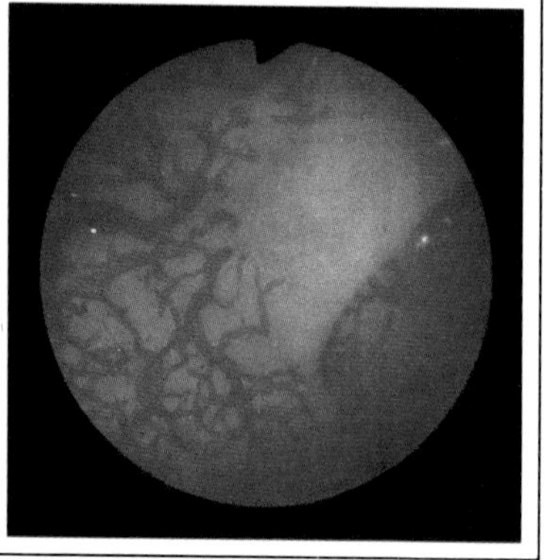

FIG. 40-5c.

FIG. 40-5. a: Ascending colon with apparent erythema. Because of its size, there is diminished illumination, especially when a low-intensity light source is used. The reflection of light from the red end of the spectrum causes the mucosa to appear erythematous, suggesting mucosal inflammation. Biopsies in this case were normal. **b:** Apparent erythema because of poor preparation. Fecal material smears the lens and decreases the delivery of light to the segment to be examined, causing the mucosa to appear erythematous. **c:** Fleet enema effect. Prior to colonoscopy a Fleet enema was used mistakenly, resulting in erythema and an accentuated vascular pattern which might suggest mucosal inflammation to the inexperienced examiner. Biopsies in this case could also show acute inflammation.

Everted Appendiceal Stump

In a patient who has had an appendectomy, eversion of the appendiceal stump may be associated with a prominent mass-like deformity (Fig. 40-4a) rather than the expected deep mouth of the appendix (Fig. 40-4b). This mass-like deformity can easily be mistaken for a submucosal polyp[9] with potentially disastrous results if polypectomy were attempted, although successful endoscopic removal of an appendiceal stump has been reported.[10] The location of a mass with apparently intact mucosa (Fig. 40-4b) in the base of the cecum in a patient with a history of an appendectomy should always raise the possibility of an everted appendiceal stump and make the examiner cautious about proceeding with an electrosurgical procedure.[9]

MUCOSAL APPEARANCES

The colonoscopist may be confronted with three nonspecific mucosal appearances which can be potentially confused with those of inflammatory bowel disease (see Chapter 43). These are: (a) mucosal erythema; (b) mucosal erosions; and (c) an absent vascular pattern.

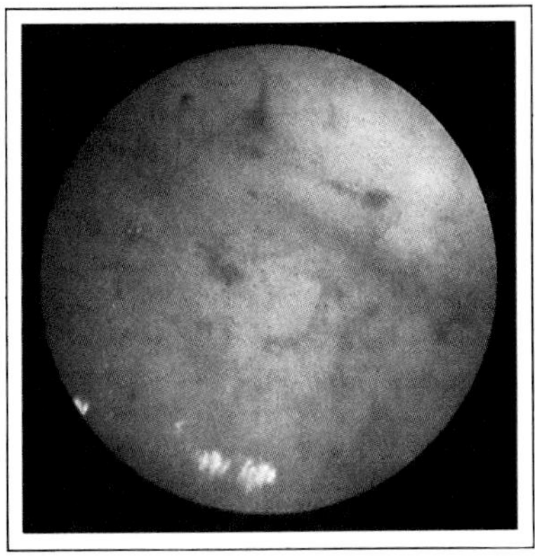

FIG. 40-6a.

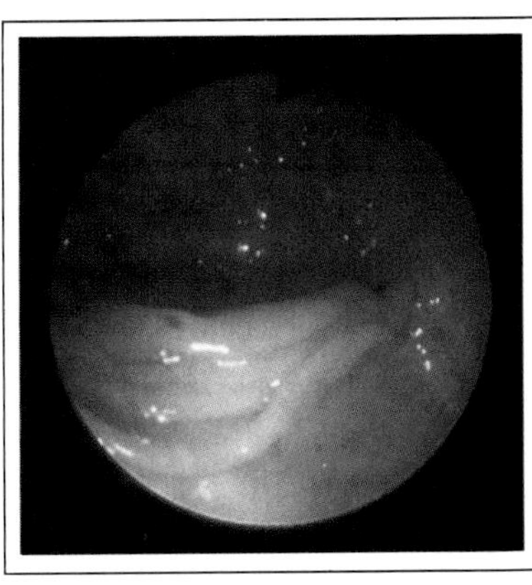

FIG. 40-6b.

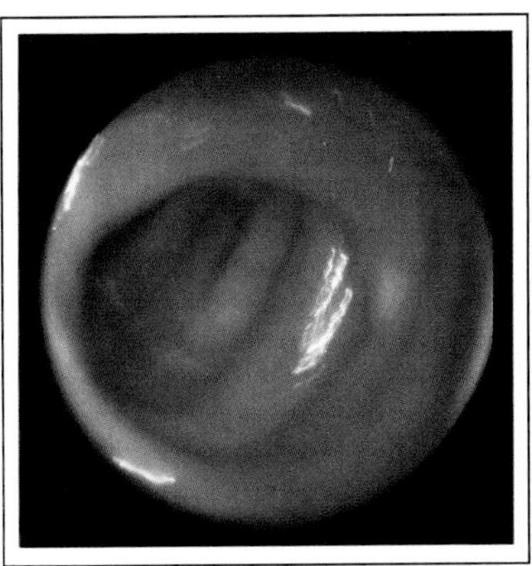

FIG. 40-6c.

FIG. 40-6. a: Endoscope-induced erythema and intramucosal hemorrhage. Because of this location in the right colon, the question of angiodysplasia was considered (see Chapter 46), although the number of small, focal red spots in a case where difficulty in intubation was encountered should always suggest instrumental artifact. **b:** Endoscope-induced intramucosal hemorrhage of the sigmoid. A solitary, perfectly round, intensely red spot in this location suggests a suction artifact, although angiodysplasia cannot altogether be excluded (see Chapter 46). **c:** Absent vascular pattern in the sigmoid. We find an absent or distorted vascular pattern for this location in 15 to 20% of patients with an otherwise normal examination. As in this case, biopsies show no histologic abnormality.

Mucosal Erythema

Mucosal erythema, a nonspecific appearance, may result from a variety of causes; however, we find two to be most often the case: (a) defective illumination; and (b) the use of irritants in preparation of the colon.

Defective Illumination

Inadequate illumination may result from any one of the following: (a) coating of the lens with stool; (b) previous radiation damage to the light guide or lens system; or (c) an inadequate light source. Alone or in combination, these result in an amount of light delivered to the lumen which does not provide adequate illumination (Fig. 40-5a). The red end of the light spectrum is thus reflected, creating the impression of diffused mucosal erythema and raising the possibility of inflammatory bowel disease or other type of colitis. In the presence of a poorly prepared colon that contains either stool or iron (Fig. 40-5b), or where the intensity of illumination is at a low level, the examiner should be exceedingly cautious about making a diagnosis of an inflammatory condition. He may wish to repeat the examination at a time when the colon is better prepared or, if possible, proceed with multiple biopsies even though preparation is poor. He should not offer a potentially confusing diagnostic impression such as "possible colitis" or "suspicious for colitis."

Use of Irritating Laxatives to Prepare the Colon

Agents such as Fleet Phospho-Soda are capable of producing mucosal erythema due to capillary dilatation.[11] The erythema may be so prominent as to obscure even the large mucosal capillaries and create the impression of both erythema and distorted vascular patterns suggestive of inflammation (Fig. 40-5c). This appearance may confuse the examiner, causing him to suspect inflammatory bowel disease if he is not aware of the effects of certain laxatives on colonic mucosa. In all cases where the changes seem to be confined to the rectum, the patient should be carefully questioned as to which laxatives were used. As histologic changes may also be associated with the use of laxatives,[11] biopsies should not be taken when there is suspicion of an acute laxative effect. The patient should simply be rescheduled and prepared in a nonirritating fashion with the use of 0.5 N saline enemas (see Chapter 39).

Mucosal Erosions

Discrete, intensely reddened areas may be found for which the term erosion is sometimes used. These may be confused with similar appearances in inflammatory bowel disease (see Chapter 43) and are thought to indicate the presence of vascular abnormalities (see Chapter 46). Two types of erosion occur which do not indicate a pathologic condition: those which are instrument-induced and those which are enema-induced.

Instrument-Induced Erosions

In the course of performing the examination, traumatic effects are common even when the examiner sees the lumen most of the time (see Chapter 39). This trauma to the mucosa results in focal intermucosal bleeding. On withdrawal, an area so traumatized shows single or multiple intensely reddened areas 3 to 10 mm in diameter or occasionally larger (Fig. 40-6a). Typically, these occur between sharply angular segments of bowel, e.g., the descending colon-sigmoid junction. The multiplicity and their location at a point where blind intubation may have proceeded should always cause the examiner to suspect this appearance to be instrument-induced (Fig. 40-6b).

Enema-Induced Erosions

The tip of the nozzle of an enema bottle or other delivery system may be associated with the production of discrete artifacts from capillary trauma and intramucosal hemorrhage. Their location in the mid-distal rectum should always cause one to consider the possibility of mucosal injury secondary to enemas.

Absent Mucosal Vascular Pattern

Distortion and/or absence of the submucosal vascular pattern when seen extensively throughout the colon is a valid sign of quiescent inflammatory bowel disease, i.e., atrophy (see Chapter 43). We have, however, already noted that within the descending colon and sigmoid the vascular pattern may be decreased or absent (Fig. 40-6c) in the face of normal histology, so that this finding is not pathognomonic of mucosal atrophy, i.e., quiescent inflammatory bowel disease. Any question about the nature of this appearance (normal versus inflammatory bowel disease) should be resolved by means of multiple biopsies taken at 10-cm intervals (see Chapter 43).

REFERENCES

1. Cowan, R. E., Gould, S. R., and Levine, D. F. (1981): An assessment of the diagnostic success of colonoscopy. *Gastroenterology,* 80:1129.
2. Nivatvongs, S., Fryd, D. S., and Fang, D. (1982): How difficult is total colonoscopy? *Gastrointest. Endosc.,* 28:140.
3. Drossman, D. A., Powell, D. W., and Sessions, J. T. (1977): The irritable bowel syndrome. *Gastroenterology,* 73:811–822.
4. Overholt, B. (1975): Colonoscope: a review. *Gastroenterology,* 68:1308–1320.
5. Nagasako, K., and Takemoto, T. (1973): Endoscopy of the ileocecal area. *Gastroenterology,* 65:403–411.
6. Lasser, E. C., and Rigler, L. G. (1955): Ileocecal valve syndrome. *Gastroenterology,* 28:1–16.
7. Seabrook, D. B., Stevens, R., and Scholl, V. (1956): Lipomatosis of the ileocecal region. *Am. J. Surg.,* 92:214–221.
8. Greenwald, R. A., Morris, S. J., and Tedesco, F. J. (1978): Ileocecal valve prolapse: confusion with carcinoma of the cecum. *Am. J. Gastroenterol.,* 70:404–406.
9. Myllarniemi, H., Perttala, Y., and Peltokallio, P. (1974): Tumor-like lesions of the cecum following inversion of the cecum following invasion of the appendix. *Am. J. Dig. Dis.,* 19:547–556.
10. Maas, L. C., Gelzayd, E. A., Uppaputhangkule, V., and Silberberg, B. (1978): Endoscopic removal of an ulcerated appendiceal stump. *JAMA,* 240:248–249.
11. Meisel, J. L., Bergman, D., Graney, D., Saudners, D. R., and Rubin, C. E. (1977): Human rectal mucosa: protoscopic and morphological changes caused by laxatives. *Gastroenterology,* 72:1274–1279.

41

COLONIC POLYPS

Colonic polyps are the commonest pathologic abnormality found at colonoscopy.[1] Polyps, principally tubular adenomas, are found in 20 to 30% of examinations in our unit and in more than half of those performed by others.[1] This high percentage reflects the prevalence in the adult population, with at least one polyp being found in as many as 50% of colons removed at autopsy.[2] Furthermore, colonic polyps are expected in up to 30% of patients with clinical findings that prompt colonoscopy, e.g., rectal bleeding,[3] a positive test for occult blood,[3] or a rectal polyp found at routine screening proctoscopy.[4] In the case of a rectal polyp, a synchronous polyp found elsewhere in the colon may be expected in up to 50% of patients undergoing colonoscopy for this indication.[4] Finally, the finding of a polyp on a well-performed double-contrast radiographic study of the colon prompted because of rectal bleeding, a positive fecal occult blood (Hemoccult) test, or nonspecific complaints is confirmed at colonoscopy in over 90% of the cases if the area in question is reached.[5] Even for patients with a negative radiologic study of the colon, especially if a single-contrast study is performed because of either gross or occult rectal bleeding, polyps are found in at least 15%.[6]

Colonic polyps may be classified in a variety of ways. The conventional classification utilized in the organization of this chapter has as its major division epithelial and nonepithelial polyps. The epithelial polyps are divided into neoplastic and nonneoplastic, with neoplastic polyps including adenomas (tubular, tubulovillous, and villous) and polypoid carcinomas. In this chapter these are discussed first. Following this, we consider nonneoplastic epithelial polyps which include the hyperplastic type, the hamartomatous (juvenile polyp) type, and the relatively infrequent inflammatory and fibrous-inflammatory polyps. Epithelial polyps may be further divided into those occurring singly or in small numbers in contrast to multiple (>50) polyps that occur as part of polyposis syndromes, which we describe separately. Finally, submucosal polyps, e.g., lipomas, leiomyomas, carcinoids, and other rare types, are discussed in the concluding section of this chapter.

EPITHELIAL POLYPS

Adenomas

Adenomas are the commonest type of polyp noted at colonoscopy as well as the most frequently encountered colonic neoplasm.[1] Histologically, one observes hyperchromic, enlarged nuclei along with stratification and mucin depletion of the neoplastic cells, which are crowded together to form glands.[7] The classification of adenomas as tubular, tubulovillous, or villous depends on the relationship of the neoplastic glands to the surface of the polyps.[7] Tubular adenomas are composed of "predominantly branching tubules embedded or surrounded by lamina propria."[7] The villous adenoma, on the other hand, is composed of "pointed or blunt finger-like processes of lamina propria covered by [neoplastic] epithelium [projecting from the surface of the polyp] which [also] reach down to the muscularis mucosa."[7] Finally, the mixed form, the tubulovillous adenoma, is composed of both tubular and villous elements.[7]

Types of Adenomas and Their Relation to Colonic Cancer

Although possibly still doubted by some, most authorities now accept the polyp-cancer sequence of Morson[8] as the most likely origin of colonic cancer. This is based on four lines of evidence: (a) that the smallest focal cancers are found in polyps rather than flat mucosa; (b) that for a given cancer there is an inverse relationship between the presence of adenomatous tissue and the cancer size and depth of invasion, suggesting that as the cancer grows it destroys the evidence of its adenomatous origin; (c) that adenomas followed over time are observed to progress to frank annular carcinomas; and (d) a study which suggested that the removal of adenomas from the rectum significantly decreases the observed incidence of rectal cancer over that expected in the general population.[8a]

Because of the existence of the polyp-cancer sequence, it is important to consider the relationship of the different types of adenoma to the likelihood of cancer. For adenomas overall, there is a 10% chance of *in situ* cancer (within the head of the polyp but without invasion of the muscularis mucosa) and a 3% chance of a focus of invasive cancer (into or through the muscularis mucosae).[7] The likelihood of invasive cancer increases with the size of the polyp. Invasive cancer is almost never found in polyps of less than 5 mm and is found in less than 1% overall for polyps 5 to 9 mm. For those 1 to 1.9 cm, the figure rises to 3%, whereas in those greater than 2 cm it is 7.5%.[7] The likelihood of invasive cancer also relates to the presence of villous elements. Although to some extent this is also related to the size of the polyp, for any given size the likelihood of cancer with a villous element present is substantially increased,[9a] probably twice that for a simple adenoma of the same size.[9] For a villous adenoma greater than 2.5 cm, the likelihood of invasive cancer approaches 50%.[10] Therefore, although the detection of any polyp of a size equal to or greater than 1.5 cm is important, finding those with villous elements, in particular villous adenomas, seems crucial to lowering significantly the risk of cancer for a given patient.

Colonoscopic Detection of Adenomas

The effective detection of adenomas at colonoscopy requires a thorough awareness of their expected endoscopic appearances. These we consider in the next section. First, however, we concern ourselves with other matters important in the detection of adenomas: (a) the role of radiology; (b) the adenomas' expected locations; (c) their differing sizes; (d) the number of adenomas expected; and (e) the relative frequency of different types of adenoma.

1. *Role of radiology.*

In several retrospective studies, colonoscopy has proven to be superior to radiology in detecting adenomas, especially lesions less than 1 cm.[11,12] This is particularly true for single-contrast examinations where the "miss rate" for adenomas is 50% overall and 25% for adenomas over 1 cm in diameter,[11] with these having the greatest likelihood of associated focally invasive cancer.[7] Although double-contrast radiographic studies of the colon are superior to single-contrast studies if they are meticulously performed, e.g., those employing the Malmo technique,[12] they may still miss up to 10% of polyps found at colonoscopy and 10% of these may be larger than 1 cm.[12] Furthermore, at some institutions what may be called a double-contrast examination may be less revealing than a single-contrast study because of the erratic mixing of air and barium when this has been performed by a technician with little or no supervision from a radiologist. Hence data derived from reports where the Malmo technique was strictly adhered to may not be applicable to every institutional setting.

Although colonoscopy may find more polyps than even a carefully performed double-contrast study, it may still miss significant adenomas of 0.5 to 1.5 cm, especially in the flexure areas (rectosigmoid, descending colon-sigmoid junction, splenic, and hepatic) as well as in segments of great surface area, e.g., the distal transverse colon.[13] In one careful study[14] the miss rate from colonoscopy was approximately 11% (6 of 56 polyps discovered by a combination of both modalities). Five of the six adenomas initially missed were found after careful inspection of the barium enema and a search at a second colonoscopy of both areas that had been suggested radiographically to contain polyps; adenomas were also found in other areas with an especially sharp angulation. In one of the six cases the polyp could not be found at all by colonoscopy but was redemonstrated radiographically. In this study the locations for hidden polyps were the splenic flexure, descending colon, rectosigmoid, and rectum. Because the potential miss rate from colonoscopy alone is 10% and probably higher, if a technically adequate air contrast barium enema is available we believe it should be performed prior to colonoscopy to give the examiner maximum information concerning any suspicious area, especially at the flexure or other areas of sharp angulation. At institutions where only single-contrast studies or a suboptimal double-contrast examination is performed, one may wish to proceed directly with colonoscopy because of the low return from this type of barium study. Even with good air contrast, some might elect to proceed directly with colonoscopy in a patient with Hemoccult-positive slides or rectal bleeding because of the increased probability of an adenoma, i.e., 15%+,[6] and a miss rate for colonoscopy that can be expected to be only 10%. In these cases one might wish to reserve colon radiology for follow-up colonoscopy (see below) where polyps, when present, tend to be smaller as well as hidden (and so missed on the first colonoscopy) or in cases where no lesion was found on colonoscopy, but where technical difficulties were encountered. Others, however, advocate double-contrast studies as a standard screening test to be performed prior to colonoscopy in all cases so that any positive finding can be thoroughly evaluated.[15] In general, we subscribe to this latter point of view.

2. *Location of adenomas.*

Several large colonoscopic studies[16,17] have indicated a distribution of adenomas to be largely left-sided, with 65% of the lesions found between the splenic flexure and rectosigmoid junction. In one of the largest reported series—

7,000 polyps removed at colonoscopy—Shinya and Wolff[16] found 77% of tubular adenomas, 79% of tubulovillous adenomas, and 75% of villous adenomas confined to the left colon, including the rectum. In this series the commonest location overall was the sigmoid (48% of tubulovillous adenomas, 47% of tubulovillous adenomas, and 46% of villous adenomas). This was followed by the descending colon, which contained 24 to 26% of each type, and lastly the rectum, containing only 14% of the villous adenomas, and 5% and 6% of the tubular and tubulovillous adenomas, respectively.[16] Even though the percentage of cancers being found on the right side of the colon has been reported to be increased, most colonoscopic studies find the bulk of adenomas to be left-sided. Still, a significant percentage of adenomas, up to 25%, as well as 10% of adenomas with focally invasive cancer were right-sided, especially in elderly patients.[18] Therefore a total colonic examination is required for any patient in whom polyps are suspected.

3. Size.

Large series such as that reported by Shinya and Wolff show most adenomas found at colonoscopy to be within the range of 5 mm to 2 cm, with one-fourth of them between 1.0 and 1.9 cm.[16] Gillespie et al.[17] found 82% of 1,049 polyps visualized to be under 2 cm, with nearly half (48%) less than 1 cm. Only 17.3% in this series were greater than 2 cm, with 35% in the 1.0 to 1.9 cm range.[17]

4. Number.

The majority of patients have a single adenoma, but Gillespie et al. found one or more in addition in 35%.[17] Of this 35%, half (17%) had just one extra, but the remainder (17% of the total) had two or more, and 10% had a total of four or more.[17] As several series have suggested, the additional lesion(s) tend to be right-sided,[4,16-18] so that total colonoscopy is necessary for their identification in up to one-third of the patients where the index of the polyp is found in the rectum or sigmoid.

5. Type.

The commonest polyp identified and removed at colonoscopy is the tubular adenoma, representing 64%[16] and 75%[17] of the total found in two large series, respectively. Tubulovillous adenomas represented 20%[17] and 27%[16] in these series, respectively, and villous adenomas, being the least common type, comprised only 5%[17] and 8%,[16] respectively.

Appearance

Only histologic examination of the polyp, ideally in its entirety, can determine both the type of adenoma—tubular, tubulovillous, or villous—and, more importantly, if it contains invasive cancer. Nevertheless, colonoscopy can provide the examiner with visual clues, both as to the type of polyp and whether it is malignant (see "Polypoid Carcinoma," this chapter). In this section we consider the features which seem to be most useful in predicting the histology of an adenoma.

Tubular adenomas.

Tubular adenomas, the commonest of all adenomas, have no one typical appearance; it varies considerably depending on the size of the polyp. One may therefore subdivide adenomas as to their appearance in relation to size: tiny adenomas (≤3 mm), small adenomas (4 to 9 mm), moderate-size adenomas (10 to 19 mm), and large adenomas (≥2 cm).

1. *Tiny adenomas* (≤3 cm): Adenomas of this size may simply appear as excrescences which have mucosa indistinguishable from that of their surroundings or be intensely erythematous in comparison (Fig. 41-1a). Adenomas of this size are almost always sessile and perfectly smooth.
2. *Small adenomas* (4 to 9 mm): These are smooth, perfectly round, sessile or pedunculated polyps (Fig. 41-1b). Like tiny adenomas, their mucosa may be indistinguishable from that of its surroundings (Fig. 41-1b) or somewhat more erythematous (Fig. 41-1c). If a pedicle is present, it is generally short (Fig. 41-1c), with a diameter of 5 mm or less.
3. *Moderate-size adenomas* (10 to 19 mm): Although these may be perfectly round, as in the case of smaller adenomas, they are often lobulated (Fig. 41-1d). The lobules tend to be on the order of 5 to 10 mm and appear as if two small tubular adenomas were fused together. The mucosa of the polyp tends to be erythematous with a somewhat irregular character to its mucosal surface. The pedicle tends to be thicker than those of the smaller adenomas, having a diameter of 1.0 to 1.5 cm and occasionally larger (Fig. 41-1d). Any polyp whose dimension is 1.5 cm or more should be considered at least potentially as having a thick pedicle, one which the prudent examiner will wish to observe, prior to proceeding with electrosurgical excision (see "Endoscopic Treatment of Colonic Adenomas," this chapter).
4. *Large adenomas* (≥2 cm): These typically are multilobulated with each lobe in excess of 5 mm (Fig. 41-2a). Again, the polyp appears as if it consists of multiple small adenomas fused together to make up one large polyp. Indeed, histologic examination of the polyp often suggests several perfect, small adenomas comprising the larger polyp.

Somewhat surprising is the pedicle of these larger polyps, especially those greater than 3 cm (Fig. 41-2b). Often its diameter is less than 1 cm so that the polyp, despite its size, can be removed easily by electrosurgical excision. Nevertheless, the examiner must define the thickness of the pedicle (Fig. 41-2c) prior to committing himself to an attempt at colonoscopic treatment (see "Visualization of an Adenoma Prior to Electrosurgical Excision," this chapter).

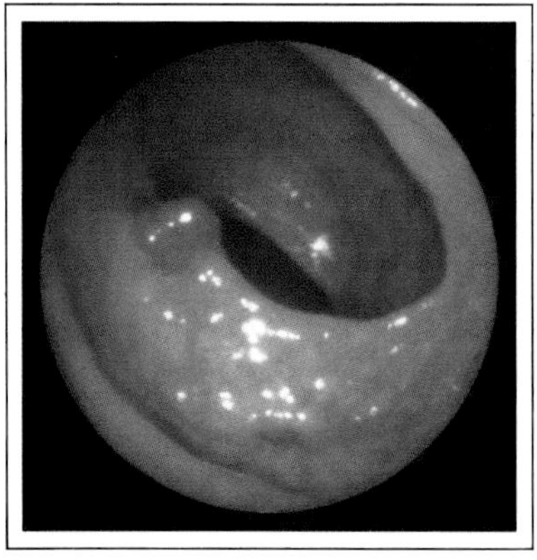
FIG. 41-1a.

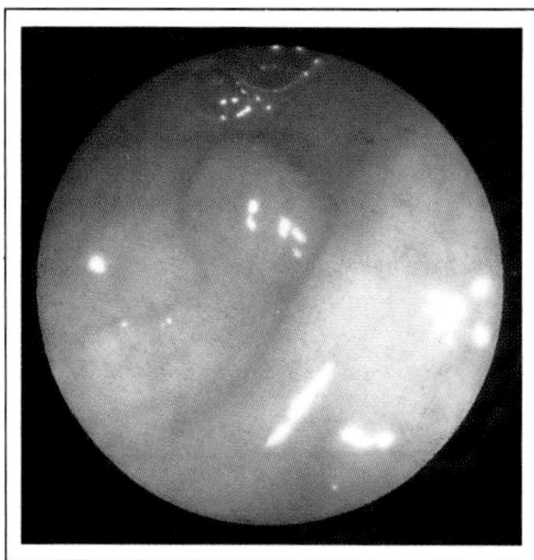
FIG. 41-1b.

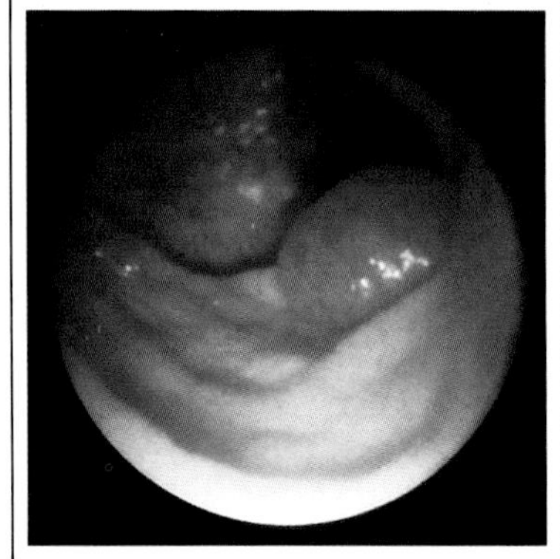
FIG. 41-1c.

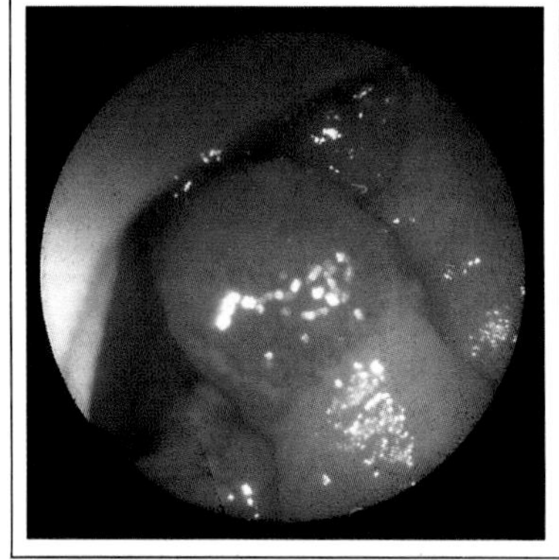
FIG. 41-1d.

FIG. 41-1. a: Adenomas, tiny. A 3-mm slightly erythematous excrescence is visualized on a sigmoid fold, as the smallest example of an adenoma generally found. **b:** Adenoma, small. A 5-mm pale lesion was found in the descending colon. Polyps of this size and location are most often adenomas[28,29] even though the color of their mucosa does not differ from that of the surroundings. **c:** Adenoma, small. A 9-mm somewhat erythematous lesion was visualized just below the splenic flexure. A tiny pedicle can be seen off toward 9 o'clock. **d:** Adenoma, moderate size. A 1.2-cm polyp (head partially obscured by a sigmoid fold) is observed on a 1-cm pedicle. At close range the mucosa of the head of the polyp is irregular, causing the light reflection to break up into tiny dots (i.e., giving it a granular appearance).

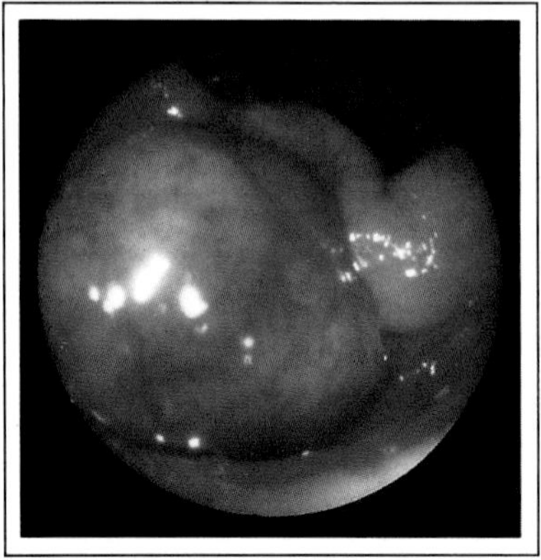
FIG. 41-2a.

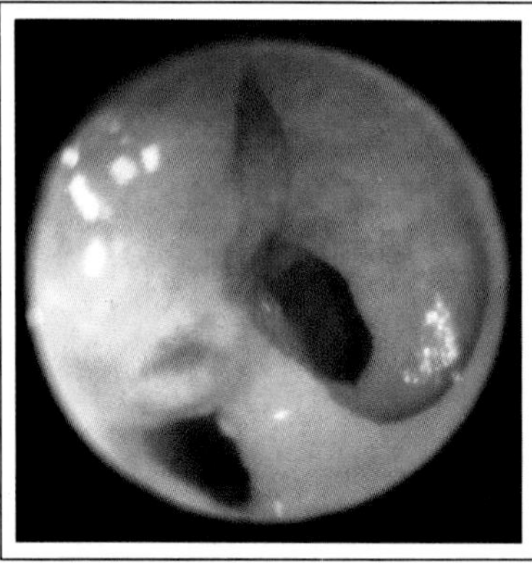
FIG. 41-2b.

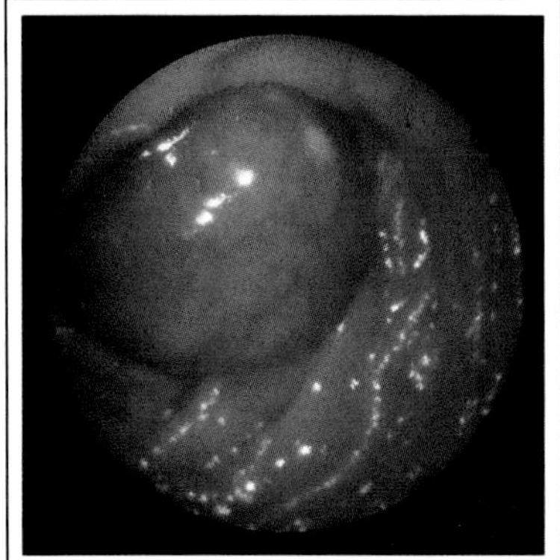
FIG. 41-2c.

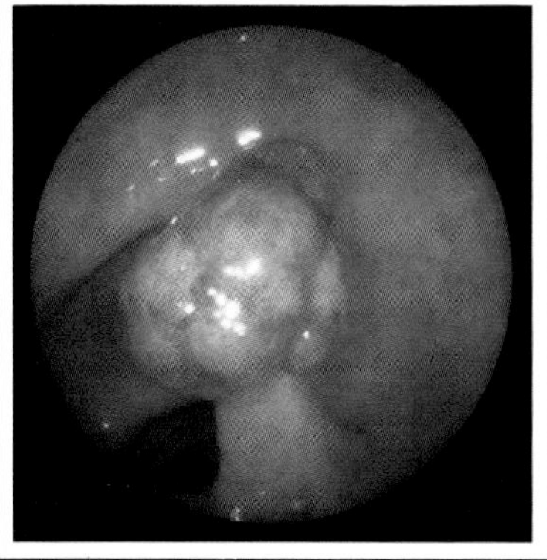
FIG. 41-2d.

FIG. 41-2. a: Adenoma, large. A 2-cm polyp with a relatively thin pedicle (off toward 3 o'clock). The polyp consists of several (approximately 1 cm) lobules, in contrast to the multiple tiny nodules of a villous adenoma (Fig. 41-3a). **b:** Adenoma, large. A 2.5-cm polyp is observed (head partially obscured) with a thin pedicle. As is true of larger polyps, the pedicle is often surprisingly thin, so that the overall size does not preclude polypectomy, so long as the pedicle is well demonstrated. **c:** Adenoma, large. A 2-cm polyp with a perfectly smooth head. **d:** Adenoma, tubulovillous type. A 1.2-cm polyp has a cauliflower appearance, being studded with tiny nodules owing to its villous component.

Tubulovillous adenomas.

Tubulovillous adenomas are generally 1 to 2 cm or larger. As this is the size range for 50% of tubular adenomas,[16,17] size alone does not differentiate these two types of adenoma. In comparison with tubular adenomas (Fig. 41-2c), the surface of the tubulovillous polyp is different, tending to be made irregular by the presence of 1- to 3-mm nodules, the visual representation of its villous component (Fig. 41-2d).

Tubulovillous adenomas may be sessile but more often are pedunculated with a tendency toward wider, shorter pedicles than tubular adenomas, possibly as a result of their villous growth pattern in which the finger-like neoplastic projection tends to grow downward into the muscularis mucosae.[7]

Villous adenomas.

Villous adenomas appear as soft, sessile lesions with a surface consisting of multiple 3- to 6-mm nodules (Fig. 41-3a) projecting off the surface for several millimeters. In some cases these projections are not pronounced, with the diagnosis of villous adenoma simply suggested by the size (>3 cm) and the irregular character of the surface (Fig. 41-3b).

Villous adenomas are, in general, large lesions with a maximum dimension exceeding 1 cm in 90%; approximately half of these are between 1 and 3 cm, and one-third are 3 to 8 cm.[10] In a series of 7,000 adenomas, Shinya and Wolff found 25% of villous adenomas to be greater than 3 cm, whereas only 10% of tubulovillous adenomas and 2.5% of tubular adenomas were of this size.[16] Any sessile polyps of 3 cm or larger therefore may be presumed to have at least a villous component, if it is not itself a villous adenoma. For large villous adenomas which exceed 3 cm, the possibility of malignant degeneration already present which occurs in up to 50%[10] must be considered, especially if the lesion appears to have a central depression or ulceration (Fig. 41-3d).

Endoscopic Treatment of Colonic Adenomas

Ultimately, only histologic examination of a completely excised polyp yields precise information concerning its type and, even more importantly, the presence of invasive carcinoma. This, because of its deep location in the head of the polyp, is not sampled in material obtained from forceps biopsy.[19] In one study in which the information derived from a single forceps biopsy was compared with that from a completely excised polyp, the biopsies failed in 26% of cases (13 of 52) to denote significant histologic features, including carcinoma in four cases.[19] Brush cytology of the surface is also not expected to yield pertinent information about the presence or absence of focal carcinomas deep

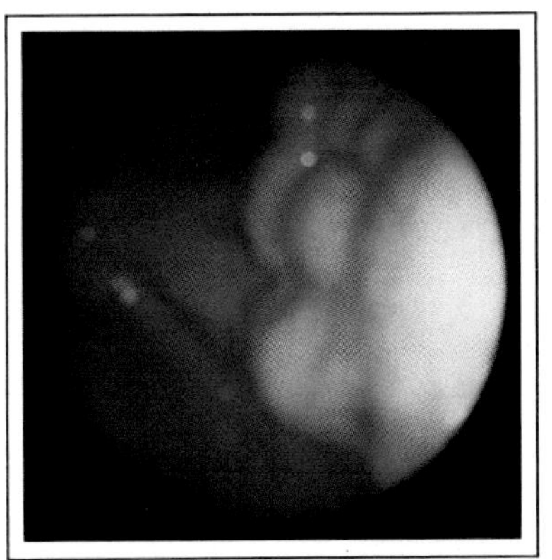

FIG. 41-3a.

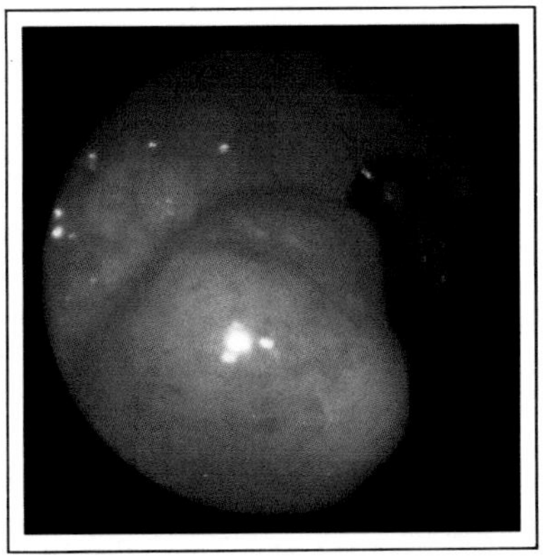

FIG. 41-3b.

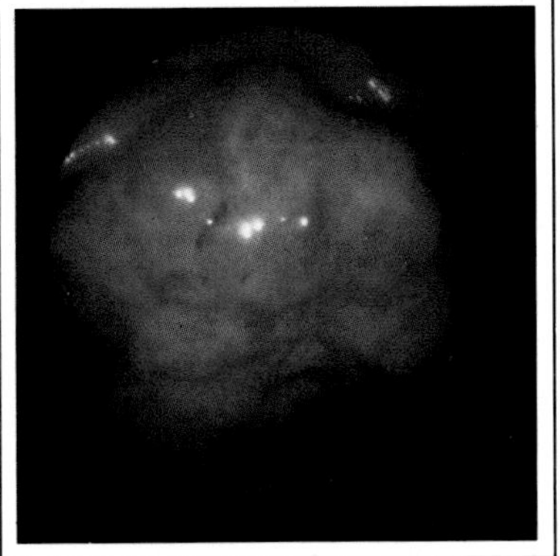

FIG. 41-3c.

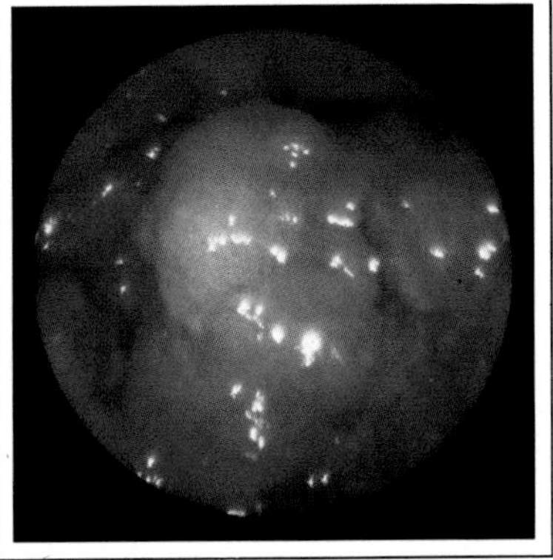

FIG. 41-3d.

FIG. 41-3. Villous adenoma. **a:** This large 3-cm sessile rectal mass has the characteristic nodular surface. The lesion itself is surprisingly soft. **b:** The size of this 3-cm sessile mass, rather than its surface, was the clue to the lesion being a villous adenoma. **c:** A close-up view of a 3-cm sessile mass (b) now reveals nodularity of the surface. **d:** With malignant degeneration. The prominent central depression (at 9 o'clock) within the 3-cm cecal mass suggested the presence of cancer, ultimately proved at surgery.

within the polyp. Worse, it might even prove misleading, if the cytologic features are interpreted as "severe atypia" or "highly suspicious for malignancy" as could be expected in 10 to 15% of large adenomas with carcinoma *in situ*. In such cases cytology might result in a decision for surgery for a polyp which could be satisfactorily treated with endoscopic excision (see "Adequacy of Colonoscopic Excision of an Adenoma with Focal Cancer," this chapter). Rather than a biopsy or brush cytology, colonoscopic polypectomy itself is the diagnostic and therapeutic maneuver of choice for evaluating and treating colonic adenomas. Most endoscopists who have performed at least 25 polypectomies under supervision find it feasible to completely excise most polyps which are less than 2 cm and many polyps 2 to 3 cm. As only 20 to 25% of the polyps are greater than 2 cm, most polyps which are identified are within the excision capability of most examiners.

Prior to performing polypectomy, the examiner should be fully cognizant of the principles of electrosurgery as well as the technique of endoscopic polypectomy. This has been reviewed extensively elsewhere and is not presented here.[20–22a] What we are concerned with in the section which follows are four other matters of concern to the colonoscopist in performing polypectomy: (a) the necessity for visualizing a polyp prior to endoscopic excision; (b) the adequacy of colonoscopic excision of an adenoma containing cancer; (c) the approach to diminutive (tiny) adenomas; and finally (d) follow-up colonoscopy in patients who have had adenomas excised colonoscopically.

Visualization of the adenoma prior to electrosurgical excision.

Before making a decision to proceed with polypectomy, the examiner should make every effort to see the polyp and its pedicle in its entirety so that he may determine whether the polyp, especially its pedicle, is of a size with which he is comfortable. Moreover, he must determine whether polypectomy should be attempted as a single excision or in a piecemeal fashion,[22a] as he would for a large sessile tubulovillous or villous adenoma.[22a,23] Finally, if the examination is performed outside a hospital, he must determine by inspection of the polyp whether the polypectomy procedure should be done in a hospital setting with prior arrangements for typing and cross-matching blood, as might be the case with a polyp on a large (>1.5 cm) pedicle.

To visualize a polyp in its entirety (Fig. 41-4a) we believe it is necessary to place the patient in at least two if not four positions (prone, supine, left and right lateral recumbent) in order to display the polyp to best advantage (Fig. 41-4b). Changing the patient's position in this way often allows determination of the safest position for polypectomy because of both better display of the pedicle (Fig. 41-4c) and the greater distance the position affords between the head of the polyp and the wall of the colon immediately opposite (Fig. 41-4d).

Adequacy of colonoscopic excision of an adenoma with focal cancer.

The histologic finding of cancer in a polyp excised at colonoscopy may be expected in approximately 10%.[7,16] More than half of these are polyps with carcinoma *in situ* (situated in the mucosa of the polyp but not invading the muscularis mucosae).[7,16] Because the lymphatics of an adenoma do not extend into the mucosa,[24] these cancers never metastasize. For these lesions, endoscopic excision is a completely effective therapy.

Invasive carcinoma is found in about 5% of adenomas removed at colonoscopy.[16,17] This is less (about 0.2%) for small adenomas (<1 cm),[17] approaching 6% for those between 1 and 2 cm and 15% for lesions over 2 cm.[17] If one considers adenomas of 2 cm or less, which account for two-thirds of the polyps removed, the expected incidence of invasive cancer is 2% overall but 6% for tubulovillous adenomas (Fig. 41-5a). There is nothing about a polyp which allows one to suspect focally invasive carcinoma other than size (a sixfold increase in incidence for polyps 1 to 2 cm compared with those of less than 1 cm) and nodularity of the surface (Fig. 41-5a), suggesting a villous component (to increase the likelihood of cancer twofold over that of a tubular adenoma of the same size[17]).

For adenomas with focally invasive cancers crossing into the muscularis mucosae, the potential for lymphatic spread is present so that polypectomy, even with an adequate margin of pedicle, may not be curative. The risk of metastasis already present in such cases is controversial, although most studies have suggested a risk of 3 to 5%[25,26] or less. One notable exception was a series reported by Colacchio et al. where 25% (6 of 24 patients) who underwent resection after polypectomy showing focally invasive cancer had evidence of metastasis.[27] As was true of the majority of patients in this study in which metastatic cancer was found, the risk of a noncurative endoscopic excision appears to be greatest if the cancer is poorly differentiated, comes within 6 mm of the margin of the resection, or already appears in blood vessels and lymphatics of the polyp. For such patients, cancer will be present at subsequent surgery, either in the wall of the colon or in lymph nodes in 20%+.[27] Even in the absence of these findings, because of the small but definitve risk (3 to 5%[25]) of colonoscopic excision being inadequate, we favor surgery for a segmental resection, especially in younger patients in whom the surgical risk is less than 1%. For elderly patients whose surgical risk[27a] might approach the risk of cancer, we do not. Unfortunately, one cannot use the appearance of the polypectomy site at 3 or 6 months after the excision as this may be entirely normal in cases where metastasis has already occurred. Only if the cancer was present in the pedicle at the margin of the resection (Fig. 41-5b) would the polypectomy site observed at a future date be likely to show evidence of residual cancer.

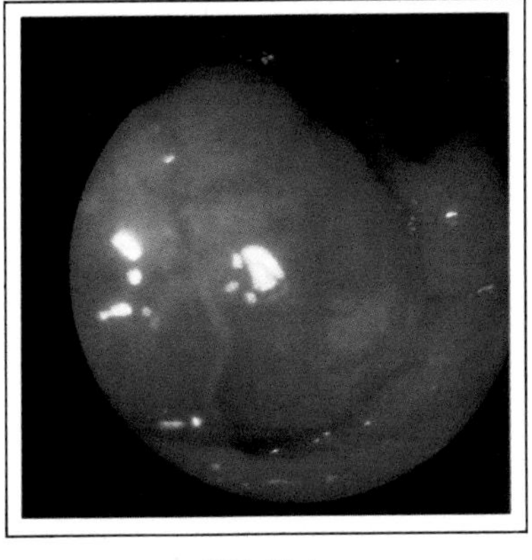

FIG. 41-4a.

FIG. 41-4b.

FIG. 41-4. a: Adenoma, incompletely visualized. Only the head is seen and not the pedicle, which would make an attempt at electrosurgical excision risky unless the pedicle (b) is demonstrated. **b:** Adenoma, better visualized. Changing the patient's position from supine to left lateral recumbency brings a pedicle into view, ensuring a safe polypectomy. **c:** Adenoma with a thick (1.5 cm) pedicle. This was demonstrated after changing the patient's position from the left lateral recumbent to the supine. The large pedicle made the examiner wish to perform the polypectomy in a hospital setting. **d:** Adenoma in relation to the colon wall. A change in the position of the patient allowed for maximum distance between the colon wall and the head of the polyp prior to electrosurgery.

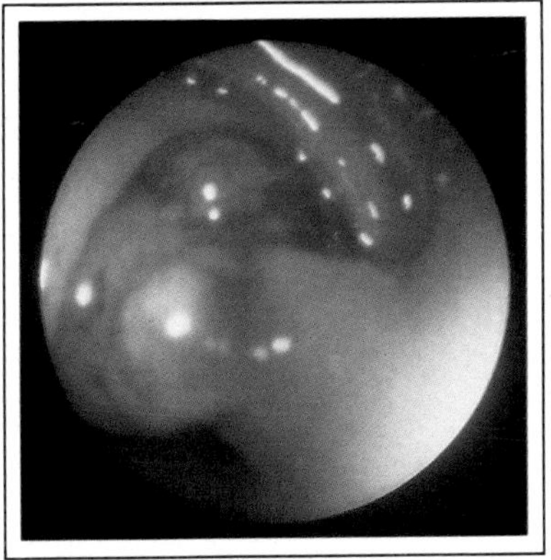

FIG. 41-4c.

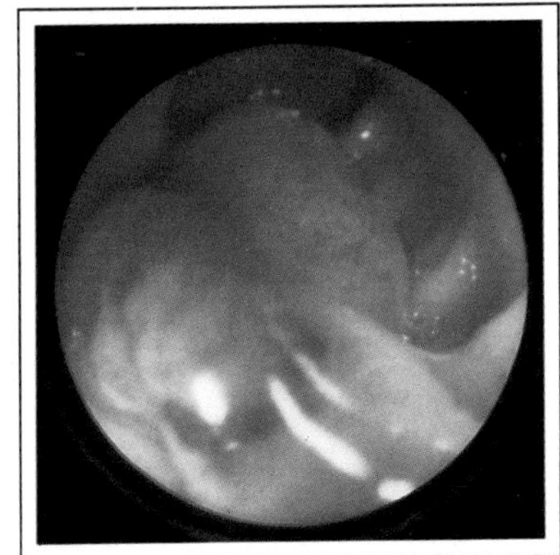

FIG. 41-4d.

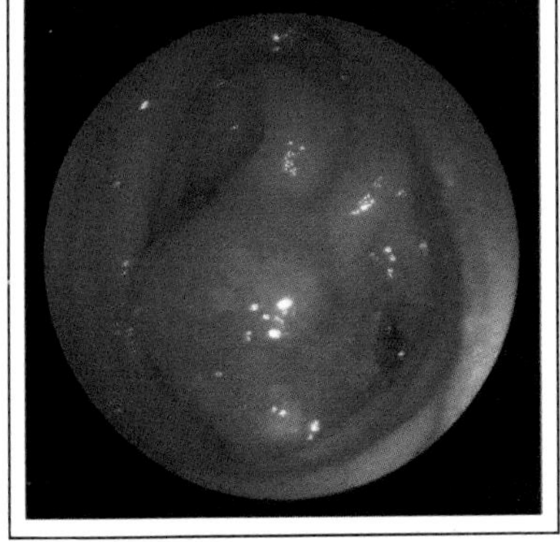

FIG. 41-5a.

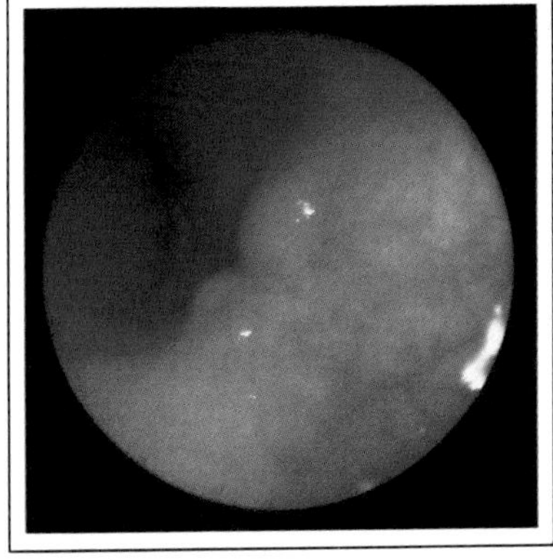

FIG. 41-5b.

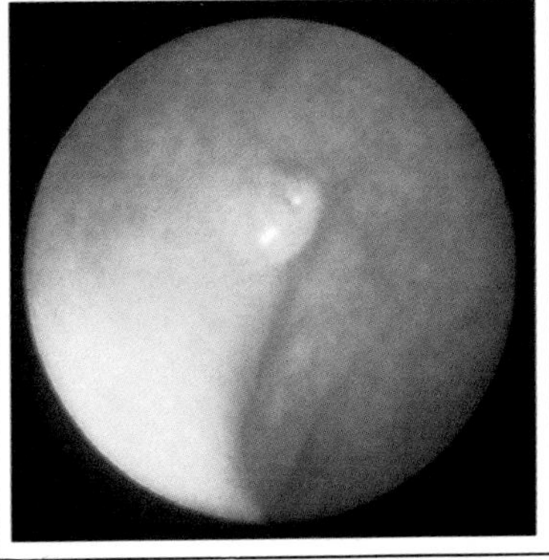

FIG. 41-5c.

FIG. 41-5. a: Tubulovillous adenoma with focally invasive carcinoma. The surface nodularity (at 6 o'clock) suggests that a villous component may be present, which would increase the likelihood of cancer from approximately 2% to 6%[9a] over that for an adenoma (Fig. 41-4c) of similar size. Even though the carcinoma was well differentiated histologically, without venous or lymphatic invasion, because of the patient's age (45) an exploration was performed, with no lymphatic spread demonstrated. **b:** Polypectomy site 6 months after excision of an adenoma, with carcinoma invading the pedicle down to the resected margin. Unlike the expected postpolypectomy appearance (c), there is a focally depressed area of mucosa suggesting residual cancer (confirmed on biopsy) necessitating a resection. **c:** Polypectomy site 6 months after electrosurgical excision of the tubular adenoma (Fig. 41-4b). The site was observed to be slightly elevated with a pale smooth mucosa without surface irregularities or depression.

For sessile villous adenomas where the risk of cancer may approach 30%,[10] the finding of cancer in a portion of the polypectomy specimen is an indication for surgery for most because of the high malignant potential of these lesions, unless there were strong medical reasons to the contrary. In such cases patients might be observed for follow-up fulguration at 2, 4, and 12 months after the initial excision, which might provide a measure of palliation if not ensure against recurrence.[23]

Treatment of diminutive (≤5 mm) adenomas.

The notion that 90% of polyps ≤5 mm are hyperplastic has recently been challenged.[28,29] In one series 50% of such polyps were found to be tubular adenomas and could not be distinguished from hyperplastic polyps on the basis of appearance.[28] In another study of 300 such polyps, 37% were tubular adenomas.[29] The largest size (4 to 5 mm) were neoplastic twice as often as polyps in the 1 to 3 mm range; moreover, patients over age 60 had a higher incidence of neoplastic polyps than younger patients.[29] Although treatment of such polyps (Fig. 41-1a) is somewhat controversial, the neoplastic potential of up to 50% of these lesions would argue that when they are encountered as many as possible should be biopsied and destroyed with coagulation using the Williams forceps.[11,20-22] This is true especially for polyps 4 and 5 mm in elderly patients, which have the greatest likelihood of being adenomatous.

Colonoscopy after electrosurgical excision.

Because 30 to 40% or more patients with one adenoma have a second one,[16,17] and the miss rate for colonoscopic detection of a single polyp is on the order of 10%,[12,14] one might expect that only 3 to 5% of patients would leave the colonoscopic examination with a significant undetected polyp, to be found at a subsequent examination within a year. Surprisingly, polyps are found on a follow-up examination in as many as 20%[30] or more.[31] That 50% of these in one study[30] were tubulovillous and 20% were villous adenomas—both types associated with an increased risk of cancer—underscores the need for a follow-up examination. We therefore recommend to patients in whom one polyp was removed to have examinations at 12- to 18-month intervals until their colons are cleared of polyps[31] and then follow-up colonoscopy at 2- to 5-year intervals or sooner if yearly stool testing for occult blood becomes positive.

Appearances Mistaken for Adenomas

Two appearances can be mistaken for adenomas: (a) mass-like folds of redundant mucosa, especially in the sigmoid; and (b) an ileocecal valve that has a polypoid appearance.

Mass-like sigmoid mucosal folds.

Large folds of redundant mucosa of the sigmoid may not be seen as such (Fig. 41-6a) but as a polypoid mass projecting into the lumen. Because they are smooth and soft and have a configuration suggesting a pedicle, they may be assumed to be adenomas warranting excision (Fig. 41-6b). Fortunately, it is rare that one actually proceeds with polypectomy because in probing further the nature of these folds becomes clear when one sees the pliant mucosa change its configuration markedly with different positions. Furthermore, the absence of any lobulation or nodularity, common features in the case of larger adenomas, also causes the examiner to suspect the "adenoma" of being either a fold or a submucosal polyp. In the latter case the change in configuration of the polyp with tenting (see Chapter 40) indicates the low likelihood of a submucosal polyp.

Polypoid ileocecal valve.

As noted elsewhere (see Chapter 39), one of the expected appearances of the ileocecal valve is that of a small polypoid mass projecting into the cecum. However, if the endoscopist is not aware of this appearance or if the valve is enlarged (see Chapter 40) (Fig. 41-6c), he may mistake it for a tubular adenoma and proceed with biopsy, or worse, attempt electrosurgical excision. Any polyp of the medial wall of the cecum should be carefully inspected and probed prior to one's resorting to any electrosurgical procedure. If seen tangentially, an effort should be made to position the endoscope tip in such a way as to obtain an *en face* view of the ileocecal valve (see Chapter 39). If there is still doubt, a forceps biopsy and then repeat colonoscopy can be done at some point if adenomatous tissue is recovered; this seems preferable to resorting immediately to an electrosurgical procedure which could have disastrous consequences if the structure were indeed the ileocecal valve.

Polypoid Carcinomas

Some polyps which resemble and therefore are mistaken for adenomas are in actuality composed largely of cancerous tissue with little or no adenomatous element. Polypoid cancers differ importantly from adenomas with focally invasive cancer in that complete electrosurgical removal of the lesion is done with less certainty, especially if the polyp is sessile.[32] Furthermore, even if the lesion seems to have been completely excised, the probability that electrosurgical treatment is curative remains to be defined, but it may be only on the order of 50%,[27] in contrast to the 75%[27] to 95%[25,26] for focally invasive cancer occurring in an adenoma.

Polypoid cancers represent only 1% of colonic polyps[16,17] and only one-fourth of "malignant" polyps.[16,17] In one large survey of 1,049 polyps, only 1% (11) were polypoid cancer,[17] being more prevalent among polyps 1 to 2 cm (2.2%) and those larger than 2 cm (2.8%). In this series the commonest location for polypoid cancer was the distal colon, i.e., rectosigmoid and sigmoid.[17]

We encountered four polypoid cancers among 375 polyps (1%) excised in our Unit over a 7-year period. All but one

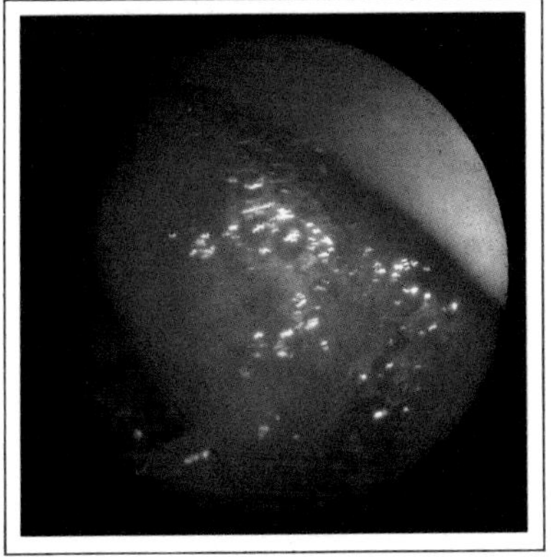

FIG. 41-6a.

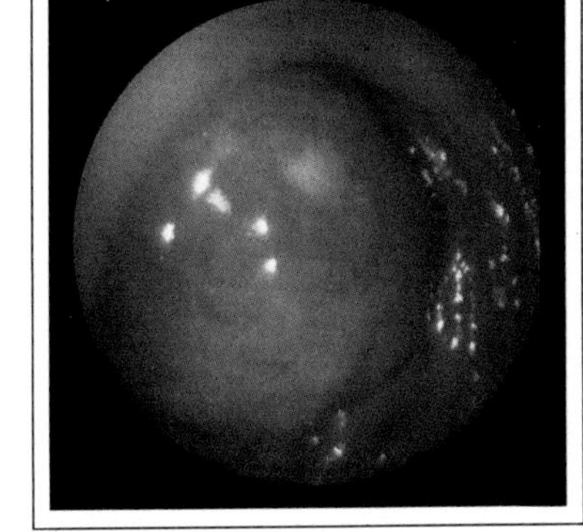

FIG. 41-6b.

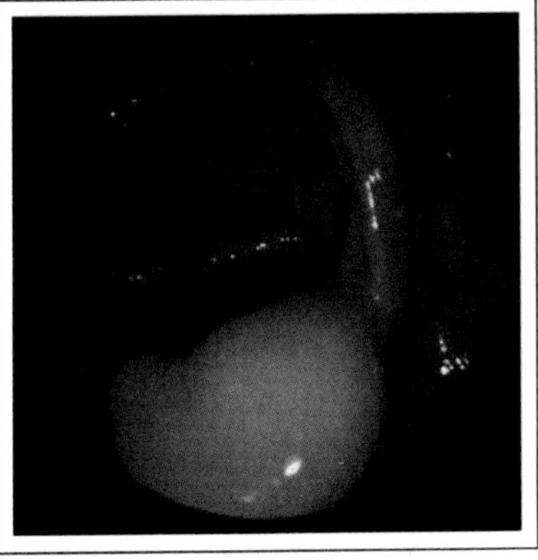

FIG. 41-6c.

FIG. 41-6. a: A prominent mucosal fold suggesting the appearance of a tubular adenoma. Prior to considering electrosurgical excision of a polyp in a case where it was not distinctly separate from a contiguous fold, one would raise it with a biopsy forceps to determine its nature more precisely. **b:** Tubular adenoma. Unlike a prominent mucosal fold (a), the polyp was seen to be separate from its surroundings. **c:** Lipoma of the ileocecal valve. Fatty infiltration of the ileocecal valve causes it to appear as a polyp. Its yellow-orange coloration, however, is a clue to its true nature. Biopsies may cause some fat to be extruded (the naked fat sign).[60]

were left-sided, the exception being a 2.5-cm polypoid cancer of the hepatic flexure.

Appearance

Of the four polypoid carcinomas found by us, three were sessile (Fig. 41-7a), with the remaining lesion having a short pedicle (Fig. 41-7b). The size range was from 1.2 to 2.4 cm. Endoscopically, one was called "benign," one was "suspicious," and two were correctly considered "malignant." Features which should have caused one to suspect malignancy in all four cases were the presence of ulceration (Fig. 41-7c), a sharp angular shape (Fig. 41-7, a and b), or a hard consistency on biopsy. These features are in contrast with the smooth, soft, regular appearance of a tubular adenoma; however, even the presence of typical features of an adenoma does not exclude polypoid carcinoma (Fig. 41-7d).

Biopsy

Although polypoid carcinoma consists entirely of malignant tissue and theoretically should be sampled adequately with forceps biopsy, this is not always true. In fact, this method of sampling proved inadequate in two of our four cases. The reason for this, we believe, is that without a larger sample the pathologist is often unable to determine with certainty whether invasion has occurred, as opposed to the lesion being simply an adenoma with mucosal atypia.[19] For a polyp in general, but especially those thought to be polypoid cancers, larger samples are recommended using the electrosurgical technique.

Endoscopic Polypectomy

Three of our four cases were referred to surgery, although in two what was thought to be complete electrosurgical excision had already been performed. One of these had no residual cancer at surgery whereas the other did have cancer remaining at the polypectomy site as well as in the lymph nodes. In the third case, a 2.5-cm sessile lesion, complete excision was not attempted, only a large-particle biopsy. In this case at surgery cancer was found in the wall but not in the lymphatics. Although our numbers are exceedingly small, they are consistent with those reported by others where for these lesions metastasis was present in 25%,[33] irrespective of whether colonoscopic excision was thought to be adequate. This fact makes many physicians inclined to refer patients with polypoid cancers for surgery, irrespective of whether the cancer was thought to be completely removed electrosurgically.[27]

Hyperplastic (Metaplastic) Polyps

Hyperplastic (metaplastic) polyps, most commonly found in the rectum, are small, sessile excrescences (≤5 mm)

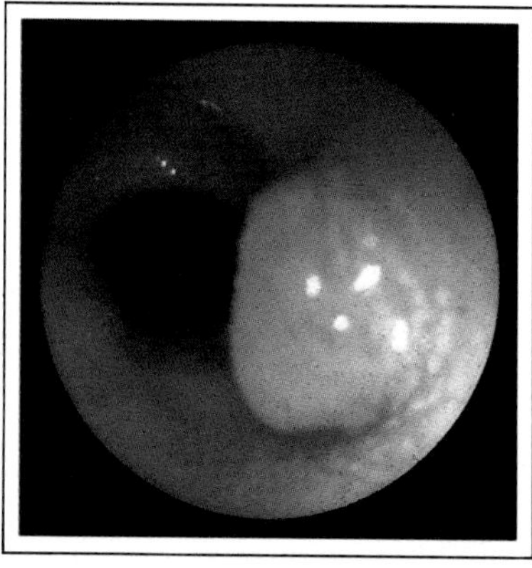

FIG. 41-7a.

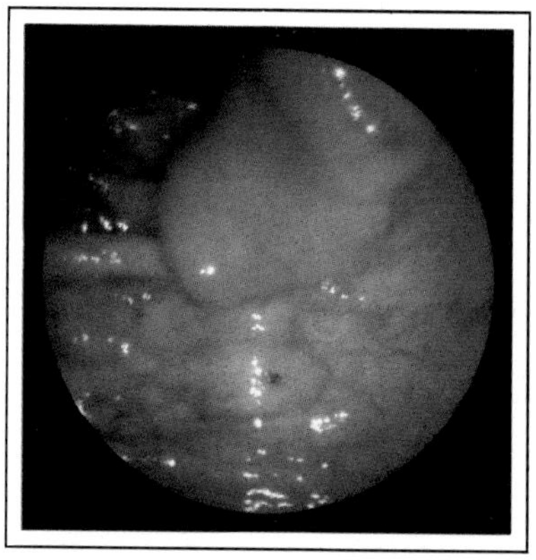

FIG. 41-7b.

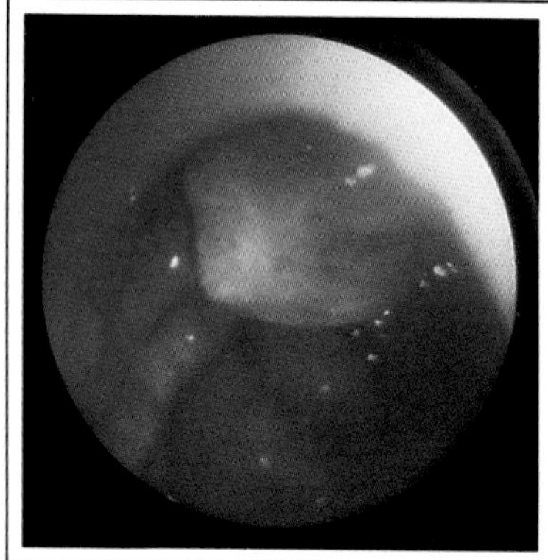

FIG. 41-7c.

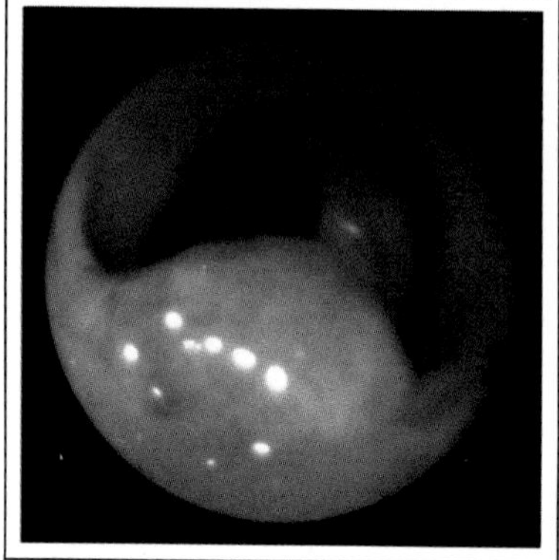

FIG. 41-7d.

FIG. 41-7. Polypoid carcinoma. **a:** This appears possibly more angulated than a tubular adenoma of comparable size (Fig. 41-2c); still, the surface is smooth and lacks ulceration to suggest carcinoma. **b:** This lesion was sharply angulated but otherwise smooth. **c:** The lesion is sharply angulated with an ulcerated surface. Biopsy of it indicated a rock-hard consistency. **d:** This lesion appears as a typical tubular adenoma without any distinguishing features.

which are nonneoplastic, and generally regarded as having no malignant potential whatsoever.[34] Recent studies suggest that they result from a delay in the shedding of surface epithelial cells rather than excessive cell proliferation[34]; hence the term metaplastic seems to be more appropriate.[7] Many workers, however, continue to use the older term, hyperplastic, in connection with these polyps.

Once thought to be the commonest type of colonic polyp, representing over 90% of diminutive or minute polyps (≤5 mm), more recent colonoscopic studies suggest that even at this size and even within the rectum, a third to one-half of these polyps are tubular adenomas.[28,29] Whereas hyperplastic polyps are composed of what has been termed "hypermature" epithelium,[35] which is not in itself neoplastic, these polyps occasionally give rise to minute adenomas,[35] even cancer,[35a] possibly under the influence of a carcinogen which affects their surface epithelium.[35]

Appearance

The characteristic finding for hyperplastic polyps is that of tiny mucosal excrescences (1 to 2 mm) or slightly larger (3 to 5 mm) mammillations, where the mucosa is slightly paler than its surroundings (Fig. 41-8a). Generally, they appear singly but up to 10% are multiple with as many as 5 to 10 or more polyps in a single segment, e.g., the rectum. In addition, one may see an exceptional patient who has, especially in the left colon, literally hundreds of hyperplastic polyps of varying size, but up to 8 mm or larger.

Although small hyperplastic polyps are invariably sessile, larger lesions (5 to 10 mm) may be pedunculated and simulate the appearance of an adenoma (Fig. 41-8b). Giant hyperplastic polyps, which are exceedingly rare, may, as in one reported case, simulate carcinoma.[36]

Differentiation from Adenomas

Using conventional colonoscopic instruments, hyperplastic (metaplastic) polyps and tubular adenomas cannot be differentiated visually, although using a specially designed lens system (with 30× magnification) and a dye-scattering technique, Nishizawa et al. observed surface mucosal detail and anticipated histologic findings.[37]

If feasible, all diminutive polyps, especially those 4 to 5 mm, in patients over the age of 60 should be excised because as many as 50% of these polyps are adenomas.[28,29] Tiny, 1 to 2 mm excrescences have only a 10 to 20% likelihood of being adneomas. If they number less than 10, excision of most or all is desirable; however, if they are more numerous, sampling of the larger of the lesions with the Williams forceps, which both biopsies and destroys a polyp, seems acceptable, especially in patients under the age of

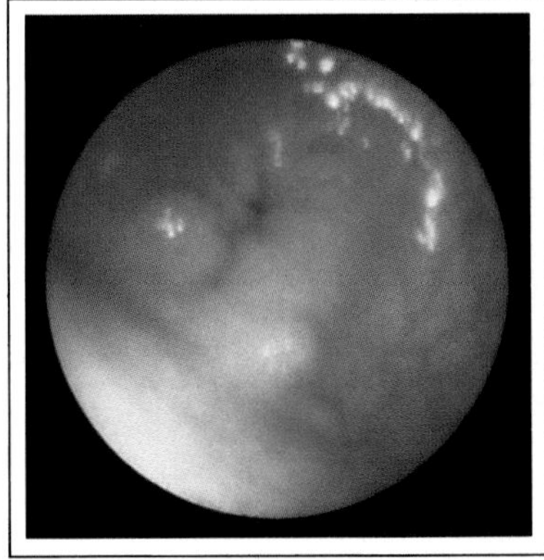

FIG. 41-8a.

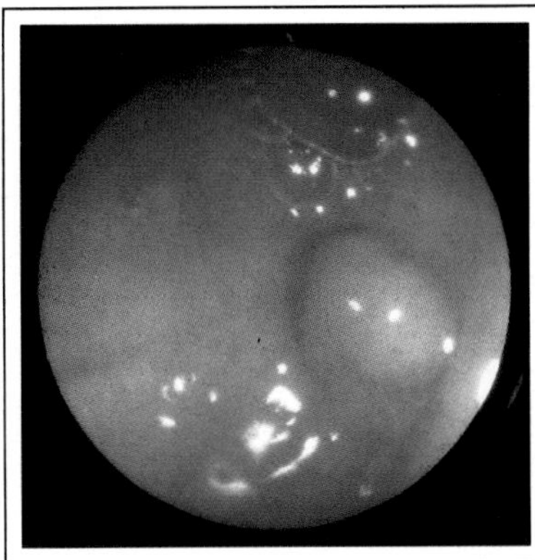

FIG. 41-8b.

FIG. 41-8. a: Hyperplastic polyp, a tiny 3-mm excrescence of the rectosigmoid. The rectum is the commonest location for this type of polyp. **b:** Hyperplastic polyp with a pedicle. Larger polyps of this type may have small pedicles and are otherwise indistinguishable from tubular adenomas (Fig. 41-1b).

60 in whom a smaller percentage of these polyps will be adenomas.

Juvenile Polyps

Although uncommon overall, juvenile polyps are the most prevalent type of polyp to be found in patients under 30, especially in children and adolescents (under 20). In one series where colonoscopy was performed in children largely for rectal bleeding, they were 12 times more common than single adenomas.[38] Most juvenile polyps are found in patients under age 30, but 15% occur in older individuals.[39]

Histologically, they are composed of mucin-filled (retention) cysts lined with glandular epithelium and lying within larger areas of a fibrous stroma and acute inflammatory cells.[7] The surface of these polyps is characteristically ulcerated, which accounts for the commonest presentation of them being recurrent lower gastrointestinal (GI) bleeding. Others with polyps located in the rectum present because of recurrent rectal prolapse.

There is no evidence that juvenile polyps are themselves precancerous, but when they occur multiply they are found together with adenomas as part of a juvenile polyposis syndrome (see below) and may be associated with adenomas and cancer elsewhere in the GI tract.

Appearance

The typical finding is that of a 1.5- to 3-cm sessile lesion[39] with an intensely erythematous, friable ulcerated surface (Fig. 41-9a), although in some the surface is nodular but not ulcerated (Fig. 41-9b) and indistinguishable from a tubulovillous adenoma of similar size (Fig. 41-9c).

Endoscopic Treatment

Up to 10% of polyps in children and young adults may be adenomatous, so that histologic examination of the excised lesion is very desirable.[38] In addition, in the case of an ulcerated juvenile polyp, excision is therapeutic with regard to lower GI bleeding and iron deficiency anemia, which may have prompted the colonoscopy. Despite their size, most juvenile polyps are readily excised electrosurgically with little or no morbidity.

Inflammatory Polyps

Most inflammatory polyps (focal, raised areas of granulation tissue) occur in the context of inflammatory bowel disease (see Chapter 43). In other patients inflammatory polyps comprise approximately 0.5 to 1% of polyps.[7] These are typically less than 1 cm, being most often diminutive (≤5 mm) (Fig. 41-10a). Histologically, they show edema, fibrosis, and a lymphocytic or neutrophilic infiltrate.[7] As is true of juvenile polyps, the surface may be ulcerated, which accounts for the occult rectal bleeding that prompts colonoscopy in some of the patients. Even when surface ulceration and irregularity are present histologically, they are usually not identified by the endoscopist, as these polyps are visually indistinguishable from other small adenomas or hyperplastic polyps. In most cases inflammatory polyps are found in the left colon. When found in the distal rectum, especially when multiple, they may occur as part of a solitary rectal ulcer syndrome (see Chapter 47).

Fibrous-Inflammatory Polyps

Some inflammatory polyps, especially those of the ileocecal area have an inflammatory as well as a fibrous component and are referred to as fibrous-inflammatory polyps.[40] When eosinophils predominate in the areas of inflammation, the term eosinophilic granuloma is sometimes used. As in the case of other inflammatory polyps, the surface may be ulcerated and account for occult or frank lower GI bleeding which may prompt investigation (Fig. 41-10b). Because of their size, which in some cases exceeds 1.5 cm, their location, and their sessile nature, the endoscopic diagnosis may be polypoid carcinoma, a fact which stresses the importance of adequate histologic sampling of these lesions.[40]

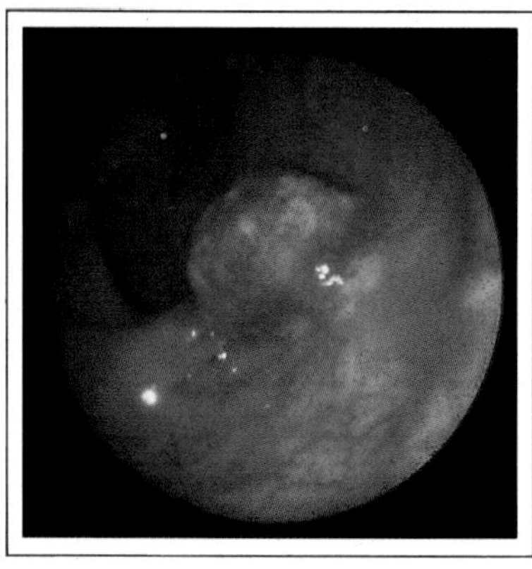

FIG. 41-9a.

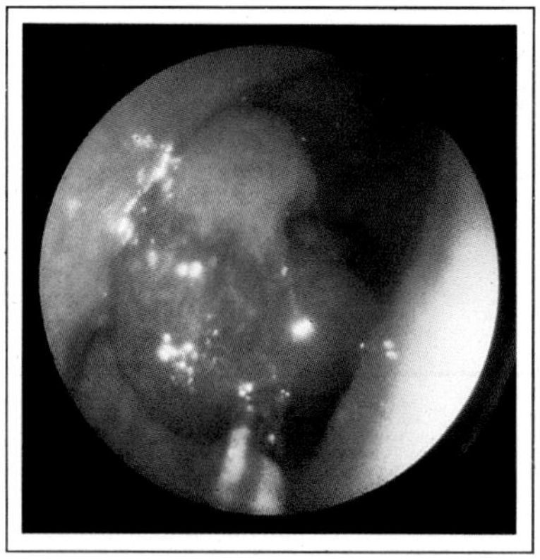

FIG. 41-9b.

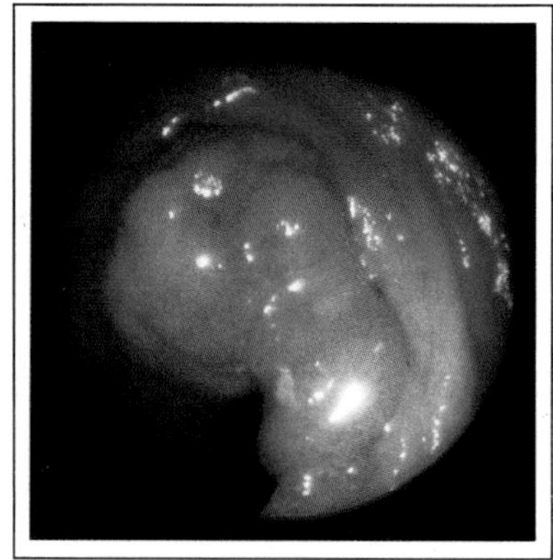

FIG. 41-9c.

FIG. 41-9. a: Juvenile polyp. A 1-cm polyp with an ulcerated surface in a 25-year-old male presenting with rectal bleeding. The age (under 30) suggested the possibility of a juvenile polyp, as did its ulcerated surface. **b:** Juvenile polyp. A larger 2-cm lesion with a pedicle and a nodular but nonulcerated surface. Although this resembles a tubulovillous adenoma or even a polypoid carcinoma, the age of this patient (20) still strongly favors its being a juvenile polyp.[38] **c:** Tubulovillous adenoma. A 1.7-cm polyp with a nodular surface has an appearance which is similar to some juvenile polyps (b).

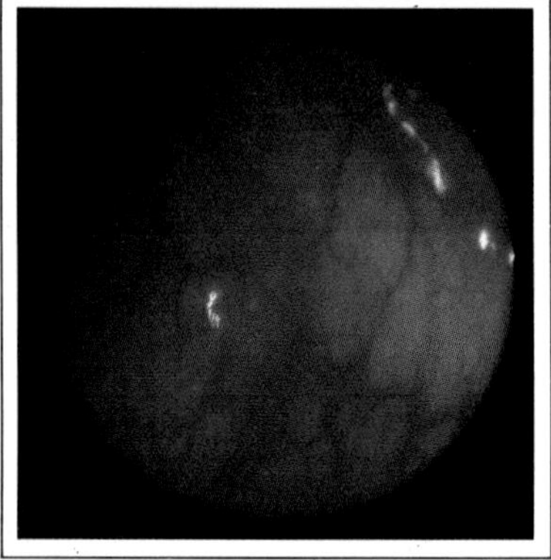

FIG. 41-10a.

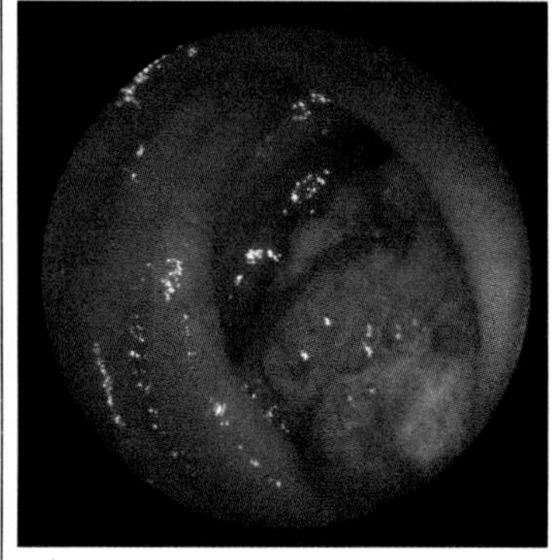

FIG. 41-10b.

FIG. 41-10. Inflammatory polyp. **a:** A small 5-mm erythematous lesion is indistinguishable from a tubular adenoma of the same size (Fig. 41-1a). **b:** A large (2 cm) lesion with a superficially ulcerated surface was thought to be a neoplasm until completely excised and submitted for histologic examination.

POLYPOSIS SYNDROMES

The various polyposis syndromes discussed in this section are all quite rare in the general population. Even the commonest, familial polyposis coli, occurs in an estimated 1 per 8,300 live births.[41] Nevertheless, they may be encountered at colonoscopy as often as one per 300 to 600 cases. We, in fact, encountered seven over a 7-year period during which 2,100 colonoscopic examinations were performed, or approximately 1 per 300 cases examined. Although this high frequency undoubtedly reflects the referral nature of our institution, the examiner, regardless of the frequency with which these syndromes are encountered, wishes to be familiar with them and the interpretive problems they present.

Patients with polyposis syndromes are often referred for colonoscopy without the condition having been suspected, or else its appearance was mistaken for the inflammatory polyps of ulcerative colitis (see below). In those cases of familial polyposis coli in which the diagnosis has already been established, patients have often been referred for cancer surveillance and appropriate endoscopic therapy, i.e., excision and/or fulguration of significant polyps (see below). In the section which follows, we consider first the adenomatous polyposis syndromes and then discuss those in which a variety of nonneoplastic polyps may be present.

Adenomatous Polyposis Syndromes

The most frequently encountered and potentially most serious because of their malignant potential are polyposis syndromes in which large numbers of adenomas are found—at least 100 but often thousands. These syndromes include: (a) familial polyposis coli, the commonest; (b) the less commonly occurring Gardner's syndrome; and (c) the exceedingly rare Turcot's syndrome.

Familial Polyposis Coli

Familial polyposis coli, the commonest polyposis syndrome, is estimated to occur in only 1 per 8,300 in the general population.[41] It is transmitted as an autosomal dominant trait, with a high degree of penetrance (90%), so that once it is detected in one family member it is usually discovered in others.[41] However, in up to 20% of the cases, no other affected family member is found. It is unclear as to whether these cases represent true mutation or whether it only appears this way because of our inability to sample all family members.

Although patients may present during infancy or even past the age of 50, most are said to become symptomatic during the fourth decade (median age 33); with the adenomas having appeared nearly 10 years before (median age 24.5).[42] In most reported series patients are diagnosed as having familial polyposis coli in their mid-thirties, with their cancers occurring when they are in their late thirties (median age 39.2), and death in untreated patients in their early forties (median age 42). The onset of colonic cancer, which almost invariably occurs in these patients, precedes that which occurs in the general population by 15 to 20 years.[43]

It is our impression that those patients who have no other affected family member tend to present with symptoms earlier, in some cases in their early twenties. In these patients we have observed locally as well as widely metastatic cancer at presentation. For these individuals, who may represent spontaneous mutation of a gene for familial polyposis, the condition as well as its malignant potential appears to be expressed early in life.

The commonest presenting symptoms are rectal bleeding and diarrhea. These taken together with the proctoscopic appearance of multiple polyps may cause the inexperienced physician to mistake these lesions for inflammatory polyps of ulcerative colitis (see below). Other symptoms include abdominal pain and a mucous discharge.[43] Barium enema, especially if done with a double-contrast method, usually shows multiple small (≤5 mm) polyps throughout the colon; however, these can be entirely missed if single-contrast studies are employed.[44] Proctoscopic examination also typically shows innumerable, small (≤5 mm) polyps which may appear to literally carpet the rectum.

In the absence of colectomy, the risk of cancer approaches 100%. For those with colectomy and preservation of the rectum and distal sigmoid, the risk of cancer is still high, approaching 30%. It is possibly less if the rectum was free of polys at the time of surgery, if the surgery included the sigmoid, and if the large majority of polyps are under 5 mm.[45] It is unclear at present if colonoscopic excision and fulguration of significant polyps (≥5 mm) further reduces the risk of cancer. In one study the cumulative incidence of cancer in such patients was still 30% over 10 years even though the majority had undergone fulguration at 6- to 9-month intervals.[45]

Appearance.

There are three distinctive appearances for familial polyposis coli: (a) a carpet of minute polyps; (b) large polyps with intervening normal mucosa; and (c) a combination of minute and large polyps.

1. *Carpet of minute polyps:* In this, the commonest appearance in our experience, there are innumerable, tiny adenomas between 1 and 3 mm; no larger polyps are found (Fig. 41-11a). As is true of small adenomas in general, these polyps are perfectly smooth and regular, with a mucosal coloration which is indistinguishable from its surroundings. As this is a common appearance of the mucosa at the time familial polyposis coli is first diagnosed, often 10 years or more before cancer is detected, it may be that polyps of this size are an early stage with a lower malignant potential than that which is associated with a finding of larger polyps, which in our experience are often seen in cases where cancer is subsequently discovered at colectomy within the same year (Fig. 41-11b).

2. *Larger polyps with intervening areas of normal mucosa:* Another distinctive, though less common, appearance is that of multiple larger polyps (4 to 8+ mm) distributed throughout the colon and rectum where areas of apparently uninvolved mucosa are seen (Fig. 41-11c). In some cases the number of polyps may actually number less than 100 (but more than 50), a presentation which may represent a *forme fruste* of familial polyposis coli. In patients with this appearance who present when they are over age 60, the malignant potential appears to be substantially less than in younger patients having this finding, although the actual risk of this subgroup has never been precisely defined.

3. *Combination of large and small polyps:* In this appearance, one sees both the mucosal surface carpeted with tiny polyps as well as the presence of larger (4 to 8+ mm) adenomas (Fig. 41-11d). It is our belief that this appearance, especially when found in younger patients (under the age of 25) with no other affected family member, is associated with a high risk that cancer is already present.

Differentiation from inflammatory polyposis.

Even though the colonoscopist will certainly biopsy, if not excise, representative polyps for histologic examination, to determine the nature of the polyposis he must still have firmly fixed in his mind features which allow visual differentiation of these two types of polyposis.

First, although inflammatory polyps, especially in ulcerative colitis, may be numerous and so resemble those of familial polyposis coli, the intervening mucosa in familial polyposis, if seen, is normal with the vascular pattern preserved (Fig. 41-12a). In the case of ulcerative colitis, one expects a distorted or absent vascular pattern (see Chapter 43). Multiple polyps in the presence of a normal vascular pattern, especially in a patient with a recent onset of rectal bleeding, causes one to strongly suspect familial polyposis. Secondly, although inflammatory polyps may be numerous (Fig. 41-12b), they rarely "carpet" the mucosa in a back-to-back fashion (Fig. 41-11a), so that there is almost always intervening mucosa. Moreover, inflammatory polyps tend to be much more pleomorphic, varying in size and shape, unlike the monotonous appearance of adenomas.

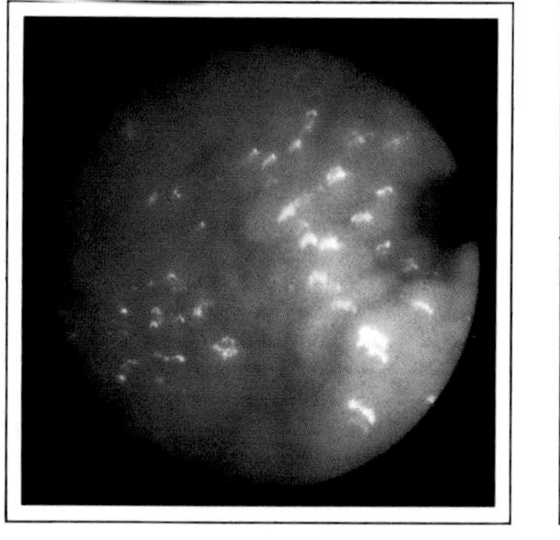

FIG. 41-11a.

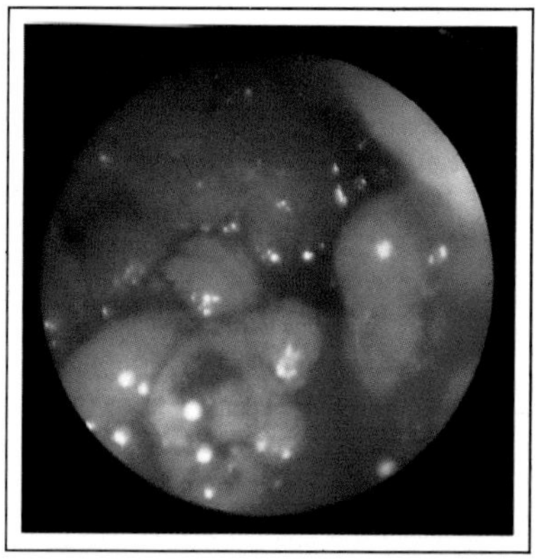

FIG. 41-11b.

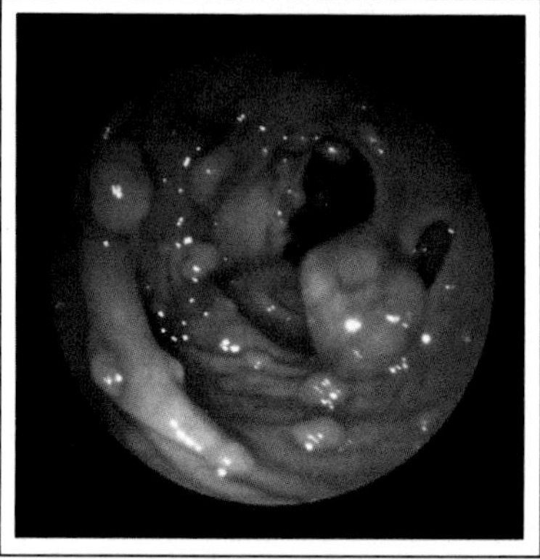

FIG. 41-11c.

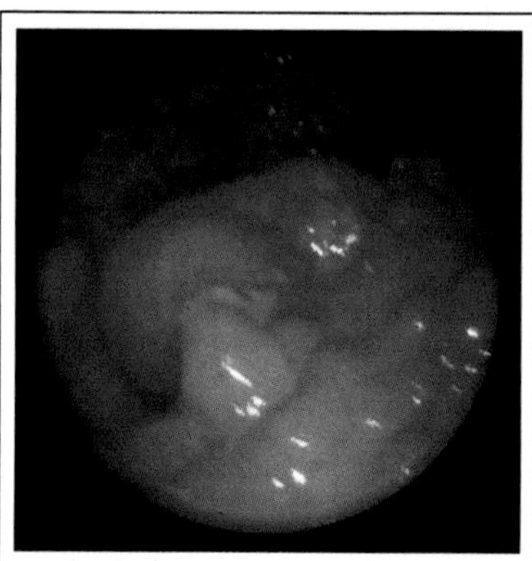

FIG. 41-11d.

FIG. 41-11. Familial polyposis coli. **a:** The mucosa of the colon is carpeted by tiny 2- to 4-mm excrescences. Biopsies showed all of these to be adenomas. **b:** Both tiny excrescences as well as larger polyps are found in a patient with a recent onset of bloody diarrhea. **c:** Multiple polyps—large and small—stud the colon, although they are not back to back (b). **d:** The presence of larger polyps in any patient should make the examiner concerned about an underlying carcinoma.

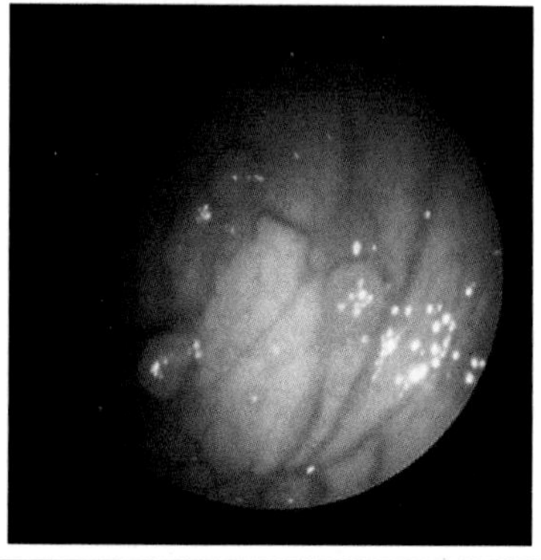

FIG. 41-12a.

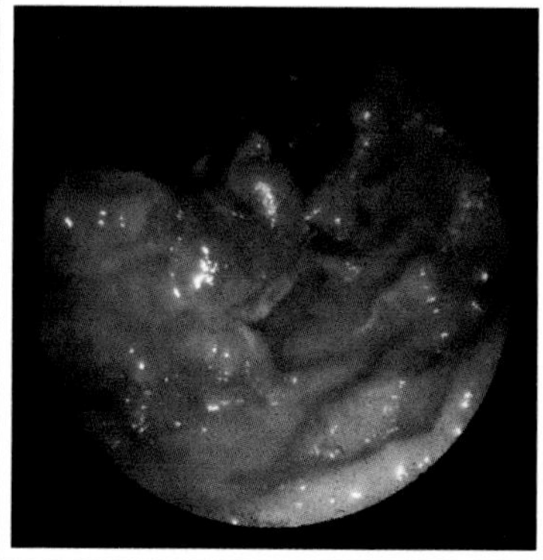

FIG. 41-12b.

FIG. 41-12. a: Familial polyposis coli. The presence of an intact vascular pattern between polyps should always suggest familial polyposis and not the inflammatory polyposis of ulcerative colitis (b). **b:** Inflammatory polyposis of ulcerative colitis. In this case the absence of a vascular pattern is an important clue to the diagnosis, which would be confirmed histologically.

Appearance of colonic cancer complicating familial polyposis coli.

Cancer in familial polyposis tends to be infiltrating rather than exophytic, so that a stricture is the expected appearance. By the time this occurs, the cancer is usually widely metastatic. Earlier dysplastic changes, even if present, tend to be obscured by the polyps themselves. A finding we have observed in association with an increased probability of malignancy in these patients is the presence of larger polyps (>9 mm) found on a background carpet of small ones (Fig. 41-13a). Any polyp, therefore, which exceeds 9 mm (Fig. 41-13a), in contrast to the appearance of multiple tiny polyps (Fig. 41-13b), particularly when associated with focal areas of narrowing, should be considered to denote a high probability of invasive cancer (Fig. 41-13c). Such patients should be strongly urged to undergo surgical exploration even if biopsies of the narrowed area or surrounding polyps fail to reveal malignancy (Fig. 41-13d).

Biopsy, excision of polyps, or fulguration?

The question of histologic sampling, electrosurgical excision of larger polyps, and fulguration of smaller ones must be considered for both untreated patients (without prior colectomy) and those having had previous surgery.

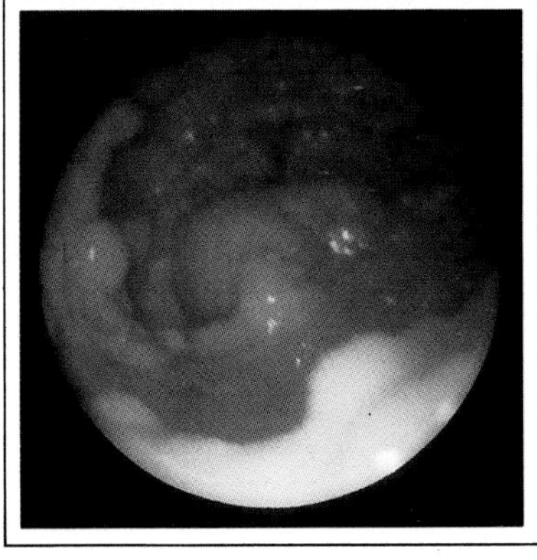

FIG. 41-13a.

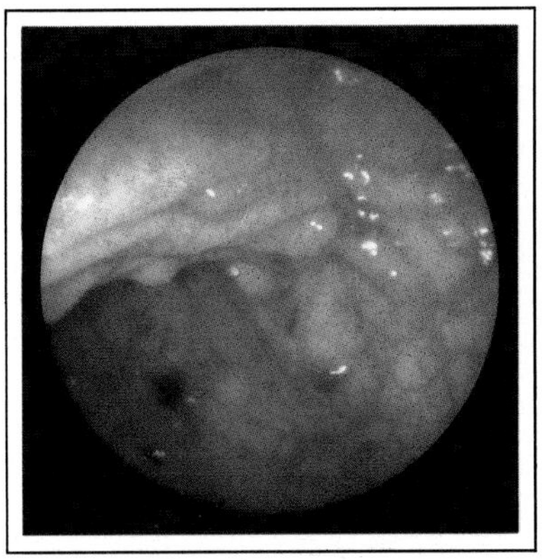

FIG. 41-13b.

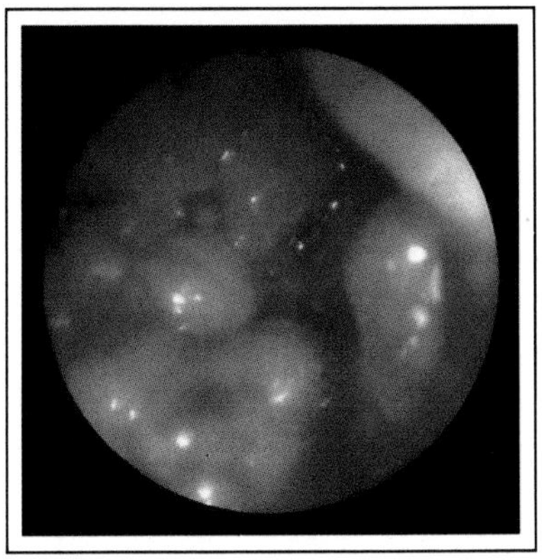

FIG. 41-13c.

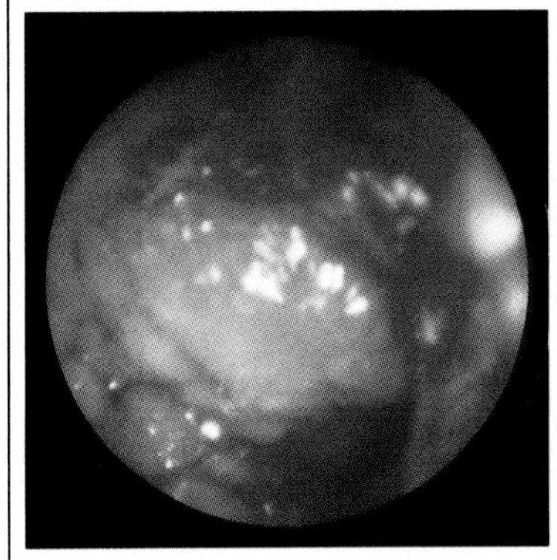

FIG. 41-13d.

FIG. 41-13. Familial polyposis coli. **a:** Complicated by carcinoma. The presence of large polyps raises the possibility of cancer already being present, confirmed in this case at colectomy. **b:** The small size of these polyps is reassuring in a patient about to undergo an ileoproctostomy; they indicate that cancer is not yet present. **c:** Complicated by carcinoma. The large polyps as well as the narrowing of the rectosigmoid (d) strongly suggested this diagnosis. Widely metastatic carcinoma was found at surgery. **d:** Complicated by carcinoma. Like the carcinomas which occur in ulcerative colitis, these tend to be infiltrating rather than exophytic lesions and appear as strictures from which biopsies may not reveal invasive carcinoma.

1. *Untreated patients:* Only colectomy with ileoproctostomy in those having a small number of rectal polyps and panproctocolectomy in others minimizes or removes altogether the high cancer risk in patients with familial polyposis coli.[45] Biopsy and/or electrosurgical excision of selected large polyps are important in establishing the diagnosis but have no effect on the cancer risk in untreated patients.
2. *Prior colectomy with preservation of the rectum or distal sigmoid:* Colonoscopy is requested for cancer surveillance, as is excision of "significant" lesions in patients previously treated with rectum sparing operations. The examiner may wish to remove electrosurgically all significant polyps (>5 mm) as well as to fulgurate as many of the smaller ones as he can. However, the efficacy of these procedures in preventing cancer has not been shown, especially where the rectum is literally carpeted by innumerable, small polyps or scores of larger (≥5 mm) lesions.[45] The lowest risk is clearly in patients who have few or no polyps at the time of initial surgery. In these patients the risk of cancer over a 5-year period is less than 5%. Whether electrosurgical excision and fulguration of multiple polyps can reduce the considerably higher risk in other patients is unclear, which in at least one study over a 5-year period was found to be over 30% in patients with multiple rectal and/or sigmoid polyps, even where fulguration had been performed as often as every 6 to 9 months.[45]

Extracolonic polyps in familial polyposis.

Gastric (see Chapter 18) and duodenal (see Chapter 30) adenomas, as well as adenomas in other locations in the small bowel, have now been well described in patients with familial polyposis coli. Upper GI endoscopy, especially with careful attention to the duodenal bulb and periampullary region, should be encouraged in all such patients.[46] Not all polyps outside the colon are adenomatous. In the terminal ileum the polyps are more likely to be the result of lymphoid hyperplasia,[47] whereas those in the fundus of the stomach are often hyperplastic.[46]

Gardner's Syndrome

In Gardner's syndrome, in addition to colonic adenomas there are a variety of mesenchymal lesions outside the GI tract, the most characteristic being osteomas of the skull and mandible, epidermoid cysts, and mesenteric fibromatosis.[48] Like familial polyposis coli, this syndrome is transmitted genetically as an autosomal dominant, but it occurs much less often than the former, with an incidence of only 1 per 14,000 live births.[42] Not all the typical features of the syndrome are found in every patient, nor do they appear at the initial presentation. Often the extracolonic manifestations are the first indication of the condition, with the colonic polyps found not because of the symptoms

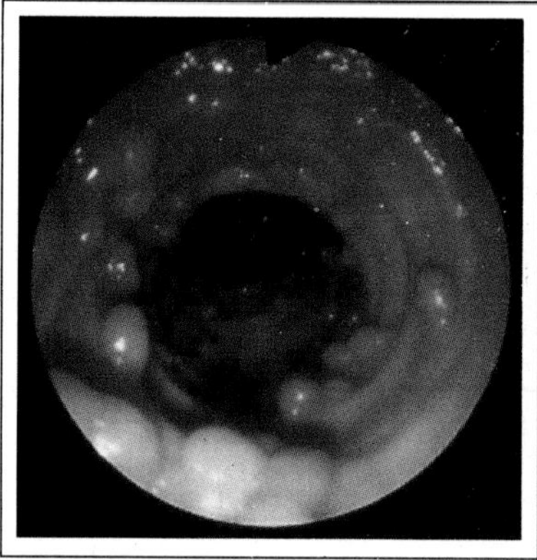

FIG. 41-14.

FIG. 41-14. Gardner's syndrome. In general, fewer adenomas are seen in this condition than in familial polyposis coli. The malignant potential is the same, however.

but as a result of Gardner's syndrome being considered and the appropriate colonic studies performed. Despite the fact that the number of polyps in Gardner's syndrome tends to be lower than that commonly found in familial polyposis (Fig. 41-14), the risk of cancer is the same, approaching 100% in untreated patients. This makes colectomy the treatment of choice, with preservation of the rectum, if a manageable number of polyps (<5) is present.[48]

Like familial polyposis, adenomas of the stomach and duodenum may be present and should be sought, especially adenomas of the ampulla of Vater (see Chapter 30) because of the increased incidence of periampullary carcinoma.[48] Whether removal of such polyps endoscopically reduces the incidence of periampullary carcinomas in these patients, however, has not been determined.

Turcot's Syndrome

Turcot's syndrome is the rarest of all adenomatous polyposis syndromes where the extracolonic manifestation is that of multiple, malignant, central nervous system tumors, including medulloblastomas and glioblastomas of the spinal cord. Patients with this condition most often succumb to the central nervous system malignancy, irrespective of whether colonic cancer is present.[49] As in Gardner's syndrome, other extracolonic GI cancers may be present.[49]

Nonneoplastic Polyposis Syndromes

The nonneoplastic polyposis syndromes include juvenile polyposis and its variant the Cronkhite-Canada syndrome, Peutz-Jeghers syndrome, and Cowden's syndrome. These are called nonneoplastic syndromes because the individual polyps are either inflammatory or hamartomatous, although in juvenile polyposis and the Peutz-Jeghers syndrome there is an association with malignancy of the GI tract.

These conditions are less common than adenomatous polyposis syndromes. For example, over a 7-year period we encountered seven adenomatous polyposis syndromes among 2,100 examinations performed (five cases of familial polyposis coli and two cases of Gardner's syndrome); however, over the same time period there were only four cases of nonneoplastic polyposis (one case of Peutz-Jeghers syndrome, two cases of juvenile polyposis in a father and son, and one case of Cowden's syndrome). We briefly consider the nonneoplastic polyposis syndromes in the section which follows.

Juvenile Polyposis

Two types of intestinal juvenile polyposis syndromes have been described. In one, juvenile polyposis coli,[50] there are multiple polyps with the same appearance as single juvenile polyps (Fig. 41-9a). These patients usually present with a history of rectal bleeding which is a result of hemorrhage from the ulcerated, friable surface of these lesions, as well as from the pedicles of those in which the polyp itself has been autoamputated.[50]

A second type of juvenile polyposis is that in which these lesions occur throughout the GI tract rather than being confined to the colon.[51] Especially in these cases, adenomas are found in association with juvenile polyps, both in the colon and elsewhere.[52] In this type where adenomas commonly occur, there is an association with GI malignancy for both the patients with juvenile polyposis and other family members.[52]

Cronkhite-Canada Syndrome

The Cronkhite-Canada syndrome is now thought to be a variant of generalized juvenile polyposis in which there are striking ectodermal manifestations: cutaneous hyperpigmentation, alopecia, and nail dystrophy.[53] The polyps are indistinguishable in appearance from juvenile polyps (Fig. 41-9a) but tend to be more numerous, especially in the stomach.[53,53a] Hypoproteinemia is often observed in this syndrome, and it is thought to be from protein losses from the ulcerated surfaces of the polyp.[53,53a] Adenomas have not been observed in this syndrome,[53] nor is there thought to be an increased cancer risk,[53a] although in occasional

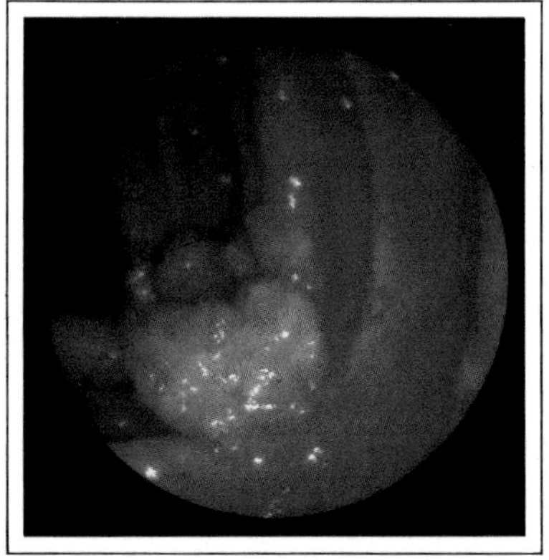

FIG. 41-15a.

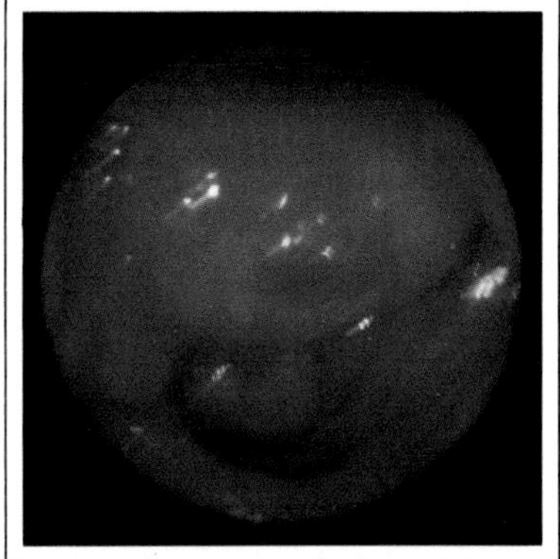

FIG. 41-15b.

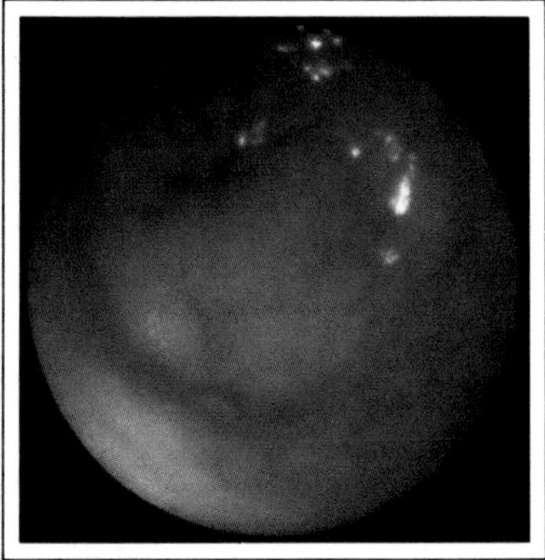

FIG. 41-15c.

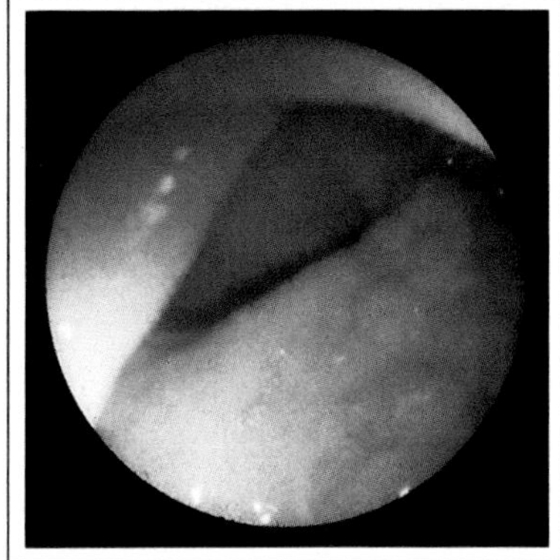

FIG. 41-15d.

FIG. 41-15. a: Peutz-Jeghers polyposis. Several pedunculated, lobulated polyps were found in a patient with the characteristic circumoral pigmentation. **b:** Peutz-Jeghers polyposis. Larger polyps (in this case 3 cm) are sometimes seen, with an erythematous lobulated or cerebriform surface. **c:** Cowden's disease. Numerous small polyps, appearing as tiny excrescences, are barely distinguishable from the surrounding mucosa. Histologically these consist of proliferation of surface epithelium along with glandular mucous cysts. **d:** Cowden's disease. These polyps are most often seen in the rectosigmoid.

cases carcinomas have been found within or in close proximity to the polyps.[53]

Peutz-Jeghers Syndrome

The polyps in patients with Peutz-Jeghers syndrome are true hamartomas, varying in size from several millimeters to 3 cm. They are characterized histologically by extensive arborization of the muscularis mucosae which courses through and divides the polyps into sectors, within which are found a variety of mature epithelial cells typical of their site of origin, e.g., parietal, chief, or goblet cells, as well as mucin-filled cysts.[7] The polyps appear throughout the GI tract with a special predilection for the small bowel, where they may become either the lead points of intussusception or the source of acute and chronic GI bleeding.[54]

The well-known extraintestinal manifestations of the Peutz-Jeghers syndrome include mucocutaneous melanotic pigmentation, clubbing, exostoses, and ovarian cysts.[7]

There is a definite increased cancer risk in patients with Peutz-Jeghers syndrome, occurring in up to 2 to 3% of these patients, with the commonest location being the gastroduodenal area, especially the periampullary region.[55] An increase risk for cervical and ovarian cancer is also present.[56] In the GI tract the origin of the cancer is uncertain, although metastatic cancer arising from within the hamartomatous polyp itself is now well described. This leads one to think that the polyps themselves, especially those situated in the gastroduodenal region are the source of the increased cancer risk.[55]

Peutz-Jeghers polyps have now been well described in the colon, being firm, lobulated, or cerebriform masses which may be sessile or pedunculated (Fig. 41-15a). Generally, few polyps are found in the colon, but in some cases 20 to 50 can be found. When they are present they tend to be less than 2 cm, although in some cases the polyps are large, with a maximum dimension of 3 cm or more (Fig. 41-15b).

Cowden's Disease

In Cowden's disease, an unusual condition, multiple hamartomas are found throughout the GI tract associated with a variety of congenital abnormalities, orocutaneous hamartomas, and malignancies, especially of the breast and thyroid.[57]

The polyps of Cowden's disease appear endoscopically as numerous small (1 to 3 mm) lesions (Fig. 41-14c), although occasionally they are larger (up to 2 cm). The typical small polyps have a smooth surface with a coloration which is indistinguishable from the surrounding mucosa (Fig. 41-15c). Histologically, they are characterized by a proliferation of surface epithelium, along with the presence of mucous cysts (cystic dilatation of glands) within or just beneath hyperplastic muscularis mucosae.[57]

Colonic involvement is less common than other sites in the GI tract. In these cases there may be numerous small, rounded, sessile polyps, generally within the rectum or rectosigmoid (Fig. 41-15d) and to a lesser extent throughout the remainder of the colon (Fig. 41-15c).

SUBMUCOSAL POLYPS

Submucosal polyps of the colon include: (a) lipomas; (b) leiomyomas and leiomyosarcomas; (c) other rare tumors, e.g., neurofibromas and carcinoids; and (d) endometrial implants which may appear as submucosal polyps. Although these lesions account for no more than 1 to 2% of colonic polyps, one nevertheless needs to be aware of their varied appearances.

Lipomas

Although lipomas are the commonest submucosal polyps of the colon, they are infrequently encountered, being seen at one center in only 1.2% of patients examined (22 of 1,827).[58] Most are discovered as incidental findings, although large lipomas may produce symptoms suggestive of recurrent intestinal obstruction or occult blood loss which prompt colonoscopy.[59] Generally only polyps greater than 2 cm are associated with symptoms. In one series none of the lipomas less than 2 cm were symptomatic, but 2% of those 3 to 4 cm and 75% of those greater than 4 cm were.[59]

At colonoscopy these are seen as soft, round sessile lesions, often greater than 2 cm,[60] largely confined to the right side of the colon (Fig. 41-16a). The overlying mucosa is usually smooth, although on occasion, especially with large lesions, it may have an irregular mucosal texture, appearing nodular or superficially ulcerated. Often there is a yellow coloration to the mucosa from the large accumulation of fatty tissue in the submucosa. As the mucosa tends to be entirely separate from the lipomatous tissue itself, it tents easily. Moreover, because of the soft nature of the fatty tissue, one can demonstrate a "cushion" effect, i.e., portions of the tumor are easily depressed when a closed biopsy forceps is applied (also referred to as the "pillow sign"[60]).

Repeated biopsy at one point or a large-particle biopsy often demonstrates one of the most striking endoscopic features of large colonic lipomas, i.e., fatty tissue actually protruding from the biopsy site.[60] This has been called the "naked fat sign" and is pathognomonic for a lipoma. Another sign in those cases in which electrosurgical excision of the lipoma is performed is flotation in fixative because of the lower density of lipomatous tissues.[61]

Although excision of 2- to 3-cm lipomas in symptomatic patients can be accomplished, it must be kept in mind that because of their size and sessile nature lipomas require more electrical current for transection, placing the patient at risk for a large burn site which could perforate or bleed.[20]

Leiomyomas/Leiomyosarcomas

Although in one recent colonoscopic series smooth muscle tumors of the colon were found as often as lipomas,[62] this has not been our experience. Of nine submucosal polyps found over a 7-year period among 500 colonic polyps, only two were leiomyomas, in contrast with six lipomas and one carcinoid. Both leiomyomas were small (<10 mm) and were thought prior to polypectomy to be tubular adenomas (Fig. 41-16c).

Like leiomyomas elsewhere in the GI tract, the commonest presenting complaint is bleeding. In these cases leiomyomas are generally large, greater than 2 cm, with central mucosal ulcerations from which the bleeding has occurred. Apart from the association with bleeding, size is also an important determinant of the likelihood of malignancy in that smooth muscle tumors greater than 4 cm may show the histologic finding of numerous mitoses as well as multinucleated and bizarre tumor cells as an indication of a predisposition to metastasis.[63]

Leiomyomas found at colonoscopy appear smooth and sessile, with a reddish appearance to the overlying mucosa; they range in size from 2 mm to 4 cm (Fig. 41-16c).[62] In both of our cases the reddish appearance of the mucosa probably contributed to our misdiagnosis of these polyps as tubular adenomas (Fig. 41-16c).

Leiomyosarcomas appear as large, sessile lesions 3 to 6 cm in greatest dimension with an ulcerated surface.[64] Although smooth muscle tumors are almost always single, recently a case of multiple leiomyomatosis of the colon was reported in which an infiltrating, multinodular myomatous growth was present, appearing as multiple sessile polyps.[64]

Carcinoids

Except for the rectum, the colon is a rare site for carcinoid tumors.[65] Surprisingly, in one series reported by Geboes et al. of submucosal tumors found at colonoscopy, carcinoids were as common as lipomas or leiomyomas.[62] In contrast, we found one carcinoid, six lipomas, and two leiomyomas. The carcinoids reported by Geboes et al. appeared at colonoscopy to be smooth, glistening, sessile lesions that were generally nonulcerating and ranging in size between 1 and 2 cm with a pale yellow cast to the mucosa.[62] A similar appearance was found for our lone carcinoid (Fig. 41-16d). Geboes et al. found that carcinoids, like other submucosal tumors, could be biopsied (large-particle technique) or removed electrosurgically without complication.[62]

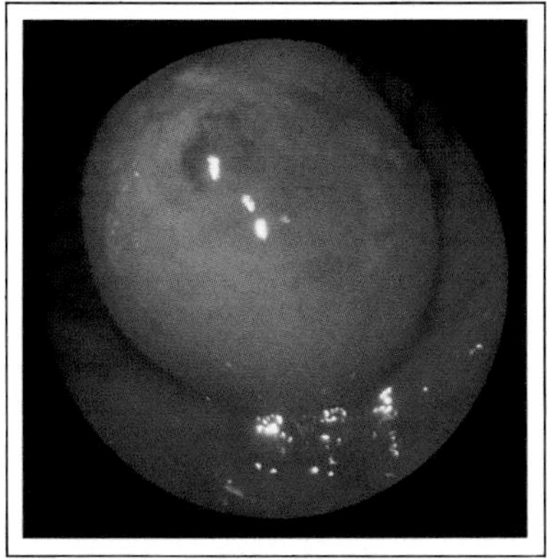

FIG. 41-16a.

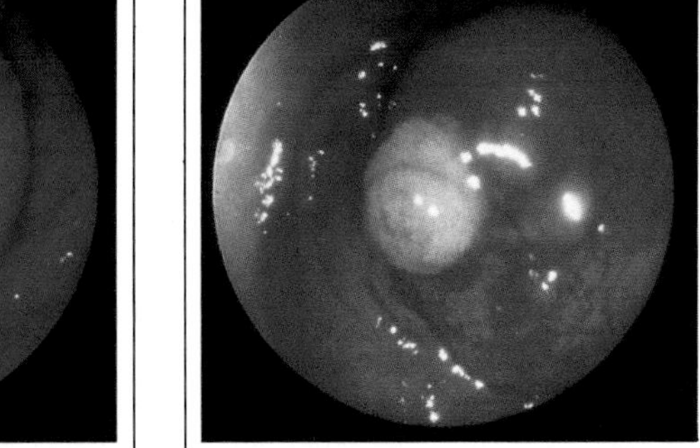

FIG. 41-16b.

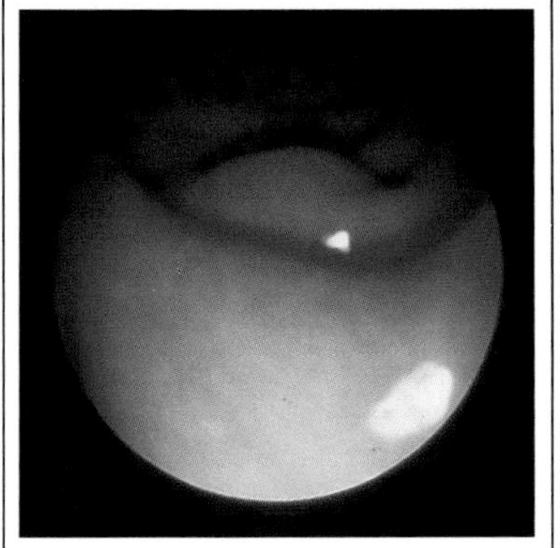

FIG. 41-16c.

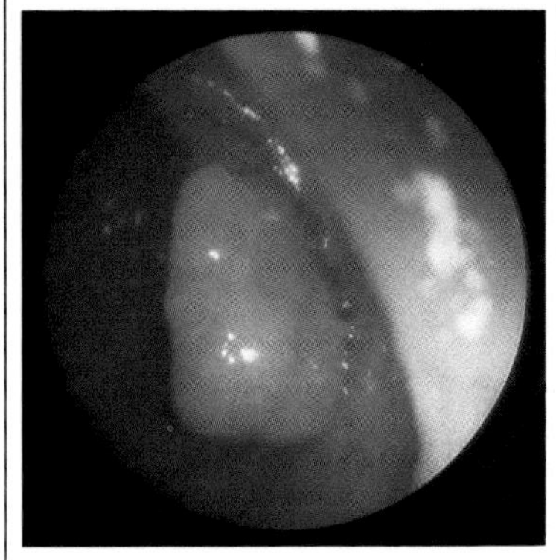

FIG. 41-16d.

FIG. 41-16. a: Lipoma. A 2- to 3-cm sessile polyp of the hepatic flexure with a somewhat erythematous surface. A definite yellow coloration is noted because of the presence of lipomatous tissue within. **b:** This lipoma after a large-particle excisional biopsy is now exuding fat (the naked fat sign). **c:** Leiomyoma. A small sessile polyp with a somewhat erythematous coloration, causing it to appear indistinguishable from a tubular adenoma. **d:** Carcinoid of the rectum. Although this had a slightly yellow coloration and smooth mucosa, it was nevertheless thought to be a common tubular adenoma.

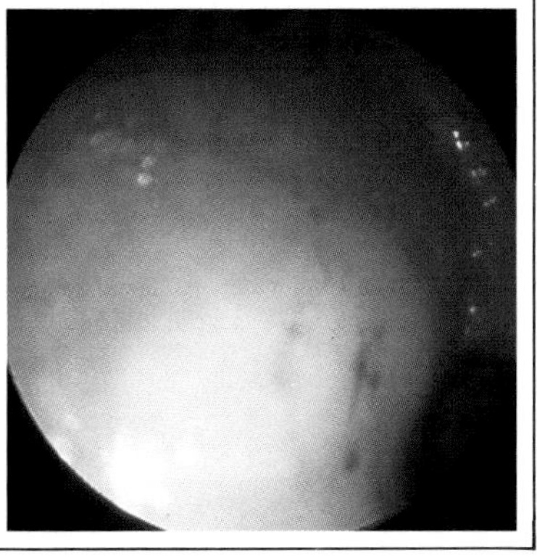

FIG. 41-17.

FIG. 41-17. Endometrial implant in the rectosigmoid junction. A discrete mass-like area of extrinsic compression was noted on the posterior (3 o'clock) wall. An endometrial implant of this area was found at surgery.

Endometrial Implants

Although obviously not derived from submucosal mesenchymal elements, an endometrial implant into the serosa of the rectum or sigmoid may appear as a submucosal polyp. Endometriosis is a relatively common condition among menstruating women, estimated to affect 8 to 15%,[66] although the actual incidence of colonic involvement with endometrial implants is unknown. Our experience suggests that these cases are exceedingly rare because over a 7-year period during which 2,100 examinations were performed only one case of an endometrial implant was encountered (Fig. 41-17).

When endometrial implants occur,[66] they may produce areas of eccentric or circumferential narrowing with obstruction rather than discrete masses. In some cases, however, they appear as discrete submucosal polyps (Fig. 41-17). Such a case has been reported where, in addition to a mass, there was a central erythematous area which proved on histologic examination of the resected specimen to be an endometrial implant which had extended through to the mucosa.[66]

REFERENCES

1. Fruhmorgen, P., Laudage, G., and Matek, W. (1981): The years of colonoscopy. *Endoscopy*, 13:162–168.
2. Rickert, R. R., Auerbach, O., Garfinkel, L., Hammond, E. C., and Frasca, J. M. (1979): Adenomatous lesions of the large bowel: an autopsy survey. *Cancer*, 43:1847–1857.
3. Gilbertson, V. A., McHugh, R., Schuman, L., and Williams, S. E. (1980): The earlier detection of colorectal cancers: a preliminary report of the results of the occult blood study. *Cancer*, 45:2899–2901.
4. Miller, C. H., Kussin, S. Z., and Winawer, S. J. (1980): Characteristics of synchronous colonic polyps. *Gastrointest. Endosc.*, 26:72.
5. Fork, F.-T. (1981): Double contrast enema and colonoscopy in polyp detection. *Gut*, 22:971–977.
6. Tedesco, F. J., Waye, J. D., Raskin, J. B., Morris, S. J., and Greenwall, R. A. (1978): Colonoscopy evaluation of rectal bleeding: a study of 304 patients. *Ann. Intern. Med.*, 89:907–909.
7. Enterline, H. T. (1976): Polyps and cancers of the large bowel. In: *Pathology of the Gastrointestinal Tract*, edited by B. C. Morson, pp. 97–142. Springer-Verlag, New York.
8. Morson, B. C. (1974): The polyp-cancer sequence in the large bowel. *Proc. Roy. Soc. Med.*, 67:451–457.

8a. Gilbertsen, V. A. (1974): Proctosigmoidoscopy and polypectomy in reducing the incidence of rectal cancer. *Cancer (suppl.)*, 34:936–939.

9. Muto, T., Bussey, H. U. R., and Morson, B. C. (1975): The evolution of cancer of the colon and rectum. *Cancer*, 36:2251–2270.

9a. Hermanek, P., Fruhmorgen, P., Guggenmoos-Holzmann, I., Altendorf, A., and Matek, W. (1983): The malignant potential of colorectal polyps—A new statistical approach. *Endoscopy*, 15:16–20.

10. Welch, J. P., and Welch, C. E. (1976): Villous adenomas of the colorectum. *Am. J. Surg.*, 131:185–191.
11. Williams, C. B., Hunt, R. H., Loose, H., Riddell, R. H., Sakai, K., and Swarbrick, E. T. (1974): Colonoscopy in the management of colon polyps. *Br. J. Surg.*, 61:673–682.
12. Thoeni, R. F., and Menuck, L. (1977): Comparison of barium enema and colonoscopy in the detection of small colonic polyps. *Radiology*, 124:631–635.
13. Miller, R. E., and Lehman, G. (1978): Polypoid colonic lesions undetected by colonoscopy. *Radiology*, 129:295–297.
14. Laufer, I., Smith, N. C. W., and Mullens, J. E. (1976): The radiological demonstration of colorectal polyps undetected by endoscopy. *Gastroenterology*, 70:167–170.
15. Dodds, W. J., Stewart, E. T., and Hogan, W. J. (1977): Role of colonoscopy and roentgenology in the detection of polypoid colonic lesions. *Am. J. Dig. Dis.*, 22:646–649.
16. Shinya, H., and Wolff, W. (1979): Morphology, anatomic distribution, and cancer potential of colonic polyps: an analysis of 7000 polyps endoscopically removed. *Ann. Surg.*, 190:679–683.
17. Gillespie, P. E., Chambers, T. J., Chan, K. W., Doronzo, F., Morson, B. C., and Williams, C. B. (1979): Colonic adenomas—a colonoscopic survey. *Gut*, 20:240–245.
18. Granqvist, S. (1981): Distribution of polyps in the large bowel in relation to age: a colonoscopic study. *Scand. J. Gastroenterol.*, 16:1025–1031.
19. Livstone, E. M., Troncale, F. J., and Sheahan, D. G. (1977): Value of a single forceps biopsy of colonic polyps. *Gastroenterology*, 73:1296–1298.
20. Cotton, P. B., and Williams, C. B. (1980): Colonoscopic polypectomy. In: *Practical Gastrointestinal Endoscopy*, pp. 129–141. Blackwell Scientific Publications, London.
21. Fruhmorgen, P. (1981): Therapeutic colonoscopy. In: *Colonoscopy*, edited by R. H. Hunt and J. D. Waye, pp. 199–235. Chapman and Hall, London.
22. Shinya, H. (1982): *Colonoscopy: Diagnosis and Treatment of Colonic Diseases.* Igaku-Shoin Medical Publishers, New York.

22a. Christie, J. P., and Shinya, H. (1982): Technique of colonoscopic polypectomy. *Surg. Clin. N. Am.*, 62:877–887.

23. Christie, J. P. (1977): Colonoscopic excision of large sessile polyps. *Am. J. Gastroenterol.*, 67:430–438.
24. Fenoglio, C., Kaye, G. I., and Lane, N. (1973): Distribution of human colonic lymphatics in normal, hyperplastic and adenomatous tissue. *Gastroenterology*, 64:52–66.
25. Shatney, C. H., Lober, P. H., Gilbertsen, V. A., and Sosin, H. (1976): Management of focally malignant pedunculated adenomatous colorectal polyps. *Dis. Colon Rectum*, 19:334–341.
26. Okike, N., Weiland, L. H., Anderson, M. J., and Adson, M. A. (1977): Stromal invasion of cancer in pedunculated adenomatous colorectal polyps. *Arch. Surg.*, 112:527–529.
27. Colacchio, T. A., Forde, K. A., and Scantlebury, V. P. (1981): Endoscopic polypectomy: inadequate treatment for colorectal carcinoma. *Ann. Surg.*, 194:704–707.

27a. Greenburg, A. G., Saik, R. P., Coyle, J. J., and Peskin, G. W. (1981): Mortality and gastrointestinal surgery in the aged. *Arch. Surg.*, 116:788–791.

28. Tedesco, F. J., Hendrix, J. C., Pickens, C. A., Brady, P. G., and Mills, L. R. (1982): Diminutive polyps: histopathology, spatial distribution, and clinical significance. *Gastrointest. Endosc.*, 28:1–5.
29. Granqvist, S., Gabrielsson, N., and Sundelin, P. (1979): Diminutive colon polyps—clinical significance and management. *Endoscopy*, 11:36–42.
30. Kronborg, O., Hage, E., and Deichgraeber, E. (1981): The clean colon: a prospective, partly randomized study of the effectiveness of repeated examinations of the colon after polypectomy and radical surgery for cancer. *Scand. J. Gastroenterol.* 16:879–884.
31. Fowler, D. L., and Hedberg, S. E. (1980): Followup colonoscopy after polypectomy. *Gastrointest. Endosc.*, 26:67.
32. Himal, H. S. (1979): The role of colonoscopic polypectomy in the management of "malignant" polyps of the colon. *Gastrointest. Endosc.*, 24:40.
33. Nivatvongs, S., and Goldberg, S. M. (1978): Management of patients who have invasive carcinoma removed via colonoscope. *Dis. Colon Rectum*, 21:8–11.
34. Hayashi, T., Yatami, R., Apostol, J., and Stemmer-Mann, G. N. (1974): Pathogenesis of hyperplastic polyps of the colon: a hypothesis based on ultrastructure and in vitro cell kinetics. *Gastroenterology*, 66:347–356.
35. Williams, G. T., Arthur, J. F., Bussey, H. J. R., and Morson, B. C. (1980): Metaplastic polyps and polyposis of the colorectum. *Histopathology*, 4:155–165.

35a. Franzin, G., and Novelli, P. (1982): Adenocarcinoma occurring in a hyperplastic (metaplastic) polyp of the colon. *Endoscopy*, 14:28–30.

36. Whittle, T. S., Varner, W., and Brown, F. M. (1978): Giant hyperplastic polyps of the colon simulating adenocarcinoma. *Am. J. Gastroenterol.*, 69:105–107.
37. Nishizawa, M., Okada, T., Sato, F., Kariya, A., Mayama, S., and Nakamura, K. (1980): A clinicopathological study of minute polypoid lesions of the colon based on magnifying fiber-colonoscopy and dissecting microscopy. *Endoscopy*, 12:124–129.
38. Habr-Gama, A., Alves, P. R. A., Gama-Rodriques, J. J., Teixeira, M. G., and Barbieri, D. (1979): Pediatric colonoscopy. *Dis. Colon Rectum*, 22:530–535.
39. Mazier, W. P., MacKeigan, J. M., Billingham, R. P., and Dignan, R. D. (1982): Juvenile polyps of the colon and rectum. *Surg. Gynecol. Obstet.*, 154:829–832.
40. Benjamin, S. P., Hawk, W. A., and Turnbull, R. B. (1977): Fibrous inflammatory polyps of the ileum and cecum: review of five cases with emphasis on differentiation from mesenchymal neoplasms. *Cancer*, 39:1300–1305.
41. Wennstrom, J., Pierce, E. R., and McKusick, V. A. (1974): Hereditary benign and malignant lesions of the large bowel. *Cancer (Suppl.)*, 34:850–857.
42. Bussey, H. J. R., Veale, A. M. O., and Morson, B. C. (1978): Genetics of gastrointestinal polyposis. *Gastroenterology*, 74:1325–1330.
43. Erbe, R. W. (1976): Inherited gastrointestinal polyposis syndrome. *N. Engl. J. Med.*, 294:1101–1104.
44. Diagnostic Oncology Case Studies (1978): Colon polyposis in cancer. *Am. J. Roentgenol.*, 131:1065–1067.
45. Bess, M. A., Adson, M. A., Elveback, L. R., and Moertel, C. G. (1980): Rectal cancer following colectomy for polyposis. *Arch. Surg.*, 115:460–467.
46. Rauzi, T., Castagnone, D., Velio, P., Bianchi, P., and Polli, E. E. (1981): Gastric and duodenal polyps in familial polyposis coli. *Gut*, 22:363–367.
47. Shull, L. N., and Fitts, C. T. (1974): Lymphoid polyposis associated with familial polyposis and Gardner's syndrome. *Ann. Surg.*, 180:319–322.

48. Naylor, E. W., and Lebenthal, E. (1980): Gardner's syndrome: recent developments in research and management. *Dig. Dis. Sci.*, 25:945–959.
49. Itoh, H., Ohsato, K., Yao, T., Iida, M., and Watanabe, H. (1979): Turcot's syndrome and its mode of inheritance. *Gut*, 20:414–419.
50. Grotsky, H. W., Rickert, R. R., Smith, W. D., and Newsome, J. F. (1982): Familial juvenile polyposis coli: a clinical and pathologic study of a large kindred. *Gastroenterology*, 82:494–501.
51. Sachatello, C. R., Pickren, J. W., and Grace, J. T. (1970): Generalized juvenile gastrointestinal polyposis: a hereditary syndrome. *Gastroenterology*, 58:699–708.
52. Stemper, J. J., Kent, T. H., and Summers, R. W. (1975): Juvenile polyposis and gastrointestinal carcinoma: a study of kindred. *Ann. Intern. Med.*, 83:639–646.
53. Daniel, E. S., Ludwig, S. L., Lewin, K. J., Ruprecht, R. M., Rajacich, G. M., and Schwabe, A. D. (1982): The Cronkhite-Canada syndrome. An analysis of clinical and pathologic features and therapy in 55 patients. *Medicine*, 61:293–309.
53a. Ali, M., Weinstein, J., Biempica, L., Halpern, A., and Das, K. M. (1982): Cronkhite-Canada syndrome: report of a case with bacteriologic, immunologic, and electron microscopic studies. *Gastroenterology*, 79:731–736.
54. McAllister, A. J., and Richards, K. F. (1977): Peutz-Jeghers syndrome: experience with twenty patients in five generations. *Am. J. Surg.*, 134:717–720.
55. Cochet, B., Carrel, J., Desbaillets, L., and Widgren, S. (1979): Peutz-Jeghers syndrome associated with gastrointestinal carcinoma: report of two cases in a family. *Gut*, 20:169–175.
56. Clement, S., Efrusy, M. E., Dobbins, W. O., and Palmer, R. N. (1979): Pelvic neoplasia in Peutz-Jeghers syndrome. *J. Clin. Gastroenterol.*, 1:341–363.
57. Weinstock, J. V., and Kawanishi, H. (1978): Gastrointestinal polyposis with orocutaneous hamartomas (Cowden's disease). *Gastroenterology*, 74:890–895.
58. DeBeer, R. A., and Shinya, H. (1975): Colonic lipomas: an endoscopic analysis. *Gastrointest. Endosc.*, 22:90–91.
59. Pemberton, L., and Manax, W. G. (1971): Complete obstruction of the colon by lipoma. *Surgery*, 69:139–141.
60. Messer, J., and Waye, J. D. (1982): The diagnosis of colonic lipomas—the naked fat sign. *Gastrointest. Endosc.*, 28:186–188.
61. Norfleet, R. G. (1979): The bobbin' polyp. *Gastrointest. Endosc.*, 25:29.
62. Geboes, K., deWolf-Peeters, C., Rutgeerts, P., Vantrappen, G., and Desmet, V. (1978): Submucosal tumors of the colon: experience with twenty-five cases. *Dis. Colon Rectum*, 21:420–425.
63. Warkel, R. L., Stewart, J. B., and Temple, A. J. (1975): Leiomyosarcoma of the colon: report of a case and analysis of the relationship of histology to prognosis. *Dis. Colon Rectum*, 18:501–506.
64. Freni, S. C., and Keeman, J. N. (1977): Leiomyomatosis of the colon. *Cancer*, 39:265–266.
65. Godwin, J. D. (1975): Carcinoid tumors: an analysis of 2837 cases. *Cancer*, 36:560–568.
66. Meyers, W. C., Kelvin, F. M., and Jones, R. S. (1979): Diagnosis and surgical treatment of colonic endometriosis. *Arch. Surg.*, 114:169–175.

42

COLONIC MALIGNANCIES

Colonoscopy is often requested because of the suspicion of colon carcinoma, the commonest gastrointestinal (GI) malignancy. A consideration of the endoscopic aspects of this cancer comprises the major portion of this chapter. In a concluding section we give brief attention to other rare but occasionally encountered malignancies, lymphoma and carcinoma metastatic to the colon, disseminated Kaposi's sarcoma, and leukemia with colonic involvement.

ADENOCARCINOMA

The large majority (90%) of colonic cancers are still discovered much as they were 50 years ago—because of symptoms[1]—despite a well-established means for diagnosis in asymptomatic patients using a standard 3-day fecal occult blood test.[2] For the minority of patients whose cancers are discovered while asymptomatic, 80%+ may still be early (Dukes' A or B), without metastasis,[3a] with 90% still at the stage where a curative resection can be performed[2] and with an overall 5-year survival approaching 80%.[4] This contrasts sharply with the prospect for the patient with symptomatic colonic cancer in which only 60% may have a curative resection[4a,5] with an overall 5-year survival of 60% or less[4,4a] and under 40% in the presence of metastasis.[4a] For symptomatic patients, matters are made even worse because diagnosis may be delayed further when neither the patient nor the physician attaches the proper importance to symptoms, e.g., a change in bowel habits or the passage of small amounts of blood, especially when mixed in with the stool. In one British study the mean delay between the onset of symptoms and the first visit to a physician was 30.5 weeks, with a mean of 38 weeks between the onset of symptoms and diagnosis.[6]

Even where symptoms are regarded seriously, if a single-contrast barium enema is used further delay could occur because of an up to 20% rate of failure to detect carcinomas actually present.[7] Also potentially adding to delay is the unwarranted faith in negative proctoscopic examination, especially with a rigid instrument. In the past up to 75% of colonic cancers were said to be within the reach of such instruments; however, because of a shift in location of cancers to the right side, fewer than 50% are currently within the reach of a rigid instrument.[8] Even the 50-cm flexible proctosigmoidoscope may fail to demonstrate one-third or more cancers, especially in patients over age 65 in whom there is an increased incidence of right-sided colonic cancers.[9]

The colonoscopist may therefore expect most examinations to be requested relatively late in the natural history of this malignancy, especially for at least 25% of symptomatic patients in whom the diagnosis is not suspected.[6] Even with a heightened awareness of the symptomatic manifestations[6] of this cancer on the part of both patient and physician, as well as greater utilization of standard fecal occult blood tests,[2] because much of the natural history of the cancer occurs prior to the onset of symptoms and even properly performed screening fecal occult blood tests may miss at least 10% of cancers present,[10] the colonoscopist still expects that over 40% of the cancers will be discovered only after they have already metastasized.[11]

Location

Rectum and Sigmoid

The commonest location for cancers found at colonoscopy is within the distal 40 cm of the colon. Tedesco et al. found this location to account for about half of 39 cancers.[12] Most of these were found in the sigmoid, possibly because colonoscopy might not have been performed in patients with obvious rectal carcinomas. The lower percentage of rectal carcinomas in this series contrasts with the predominance of rectal over sigmoid cancers in epidemiologic studies.[13]

TABLE 42-1. *Colonic cancers—51 cases (1976–1980)*

Location	No.	Percent of total	No. with appearance: Ulcerated mass	Polypoid	Annular	Plaque	Stricture
Rectum	4	8	2	1	—	1	—
Rectosigmoid (15–20 cm)	10	19	4	3	2	—	1
Sigmoid colon	12	23	3	6	2	—	1
Descending colon	7	14	4	—	—	1	2
Splenic flexure	4	8	3	—	1	—	—
Transverse colon	4	8	2	1	1	—	—
Ascending colon	5	10	2	2	1	—	—
Cecum	5	10	4	1	—	—	—
Total	51	100	24 (46)[a]	14 (28)[a]	7 (14)[a]	2 (4)[a]	4 (8)[a]

[a] Percent of total.

Our own experience (Table 42-1) is similar to that reported by Tedesco et al.[12] Of 51 patients with colorectal cancer examined by us over a 5-year period, only four (8%) had their cancer in the rectum or the low sigmoid, less than 18 cm from the anal verge. The rectosigmoid (15 to 20 cm) and sigmoid were the next commonest location, accounting for 42% of the cases (22 of 51).

Descending Colon and Splenic Flexure

Cancers in the descending colon and splenic flexure have been reported to account for approximately 15% of the total.[12] In our own series, these represented 22% of the total (11 of 51), but nearly half (11 of 25) of those were proximal to the sigmoid (Table 42-1).

Transverse and Right Colon

The transverse and right colon may account for nearly 30% of the total locations,[12] with 15 to 20% of these being purely right-sided (cecum and ascending colon). In our series 20% were in the right colon (cecum and ascending colon) with the remaining 10% distributed within the transverse colon (Table 42-1).

Appearance

There are five appearances for colonic cancers. These are: (a) a centrally ulcerated mass; (b) a polypoid mass (without ulceration); (c) an annular (circumferential) mass; (d) a raised plaque-like mass; and (e) a stricture without a mass. These appearances bear some relationship to the gross features of carcinomas as seen in the resected specimen but are at considerable variance because the lesion at colonoscopy is often incompletely visualized. Therefore we believe it is correct to regard these as essentially colonoscopic designations although related in some part to the actual pathologic appearance.

Ulcerated Mass

The appearance of an ulcerated mass accounted for nearly half (45%) of our cases, which probably more than any other appearance reflects the exophytic growth pattern of colonic cancer, being found when the cancer is discovered at a relatively late stage. This is evidenced by the fact that only half of these cases are operable and, of these, local or distant metastases are found in more than half.[14]

Among our cases, 24 had this appearance. Only 10 were operable, and of these only five patients had curative resections (Table 42-2), the others already having metastasized.

TABLE 42-2. *Colonoscopic appearance of 51 cancers in relation to surgical outcome*

Colonoscopic appearance	No.	No. not resected	Outcome in patients with resection attempted Dukes' (Modified Astler-Coller) stage: B_1	B_2	C_2	D	Total No. resected
Ulcerated mass	24	14	—	5	4	1	10
Polypoid	14	6	4	2	2	—	8
Annular	7	—	—	4	3	—	7
Plaque	2	—	—	1	1	—	2
Stricture	4	1	—	1	2	—	3
Total	51	21	4	13	12	1	30

In these cases the appearance is that of a large (≥4 cm) centrally ulcerated tumor mass with the ulceration being deep (Fig. 42-1a). Smaller masses (≤3 cm) may be only superficially ulcerated. The mass itself is generally hard with a surface of grayish-pink, friable tissue (Fig. 41-1b).

Polypoid Mass

The polypoid mass is the next commonest appearance, representing about one-third of the cancers found by us (Table 42-2). That cancers of this appearance may represent an earlier stage of colonic cancer growth is suggested by the fact that the majority of these, unlike those having the ulcerated mass appearance, are operable (Table 42-2); and of these, most were still without metastasis at the time of surgery, resulting in curative resections in almost half the patients found with this appearance.

The colonoscopic features of the polypoid mass of colonic cancer were discussed elsewhere (see Chapter 41). The typical lesion is that of a small, raised sessile mass having an ulcerated surface or sharply angulated borders that suggest the diagnosis of cancer (Fig. 42-2a). In some cases the mass itself is subtle, especially when it appears as only a focal enlargement of a fold (Fig. 42-2b).

Annular Mass

The annular mass is in reality a large ulcerated mass (Fig. 42-3a) which has simply spread circumferentially so as to envelope the entire wall of the colon as well as penetrate through it (Fig. 42-3b). Although many prove resectable, as in the case of the ulcerating mass, most often these are late lesions as evidenced by the high percentage found with metastasis, as well as a decreased 5-year survival for those undergoing resection.[15] Among our cases, this appearance accounted for approximately 15%. Although all were operable, 40% (three of seven) had already metastasized at the time of surgery.

Generally, only part of the mass is seen by the colonoscopist, i.e., the distal margin, although he may obtain a glimpse of the central ulceration. Because of the narrow caliber of the sigmoid, any mass in it may take on a circumferential or annular appearance, so that for the sigmoid (Fig. 42-3a) as well as the rectosigmoid there is sometimes a considerable discrepancy between what the endoscopist sees and where the lesion actually appears when the surgical specimen is opened (Fig. 42-3b). Often the apparently circumferential "napkin ring" (Fig. 42-3c) carcinoma turns out to be simply an ulcerated mass set in the narrow sigmoid-rectosigmoid area.

Plaque-Like Mass

The appearance of a slightly raised, flat or discoid mass with a central umbilication or ulceration (Fig. 42-4) is distinctly uncommon but is a characteristic appearance for carcinoma near open areas such as the rectum or ascending colon (Fig. 42-4a). Other areas, including the sigmoid, can be involved. The low-set nature of this lesion along with its central umbilication accounts for its saddle shape, observed radiographically (Fig. 42-4b).[16]

We observed this type of appearance in only 2 of 51 cases (Table 42-2), indicating its rarity. It has been suggested that cancers with this configuration are relatively indolent in that 50% of these lesions are not associated with metastasis at surgery even when they are initially missed radiologically (but noted in retrospect), being detected after progressing to an annular appearance.[16]

Stricture

As the growth pattern of colonic carcinoma is exophytic, cancer appearing endoscopically as a stricture, i.e., an abrupt termination of the lumen without an obvious tumor mass, is uncommon (Fig. 42-5a). Among our 51 cancers, only four appeared as strictures (Table 42-2). Of the three that underwent resection, two proved to have an exophytic growth pattern even though appearing as a stricture. In only one of four cases was the growth pattern true infiltrative, i.e., colonic linitis plastica,[17] similar to the malignant appearance which occurs in ulcerative colitis (see Chapter 43). In the two other cases the stricture was a result of complete obstruction of the lumen by an exophytic mass (Fig. 42-5a), so that all that could be seen was heaped-up, though endoscopically normal, mucosa projecting out from the lumen. In one case, with a change in the patient's position, the exophytic nature of the carcinoma became clear (Fig. 42-5b) with the observation of a rim of tumor at the mouth of the stricture although the annular cancer was never seen in its entirety (Fig. 42-5c). In the case of the truly infiltrative carcinoma (or colonic linitis plastica), no such rim of tumor is apparent. A final cause of the stricture appearance is where the lumen has been narrowed by the presence of the extension of tumor into pericolic fat, with compression of the colon distally so that the exophytic mass cannot be observed.

Synchronous Adenomas

As colonic cancers are for the most part derived from preexisting adenomas (see Chapter 41), it is not surprising that adenomas should be found in association with cancer (Fig. 42-6). In a large series from Malmö, Sweden, based on double-contrast radiography, proctoscopy, and autopsy, coexisting adenomas were found in 22% of 960 patients with cancer.[18] Among our 51 patients with cancer having colonoscopy, adenomas were found in 13, a similar proportion (26%). In most, the polyps are single but as was true in the Malmö study they may be multiple (≥3) in 25%.[18] Similarly,

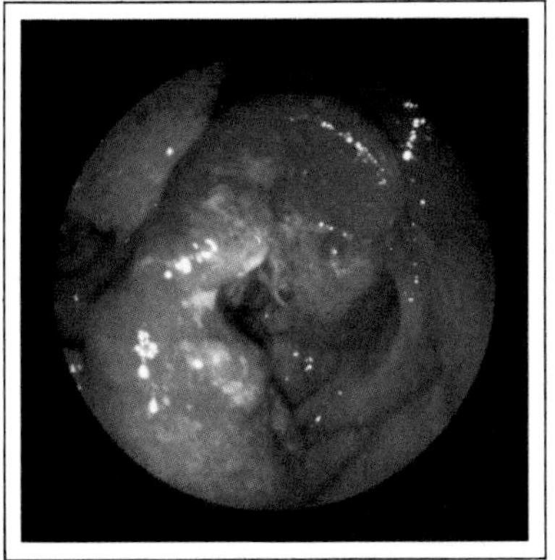

FIG. 42-1a.

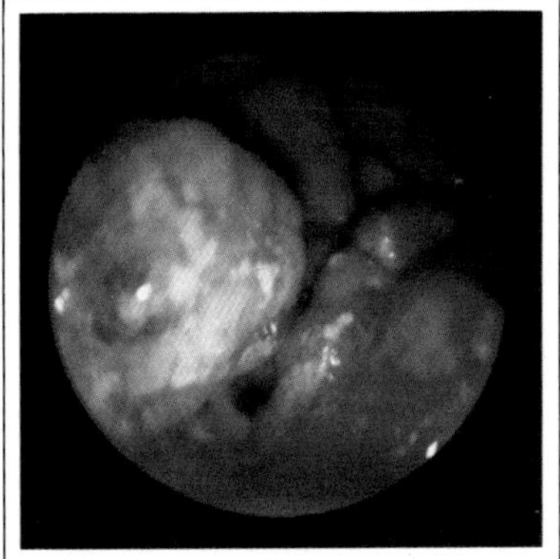

FIG. 42-1b.

FIG. 42-1. Adenocarcinoma, ulcerated mass. **a:** The endoscopic finding was a 3 × 4 cm polypoid mass with a central excavation and ulceration. This is the commonest endoscopic appearance of colonic cancer, accounting for nearly 50% of our cases (Table 42-1). **b:** A close-up view of a large lesion (a) shows the centrally excavated ulcerated portion which is entirely carcinoma. Its rock hard consistency was appreciated when biopsies were performed.

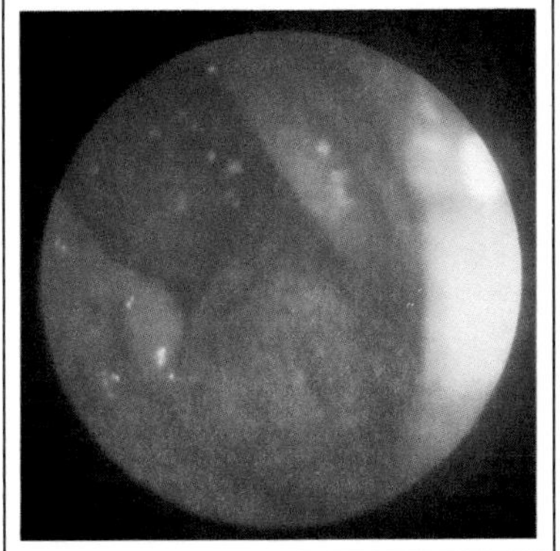

FIG. 42-2a.

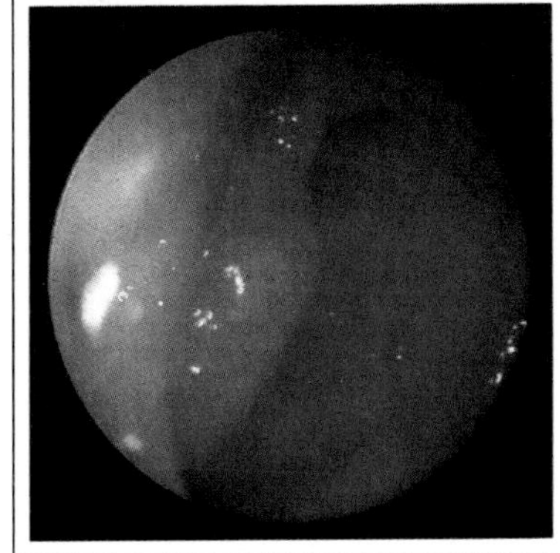

FIG. 42-2b.

FIG. 42-2. Adenocarcinoma, polypoid mass. **a:** The mass with its dull surface character is distinctly seen in relation to the glistening mucosa of the adjacent intrahaustral folds. **b:** A 1.5-cm polypoid mass. This sessile lesion is the smallest cancer that one may expect to find at colonoscopy outside of a malignant focus within an adenoma. In this case it was seen as focal enlargement of a mucosal fold within the sigmoid.

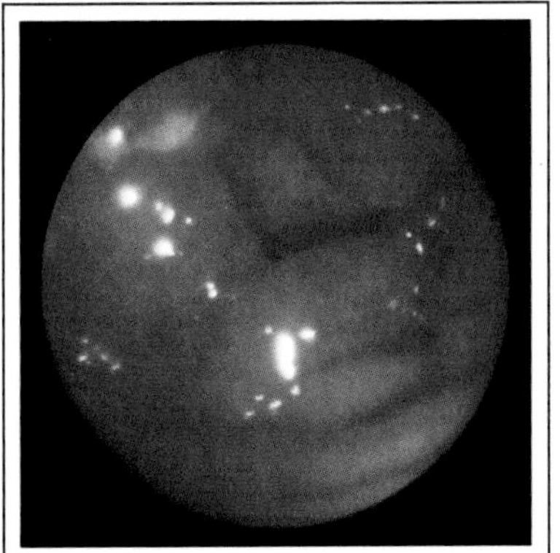

FIG. 42-3a.

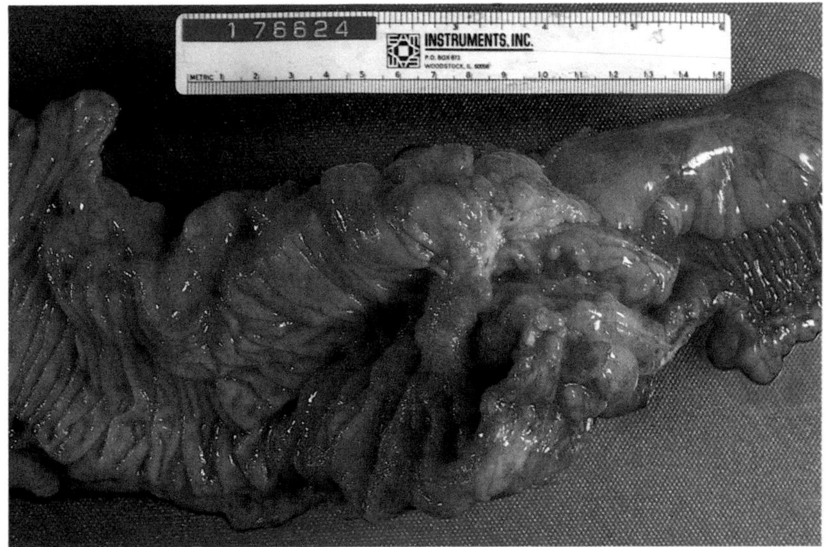

FIG. 42-3b.

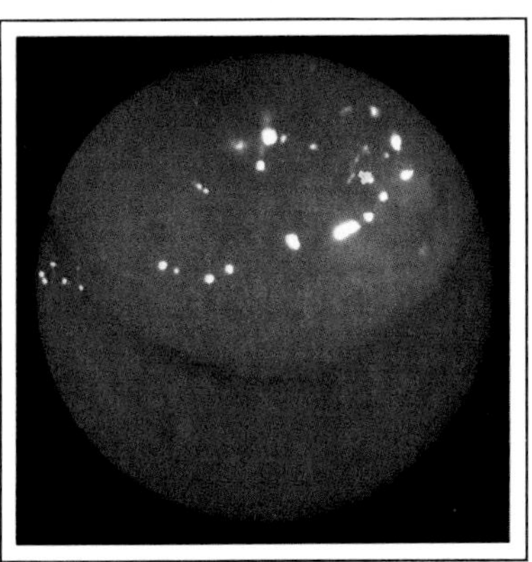

FIG. 42-3c.

FIG. 42-3. Adenocarcinoma, annular mass. **a:** The mass encircles the sigmoid, compromising the lumen. Its ulcerated center was not apparent at endoscopy but was clearly shown in the dissected specimen (b). **b:** The resected specimen in this case shows a central ulcerated portion of what appeared at colonoscopy to be only a circumferential tumor mass (a). **c:** The circumferential tumor mass (pinpoint narrowing of the lumen in a patient presenting with obstruction).

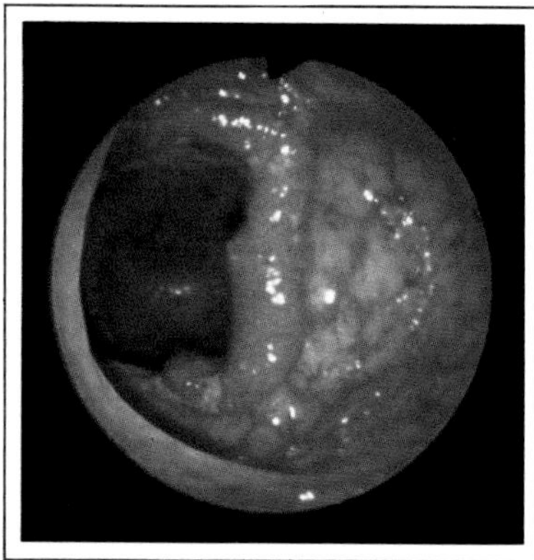

FIG. 42-4a.

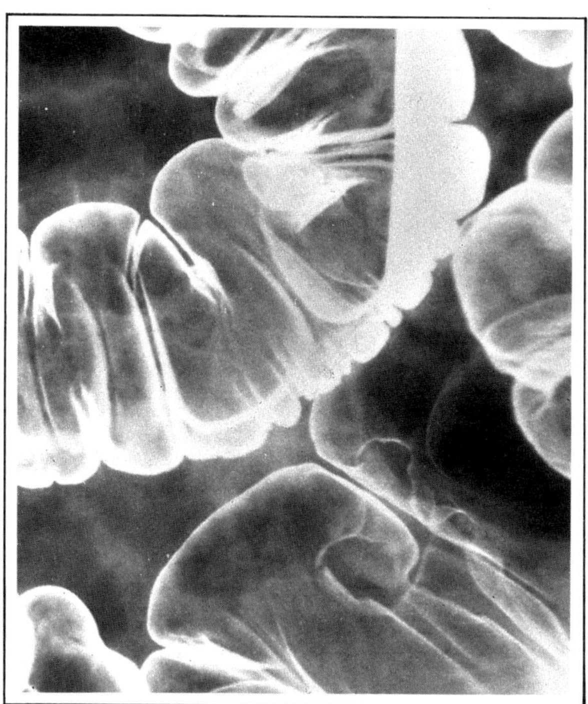

FIG. 42-4b.

FIG. 42-4. a: Adenocarcinoma, plaque-like mass. The lesion located proximal to the cecum (on the posterior wall at 3 o'clock) appears as a slightly raised, discrete mass with central depressions. **b:** Plaque-like adenocarcinoma, radiographic appearance. The lesion (left lower quadrant) is seen with raised margins around a central depression, giving the appearance of a saddle.[16]

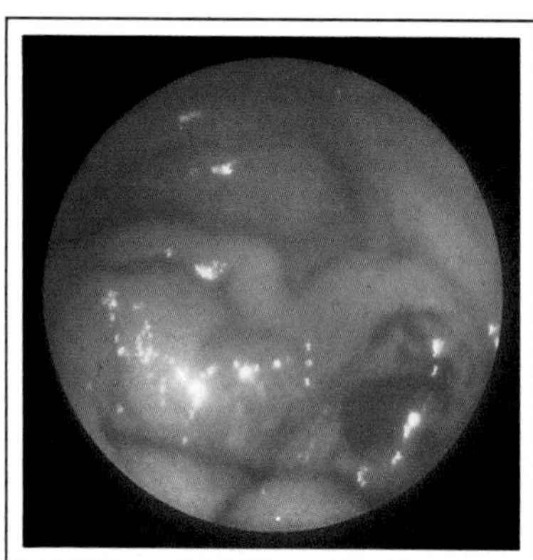

FIG. 42-5a.

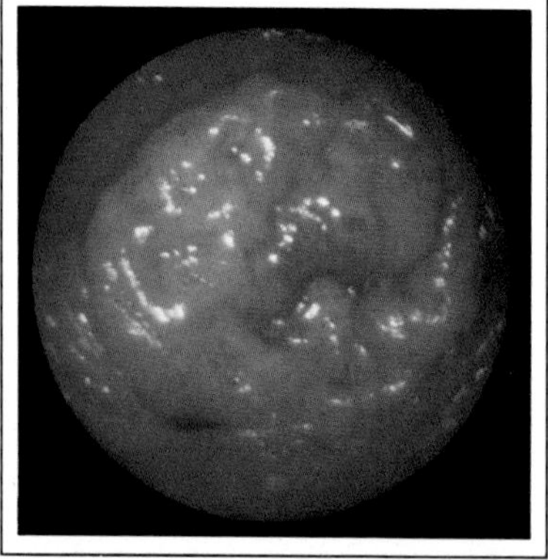

FIG. 42-5b.

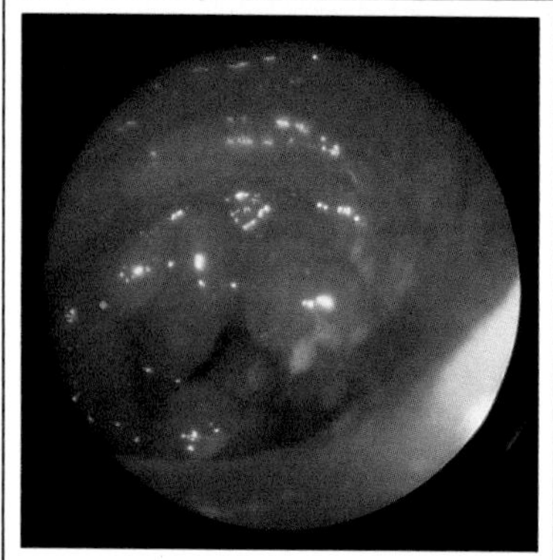

FIG. 42-5c.

FIG. 42-5. a: Adenocarcinoma, stricture. Folds radiate to a pinpoint narrowing. The intact overlying mucosa suggests an infiltrating, rather than an exophytic, growth pattern. Biopsies of the mouth of the stricture were negative, but brushing cytology was positive, emphasizing its usefulness with this type of appearance. **b:** Adenocarcinoma, stricture. A mass effect is apparent, suggesting that this lesion may have an exophytic-type growth pattern. For the most part, the mucosa is intact [as in (a)], except for a small rim at the mouth of the stricture. **c:** Adenocarcinoma, annular mass. In this case the stricture is entirely the result of this tumor, which has broken through at the point of luminal narrowing.

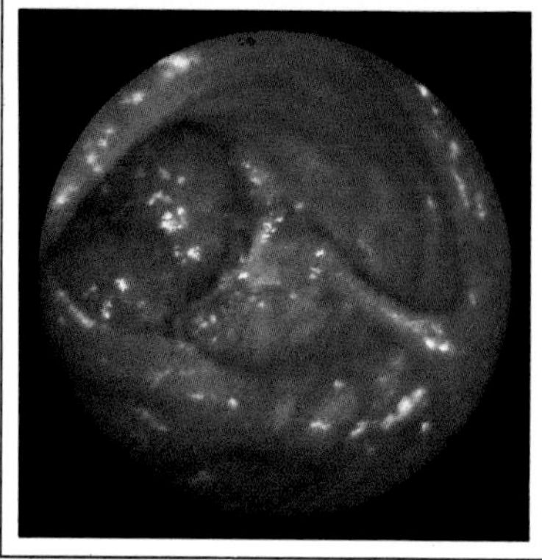

FIG. 42-6.

FIG. 42-6. Adenocarcinoma, sigmoid with synchronous (sentinel) adenoma. A cancer with an ulcerated mass appearance was found at the splenic flexure (in the distance at 3 o'clock). Just distal to this in the proximal descending colon a pedunculated polyp is noted as a sentinel neoplasm. The possibility of other adenomas or even cancers being present in this colon suggests the need to perform a colonoscopy 6 to 12 months after a curative resection for this malignancy.

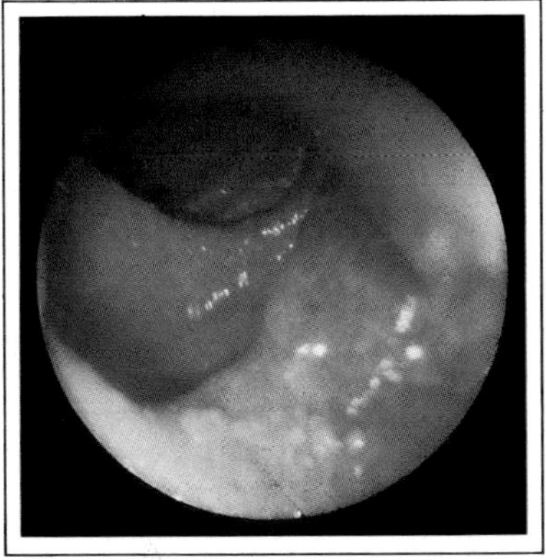

FIG. 42-7a.

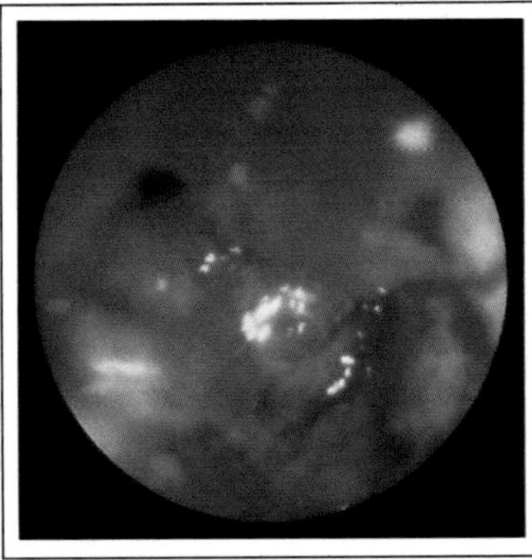

FIG. 42-7b.

FIG. 42-7. a: Synchronous carcinoma of the sigmoid. An asymmetrical, focally enlarged fold was noted in a patient in which a large carcinoma was found at the hepatic flexure (b). Because the possibility of a second carcinoma was considered, the asymmetrical fold was aggressively biopsied, which proved it to be a small adenocarcinoma. This case emphasizes the need for a careful examination of the colon for a second neoplasm once carcinoma is found. **b:** Adenocarcinoma, hepatic flexure. A large 3 × 5 cm polypoid mass was first identified in a patient with a small synchronous carcinoma of the sigmoid (a).

among our 13 patients with adenomas, three (23%) had multiple lesions, including one patient with 50 polyps! Of interest is the incidence of multiple adenomas (≥3), which appears to be somewhat higher in patients with cancer than those without, as evidenced in one large colonoscopy series (more than 1,000 polyps removed) where only 16% were mutiple (≥3).[19] Recently, an even higher proportion (62%) of patients with cancer having synchronous polyps was reported in which a third of the polyps were larger than 1 cm.[20]

Synchronous Cancers

Colonic Cancers

The finding of a second cancer at colonoscopy at the time the first is discovered may be expected in up to 10% of the cases, although in most series this has ranged between 3 and 7.6%.[20,21] Among our 51 patients, two additional cancers (3.9%) were found at colonoscopy. In one case, a 2-cm polypoid cancer of the sigmoid (Fig. 42-7a) was found in a patient with a large circumferential mass of the ascending colon (Fig. 42-7b), whereas in another with carcinoma of the splenic flexure and multiple (>15) polyps distal to this, a 1.5 × 2 cm villous adenoma with focally invasive cancer was found in the sigmoid.

Other Cancers

Two out of the 51 (3.9%) cancers in our series were discovered prior to esophago-gastrectomy. In these cases, colonoscopy was done because of a suspicious lesion found on an air-contrast barium enema performed prior to colonic interposition. The predisposition for a second cancer in a patient already having one cancer is well known. Based on our experience, we recommend an air-contrast barium enema in patients undergoing surgery for esophageal or cardial carcinoma, as these patients seem to be at increased risk for colonic cancer compared with the general population.[22]

Biopsy and Cytology

Biopsy

One would expect that with an exophytic growth pattern of colonic cancer simple forceps biopsy would be a relatively high-yield procedure, but this has not proved to be the case. In one study of 40 carcinomas[23] in which the majority of colonoscopic lesions were considered to be exophytic—the typical appearance of colonic cancer (Fig. 42-8a)—the yield was only 72%. This was even lower when only thickened folds were seen (Fig. 42-8b) and in others where the growth pattern was considered to be possibly infiltrative (Fig. 42-8c). In these cases the yield was only 44%, whereas for the group as a whole the yield was 60%.

The relatively low yield even for exophytic-appearing lesions is not difficult to understand once the technical difficulties of sampling are considered. Often this is simply a matter of not being able to position the instrument tip in a way that causes it to be perfectly *en face* with the lesion. Should the lesion be seen tangentially, the biopsy forceps cannot be positioned in such a way that it necessarily samples the surface of the cancer where it has clearly broken through the mucosa and stands in the lumen (Fig. 42-8a). Even when the carcinoma is in a position to be effectively sampled, another problem of superficial forceps biopsy is their failure to provide a deep enough sample to allow a diagnosis of invasive cancer rather than simply one of *in situ* carcinoma or neoplastic tissue suggestive of severe atypia. Some may wish to obviate this problem by providing deeper sections using the large-particle technique in which an excisional biopsy of the lesion is performed electrosurgically. However, in the usual clinical setting of a symptomatic patient with an annular-constricting lesion seen radiographically, the additional confirmatory evidence, beyond the demonstration of a mass and its neoplastic nature, seems unnecessary. Whereas large-particle biopsy could be a way of obtaining deeper samples, the potential for complications is also increased without an increased benefit in most cases. Clearly for strictures or other annular lesions

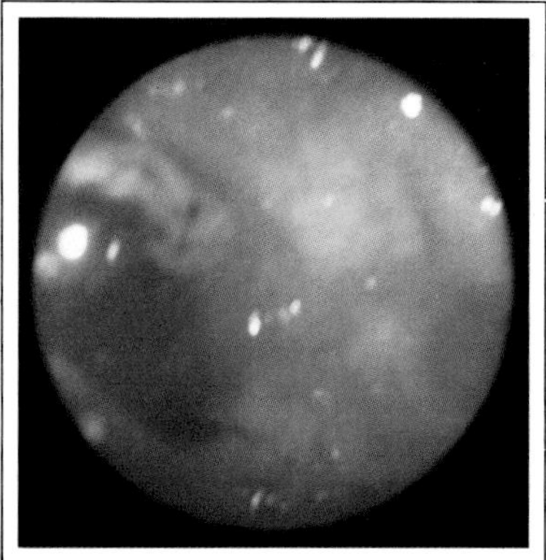

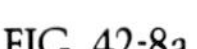

FIG. 42-8a.

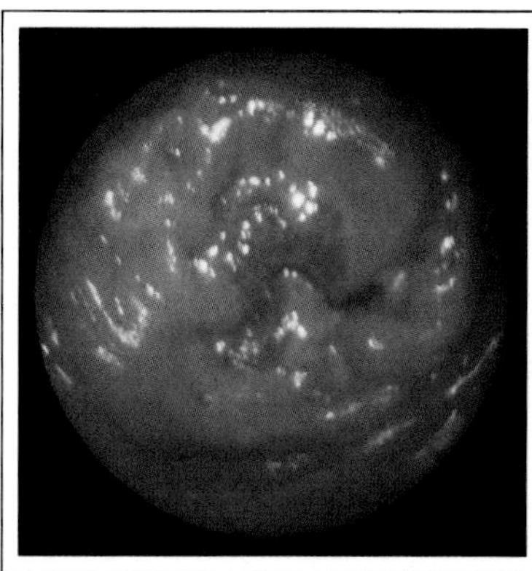

FIG. 42-8b.

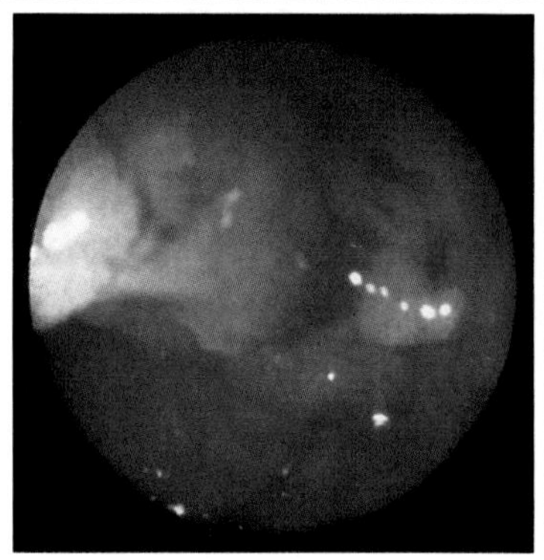

FIG. 42-8c.

FIG. 42-8. Adenocarcinoma. **a:** Exophytic-type lesion. The yield from biopsy of this type of lesion is reasonably high (70%+)[23] but only if the cancer is biopsied at the point of mucosal breakthrough (in this case at 3 o'clock). Because of the potential difficulty in establishing an *en face* view to maximize the yield from biopsy, a brushing cytology is recommended as well. **b:** Exophytic-type lesion, appearing as a stricture. Although the tumor breakthrough at the mouth of the stricture makes this an exophytic-type lesion, biopsy might fail because of the stricture decreasing the high-yield surface area where the tumor has broken through. In such a case, brushing cytology from the mouth as well as within the stricture is strongly recommended. It may be that this stricture-like annular type of appearance accounts for the lower yield (70%+)[23] for the exophytic-type growth pattern, which based on its appearance in the resected specimen (Fig. 42-3b), one would think ought to be higher, i.e., approach 90%+ as in gastric carcinomas (see Chapter 16). **c:** Infiltrative type. A small area of tumor breakthrough may have occurred within the stricture but nowhere else. Biopsies of the mouth of the stricture would have an exceedingly low yield, whereas brushing cytology from within the stricture may be positive.

where the mucosa appears heaped-up but intact, one does not wish to risk perforation of the segment of noncancerous colon adjacent to the carcinoma.

Cytology

The addition of brush cytology, especially if brushes are protected by a Teflon sheath, seems to increase the yield over biopsy alone.[23] In the study previously mentioned,[23] for exophytic lesions the yield increased from 72% to 94%, whereas for infiltrating tumors a positive result was obtained in 78% with combined modalities, in contrast with 44% for biopsy alone. The overall yield for the combined modalities was 80%+, contrasted with 60% for biopsy alone. The cases where cytology has the greatest impact on diagnosis are those where the colonoscope tip position fails to allow adequate technical control of the portion of the lesion where the cancer has broken through the mucosa. Furthermore, in cases where the appearance is either annular or that of a stricture, brushing within the stenotic portion of the lesion recovers neoplastic cells even where the adjacent mucosa shows no sign of carcinoma.

Differentiation of Cancer from Other Appearances

For the most part, the distinctive appearances of colonic cancer do not cause interpretive difficulties. However, in several instances one may wrongly suspect a lesion of being colonic cancer. These include the following appearances: (a) an incompletely visualized sessile adenoma, especially in the presence of diverticular disease; (b) inflammatory strictures associated with diverticular disease; and (c) other mass-like deformities, e.g., an enlarged ileocecal valve.

Incompletely Visualized Adenoma in Association With Diverticular Disease

The sigmoid is the commonest location for both adenomas (see Chapter 41) and carcinomas (Table 42-1). It is also the narrowest segment of the colon and one which commonly has prominent valvulae, making the lumen seem even narrower (Fig. 42-9a). A sessile adenoma of the sigmoid may therefore be mistaken for carcinoma if it is incompletely visualized because of associated diverticular disease. Furthermore, large adenomas which often have a villous component may show enough surface irregularity and friability to add to the endoscopist's confusion. The examiner's recourse is to inspect the portion of the mass available to him as best he can. If it is soft and easily compressed by the biopsy forceps, it is less likely to be carcinoma, although this feature does not exclude the diagnosis—nor would a forceps or even large-particle biopsy showing "adenomatous tissue" (Fig. 42-9b). In many cases

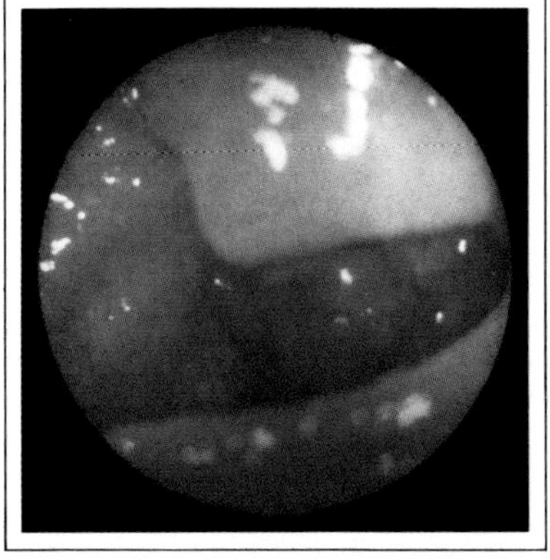

FIG. 42-9a.

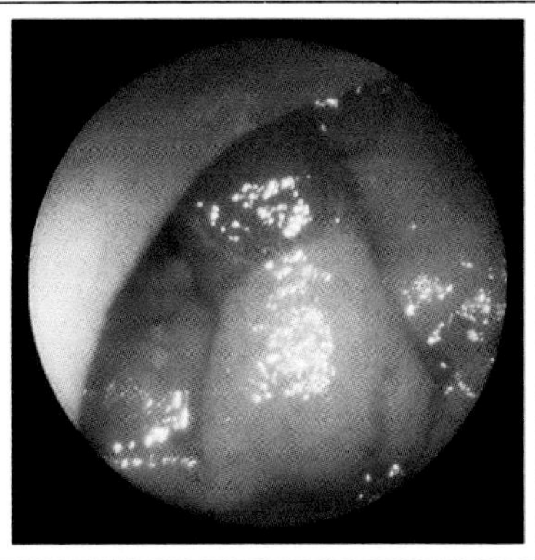

FIG. 42-9b.

FIG. 42-9. Adenoma of the sigmoid. **a:** Because of apparent luminal narrowing, it was initially mistaken for carcinoma. Because the pedicle was not appreciated, this lesion in the context of a narrowed lumen was thought to represent carcinoma. Further confusion would be expected from biopsies taken from an adenoma showing neoplastic tissue. **b:** Because of luminal narrowing, the pedicle was difficult to visualize (a), although with a change in position this is now clearly seen to be an adenoma, rather than a carcinoma.

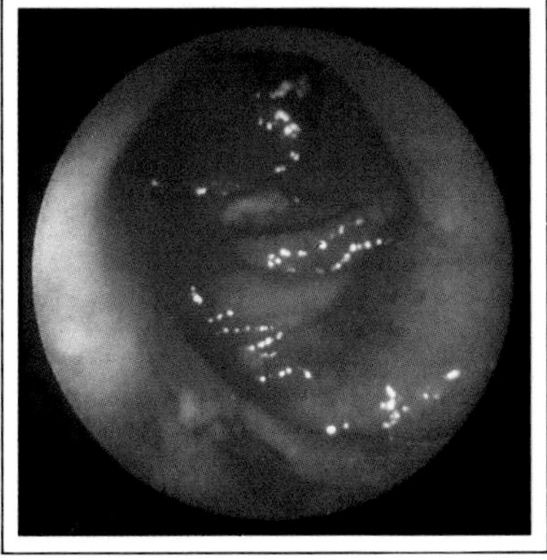

FIG. 42-10a.

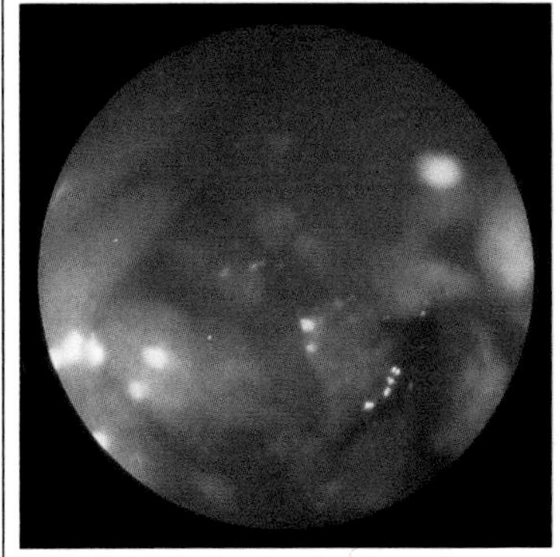

FIG. 42-10b.

FIG. 42-10. a: Diverticular stricture of the sigmoid. The lumen becomes markedly narrow at 12 o'clock. Because of mucosal friability, the examiner's impression was that of a malignant stricture [similar to that in (b)]. Biopsies and brushing cytology were negative, but because of the clinical suspicion surgical resection was performed, showing the lesion to be a diverticular stricture. **b:** Malignant stricture of the sigmoid. The mouth of the stricture (going off to 5 o'clock) shows friability as well as nodularity. Nevertheless, it is similar in appearance to a diverticular stricture (a).

it is possible to remove such adenomas using the piecemeal technique at several sittings so that the endoscopist may choose to submit a large portion of the lesion for histologic examination to determine its nature. In cases where the piecemeal technique cannot be employed and considerable doubt remains as to the nature of the lesion, one may have no recourse but to recommend surgical excision, both to determine the nature of the mass as well as to completely remove its malignant potential.

Diverticular Strictures

As colonic radiology is often equivocal or in error (up to 20%) concerning the nature of a stricture associated with diverticular disease,[24] colonoscopy is not infrequently requested with the hope of determining its true nature (Fig. 42-10a). Although the accuracy of colonoscopy in differentiating benign from malignant strictures appears to be high from retrospective studies, a prospective evaluation has not yet been reported. Colonoscopy combined with biopsy, especially cytology, seems at present to provide the best information concerning any stricture, assuming that a stricture can be reached. However, apart from examinations which fail to reach the stricture and therefore can provide no information, the colonoscopist may still have problems in differentiation, which may approach 10%, where an erroneous diagnosis of cancer is made in the presence of diverticular stricture or vice versa.

The commonest appearance of a diverticular stricture which causes confusion is that of marked luminal narrowing in association with circular muscle hypertrophy (see Chapter 45). The valvulae which form the mouth of the diverticular stricture are perfectly regular and symmetrical, appearing similar to other valvulae which do not compromise the lumen. Unlike an annular carcinoma which projects out into the lumen, the valvulae are perfectly flat (Fig. 42-10a). Also unlike many carcinomas (Fig. 42-10b), the mucosa overlying the mouth of the stricture is intact. In the case of carcinoma, even when the malignancy has not been through the mucosa around the mouth of the stricture, the folds are distinctly irregular and heaped-up in comparison to the surrounding folds (Fig. 42-10b).

In cases where one cannot be certain, even by looking at the stricture as to its nature, brush cytology from within the stricture as well as biopsy of the mouth is indicated, although a negative result never excludes a diagnosis of cancer. One may expect that in 5 to 10% of the cases endoscopy will be indeterminate with benign as well as malignant features, so that laparotomy and segmental resection may ultimately be necessary to determine the nature of stricture.

Mass-Like Deformities Including Ileocecal Valve Enlargement

Any area of redundant colonic mucosa (see Chapter 40), especially in flexure areas (particularly after blind intubation causes the mucosa to become erythematous), may take on a mass-like appearance (Fig. 42-11a) and suggest the presence of cancer (Fig. 42-11b). The commonest such deformity is the ileocecal valve itself protruding out into the lumen, especially when it assumes its polypoid configuration (see Chapter 39). In cases where enlargement of the ileocecal valve occurs (see Chapter 40), an even more striking resemblance to carcinoma may be observed. In addition, other submucosal polypoid masses (see Chapter 41) may be mistaken for polypoid cancer, especially if surface irregularity is present. This we have encountered in a case where a large (5 cm) lipoma of the transverse colon impressed the examiner as being "rock hard" and nodular. Surgical removal of it revealed it to be entirely lipomatous with surface erosions and ulcerations (thought to be from mucosal wear and tear from such a large mass protruding into the lumen), which caused the examiner to mistake it for a carcinoma. For any mass, especially one suggestive of a submucosal origin, deeper biopsies might be obtained using a large-particle technique to establish the nature of the lesion. In a case where one is uncertain, even as to whether the lesion is a mass (or a mass-like redundant fold of the mucosa), large-particle biopsy should be avoided because of the possibility of perforation. Instead, one examines such masses in different positions and attempts to tent the mucosa to see if its configuration changes as the mucosa is drawn out into the lumen, as would be the case with a mass-like fold of redundant mucosa (see Chapter 40).

Follow-up Colonoscopy

Screening for Other Neoplasms

Because up to 60% of patients with colonic cancer have at least one synchronous adenoma[20] and because 3 to 8% have a second cancer, either at the time of the original surgery[20] or discovered over the next 4 years,[20] all patients after resection (especially if it is thought to be curative) should have colonoscopy within a year of surgery to look for additional lesions. This is particularly important for patients whose examination at the time of surgery was not complete, because of an obstructing left sided or transverse colon cancer. Still, because of the 10% potential miss rate of colonoscopy for polyps (see Chapter 41), colonoscopy at 1 year should be mandatory for all patients (Fig. 42-12), even those having a "complete" examination at the time of the diagnosis of cancer. This should be performed irrespective of whether a barium enema shows a polyp or a fecal occult blood is positive. If no polyps are found, the patient is placed in the same category as others having single polyps removed; he should have yearly tests for stool occult blood and repeat colonoscopy within 3 to 5 years or sooner should occult blood be detected or other symptoms appear that raise the suspicion of recurrent carcinoma.

Suspicion of Recurrent Carcinoma

Colonoscopy may be requested because of a question of recurrent cancer at the anastomotic site, the location for recurrence in 10% of patients having prior surgical resection.[24a] In a case where recurrent carcinoma is suspected, a barium enema will routinely be performed, in addition prompting colonoscopy because of nonspecific radiologic appearances of the anastomotic site, such as stenosis or a mass-like deformity—cases where recurrent cancer cannot be excluded.[25]

While cancer may recur at the suture line,[24a] most recurrences are found in lymphatics, or other sites outside the colon, not removed at the time of the original surgery.[26] As the tumor in these cases is located at some distance from the mucosa, colonoscopy is generally unhelpful in determining whether recurrence is present. For the most part the examiner observes mucosal breakthrough of cancer only in the case of suture line recurrences, which probably account for no more than 30% of total cases of recurrence.[26] Although these may occur in any location, they are rare except for the rectum and rectosigmoid,[24a] where the completeness of the initial resection may have been compromised because of the technical difficulties of working within the pelvis.[24a,25] Here the examiner may find visual evidence of carcinoma as rock hard, friable tumor mass (Fig. 42-13a). For the large majority of anastomoses the examiner encounters in patients with previous resections for carcinoma, however, even those with recurrences of regional lymph nodes show a variety of nonspecific appearances centering around nodularity (Fig. 42-13b) which occurs because interrupted sutures were used to form the anastomosis. In some cases a nodule may become sizable because of tissue reaction to the suture material, resulting in the formation of a suture granuloma (see Chapter 47); in most cases this type of nodularity, even if asymmetrical, is not confused with the rock-hard, sessile, ulcerated mass which occurs in and around an anastomotic site (Fig. 42-13a) which would cause one to suspect recurrence, especially in the rectum or rectosigmoid area.

COLONIC LYMPHOMA

Colonic lymphomas are uncommon, with lymphoma from all sites occurring only one-fifth as often as colonic carcinoma[27] and colonic involvement occurring in only 2% of lymphomas.[28] The expected ratio of colonic lymphoma to carcinoma is therefore 1 case per 250 carcinomas ($1/5 \times 1/50 = 1/250$). At our hospital, which is a referral center for lymphoma, the prevalence for lymphoma in

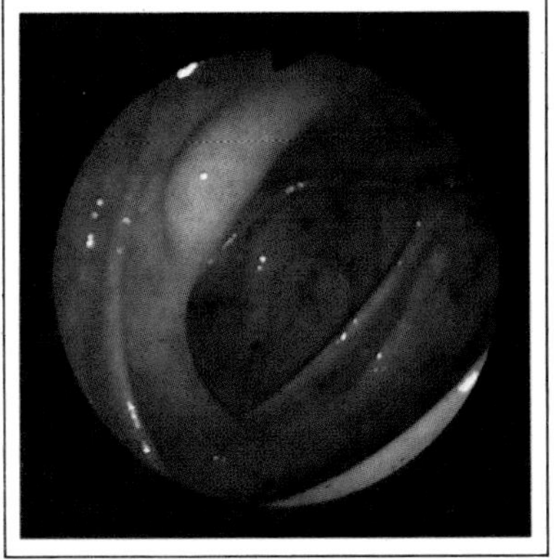
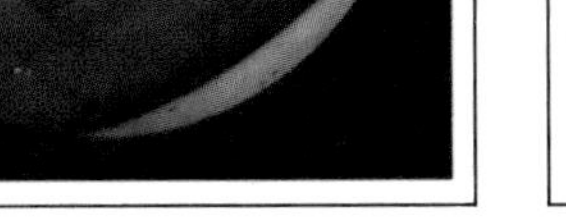

FIG. 42-11a.

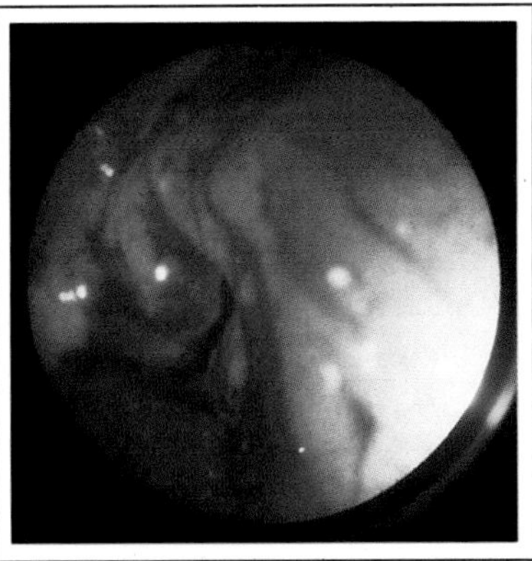
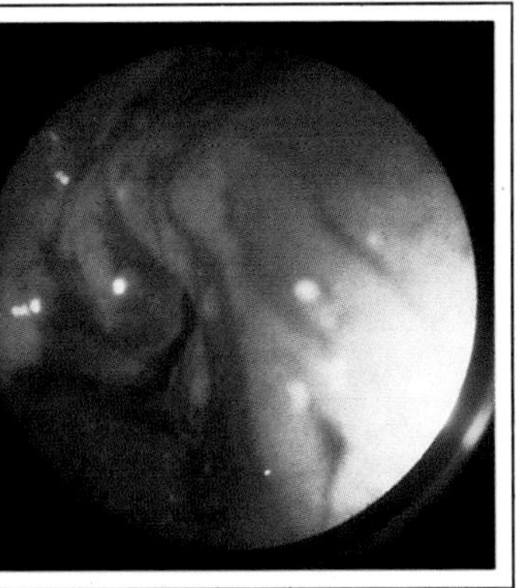

FIG. 42-11b.

FIG. 42-11. a: Prominent ileocecal valve. A focal area of thickening somewhat resembles the appearance of a small polypoid carcinoma (Fig. 42-7a). In this case the location is appropriate for the ileocecal valve. A forceps biopsy rather than one of the large-particle, excisional type (which could injure the ileocecal valve) is indicated. **b:** Carcinoma of the ileocecal valve with an *en face* view of the ileocecal valve in an irregular mass with central excavation-ulceration is noted. It strongly suggests malignancy (which was confirmed by forceps biopsy).

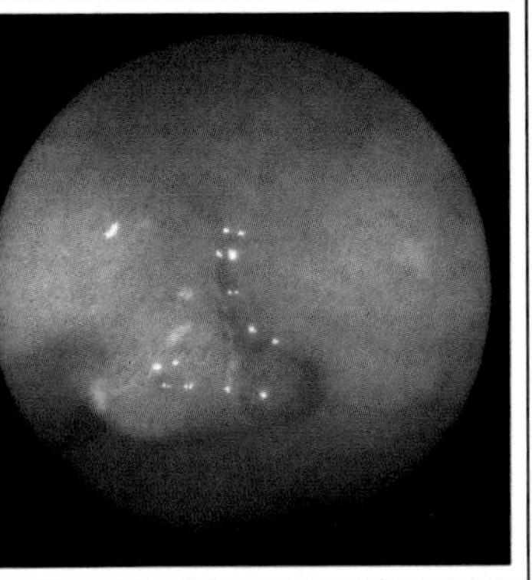

FIG. 42-12.

FIG. 42-12. Synchronous adenoma in a patient with ileocecal valve carcinoma (Fig. 42-11b). Careful examination of the remainder of the colon in this patient revealed a semipedunculated adenoma which was removed prior to surgery. Follow-up colonoscopy within 6 months to a year is advisable.

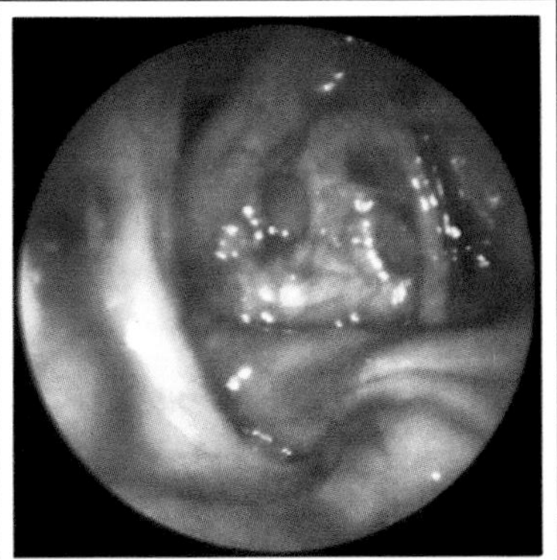

FIG. 42-13a.

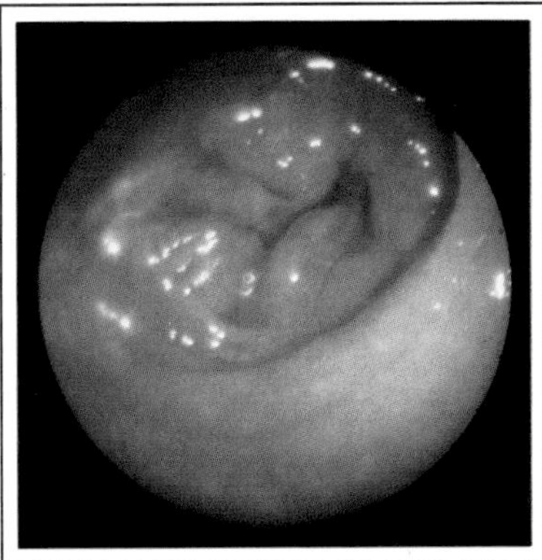

FIG. 42-13b.

FIG. 42-13. a: Recurrent rectosigmoid carcinoma. The anastomosis, which appears asymmetrical because of the location (the rectosigmoid), and the somewhat indurated nature of this fold suggest recurrence, which was confirmed by biopsy. **b:** An anastomotic site after resection for sigmoid carcinoma. The symmetrical, nodular appearance derives from the use of interrupted sutures.

relation to carcinoma is considerably higher. Over a 5-year period, we observed five colonic lymphomas in contrast to 51 carcinomas, the lymphoma occurring on the order of 1 per 10 carcinomas rather than the expected 1 per 250. Of the five cases of colonic lymphoma, three were asymptomatic or had nonspecific symptoms and were studied because of a lymphoma protocol or GI bleeding after the initiation of cytotoxic agents. In the past, such asymptomatic involvement of the colon would not likely have been noted until autopsy. In general, autopsy series reveal a higher incidence of GI involvement (up to 65%)[29] and colonic involvement (11% of GI or 6.5% of the total) in contrast with the generally stated figure of 1 to 2%[28] for colonic involvement in patients who were evaluated because of specific symptoms referable to the colon.

Although most colonic lymphomas at autopsy are found as part of generalized abdominal involvement,[29] a variable percentage of symptomatic patients at a referral center have primary colonic lymphoma, i.e., associated with lymphoma elsewhere.[30] Of 69 patients with histologically proved colonic lymphoma seen at the Mayo Clinic over a 57-year period (1907 through 1964), 50 had primary lymphoma whereas only 19 had the secondary type.[30] The reported experience from our institution, however, was the reverse, in that, of 33 patients with colonic lymphoma where a barium enema had been suggestive of the diagnosis, 13 were primary, and 21 were secondary. Unlike the patients in the Mayo Clinic study, the indication for barium enema was not always symptoms; more often barium enemas were done as part of a group of studies performed prior to randomization to a treatment protocol, making this group more like an autopsy series with a high percentage of colonic involvement in asymptomatic patients with generalized abdominal lymphoma.[31]

Clinical Features

Symptoms found in association with either primary or secondary colonic lymphoma are fever, pain, weight loss, the presence of an abdominal mass, diarrhea, and rectal bleeding.[29,31] It is important to bear in mind that the symptoms of colonic lymphoma and the radiologic appearance may suggest inflammatory bowel disease.[32] Moreover, colonic lymphoma may occur in patients with longstanding ulcerative colitis, although this is rare, with fewer than 32 cases having been reported up to 1980,[33] including one from our institution.[34]

Histologic Type

The commonest type of primary or secondary lymphoma in recent reports has been either poorly differentiated lymphoma (in the older classification, lymphosarcoma) or histiocytic lymphoma (also known as reticulum cell sarcoma).[29] In a report from our institution, all 13 primary and 19 of 21 secondary lymphomas were of one or the other of these cell types, generally poorly differentiated lymphomas.[31] Curiously, in the older Mayo Clinic study these two types accounted for only half the primary and secondary lymphomas, with the remainder made up of different cell types including Hodgkin's disease.[30] In contrast to other presentations where the histiocytic type is in the minority, in the cases of lymphoma complicating ulcerative colitis this has been the predominant type in nearly all the reported cases,[33,34] with this type exhibiting an extremely poor prognosis. It has a 1-year mortality close to 50%, contrasted with 25% or less for the other types.[31]

Location

The location tends to relate to whether the colonic lymphoma is primary or secondary.

Primary Lymphoma

The commonest location of the primary lesions is the ileocecal area. In the University of Chicago radiology series, 9 of 13 primaries had this location in contrast to only 4 of 21 of the secondary type. In 4 of the 13 patients with primary lymphoma, there were two separate areas, most often the cecum and transverse colon. The left colon and rectum were involved in less than half of these cases (5 of 13).[31]

Secondary Lymphomas

In the University of Chicago series, the rectum and left colon were the principal sites in 14 of 21 cases in which colonic lymphoma appeared as part of generalized disease, with the ileocecal area involved in only 7 of 19.[31] A similar distribution was found in the older Mayo Clinic series, with the ileocecal area being involved in only 6 of the 19 cases of this type.[30]

Appearance

The few reported cases of colonic lymphoma studied by colonoscopy suggest a pattern similar to that found in radiologic series with three types of appearance: (a) polypoid mass(es); (b) diffuse involvement; and (c) an annular appearance.

Polypoid Mass(es)

The typical appearance for colonic lymphoma is that of single, or more commonly multiple, sessile, hard, rubbery polypoid masses.[35] These range in size from 5 mm to 2 to 3 cm (Fig. 42-14a). They are markedly erythematous, granular, and friable, and occasionally are large enough to fill the entire colonic lumen, especially in the sigmoid.[35]

Diffuse (Infiltrative) Appearance

Fewer than 10% of colonic lymphomas are found with the diffuse (infiltrative) appearance when the mucosa is diffusely erythematous and friable so as to suggest inflammatory bowel disease.[33,36] One patient in our series with left-sided involvement originally had this colonoscopic appearance with biopsies which were mistakenly interpreted as Crohn's disease, whereas in reality poorly differentiated lymphoma was present (Fig. 42-14b). He was recolonoscoped 2.5 years later, and repeat biopsies clearly showed lymphoma.

Annular Appearance

In an occasional case (one of our five patients) the appearance is that of a malignant stricture with a prominent exophytic component which is indistinguishable from the common adenocarcinoma.[37]

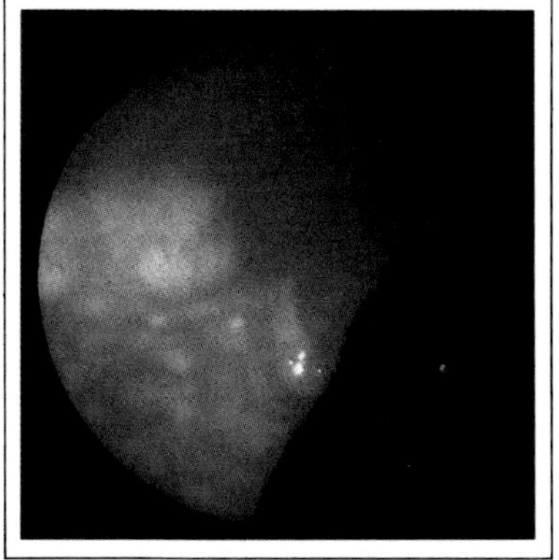

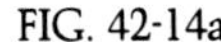

FIG. 42-14a.

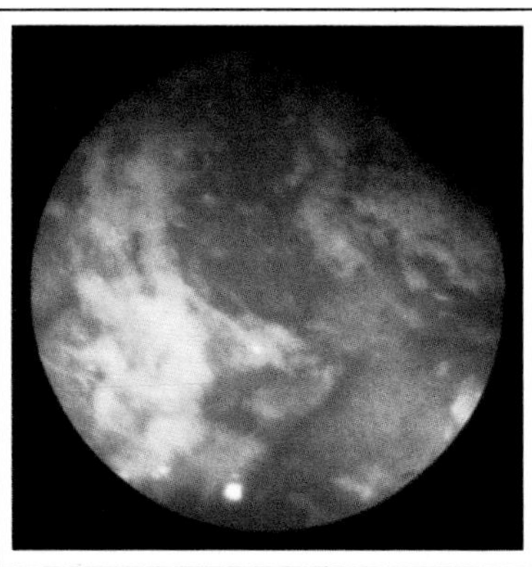

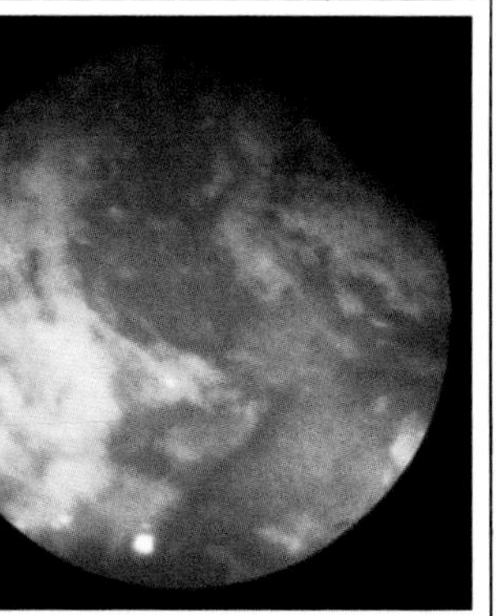

FIG. 42-14b.

FIG. 42-14. a: Lymphoma. Multiple polyps of the cecum in a patient with abdominal lymphoma always suggests involvement of this segment, even in an asymptomatic patient. **b:** Lymphoma simulating ulcerative colitis. Ulcerations and friability in this patient presenting with watery diarrhea caused this appearance, which was initially mistaken for inflammatory bowel disease. Biopsies, however, showed poorly differentiated lymphoma.

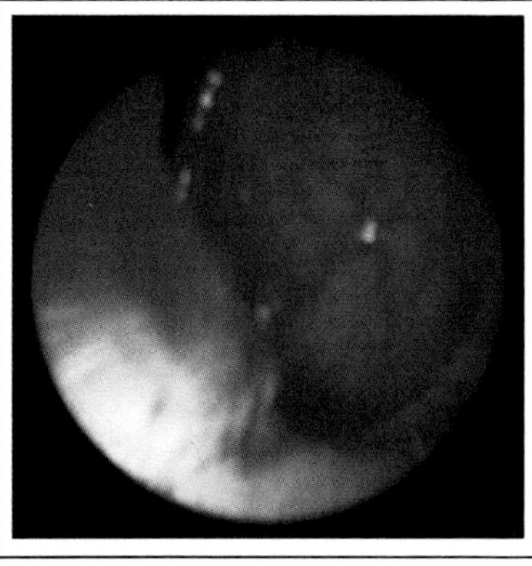

FIG. 42-15.

FIG. 42-15. Metastatic carcinoma to the colon from a cervical primary. Local spread produced a mass and cervical narrowing at the rectosigmoid junction. Biopsies showed squamous carcinoma similar to that found in the original cervical carcinoma.

Biopsy and Cytology

Biopsy

Biopsy is generally effective in establishing the diagnosis if the lesion can be reached. Often forceps biopsies prove sufficient, as the lymphoma cells are often within the lamina propria of the mucosa.[35] As lymphomas tend to be deep-seated, replacing much of the wall of the colon, theoretically one might risk perforation with deep large-particle biopsies without substantially adding to the diagnostic yield.

Cytology

As in gastric lymphomas, cytology can be helpful especially where there is not enough technical control of the lesion to permit directed forceps biopsies. The finding of atypical lymphocytes in the presence of a polypoid mass strongly suggests a diagnosis of colonic lymphoma.

METASTATIC CARCINOMA TO THE COLON

Metastatic carcinomas in the colon are unusual, accounting for less than 1% of colonic cancers. They may arise from neighboring pelvic organs (cervix, uterus, ovaries) or from distant primaries, i.e., breast,[38] lung,[39] and skin melanomas,[40] and occasionally the pancreas, kidney, or stomach.

Appearance

The appearance of metastatic cancer to the colon largely depends on whether the cancer involves the colon by direct extension or by spread from a distant primary.

Direct Extension

The usual appearance for involvement of the colon by direct extension is that of a tight stricture of the rectosigmoid colon (Fig. 42-15). The mucosa of the mouth of the stricture may show nonspecific changes, e.g., erythema and some friability, with the cancer itself being on the serosal aspect or within the wall; it rarely breaks through the mucosa.

Distant Primaries

In the case of a distant primary, as in the upper small bowel, hematogenous spread of tumor produces implants within the wall which may assume an exophytic growth pattern, thereby breaking through into the lumen. As such, it may be observed at colonoscopy as a 1- to 2-cm polypoid mass with central depressions or ulceration. In the particular case of metastatic melanoma, small mucosal implants tend to be dark brown or black; however, when they appear as larger masses (>1.5 cm) they may, as in the stomach and duodenum, appear amelanotic, especially when ulcerated.

Breast carcinoma metastatic to the colon may produce an unusual type of annular carcinoma with stricture formation, in which the mouth of the stricture contains irregular, friable, nodular tissue suggestive of carcinoma.[38]

DISSEMINATED KAPOSI'S SARCOMA

The disseminated form of Kaposi's sarcoma, which is increasingly being recognized in homosexual males,[41] is found with colonic involvement[42,43] in over 40 to 50% of the cases when these individuals are subjected to colonoscopy.[42] This is similar to the proportion (47%) with gastric involvement[42] (see Chapter 16).

Two types of colonic appearance have been reported. The first of these, which is found in all reported cases,[41–43] is that of a focal, slightly raised erythematous macular lesion with stellate-type projections from the center of the lesion, causing it to resemble angiodysplasia[43] (see Chapter 46).

A second type of lesion is that of a small (<1 cm) erythematous polyp[42] which resembles inflammatory polyps of ulcerative colitis. We have observed one case of disseminated Kaposi's sarcoma in a patient with long-standing ulcerative colitis where biopsies of typically appearing inflammatory polyps all showed neoplastic spindle cells and proliferating vessels, similar to other involved tissues.

LEUKEMIA WITH COLONIC INVOLVEMENT

While leukemia infiltrates may be found in the colon in up to 10% of autopsy cases,[44] patients with leukemia are rarely, if ever, subjected to colonoscopy; so descriptions of the colonoscopic findings associated with leukemia infiltrates have been rare.[45] In one recent report[45] of a patient with untreated chronic lymphocytic leukemia (wbc = 270,000/mm^3), where colonoscopy was performed because of chronic diarrhea, the findings were suggestive of acute ulcerative colitis (see Chapter 43), with plaque-like exudates, marked mucosal friability, granularity, and loss of mucosal vascular pattern.[45] Biopsies showed dense leukemic infiltrates. A similar endoscopic picture may be seen in profoundly neutropenic patients (absolute neutrophil count less than 1,000/mm^3) who develop the picture of necrotizing colitis following treatment of leukemia with cytotoxic agents (see Chapter 44).

REFERENCES

1. De Peyster, F. A. (1975): Pathogenesis and manifestations (of colon carcinoma). *JAMA,* 231:643–645.
2. Winawer, S. J. (1980): Screening for colorectal cancers: an overview. *Cancer,* 45:1093–1098.
3. Gilbertsen, V. A., McHugh, R., Schuman, L., and Williams, S. (1980): The earlier detection of colorectal cancers: a preliminary report of the results of the occult blood study. *Cancer,* 45:2899–2901.

3a. Hardcastle, J. D., Farrands, P. A., Balfour, T. W., Chamberlain, J., Amar, S. S., and Sheldon, M. G. (1983): Controlled trial of faecal occult blood testing in the detection of colorectal cancer. *Lancet,* 2:1–4.

4. Murrary, D., Hreno, A., Dutton, J., and Hampson, L. G. (1975): Prognosis in colon cancer: a pathologic reassessment. *Arch. Surg.,* 110:908–913.

4a. Miller, D. R., and Allbritten, F. F. (1976): Carcinoma of the colon and rectum. A review of surgical treatment in 164 patients. *Arch. Surg.,* 111:692–696.

5. Diggs, C. H. (1979): Carcinoma of the colon: epidemiology, etiology, diagnosis and treatment. *Am. J. Med. Sci.,* 277:4–16.
6. Holliday, H. W., and Hardcastle, J. D. (1979): Delay in diagnosis and treatment of symptomatic colorectal cancer. *Lancet,* 1:309–311.
7. Miller, R. E. (1974): Detection of colon carcinoma and the barium enema. *JAMA,* 230:1195–1198.
8. Blasset, M. L., Bennett, S. A., and Goulston, K. J. (1979): Colorectal cancer: a study of 230 patients. *Med. J. Aust.,* 1:589–592.
9. Synder, D. N., Heston, J. F., Meigs, J. W., and Flannery, J. T. (1977): Changes in the site distribution of colorectal carcinoma in Connecticut, 1940–1973. *Am. J. Dig. Dis.,* 22:791–797.
10. Macrae, F. A., and St. John, D. J. B. (1982): Relationship between patterns of bleeding and Hemoccult sensitivity in patients with colorectal cancers or adenomas. *Gastroenterology,* 19:891–898.
11. Porter, F. R., Strickland, R. G., and Volpicelli, N. A. (1978): Increased yield of Dukes' A colon cancer in symptomatic patients following introduction of colonoscopy. *Gastroenterology,* 74:1080.
12. Tedesco, F. J., Waye, J. D., Avella, J. R., and Villalobos, M. M. (1980): Diagnostic implications of the spatial distribution of colonic mass lesions (polyps and cancers): a prospective colonoscopic study. *Gastrointest. Endosc.,* 26:95–97.
13. Rhodes, J. B., Holmes, F. F., and Clark, G. M. (1977): Changing distributions of primary cancers in the large bowel. *JAMA,* 238:1641–1643.
14. Spratt, J. S., and Spjut, H. J. (1967): Prevalence and prognosis of individual clinical and pathological variables associated with colorectal carcinoma. *Cancer,* 20:1976–1985.
15. Buckwalter, J. A., and Kent, T. H. (1973): Prognosis and surgical pathology of carcinoma of the colon. *Surg. Gynecol. Obstet.,* 136:465–473.
16. Dreyfuss, J. R., and Benacerraf, B. (1978): Saddle cancers of the colon and their progression to annular carcinomas. *Radiology,* 129:289–293.
17. Lydon, S. B., Wu, W., and Dodds, W. I. (1976): Segmental narrowing of the sigmoid colon. *Am. J. Dig. Dis.,* 21:44–46.
18. Ekelund, G., and Lindstrom, C. (1974): Histopathological analysis of benign polyps in patients with carcinoma of the colon and rectum. *Gut,* 15:654–663.
19. Gillespie, P. E., Chambers, T. J., Chan, K. W., Doronzo, F., Morson, B. C., and Williams, C. B. (1979): Colonic adenomas—a colonoscopic survey. *Gut,* 20:240–245.
20. Reilly, J. C., Rusin, L. C., and Theuerkauf, F. J. (1982): Colonoscopy: its role in cancer of the colon and rectum. *Dis. Colon Rectum,* 25:532–538.
21. Burns, F. J. (1980): Synchronous and metachronous malignancies of the colon and rectum. *Dis. Colon Rectum,* 23:578–579.
22. Spratt, J. S. (1977): Multiple primary cancers: review of clinical studies from two Missouri hospitals. *Cancer,* 40:1806–1811.
23. Winawer, S. J., Leidner, S. D., Hajdu, S. I., and Sherlock, P. (1978): Colonoscopic biopsy and cytology in the diagnosis of colon cancer. *Cancer,* 42:2849–2853.
24. Schnyder, P., Moss, A. A., Thoeni, R. F., and Margulis, A. R. (1979): A double-blind study of radiologic accuracy in diverticulitis, diverticulosis, and carcinoma of the sigmoid colon. *J. Clin. Gastroenterol.,* 1:55–66.

24a. Manson, P. N., Corman, M. L., Coller, J. A., and Veidenheimer, M. C. (1976): Anastomatic recurrence after anterior resection for carcinoma. Lahey Clinic experience. *Dis. Colon Rectum,* 19:219–224.

25. Gabrielsson, N., Granqvist, S., and Ohlsen, H. (1976): Recurrent carcinoma of the colon in anastomosis diagnosed by roentgen examination and colonoscopy. *Endoscopy,* 8:47–52.

26. Vassilopoulos, P., Ledesma, E., Yoon, J. E., Jung, O., and Mittleman, A. (1981): Surgical treatment of metastatic colorectal adenocarcinoma. *Dis. Colon Rectum,* 24:265–271.
27. American Cancer Society (1981): *82 Facts and Figures.* ACS, New York.
28. Burgener, F. A., and Hamlin, D. J. (1981): Histiocytic lymphoma of the abdomen: radiographic spectrum. *Am. J. Roentgenol.,* 137:337–342.
29. Ehrlich, A. N., Stalder, G., Geller, W., and Sherlock, P. (1968): Gastrointestinal manifestations of malignant lymphoma. *Gastroenterology,* 54:1115–1121.
30. Wychulis, A. R., Beahrs, O. H., and Woolner, L. B. (1966): Malignant lymphoma of the colon: a study of 69 cases. *Arch. Surg.,* 95:215–115.
31. O'Connell, D. J., and Thompson, A. J. (1978): Lymphoma of the colon: the spectrum of radiologic changes. *Gastrointest. Radiol.,* 2:377–385.
32. Parnes, I. H., Pichel Warner, R. R., Berman, R., and Sanders, M. (1974): Diffuse lymphoma of the colon simulating ulcerative colitis. *Mt. Sinai J. Med. (N.Y.),* 41:802–806.
33. Bashiti, H. O., and Kraus, K. T. (1980): Histocytic lymphoma in chronic ulcerative colitis. *Cancer,* 46:1695–1700.
34. Wagonfeld, J. B., Platz, C. E., Fishman, F. L., Sibley, R. K., and Kirsner, J. B. (1977): Multicentric colonic lymphoma complicating ulcerative colitis. *Am. J. Dig. Dis.,* 22:502–508.
35. Ruppert, G. B., and Smith, V. M. (1979): Multiple lymphomatous polyposis of the gastrointestinal tract. *Gastrointest. Endosc.,* 25:67–69.
36. Weir, A. B., Poon, M.-C., Groarke, J. F., and Wilkerson, J. A. (1980): Lymphoma simulating Crohn's colitis. *Dig. Dis. Sci.,* 25:69–72.
37. Greene, F., Livstone, E. M., McAllister, W. B., Passarelli, N. M., and Troncale, F. J. (1974): Reticulum cell sarcoma of the large intestine: the role of fiberoptic colonoscopy. *Am. J. Dig. Dis.* 19:379–384.
38. Fayemi, A., Ali, M., and Braun, E. V. (1979): Metastatic carcinoma simulating linitis plastica of the colon. *Am. J. Gastroenterol.,* 71:311–314.
39. Brown, K. L., Beg, R. A., Demany, M. A., and Lacerna, M. A. (1980): Rare metastasis of primary bronchogenic carcinoma to sigmoid colon. *Dis. Colon Rectum,* 23:343–345.
40. Sacks, B. A., Jaffe, N., and Antonioli, D. A. (1977): Metastatic melanoma presenting clinically as multiple colonic polyps. *Am. J Roentgenol.,* 129:511–513.
41. Friedman-Kien, A. E., Laubenstein, L. J., Rubinstein, P., Buimovici-Klein, E., Marmor, M., Stahl, R., Spigland, I., Kim, K. S., and Zolla-Pazner, S. (1982): Disseminated Kaposi's sarcoma in homosexual men. *Ann. Intern. Med.,* 96:693–699.
42. Rose, H. S., Balthazar, E. J., Megibow, A. J., Horowitz, L., and Laubenstein, L. J. (1982): Alimentary tract involvement in Kaposi sarcoma: Radiographic and endoscopic findings in 25 homosexual men. *Am. J. Roentgenol.,* 139:661–666.
43. Weprin, L., Zollinger, R., Clausen, K., and Thomas, F. B. (1982): Kaposi's sarcoma: Endoscopic observations of gastric and colonic involvement. *J. Clin. Gastroenterol.,* 4:357–360.
44. Prolla, J. C., and Kirsner, J. B. (1964): The gastrointestinal lesions and complications of leukemias. *Ann. Intern. Med.,* 61:1084–1103.
45. Scharschmidt, B. F. (1978): Chronic lymphocytic leukemia presenting as colitis. Report of a case with proctoscopic and colonoscopic findings. *Dig. Dis. Sci.,* 23(Suppl.): 9S–12S.
46. Dosik, G. M., Luna, M., Valdivieso, M., McCredie, K. B., Gehan, E. A., Gil-Extremera, B., Smith, T. L., and Bodey, G. P. (1979): Necrotizing colitis in patients with cancer. *Am. J. Med.,* 67:646–656.

43

INFLAMMATORY BOWEL DISEASE

THE INDICATIONS FOR COLONOSCOPY

Endoscopic examination of the entire colon is a powerful tool for collecting visual and histologic information in patients with inflammatory bowel disease. Some indication of its potential impact can be appreciated from the fact that in up to 20% of the cases colonoscopic findings are at variance with the clinical assessment as to the extent of the disease, its activity, or its type.[1] Still, even though colonoscopy may provide a more precise determination of the extent of activity than the standard examinations—proctoscopy and barium enema—this does not necessarily alter the clinician's approach to the disease, especially management decisions, in many if not the majority of cases. At the same time, colonoscopy should not be considered an entirely benign procedure, especially in patients who are at the most severe end of the clinical spectrum with fever, marked leukocytosis, and rectal bleeding. Like a barium enema, colonoscopy in such patients can precipitate toxic megacolon or can lead to perforation.[2]

We believe that the decision to perform colonoscopy should always take into account the specific diagnosis and/or therapeutic issues which the procedure may be asked to resolve. These we discuss under the following headings: (a) establishing the diagnosis; (b) activity of the disease; (c) extent of involvement; (d) type of disease; and (e) suspicion of cancer and cancer surveillance.

Establishing the Diagnosis

Using a combination of proctoscopy with rectal biopsy[3] and barium enema,[4] one can reasonably expect to establish the diagnosis and correct type of inflammatory bowel disease in at least 60 to 70% of cases.[3,4] Colonoscopy, because it can provide visual and histologic sampling, can be expected to provide accurate diagnostic information in more than 90% of the cases.[5]

Although ideally the increased accuracy of colonoscopy over other diagnostic procedures should allow one to tailor therapy more precisely, because of the limited therapeutic options in inflammatory bowel disease it usually does not. The major medical decisions can generally be made correctly from the less elegant but highly serviceable proctoscopic examination with biopsy plus barium enema. We believe that the indication for colonoscopy and the diagnosis of inflammatory bowel disease should be based on an equivocal or unrevealing proctoscopic examination (with rectal biopsies) or barium contrast studies[6]; this is especially true when there is a disparity between the clinical presentation and the findings of these studies. For example, a patient with arthritis, fever, and diarrhea, which suggest inflammatory bowel disease, may have proctoscopic and barium enema findings that are interpreted as "normal" or show only nonspecific changes, e.g., the presence of edema.

Activity of the Disease

Although proctoscopy[7] and barium enema, especially with the single-contrast technique,[8] may in a given case correlate poorly with the colonoscopic assessment of activity, we find that in a majority of patients sufficient information is provided from these studies to make therapeutic decisions, e.g., the use of systemic rather than rectal steroids based on finding colitis that involves the proximal colon. In such cases we do not recommend colonoscopy, especially if treatment has not yet been instituted. On the other hand, if such treatment has been started, or in cases of Crohn's disease if surgery had been performed, and doubt arose as to whether the present symptoms were from inflammatory bowel disease or other functional causes, the determination of activity by colonoscopy is valuable. Certainly in cases where surgery is contemplated, one is especially anxious to perform colonoscopy if there is any uncertainty as to the cause of the symptoms.

Extent of Involvement

The extent of involvement as assessed by colonic radiology may differ from that determined by colonoscopy and biopsy in 20 to 30% of cases.[4] Does this really matter? Like information concerning activity, a precise determination of the extent has its greatest impact where a therapeutic change is contemplated, e.g., the addition of systemic steroids in a patient already receiving steroid enemas, or the addition of azathioprine for a patient with symptoms which can be controlled only with high doses of systemic steroids. In the latter case the physician might be more likely to continue with a medical program for active disease confined to the left side, with preservation of the remainder, than for total colonic involvement, where the case for surgery is more compelling.

Type of Disease

Clinical features and proctoscopic and radiologic findings lead to a correct determination of the type of inflammatory bowel disease—ulcerative colitis or Crohn's disease—in 60 to 70% of the cases.[3,4] Because medical management of these two conditions does not differ substantially and might not be influenced by more accurate typing, which is available from colonoscopic visual and histologic data, colonscopy for the purposes of determining the type of disease offers, on the whole, little that would change the medical management or its outcome. However, in cases where standard medical management (sulfasalazine, rectal and/or systemic steroids) has failed to control symptoms and surgery is contemplated, colonoscopy could play an important role in the ultimate decision. Because Crohn's colitis treated by proctocolectomy is associated with a nearly 40% cumulative incidence of recurrence, compared with a less than 10% likelihood of ileal dysfunction after resection for ulcerative colitis,[9] with colonoscopy establishing a diagnosis of Crohn's disease, the physician might wish to pursue an even more intensive medical program; thus in selected cases he might add azathioprine[10] or 6-mercaptopurine to the regimen.[10,11] In contrast, for a patient in whom colonoscopic examination with biopsy establishes the diagnosis of ulcerative colitis, because of its greater malignant potential (see below), in the face of comparable severity the physician would seriously consider surgery rather than continued attempts at medical management.

Suspicion of Cancer and Cancer Surveillance

Patients with ulcerative colitis[12] and Crohn's disease[13] are at increased risk for developing colonic cancer. For patients with ulcerative colitis that involves the entire colon, the risk is 20- to 50-fold over that for the general adult population.[12] For these patients, especially those with ulcerative colitis of more than 10 years' duration that involves the entire colon, colonoscopy may be requested because new clinical activity after a long quiescent phase prompts concern about malignancy, especially when a barium contrast study shows a mass or stricture. For other asymptomatic patients with longstanding ulcerative colitis, the referring physician wishes to determine which individuals stand the greatest likelihood of either already having cancer or developing it over the next calendar year (see below), with the hope that these patients might be encouraged to undergo proctocolectomy while the cancer is still in an early stage.[14,14a] Colonoscopy has been found to be a means by which high-risk patients with longstanding, extensive ulcerative colitis can be identified. This has been accomplished by means of sampling both flat mucosa[14,14a] and discrete, raised areas[15] for evidence of neoplastic transformation, i.e., dysplasia. The finding of high-grade dysplasia (see below) on biopsies of flat mucosa identifies a group of patients at high risk who require follow-up colonoscopy within 3 to 6 months, if not colectomy,[14] because carcinoma is ultimately found in up to 40% of them.[14] The finding of dysplasia of any degree in association with a polypoid mass, especially one 1.5 cm or larger, identifies yet another group among whom up to 60% will have cancer, making this finding a compelling indication for colectomy.

ULCERATIVE COLITIS

Colonoscopy in patients with ulcerative colitis is not performed in the abstract but is done to answer specific question(s) posed by the clinical indication. Our presentation of the colonoscopic appearance in the sections which follow is therefore organized around the indications for it in these patients (Table 43-1).

Among 305 patients examined in our Unit over a 5-year period with a diagnosis of ulcerative colitis, the indications were as follows: For 45% (135 of 305) colonoscopy was performed to determine the extent and/or activity of the disease in patients who were considered to be in poor symptomatic control. For 35% (110 of 305) the indication was cancer surveillance or the actual suspicion of cancer, with the high percentage in this category undoubtedly a reflection of our ongoing surveillance study.[15] In 15% (45 of 305)

TABLE 43-1. *Indications for colonoscopy in 305 patients with ulcerative colitis (1976–1980)*

Indication	No.	%
Extent and/or activity	135	45
Suspicion of cancer/cancer surveillance	110	35
Differentiation from Crohn's disease	45	15
Clinical suspicion of ulcerative colitis	15	5
Total	305	100

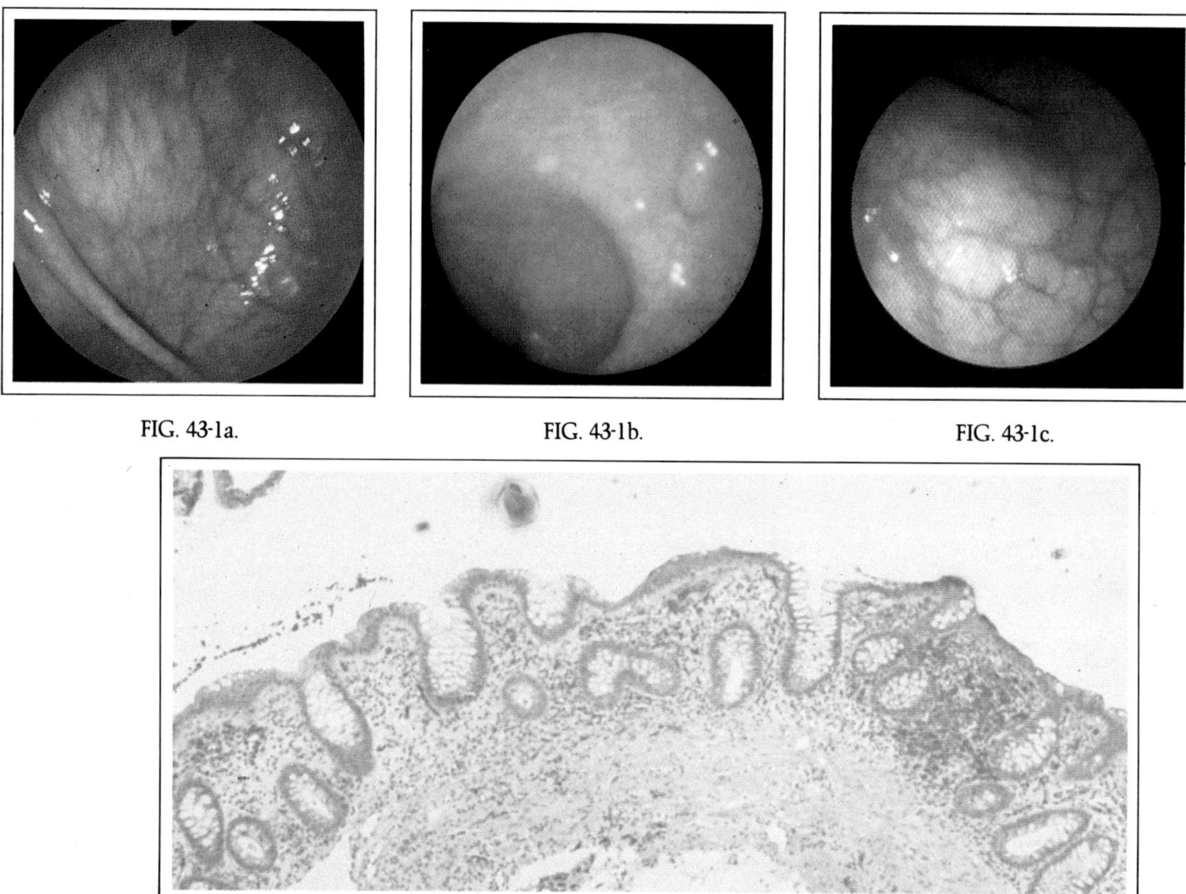

FIG. 43-1a. FIG. 43-1b. FIG. 43-1c.

FIG. 43-1d.

FIG. 43-1. a: Ulcerative colitis, distortion (blunting) of the mucosal vascular pattern (MVP). We find that this is the least altered mucosal appearance that suggests histologic involvement. Here one expects the biopsy to show mucosal atrophy [similar to that in (d)]. **b:** Ulcerative colitis, loss of MVP. No vascular pattern is seen. In addition, there is an inflammatory polyp noted at 3 o'clock. Biopsy showed mucosal atrophy [similar to that in (d)]. **c:** Normal rectal mucosa with vessels that show obvious branching. **d:** Ulcerative colitis, clinically quiescent. A biopsy was taken from an area that showed only a distorted MVP [similar to that in (a)]. Histologically, mucosal atrophy is seen with loss of crypts and thickening of the muscularis.

colonoscopy was performed to determine the type of inflammatory bowel disease—ulcerative colitis or Crohn's disease—and in 5% (15 of 305) the indication was the clinical suspicion of ulcerative colitis in the absence of previously established disease.

In this section we consider the colonoscopic appearance of ulcerative colitis in relation to the two indications which predominated in our patients: (a) the determination of extent or activity; and (b) cancer surveillance and/or the clinical suspicion of malignancy. These are presented under the headings: extent of involvement, disease activity, and malignancy in ulcerative colitis. The differentiation of ulcerative colitis from Crohn's disease is taken up as part of our treatment of the colonoscopic aspects of Crohn's disease itself in the latter part of the chapter.

Extent of Involvement

An accurate determination of extent depends first on intubation of the cecum. Because of the foreshortening of the colon in ulcerative colitis and tubularization (see below), even a relatively inexperienced examiner, we find, can succeed in 70 to 80% of the cases[15] if not more. Apart from performing a complete examination, the determination of extent depends on an awareness of the following: (a) the spectrum of appearances for involved mucosa, including minimal changes; (b) structural changes associated with mucosal involvement; and (c) the patterns of involvement, whether universal, left-sided, etc.; and finally (d) the role of biopsy.

Mucosal Appearances Denoting Involvement

Because the endoscopic features denoting involvement in ulcerative colitis may be primarily a mucosal change (e.g., ulceration) or a structural change (e.g., stricture formation), we consider these separately, with this section devoted to mucosal appearances and the succeeding sections to structural ones. We also find it useful, although somewhat arbitrary, to consider mucosal changes as a spectrum

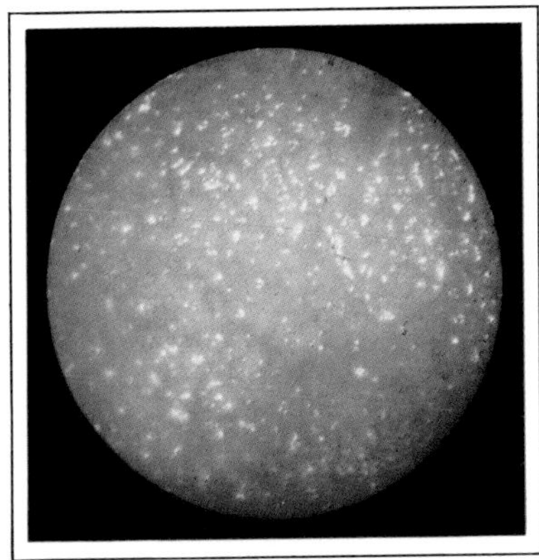

FIG. 43-2a.

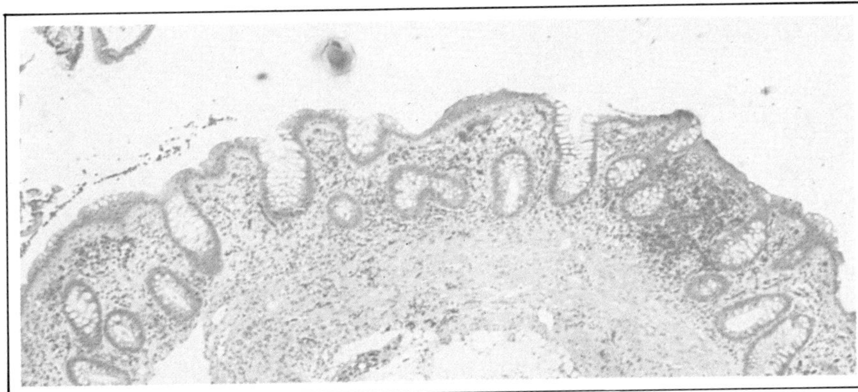

FIG. 43-2b.

FIG. 43-2. a: Ulcerative colitis, granularity. The light reflex is broken up into a myriad of tiny dots, giving the mucosa a coarsened or granular appearance. Surface mucosa irregularity from regenerative changes [such as those seen in (b)] may account for this appearance. **b:** Ulcerative colitis, histologic appearance of a mucosal surface that shows granularity. The biopsy shows atrophy as well as regenerative changes of the remaining crypts, i.e., budding and branching.

of appearances from what we call "minimal changes," which are sometimes noted only with great difficulty compared to the more obvious ulcerations and inflammatory polyps. We find it useful when presenting these appearances to work our way up from minimal changes to the more striking abnormalities, recognizing that more often than not these features coexist in the same patient.

Minimal changes—distortion or loss of the normal mucosal vascular pattern.

It is our impression that distortion (Fig. 43-1a) or loss (Fig. 43-1b) of the normal mucosal vascular pattern (MVP) (Fig. 43-1c) is the least altered appearance that denotes the presence of histologic abnormalities, i.e., quiescent colitis. However, there are no studies of which we are aware that have established this truly as the minimal visual feature. The cause of vascular distortion is unknown, but as biopsies with this appearance often show both mucosal atrophy (Fig. 43-1d) and thickening of the muscularis mucosae[16] we believe that the endoscopic findings relate to the presence possibly of both an altered relationship of the mucosal capillaries to the crypts, causing a distorted vascular appearance, as well as a decreased transparency of the mucosa so that even larger submucosal vessels may not be seen at all. Distortion of the MVP appears as "blunting," i.e., where the vessels appear not to branch at all, contrasted to normal vessels which branch out to a second or third division (Fig. 43-1c) (see Chapter 39). In other cases no vascular pattern is found (Fig. 43-1d).

The presence of a distorted or absent MVP may occur with an otherwise normal appearance, with the altered vascular pattern the only visual manifestation of the quiescent or healed stage of ulcerative colitis.

Granularity.

Another minimal change which can occur alone or with alteration of the MVP is the appearance of granularity, where the mucosal texture, which is normally smooth (Fig. 43-1c), becomes coarsened (Fig. 43-2a). In such cases the light reflex, which is normally homogeneous, is broken up into multiple tiny zones of light (Fig. 43-2a). There has never been a satisfactory explanation for this appearance. Histologically, one notes that with the endoscopic appearance of granularity alone there is atrophy with regenerative changes (budding or branching) of the crypts (Fig. 43-2b). Granularity therefore could be the visual manifestation of the surface irregularity which might be expected to accompany a distortion in mucosal architecture seen with these histologic changes.

Erythema and friability.

As was noted elsewhere (see Chapter 40), erythema can be entirely unrelated to mucosal disease, being simply a reflection of deficient illumination and/or the use of chemical irritants, e.g., sodium phosphate (Fleet enema), when preparing the patient for colonoscopy (see Chapter 40). However, with a history compatible with ulcerative colitis, one regards erythema, especially if it is seen in association with granularity and a distorted or absent vascular pattern (Fig. 43-3a), as indicative of mucosal involvement. In contrast to alterations of the MVP or the presence of granularity, which are most often found in association with biopsy evidence of only atrophy (Fig. 43-2b), erythema is generally found with histologic evidence of activity (i.e., the presence of acute inflammatory cells in the lamina propria) or as crypt abscesses (Fig. 43-3b). Here the erythema may be the result of mucosal capillary dilatation seen in response to acute inflammation (Fig. 43-3b).[16] When present, erythema is usually diffuse (Fig. 43-3a), although occasionally one finds it focally (Fig. 43-3c). In the latter case, the erythema is sometimes referred to as erosions, although because biopsies typically show intact surface epithelium we prefer the term "focal erythema" for this appearance (Fig. 43-3c).

Usually accompanying erythema, and very likely also the result of mucosal capillary dilatation, is the finding of

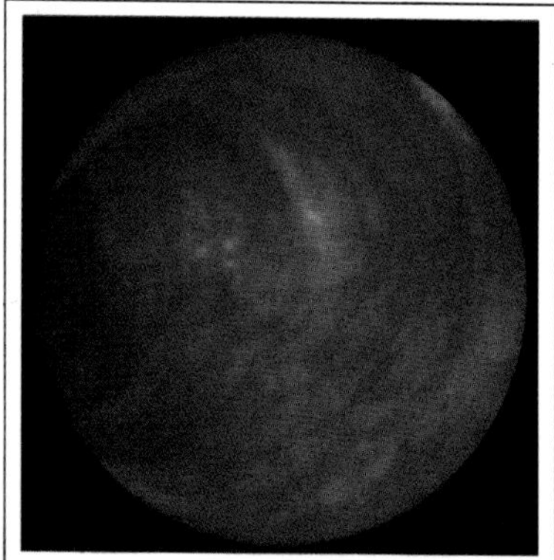

FIG. 43-3a.

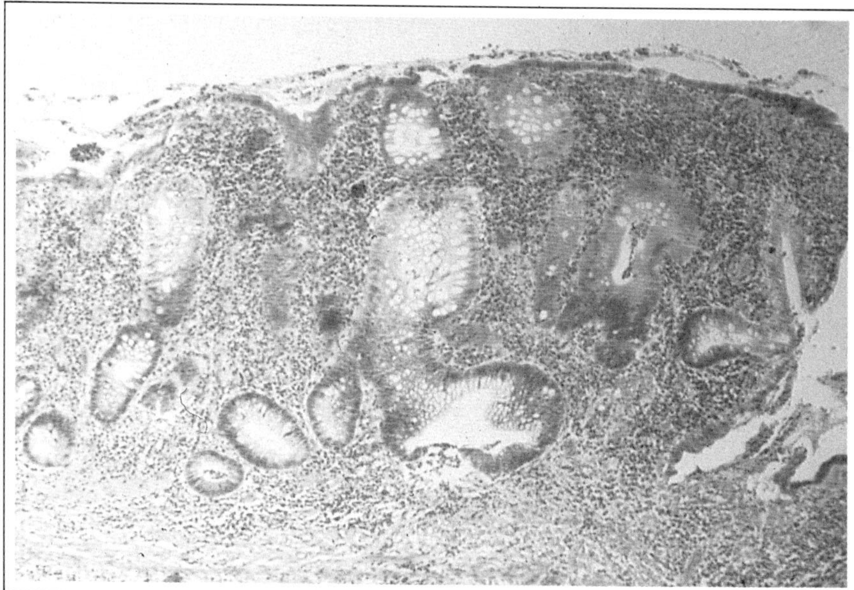

FIG. 43-3b.

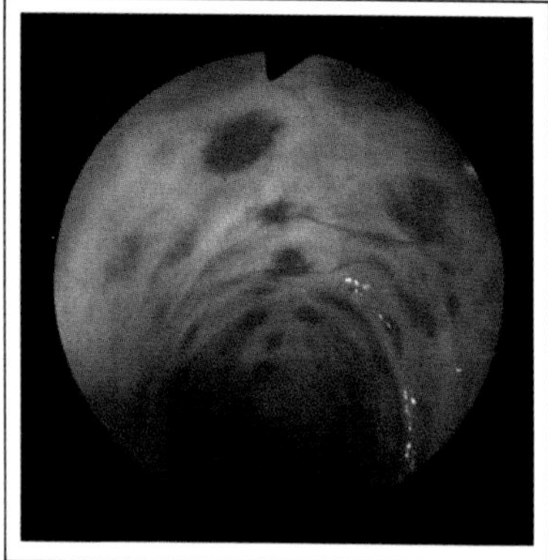

FIG. 43-3c.

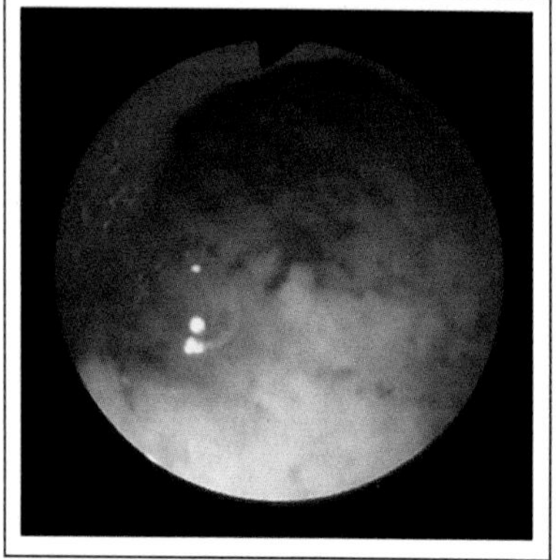

FIG. 43-3d.

FIG. 43-3. Ulcerative colitis. **a:** Erythema (diffuse mucosal reddening) is seen within the sigmoid. Unlike a distorted MVP (Fig. 43-1a) or granularity (Fig. 43-2a), which do not imply activity, the finding of erythema may be associated histologically with acute inflammation (b). **b:** Acute inflammation. Biopsy from mucosa with erythema showed acute inflammatory cells along with capillary dilatation and some mucin depletion, which accounts for the reddened appearance. **c:** Focal erythema. Discrete zones of reddening may be accounted for by focal capillary ectasia and hemorrhage as a response to inflammation. Focal erythema is much less commonly observed in ulcerative colitis than the diffuse form (a). **d:** Erythema and friability. Friability (also known as touch bleeding) is probably the result of capillary dilatation, commonly found histologically with the erythematous appearance.

friability (Fig. 43-3d), i.e., the appearance of mucosal hemorrhage following trivial amounts of pressure applied to the mucosa. The most consistent histologic finding from areas showing friability is vascular congestion, usually seen in association with evidence of acute inflammation (Fig. 43-3b).

Mucopurulent exudate.

Indicative of more marked activity than erythema is the presence of a loosely adherent, yellow-brown exudate (Fig. 43-4a). The inexperienced examiner may dismiss this as liquid stool or barium (especially if a barium enema has been performed recently). However, its stringy nature and its yellow coloration should always raise the possibility of a mucopurulent exudate. If still in doubt, the examiner may aspirate some of it using a Teflon cannula and examine it under the microscope using the methylene blue staining technique for fecal leukocytes. Biopsies taken from areas that show mucopurulent exudate typically have crypt abscesses, so that one is justified in regarding mucopurulent exudate as the discharge from such crypts (Fig. 43-4b).

Single or multiple ulcerations.

Single or multiple ulcerations are an expected finding in active ulcerative colitis (Fig. 43-5a). Common to the visual finding of ulceration, mucopurulent exudate and in some

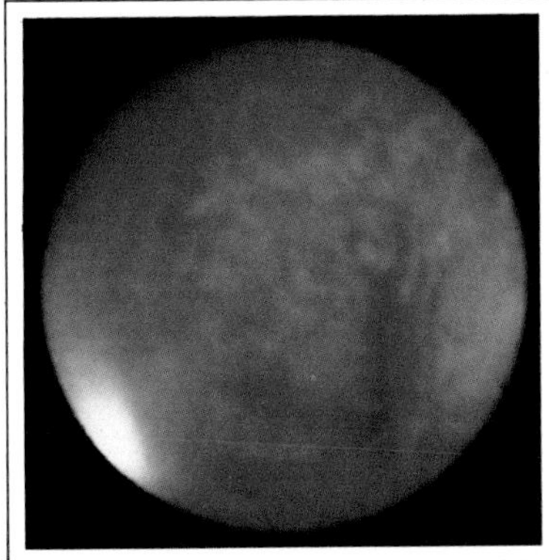

FIG. 43-4a.

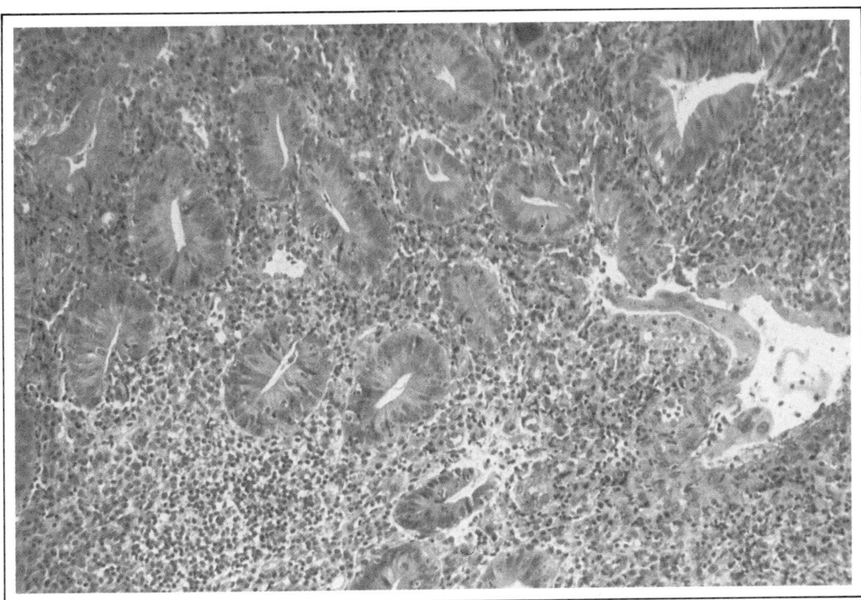

FIG. 43-4b.

FIG. 43-4. Ulcerative colitis. **a:** Mucopus. This acute inflammatory exudate, which is easily mistaken for fecal matter, can be the visual presentation of crypt abscesses noted histologically (b). **b:** Biopsy from mucosa showing mucopurulent exudate. Crypt abscesses are also seen which may "explode" into the lumen, giving rise to the mucopurulent exudate (a).

cases erythema is the histologic appearance of crypt abscesses. It has been suggested that ulceration occurs as a result of these abscesses, which have broken into the surrounding lamina propria; this results in an undermining of an area of mucosa, causing it to slough with resultant ulceration (Fig. 43-5c).[16] Seen endoscopically, the ulcers are pleomorphic, varying in size from 5 mm (Fig. 43-5a) to several centimeters (Fig. 43-5b). They may be linear, serpiginous, circinate, or ovoid. Whatever their form, their single most characteristic feature is their being set in abnormal mucosa (Fig. 43-5d), which is characteristically erythematous and friable.

Ulcerations with intervening inflammatory polyps—cobblestone effect.

In cases of ulcerations with intervening inflammatory polyps, rather than flat (though inflamed) mucosa between ulcerations, this appears nodular, particularly in the presence of sizable (often up to 1.5 cm) inflammatory polyps (Fig. 43-6a). What is characteristic about the cobblestone appearance in ulcerative colitis is that the mucosa surrounding the ulceration is abnormal, with especially marked erythema and friability, in contrast to the cobblestone appearance in Crohn's disease where the mucosa is only slightly erythematous or even normal with a preserved vascular pattern (see Fig. 43-22a).

Inflammatory polyps.

Inflammatory polyps are thought to form from focal areas of epithelium which remain at the margin of deep ulceration (Fig. 43-5c), probably similar to those areas which produce the cobblestone effect (Fig. 43-6a). As the ulcerations heal and the acute inflammation subsides, or possibly because of some ongoing acute inflammation, focally nodular areas enlarge, resulting in the formation of inflammatory polyps (Fig. 43-6b). These range in size from little more than mucosal excrescences (1 to 2 mm) to several centimeters or more (Fig. 43-6c). They are pedunculated or sessile and are soft, easily compressible with friable, eroded or ulcerated tips if larger than 1 cm (Fig. 43-6c). Some grow to great size (>3 cm or even 6 cm) and may be regarded radiographically or even endoscopically as suspicious for malignancy.[17] Biopsies, however, show these to be inflammatory rather than neoplastic (Fig. 43-6d). In general, inflammatory polyps are multiple small lesions less than 1 cm, although single larger lesions (1.5 cm or more) may account for up to 25% of the cases.[17] Ulceration of the larger inflammatory polyps is expected (Fig. 43-6c), and its absence should make the examiner suspect a neoplastic rather than an inflammatory process (see "Malignancy in Ulcerative Colitis," this chapter).

An unusual appearance for inflammatory polyps is one in which the polyps are interconnected by bridging mucosal folds (Fig. 43-7). These probably form in the wake of undermining ulcers (as in Fig. 43-5b) which leave a latticework of mucosa, ultimately becoming hyperplastic polyps with bridging folds.

Structural Abnormalities Associated With Mucosal Changes

To a large extent, structural abnormalities are a reflection of the acute inflammatory changes within the mucosa. For

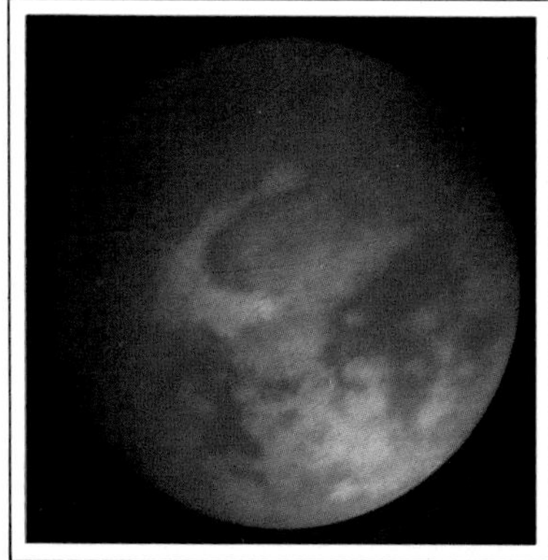

FIG. 43-5a.

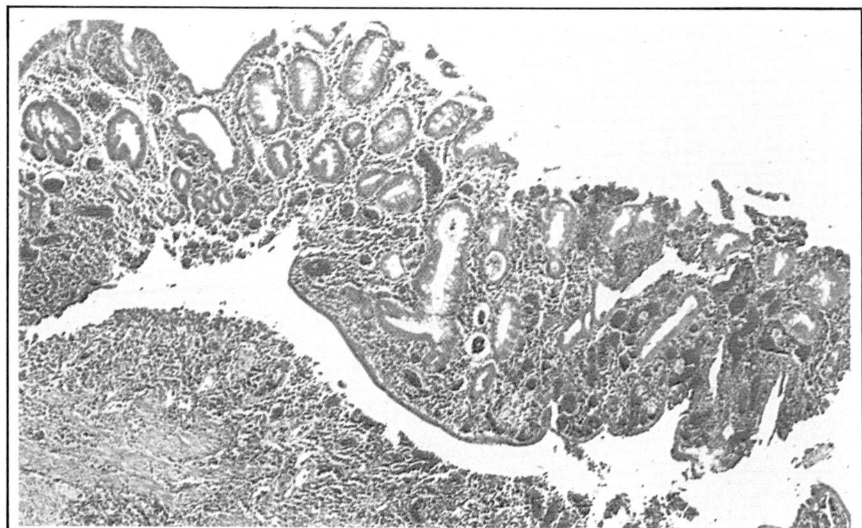

FIG. 43-5c.

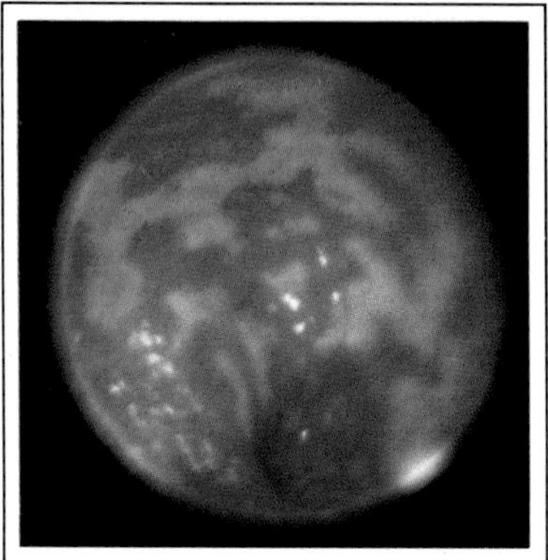

FIG. 43-5b.

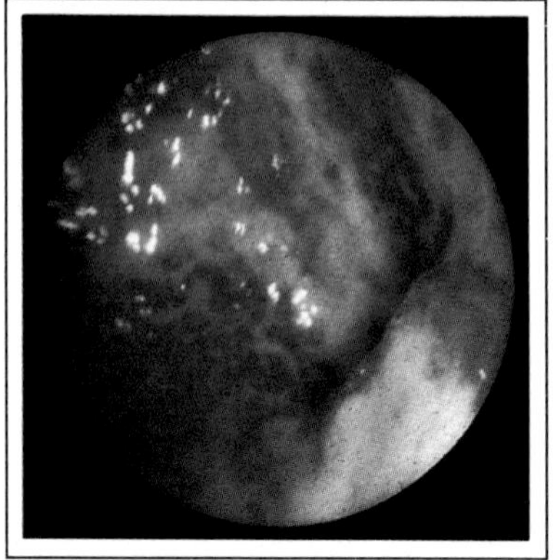

FIG. 43-5d.

FIG. 43-5. Ulcerative colitis. **a:** Ulceration on a background of abnormal mucosa showing erythema and friability as evidence of acute inflammation. **b:** Multiple confluent ulcerations. The background of erythematous friable mucosa is still apparent and has a superficial similarity to the cobblestone appearance of Crohn's disease (Fig. 43-23a) in that there are raised areas between the ulcerations. Unlike the cobblestone appearance in Crohn's disease, however, where this is edematous or hyperplastic mucosa, in ulcerative colitis the mucosa is acutely inflamed (c). **c:** Colectomy specimen showing part of an ulcer in relation to its surrounding mucosa. The crypt abscesses, which are adjacent to the ulcer, may play a role in its formation.[16] **d:** These ulcerations occur along with a mucopurulent exudate (mucopus), which is itself an ulcer-equivalent.

disease activity which may be considered severe (see "Grading the Activity of Ulcerative Colitis," this chapter), the structural abnormalities may be marked, particularly diffuse luminal narrowing or stricture formation. Should the mucosal activity subside and the disease enter the quiescent or inactive phase, there may be a reversal of the structural abnormalities back to normal luminal, valvular, and haustral appearances—a progression which can be noted on serial radiographic examination of the colon.[17a] We therefore believe that many of the structural changes associated with acute inflammation are largely the result of edema, an increase in cellularity, and muscle hypertrophy—all noted histologically in association with crypt abscesses and other evidence of acute inflammation in the mucosa.[16] These changes, including muscle hypertrophy, are all potentially reversible.[18,19]

The principal structural abnormalities seen in association with acute mucosal inflammation are discussed in this section. They are: (a) edema (thickening and blunting) of the valvulae; (b) loss of the expected haustral pattern; (c) diffuse luminal narrowing with the emergence of a narrow tubular appearance; (d) stricture formation; (e) the presence of bridging (mucosal interconnections); and (f) effacement of the ileocecal valve.

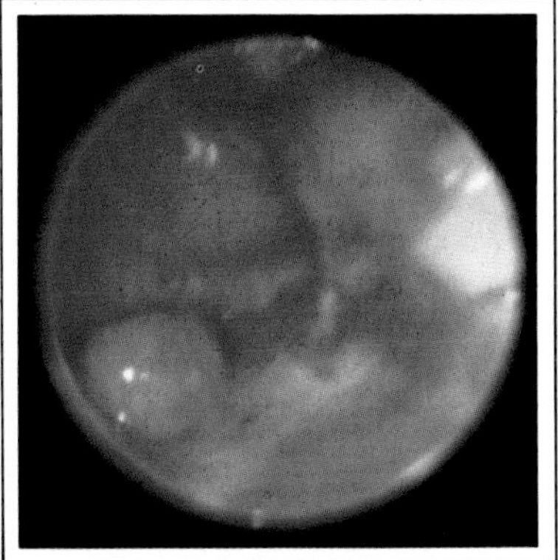

FIG. 43-6a.

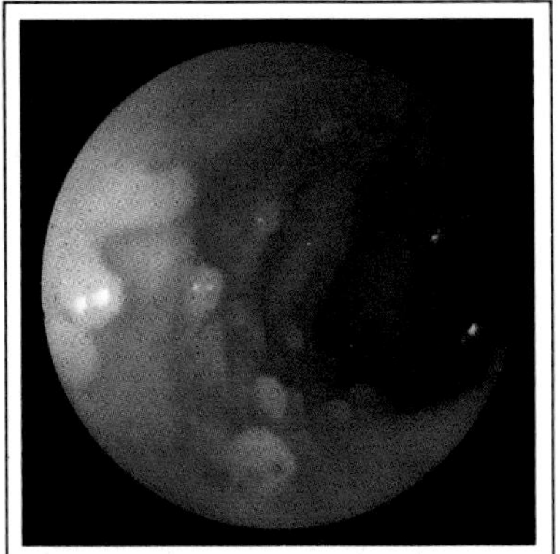

FIG. 43-6b.

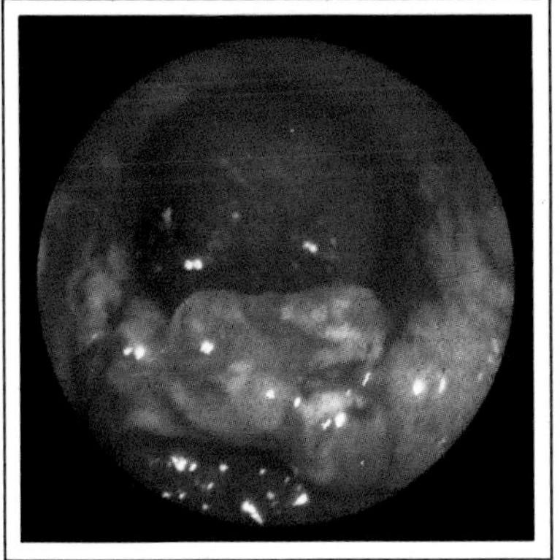

FIG. 43-6c.

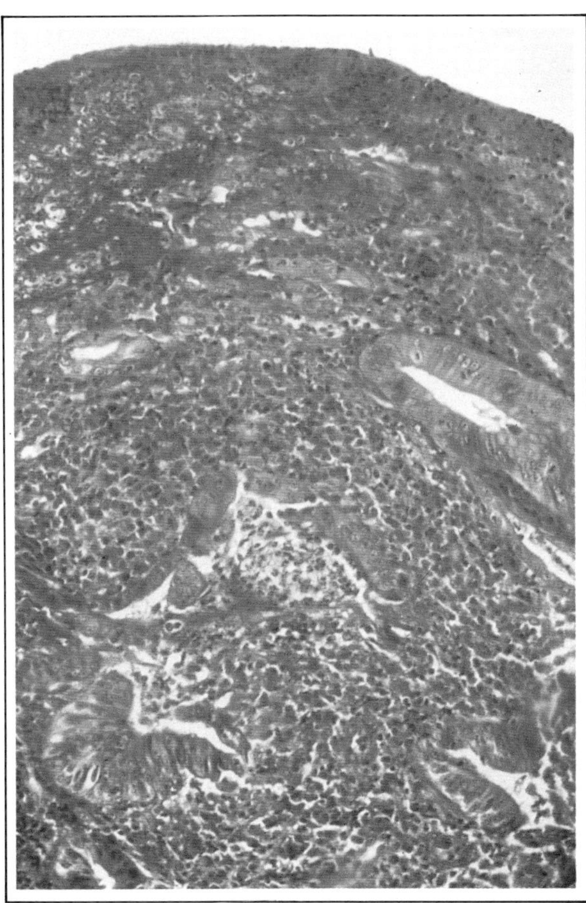

FIG. 43-6d.

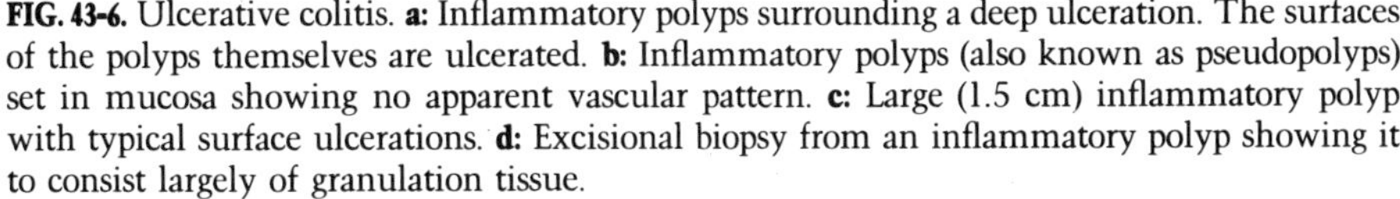

FIG. 43-6. Ulcerative colitis. **a:** Inflammatory polyps surrounding a deep ulceration. The surfaces of the polyps themselves are ulcerated. **b:** Inflammatory polyps (also known as pseudopolyps) set in mucosa showing no apparent vascular pattern. **c:** Large (1.5 cm) inflammatory polyp with typical surface ulcerations. **d:** Excisional biopsy from an inflammatory polyp showing it to consist largely of granulation tissue.

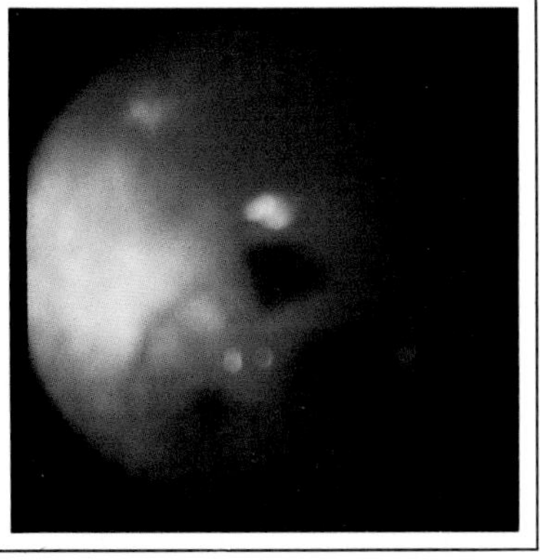

FIG. 43-7.

FIG. 43-7. Ulcerative colitis, inflammatory polyps connected by mucosal bridging. Deep ulcerations of the type associated with the formation of inflammatory polyps undermine adjacent mucosa and produce mucosal bridges. These are seen in both ulcerative colitis and Crohn's disease (Fig. 43-25a).

Edema of the valvulae.

The first noticeable structural abnormality in the face of mucosal inflammation is that of loss of the sharp terminations of the valvulae, causing them to appear thickened or blunted (Fig. 43-8a). This has been termed edema; however, histologically acute inflammation along with some edema is expected.[16] This endoscopic feature is most noticeable in an area such as the transverse colon where the expected sharp, thin, triangular folds (Fig. 43-8b) are rounded and thickened (Fig. 43-8a).

Loss of interhaustral folds.

The interhaustral fold pattern is generally thought to result from contraction of the teniae coli. With mucosal inflammation there is muscle hypertrophy, which is noted histologically[16] as hypertrophy of the muscularis mucosae.[16] This hypertrophy prevents the formation of haustrae, resulting in a lumen which appears continuous (Fig. 43-8c).

Diffuse luminal narrowing—tubularization.

With muscle hypertrophy, the width of the lumen decreases from 6 cm or more (as in the right colon) to less than 13 mm, a diameter which may just barely admit the colonoscope (Fig. 43-8d). With the loss of haustrae and the luminal narrowing, the overall appearance of the colon resembles that of a long narrow tube—hence the term tubularization.

Stricture formation.

In some cases muscle hypertrophy does not lead to diffuse luminal narrowing (see above) but to a focal reaction which appears endoscopically and radiographically as stricture formation. In ulcerative colitis, inflammatory strictures tend to be composed largely, if not exclusively, of hypertrophic smooth muscle, in contrast with Crohn's disease where they are fibrotic.[19] Generally, in and around the inflammatory strictures seen in ulcerative colitis one finds mucosal ulceration (Fig. 43-9a). Such ulcerations may play a role in the formation of these strictures by, in some way, inducing the focal muscle hypertrophy. Along with the ulcerations, one may find the cobblestone appearance of the intervening mucosa (Fig. 43-9b). In the absence of ulceration, the mouth of the stricture appears quite regular (Fig. 43-9c). The mucosal texture and granularity are coarsened, but the mucosa is soft, being easily compressed with a biopsy forceps. The most characteristic appearance for the mouth of an inflammatory stricture is superficial or deep ulceration with markedly erythematous, friable intervening mucosa (Fig. 43-9d). The absence of ulceration with nodular indurated mucosa is an atypical appearance and makes the examiner suspect malignancy (see "Malignancy in Ulcerative Colitis," this chapter).

Inflammatory strictures are generally short (Fig. 43-9d), so the mucosa can be easily sampled with multiple biopsies. Many strictures can be entered directly especially if a narrow-caliber ($\leq$9 mm) endoscope is employed. Some strictures in ulcerative colitis are somewhat longer, up to 2 to 3 cm; however, any stricture which is longer than 5 cm, especially one whose mouth has atypical features, should cause the examiner to strongly suspect malignancy.

Bridging.

Areas of the colon may show mucosal interconnections which result from healing of undermining ulcerations with re-epithelialization after the resolution of acute activity (Fig. 43-7). Bridging is found to interconnect areas of flat mucosa as well as inflammatory polyps, where they appear as interconnecting folds (Fig. 43-7).

Effacement of the ileocecal valve.

Probably as a result of muscle hypertrophy, the ileocecal valve becomes completely effaced, appearing patulous with a diameter which approximates that of the terminal ileum. This allows the endoscope to enter the terminal ileum easily (Fig. 43-10), which may itself show evidence of acute inflammation (see Chapter 48).

Patterns of Involvement

Characteristic of ulcerative colitis is its continuous nature from the rectum to the point of farthest extent. Five distinct patterns of involvement based on extent may be observed in colonoscopy. These are, in order of frequency: (a) universal involvement; (b) subtotal (left-sided) and transverse colon involvement; (c) left-sided involvement; (d) rectosigmoid involvement only; and (e) rectal involvement only.

Universal involvement.

Universal involvement is the commonest pattern seen at our institution, accounting for nearly 50% of the cases (Table 43-2). In approximately half of these the disease is clinically inactive, with patients undergoing colonoscopy because of cancer surveillance (see below). Here, except for a distorted mucosal vascular pattern or granularity, the mucosal appearance is normal, as are the structural features, e.g., the lumen and valvulae. For the remainder that showed

TABLE 43-2. *Pattern of involvement at colonoscopy in 305 patients with ulcerative colitis (1976–1980)*

Type of involvement	No.	%
Universal	145	47
Subtotal (to hepatic flexure)	75	25
Left-sided (to splenic flexure)	45	15
Proctosigmoiditis	30	10
Proctitis	10	3
Total	305	100

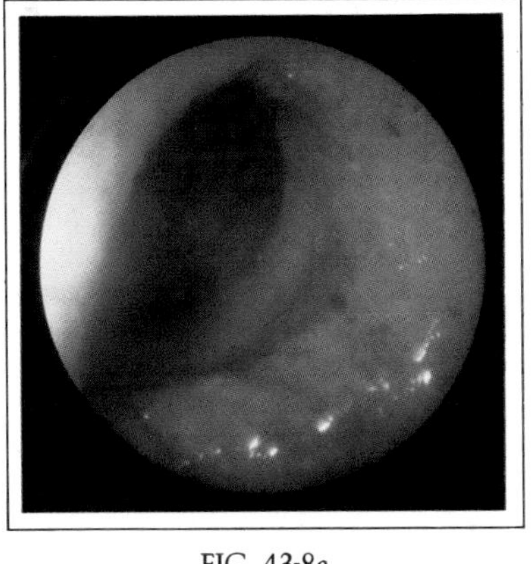

FIG. 43-8a.

FIG. 43-8b.

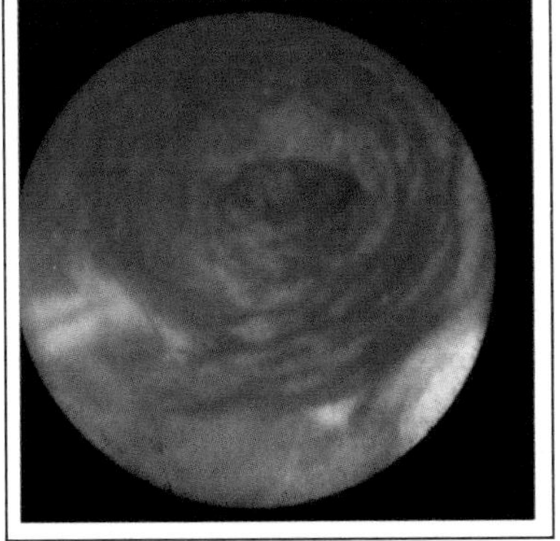

FIG. 43-8c.

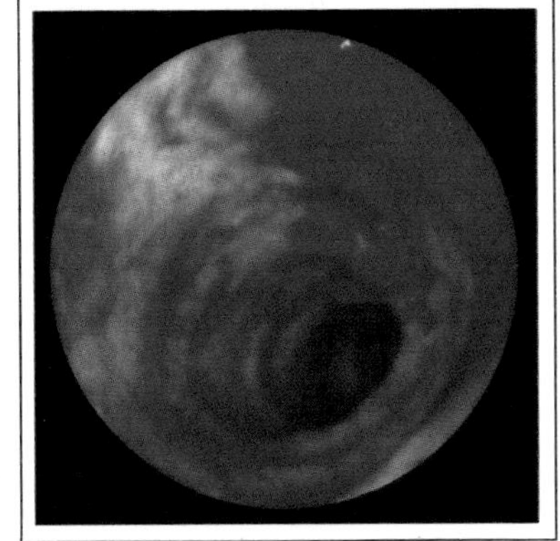

FIG. 43-8d.

FIG. 43-8. a: Ulcerative colitis, blunting of interhaustral folds. This is thought to be secondary to acute inflammation, edema, and muscle hypertrophy.[19] **b:** Normal interhaustral folds in the transverse colon. These are characteristically tall and sharply demarcated. **c:** Ulcerative colitis with loss of interhaustral folds. The activity in this case (ulceration and mucopus) may be associated with diffuse muscle hypertrophy, decreasing their contractility such that the usual haustral pattern (which requires contraction of the muscularis) is lost. **d:** Ulcerative colitis, tubularization, with acute mucosal inflammation and muscularis hypertrophy.

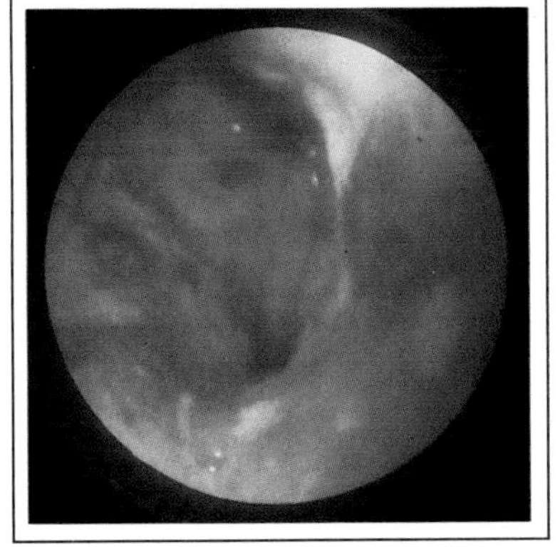

FIG. 43-9a.

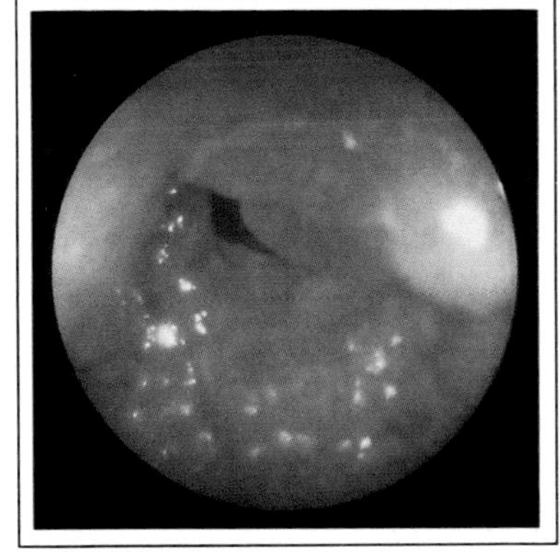

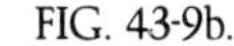

FIG. 43-9b.

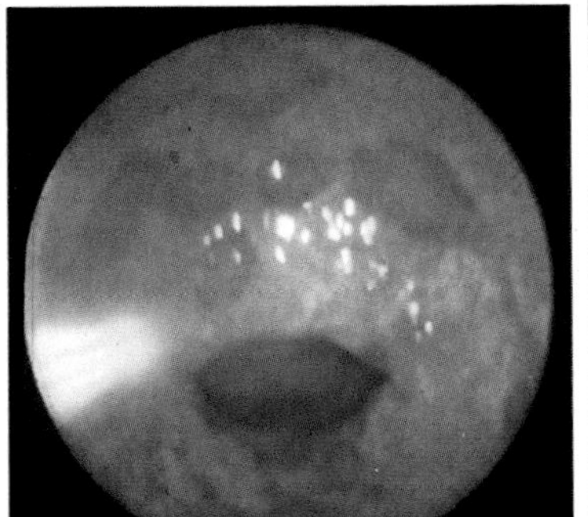

FIG. 43-9c.

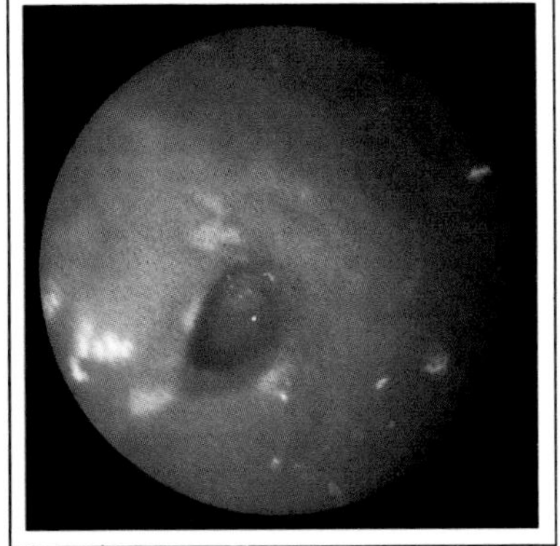

FIG. 43-9d.

FIG. 43-9. Ulcerative colitis. **a:** Stricture formation. The marked luminal narrowing which results in the formation of a stricture is thought to be focal muscle hypertrophy at a site of marked mucosal inflammation.[19] In this case acute activity is indicated at the mouth of the stricture by the presence of mucopus. **b:** Stricture formation with inflammatory polyps. The polyps result from previous ulceration in and around the mouth of the stricture. Should the ulceration itself disappear, the irregularity caused by the inflammatory polyps results in an appearance similar to that of a malignant stricture (Fig. 43-14b). **c:** Stricture. The smooth, slightly ulcerated mouth is characteristic of an inflammatory stricture. **d:** Short inflammatory stricture with ulceration.

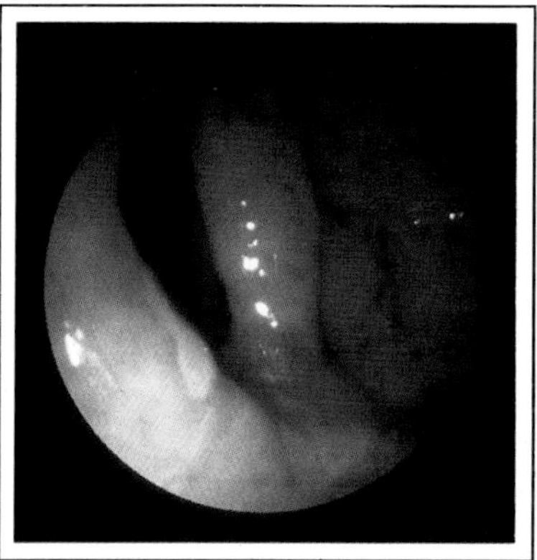

FIG. 43-10. Ulcerative colitis, patulous ileocecal valve. This finding is typical of universal involvement. It allows easy entry into the terminal ileum to biopsy for "backwash ileitis" (see Chapter 48).

FIG. 43-10.

activity, in most cases this was more severe distally, especially in the distal descending colon, sigmoid, and rectum; however, in about one-fourth of those showing activity, this was seen throughout the colon, with the activity greatest in the proximal colon in a few patients.

Subtotal involvement.

For 25% of our cases the involvement terminates at the hepatic flexure, with the right side being entirely normal by both appearance and histologic sampling. As with universal involvement, activity tends to be more marked distally, although in 20% of these cases the activity is uniform throughout.

Left-sided involvement.

For 15% of our cases the involvement stops at or just proximal to the splenic flexure, where a relatively sharp demarcation can be seen between the involved and uninvolved portions. Generally with this pattern there is mild to moderate activity (erythema or mucopurulent exudate) within the splenic flexure area, with the activity becoming more marked (with ulcerations) distally.

Proctosigmoiditis.

For 10% the disease is confined to the rectosigmoid. There is some activity in virtually all these cases. This may be either uniformly distributed or appear more marked in the sigmoid.

Proctitis.

For 3% the involvement is in the rectum only, with a sharp demarcation between the rectum and sigmoid both visually and histologically. The degree of activity varies, although in at least one-third of the cases the proctitis appears severe with marked friability and ulceration.

Role of Biopsy in Determining Extent

Although the visual assessment of involvement is borne out histologically in the majority of cases, there are some features that cause the examiner to err concerning the extent. This occurs, for example, in a visually normal proximal colon, where definite mucosal activity is sometimes seen histologically (crypt abscesses and/or the presence of inflammatory cells). In most patients in whom there is a discrepancy, one sees only histologic evidence of healed disease (atrophy and regenerative changes), or histology disproves a visual suggestion of involvement that was suggested by the presence of a distorted mucosal vascular pattern, granularity, or erythema. Altogether, we find that in up to 30% of the cases histologic sampling may differ from the visual assessment in determining the true extent of the disease. Whether the more precise determination of extent resulting from biopsy is of clinical significance is unsettled.

Grading the Activity of Ulcerative Colitis

There is no universally accepted system for grading the activity of ulcerative colitis by colonoscopy. Still, one would like to have a system which allows for some consistency from one examination to another. The one we present in this section has evolved from a conscious effort to correlate the visual assessment of activity from mucosal appearances to that which is found histologically. In our system, the degree of activity (Table 43-3) relates the number and size of ulceration in a given area, as well as the presence or absence of spontaneous bleeding. As is true with proctoscopic appearances, these visual assessments do not necessarily correlate with clinical activity.[7] The virtue of this system is that it can be applied to a single patient who has sequential examinations as well as be used to compare activity in different patients.

In our system (Table 43-3) four categories of activity are used, ranging from no activity (i.e., quiescent disease) to marked activity, (i.e., severe colitis). The four categories are: (a) quiescent colitis; (b) mildly active colitis; (c) moderately active colitis; and (d) severe colitis.

Quiescent Colitis

In cases of quiescent colitis, except for an altered mucosal vascular pattern (MVP) or the presence of granularity (see

TABLE 43-3. *Grading activity in ulcerative colitis*

Activity	Appearance
Quiescent	1. Distorted or absent mucosal vascular pattern 2. Granularity
Mildly active	1. Continuous or focal erythma 2. Friability (touch bleeding)
Moderately active	1. Mucopurulent exduate (mucopus) 2. Single or multiple ulcers (<5 mm); fewer than 10 per 10-cm segment
Severe colitis	1. Large ulcers (>5 mm); more than 10 per 10-cm segment 2. Spontaneous bleeding

above), the mucosal appearance is normal (Fig. 43-11a). As we have already noted (see above), alteration of the MVP and granularity correlate best with the presence of mucosal atrophy and regenerative changes of the crypts, with acute inflammation generally being absent. With an altered MVP, one may also note friability (Fig. 43-11b), i.e., touch bleeding, which correlates histologically, in the absence of erythema, only with atrophy. None of these findings, particularly friability in the absence of erythema, implies clinical activity.[7]

Mildly Active Colitis

Erythema, either diffuse (Fig. 43-11c) or focal (Fig. 43-11d), is the first finding to denote histologic activity. Clinically, patients with this as their maximum grade of activity may be indistinguishable from those with quiescent colitis.[7] The MVP appears either distorted or absent because the erythema itself obscures the mucosal capillaries or there are underlying chronic mucosal changes, i.e., atrophy which itself is associated with a distorted MVP (see above). Histologically, one finds evidence of acute inflammation in the lamina propria, but crypt abscesses are seen less often (in only 10 to 15% of the cases).

Moderately Active Colitis

We include under the designation "moderately active colitis" single (Fig. 43-12a) or scattered (Fig. 43-12b) ulcerations of less than 5 mm maximum dimension with fewer than 10 of these ulcers occurring over a 10-cm segment. Along with the finding of small ulcers, we include mucopurulent exudate (Fig. 43-12c), which we regard as an ulcer-equivalent (Fig. 43-12d). With either finding—ulceration or mucopurulent exudate—we expect to find crypt abscesses histologically in the majority (80%) of the cases. As the formation of crypt abscesses is probably central to

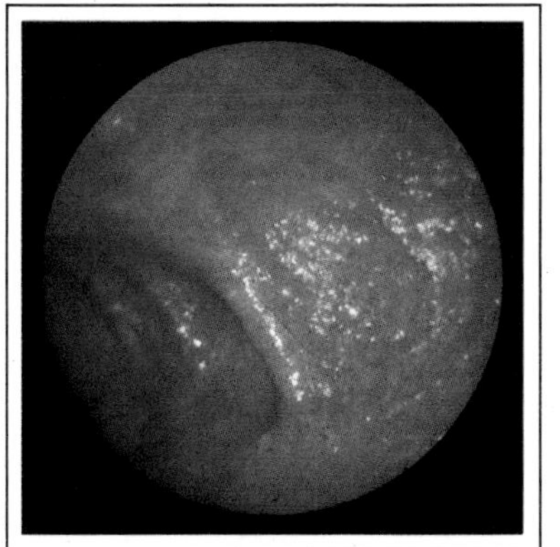

FIG. 43-11a.

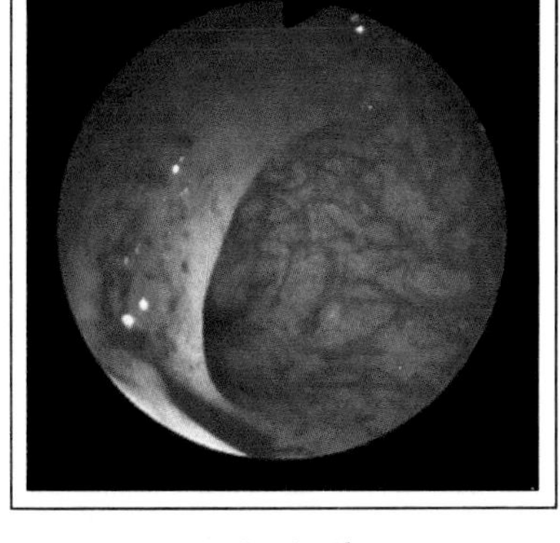

FIG. 43-11b.

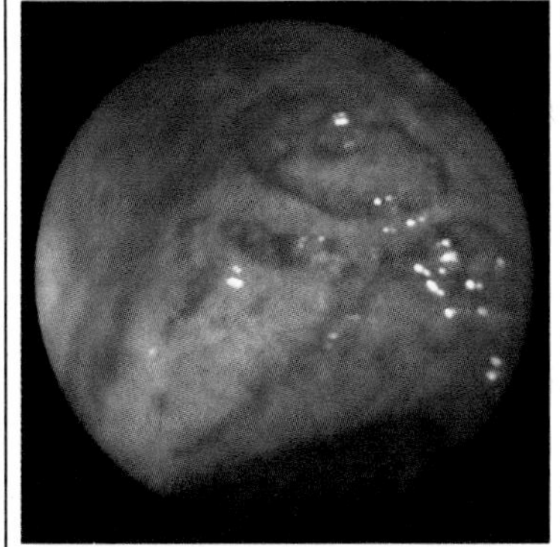

FIG. 43-11c.

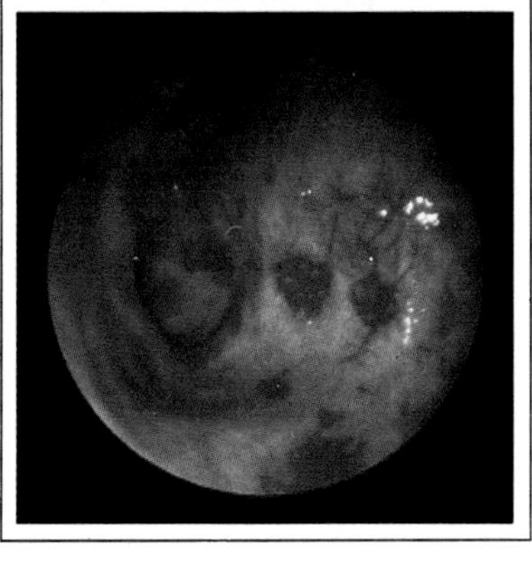

FIG. 43-11d.

FIG. 43-11. Ulcerative colitis. **a:** Quiescent. The visual features are a loss of the mucosal vascular pattern and granularity. Biopsies revealed only mucosal atrophy (similar to that in Fig. 43-1d). **b:** Quiescent. Some friability is noted in addition to a blunted mucosal vascular pattern. There was no erythema, and biopsies showed only mucosal atrophy. **c:** Mildly active. Erythema, diffuse or focal (d), is the first visual sign we find to verify the acute inflammation observed histologically. **d:** Mildly active. The focal erythema present here was associated with minimal acute inflammation histologically (Fig. 43-3b).

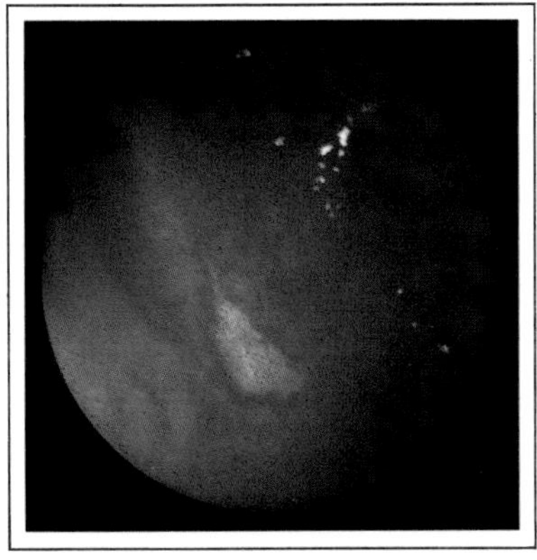

FIG. 43-12a.

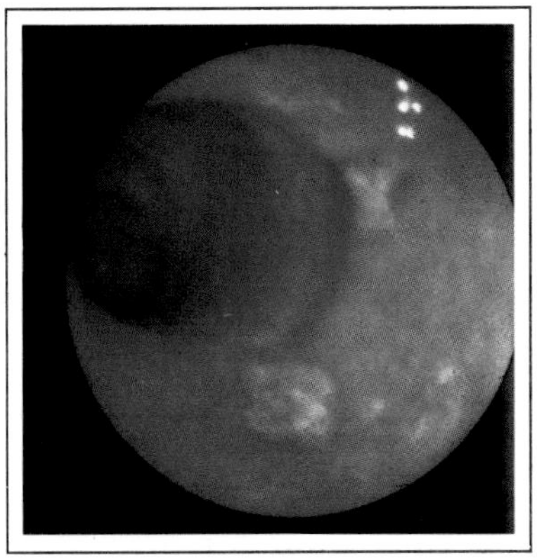

FIG. 43-12b.

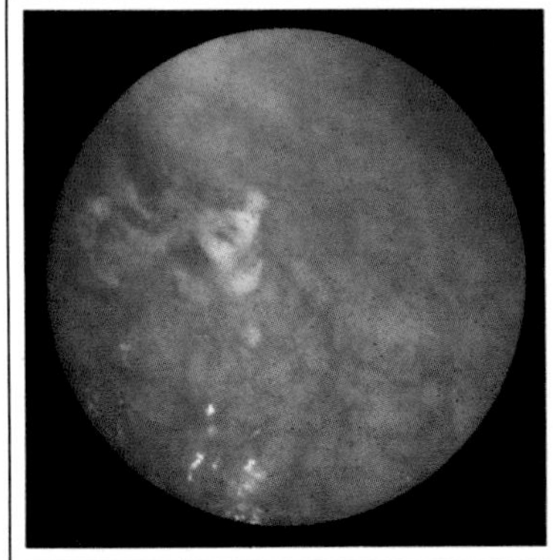

FIG. 43-12c.

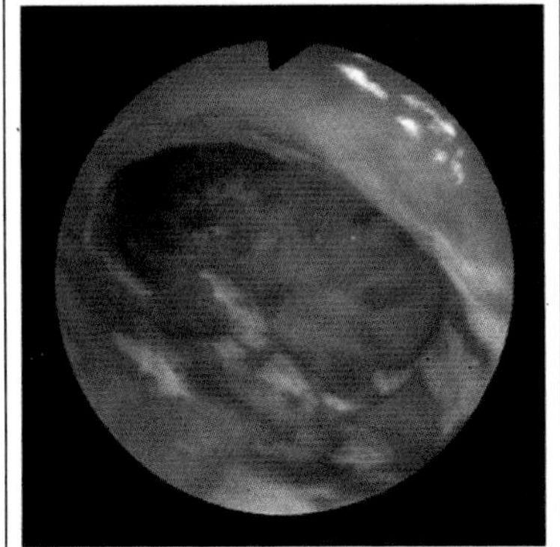

FIG. 43-12d.

FIG. 43-12. Ulcerative colitis. **a:** Moderately active. One of several small (<5 mm) ulcerations noted over a 10-cm segment. This appearance we arbitrarily assign a "moderate" grade of activity. **b:** Moderately active. Two small discrete ulcers were seen over a 10-cm segment in the area of maximim activity, causing us to assign a grade of "moderately active" colitis. **c:** Moderately active. For mucopus, considered by us an ulcer-equivalent, we assign a grade of "moderately active." **d:** Moderately active to severe colitis. Both the size and small number of ulcers caused us to grade the activity "moderately active"; however, the number and size increased distally (in the foreground) and received a grade of focally "severe colitis."

the mechanism of mucosal ulceration,[16] and as mucopurulent exudate probably derives from crypt abscesses, we believe this to be a preulcer stage if not a true ulcer-equivalent, deserving of the same activity status as small ulcers themselves. The clinical activity seen in patients with moderately active colitis colonoscopically is variable. Although it is our impression that patients with this finding tend to have more clinical activity than those with the finding of quiescent colitis alone, this has not been confirmed by any study to date.

Severe Colitis

Ulcers larger than 5 mm (Fig. 43-13a) or more than 10 ulcers of any size per 10-cm segment (Fig. 43-13b), along with the appearance of sponanteous bleeding (Fig. 43-13c), we regard as evidence of severe colitis. These findings at sigmoidoscopy, especially that of spontaneous bleeding,[7] correlate with increased clinical severity compared to patients without spontaneous bleeding (Fig. 43-13d) who we would probably classify as having either quiescent colitis, mildly active, or only moderately active colitis. Furthermore, the appearances which we consider to be indicative of severe colitis are found in colectomy specimens removed from patients who have proved to be refractory to medical management. We therefore believe that we are on reasonably secure ground in regarding this appearance as severe, even though studies correlating this appearance with clinical activity have not been performed. Curiously, approximately 10% of our patients with colonoscopic findings of severe colitis, especially those with exclusively distal involvement, are only mildly symptomatic or without symptoms altogether.

Malignancy and Ulcerative Colitis

The overall risk of cancer in patients with ulcerative colitis is 3 to 5%,[20] with increasing risk for patients with universal involvement and those having had their disease for more than 8 years, and especially in excess of 20 years. In such patients the risk may be as high as 30 to 40%, particularly in those in whom the disease began during childhood.[12]

For asymptomatic patients with universal ulcerative colitis for 10 years' duration or more, colonoscopy has proved to be an effective means for providing cancer surveillance with the opportunity for detecting early cancer while it is still curable.[14,14a] One hopes that with the availability of colonoscopic surveillance an increasing number of colitic cancers will be detected at a curable stage, in contrast to the present situation where patients present with rectal bleeding or weight loss and in whom the malignancy at surgery, similar to the case in noncolitics, is often found to be metastatic, with a 5-year survival of only 30%.[21,21a]

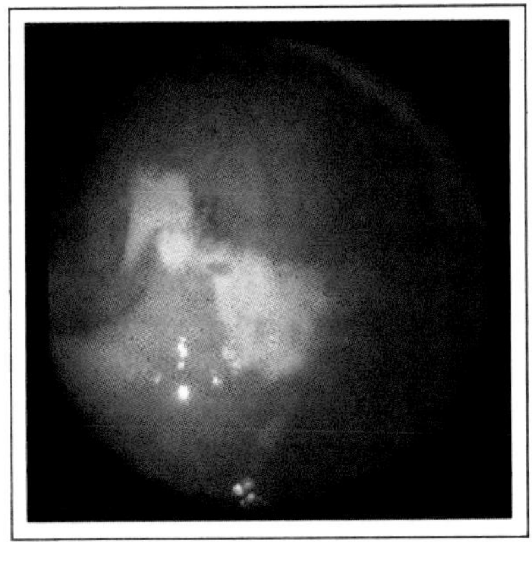

FIG. 43-13a.

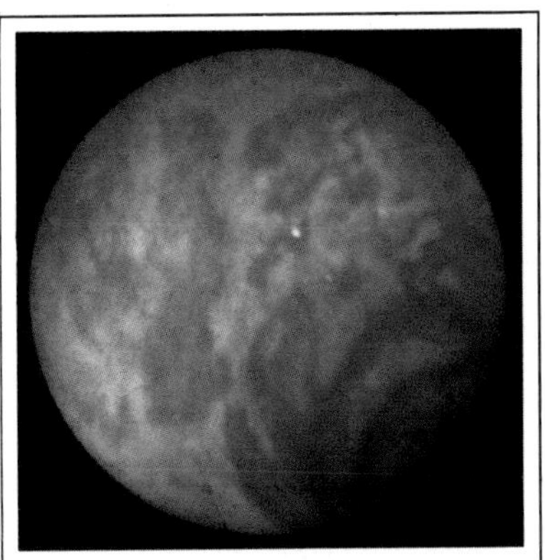

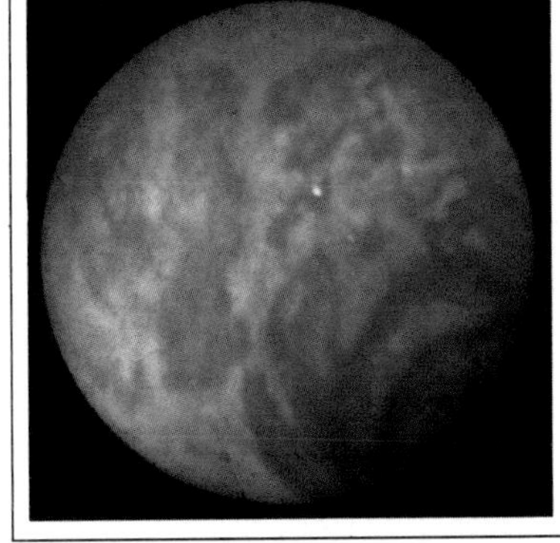

FIG. 43-13b.

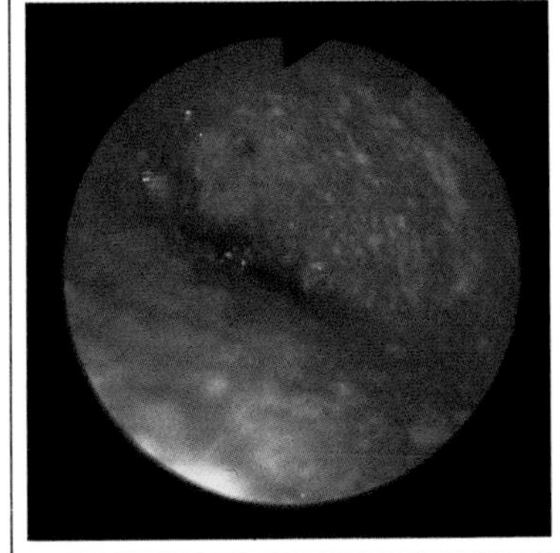

FIG. 43-13c.

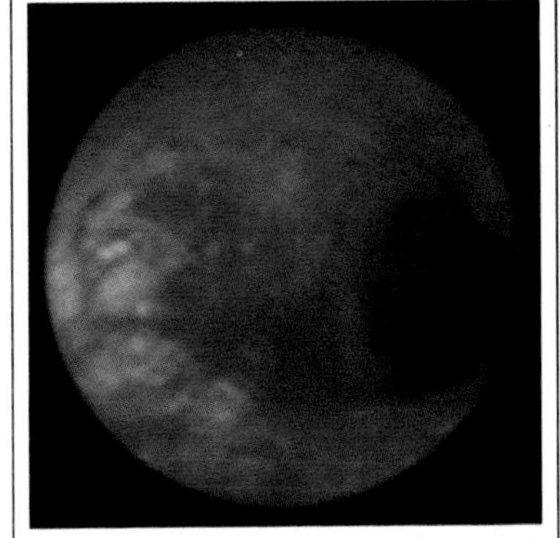

FIG. 43-13d.

FIG. 43-13. Ulcerative colitis. **a:** Severe. One of several long (>1.5 cm) serpiginous ulcers noted over a 10-cm area caused us to assign a "severe" grade of activity. **b:** Severe. The extensive confluent ulceration with little intervening mucosa is another appearance which we feel is deserving of a grade of "severe." **c:** Severe. Spontaneous bleeding with boggy erythematous mucosa is also indicative of marked activity and so receives the grade "severe." Spontaneous bleeding in one proctoscopic study was associated with an increase in severity of symptoms over those associated with appearances which lacked this finding.[7] **d:** Moderately active, in an asymptomatic patient. Mucopus and friability (touch bleeding) were present, but not spontaneous bleeding [as in (c)].

In the section which follows we consider carcinoma and ulcerative colitis first in symptomatic patients, its commonest setting at present. This is followed by a discussion of its detection by means of periodic colonoscopy for cancer surveillance in symptomatic patients. We conclude with a brief presentation of the rare case of lymphoma complicating ulcerative colitis.

Carcinoma in Symptomatic Patients

Location.

A significant difference between colitic and noncolitic cancer is the shift in distribution of colitic cancer to the right side. Although only about 20% of noncolitic cancers are proximal, half or more of those found in ulcerative colitis may be located proximal to the splenic flexure.[22,23] In a study reported by Cook and Goligher,[22] 14 of 26 cancers (53%) found at colectomy were in the transverse colon (incuding the splenic flexure) or right colon.[22] A study from our institution reported that 15 of 33 cancers (45%) resected over an 18-year period were located proximal to the splenic flexure.[23]

Appearance.

Unlike cancer in noncolitic patients, which typically displays an exophytic growth pattern and appears as an ulcerated mass (Fig. 43-14a), colitic cancers are infiltrating. Although one might expect these cancers to uniformly appear as strictures, a variety of endoscopic findings may be encountered with this growth pattern, including slightly elevated plaque-like lesions, single nonulcerated sessile masses, or multiple smaller, indurated polypoid masses. In the uncommon case where the growth pattern is exophytic, an ulcerated mass indistinguishable from noncolitic cancer may be found.

1. *Malignant strictures:* Although the expected endoscopic appearance for infiltrating carcinoma is a stricture, somewhat surprisingly the cancers with this growth appearance accounted for less than one-third (6 of 21) of the cancers found by Cook and Goligher in a study of surgically resected specimens.[22] At colonoscopy one finds abrupt tapering of the lumen to form the stricture, with the mouth appearing nodular and friable but typically nonulcerative (Fig. 43-14b). As colitic cancers tend to be scirrhous, biopsies taken from the mouth of the stricture give the impression of a rock-hard surface.

2. *Plaque-like lesions:* A focal, rather than more diffusely infiltrating, carcinoma gives rise to this appearance. At colonoscopy the lesion is seen as a slightly raised, flat, nodular mass with ill-defined edges (Fig. 43-14c). In the Cook and Goligher study these lesions were found in an incidence similar (7 of 21) to that of malignant strictures (see above).[22]

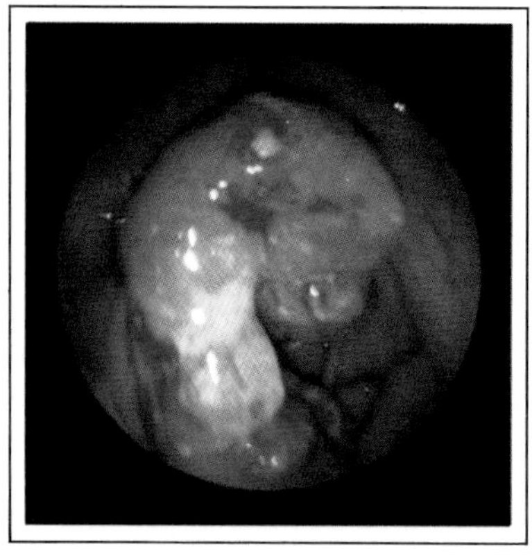

FIG. 43-14a.

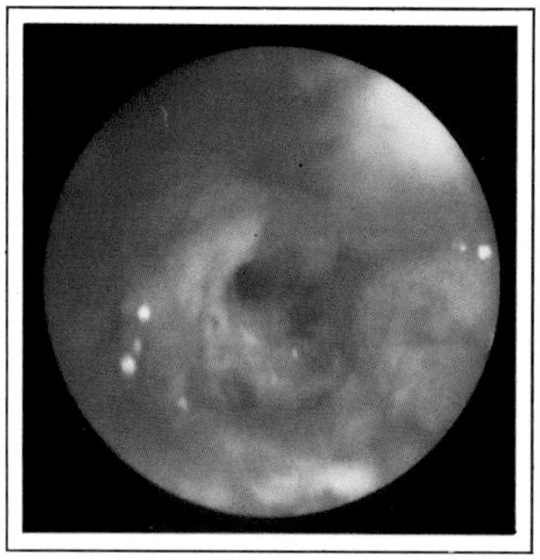

FIG. 43-14b.

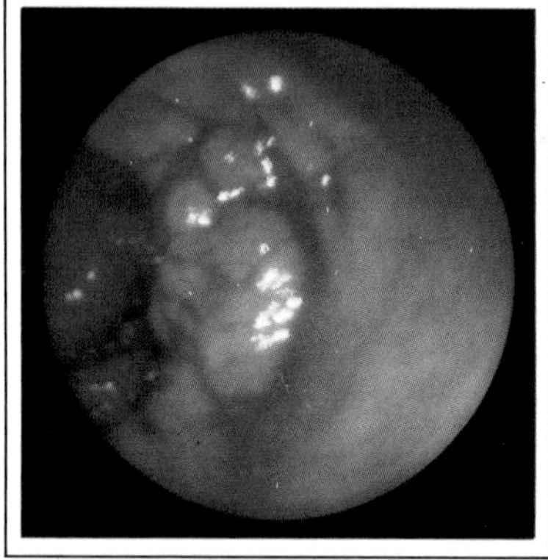

FIG. 43-14c.

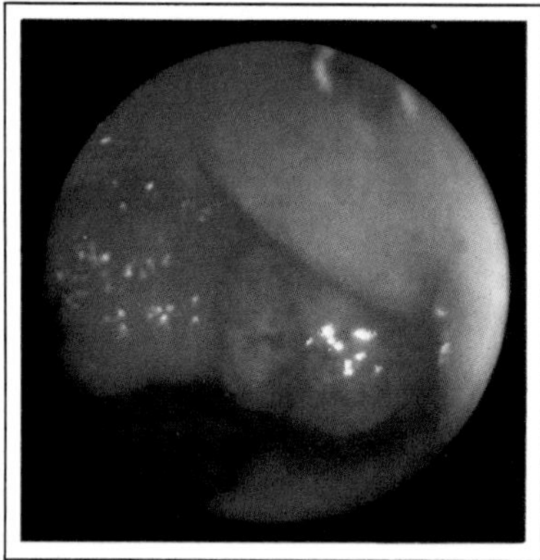

FIG. 43-14d.

FIG. 43-14. Carcinoma. **a:** In a noncolitic patient (see Chapter 42). With the characteristic exophytic-type growth pattern of noncolitic cancer, there is a large mass with central ulceration. **b:** In ulcerative colitis. With the characteristic infiltrating, rather than exophytic, growth pattern, carcinoma may appear as a stricture with an asymmetrical, irregular mouth. **c:** In ulcerative colitis. A focally elevated, plaque-like mass is seen and is associated with focal infiltration histologically. Biopsy of this lesion revealed carcinoma. **d:** In ulcerative colitis. Here the carcinoma appears as a nonulcerated polypoid mass, similar to the appearance of polypoid cancer in that it is noncolitic.

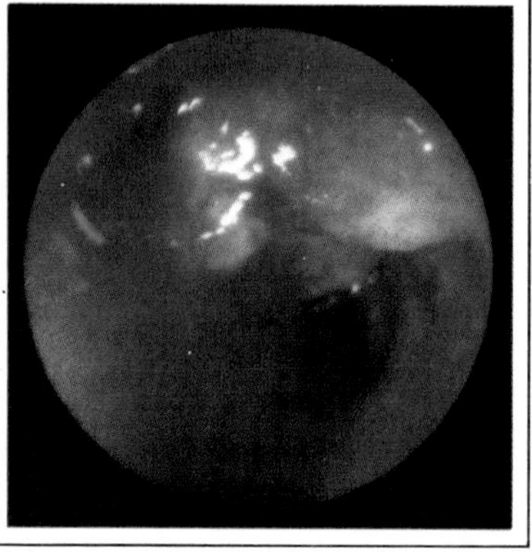

FIG. 43-15.

FIG. 43-15. Cancer in ulcerative colitis. In this case a sessile mass was observed with central ulceration, similar to the exophytic type of lesions found in noncolitic cancer (Fig. 43-14a).

3. *Single polypoid masses:* This is the commonest appearance of colitic cancer at our institution (Fig. 43-14d) representing nearly half the cases.[23] In the Cook and Goligher surgical study, however, it accounted for only 14% (3 of 21). We find these masses to range in size between 2 and 4 cm. The surface mucosa is nonulcerated, being either smooth or slightly irregular (Fig. 43-14d).

4. *Multiple polypoid masses:* Another common appearance at our institution, accounting for nearly 40% of the cases,[23] was that of multiple (1 to 2 cm) sessile polyps with friable though nonulcerated surface mucosa (Fig. 43-15). The absence of ulcerations along with the hard, rubbery consistency, best appreciated on biopsy, distinguishes these from inflammatory polyps (Fig. 43-6a).

5. *Ulcerated mass lesions:* This appearance, which is indistinguishable from that of noncolitic carcinoma (Fig. 43-14a), is rare at our institution. Only one case of colitic cancer observed by us over a 7-year period was of this type, consisting of a large 4- to 5-cm mass with central ulceration. However, in the Cook and Goligher surgical series[22] nearly 25% were said to be "indistinguishable" from ordinary carcinoma, which is a mass with central ulceration. This experience, however, has not been widely reported by others.

Biopsy and brushing.

Because of the infiltrating nature of colitic carcinoma, biopsy may fail to provide evidence of cancer; we find this to be true in two-thirds or more of our cases. Biopsies taken from these lesions reveal neoplastic tissue (or epithelial dysplasia—see below) but not cancer. Still, finding a lesion at colonoscopy that has an appearance suggestive of cancer with a biopsy that shows the lesion to be neoplastic should make it highly suspicious for carcinoma. In a series from our institution where nine patients were subjected to colectomy because of a macroscopic appearance compatible with colitic cancer but with biopsies showing only dysplasia (and not cancer), six nevertheless proved to be malignant.[15] Whether the large-particle technique would increase the yield of biopsy without additional risk remains to be determined, although one would still wish to subject all such patients to colectomy, irrespective of whether a histologic diagnosis of cancer had been obtained.

In cases where a stricture is present which cannot easily be biopsied, brushing or even lavage cytology[24] has been a useful procedure. In these cases, at the mouth of the stricture or within it there may be some part of the cancer which has broken through the mucosa and can be sampled by the brushing technique. Brushing plays a secondary role for sessile masses, being reserved for lesions which cannot be readily biopsied; brushing is unlikely to sample the cancer, which may be situated deep within the lesion.

Cancer Surveillance in Asymptomatic Patients

The patient with universal, subtotal, or even left-sided ulcerative colitis[25] of more than 10 years' duration is now recognized to have a cancer risk which is 20 to 50 times that of the normal population.[20] Such patients are referred to colonoscopy for cancer surveillance. For these patients the examiner tries to inspect as much of the surface area of the colon as possible, looking for the macroscopic appearances of colitic cancer (see above) as well as taking biopsies at 10-cm intervals for examination by pathologists for histologic evidence of epithelial dysplasia, defined as a disordered cell pattern in the crypts indicative of neoplastic transformation.[26] Any dysplasia found is now graded (Table 43-4) as "high grade" (previously called "severe," "precancer," or "moderate" dysplasia) or "low grade" (previously called "mild" dysplasia).[27]

The significance of dysplasia in biopsies of flat mucosa lies in the finding of the high-grade type, particularly what in the past had been called severe dysplasia or precancer. This finding, especially if present on more than one examination or in several locations,[14] carries a 30 to 40% likelihood of cancer.[28] Because these cancers may still be in an intramucosal (Duke's A) stage,[14,14a] they could easily escape detection if one inspects the mucosa only for the macroscopic features (see above) of colitic cancer.[29]

TABLE 43-4. *Grading of epithelial dysplasia in ulcerative colitis*

New system[27]	Old system[15]	Criteria[15]
High grade	Severe	Hyperchromatic nuclei; mucin depletion; cell stratification; numerous nuclei close to surface
	Moderate	Nuclei more hyperchromatic, with increased cell stratification; mucin depletion more marked than for mild type
Low grade	Mild	Open vesicular nuclei; some reduction of mucus; mild but definite nuclear stratification
Indefinite	Borderline	Large, open vesicular nuclei; cells contain normal amount of mucin

In addition to finding dysplasia in random biopsies taken from flat mucosa, it may be found in association with a mass or other macroscopic lesion.[15] Here the cancer risk for either high-grade or low-grade dysplasia may approach 60%.

In the section which follows we discuss separately the dysplasia that occurs with subtle or no mucosal features (flat dysplasia) and that which occurs in association with polypoid masses or other macroscopic lesions (macroscopic dysplasia).

Flat dysplasia.

Definite dysplasia may be found in random biopsies in up to 20% of patients with longstanding ulcerative colitis, especially those with universal involvement.[26] There may be no macroscopic feature to indicate that dysplasia might be found histologically; however, a low villous appearance has been described[26] and observed by us (Fig. 43-16a) that can be recognized colonoscopically and differentiated by its focal nature from simply the granular-type mucosal appearance (Fig. 43-16b) associated with the quiescent stage of ulcerative colitis (see "Activity of the Disease," this chapter). In our experience, most flat dysplasia is of the low-grade type, with cancer being seen infrequently. In our reported experience[15] only 1 of 27 patients with flat dysplasia was found to have cancer over a 4-year period, a follow-up that included six patients who underwent colectomy. (Subsequently, a second patient did develop cancer, making the overall risk for this group approximately 10%.)

Macroscopic dysplasia.

We find dysplasia in association with a polypoid mass or other macroscopic appearance (dysplasia-associated lesion

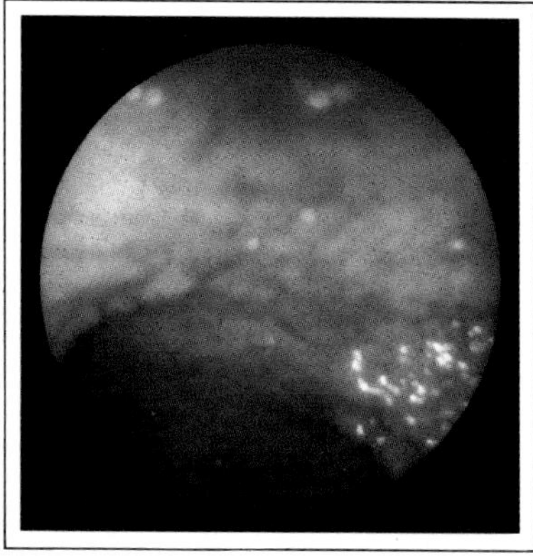

FIG. 43-16a.

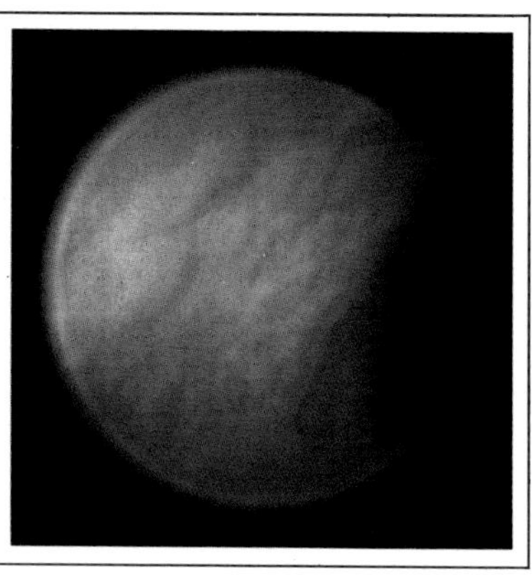

FIG. 43-16b.

FIG. 43-16. a: Flat dysplasia in a patient with longstanding ulcerative colitis. Biopsies from this zone showing focal nodularity revealed definite low-grade dysplasia (Table 43-4). This so-called low villous[26] appearance of flat dysplasia may be difficult to differentiate from simple granularity (b). Any area of irregular mucosa, especially if found as in this case, should be biopsied to determine if dysplasia is present. **b:** Ulcerative colitis, mucosal granularity. The diffuse, rather than focal, nature of this abnormality, even though giving the mucosa a nodular appearance, makes one suspect granularity rather than flat dysplasia with a low villous type of appearance.[26]

or mass; DALM) in up to 10% of patients with longstanding ulcerative colitis. In a retrospective review of 112 such patients colonscoped at our institution over a 4-year period, 12 (10.7%) had DALM.[15] Seven proved to have cancers, although in no case was this found on forceps biopsies taken from the DALM. Furthermore, the degree of dysplasia was high grade in only four (severe in two and moderate in two), whereas it was low grade in three, thus making the presence of DALM itself rather than the grade of dysplasia the feature which best denotes the presence of cancer.

In 6 of the 12 patients with DALM, including one of the seven cancers, studies were undertaken for cancer surveillance; in the remainder, all of whom had cancer, investigations were performed for symptoms, the most common being rectal bleeding (four of six). This seems to indicate that a DALM detected in a symptomatic patient stands the greatest likelihood (67% in our series) of being a cancer, and those detected in asymptomatic patients to be less likely (17%) but still indicating a substantial risk of cancer compared with patients with flat dysplasia (approximately 3% overall).[15]

1. *Single polypoid mass:* These constituted nearly half of the DALM lesions in our series (5 of 12) and were found in all but two of the seven patients with cancer. Typically, the DALM appearing as a single polypoid mass was a 2- to 4-cm sessile lesion with a slightly irregular though nonulcerated surface (Fig. 43-17a). As we have already noted (see "Carcinoma in Symptomatic Patients," this chapter), this is one of the typical appearances of colitic cancer (Fig. 43-17b). Although many, if not most, of these lesions are in fact cancers, we consider them to be examples of DALM because biopsies reveal only dysplasia. In two of the five cases, this was low grade (previously called mild).

2. *Multiple polyps:* Another common appearance (5 of 12 cases) was that of 5- to 15-mm, rubbery, sessile polypoid masses located in a discrete 5- to 10-cm segment (Fig. 43-17c). Two of these five cases proved to be carcinoma. Again biopsies taken from these lesions failed to reveal malignancy, with dysplasia in one case being low grade (mild).

3. *Plaque-like lesion:* The least common type of DALM, occurring in only 2 of the 12 cases, was called plaque-like; it had the appearance of a slightly raised, nodular area that extended over a finite distance (Fig. 43-17d). Although in neither case was invasive cancer found at colectomy, in one of the two (not shown) there was a 9-cm raised lesion present with foci of cancer *in situ* in a 49-year-old man with a 35-year history of ulcerative colitis, indicative of a high probability of a frank malignant change at a future time had not the surgery been performed.

4. *Differentiation of DALM from inflammatory polyps:* As larger inflammatory polyps may achieve a size in excess of 2 cm (Fig. 43-18a),[17] these could be confused with the sessile polypoid-type DALM. Inflammatory polyps (see above), especially large ones, are characteristically ulcerated with an erythematous, friable, overlying mucosa, and they are often adjacent to ulcerations (Fig. 43-18b). In contrast, the polypoid-type DALM has a smooth, slightly irregular (or nodular) but nonulcerated surface (Fig. 43-18c) with nonulcerated surrounding mucosa. For any large (>1.5 cm) sessile mass, multiple biopsies are necessary to establish its nature, whether neoplastic or inflammatory.

5. *Differentiation of DALM from tubular adenomas:* Single or multiple tubular adenomas (see Chapter 41) may be found in patients with longstanding ulcerative colitis; in and of themselves they do not indicate the presence of cancer (Fig. 43-18d). Because the smallest polypoid cancer we found in our series was 2 cm, we believe it is safe to remove small (<1 cm) adenomas colonoscopically (Fig. 43-18d). One may consider this treatment to be adequate if multiple biopsies of the surrounding flat mucosa show that the adenoma was not part of a larger area of dysplasia, in which case local excision is not adequate treatment.

Follow-up colonoscopy versus colectomy for patients with dysplasia.

1. *Flat dysplasia:* Because the low overall risk (5 to 10%) of cancer actually found in patients with flat dysplasia (Fig. 43-19a) is possibly no greater than for the ulcerative colitis population as a whole,[19] we believe that colonoscopic follow-up in these patients is appropriate, so long as the dysplasia is not high grade (Fig. 43-19b). In this case, if found on at least two examinations within 6 to 12 months of each

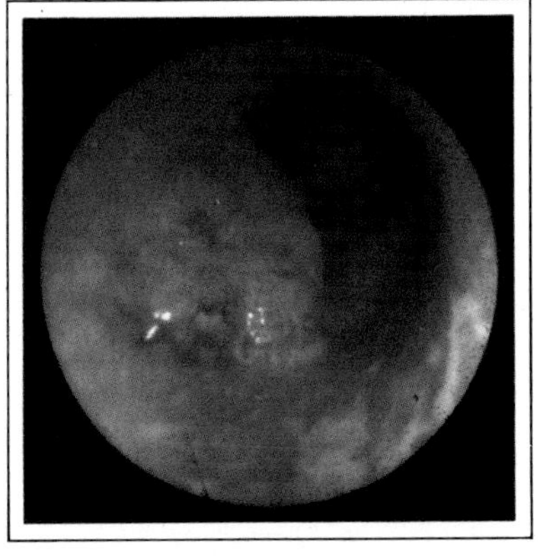

FIG. 43-17a.

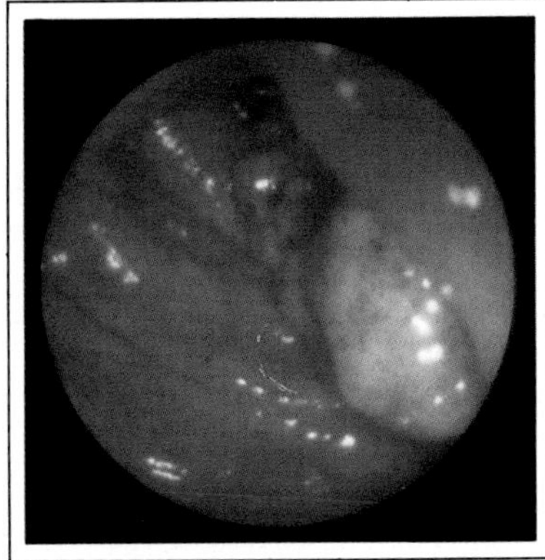

FIG. 43-17b.

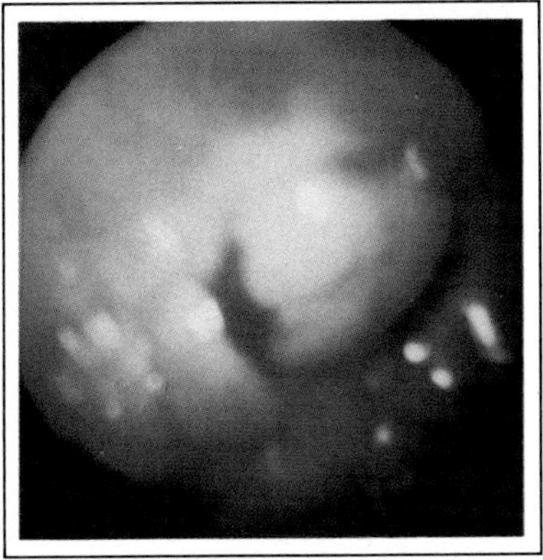

FIG. 43-17c.

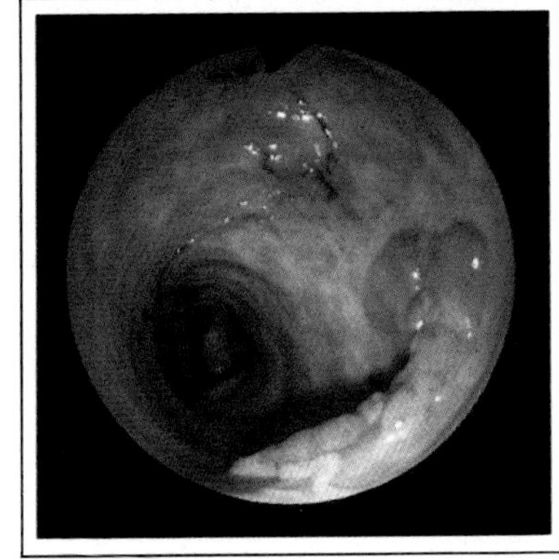

FIG. 43-17d.

FIG. 43-17. Ulcerative colitis. **a:** Dysplasia-associated polypoid mass. The appearance of this 2-cm sessile mass is indistinguishable from the polypoid carcinoma that occurs with ulcerative colitis (b). Although biopsy showed only dysplasia, this nevertheless proved to be malignant at surgery. Even though biopsy fails to reveal carcinoma, 60% or more of patients with this appearance studied by us already have cancer.[15] **b:** Polypoid carcinoma. A biopsy from this mass revealed carcinoma, but its appearance is indistinguishable from that of the dysplasia-associated polypoid mass where biopsy does not reveal invasive carcinoma (a). **c:** Dysplasia associated with sessile polyps. Numerous, rubbery, sessile polyps (0.5 to 1.5 cm) were seen over a 10-cm area. Biopsy showed high grade dysplasia, with infiltrating carcinoma found at colectomy. **d:** Dysplasia associated with a plaque-like mass. This mass is easily recognized as it stands out in an otherwise featureless lumen. In this case the biopsy showed high-grade dysplasia, with a villous adenoma being found in the colectomy specimen.

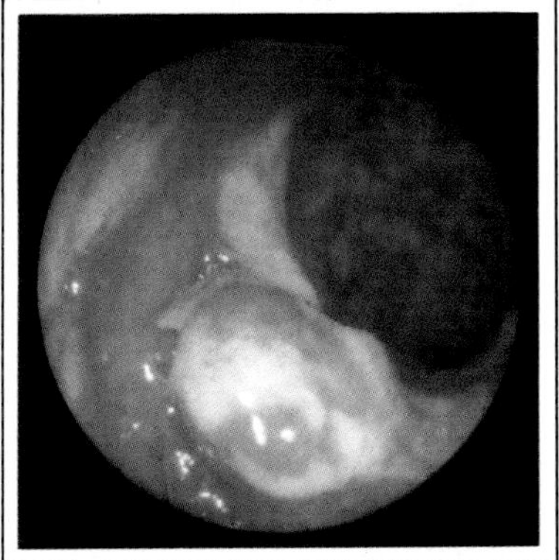

FIG. 43-18a.

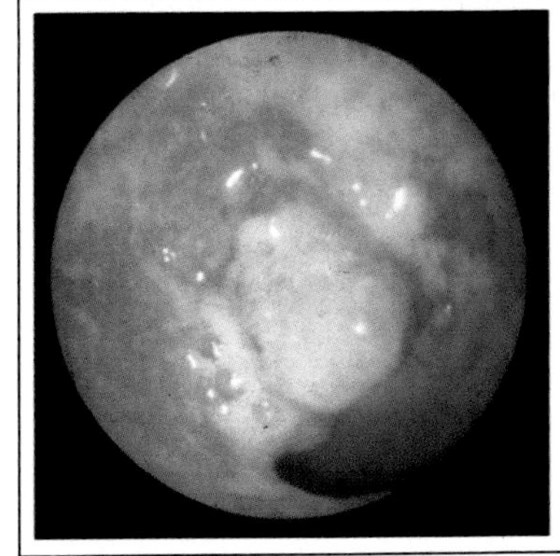

FIG. 43-18b.

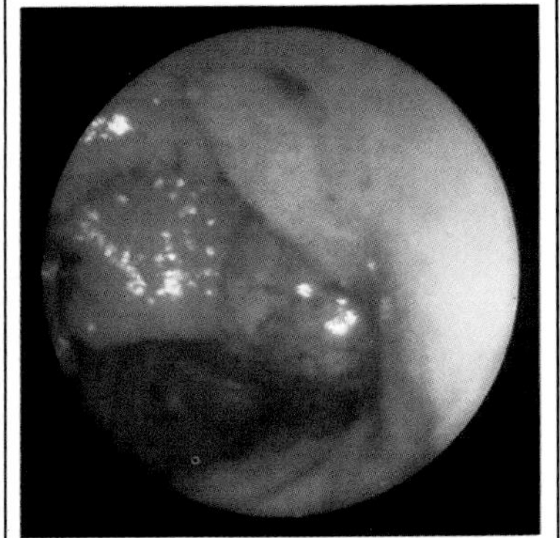

FIG. 43-18c.

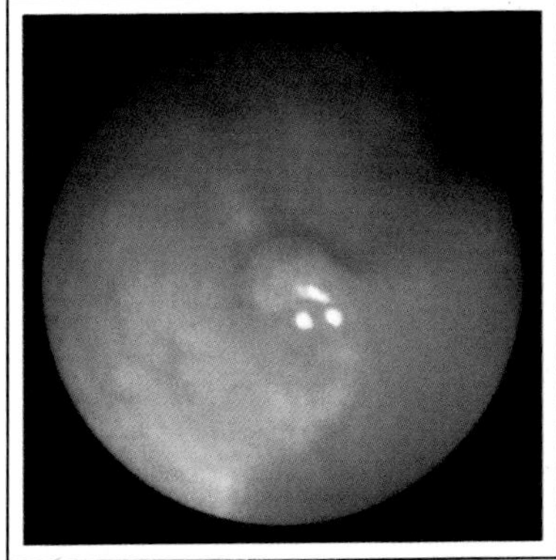

FIG. 43-18d.

FIG. 43-18. Ulcerative colitis. **a:** Inflammatory polyp. In contrast to the dysplasia associated with a polypoid mass (Fig. 43-17b), which the lesion resembles, its surface is ulcerated. Biopsies show it to be composed of granulation tissue with no dysplasia (similar to that in Fig. 43-6d). **b:** Inflammatory polyp. Another clue to a lesion's being an inflammatory polyp as opposed to dysplasia associated with a polypoid mass (Fig. 43-19a) is the presence of ulcerated mucosa surrounding it. **c:** Polypoid carcinoma. A single, nonulcerated, sessile polypoid mass is observed (at 3 o'clock). Even if biopsies had not shown carcinoma, but only dysplasia, colectomy would have been strongly advised because of the high likelihood (60%+) of the mass being carcinoma.[15] **d:** Tubular adenoma. The size of this lesion (5 mm) and the absence of dysplasia in the surrounding mucosa argues for simple excision rather than colectomy. Periodic colonoscopic surveillance (at yearly intervals) is still necessary in this patient with longstanding (>10 years) ulcerative colitis.

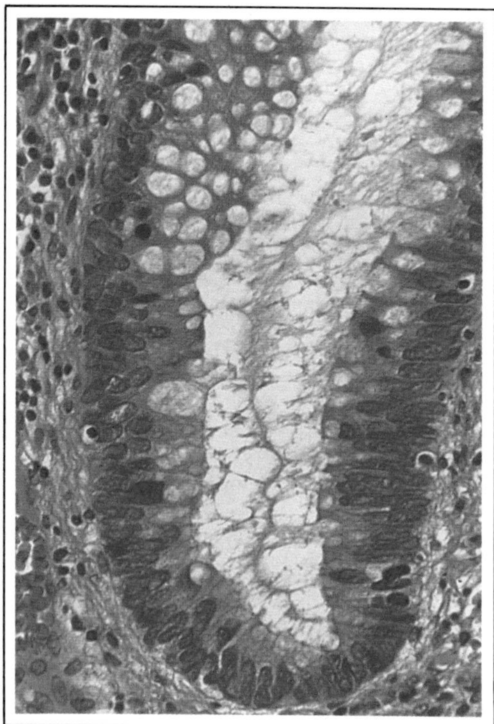

FIG. 43-19a.

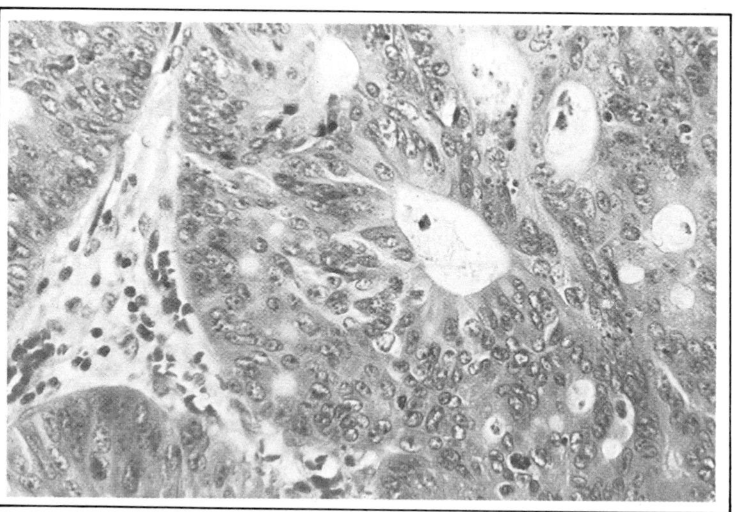

FIG. 43-19b.

FIG. 43-19. Ulcerative colitis. **a:** Biopsy showing low-grade dysplasia. This is evidenced by the presence of hyperchromatic nuclei with some stratification and mucin depletion (Table 43-4). In this case the low-grade dysplasia was found in random biopsies. The probability of cancer being found at colectomy in a patient with flat dysplasia of this grade is probably no greater than the probability of cancer overall in patients with longstanding ulcerative colitis, i.e., 5 to 10%.[20] **b:** Biopsy showing high-grade dysplasia. This is evidenced by the presence of back-to-back glands showing hyperchromatic, stratified nuclei which abut into the lumen. If high-grade dysplasia especially with changes approaching cancer *in situ* (precancer),[28] is found in random biopsies of flat mucosa, there is a 30 to 40% likelihood of discovering carcinoma,[28] often of an intramucosal or early type (Dukes' A).[14]

other, or at two locations within the colon on the same examination, the risk of an early (intramucosal) cancer approximates 30 to 40%,[14] which we believe justifies colectomy.

2. *Macroscopic dysplasia:* The presence of DALM, especially with the appearance of a polypoid mass (Fig. 43-20a) in a symptomatic patient, indicates a high likelihood of cancer being already present; this incidence in our study was 60 to 70%.[15] This is almost twice the risk of cancer observed for dysplasia found in biopsies taken from flat mucosa even if it is high grade (Fig. 43-20b)—estimated to be 30 to 40%.[28] The association of DALM and cancer causes us to regard its presence as the strongest surveillance indication for colectomy irrespective of the grade of dysplasia.

Colonic Lymphoma

Colonic lymphoma complicating ulcerative colitis is uncommon, with only 20 reported cases to 1981[30] including one patient with multicentric lymphoma from our institution.[31] Almost all of the cases are of the non-Hodgkin's type. Patients are referred to colonoscopy because of colitic-type symptoms, which, as in the case of colitic carcinoma, have worsened over the preceding year. The colonoscopic appearance may be indistinguishable from that of active ulcerative colitis (Fig. 43-21) with only the biopsies revealing lymphoma. In other cases one expects single or multiple polypoid masses, similar to the appearance of colonic lymphoma in noncolitic patients (see Chapter 42).

CROHN'S DISEASE OF THE COLON

Colonic involvement in Crohn's disease is principally of two kinds. The commonest ileocecal involvement occurs in up to half the cases (41%[32] to 55%[33]). Less commonly (5%[33] to 25%[32]) there is colonic Crohn's disease without small bowel involvement. Some colonic involvement therefore is expected in two-thirds of the patients with Crohn's disease.[32,33]

Patients with Crohn's disease undergo colonoscopy for different reasons than those with ulcerative colitis. Because the rectum may be spared or show only nonspecific changes, a much greater percentage of patients with Crohn's disease are referred for primary diagnosis. As is true for ulcerative colitis, the majority of examinations performed on patients with Crohn's disease are to determine the extent and the activity. In about one-third of the cases, the referring physician wishes to know whether the patient does in fact

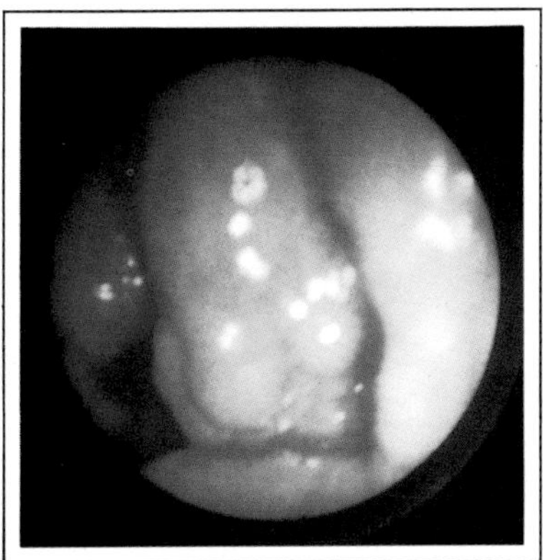

FIG. 43-20a.

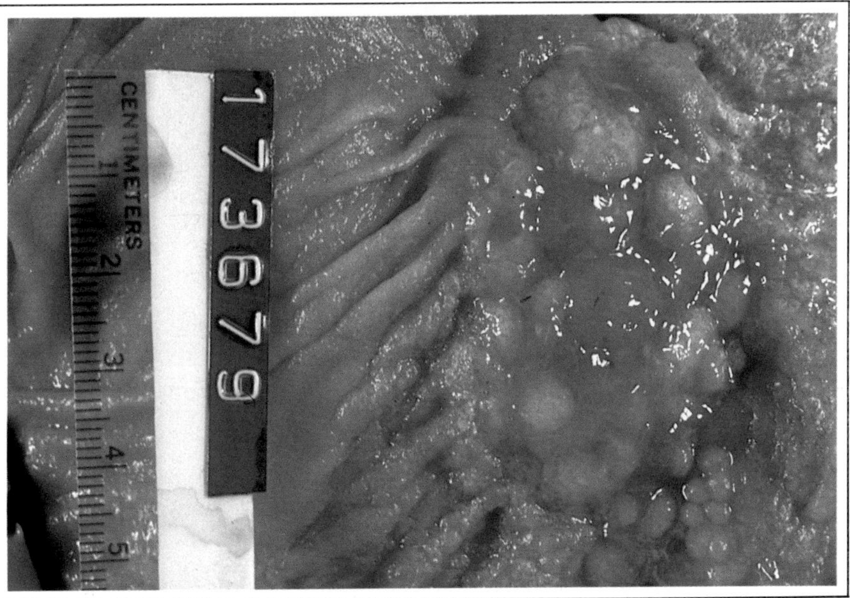

FIG. 43-20b.

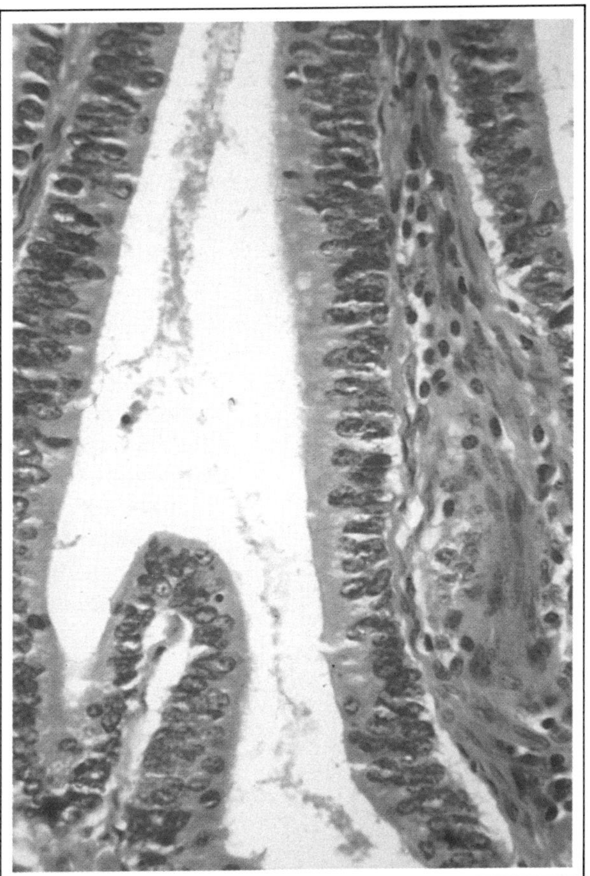

FIG. 43-20c.

FIG. 43-20. Ulcerative colitis. **a:** Dysplasia-associated polypoid mass. Biopsy showed only dysplasia, although it was high grade (c). At surgery this proved to be part of a colloid carcinoma (b). **b:** Polypoid carcinoma, 3 × 4 cm. A dysplasia-associated polypoid mass (a) noted at colonoscopy was in actuality this carcinoma. **c:** Biopsy of a dysplasia-associated polypoid mass (a) showing high-grade dysplasia. Irrespective of the degree of dysplasia, with a mass or other dysplasia-associated lesion, there is a high probability (60%) of cancer being found at colectomy.[15]

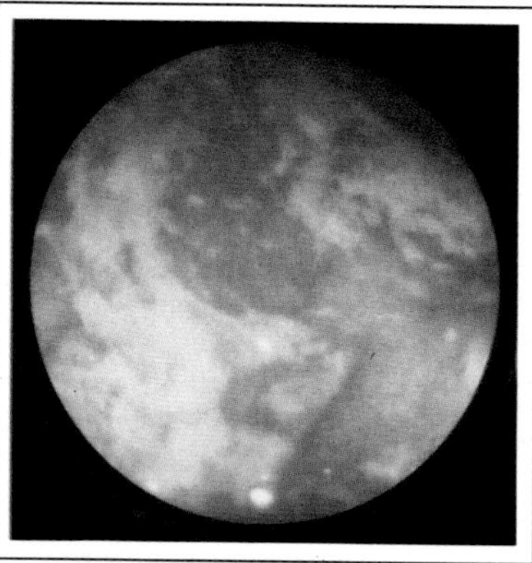

FIG. 43-21. Ulcerative colitis, complicated by lymphoma. Biopsies showing histiocytic lymphoma were entirely unexpected in a patient with longstanding ulcerative colitis and increased clinical activity over the preceding year.

FIG. 43-21.

have Crohn's disease or ulcerative colitis. Finally, a very small number of patients are referred for an assessment of the malignant potential of Crohn's disease, which is increased over the general population by three- to tenfold.[13] In this section we consider the colonoscopic aspects of Crohn's colitis from the standpoint of the principal indications for the procedure, as: (a) determining the presence, extent and severity of involvement; (b) differentiation from ulcerative colitis; and (c) the appearance of carcinoma in Crohn's disease.

Determining the Presence, Extent, and Severity of Crohn's Colitis

The assessment of colonic involvement in Crohn's disease requires an appreciation of: (a) the characteristic mucosal findings which denote Crohn's disease, including the grade of activity; (b) the structural alterations which accompany mucosal changes; and (c) the patterns of involvement.

Characteristic Mucosal Findings

Aphthous ulcerations.

Aphthous ulcerations are generally regarded as the first specific endoscopic finding in Crohn's disease (Fig. 43-22a)[34]; this results from partial or total destruction of the crypt and surrounding surface epithelium in areas where previously focal inflammation had existed. Recently, a preaphthous ulcer phase (Fig. 43-22b) has been described, with the appearance of focal erosions called erythematous mucosal plaques[35] similar to the focal erosions seen in ulcerative colitis (Fig. 43-11d). In these cases the plaque consists of intramucosal hemorrhage associated with focal crypt abscesses and destruction of the crypt epithelium.

Unlike ulcerative colitis, the ulcerations are set in a background of normal-appearing mucosa (Fig. 43-22a), reflecting the focal nature of Crohn's disease.[34,36]

By the term aphthous, one means small, 1- to 3-mm ulcers (no larger than 5 mm) which are flat or just slightly depressed and have a characteristic small rim of erythema, in the absence of a raised margin.[34] They may be segmentally located or appear diffusely throughout the colon. Biopsies taken from their centers may reveal, along with the acute inflammatory cells, characteristic microgranulomas.[16,36]

Larger ulcerations.

The commonest ulcers found in Crohn's disease are larger (>5 mm) and deeper (Fig. 43-22c) than the aphthous type (Fig. 43-22a). We find these larger ulcers in as many as 75% of our cases. They may be up to 3 cm in greatest dimension or even larger (Fig. 43-22d). They appear in a variety of shapes and sizes, ranging from small, flat ulcers to deep, irregular tortuous ones to which the term serpiginous is sometimes applied. Some investigators maintain that the greater than 1 cm, deep, serpiginous type (Fig. 43-22c) is more characteristic of Crohn's disease[34]; however, this has not been our experience, as similar ulcers are present with equal frequency in ulcerative colitis (Fig. 43-13a). Although there is a distinct margin to these ulcers because of their depth (Fig. 43-22b), there is surprisingly little reactive change around them, again emphasizing their focal nature, being set in what appears to be normal mucosa.

Cobblestone appearance.

Rather than intact flat mucosa between ulcerations, the cobblestone appearance shows hyperplastic, edematous though otherwise normal-appearing mucosa between interconnecting ulcerations (Fig. 43-23a). These intervening areas may appear as large inflammatory polyps (Fig. 43-23b), creating the cobblestone feature.[34] Although the mucosa of the cobblestone areas between ulcerations may be somewhat pinker than the surrounding epithelium, it is typically not friable, suggesting the absence of acute inflammation with accompanying capillary dilatation that causes contact bleeding, or friability.

Because involvement with Crohn's disease tends to be focal, the cobblestone appearance is also contained in segments of less than 5 cm. It is particularly common at the mouth of inflammatory strictures (see below).

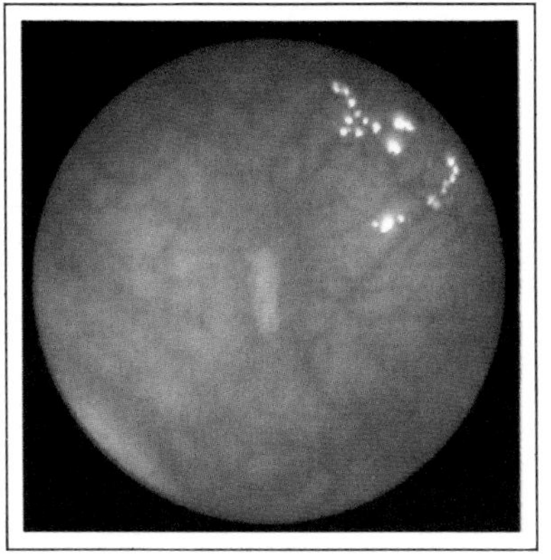

FIG. 43-22a.

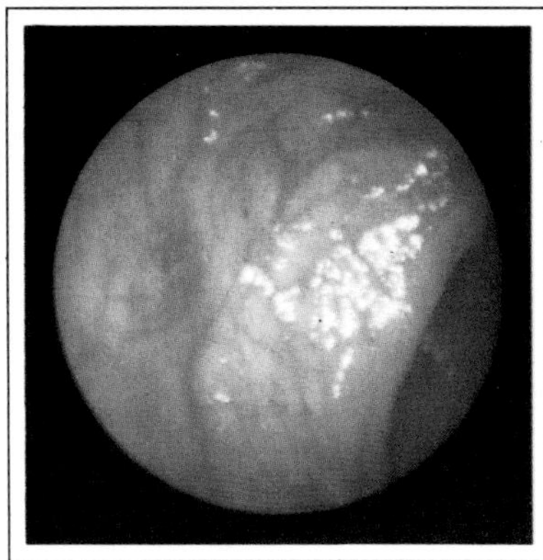

FIG. 43-22b.

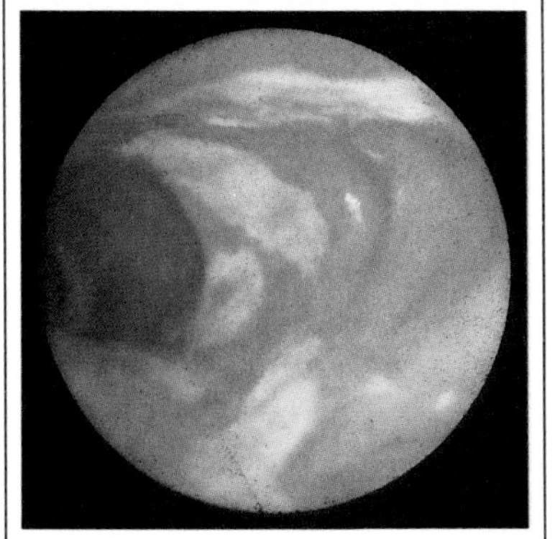

FIG. 43-22c.

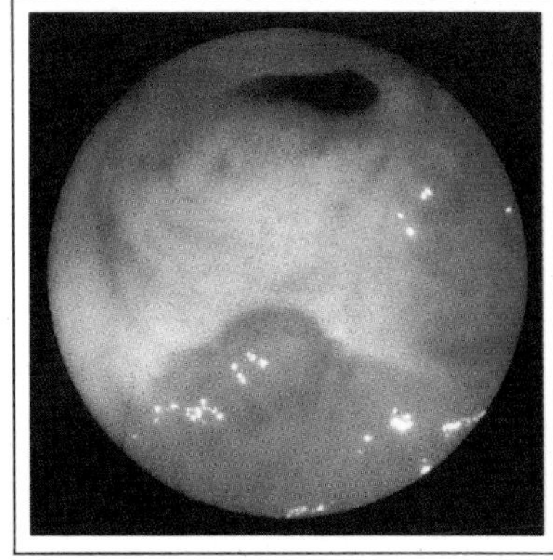

FIG. 43-22d.

FIG. 43-22. Crohn's colitis. **a:** Aphthous ulcer. A 2-mm ulcer is observed on the background of normal mucosa (with a preserved mucosal vascular pattern). **b:** Erythematous mucosal plaque. This small raised zone of focal erythema may be a precursor lesion to the aphthous ulcer,[35] where histologically one observes hemorrhage and focal crypt abscesses. As such, this represents the earliest visual sign of mucosal activity in Crohn's disease. **c:** Multiple ulcerations. These vary in size (5 to 10 mm) and shape. Characteristically, they are set in a background of essentially normal mucosa. **d:** With extensive (10 cm) ulceration of one surface (the 6 o'clock wall) of the descending colon-sigmoid junction. Sparing of the opposite wall is typical of the asymmetrical distribution of Crohn's involvement within a segment. In addition, a hyperplastic polyp is seen at the margin of the ulcer, possibly as an early cobblestone effect.

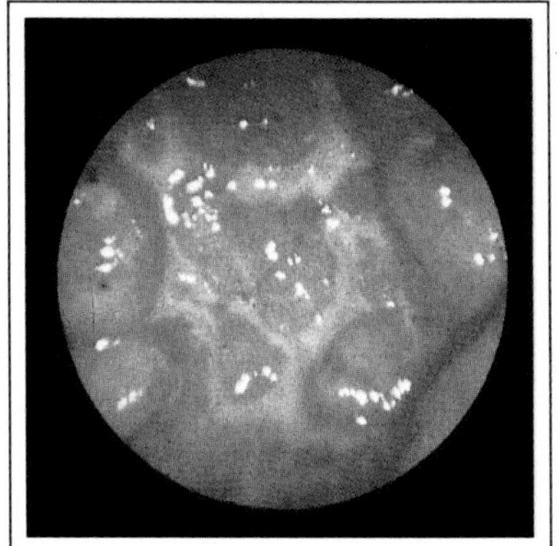

FIG. 43-23a.

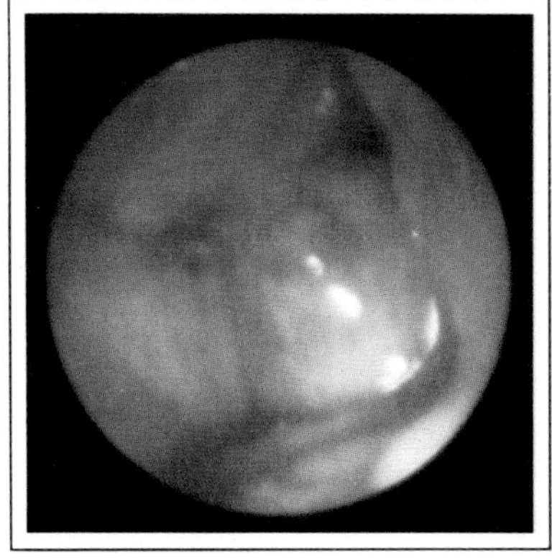

FIG. 43-23b.

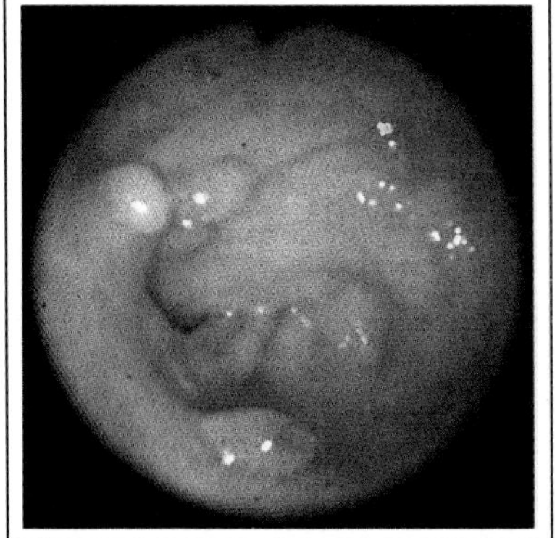

FIG. 43-23c.

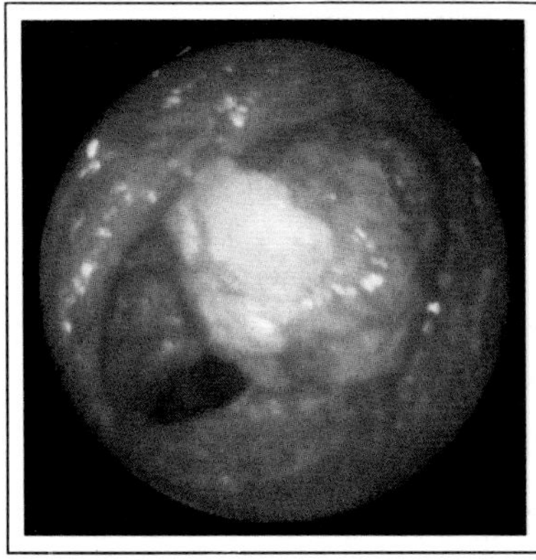

FIG. 43-23d.

FIG. 43-23. Crohn's colitis. **a:** Cobblestone appearance. Zones of hyperplastic mucosa (the cobblestones) surround ulcerations, giving rise to this appearance. Biopsies from the cobblestones show them to be hyperplastic and/or edematous but not acutely inflamed as would be the case in ulcerative colitis (Fig. 43-5b). **b:** Large (1.5 cm) inflammatory polyp with adjacent ulcer (at 6 o'clock). Asymmetrical involvement in this segment is evidenced by the largely uninvolved opposite wall (except for a single aphthous ulcer). **c:** Multiple inflammatory polyps. These are indistinguishable from those of ulcerative colitis (Fig. 43-5b). **d:** With a large (2 cm) inflammatory polyp with adherent barium from a recent contrast study.

Inflammatory polyps.

In our experience and that of others,[5,34] inflammatory polyps are commonly found in Crohn's disease. They tend to be focal, confined to a segment, although within the segment they are multiple (Fig. 43-23c). Generally the polyps themselves are less than 1.5 cm in greatest dimension, but occasionally they enlarge to exceed 4 cm (Fig. 43-23d), giving rise to giant inflammatory polyps which may simulate carcinoma radiologically.[37]

Grading of activity.

As in the case of ulcerative colitis, there is no universally accepted system for grading activity in Crohn's disease. The system we use based on the presence, size, and number of ulcerations (Table 43-5) has evolved as one which seems to correlate with clinical activity. As in the case of ulcerative colitis, a dissociation is to be expected between clinical severity and activity as judged by colonoscopy.

In our system, as in the case of ulcerative colitis, distortion of the vasculae pattern or granularity indicate quiescent colitis. Erythema, focal or confluent, but without the appearance of ulcerations, would receive a designation of mildly active or possibly active. For the finding of aphthous or other ulcers that have a maximum dimension of less than 5 mm and fewer than five ulcers per 10-cm segment, we use the term "moderate" activity. In cases where there are larger ulcers with a maximum dimension of greater than 5 mm and/or more than five ulcers per 10 cm, we use the term "severe colitis."

Structural Alterations in Crohn's Disease

As in ulcerative colitis, structural alterations accompany mucosal abnormalities. However, in Crohn's disease these tend to be more varied. In keeping with the transmural nature of Crohn's disease, deep ulcerations and fissures are commonly found in pathologic specimens,[16] unlike the more superficial mucosal ulcerations of ulcerative colitis which are associated with muscle hypertrophy,[16] the structural alteration associated with the deeper ulcerations of Crohn's disease tend to be associated with fibrosis.[16] It is the fibrosis that causes them to be permanent, remaining long after the activity has disappeared.[19] Another permanent change occurs when deep ulceration causes undermining of the surrounding mucosa. When the activity subsides and the ulcers re-epithelialize, mucosal bridging results. Furthermore, we find prior surgery involving the colon to have been performed in up to one-third to one-half of the cases coming to colonoscopy.[32,33] The surgery itself creates new structures, i.e., anastomoses with a wide variety of possible appearances. Finally, colonic fistulas may be expected in nearly 10% of patients with colonic involvement,[33] and these may be apparent at colonoscopy.

TABLE 43-5. *Grading activity in Crohn's colitis*

Activity	Appearance
Quiescent	Distorted or absent mucosal vascular pattern; granularity
Mildly active	Focal (or diffuse) erythema
Moderately active	Aphthous or small (<5 mm) ulcerations; fewer than five per 10-cm segment
Severe colitis	Multiple larger (>5 mm) ulcerations; more than five per 10-cm segment

In this section we discuss the structural alterations associated with: (a) acute inflammation; (b) stricture formation; (c) mucosal bridging; (d) postsurgical anastomotic changes; and (e) fistula formation.

Changes associated with acute inflammation.

1. *Edematous folds:* Ulceration in Crohn's disease, apart from the aphthous type, is characteristically deep in the submucosa; it is often associated with lymphangiectasia, which leads to submucosa edema and fibrosis.[16] Not surprisingly, the valvulae in segments in which there are ulcerations appear thickened and blunted as a result of the submucosal edema and fibrosis (Fig. 43-24a). Often, because of the submucosal changes the haustral pattern may be lost. In one colonoscopic study the interhaustral fold pattern was abnormal in Crohn's disease in three-fourths of the cases examined.[36]

2. *Luminal narrowing:* As a consequence of thickening of the interhaustral folds and the intervening wall (Fig. 43-24b), there is a decrease in luminal diameter, giving it a narrowed appearance. Although not rare, this is found less often than simple edematous folds. In our experience, luminal narrowing occurs in less than half of the patients with Crohn's disease of the colon.

3. *Stricture formation:* Crohn's disease is a well-known setting for strictures found at colonscopy, accounting for 15% of the cases in one recent series.[38] In these cases there are focal areas of intense activity with ulceration and deep fissuring into the submucosa (Fig. 43-24c). The strictures that result are typically longer than those seen in ulcerative colitis—often greater than 3 cm and sometimes up to 10 cm, although in a common location for stricture formation, the rectosigmoid junction, they tend to be shorter (<3 cm).

Strictures vary as to the degree to which the lumen is compromised and may be graded accordingly. For a low-grade stricture, the diameter is 10 to 15 mm (Fig. 43-24d); a moderate stricture has a diameter of 5 to 10 mm, and a high-grade stricture has a diameter of less than 5 mm (Fig. 43-24c). For nearly all low-grade and many moderate strictures, a 9-mm pediatric-type endoscope can be used to examine within and beyond the strictures in cases where the

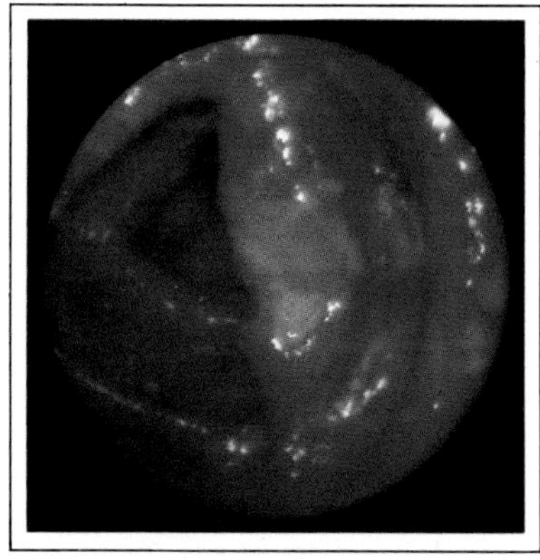
FIG. 43-24a.

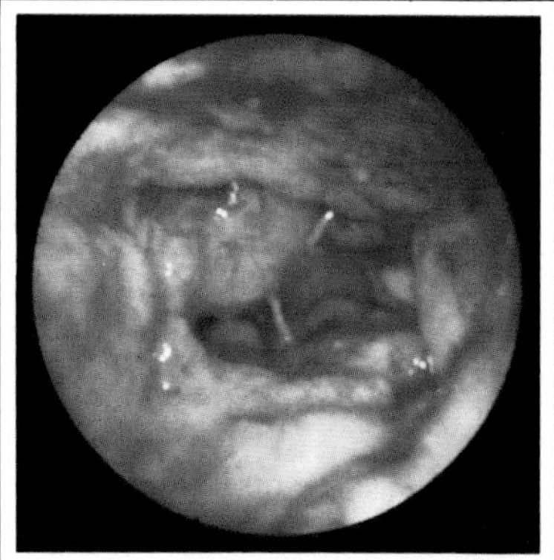
FIG. 43-24b.

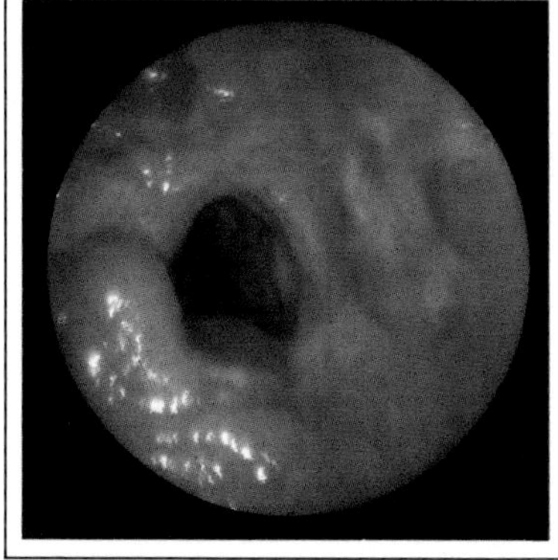
FIG. 43-24c.

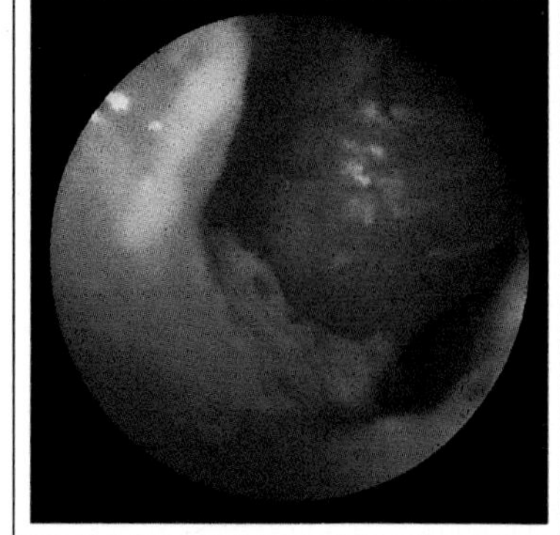
FIG. 43-24d.

FIG. 43-24. Crohn's colitis. **a:** Asymmetrical involvement of the transverse colon. Here there is involvement of one wall (edema and ulceration of an interhaustral fold) with sparing of the adjacent folds. **b:** Confluent (circumferential) involvement. The acute inflammatory changes (edema and ulceration) are superimposed on longstanding intramural fibrosis leading to narrowing of the lumen. **c:** High-grade stricture, with extensive ulceration at its mouth. A biopsy taken from the enlarged but nonfriable fold between 6 and 9 o'clock showed hyperplastic, rather than acutely inflamed mucosa—in contrast to a similar-appearing stricture in ulcerative colitis (Fig. 43-9c) where the mucosa is acutely inflamed. **d:** Low grade stricture. Some ulceration is seen at its mouth on the 3 o'clock aspect which contributes to the modest narrowing of the lumen (to approximately 13 mm), which just admits the colonoscope.

standard (13 mm) colonoscope cannot be used. Often activity, as evidenced by single or multiple interconnected ulcerations, is found within the stricture, especially around its mouth (Fig. 43-24c), commonly with a cobblestone appearance (see above).

Mucosal bridging.

As in ulcerative colitis, an extensive undermining ulceration may result in the formation of mucosal bridges once the activity has subsided and re-epithelialization has occurred (Fig. 43-25a). In contrast to some authors,[34] we have seen this only on rare occasions. In one case (Fig. 43-25b) the mucosal bridge caused luminal obstruction and required electrosurgical excision (Fig. 43-25c).

Postsurgical appearances.

We find that approximately one-third of the patients undergoing colonoscopy for Crohn's disease have had previous surgery. As right-sided colonic involvement is twice as common as that of the entire colon,[33] most often the previous surgery involved a right hemicolectomy with a variable length of terminal ileum resected and ileotransverse colon anastomosis. About one-fourth had a subtotal colectomy with an ileum-descending sigmoid or rectal anastomosis.

Recurrent Crohn's disease is common in and around the anastomosis (Fig. 43-26a). Evidence of recurrent disease includes discrete ulcerations, often of the aphthous type, within the anastomosis. Frequently the ulcerations are deep, with the intervening mucosa being edematous and hyperplastic, accentuating the basic nodular character (Fig. 43-25b) of the anastomosis caused by its construction with interrupted sutures (Fig. 43-25c), so that it takes on a cobblestone appearance (Fig. 43-25b). In these cases the deep ulcerations themselves seem to follow the lines of previous sutures. With extensive ulceration the intervening mucosa may disappear altogether, and the anastomosis appears as one continuous area of ulceration. This type of ulceration leads to an intense submucosal tissue reaction, with edema, fibrosis, and ultimately conversion of the anastomosis into a high-grade stricture (Fig. 43-25c).

Fistula formation.

A variety of fistulas may form in as many as 8% of patients with Crohn's colitis.[33] They may be colocutaneous, enteric, or vesicular. Although the fistula itself is usually not examined at any length because of the possibility of perforation, the examiner may observe the orifice as a deep, rounded, ulcer-like cavity often just proximal to a stricture. After identification of the orifice, one could inject it with

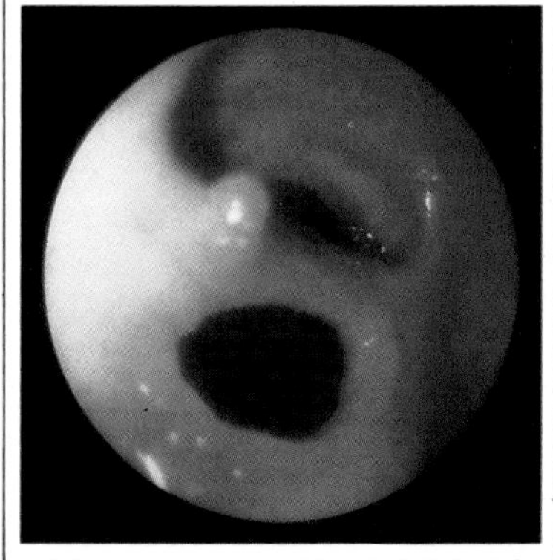

FIG. 43-25a.

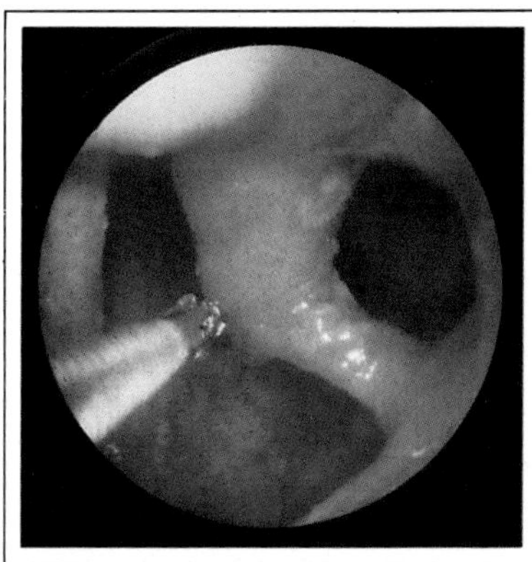

FIG. 43-25b.

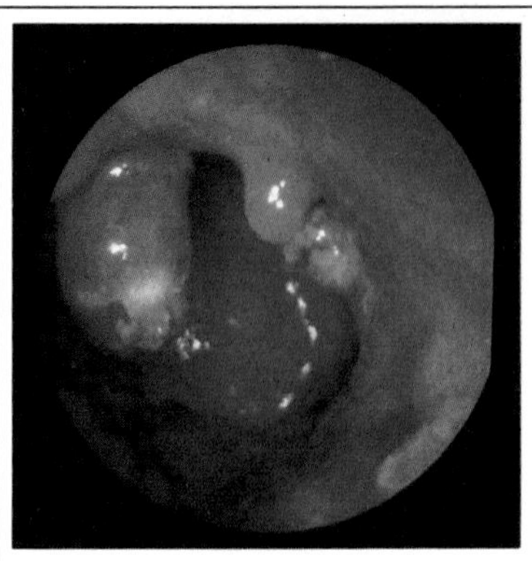

FIG. 43-25c.

FIG. 43-25. Crohn's colitis. **a:** Mucosal bridging. This bisects the transverse colon in a patient with only diarrhea. **b:** Mucosal bridge. In this case intermittent obstructive symptoms were relieved after electrosurgical transection of the mucosal bridge. This was accomplished by repeated applications of a Williams' forceps to the bridge until it is transected (c). **c:** Mucosal bridge, after electrosurgical transection (b) in a symptomatic patient.

contrast material, i.e., Gastrografin, to determine its anatomy, but it would not be advisable to attempt to enter the fistula (Fig. 43-26d).

Patterns of involvement.

The examiner encounters four patterns of involvement in Crohn's disease. They are not mutually exclusive, with several or all being encountered in any given patient. These are: (a) rectal-sparing; (b) right-sided involvement; (c) segmental involvement with skip areas; and (d) asymmetrical involvement within a segment.

1. *Rectal-sparing:* This well-known pattern of involvement in colonic Crohn's disease is found in fewer than half the cases.[33] The rectum and adjacent sigmoid are either normal, or there is involvement beginning at the rectosigmoid junction, often with stricture formation and deep ulceration, but with sparing of the rectum itself. Another pattern in which there is relative rectum sparing is one where there is involvement of the anus and 3 to 5 cm of distal rectum with ulceration and stricture formation (Fig. 43-27a), with abrupt transition above this point to uninvolved rectum. In some cases where the rectum is involved throughout, this may be minimal, i.e., only by virtue of a loss of normal vascular pattern and enlargement of the folds, with the degree of activity entirely unreflective of the severity of the disease proximally (Fig. 43-27b). We find in only 5 to 10% of the cases of Crohn's disease that involve the colon is the activity within the rectum severe, with extensive and interconnecting ulcerations, and the intervening mucosa is noted to be hyperemic and friable. In these cases, the appearance is indistinguishable from that of severe ulcerative colitis (Fig. 43-5b).

2. *Right-sided involvement:* The commonest site of involvement for Crohn's disease is the ileocecal area, with 40%[32] to 55%[33] of the cases displaying this pattern of involvement (Fig. 43-27c). In an additional 20 to 30%[32,33] the colon is involved exclusively, but in the majority of these cases the disease still tends to be right-sided. As a result of these two patterns of involvement, nearly 70% of the patients coming to colonoscopy have largely, if not exclusively, right-sided involvement, including the ileocecal valve and distal terminal ileum. About one-third of these have left-sided involvement in addition, especially at the rectosigmoid junction and within the distal rectum and anorectal area.

3. *Segmental involvement (skip areas):* In the large majority of cases of Crohn's disease of the colon, segmental involvement is the rule, with skip areas in which normal mucosa is preserved between other areas of disease[5,34] (Fig. 43-29b). Because the left colon seems to be less involved than the right, these skip areas tend to be noted in left-sided segments because of the characteristic focal areas of involvement, e.g., the distal rectum, rectosigmoid junction, descending colon-sigmoid junction, and splenic flexure. On

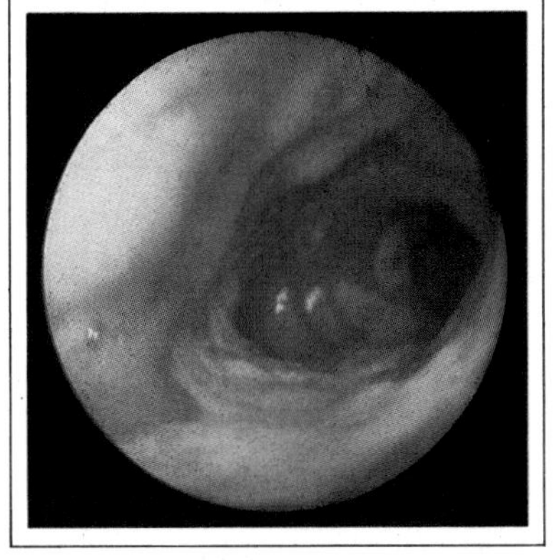

FIG. 43-26a.

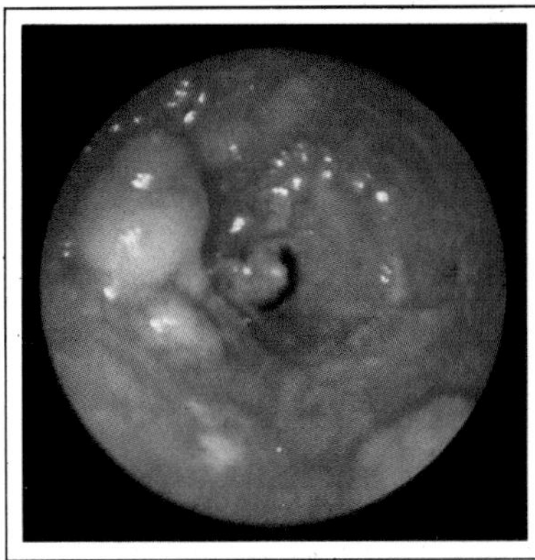

FIG. 43-26b.

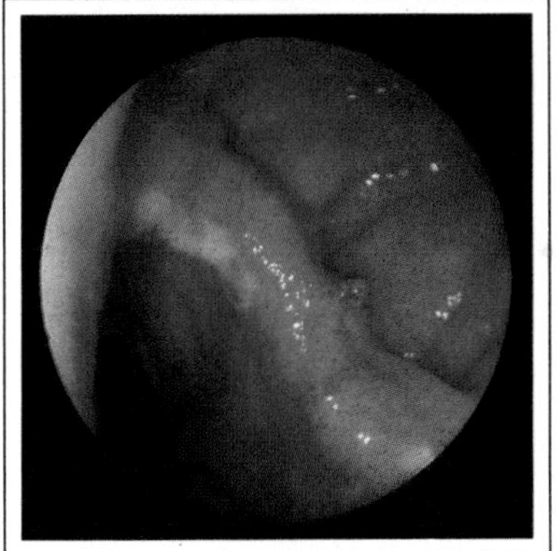

FIG. 43-26c.

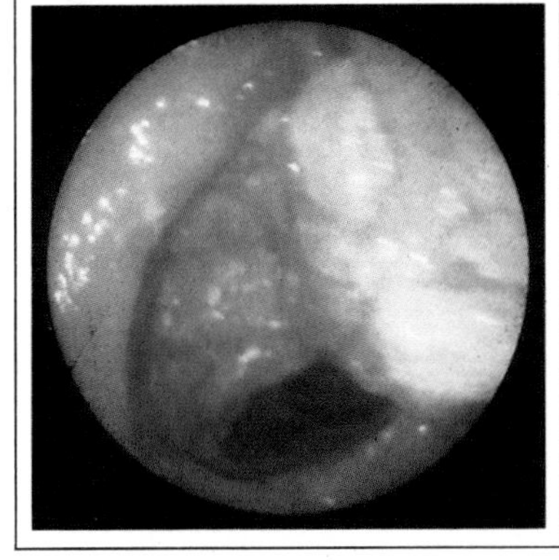

FIG. 43-26d.

FIG. 43-26. Crohn's colitis. **a:** Recurrent disease at the ileocolic anastomosis. A common site of recurrence after previous surgery is at the anastomosis, with activity indicated here by the presence of ulcerations within both the terminal ileum and the proximal transverse colon at and just beyond the anastomosis. **b:** Recurrent disease at the ileocolic anastomosis. Inflammatory polyps at the anastomosis markedly accentuate its usual slightly nodular character (c). Some stricturing is also apparent in this case, although the patient's only complaint was that of a modest increase in bowel frequency (four to six motions a day). **c:** Recurrent disease at the anastomosis. The ring-like deformity at the anastomosis is expected, as is its slightly nodular character due to the presence of interrupted sutures. Some scattered ulcerations mark the recurrence in this case where the patient was entirely asymptomatic. **d:** With an ileosigmoid fistula. The mouth of the fistula, marked by granulation tissue, is apparent at 3 o'clock.

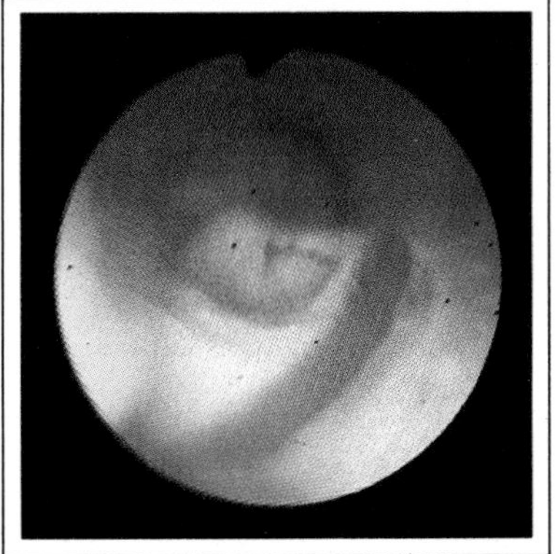

FIG. 43-27a.

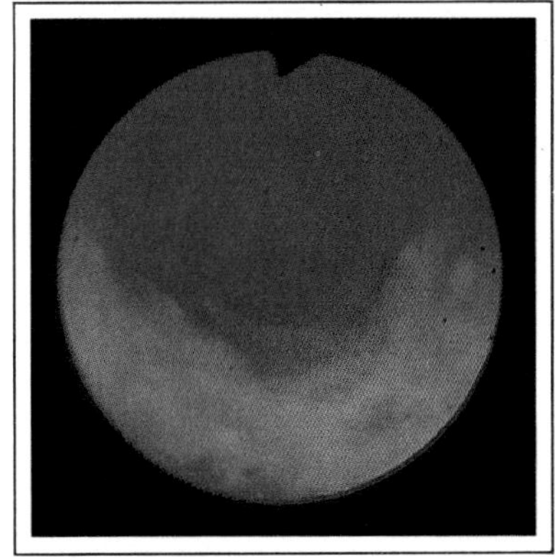

FIG. 43-27b.

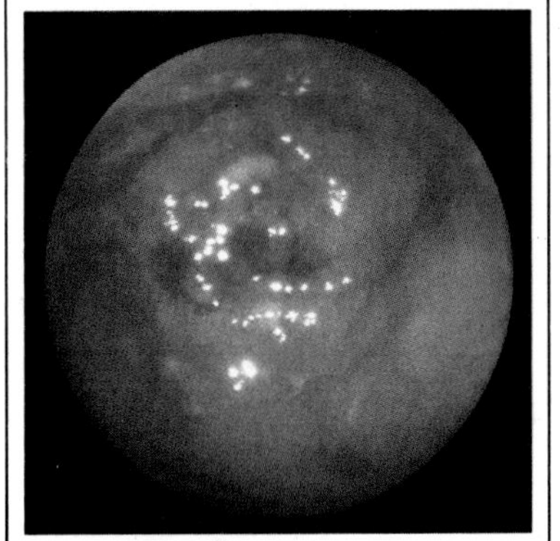

FIG. 43-27c.

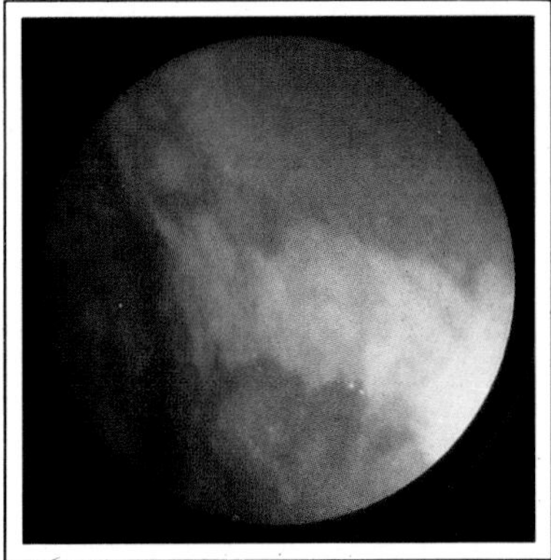

FIG. 43-27d.

FIG. 43-27. Crohn's colitis. **a:** With perianal involvement. Note the perianal ulceration, with the rectum above the distal 5 cm being largely spared. **b:** With relative rectum sparing. Only some nonspecific focal erythema is present above a distal rectal area of intense activity (ulceration and fistual formation). **c:** Ileocecal valve stricture and ulceration. This stands in contrast to patulous (even if ulcerated) appearance of the ileocecal valve in ulcerative colitis (Fig. 43-28d). **d:** Long serpiginous ulcerations set in otherwise normal mucosa.

the left side, skip areas may be 15- to 20-cm segments, whereas on the right they tend to be shorter.

4. *Asymmetrical segmental involvement:* The focal nature of colonic involvement with Crohn's disease is even more striking in the pattern of asymmetrical involvement within a segment (Fig. 43-27d). This pattern is seen as ulcerations exclusively on one colonic surface, with the opposite wall completely free of disease.[5]

Differentiation of Ulcerative Colitis from Crohn's Disease

Fifteen percent of our patients with Crohn's disease are referred for colonoscopy specifically to determine the type of inflammatory bowel disease present—whether Crohn's disease or ulcerative colitis. In such patients the type of inflammatory bowel disease remains unclear from clinical, proctoscopic, and radiologic findings. The differentiation of ulcerative colitis from Crohn's disease, if possible, is especially important to the referring physician if a colectomy is contemplated; for example, with relative rectal sparing and a diagnosis of Crohn's disease, an ileorectal anastomosis might be performed, in contrast to the case of ulcerative colitis where because of the malignant potential of a retained rectum,[20a] proctectomy would be considered mandatory. Even when the patient is not specifically referred for this type of determination, it is still desirable for the examiner to make the differentiation.

In this section, we consider the differentiation of ulcerative colitis from Crohn's disease based on endoscopic appearance and finally the role of biopsy in this determination.

Differentiation Based on Endoscopic Appearance

No prospective study has been reported which validates any of the endoscopic findings which many authorities consider useful. These have been called "valuable signs, differentiating IUC (idiopathic ulcerative colitis) and Crohn's disease"[39] even though they have never been tested. Nevertheless, this does not detract from the apparent usefulness of some of these findings to guide the examiner to a correct determination of type in what is, in our impression, a high (although as yet uncertain) percentage of cases. The examiner, however, should be aware of the fact that visual diagnosis is only a gross estimate of the probability of one or the other condition, and he should expect an error rate of at least 15 to 20% even when the final histologic diagnosis from proctocolectomy is known.

Features favoring a diagnosis of ulcerative colitis.

1. *Ulcerations set in a background of a diffuse mucosal abnormality:* This finding most often, in our experience, allows one to correctly differentiate ulcerative colitis from Crohn's disease (Table 43-6). Rather than any characteristic of the ulcer itself, i.e., size, shape, or depth, it is the background mucosal abnormality which is most important (Fig. 43-28a)—marked erythema and friability indicating acute mucosal inflammation as the setting of the ulceration (Fig. 43-28b).

TABLE 43-6. *Colonoscopic differentiation of ulcerative colitis from Crohn's disease*

Feature	Favoring ulcerative colitis	Favoring Crohn's disease
Background of ulceration	Ulcer set in erythematous, friable mucosa	Ulcer set in normal mucosa
Pattern of mucosal involvement	Continuous	Asymmetrical segmental
Rectal involvement	Present and continuous	Absent or segmental
Ileocecal valve	Patulous, free of ulceration	Stenotic and ulcerated

2. *Continuous mucosal involvement:* Although the degree of activity may not be uniform, the mucosa is abnormal for the extent of the involvement (Fig. 43-28b)—whether universal or only rectal. Within the segments involved, there are changes at least suggestive of quiescent colitis if not signs of inflammation, e.g., focal and diffuse erythema, friability, mucopurulent exudate, or ulceration.

3. *Rectal involvement:* Some evidence of mucosal involvement of the rectum is present in 95% of the cases, although this may not be striking (Fig. 43-28c), even in the face of marked clinical activity.[40] Still, even in such cases the rectum is not entirely normal; one expects to see at least a distorted or absent vascular pattern, granularity, and some (although not necessarily striking) erythema. A completely normal rectal appearance endoscopically favors the diagnosis of Crohn's disease.[5,34,39]

4. *Patulous ileocecal valve:* In almost half of the patients who have colonoscopy, we find universal involvement (Table 43-2). In one-half to two-thirds of these we observe effacement of the ileocecal valve, so that its opening is widely patent (Fig. 43-28d). This finding depends on a structural loss of the ileocecal valve, presumably from circular muscle hypertrophy occurring in the cecum as a response to acute inflammation. Often there is evidence of acute inflammation—either focal or diffuse erythema, and ulcerations—in and around the ileocecal valve (Fig. 43-28d). Because this finding depends on the activity status of the right colon, especially around the ileocecal valve, the presence of a normal ileocecal valve in the absence of acute inflammation does not necessarily favor the diagnosis of Crohn's disease. On the other hand, the presence of extensive ulceration around a closed, especially a stenotic, ileocecal valve (see below) militates against a diagnosis of ulcerative colitis.

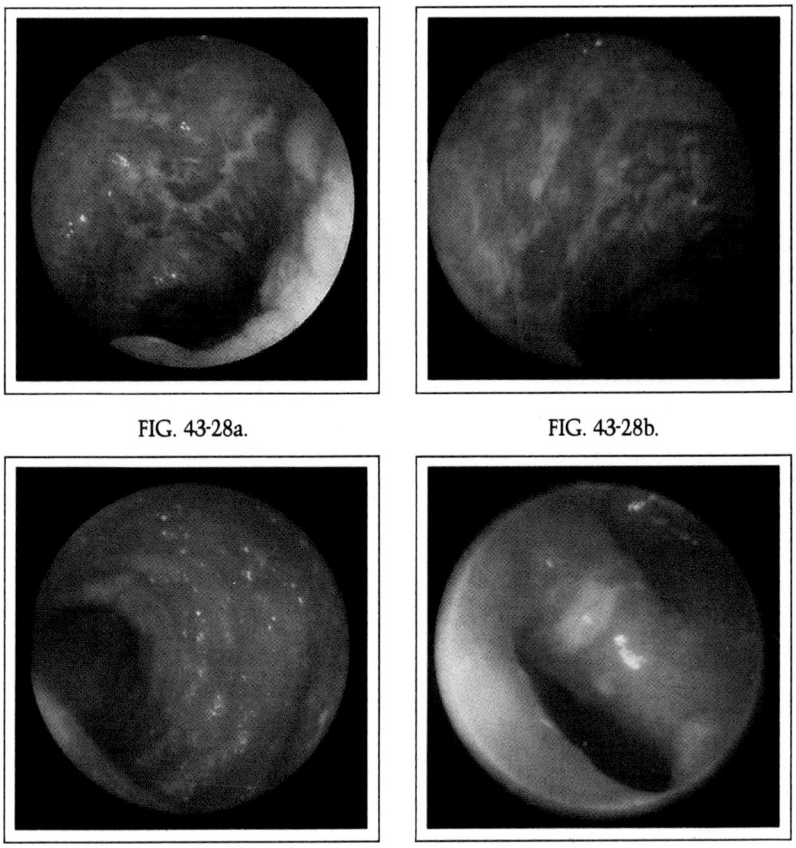

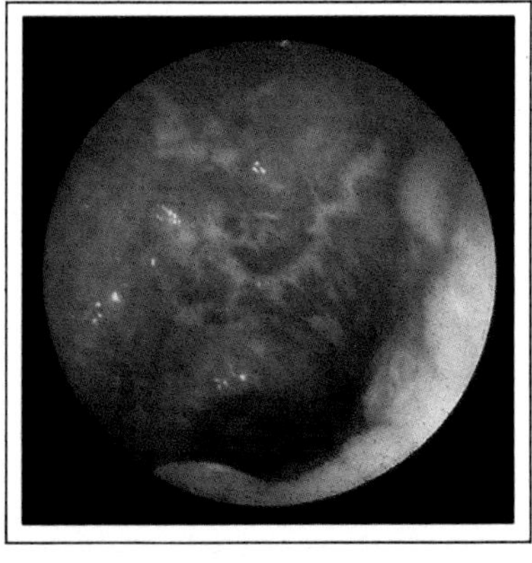

FIG. 43-28a.

FIG. 43-28b.

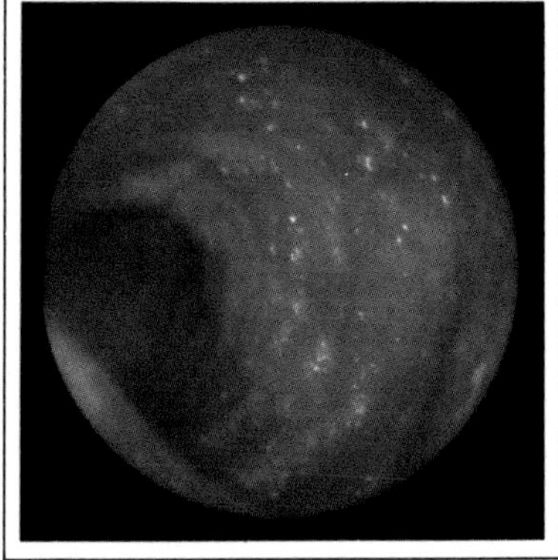

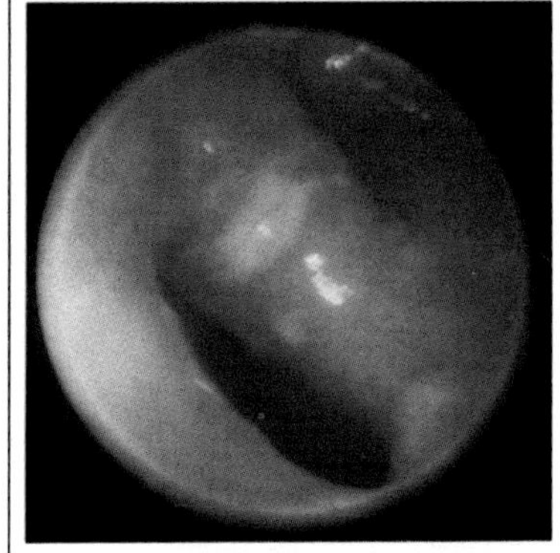

FIG. 43-28c.

FIG. 43-28d.

FIG. 43-28. Ulcerative colitis. **a:** Ulcerations. These are found with a background of mucosa showing inflammation: mucopurulent exudate (mucopus), erythema, and friability **b:** Extensive confluent ulcerations. Again these are set on a background of mucosa that shows acute inflammation (intense erythema and mucopus). **c:** Mucopus on a background of erythematous mucosa with no apparent vascular pattern. The background mucosal abnormality favors a diagnosis of ulcerative colitis. **d:** Patulous ileocecal valve. The open ileocecal valve is characteristic of ulcerative colitis, in contrast to Crohn's disease where it may be stenotic (Fig. 43-27c).

Features favoring a diagnosis of Crohn's colitis.

1. *Ulcerations set in normal mucosa:* The ulcers of Crohn's disease do not markedly differ from those found in ulcerative colitis, although deep, extensive ulcerations seem to be more characteristic of Crohn's disease (Fig. 43-29a). We find that the commonest ulcerations in both conditions are small, linear or serpiginous connecting ulcers, so that something is required in addition to the ulcer itself for differentiation. Again, as in ulcerative colitis, the background mucosa in which the ulcer is set is the key. In Crohn's disease, unlike ulcerative colitis, the background is normal with a preserved vascular pattern, or if this is not apparent there is no sign of acute inflammation (erythema, friability, and/or mucopurulent exduate). This is especially true when the adjacent mucosa shows the cobblestone appearance (Fig. 43-23a), where the mucosa, although heaped-up, nodular, and slightly pink, is not friable.

2. *Discontinuous (segmental) mucosal involvement:* The segmental distibution of Crohn's activity provides a useful sign, if present, to assist the colonoscopist at differentiation (Fig. 43-29b). Finding areas of apparently normal mucosa (Fig. 43-29c) between others where ulcerations are present causes one to suspect Crohn's disease, as does an asymmetrical distribution of ulcerations within a segment, i.e., ulcerations on one surface with the opposite side being uninvolved.

3. *Absence of rectal involvement:* In at least 30%[33] of the cases of Crohn's disease that involve the colon, the rectum is free of disease visually. When the rectum is involved in Crohn's disease grossly, it is generally part of rectosigmoid or perianal involvement, so that a large portion of the rectum may still show normal mucosa. The presence of diffuse erythema or the absence of a vascular pattern in the rectum may be found in either Crohn's disease or ulcerative colitis. As such, they have no value in the differentiation.

4. *Stenosis of the ileocecal valve:* With involvement of the right colon (as occurs in 75%) and of the terminal ileum (which occurs in two-thirds of cases), one expects either ulcerations alone or in combination with stenosis or distortion of the ileocecal valve (Fig. 43-29d). The presence of ulcerations and stenosis of the ileocecal valve, along with a predominant right-sided involvement, strongly suggests Crohn's disease.[36]

Role of Biopsy

Although the endoscopic features that suggest either Crohn's disease or ulcerative colitis are useful, we find

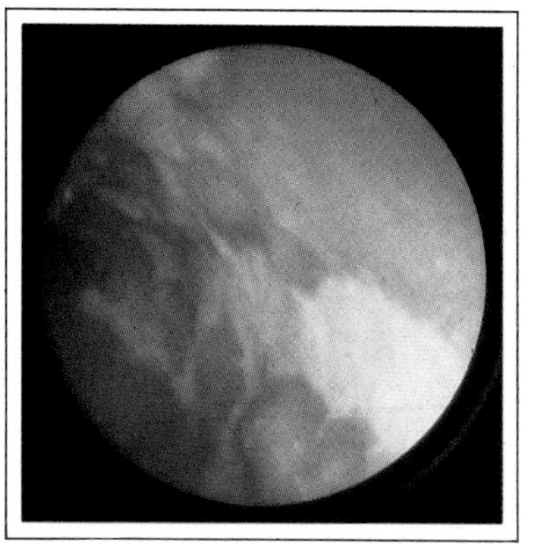

FIG. 43-29a.

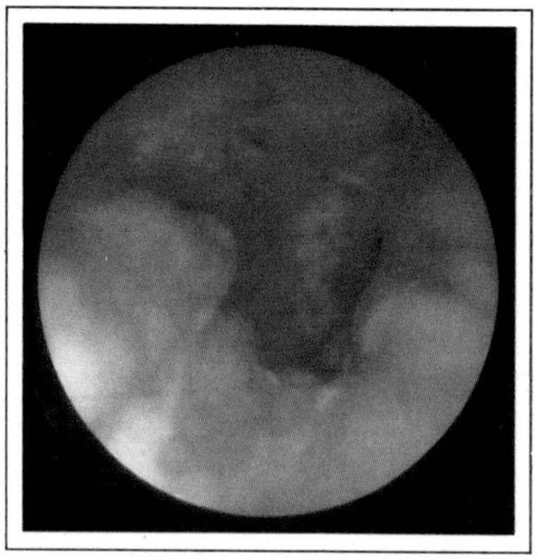

FIG. 43-29b.

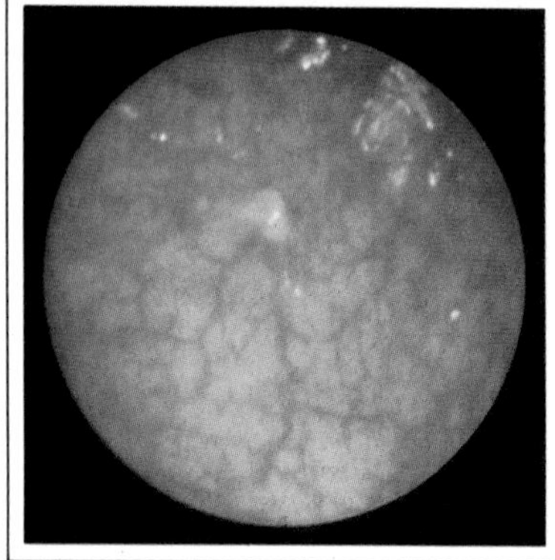

FIG. 43-29c.

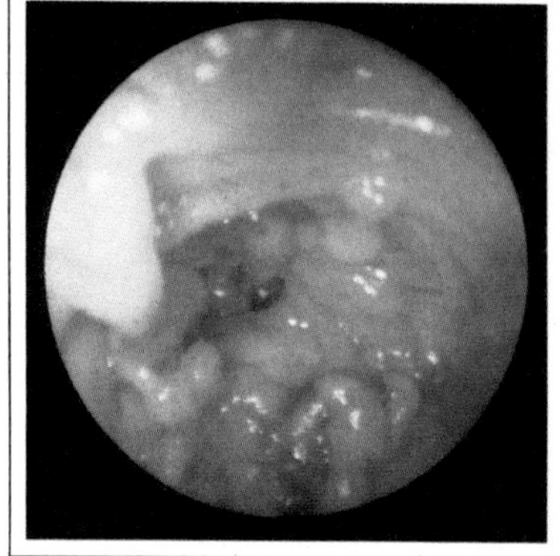

FIG. 43-29d.

FIG. 43-29. Crohn's colitis. **a:** With a long ulceration on a background of normal-appearing mucosa. The uninvolved mucosa adjacent to the ulceration favors a diagnosis of Crohn's disease. **b:** Focal involvement proximally with a skip area in the distance. In the involved portion (distal rectum) there are enlarged ulcerated folds. **c:** Aphthous ulcers set on a background of perfectly normal mucosa. **d:** Ileocecal valve stricture. The presence of inflammatory polyps give it a nodular appearance. The presence of a stricture, especially with ulcerations within it (Fig. 43-27c) strongly favors a diagnosis of Crohn's disease.

them at variance with the final diagnosis from surgically resected specimens in up to 20% of cases. This makes it advisable if not imperative to supplement the visual impression with histologic sampling obtained at 10-cm intervals. In this way, histologic features may be combined with visual criteria, which one would expect would ultimately increase the agreement of the preoperative colonoscopic assessment with the final diagnosis. To what extent this actually occurs is unknown. In this regard, the biopsy finding of multiple crypt abscesses in the presence of epithelial cells that show a diminished mucin content with a continuous pattern of activity favors a diagnosis of ulcerative colitis.[37] On the other hand, the presence of microscopic skip areas, few crypt abscesses, and an intact mucous content within the crypts, especially in the presence of microgranulomas, favors the diagnosis of Crohn's disease.[37]

Indeterminate Cases

In at least 5% of examinations, even the colonoscopic appearances plus the histologic findings are insufficient to allow differentiation of ulcerative colitis from Crohn's disease. Many of these cases remain indeterminate even after proctocolectomy.[41] Generally, there are well-demarcated ulcers that are often deep with intervening mucosa and which show only minimal vascular distortion, granularity, or erythema; hence on visual grounds Crohn's disease seems probable. Yet histologically the biopsies may show only a nonspecific pattern of inflammation with no definite features of Crohn's diseases, e.g., lymphoid aggregates, submucosal fibrosis, or granulomas. One can only hazard a guess as to whether such cases will behave similarly to Crohn's disease even though they lack features which establish the diagnosis with certainty.

Colonic Carcinoma in Crohn's Disease

As with ulcerative colitis, there is an increased incidence of colonic cancer in patients with Crohn's disease. Its incidence here is 5 to 10 times that in the general population, and it may be even higher.[13] This seems to be especially true of patients with extensive colonic involvement,[13] with a diagnosis made before the age of 21,[42] and with previous surgery that bypassed or excluded an intestinal loop.[43] The cancers are characterized by their occurrence in the relatively young patient (fourth to fifth decade), their right-sided distribution, and their preferential location in areas of fistula formation.[44,45] As with ulcerative colitis, the cancers associated with Crohn's disease display an infiltrative

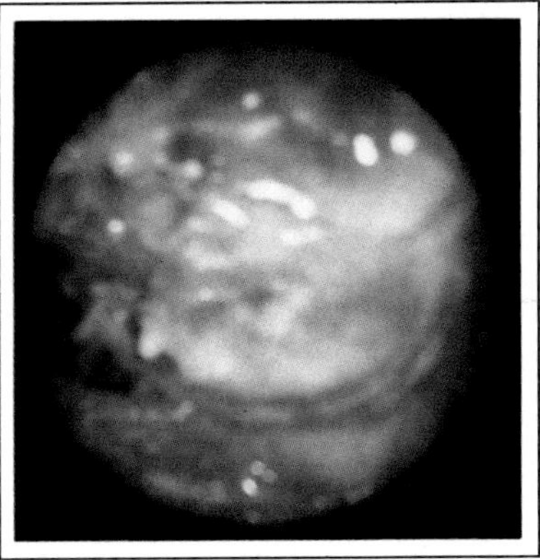

FIG. 43-30. Crohn's colitis, with carcinoma appearing as an inflammatory mass. At colonoscopy the mass was thought to be inflammatory. The dysplasia present, which was low grade, was thought to be reactive. After colectomy, sectioning of the mass and histologic examination revealed infiltrating carcinoma.

FIG. 43-30.

rather than an exophytic type of growth pattern, causing them to appear as either low or flat, plaque-like, nodular or sessile, polypoid masses.[44,45] They are not always suspected at surgery or on gross inspection by the pathologist[45] but only on meticulous histologic examination.[46] In patients with ulcerative colitis cancers typically occur in the setting of quiescent or healed disease, so that the cancer stands out as an isolated polypoid mass (Fig. 43-14d)—a discrete segment containing multiple, sessile, rubbery polypoid masses or an atypical stricture (see above). In Crohn's disease these same gross appearances of infiltrating-type colitic cancer tend to be obscured by the macroscopic features of Crohn's disease itself, i.e., strictures, cobblestone mucosal appearances between ulcerations, and luminal narrowing.[44,45]

Because patients with Crohn's disease of the colon constitute a high-risk group, some means of cancer surveillance is desirable so that, as in the case of ulcerative colitis, cancer could be detected while the patient is still asymptomatic. This would lead to a higher percentage of 5-year survivals, in contrast to the present situation where cancers are detected in symptomatic patients.[45]

Recently dysplastic (precarcinomatous) changes have been found in surgically resected specimens in areas contiguous with the cancer, suggesting the possibility of surveillance.[46] One could therefore consider colonoscopy for cancer surveillance in patients with Crohn's disease in which multiple biopsies would be taken at 10-cm intervals, as is currently done in patients with ulcerative colitis. As yet, however, in no reported case was the finding of dysplasia, detected preoperatively by means of colonoscopic biopsy, a key factor in the decision to operate, as has been true for ulcerative colitis. Therefore the efficacy of such surveillance is at present entirely unknown, although a finding of unequivocal dysplasia in an area associated with structural change, e.g., at a stricture or the mouth of a fistula, would make one seriously consider resection.[46] Prospective studies are necessary to determine the efficacy of cancer surveillance, especially in view of the potential problems of visually and histologically differentiating inflammatory from neoplastic lesions.

Appearance

We are unaware of carcinoma complicating Crohn's disease diagnosed preoperatively by colonoscopy. Several of the patients reported from our institution[45] had colonoscopy, but in no case was the diagnosis established. In one of the cases an inflammatory mass was found (Fig. 43-30), but biopsies revealed neither cancer nor dysplasia. Subsequently the patient underwent colectomy, and a focus of cancer was found deep within the inflammatory mass. This case points up a major difficulty in diagnosing cancer complicating Crohn's disease with a location deep within areas of inflammation.[45]

REFERENCES

1. Gabrielsson, N., Granqvist, S., Sondelin, D., and Thorgeirsson, T. (1979): Extent of inflammatory lesions in ulcerative colitis, assessed by radiology, colonoscopy, and biopsies. *Gastrointest. Radiol.*, 4:395–400.
2. Hartong, W. A., Arvanitakis, C., Skibba, R. M., and Klotz, A. P. (1977): Treatment of toxic megacolon: a comparative review of 29 patients. *Am. J. Dig. Dis.*, 22:195–280.
3. Korelitz, B. I., and Sommers, S. C. (1974): Differential diagnosis of ulcerative and granulomatosis colitis by sigmoidoscopy, rectal biopsy and cell counts of rectal mucosa. *Am. J. Gastroenterol.*, 61:460–469.
4. Laufer, I., and Hamilton, J. (1976): The radiological differentiation between ulcerative and granulomatous colitis by double contrast radiology. *Am. J. Gastroenterol.*, 66:259–269.
5. Waye, J. D. (1977): The role of colonoscopy in the differential diagnosis of inflammatory bowel disease. *Gastrointest. Endosc.*, 23:150–154.
6. Elliott, P. R., Williams, C. B., Lennard-Jones, J. E., Dawson, A. M., Bartram, C. I., Thomas, B. M., Swarbrick, E. T., and Morson, B. C. (1982): Colonoscopic diagnosis of minimal change colitis in patients with a normal sigmoidoscopy and normal air-contrast barium enema. *Lancet*, 1:650–651.
7. Powell-Tuck, J., Day, D. W., Buckell, N. A., Wadsworth, J., and Lennard-Jones, J. E. (1982): Correlations between defined sigmoidoscopy appearances and other measures of disease activity in ulcerative colitis. *Dig. Dis. Sci.*, 17:533–537.
8. Laufer, I., Mullens, J. E., and Hamilton, J. (1976): Correlation of endoscopy and double-contrast radiography in the early stages of ulcerative and granulomatous colitis. *Radiology*, 118:1–5.
9. Vender, R. J., Rickert, R. R., and Spiro, H. M. (1979): The outlook after total colectomy in patients with Crohn's colitis and ulcerative colitis. *J. Clin. Gastroenterol.*, 1:209–217.
10. Lennard-Jones, J. E. (1981): Azathioprine and 6-mercaptopurine in the treatment of Crohn's disease. *Dig. Dis. Sci.*, 26:364–386.

11. Present, D. H., Korelitz, B. I., Wisch, N., Glass, J. L., Sachar, D. B., and Pasternack, B. S. (1980): Treatment of Crohn's disease with 6-mercaptopurine: a long-term, randomized, double-blind study. *N. Engl. J. Med.*, 302:981–987.
12. Devroede, G. J., Taylor, W. F., Sauer, W. G., Jackman, R. J., and Stickler, G. B. (1971): Cancer risk and life expectancy of children with ulcerative colitis. *N. Engl. J. Med.*, 285:17–21.
13. Gyde, S. N., Prior, P., Macartney, J. C., Thompson, H., Waterhouse, T. A. H., and Allan, R. N. (1980): Malignancy in Crohn's disease. *Gut*, 21:1024–1029.
14. Lennard-Jones, J. E., Morson, B. C., Ritchie, J. K., Shove, D. C., and Williams, C. B. (1977): Cancer in colitis: assessment of the individual risk by clinical and histological criteria. *Gastroendoscopy*, 73:1280–1289.
14a. Lennard-Jones, J. E., Morrison, B. C., Ritchie, J. K., and Williams, C. B. (1983): Cancer surveillance in ulcerative colitis. Experience over 15 years. *Lancet*, 2:149–153.
15. Blackstone, M. O., Riddell, R. H., Rogers, B. H. G., and Levin, B. (1981): Dysplasia-associated lesion or mass (DALM) detected by colonoscopy in long-standing ulcerative colitis: an indication for colectomy. *Gastroenterology*, 80:366–374.
16. Morson, B. C., and Dawson, I. M. P. (1979): Inflammatory disorders. In: *Gastrointestinal Pathology*, pp. 513–542. Blackwell Scientific Publishers, London.
17. Teague, R. H., and Read, A. E. (1975): Polyposis in ulcerative colitis. *Gut*, 16:792–795.
17a. Marshak, R. H., and Lindner, A. E. (1977): Ulcerative colitis (radiologic findings). *Practical Gastroenterol.*, Sept./Oct.:35–43.
18. Lennard-Jones, J. E., Lockhart-Mummery, H. E., and Morson, B. C. (1968): Clinical and pathological differentiation of Crohn's disease and proctocolitis. *Gastroenterology*, 54:1162–1170.
19. Goulston, S. J. M., and McGovern, V. J. (1969): The nature of benign stricture in ulcerative colitis. *N. Engl. J. Med.*, 292:290–295.
20. Sherlock, P., and Winawer, S. J. (1978): Cancer in inflammatory bowel disease: risk factors and prospects for early detection. In: *Gastrointestinal Cancer*, edited by M. Lipkin, R. W. Good, and S. Day, pp. 479–478. Plenum, New York.
20a. Kurtz, L. M., Flint, G. W., Platt, N., and Wise, L. (1980): Carcinoma in the retained rectum after colectomy for ulcerative colitis. *Dis. Colon Rectum*, 23:346–350.
21. Van Heerden, J. A., and Beart, R. W. (1980): Carcinoma of the colon and rectum complicating chronic ulcerative colitis. *Dis. Colon Rectum*, 23:155–159.
21a. Ohman, V. (1982): Colorectal carcinoma in patients with ulcerative colitis. *Am. J. Surg.*, 144:344–349.
22. Cook, M. G., and Goligher, J. C. (1975): Carcinoma and epithelial dysplasia complicating ulcerative colitis. *Gastroenterology*, 68:1127–1136.
23. Hughes, R. G., Hall, T. J., Block, G. E., Levin, B., and Moossa, A. R. (1978): The prognosis of carcinoma of the colon and rectum complicating ulcerative colitis. *Surg. Gynecol. Obstet.*, 146:46–48.
24. Katz, S., Katzka, I., Platt, N., Hajdu, E. O., and Bassett, E. (1977): Cancer in chronic ulcerative colitis: diagnostic role of segmental colonic lavage. *Am. J. Dig. Dis.*, 22:355–364.
25. Greenstein, A. J., Sachar, D. B., Smith, H., Pucillo, A., Papatestas, A. E., Kreel, I., Geller, S. A., Janowitz, H. D., and Aufses, A. H. (1979): Cancer in universal and left sided ulcerative colitis: factors determining risk. *Gastroenterology*, 77:290–294.
26. Riddell, R. H. (1976): The precarcinomatous phase of ulcerative colitis. In: *Topics in Pathology*, edited by B. C. Morson, pp. 179–219. Springer-Verlag, New York.
27. Riddell, R. H., Goldman, H., Ransohoff, D. F., Appelman, H. D., Fenoglio, C. M., Haggitt, R. C., Ahren, C., Correa, P., Hamilton, S., Morson, B. C., Sommers, S. C., and Yardley, J. H. (1983): Dysplasia in inflammatory bowel disease: Standardized classification with provisional clinical implications. *Hum. Pathol.*, 14:931–968.
28. Dobbins, W. O. (1977): Current status of the precancer lesion in ulcerative colitis. *Gastroenterology*, 73:1431–1433.
29. Crowson, T. D., Ferrante, W. F., and Gathjright, J. B. (1976): Colonoscopy: inefficacy for early carcinoma detection in patients with ulcerative colitis. *JAMA*, 236:2651–2652.
30. Bartolo, D., Goepel, J. R., and Parsons, M. A. (1982): Rectal malignant lymphoma in chronic ulcerative colitis. *Gut*, 23:164–168.
31. Wagnonfeld, J. B., Platz, C. E., Fishman, F. L., Sibley, R. K., and Kirsner, J. B. (1977): Multicentric colonic lymphoma complicating ulcerative colitis. *Am. J. Dig. Dis.*, 22:502–508.
32. Farmer, R. G., Hawk, W. A., and Turnbull, R. B. (1975): Clinical patterns in Crohn's disease: a statistical study of 615 cases. *Gastroenterology*, 68:627–635.
33. Mekhjian, H. S., Switz, D. M., Melnyk, C. S., Rankin, G. B., and Brooks, R. K. (1979): Clinical features and natural history of Crohn's disease. *Gastroenterology*, 77:898–906.
34. Hogan, W. J., Hensley, G. T., and Geenen, J. E. (1980): Endoscopic evaluation of inflammatory bowel disease. *Med. Clin. North Am.*, 64:1083–1102.
35. Watier, A., Devroede, G., Perey, B., Haddad, H., Madarnas, P., and Grand-Maison, P. (1980): Small erythematous mucosal plaques: an endoscopic sign of Crohn's disease. *Gut*, 21:835–839.
36. Meuwissen, S. G. M., Pape, K. S. S. B., Agenant, D., Oushoorn, H. H., and Tytgat, G. N. J. (1976): Crohn's disease of the colon: analysis of the diagnostic value of radiology, endoscopy, and histology. *Am. J. Dig. Dis.*, 21:81–88.
37. Fishman, R. S., Fleming, C. R., and Stephens, D. H. (1978): Roentgenographic simulation of colonic cancer by benign masses in Crohn's colitis. *Mayo Clin. Proc.*, 53:447–449.
38. Aste, H., Pugliese, V., Munizzi, F., and Giacchero, A. (1983): Left-sided stenosing lesions in colonoscopy. *Gastrointest. Endosc.*, 29:18–20.
39. Banche, M., Rossini, F. P., Ferrari, A., Roatta, L., Gilli, E., and Cirillo, R. (1976): The role of coloscopy in the differential diagnosis between idiopathic ulcerative colitis and Crohn's disease of the colon. *Am. J. Gastroenterol.*, 65:539–545.
40. Burnham, W. R., Ansell, I. D., and Langman, M. J. S. (1980): Normal sigmoidoscopic findings in severe ulcerative colitis: an important and common occurrence. *Gut*, 21:A460.
41. Lee, K. S., and Medline, A. (1979): Indeterminate colitis in the spectrum of inflammatory bowel disease. *Arch. Path. Lab. Med.*, 103:173–176.
42. Weedon, D. D., Shorter, R. G., Ilstrup, D. M., Huizenga, K. A., and Taylor, W. F. (1973): Crohn's disease and cancer. *N. Engl. J. Med.*, 289:1099–1103.
43. Greenstein, A. J., and Janowitz, H. D. (1975): Cancer in Crohn's disease: the danger of a by-passed loop. *Am. J. Gastroenterol.*, 64:122–124.
44. Keighley, M. R. B., Thompson, H., and Alexander-Williams, J. (1975): Multifocal colonic carcinomas and Crohn's disease. *Surgery*, 78:534–537.
45. Traube, J., Simpson, S., Riddell, R. H., Levin, B., and Kirsner, J. B. (1980): Crohn's disease and adenocarcinoma of the bowel. *Dig. Dis. Sci.*, 939–944.
46. Simpson, S., Traube, J., and Riddell, R. H. (1981): The histologic appearance of dysplasia (precarcinomatous change) in Crohn's disease of the small and large intestine. *Gastroenterology*, 81:492–501.

44

ACUTE DIARRHEAL ILLNESSES AND UNCOMMON TYPES OF COLITIS

Although ulcerative colitis and Crohn's disease (see Chapter 43) account for the large proportion of patients with diarrhea and an altered mucosal appearance at colonoscopy, other conditions are encountered which because of similar appearances can be mistaken for inflammatory bowel disease. In this chapter we consider these conditions under two main headings: (a) acute diarrheal illnesses; and (b) uncommon types of colitis.

ACUTE DIARRHEAL ILLNESSES

Viral Gastroenteritis

Viral gastroenteritis, an extremely common illness, affects all age groups. It produces a self-limited watery diarrhea associated with nausea and vomiting and in most cases lasts only 24 to 48 hr, particularly if the Norwalk-like virus is responsible.[1] In cases where the diarrhea is caused by rotoviruses,[2] it may last up to a week, but it is unlikely that colonoscopy would be performed because of a week's course of diarrhea alone. However, the diarrhea may cause the patient to have blood in the stool from another condition, e.g., hemorrhoids, which may prompt an examination of at least the sigmoid if not the entire colon.

Appearance

The colonic mucosa may be entirely normal or show nonspecific features, e.g., loss of the normal vascular pattern, causing the mucosa to appear pale (Fig. 44-1a). In the same way, the valvulae may show nonspecific edema and appear blunt. In some cases friability (touch bleeding) is present. With the termination of the diarrhea, these changes completely resolve (Fig. 44-1b).

Biopsy

We have noted nonspecific edema of the lamina propria as well as an increase in chronic inflammatory cells in some cases which have been biopsied.

Campylobacter Colitis

Campylobacter fetus, subspecies *jejuni,* is emerging as the commonest cause of bacterial diarrhea, overtaking *Salmonella* and *Shigella.*[3] It may now account for up to 5 to 10% of all cases of acute diarrhea and 30 to 40% of those which are bacterial.[4]

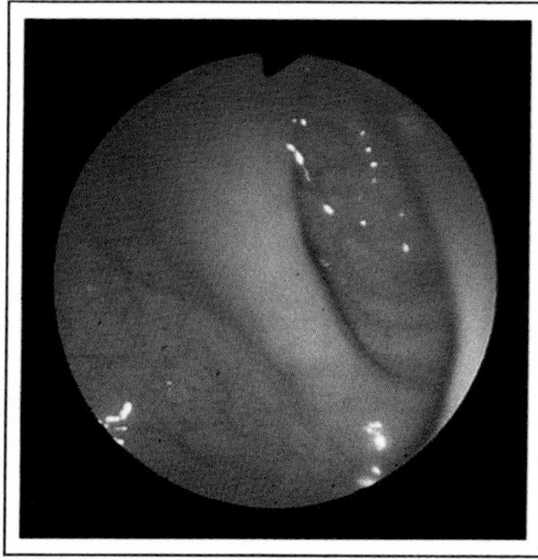

FIG. 44-1a.

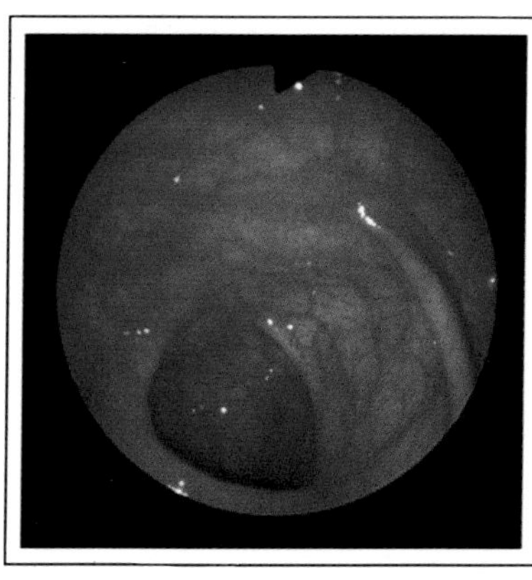

FIG. 44-1b.

FIG. 44-1. a: Viral gastroenteritis. Nonspecific enlargement of the sigmoid valvulae and a decrease in mucosal vascular pattern was observed in a middle-aged man with a 1-week history of diffuse watery diarrhea (stool negative for fecal leukocytes and enteric pathogens). Acute and convalescent viral serology suggested a rotovirus as the etiologic agent. Repeat examination 1 month later showed an entirely normal mucosal appearance (b). **b:** Normal sigmoid in a patient with prior nonspecific changes associated with protracted viral diarrhea.

The clinical presentation in these cases is frequent diarrhea (more than eight stools per day) which are bloody in half the cases.[3,4] Early, the bleeding may be massive.[5] Because of the bleeding the picture can be confused with that of ulcerative colitis, especially when the illness lasts longer than 1 week or, as in 20%, where there is a clinical relapse after an initial period of improvement.[3,4] In the majority of cases, no predisposing epidemiologic feature is found, e.g., the use of unpasteurized cows' milk, exposure to sick animals, or ingestion of meat scraps or spoiled meat, which would suggest the diagnosis of *Campylobacter* colitis prior to colonoscopy.[3,4]

Appearance

There may be either a diffusely abnormal mucosa that shows marked edema, hyperemia, or ulceration, which is indistinguishable from that of ulcerative colitis (see Chapter 43), or segmental involvement (Fig. 44-2a) that resembles Crohn's disease[6] with patchy areas of erythematous friable and ulcerated mucosa. In some cases mucopurulent exudate, rather than true ulcerations, is noted. Also, ulceration with adjacent hyperplastic mucosa showing a cobblestone effect may be found within involved areas.[6] Another distinctive feature is the presence of large (3 to 4 cm) shaggy ulcers with markedly friable mucosa comprising their margin.[3,4] All colonoscopic findings disappear in time, possibly hastened with treatment (erythromycin).[3,4]

Biopsy

Biopsies typically show an acute inflammatory infiltrate in the lamina propria with polymorphonuclear leukocytes predominating, but with plasma and mononuclear cells also present.[4a] The finding of crypt abscesses in these cases as well as a diminished number and a regular distribution of crypts bears a resemblance to biopsies of active ulcerative colitis (see Chapter 43). Nevertheless, true crypt distortion characterized by the presence of branching or budding crypts is not observed.[4a,4b] Its presence would indicate underlying ulcerative colitis.[4b]

Shigella

At one time *Shigella* was the commonest cause of bacterial diarrhea, but it is now decreasing in importance.[7] It is still recognized among elderly patients in nursing homes,[8] however, and recently it has been found as a common cause of bacterial diarrhea among homosexuals.[9] Of the four strains of *Shigella* recognized in the United States, *S. flexneri* and *sonnei* are the commonest.[10] This organism elaborates a cytotoxin that is responsible for mucosal penetration and invasion, which leads to intraepithelial multiplication and results in mucosal inflammation and destruction.[7] The symptoms resulting from mucosal invasion are those of dysentery, consisting of urgency, tenesmus, and bloody diarrhea[7]—a picture which simulates acute ulcerative colitis. Colonoscopy may be requested with such a presentation, especially if a barium enema shows deep, collar-button-type ulcerations,[11] further simulating bowel disease. Another presentation is simply a protracted course of diarrhea, to which elderly patients are especially prone, where the diarrhea may last up to 3 weeks.[8] Like *Salmonella* (see below), *Shigella* may be superimposed on quiescent or subclinical ulcerative colitis, causing an acute episode.

Appearance

The colonoscopic features of 4 cases of *Shigella* infection were reported by Rutgeerts et al.[11a] Three had focal aphthoid ulcers confined to the rectosigmoid region, while in the fourth those were found throughout the colon. We have observed one case, with the stool culture positive for *Shigella* in which there were punched-out ulcerations on a background of erythematous mucosa, resembling left-sided ulcerative colitis (Fig. 44-2b). This appearance completely resolved over a 3-week period (Fig. 44-2c), a characteristic feature of an acute bacterial colitis.

Biopsy

Preservation of the underlying crypt architecture and number in the face of acute inflammatory changes with crypt abscesses is consistent with a bacterial diarrhea from an invasive organism such as *Shigella*.[4b,11a] Biopsies should therefore be obtained in all cases, as patients may present late and cultures then may fail to grow *Shigella*. Conversely, although one may see crypt abscesses and a diminished number of crypts in a bacterial colitis, as in the case of *Campylobacter* (see above), this finding on biopsy especially with crypt distortion would suggest a bacterial diarrhea superimposed on longstanding ulcerative colitis.[11a] In this case one advises a follow-up examination of the left colon 3 to 4 weeks later to determine if there has been a return of the mucosa, both visually and histologically, to normal appearances, as would be the case for *Shigella* colitis alone.

Salmonella

Salmonella infection of the gastrointestinal (GI) tract is the commonest cause of bacterial diarrhea among pediatric patients (under 10 years) and elderly patients in nursing homes.[7] In these cases the diarrhea is often protracted and

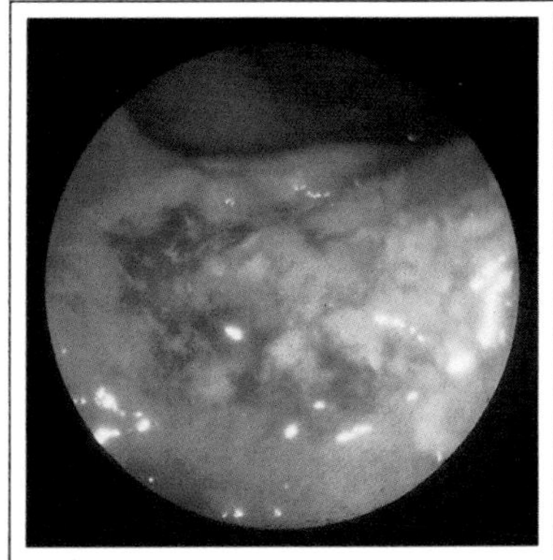

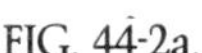

FIG. 44-2a.

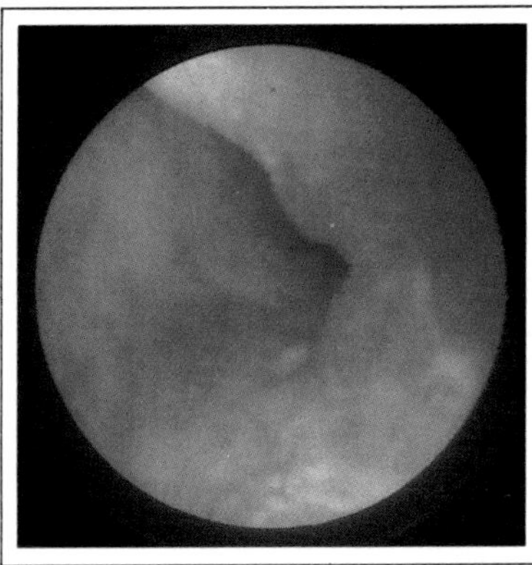

FIG. 44-2b.

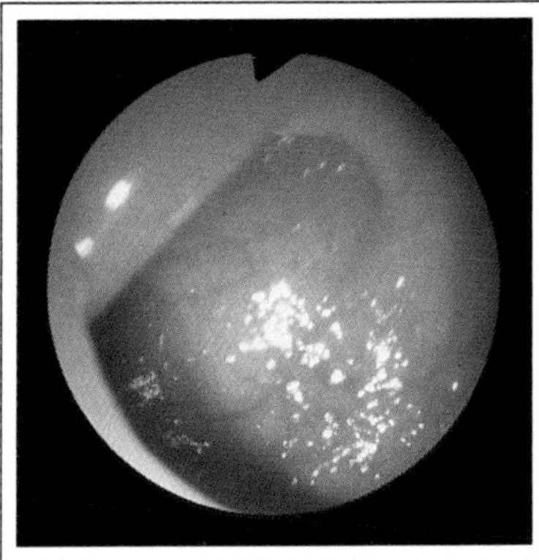

FIG. 44-2c.

FIG. 44-2. a: *Campylobacter* colitis. One of the multiple focal ulcerative-exudative lesions in a patient with a 2-week history of bloody diarrhea (stool positive for *Campylobacter fetus ss. jejuni*). This segmental type of involvement, noted by others,[6] is similar to that found in Crohn's disease (see Chapter 43). **b:** *Shigella* colitis. Beginning in the descending colon, down to and including the rectum, there was diffuse erythema, enlargement of folds, narrowing of the lumen, and the presence of mucopurulent exudate, suggesting ulcerative colitis. A stool culture was positive for *Shigella*. Repeat examination 3 weeks later showed a return to a normal appearance (c). **c:** Normal sigmoid after *Shigella* colitis.

severe, especially if *S. typhimurium* is involved, the commonest serotype identified.[7] The strain produces mucosal invasion with penetration of the submucosa; involvement is preferentially on the right side but in some cases includes the entire colon.[7,10] Prior gastric surgery seems to predispose to *Salmonella* infection.[12] The resulting infection is usually self-limited, lasting 12 to 24 hr with nausea, vomiting, bloody diarrhea, and fever,[10] but it may last up to 1 week and thus prompt colonoscopy.[13] Like *Shigella* infection, that caused by *Salmonella* may be superimposed on ulcerative colitis or Crohn's disease[11a]—always a consideration in cases where the course is protracted (10 days to 2 weeks).[14]

Appearance

The colonoscopic appearance for 6 cases of *Salmonella* infection was reported by Rutgeerts et al.[11a] Consistent with older case reports utilizing barium studies and proctoscopy these workers found the appearance to be a pancolitis with diffuse, erythematous mucosa, granularity, friability, and petechial hemorrhages similar to ulcerative colitis.[13] As predominant right-sided involvement and skip areas may occur,[13] the colonoscopic appearance of *Salmonella* infection could resemble that of Crohn's disease. Rapid reversal over a 3- to 4-week period is an important finding that rules against a diagnosis of Crohn's disease and in favor of a *Salmonella* infection, even if stool cultures fail to demonstrate this organism.

Biopsy

Biopsy shows, as in *Shigella* infections, acute colitis superimposed on generally normal mucosa with preserved crypts.[11a] As with *Shigella*, a *Salmonella* infection may be superimposed on underlying inflammatory bowel disease, especially ulcerative colitis, the latter being reflected in the biopsy as a decrease in number and distorted appearance of the remaining crypts.[11a,14]

UNCOMMON TYPES OF COLITIS

Somewhat arbitrarily we have singled out five types of colitis to be presented first which are at least better known although infrequently observed. These are: (a) antibiotic colitis; (b) amebic colitis; (c) ischemic colitis; (d) contraceptive-associated colitis; and (e) radiation colitis. In the final section of this chapter we present eight truly rare conditions: (a) Behçet's disease; (b) hemolytic-uremic syndrome; (c) malakoplakia; (d) schistosomiasis; (e) colonic tuberculosis; (f) *Yersinia* enterocolitis; (g) cytomegalovirus colitis; (h) drug-induced colitis; and (i) necrotizing enterocolitis and typhlitis of leukemia.

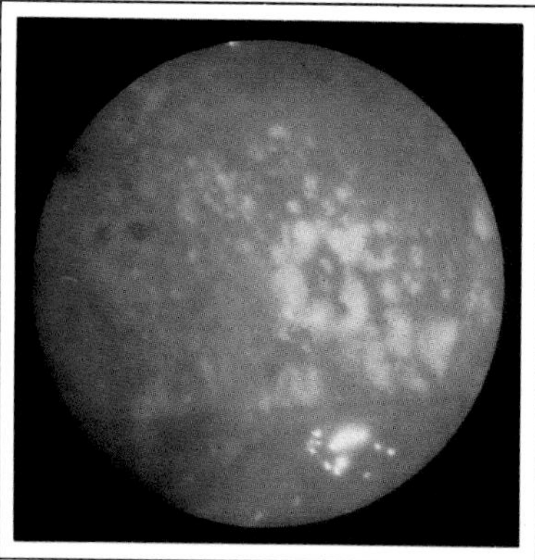

FIG. 44-3.

FIG. 44-3. Antibiotic colitis. Discrete exudates (pseudomembranes) are observed in the rectum and sigmoid 5 days after the onset of perfuse watery diarrhea during the course of clindamycin administration. The stools were strongly positive for *Clostridium difficile* toxin.

Well-Known Though Infrequently Observed Types of Colitis

Antibiotic Colitis

The use of certain antibiotics predisposes to the emergence of *Clostridium difficile,* leading in some cases to severe pseudomembranous colitis. These antibiotics are clindamycin and ampicillin in particular, but lincomycin, the cephalosporins, erythromycin, and Bactrim have also been implicated.[15] The *C. difficile* which emerges elaborates a cytotoxin which in the appropriate concentrations leads to focal necrosis along with an acute inflammatory exudate which is the pseudomembrane. *C. difficile* is a ubiquitous organism in the colon and does not always need antibiotics to trigger its overgrowth, as the same clinical picture has been described in patients who have not received antibiotics.[16]

Patients with antibiotic colitis present with cramping abdominal pain, a watery diarrhea which becomes bloody in 5 to 10% of cases, fever, leukocytosis, and rebound tenderness.[17] In most cases the patient becomes symptomatic while taking antibiotics, but for up to 20% this occurs 5 to 10 days after antibiotics have been discontinued.[17]

The illness is usually self-limited, resolving within 49 to 72 hr after the antibiotic is stopped. In cases where the diarrhea begins after the medication was stopped, or if antibiotics are continued, the diarrhea and/or rectal bleeding become intractable.[17]

Because in most cases the diagnosis is obvious from the history, from the *C. difficile* toxin titers in stool, and from proctoscopy, colonoscopy is usually not requested prior to instituting treatment, which is now vancomycin[18] or metronidazole.[19] Because positive *C. difficile* stool titers have been reported in (a) patients with inflammatory bowel disease,[20] (b) patients with bloody diarrhea which has proved refractory to treatment so as to suggest ulcerative colitis, or (c) those without rectal involvement thereby simulating Crohn's disease, some cases may be referred for colonoscopy with the hope that it can differentiate antibiotic colitis from inflammatory bowel disease.

Appearance.

The colonoscopic findings in antibiotic colitis seem to occur in four distinctive patterns[21,22]: (a) mild; (b) severe; (c) rectum-sparing; and (d) right-sided.

1. *Mild:* In up to one-third of the cases there may be only erythema and edema, with no pseudomembrane formation. Biopsy in these cases may show only nonspecific mucosal edema.

2. *Severe:* In the majority of the cases (up to two-thirds), large confluent pseudomembranes may be present along with erythema and edema (Fig. 44-3). The pseudomembranes appear as 1- to 5-mm yellow plaques, with their size apparently depending on the timing of colonoscopy in relation to the onset of diarrhea. Within the first 18 hr the plaques may be tiny (1 to 3 mm) and minimally raised. After 72 hr they become larger and tend to be more confluent, with still larger plaques being observed (4 to 5 mm) after 6 days, especially if the antibiotic is continued.[17] Generally, the involvement is distal or left-sided, but it may be universal, especially if large plaques are observed.

3. *Rectum-sparing:* In a variable percentage of cases, possibly up to 20 to 30%,[21] the rectum may be entirely spared or show only nonspecific erythema. In most of these cases the offending antibiotic is clindamycin, with ampicillin and cephalosporins accounting for the remainder of the cases. In about one-third of the cases where the rectum is spared, there is no involvement of the sigmoid as well. In these cases colonoscopy may be crucial for establishing the presence of pseudomembranous colitis.

4. *Right-sided involvement:* Least common overall, but one which has been noted for ampicillin,[22] is involvement confined to the right colon. In these cases colonoscopy may be decisive for establishing the diagnosis.

Amebic Colitis

Although the prevalence of *Entamoeba histolytica* is estimated to be 5% in the general population,[23] it is an infrequent cause of colitis, existing in most cases as an

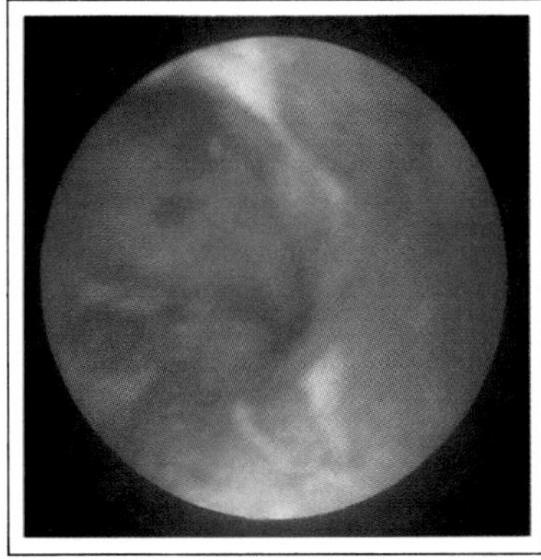

FIG. 44-4a.

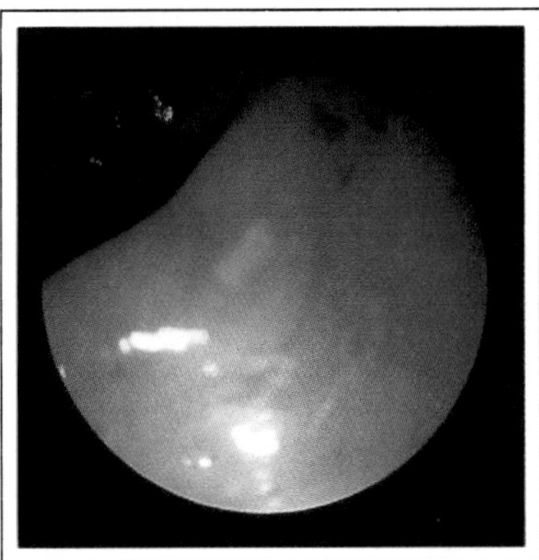

FIG. 44-4b.

FIG. 44-4. Amebic colitis. **a:** Acute. Colonoscopy was performed 3 months after the onset of bloody diarrhea, cramping abdominal pain, tenesmus, mucopurulent exudate, ulceration, erythema, and friability. Biopsies from the ulcerated areas showed amebic trophozoites. An amebic serology (indirect hemagglutination) was positive for the titer 1:512. The close similarity between acute amebic colitis and active ulcerative colitis (see Chapter 43) is apparent from this case. **b:** Subacute. Multiple discrete small ulcerations were noted in a patient with a 1-year history of diarrhea. Biopsies of the ulcers showed amebic trophozoites. These focal ulcerations are similar to the aphthous ulcerations of Crohn's disease (see Chapter 43).

unobtrusive saprophyte in equilibrium with the normal intestinal flora. In those who become freshly exposed to the organism, e.g., those who travel to endemic areas, it is occasionally a cause of prolonged traveler's diarrhea.[24] Another group in whom the organism is being increasingly recognized is homosexuals, who present with a recent onset of bloody diarrhea and tenesmus that suggests ulcerative colitis.[25] Finally, the diagnosis is always a consideration in elderly patients who are referred from nursing homes with new-onset diarrhea.[8]

In addition to the above, one must always consider a diagnosis of amebic colitis in any fresh case of ulcerative colitis because of the similarity in clinical presentation, with bloody diarrhea and cramping abdominal pain common to both.[26] The use of steroids in patients with amebic colitis erroneously diagnosed as ulcerative colitis places the patient at risk of disastrous complications, e.g., amebic metastasis to the liver or intestinal wall (amebomas) or even free perforation. It is hoped that such cases of mistaken identity will become rare with the widespread availability of amebic serology (immunodiffusion and indirect hemagglutination),[27] where a positive result (titer 1:128) strongly points to a diagnosis of intestinal amebiasis in the clinical context of acute colitis.

Appearance.

One may speak of three distinct endoscopic appearances for colonic amebiasis[27]: (a) acute amebic colitis of the rectosigmoid; (b) subacute colonic involvement; and (c) right-sided (cecal) involvement.

1. *Acute type:* This is a common proctoscopic appearance which is to be expected at colonoscopy.[28] Here the mucosa of the rectum and sigmoid shows mucopurulent exudate or ulcerations, erythema, and friability which is indistinguishable from that of acute ulcerative colitis[11a] (Fig. 44-4a). Smears made from the exudate reveal trophozoites as do biopsies taken from the ulcerations themselves.

2. *Subacute type:* With this appearance, which reflects a more chronic mucosal involvement, discrete 3- to 5-mm ulcerations (Fig. 44-4b) are observed surrounded by mucosa which may appear normal or show nonspecific changes, e.g., loss of the mucosal vascular pattern or blunting of the folds (edema).[29] The ulcerations are reminiscent of the aphthous ulcers seen in Crohn's disease with which they may be confused. Another subacute appearance which could cause confusion is that of inflammatory polyps (pseudopolyps).[30] As is true of inflammatory polyps in ulcerative colitis or Crohn's disease, there may be adjacent ulcers. These are important for diagnosis as biopsies taken from amebic ulcers have been reported to show trophozoites in up to 90% of the cases.[21]

3. *Right-sided cecal involvement:* This is the least common appearance, being expected in less than 5% of cases. In these, colonoscopy reveals cecal erosions, ulcerations, or submucosal ulcerating masses (amebomas) which radiographically may have suggested carcinoma. As in the case of subacute left-sided involvement, biopsies of the ulcerations may show amebic trophozoites.[31]

Ischemic Colitis

Ischemic colitis is being increasingly recognized clinically in elderly patients (over age 60) who present with their first episode of colitis as lower abdominal pain and rectal bleeding. In fact, ischemic colitis, rather than ulcerative colitis, may be the commonest cause of such episodes in the elderly.[32]

The etiology of ischemic colitis best relates to inadequate tissue perfusion of the mesenteric arterial circuit.[33] Generally this is nonocclusive, being associated with a low-flow states where there is reduced cardiac output, e.g., dehydration or cardiogenic shock.[33] In a small percentage of the cases, ischemic colitis is secondary to occlusion of the inferior mesenteric artery; or it may be seen when the mesenteric artery is resected as part of an abdominal aortic reconstruction and the major collateral artery of the superior mesenteric circuit (the marginal artery of Drummond) is not patent.[34] Similarly, abdominoperineal resection of the rectum for carcinoma which requires dissection and removal of the inferior mesenteric artery may also lead to ischemic colitis because of the lack of adequate collateral circulation from the superior mesenteric circuit.[35,36] Finally, ischemic colitis may occur secondary to vasculitis,[37] the use of oral contraceptives (see below), and intravascular hemolysis in the hemolytic-uremic syndrome (see below).

The typical presentation[32] is that of an elderly patient with left lower quadrant abdominal pain and bloody diarrhea, although in some cases there is only a small amount of blood mixed with stool. Plain abdominal radiographs may show pronounced thickening of the interhaustral folds from intramucosal hemorrhage. This may give the wall of the colon a scalloped appearance, i.e., thumbprinting on a plain abdominal radiograph (Fig. 44-5d). A barium enema, if performed, may show similar thickening of the intrahaustral folds and thumbprinting.[32]

Appearance.

The largest series of patients to date (15 cases) with ischemic colitis who were colonoscoped was reported by Scrowcroft et al.[38] The colonoscopic findings were abnormal in all 15 cases. This contrasted with the protoscopic results which were normal in 6 of the 15 cases, and barium enema, which was unrevealing in 9 of the 15. No untoward effects followed colonoscopy. From these examinations, Scrowcroft et al. recognized three distinctive appearances: (a) the acute stage; (b) the subacute stage; and (c) the chronic or healing stage.

1. *Acute stage (first 72 hr):* Initially (within the first 24 hr), patchy areas of hyperemic mucosa alternate with pale areas, which are thought to result from transient blanching of mucosal blood vessels. Over the next 24 hr the erythema coalesces which, according to Scrowcroft et al.,[38] occurs "as the zone of relative ischemia spreads to involve more mucosal surface area." At this point, superficial ulcers ranging in size from 2 to 4 mm are found (Fig. 44-5a), and there is evidence of submucosal bleeding manifested by "pinpoint petechiae or . . . submucosal hemorrhage" (Fig. 44-5b). In addition, the interhaustral folds are thickened because of edema or submucosal hemorrhage (Fig. 44-5c) and correlate with the thumbprinting appearance noted radiographically (Fig. 44-5d).

2. *Subacute stage (72 hr to 7 days):* During this stage ulcerations are found which are elongated and serpiginous. Because of the nonspecific character of the mucosa surrounding them, the presence of these ulcers suggests a diagnosis of Crohn's disease. In some cases acute inflammatory exudate rather than ulceration appears. Biopsies taken from the ulcer or exudates show acute inflammation with crypt abscesses and destruction of the normal glandular architecture, presumably from ischemic necrosis. Pseudomembranes are also found along with evidence of intramural hemorrhage by virtue of hemosiderin-laden macrophages. In cases where only crypt abscesses and destruction of the glandular architecture are observed, the histologic picture is likely to be confused with that of inflammatory bowel disease (see below).

3. *Chronic stage (2 weeks to 3 months):* As noted by Scrowcroft et al.,[38] there may be progression to complete healing within the first 2 weeks or it may occur as late as 3 months. In most patients healing was observed within 6 weeks.[38] Colonoscopy at this time showed either completely normal mucosa or some residual granularity. Of the 15 patients with ischemic colitis studied, stricture formation occurred in four. Histologically corresponding to healing was mucosal atrophy, loss of mucosal thickness, and submucosal granulation tissue.[38]

Sites of involvement.

Scrowcroft et al.[38] found that the two commonest patterns were rectosigmoid involvement alone or generalized left-sided involvement. Of the 15 cases, the right colon was involved alone in only one case and the transverse colon including the splenic flexure in only three cases. Hagihara et al.,[34] by means of proctoscopy and barium enema alone, found that left-sided involvement which excluded the rectum was the most common pattern in patients requiring surgery and those treated conservatively. This contrasts with the experience of Scrowcroft et al., who found rectal involvement in 9 of their 15 cases.[38]

Differentiation from inflammatory bowel diseases.

Scrowcroft et al. believed that ischemic colitis could be differentiated from inflammatory bowel disease. Features which were most suggestive of ischemia among their patients were advanced age (>60 years), segmental distribution of the disease, and especially rapid evolution to healing within 6 weeks, particularly in patients with rectal involvement.[38] They did not believe that ischemic colitis in inflammatory bowel disease could be differentiated histologically.[38]

Contraceptive (Estrogen-Containing) Associated Colitis

Acute, reversible colitis with features suggestive of ischemic colitis has been reported in young adult females (under age 40) who have used estrogens,[39] especially estrogen-containing contraceptives,[40–42] and in one instance, progesterone.[42] The duration of such usage in these patients ranged from 1 day to more than 3 years. Their symptoms varied but generally included abdominal pain, bloody diarrhea, and fever.[40–42] The mechanism of the estrogenic effect is uncertain, although it has been proposed that its use in susceptible patients results in a hypercoagulable state in

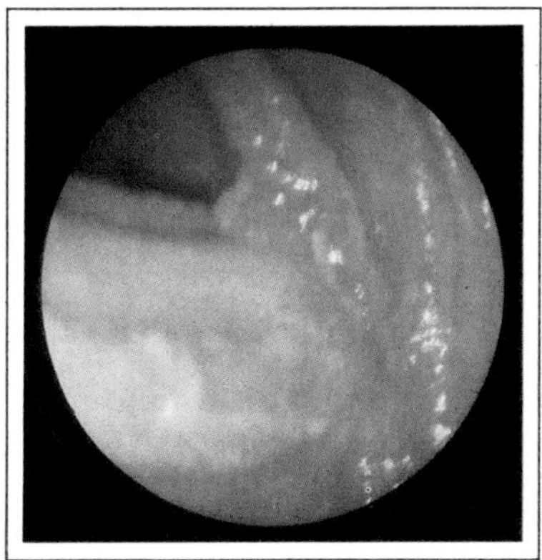

FIG. 44-5a.

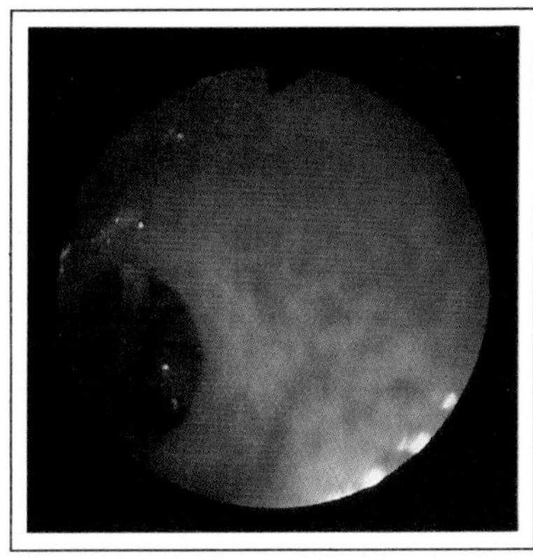

FIG. 44-5b.

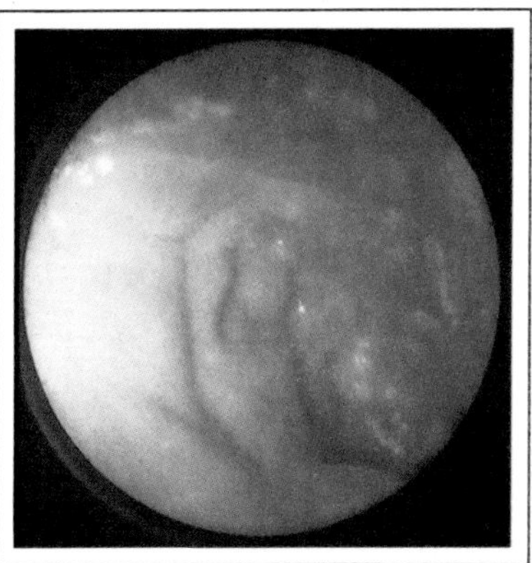

FIG. 44-5c.

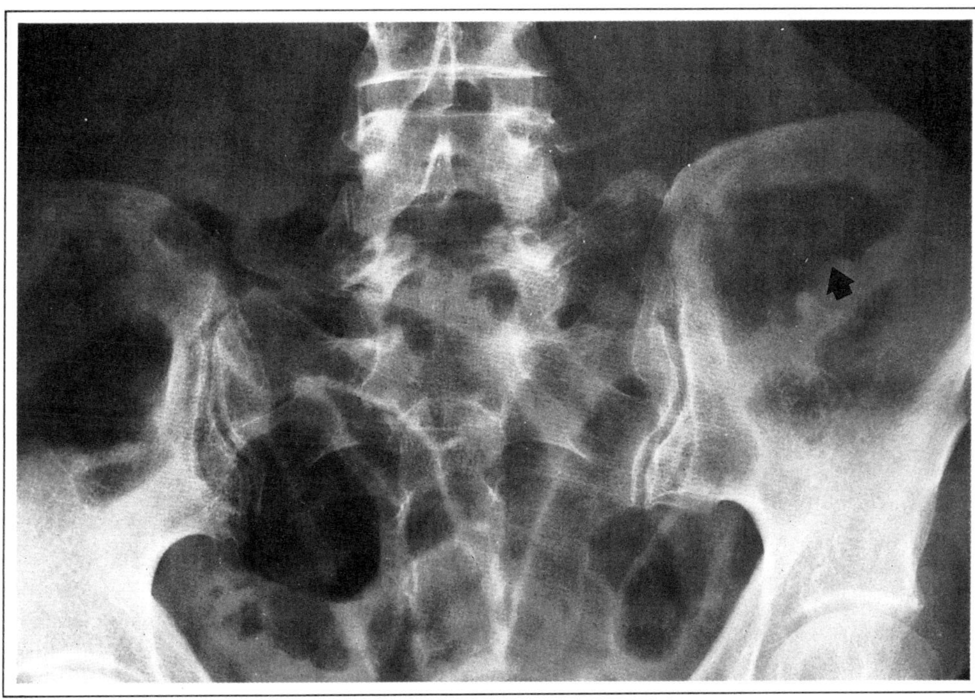

FIG. 44-5d.

FIG. 44-5. Ischemic colitis. **a:** Focal ulcerations were observed in a 65-year-old patient presenting with acute onset of bloody diarrhea for approximately 1 week (negative for enteric pathogens) and leukocytosis. Over the next week the diarrhea completely abated. Repeat examination 4 weeks after the first was entirely normal. The rapid resolution in this case favors the diagnosis of ischemia colitis over inflammatory bowel disease. **b:** Erythema, friability, and diffuse petechiae (probably from intramucosal hemorrhage) in an elderly patient with a recent onset of rectal bleeding. Because of continued massive bleeding, colectomy was ultimately performed, with ischemic colitis proved histologically. **c:** Enlargement of the intrahaustral folds occurs because of intramucosal hemorrhage. **d:** Radiographic appearance. Thumbprinting is best seen at the margin (*arrow*) of the transverse colon.

which intravascular clotting occurs, or that in some other way its use leads to a low-flow state.

Like ischemic colitis, the principal feature which allows differentiation from inflammatory bowel disease is rapid resolution of symptoms and colonoscopic findings—in this case after the discontinuation of contraceptives. The site of involvement in contraceptive-associated colitis is variable, although in at least two reports[41,42] it was proximal to the descending colon; in a third report[40] the left colon was primarily involved. The rectum has been spared in most cases reported to date.

Appearance.

The colonoscopic findings in five patients with contraceptive colitis have been reported as localized areas of intense friability, erythema, and edema.[42] Discrete ulcers were noted in three of the five cases; two of the five patients underwent resection, and findings thought to be consistent with Crohn's disease of the right colon were observed. The remainder, however, showed complete resolution within days after discontinuation of the contraceptive.[42]

Radiation Colitis

Radiation colitis is not an uncommon complication of radiotherapy for malignant tumors of pelvic organs, occurring in 5 to 10% of patients who have received 3,000 rads or more.[43] Of those who develop this condition, 50% will have had irradiation because of cervical carcinoma, reflecting the prevalence of this malignancy in the general population. The remainder will have had treatment for vaginal, ovarian, rectal, or prostate malignancies.[44] Predisposing to intestinal injury are the age of the patient (>60 years), evidence of arteriosclerosis, and previous pelvic surgery,[44] with these factors independently and together increasing the sensitivity of blood vessels in the field of radiation to injury (endarteritis). This vascular injury ultimately leads to chronic ischemia of the affected colonic segment. Because most radiation in these cases is for cervical cancer, lying in close proximity to the rectosigmoid junction (proximal rectum and distal sigmoid), this is the most commonly involved segment.[44,45]

Two types of presentation occur with radiation injury. An acute presentation is seen during the course of irradiation and lasting 6 weeks thereafter, with the patient complaining of diarrhea and tenesmus. Delayed effects of irradiation begin 6 to 12 months later and most commonly include rectal bleeding, pain, and diarrhea.[46] Such symptoms may prompt colonoscopy. In our Unit approximately 1% of examinations per year are performed in symptomatic patients who have had previous pelvic irradiation, an experience similar to that of others.[47]

Appearance.

The largest series of colonoscopic findings in radiation colitis was reported by Reichelderfer and Morrissey,[47] who found 13 cases among 1,200 colonoscopic examinations performed over 8 years, or approximately 1 per 1,000 examinations. In 12 of the 13, a barium enema had been performed, with a suggestion of a stricture in eight. In common in eight patients was the finding of a stricture, most often located at the rectosigmoid (Fig. 44-6a). Mucosal changes varied from the presence of either "pale and opaque mucosa," suggesting submucosal edema and/or fibrosis,[47] or the presence of telangiectatic mucosal vessels (Fig. 44-6b). In addition to these changes, which were the commonest, acute mucosal inflammation was noted in several patients with friability, erythema, and granularity (Fig. 44-6c); in one patient this was observed 6 years after treatment. The finding of discrete ulceration was unusual, however, and was not seen in any of the original 13 patients, although it was found in one subsequent patient.

Strictures tended to appear in association with either pale mucosa or telangiectasis (Fig. 44-6a). These mucosal features tend, in our experience, to support a diagnosis of radiation stricture although they do not rule out either tumor recurrence or a second primary colonic cancer arising in the irradiated portion.

RARE TYPES OF COLITIS

Behçet's Disease

Behçet's disease is an unusual condition characterized by oral and genital ulcers, ocular inflammation, skin lesions, and arthritis. In cases where GI ulcerations occur, they tend to be colonic.[48] It is, in general, a disease of young patients (under age 40) with similarities to Crohn's disease, i.e., the age of the patient at presentation, the extraintestinal manifestations (e.g., iritis, arthritis that involves single large joints, erythema nodosum and other skin lesions), and the occurrence of rectovaginal fistulas.[48] Furthermore, within the colon the presence of focal areas of involvement characterized by ulcers set in apparently normal mucosa is reminiscent of aphthous ulcers of Crohn's disease from which they cannot visually be differentiated (see below).

However, several features do set Behçet's disease apart from Crohn's disease. These are recurrent thrombophlebitis reported in about one-fourth of the cases of Behçet's disease and neurologic findings referable to the central nervous system in 20%[48]—both manifestations being unusual in Crohn's disease. Still, the other features are similar enough to Crohn's disease to make one think that Behçet's disease may be a variant rather than a different entity altogether.

Appearance

Colonic involvement occurs in only one-third of the cases at most,[49] with no involvement also being reported,[48] although in this study neither colonoscopy nor the sensitive double-contrast barium enema technique was employed which would be necessary to detect small discrete ulcers. Where colonoscopy has been utilized, the finding is characteristically that of discrete, punched-out ulcerations (Fig. 44-7) set on a background of mucosa which either appears normal or shows nonspecific erythema or granularity.[50] The location may be predominantly right-sided or involve the colon diffusely. Rectal involvement is variable,[49,50] but Smith et al., in a series of 14 patients, found some abnormality, especially ulcerations, within the rectum in all but one.[50]

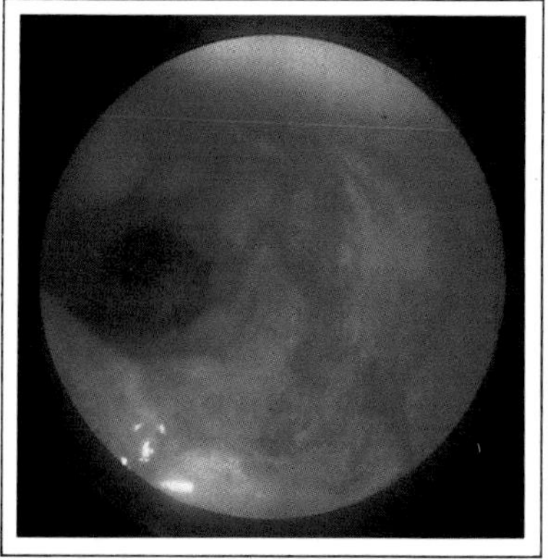

FIG. 44-6a.

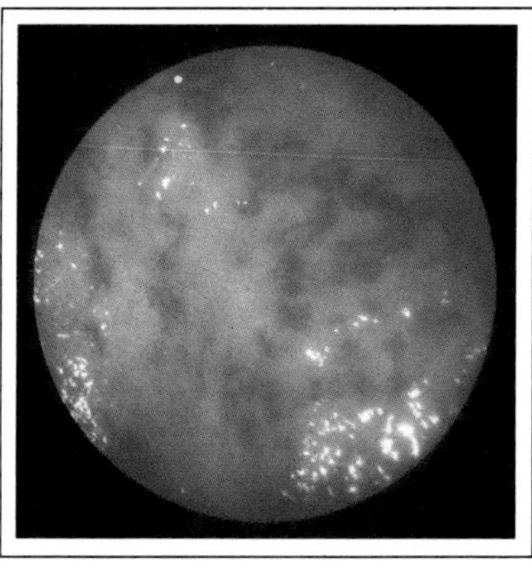

FIG. 44-6b.

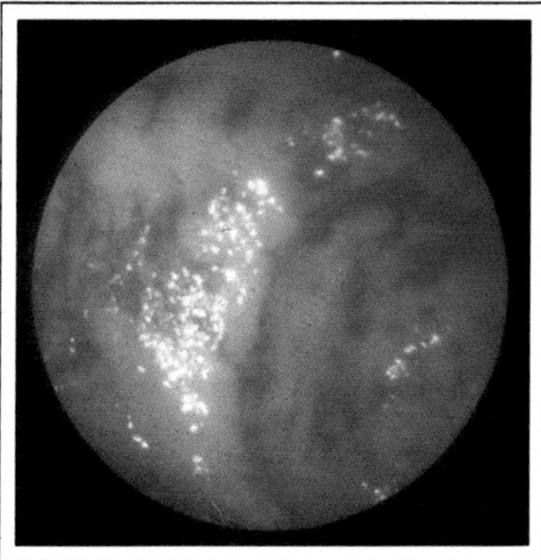

FIG. 44-6c.

FIG. 44-6. Radiation colitis. **a:** A rectosigmoid stricture with erythema, friability, and telangiectatic vessels 1 year after administration of 4,000 rads for cervical carcinoma. **b:** Telangiectatic vessels are superimposed on what otherwise appears to be pale and opaque mucosa, with the latter feature possibly reflecting the presence of submucosal fibrosis. **c:** Thickening (enlargement) of the intrahaustral folds of the rectosigmoid junction secondary to submucosal fibrosis (proved histologically).

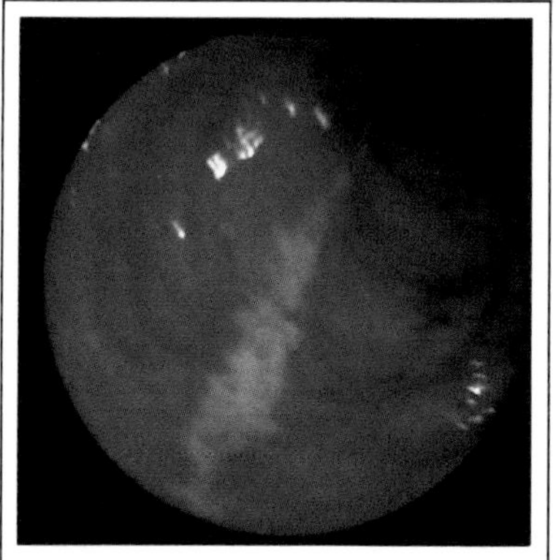

FIG. 44-7a.

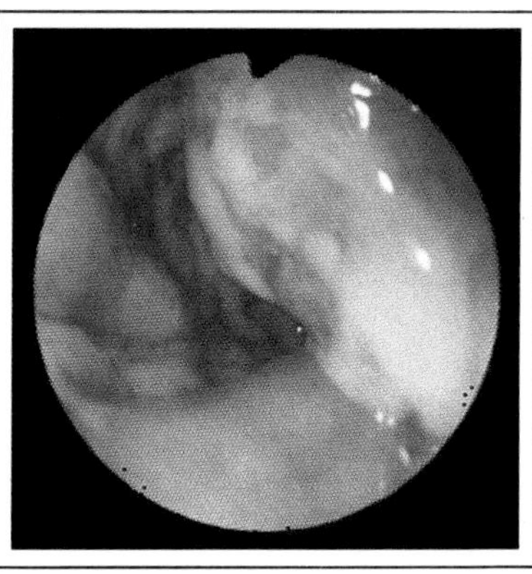

FIG. 44-7b.

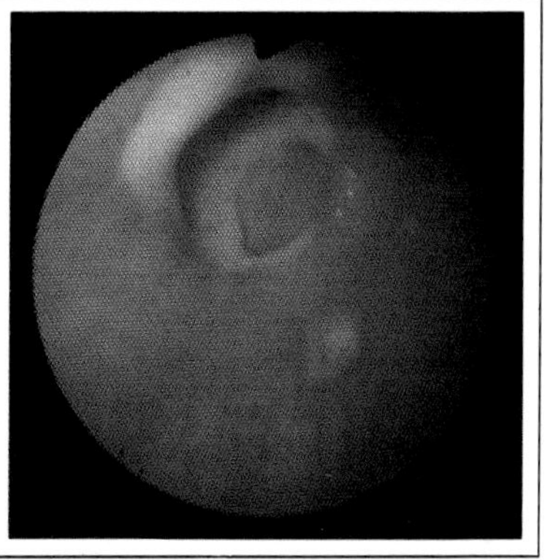

FIG. 44-7c.

FIG. 44-7. Behçet's disease involving the colon. **a:** A discrete, long, linear ulceration set in a background of nonspecific erythema. This was observed in a patient with oral and vaginal ulcerations, along with iritis—the clinical constellation of Behçet's disease. **b:** A discrete deep ulceration of the sigmoid in a patient with clinical features favoring Behçet's disease. The endoscopic appearance, however, does not allow differentiation from Crohn's disease, although colonic biopsies with evidence of vasculitis (lacking in this case) would have strongly favored Behçet's disease.[50] **c:** Discrete deep punched-out ulcerations are typical of colonic involvement in Behçet's disease, not unlike those found in Crohn's colitis.

Biopsy

Although it has been suggested that inflammatory infiltrate around vessels on colonic mucosal biopsies, similar to their appearance in other tissues, is specific for Behçet's disease, this may occur in only half the cases where biopsies are obtained. In other cases the appearance is similar to that of Crohn's disease, even with granulomas and giant cells being found.[50]

Hemolytic-Uremic Syndrome

The hemolytic-uremic syndrome, although generally seen in children, can also occur in adults, especially women on oral contraceptives or in the immediate postpartum state after deliveries complicated by eclampsia or abruptio placentae, or requiring cesarean section.[51]

The onset of hemolytic-uremic syndrome is often preceded by nonspecific symptoms, e.g., pain, nausea, vomiting, and diarrhea, after delivery or in a patient on oral contraceptives.[51] This is followed by anemia, GI bleeding, and renal failure, which denote the full-blown syndrome.[51,52] Such patients show a decreasing hematocrit and platelet count with rising blood urea nitrogen and white blood cell and reticulocyte counts. Barium enema performed in such patients may show features suggestive of ischemic colitis, with diffuse mucosal edema, luminal narrowing, thumbprinting, and pseudotumors—all an indication of submucosal hemorrhage.[52]

The colonoscopic findings in this syndrome have not yet been reported; however, from the radiologic appearance (see above) one expects at colonoscopy a picture similar to that of acute ischemic colitis (see above), with the presence of mucosal hyperemia, edema, and petechiae or ecchymosis as evidence of submucosal hemorrhage. This appearance could be confused with that of acute ulcerative colitis,[53] although the presentation and relationship of the colitis to the uremic state serve to differentiate these conditions clinically.

Malakoplakia

Malakoplakia is a rare type of granulomatous condition that involves various organ systems of the body primarily within the genitourinary system and, much less often, the GI tract. In this regard, up to 1979 there had only been 30 reported cases in which there was GI involvement.[54]

The condition occurs in debilitated patients with infections or neoplastic disease, often with an associated immune deficiency state.[54] Histologically, the lesion consists of an accumulation of histiocytes infiltrating the involved organ system. There is a pathognomonic histologic finding—the Michaelis-Gutmann body, a cytoplasmic inclusion which is PAS-positive and diastase-resistant, and contains calcium and often iron (Fig. 44-8b). Studies concerning the pathogenesis of these inclusion bodies indicate that they result from an accumulation of partially digested gram-negative bacteria, possibly *Escherichia coli*, which suggests a defect in the handling of ingested bacteria by the histiocytes.[54,55]

Appearance

We have observed one case of malakoplakia in a 39-year-old black man who had been treated 7 years before for Hodgkin's disease involving the stomach, liver, and regional lymph nodes. In addition, at the time of presentation hypogammaglobulinemia was found [involving immunoglobulin G (IgG), IgA, and IgM] in conjunction with nodular lymphoid hyperplasia and giardiasis of the duodenum (see Chapter 28).

In this patient, colonoscopy revealed uniform involvement of the entire colon with hundreds of 2- to 5-mm, slightly raised erythematous, nodular lesions, many of which were partially ulcerated (Fig. 44-8a). The mucosa adjacent to the lesions was somewhat erythematous but otherwise normal (Fig. 44-8c). In addition to the smaller lesions was a 2.5-cm polypoid rectal mass (Fig. 44-8d). Biopsies from the nodular lesion and rectal mass showed characteristic Michaelis-Gutmann bodies (Fig. 44-8b). The lesions in this case had nodules 3 mm to 1 cm in size with central umbilication or ulceration and were similar to those reported by others.[54]

Schistosomiasis

Schistosomiasis, although affecting 200 million persons throughout the world, is extremely rare in the United States and other western countries. Still, with emigration from endemic areas such as the Caribbean, an endoscopist in the United States may actually encounter a case.[56]

Colonic complications of schistosomiasis are directly related to the deposition of schistosomal eggs (generally *Schistosoma mansoni*) in terminal portal venules within colonic mucosa as part of the life cycle of a schistosomal organism.[56] The presence of these eggs leads to a local tissue reaction to the protein of the egg wall, and this is associated with mucosal changes, e.g., focal ulcerations and the presence of multiple inflammatory polyps.[56,57]

Appearance

The colonoscopic features which have been described for schistosomiasis, including focal ulcerations, mucosal thickening, luminal narrowing, and stricture formation, simulate those of inflammatory bowel diseases, especially ulcerative colitis.[56,57] A further similarity with ulcerative colitis is the appearance of inflammatory polyps which range in size from 2 to 20 mm and are largely in the rectum and sigmoid.[56,57] Their characteristic feature is a central ulceration or exudate. Of interest is the resolution of these polyps that can be seen with treatment.[57] Biopsies from these lesions have revealed *Schistosoma* egg granulomas.[56,57]

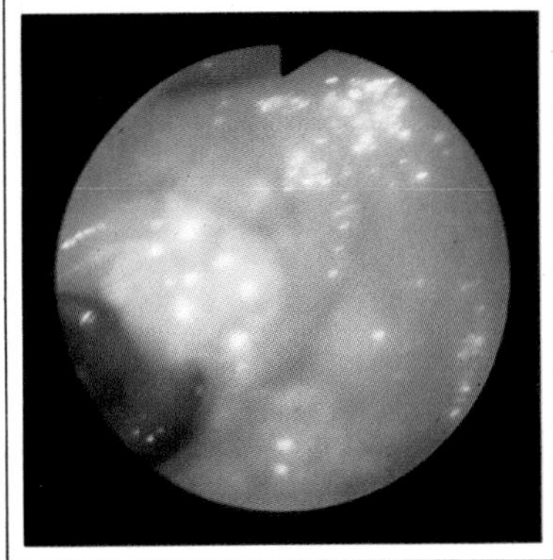

FIG. 44-8a.

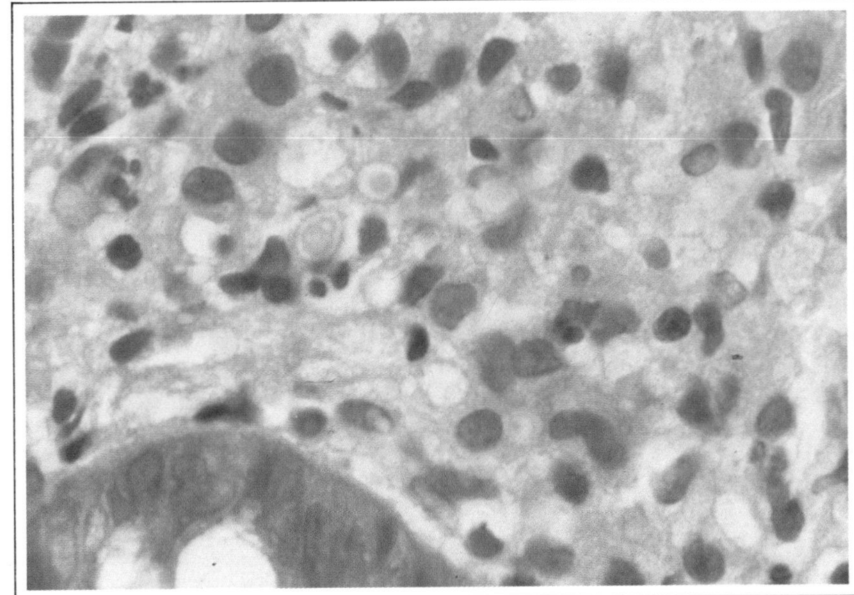

FIG. 44-8b.

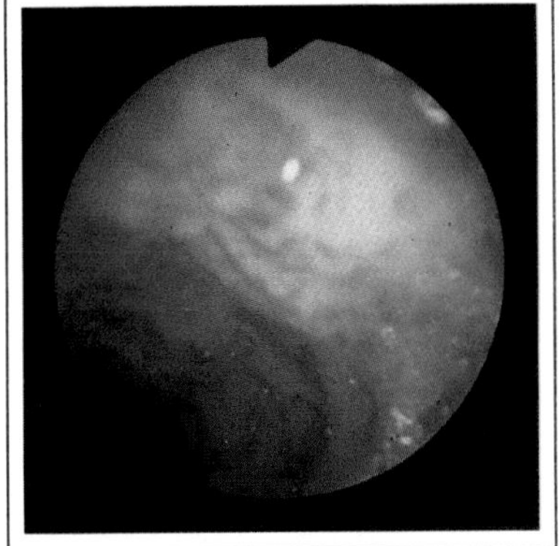

FIG. 44-8c.

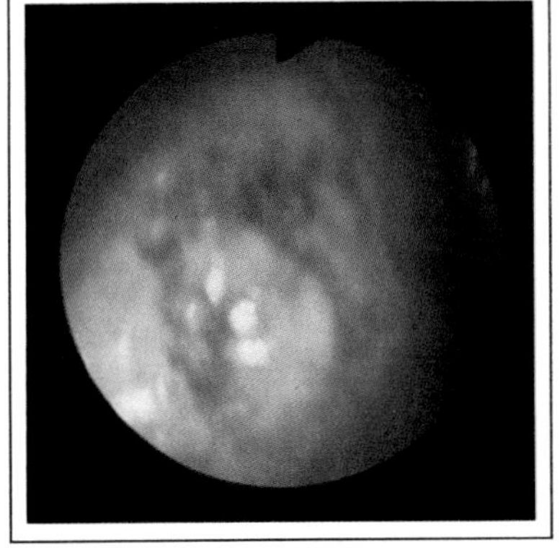

FIG. 44-8d.

FIG. 44-8. Malakoplakia of the colon. **a:** Focal, raised, superficially ulcerated lesions are seen in this rare type of granulomatous colitis. In this case the patient had hypogammaglobulinemia and had had previous irradiation and chemotherapy before abdominal Hodgkin's disease. Biopsies of these lesions showed typical histologic appearances (b). **b:** Histologic appearance. Sheets of histiocytes are seen within the lamina propria and submucosa; they contain pale blue Michaelis-Gutmann bodies. **c:** Focal, raised ulcerated lesions were seen throughout [same case as in (a)]. **d:** Enlarged (2 cm) focal lesion in the rectum in a patient with diffuse smaller lesions (c) elsewhere in the colon.

Colonic Tuberculosis

Although colonic tuberculosis is a rare condition, an awareness of it is essential, especially in inner city settings (municipal and county hospitals)[58] where tuberculosis is still endemic, and in parts of the southwestern United States.[59] The tuberculosis is secondary to the ingestion of tubercle bacilli which have been expectorated from cavitary lung lesions and then swallowed. Therefore the finding of active tuberculosis on a chest radiograph is expected.[58,59] Predisposing to intestinal tuberculosis is a history of gastric surgery or known achlorhydria, allowing access of organisms to the small bowel, which would likely have been inactivated by gastric acidity.[60] The most common sites of tuberculosis within the colon are the right side, especially the ileocecal area, which is the richest in lymphatics where the organisms tend to be attracted.[58,59] Here they infiltrate through the lymphatics into the submucosa where an intense inflammatory reaction occurs associated with caseating necrosis, particularly around lymphatic channels.[58,59] This results in a circumferential distribution of involvement so that a relatively discrete, annular type of lesion can be expected. Because of this, barium enema performed in such patients may suggest annular carcinoma of the cecum or ascending colon.[51] In addition, the involved mucosa in an area of active tuberculosis appears irregular. This is true for several reasons. First, with the intense submucosal inflammation there is edema and some hypertrophy of the mucosa, causing it to appear thickened.[58] Secondly, with submucosal caseating necrosis, there is lymphangitis and endarteritis which can be associated with mucosal ulcerative changes.[58] These tend to occur within areas of mucosal edema, creating a cobblestone appearance, also referred to as the ulcerohypertrophic form of colonic tuberculosis.[58,59]

One may expect patients with colonic tuberculosis to present for colonoscopy in the absence of a prior diagnosis with a picture which suggests either Crohn's disease or carcinoma of the right colon.[61] In the majority of patients symptoms include abdominal pain, largely periumbilical; vomiting, constipation, or diarrhea; and fever.[58–61] Also similar to Crohn's disease is the fact that the symptoms can be of long duration (1 to 3 years) prior to diagnosis.[58,59]

Appearance

The typical location for colonic tuberculosis is within the ileocecal valve, which shows thick, nodular ulcerated mucosal folds (Fig. 44-9).[62–64] In contrast to that in Crohn's disease the ileocecal valve is typically gaping, but unlike ulcerative colitis where this also occurs, the surrounding folds are heaped-up and ulcerated.[62–64] Biopsies taken from these areas often reveal the caseating granulomas of tuberculosis.[62–64]

In some cases the changes are in the cecum or the ascending colon away from the ileocecal valve. Still, one expects to find focal stenotic areas which are deeply ulcerated (Fig. 44-9). Because such focal involvement can occur in Crohn's disease, biopsy of such lesions is essential, especially if the clinical diagnosis is Crohn's disease and treatment with steroids is contemplated,[62] which would be disastrous in patients with colonic tuberculosis. In older patients the appearance of such focal stenotic areas can be mistaken for carcinoma, and again biopsy can be expected to play a crucial role in their differentiation.[61]

In one case we observed a diffuse lesion of the entire colon, rather than focal involvement of the right side. This patient had multiple, focal erythematous nodular lesions containing areas of ulceration from which biopsies showed typical tuberculosis organisms.

Yersinia Enterocolitis

Yersinia enterocolitica, a gram-negative rod, has been known for some time to cause acute diarrhea, mainly in infants and young children.[65] It may also present as right lower quadrant pain and fever suggestive of acute appendicitis, in which case either mesenteric lymphadenitis or acute terminal ileitis is found at surgery.[65]

More recently, a picture of chronic diarrhea that lasts 2 to 6 weeks, sometimes longer, was described initially in Europe,[65] and it is now becoming recognized in the United States.[66] In a report from Wisconsin of 28 symptomatic patients, 26 of whom had diarrhea, 14 remained symptomatic for more than 2 weeks.[66] In addition, such patients often have abdominal pain and fever which mimic Crohn's disease, as well as, in a minority, erythema nodosum, arthritis, and intra-abdominal abscess formation. Further adding to the confusion could be the radiologic picture of thickened folds and a nodular pattern within the terminal ileum and throughout the colon as well as aphthous ulcerations, suggesting Crohn's disease. Because of this similarity in presentation and radiologic appearance, colonoscopy may be requested in such patients, especially in the absence of a bacteriologic diagnosis.

Appearance

The endoscopic features of *Yersinia* enterocolitis have been described by Vantrappen and his co-workers.[11a,65] The characteristic finding is that of multiple 1- to 2-mm, shallow, aphthous ulcerations situated in the center of a surrounding 1- to 2-mm circumferential zone of erythema. In contrast to Crohn's disease, where the ulcers are of variable size and shape, those of *Yersinia* enterocolitis tended to be small and uniform.[11a,65] The involvement was right-sided in 20%, cecum to rectosigmoidal in 30%, and the entire colon, including the rectum, in 50%.[11a] In these latter patients the mucosa is diffusely involved, being described as erythematous, friable, and appearing "swollen."[65]

The response to antibiotic treatment, as observed by Vantrappen et al.,[65] was the disappearance of the ulcers within 4 to 5 weeks of the initiation of therapy.

Cytomegalovirus Colitis

Cytomegalovirus (CMV) colitis is now recognized in two settings with differing patterns of colonic involvement. Best known is a limited form that occurs in renal transplant recipients presenting with colonic bleeding who are generally found to have at least one large (≥1 cm), right colonic ulcer (see Chapter 47, "Colonic Ulcers in Renal Transplant Recipients").

Recently, a pattern of multiple, diffuse, small (1 to 6 mm) ulcerations, largely right sided, but occurring throughout the colon, was reported in a homosexual patient with the acquired immunodeficiency syndrome (AIDS) who was hospitalized because of fever and opportunistic infection. In this case, typical CMV inclusions were found in biopsies taken from the ulcers.[66a] We have observed yet another type of appearance and pattern of involvement in a homosexual patient with AIDS and a 9 month history of diarrhea with combined cryptosporidia and *Giardia lamblia* intestinal infestation. In our case, no ulcerations were observed; instead, multiple, discrete zones of intense erythema were present, ranging in size from 2 to 4 mm up to 2 cm

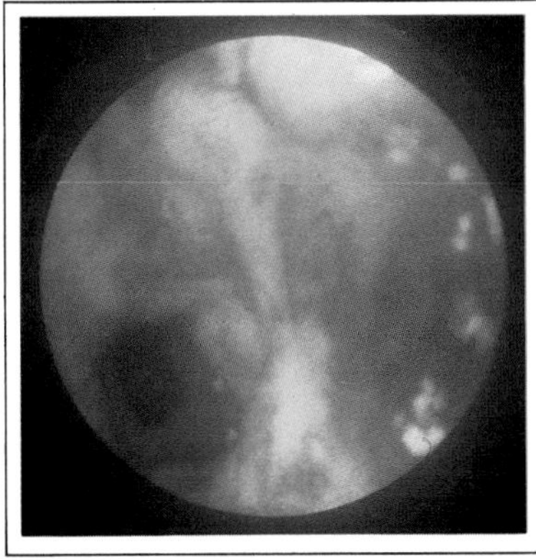

FIG. 44-9.

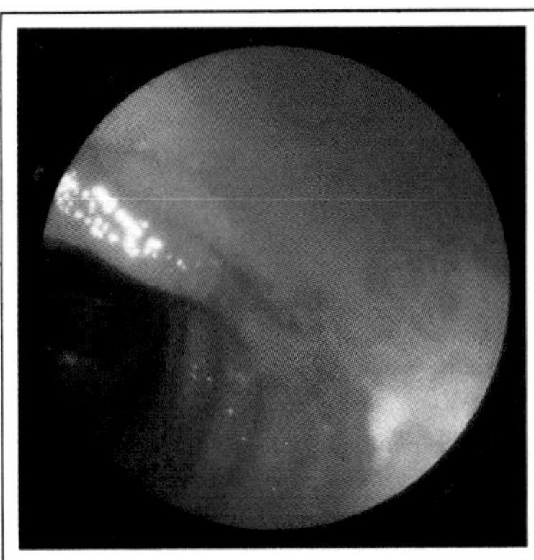

FIG. 44-10.

FIG. 44-9. Colonic tuberculosis. Scattered ulcerations and narrowing of the cecum in a patient with a known cavitary pulmonary type of tuberculosis. The biopsy shows caseating granulomas with typical Langhan's giant cells.

FIG. 44-10. Drug-induced (Tegafur) colitis. Perfuse, watery diarrhea began 16 days after administration of the furanidyl derivative of 5-fluorouracil. At colonoscopy multiple scattered ulcerations were seen from the splenic flexure down to the site of the prior sigmoid resection (for carcinoma). The diarrhea (and accompanying stomatitis) disappeared entirely on withdrawal of the Tegafur.

with most lesions between 5 and 15 mm. These were found mainly in the transverse and descending colon. Between the lesions, the interhaustral folds were thickened and the mucosa pale, being devoid of its normal vascular pattern, giving an overall appearance similar to that of ulcerative colitis with focal erythema (see Chapter 43, Fig. 43-3c). Biopsies from all involved areas showed typical CMV inclusions.

Drug-Induced Colitis

We have already considered the commonest type of drug-induced colitis—that which follows the use of antibiotics, especially clindamycin (see "Antibiotic Colitis," this chapter). In this section we consider briefly three other drugs capable of producing colitis. These are: (a) gold salts, used in the treatment of rheumatoid arthritis; (b) methyldopa, widely used as an antihypertensive agent; and (c) Tegafur, a 5-fluorouracil derivative used as an antineoplastic agent.

Gold Salts

An acute colitis[67,68] has been described in association with the (intra-articular) administration of gold salts in an accumulative dosage of 200 to 250 mg. Generally, the colitis is seen within a month of such administration, with the patient presenting with protracted vomiting and diarrhea.

Although a single characteristic colonoscopic appearance has not been described, from the radiologic picture[67,68] one would expect marked mucosal hyperemia along with blunting of the folds (edema) especially involving the right colon and terminal ileum. Biopsies would be expected to show acute, intense inflammatory reaction, especially with an increased number of eosinophils, producing a histologic picture similar to that of eosinophilic gastroenteritis.[68] The finding of eosinophils has suggested treatment with cromolyn, which (by inhibiting the degranulation of sensitized mast cells) may blunt mucosal injury caused by the sensitization of the mucosa to food (or other) allergens resulting in some way from administration of gold salts.[68]

Methyldopa

Rare cases of methyldopa colitis have been reported. In one, it was seen in association with liver injury,[69] although other cases have been reported subsequently with no liver involvement.[70] The clinical picture is that of an acute, watery diarrhea with high fever and shaking chills usually beginning within 2 weeks after initiation of methyldopa.[69,70]

The expected mucosal appearance is that of hyperemic, friable mucosa with many small petechiae.[69,70] Biopsies may be expected to show evidence of an acute colitis with crypt abscesses.[69]

Tegafur (Furanidyl-5-fluorouracil)

Despite the potential for colonic injury from potent cytotoxic agents, reports for such are infrequent.[71] One agent which has been known for some time to produce colonic toxicity when given in large doses is 5-fluorouracil.[72] Recently we observed a case where Tegafur, the furanidyl-5-fluorouracil derivative, was associated with an acute colitis which began 16 days after initiation of the drug, after a total dose of 2.0 g/m^2. This rapidly progressed to chills, fever, and worsening of diarrhea with 12 to 20 stools per day. Stomatitis also became apparent at this time.

A colonoscopic examination performed 20 days after initiation of the drug showed mucosal involvement with patchy erythema, edema, and ulceration beginning in the mid-transverse colon running down to the site of a sigmoidectomy for colonic cancer performed 3 years before (Fig. 44-10). The biopsies in this case showed changes of an acute colitis with ulceration, which was especially marked around the splenic flexure, along with regenerative changes. Upon withdrawal of the Tegafur, the clinical picture of acute colitis resolved entirely over the next 10 days.

Necrotizing Enterocolitis and Typhlitis in Leukemia

Patients with leukemia, generally of the acute myelogenous type, may develop necrotizing colitis with ulcerations of varying depth, generally containing bacteria.[73,74] Some of these ulcerations are associated with a pseudomembrane and resemble the picture either of antibiotic colitis (Fig. 44-3)[74] or leukemia with colonic involvement (see Chapter 42). The colonic involvement may be widespread, as enterocolitis,[73,74] or confined to the cecum, as typhlitis.[75] In either case the patient presents with fever, abdominal pain, and tenderness along with diarrhea which may be bloody.

The cause of this condition is unclear, but it is probably multifactorial, relating to the effects of the cytotoxic agents, ischemia, and the emergence of *Clostridium difficile* (see "Antibiotic Colitis," this chapter) with or without prior antibiotics. In this regard, one case of necrotizing enterocolitis was successfully treated with vancomycin,[76] as in cases of antibiotic colitis associated with *C. difficile*. Finally, the neutropenic state itself may be a factor that allows bacterial colonization of the ulcers, similar to an effect we have observed in esophagitis associated with chemotherapy and neutropenia (see Chapter 3).

Although colonoscopy might be thought of as particularly dangerous in patients with this condition, it has been performed without incident.[75,77] Experience remains quite limited, as yet, but the importance of colonoscopy may lie in its ability to determine both the extent of the necrotizing colitis, as well as the depth of individual lesions. Patients with principally focal right-sided involvement[75] and superficial-appearing lesions might be considered for medical (vancomycin) treatment,[76] whereas those with more extensive disease[73,74] or deep ulcerations may require resection for a type of involvement that has been reported to be almost uniformly fatal without surgery.[73] For those in whom medical treatment has been instituted, colonoscopy might also be used to assess whether any improvement has occurred.

Appearance

The colonoscopic findings have been reported in two cases. In the first, where the involvement was confined to the ascending colon and cecum (typhlitis),[75] several superficial, discrete ulcerations were seen. In another case with massive cecal dilatation, colonoscopy revealed the cecum to have an "ulcerated base" with "necrotic debris in the ulcers."[77] We ourselves have observed one case of necrotizing enterocolitis where colonoscopy was performed because of massive colonic bleeding; this was a patient with leukemia in "blast crisis" who had been treated with vincristine 2 weeks before, as well as Adriamycin plus cytosine arabinoside just prior to the onset of rectal bleeding. Discrete pseudomembranous plaques were seen at the rectosigmoid junction (but not in the rectum itself) and in the sigmoid colon just above. A *C. difficile* toxin titer of 1:20,000 was also noted. Because of the continued bleeding, the patient came to colectomy, where in addition to ulcerations of the rectosigmoid there were deep, shaggy ulcers of the right and transverse colon with near perforation. The histology of the resected specimen was consistent with necrotizing enterocolitis.

REFERENCES

1. Kaplan, J. E., Gary, W., Baron, R. C., Singh, N., Schonberger, L. B., Feldman, R., and Greenberg, H. B. (1982): Epidemiology of Norwalk gastroenteritis and the role of Norwalk virus in outbreaks of acute nonbacterial gastroenteritis. *Ann. Intern. Med.*, 96:756–761.
2. Wolf, J. L., and Schrieber, D. S. (1982): Viral gastroenteritis. *Med. Clin. North Am.*, 66:575–595.
3. Blaser, M. J., Berkowitz, I. D., LaForce, F. M., Cravens, J., Reller, B., and Wang, W.-L. L. (1979): Campylobacter enteritis: clinical and epidemiologic features. *Ann. Intern. Med.*, 91:179–185.
4. Blaser, M. J., and Reller, L. B. (1981): Campylobacter enteritis. *N. Engl. J. Med.*, 305:1444–1451.
4a. Blaser, M. J., Parsons, R. B., and Wang, W-L. L. (1980): Acute colitis caused by *campylobacter fetus ss. jejuni*. *Gastroenterology*, 78:448–453.
4b. Kumar, N. B., Nostrant, T. T., and Appleman, H. D. (1982): The histopathologic spectrum of acute self-limited colitis (acute infectious-type colitis). *Am. J. Surg. Pathol.*, 6:523–529.
5. Michalak, D. M., Perrault, J., Gilchrist, M. J., Dozois, R. R., Carney, J. A., and Sheedy, P. F. (1980): Campylobacter fetus ss jejuni: a cause of massive lower gastrointestinal hemorrhage. *Gastroenterology*, 79:742–745.
6. Loss, R. W., Mangla, J. C., and Pereira, M. (1980): Campylobacter colitis presenting as inflammatory bowel disease with segmental colonic ulcerations. *Gastroenterology*, 79:138–140.
7. Plotkin, G. R., Kluge, R. M., and Walamon, R. H. (1979): Gastroenteritis: etiology, pathophysiology and clinical manifestations. *Medicine*, 58:95–114.
8. Donta, S. T. (1975): Changing concepts in infectious diarrheas. *Geriatrics*, 30:123–126.
9. Drusin, L. M., Genvert, G., Topf-Olstein, B., and Levy-Zombek, E. (1976): Shigellosis: another sexually transmitted disease? *Br. J. Vener. Dis.*, 52:348–350.
10. Grady, G. F., and Keusch, G. T. (1971): Pathogenesis of bacterial diarrhea. *N. Engl. J. Med.*, 285:831–846.
11. McElfatrick, R. A., and Wurtzebach, L. R. (1973): Collar-button ulcerations of the colon in a case of shigellosis. *Gastroenterology*, 65:303–307.
11a. Rutgeerts, P., Geboes, K., Ponette, E., Coremans, G., and Vantrappen, G. (1982): Acute infective colitis caused by endemic pathogens in Western Europe: Endoscopic features. *Endoscopy*, 14:212–219.
12. Buchin, P. J., Andriole, V. T., and Spiro, H. M. (1980): Salmonella infection and hypochlorhydria. *J. Clin. Gastroenterol.*, 2:133–138.
13. Saffouri, B., Bartolomeo, R. S., and Fuchs, B. (1979): Colonic involvement in salmonellosis. *Dig. Dis. Sci.*, 24:203–208.
14. Dronfield, M. W., Fletcher, J., and Langman, M. J. S. (1974): Coincident salmonella infections and ulcerative colitis: problems of recognition and management. *Br. Med. J.*, 1:99–100.
15. Lishman, A. H., Al-Jumaili, I. J., and Record, C. O. (1981): Spectrum of antibiotic-associated diarrhea. *Gut*, 22:34–37.
16. Peikin, S. R., Galdibini, J., and Bartlett, J. G. (1980): Role of Clostridium difficile in a case of nonantibiotic associated pseudomembranous colitis. *Gastroenterology* 79:948–951.
17. Tedesco, F. J. (1976): Clindamycin-associated colitis: review of the clinical spectrum of 47 cases. *Am. J. Dig. Dis.*, 21:26–32.
18. Silva, J., Batts, D. H., Fekety, R., Plouffe, J. F., Rifkin, G. D., and Baird, I. (1981): Treatment of Clostridium difficile colitis and diarrhea with vancomycin. *Am. J. Med.*, 71:815–822.
19. Cherry, R. D., Portnoy, D., Jabbari, M., Daly, D. S., Kinnear, D. G., and Goresky, C. A. (1982): Metronidazole: an alternative therapy for antibiotic-associated colitis. *Gastroenterology*, 62:849–851.
20. Trnka, Y., and LaMont, J. T. (1981): Association of Clostridium difficile toxin with symptomatic relapse of chronic inflammatory bowel disease. *Gastroenterology*, 80:693–696.
21. Seppala, K., Hjelt, L., and Sipponen, P. (1981): Colonoscopy in the diagnosis of antibiotic-associated colitis. *Scand. J. Gastroenterol.*, 16:465–468.
22. Sakurai, Y., Tsuchiya, H., Ikegami, F., Funatomi, T., Takasu, S., and Uchikoshi, T. (1979): Acute right-sided hemorrhagic colitis associated with oral administration of ampicillin. *Dig. Dis. Sci.*, 24:910–915.
23. Pittman, F. E. (1980): Intestinal amebiasis. *Practical Gastroenterol.*, 4(March):33–39.
24. Banwell, J. G., and Kisller, L. A. (1980): Traveler's diarrhea. *Practical Gastroenterol.*, 4(April):20–29.

25. Burnham, W. R., Reeve, R. S., and Finch, R. G. (1980): Entamoeba histolytica infection in male homosexuals. *Gut,* 21:1097–1099.
26. Tucker, P. C., Webster, P. D., and Kilpatrick, Z. M. (1975): Amebic colitis mistaken for inflammatory bowel disease. *Arch. Intern. Med.,* 135:681–685.
27. Krogstad, D. J., Spencer, H. C., and Healy, G. R. (1978): Amebiasis. *N. Engl. J. Med.,* 295:262–265.
28. Pittman, F. E., El-Hashimi, W. K., and Pittman, J. C. (1973): Studies of human amebiasis. I. Clinical and laboratory findings in eight cases of acute amebic colitis. *Gastroenterology,* 65:581–587.
29. Kaplan, L. R., and Pries, J. M. (1979): A case of endemic amebic colitis: diagnosis with colonoscopic biopsy. *Dis. Colon Rectum,* 22:573–574.
30. Berkowitz, D., and Bernstein, L. H. (1975): Colonic pseudopolyps in association with amebic colitis. *Gastroenterology,* 68:786–789.
31. Crowson, T. D., and Hines, C. (1978): Amebiasis diagnosed by colonoscopy. *Gastrointest. Endosc.,* 24:250–255.
32. Eisenberg, R. L., Montgomery, C. K., and Margulis, A. R. (1979): Colitis in the elderly: ischemic colitis mimicking ulcerative and granulomatous colitis. *Am. J. Roentgenol.,* 133:1113–1118.
33. Marston, A., Pheils, M. T., Thomas, M. L., and Morson, B. (1966): Ischaemic colitis. *Gut,* 7:1–15.
34. Hagihara, P. F., Ernst, C. B., and Griffen, W. O. (1979): Incidence of ischemic colitis following abdominal aortic reconstruction. *Surg. Obstet. Gynecol.,* 149:571–573.
35. Lea Thomas, M., and Wellwood, J. M. (1973): Ischaemic colitis and abdominoperineal excision of the rectum. *Gut,* 14:64–67.
36. Wittenberg, J., O'Sullivan, P., and Williams, L. (1975): Ischemic colitis after abdominoperineal resection. *Gastroenterology,* 69:1321–1325.
37. Wood, M. K., Read, D. R., Kraft, A. R., and Barreta, T. M. (1979): A rare cause of ischemic colitis: polyarteritis nodosa. *Dis. Colon Rectum,* 22:428–433.
38. Scrowcroft, C. W., Sanowski, R. A., and Kozarek, R. A. (1981): Colonoscopy in ischemic colitis. *Gastrointest. Endosc.,* 27:156–161.
39. McClennan, B. L. (1976): Ischemic colitis secondary to Premarin: report of a case. *Dis. Colon Rectum,* 19:618–620.
40. Barcewicz, P. A., and Welch, J. P. (1980): Ischemic colitis in young adult patients. *Dis. Colon Rectum,* 23:109–114.
41. Bernardino, M. E., and Lawson, T. L. (1976): Discrete colonic ulcers associated with oral contraceptives. *Am. J. Dig. Dis.,* 21:503–506.
42. Tedesco, F. J., Volpicelli, N. A., and Moore, F. S. (1982): Estrogen- and progesterone-associated colitis: a disorder with clinical and endoscopic features mimicking Crohn's colitis. *Gastrointest. Endosc.,* 28:247–249.
43. Stockbrine, M. F., Hancock, J. E., and Fletcher, G. H. (1970): Complications in 831 patients with squamous cell carcinoma of the intact uterine cervix treated with 3000 rads or more whole pelvis irradiation. *Am. J. Roentgenol.,* 108:293–304.
44. Loludice, T., Baxter, D., and Balint, J. (1977): Effects of abdominal surgery on the development of radiation enteropathy. *Gastroenterology,* 73:1093–1097.
45. Kwitko, A. O., Pieterse, A. S., Hecker, R., Rowland, R., and Wigg, D. R. (1982): Chronic radiation injury to the intestine: a clinico-pathological study. *Aust. N.Z. J. Med.,* 12:272–277.
46. Novak, J. M., Collins, J. T., Donowitz, M., Ferman, J., Sheahan, D. G., and Spiro, H. M. (1979): Effects of radiation on the human gastrointestinal tract. *J. Clin. Gastroenterol.,* 1:9–39.
47. Reichelderfer, M., and Morrissey, J. F. (1980): Colonoscopy in radiation colitis. *Gastrointest. Endosc.,* 26:41–43.
48. Chajek, T., and Fainaru, M. (1975): Behçet's disease: report of 41 cases and review of the literature. *Medicine,* 54:179–196.
49. O'Duffy, J. D., Carney, J. A., and Deodhar, S. (1971): Behçet's disease: report of 10 cases, 3 with new manifestations. *Ann. Intern. Med.,* 75:561–570.
50. Smith, G. E., Kime, L. R., and Pitcher, J. L. (1973): The colitis of Behçet's disease: a separate entity? Colonoscopic findings and literature review. *Am. J. Dig. Dis.,* 18:987–1000.
51. Ponticelli, C., Rivolta, E., Imbasciati, E., Rossi, E., and Mannucci, P. M. (1980): Hemolytic-uremic syndrome in adults. *Arch. Intern. Med.,* 140:353–357.
52. Whitington, P. E., Friedman, A. L., and Chesney, R. W. (1979): Gastrointestinal disease in hemolytic-uremic syndrome. *Gastroenterology,* 76:728–733.
53. Yates, R. S., and Osterholm, R. K. (1980): Hemolytic-uremic syndrome colitis. *J. Clin. Gastroenterol.,* 2:359–363.
54. Chaudhry, A. P., Saigal, K., Intengan, M., and Nickerson, P. A. (1979): Malakoplakia of the large intestine found incidentally at necropsy: light and electron microscopic features. *Dis. Colon Rectum,* 22:73–81.
55. Stanton, M. J., and Maxted, W. (1981): Malacoplakia: a study of the literature and correct concepts of pathogenesis, diagnosis, and treatment. *J. Urol.,* 125:139–146.
56. Gambescia, R. A., Kaufman, B., Noy, J., Young, J., and Tedesco, F. J. (1976): Schistosoma mansoni infection of the colon: a case report and review of late colonic manifestations. *Am. J. Dig. Dis.,* 21:988–991.
57. Nebel, O. T., El Masry, A., Castell, D. O., Farid, Z., Fornes, M. F., and Sparks, H. A. (1974): Schistosomal disease of the colon: a reversible form of polyposis. *Gastroenterology,* 67:939–943.
58. Sherman, S., Rohwedder, J. J., Ravikrishnan, K. P., and Weg, J. G. (1980): Tuberculosis enteritis and peritonitis: report of 36 general hospital cases. *Arch. Intern. Med.,* 140:506–508.
59. Tabrisky, J., Lindstrom, R. R., Peters, R., and Lachman, R. S. (1975): Tuberculosis enteritis: review of a protean disease. *Am. J. Gastroenterol.,* 63:49–57.
60. Steiger, Z., Nickel, W. O., Shannon, G. J., Nedwicki, E. G., and Higgins, R. F. (1976): Pulmonary tuberculosis after gastric resection. *Am. J. Surg.,* 131:668–671.
61. Murillo, J., Wells, G. M., Barry, D. W., and Calia, F. M. (1978): Gastrointestinal tuberculosis mimicking cancer—a reminder. *Am. J. Gastroenterol.,* 70:76–78.
62. Aoki, G., Nagasako, K., Nakae, Y., Suzuki, H., Endo, M., and Takemoto, T. (1975): The fibercolonoscopic diagnosis of intestinal tuberculosis. *Endoscopy,* 7:113–121.
63. Bretholz, A., Strasser, H., and Knoblauch, M. (1978): Endoscopic diagnosis of ileocecal tuberculosis. *Gastrointest. Endosc.,* 244:250–251.
64. Franklin, G. O., Mohapatra, M., and Perrillo, R. P. (1979): Colonic tuberculosis diagnosed by colonoscopic biopsy. *Gastroenterology,* 76:362–364.
65. Vantrappen, G., Geboes, K., and Ponette, F. (1982): Yersinia enteritis. *Med. Clin. North Am.,* 66:639–653.
66. Snyder, J. D., Christenson, E., and Feldman, R. A. (1982): Human Yersinia and enterocolitis infections in Wisconsin: clinical, laboratory and epidemiologic features. *Am. J. Med.,* 72:768–774.
66a. Gertler, S. L., Pressman, J., Price, P., Brozinsky, S., and Miyai, K. (1983): Gastrointestinal cytomegalovirus infection in a homosexual man with severe acquired immunodeficiency syndrome. *Gastroenterology,* 85:1403–1406.
67. Stein, H. B., and Urowitz, M. B. (1976): Gold-induced enterocolitis: case report and literature review. *J. Rheumatol.,* 3:21–26.
68. Martin, D. M., Goldman, J. A., Gilliam, J., and Nasrallah, S. M. (1981): Gold-induced eosinophilic enterocolitis: response to oral cromolyn sodium. *Gastroenterology,* 80:1567–1570.
69. Bonkowsky, H. L., and Brisbane, J. B. (1976): Colitis and hepatitis caused by methyldopa. *JAMA,* 236:1602–1603.
70. Graham, C. F., Gallagher, K., and Jones, J. K. (1981): Acute colitis with methyldopa. *N. Engl. J. Med.,* 304:1044–1045.
71. Motolo, N. M., Garfinkle, S. E., and Wolfman, E. F. (1976): Intestinal necrosis and perforation in patients receiving immunosuppressive drugs. *Am. J. Surg.,* 132:753–754.
72. Milles, S. S., Muggin, A., and Spiro, H. M. (1962): Colonic histologic changes induced by 5-fluorouracil. *Gastroenterology,* 43:391–399.
73. Steinberg, D., Gold, J., and Brodin, A. (1973): Necrotizing enterocolitis in leukemia. *Arch. Intern. Med.,* 131:538–543.
74. Dosik, G. M., Luna, M., Valdivieso, M., McCredie, K. B., Gehan, E. A., Gil-Extremera, B., Smith, T. L., and Bodey, G. P. (1979): Necrotizing colitis in patients with cancer. *Am. J. Med.,* 67:646–656.
75. Dworkin, B., Winawer, S. J., and Lightdale, C. J. (1981): Typhlitis: report of a case with long-term survival and a review of the recent literature. *Dig. Dis. Sci.,* 26:1032–1037.
76. Freeman, H. J., Rabeneck, L., and Owen, D. (1981): Survival after necrotizing enterocolitis of leukemia treated with oral vancomycin. *Gastroenterology,* 81:791–794.
77. Cronin, T. G., Calandra, J. D., and Del Fava, R. L. (1981): Typhlitis presenting as toxic cecitis. *Radiology,* 138:29–30.

45

DIVERTICULAR DISEASE AND OTHER CAUSES OF SIGMOID NARROWING

As colonic diverticula can be demonstrated radiographically in 30 to 40% of patients over the age of 70[1] and for a similar percentage at autopsy in individuals over the age of 60,[2] it is not surprising that they are commonly found in patients undergoing colonoscopy. Overall, we find diverticula in a constant 20% of patients undergoing colonoscopy in our Unit. In half of these cases the diverticula are the only finding.

Patients with diverticula may have irritable digestive tract type symptoms which prompt colonoscopy. These have led some to consider the irritable digestive tract syndrome as a prediverticular condition.[3] These symptoms include flatulence, lower abdominal pain of a colicky nature, diarrhea alternating with constipation, mucus in the stool, and tenesmus. In these cases one expects to find simply diverticula, possibly along with enlarged sigmoid valvulae which result from smooth muscle hypertrophy and are common to patients with diverticula as well as those with irritable digestive tract symptoms alone (see Chapter 40). In other cases colonoscopy is performed because of obstructive symptoms, especially where a barium enema was indeterminate regarding the presence of a malignancy.[4] When obstructive symptoms occur in the context of left lower quadrant pain, fever, and leukocytosis, the colonoscopist may find evidence of acute diverticulitis.[5] In cases where the examination was prompted by a history solely of increasing constipation, a diverticular stricture may be found.

In this chapter we present the colonoscopic appearances of diverticular disease in the context of three clinical presentations: (a) diverticulosis, either asymptomatic or with irritable digestive tract symptoms; (b) acute diverticulitis; and (c) diverticular strictures. In regard to the latter appearance we touch on other causes of colonic narrowing of the sigmoid which need to be considered in a differential diagnosis of diverticular strictures.

DIVERTICULOSIS

Colonic diverticula, along with polyps (see Chapter 41), constitute the commonest abnormality encountered at colonoscopy. Their importance to the colonoscopist lies first in the technical difficulty they create for performing a complete and safe examination. Diverticula have an additional significance, particularly in patients with rectal bleeding in that their presence may compromise even a carefully performed air contrast barium enema to the point where colonic adenomas and carcinomas are missed by this examination and detected only at colonoscopy.[5a] For these reasons, it is especially important for the examiner to be cognizant of the various appearances of diverticula so that technical mishaps can be avoided. In this section we present first a brief discussion of their pathogenesis, which we believe provides the reader with a better appreciation of them. After this, we consider their appearance, especially regarding the differentiation of the mouth of a diverticulum from the lumen.

Pathogenesis

Colonic diverticula are protrusions of mucosa with a thin covering of muscularis appearing at the point where the nutrient artery penetrates the muscular wall to reach the mucosa.[6,7] Diverticula are thought to occur because of increased luminal pressure transmitted to the haustrae, causing mucosa to prolapse into the sites of penetrating arteries. It has been suggested that the cause of the increased luminal pressure is a marked increase in the size of the circular and transverse muscle layer, generating higher intraluminal pressures for any given stimulus or contraction.[6] It is believed that the origin of the muscle hypertrophy is the result of delayed colonic transit of smaller, harder stools which, because of their low residue content (from diets common in Western societies), hold less fecal water.[7]

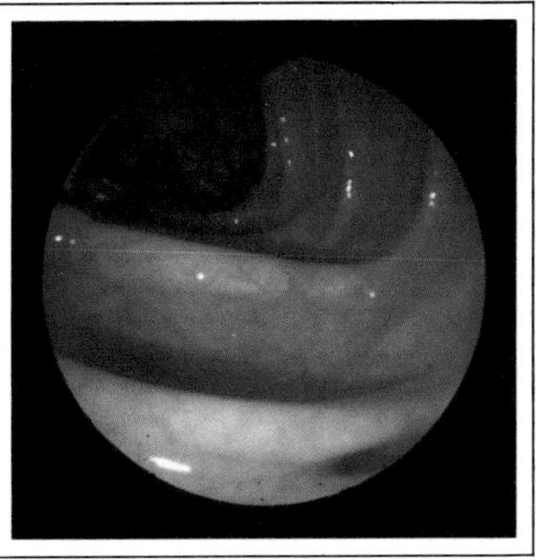

FIG. 45-1.

FIG. 45-1. Single colonic diverticulum. The lone sigmoid diverticulum in this case (just visible at 5 o'clock) was the only finding in a patient with a positive test for fecal occult blood.

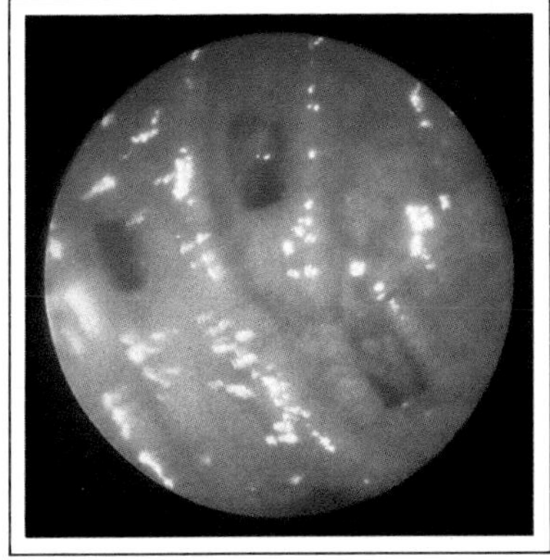

FIG. 45-2a.

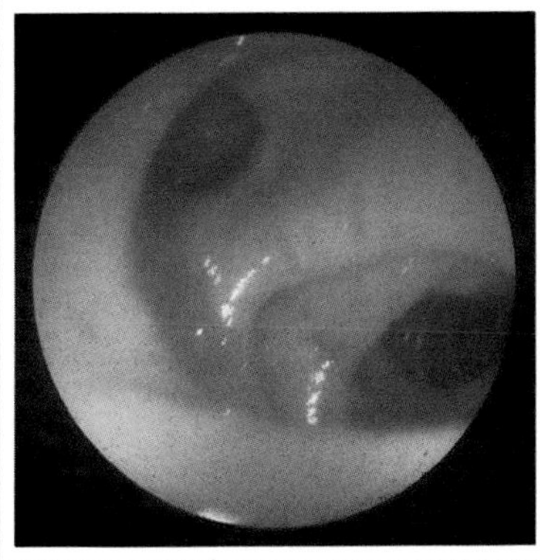

FIG. 45-2b.

FIG. 45-2. a: Multiple colonic diverticula. In this case two diverticula are found within one haustral segment (best seen at 6 o'clock and 10 o'clock), occurring at the midpoint between the valvulae, presumably at the point of entry of penetrating arteries (from the serosa to the mucosa). **b:** Colonic diverticulum in relation to the lumen. The diverticulum is noted at 11 o'clock, being recessed between two sigmoid valvulae; the lumen is denoted by the convergence of valvulae rather than as an opening between them.

Appearance

Single Diverticula

Single diverticula are found as 2- to 5-mm outpouchings during examination of the sigmoid or other segments of the colon, where they represent a focal weakness of the colonic wall in the area of a penetrating vessel (Fig. 45-1). In these cases the valvulae are not prominent (Fig. 45-1). Most single diverticula are small (having a diameter of ≤5 mm). Rare diverticula have been reported to attain a considerable size (with a diameter exceeding 2 cm).[8]

Multiple Diverticula

A commoner finding than the single diverticulum is the appearance of multiple diverticula in the sigmoid or even the entire colon. Within the sigmoid, which is their commonest location, they are recognized as 3- to 5-mm circular openings in the central portion of a short haustral segment, situated between enlarged valvulae (Fig. 45-2a). Although the diverticula actually form the deepest point of the haustra, this may not be apparent endoscopically where one sees simply a circular opening between valvulae. Generally, there is one diverticulum per haustral segment, although on occasion two may be noted (Fig. 45-2a). The diverticula themselves are surprisingly clear of debris in a well-cleaned colon, although in a poorly prepared patient they may either be impacted with stool or barium (even if radiographic studies were performed months earlier).

Differentiation of the Mouth of a Diverticulum from the Lumen

Colonic diverticula are for the most part incidental findings. Their importance as far as the colonoscopic examination is concerned derives from the fact that their openings can be confused with the lumen, making the examiner reluctant to proceed. This is especially the case with multiple diverticula in association with prominent valvulae (Fig. 45-2b), where the examiner is continually concerned about whether the opening entered is the mouth of the larger diverticulum or the lumen (Fig. 45-2b). If he cannot be assured that it is the lumen, quite correctly he stops the examination rather than risk perforation. However, even in the face of multiple diverticula, a somewhat narrowed sigmoid can be negotiated so long as any given opening can be seen in relation to the valvulae. Diverticula are observed as openings between valvulae (Fig. 45-2a), whereas the lumen is seen as an opening at which two valvulae

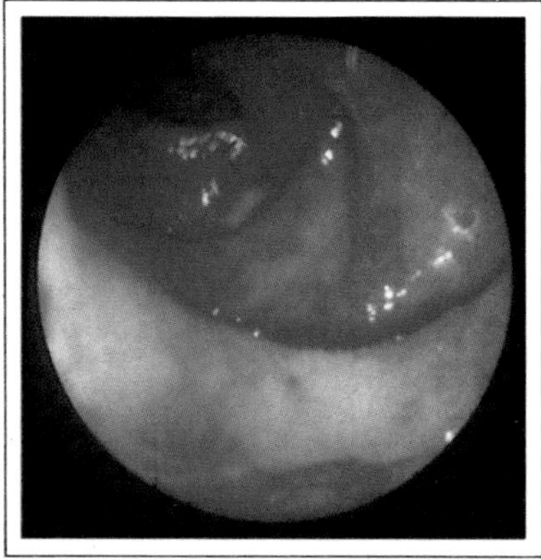

FIG. 45-3a.

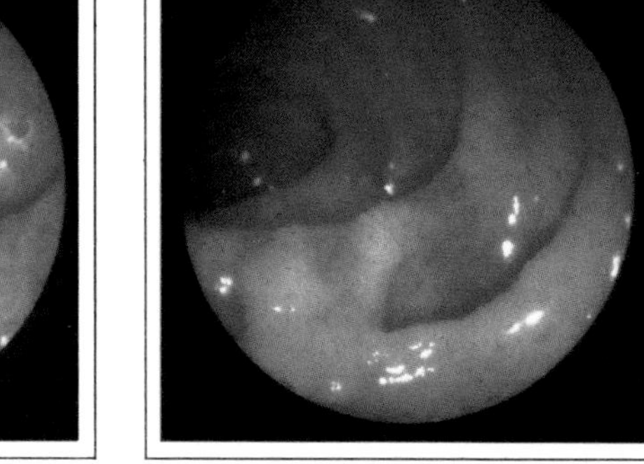

FIG. 45-3b.

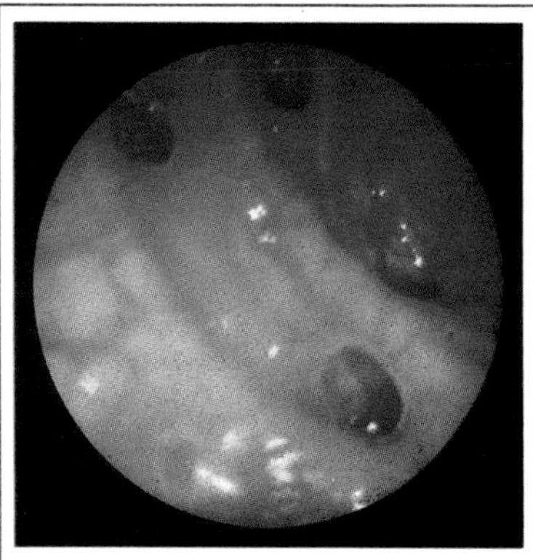

FIG. 45-3c.

FIG. 45-3. a: Acute diverticulitis, resolving. This patient was examined 2 weeks after the onset of fever and left lower quadrant pain because of a barium enema which could not exclude malignancy. Colonoscopy showed enlarged sigmoid valvulae (in comparison with Fig. 44-2b), with mucosal erythema. These changes completely disappeared within the next month (c). **b:** Acute diverticulitis, with a diverticulum exuding a purulent exudate. A close-up view in a patient with acute diverticulitis (a) shows purulent material exuding from an intrahaustral segment, possibly from the perforated diverticulum that initiated the clinical episode. **c:** Colonic diverticulosis after complete resolution of acute diverticulitis (b). The diverticula are easily seen now, without mucosal erythema or enlargement of the valvulae.

converge (Fig. 45-2b). In general, it is this convergence of valvulae which gives the examiner the confidence to proceed (Fig. 45-2b). Should the examiner have any doubt, however, the prudent measure is to withdraw first and reestablish the general direction of the valvulae rather than to proceed blindly into what might be a larger diverticulum with the potential for perforation.

ACUTE DIVERTICULITIS

The pathologic basis for acute diverticulitis is that of a perforation within a single diverticulum.[9] This is thought to result from the presence of a fecolith within the diverticulum which abrades the mucosal lining, ultimately extending through the thin wall of the diverticulum with the formation of a pericolic abscess. In some cases the abscess can extend for a short distance along the bowel wall, forming a dissecting abscess as part of an inflammatory mass.[9] Not surprisingly, a barium enema performed within the first 2 weeks after the onset of acute diverticulitis may suggest a diagnosis of an obstruction neoplasm and prompt colonoscopy, although the endoscopist should be most reluctant to perform an examination at a time when there is some danger of adversely affecting the outcome, especially by direct instrumental injury, i.e., perforation.[5] Still, in cases where there was a strong suspicion of malignancy, we have performed colonoscopy without incident before a clinical episode of acute diverticulitis has entirely resolved.

Appearance

Although only one diverticulum needs to perforate to result in an acute clinical episode, a segment often up to 5 cm may be involved because of the pericolic dissecting abscess type inflammatory mass.[9] This area immediately becomes apparent to the endoscopist because of spasm, marked narrowing of the lumen, and large valvulae (Fig. 45-3a). Depending on how close to the beginning of the acute clinical episode the examination is performed, one sees erythema of the valvulae which may be marked (Fig. 45-3a). In some cases, although it is uncommon, purulent material may be seen to extrude from the mouth of the perforated diverticulum (Fig. 45-3b). After resolution of the acute clinical episode, the erythema, luminal narrowing, and edema of the valvulae may entirely disappear from the picture, which returns to simply multiple diverticula (Fig. 45-3c).

DIVERTICULAR STRICTURES

Apart from rectal bleeding (see Chapter 46), the commonest indication for colonoscopy that arises from diver-

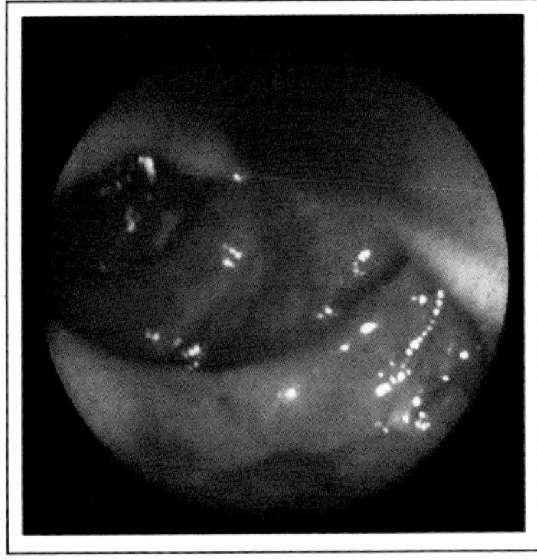

FIG. 45-4a.

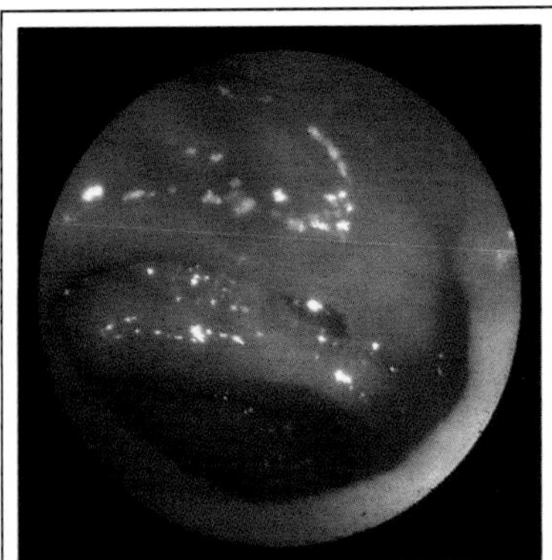

FIG. 45-4b.

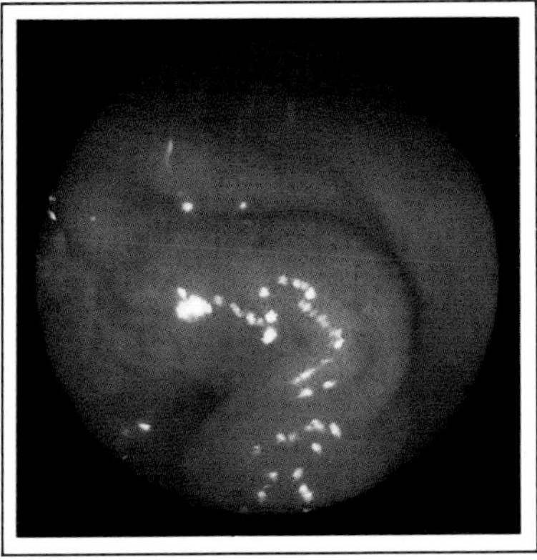

FIG. 45-4c.

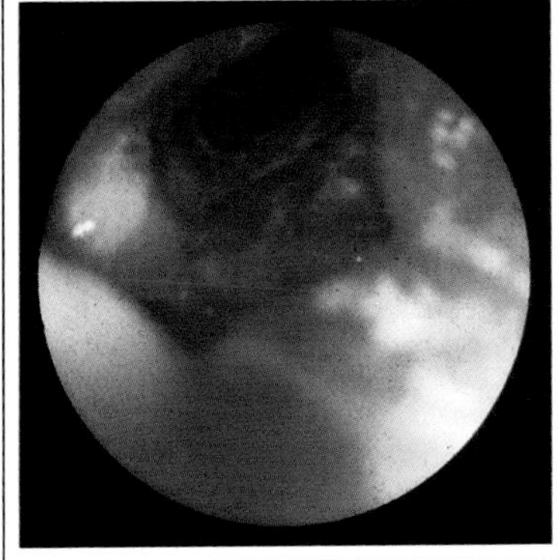

FIG. 45-4d.

FIG. 45-4. a: Acute diverticulitis with stricture. The valvulae are enlarged because of circular muscular hypertrophy and acute inflammatory changes which accompany the clinical episode of acute diverticulitis (same case as Fig. 45-3b). The enlargement of the valvulae results in luminal narrowing (stricture formation) at 10 o'clock which could not, at this time, be traversed. One month later (Fig. 45-3c), with the return of the valvulae to normal size, the stricture had entirely disappeared. **b:** Acute diverticulitis with stricture. An eccentric appearance of the lumen is expected because of the presence of a pericolonic inflammatory mass that forms around the diverticulum which has perforated. The valvulae within the stricture are intact and have a regular appearance in contrast with their appearance with carcinoma (c). **c:** Malignant stricture in association with diverticula (not shown). An asymmetrical, enlarged valvular fold that becomes entirely disrupted at the point at which the stricture begins (at 8 o'clock). This strongly suggests carcinoma. **d:** Malignant stricture (recurrent carcinoma) of the sigmoid. A symmetrical narrowing (from the 6 o'clock wall) is noted with mucosal erythema and friability. The mucosa and valvular appearance of the opposite wall are preserved. This appearance was considered by the examiner to be "indeterminate" in terms of malignancy. Even though biopsies and brushings were negative,[12] a second-look operative procedure was performed, at which time recurrent carcinoma within regional lymph nodes and invading the wall of the sigmoid was discovered.

ticular diseases is the assessment of strictures which are noted radiographically.[10] As clinical features are similar in patients with diverticular disease alone and those with carcinoma,[4] these cannot be used to differentiate the two conditions. Because the barium enema itself, even if done with air contrast, has an overall error rate in the face of diverticular disease of at least 20%[4] and approaches 50% in the presence of neoplasms (either polyps or cancer),[4] colonoscopy has now become the method of choice for determining whether a neoplasm is present in patients with diverticula and, even more importantly, if a given stricture is malignant.[5,10,11]

Appearance

Colonoscopy allows differentiation between: (a) a benign (inflammatory) diverticular stricture; and (b) malignant strictures found in association with diverticular disease.

Benign (Inflammatory) Diverticular Strictures

The colonic narrowing associated with diverticular disease largely results in compromise of the lumen because of thickening of the circular and longitudinal muscle layers. This is particularly apparent in the increased thickness of the valvulae (Fig. 45-4a). Further compromise of the lumen can result from a superimposed pericolic inflammatory mass, as is expected in acute diverticulitis (see above) as well as pericolic fibrosis once the acute inflammation has resolved.[6] In these cases the lumen becomes quite narrow (Fig. 45-4b), although the overlying mucosa is still intact and the valvulae themselves appear symmetrical and regular (Fig. 45-4a). Because the lumen is compromised and the valvulae themselves are enlarged and not easily negotiated and thus appear "spastic," they may be seen only tangentially, so that their symmetry cannot be appreciated (Fig. 45-4a). The valvulae which can be seen, however, maintain their basic shape (Fig. 45-4b), with intact mucosa, which favors the diagnosis of a diverticular stricture[12] rather than carcinoma, which would both obliterate and distort parts of the involved valvulae (Fig. 45-4c). Even in the face of acute diverticulitis with extrinsic compression from a pericolic mass (Fig. 45-4b), within the area giving rise to the distortion the valvulae are intact—in contrast to the malignant stricture, where within the asymmetrical portion the valvulae are obliterated (Fig. 45-4c). Still, carcinoma cannot be excluded by any endoscopic appearance in the face of narrowing, even one where the mucosa appears to be intact. Aste et al. found malignancy in 30% (12 of 41) of such cases.[12]

Malignant Strictures in Association with Diverticular Disease

The loss of the regular, uniform appearance of the valvulae which form the mouth of the stricture is a highly suspicious feature for malignancy (Fig. 45-4c), along with a rock-hard consistency to the folds of the mouth of the malignant stricture. The cardinal feature is the appearance of exophytic tumor masses (Fig. 45-4d). Aste et al.[12] found carcinoma to be associated with this appearance in almost 90% (71 of 81) of cases and found this endoscopic appearance to be the commonest one of colonic cancer associated with stenosis (71 of 82 cases).[12]

Biopsy and Cytology

Biopsy

During biopsy the colonoscope is advanced to a point as close to the narrowed opening as possible (Fig. 45-4d). At least four but preferably six or more biopsies are taken from the mouth of the stricture. Even with biopsy aggressively pursued, it may fail in up to 20% of cases overall and most if not all cases where tumor has not broken through the mucosa.[12] Even for lesions which have broken through, there are still inherent technical difficulties in performing targeted biopsies tangentially within the tubular sigmoid, especially in the face of additional deformity from preexisting diverticular disease.

Cytology

Because of the difficulties mentioned above in obtaining complete technical control for biopsying not only the mouth of the stricture but ideally the portion within, brushing cytology seems to be the desirable adjunctive modality by which the mucosa of a suspicious lesion could be sampled. Several brushings are taken from within the stricture as well as around its mouth with the hope of increasing its yield, especially from the irregular friable surface.[13] Aste et al.[12] found that cytology was as effective as biopsy for this type of exophytic lesion, with either modality having a yield of 95%. For pure infiltrating malignancies where the mucosa appears intact, cytology did not improve the yield, being only 18%, in contrast with cytology for strictures in other locations, e.g., gastric cardia (see Chapter 10), where its yield approaches 70%.[14]

OTHER CAUSES OF SIGMOID NARROWING IN PATIENTS WITH DIVERTICULA

Although diverticular disease and carcinoma (see Chapter 42) account for the large majority of cases, other conditions are observed which would cause narrowing of the sigmoid lumen. These are: (a) extrinsic compression; (b) inflammatory bowel disease; (c) ischemic strictures; (d) radiation strictures; (e) postoperative strictures; and (f) lymphogranuloma venereum. Because of their prevalence in the general population, especially for individuals over the age of 50, incidental diverticula may be found and may create some diagnostic confusion.

Extrinsic Compression

An enlarged (fibroid) uterus or ovary may compress an adjacent wall of the sigmoid, distort the lumen, and create a stricture-like appearance (Fig. 45-5a). This may raise the question of malignancy, especially if not enough of the narrowed area is seen to determine that the valvulae are intact (Fig. 45-5a). If these are intact in the absence of clinically significant diverticular disease (see above), an asymmetrical appearance makes the examiner suspect extrinsic compression and recommend that other studies such as pelvic ultrasound or an abdominal computerized tomographic (CT) scan be obtained in an attempt to determine both if an extrinsic mass is present and its nature. In some cases surgery is required to relieve obstructive symptoms which may have prompted the investigations and to eliminate any lingering suspicion of underlying malignancy.[12]

Inflammatory Bowel Disease

Ulcerative colitis and Crohn's disease especially may coexist with diverticular disease.[15] In one study of resected specimens, histologic evidence of diverticulitis was found in nearly half the cases.[15] Clinically, the presentation of Crohn's colitis with complicating acute diverticulitis is similar to that of Crohn's colitis alone, with fever and pain predominating in either condition.[15] Moreover the radiologic finding of a longitudinal fistulous tract, while once thought pathognomonic of Crohn's (granulomatous) colitis,[16] is now well recognized to occur in diverticulitis alone.[16a]

We regard the finding of erythema, friability, enlarged valvulae, and mucopurulent exudate confined to the sigmoid, in the face of diverticular disease, as evidence of acute diverticulitis alone (Fig. 45-3b) and not Crohn's disease unless typical features of the latter (focal ulcerations, cobblestone appearance, etc.—see Chapter 43) are seen elsewhere. Further support for the appearance being that of acute diverticulitis, rather than inflammatory bowel disease, is a return to a normal appearance (except for diverticula) at colonoscopy performed within 1 month of the first examination (Fig. 45-3c).

Ischemic Strictures

The presence of diverticular disease does not preclude ischemic colitis and the formation of a stricture as a man-

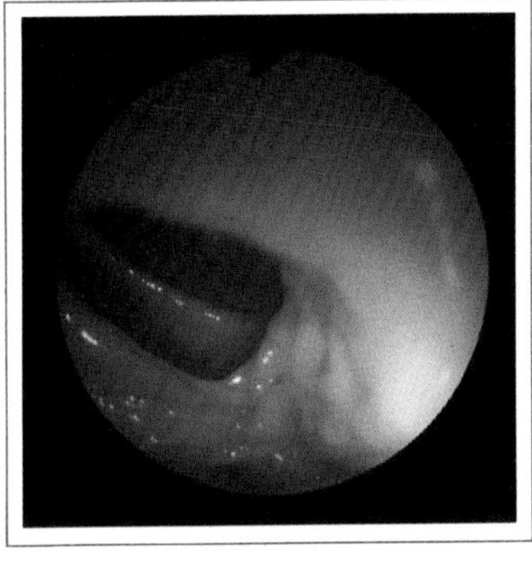

FIG. 45-5a.

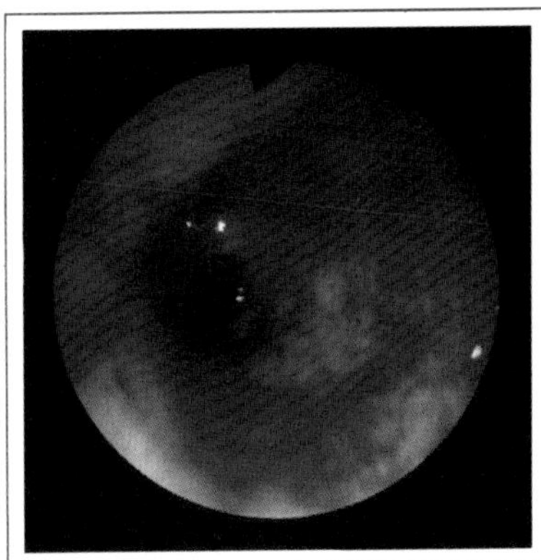

FIG. 45-5b.

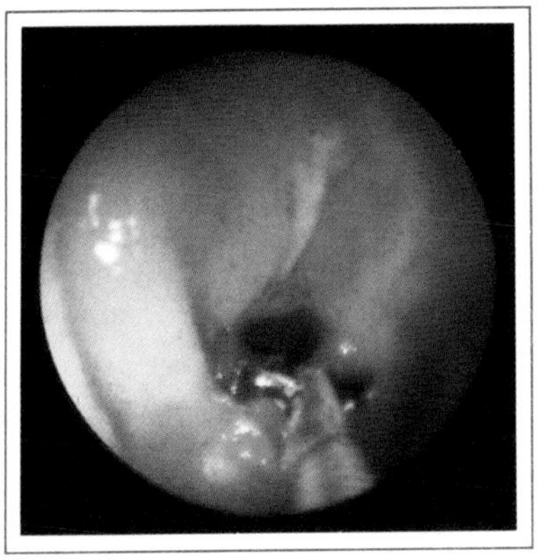

FIG. 45-5c.

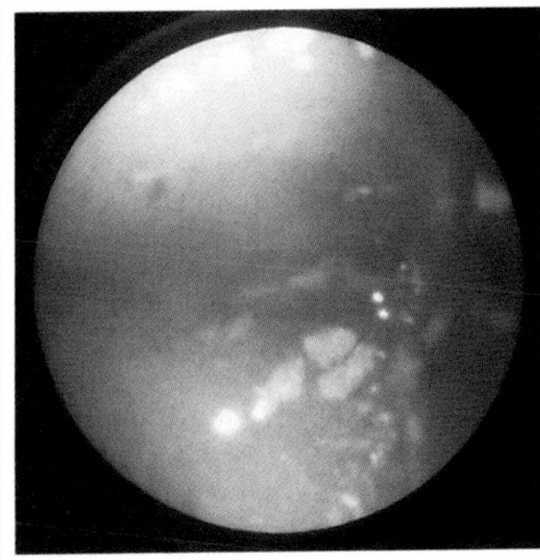

FIG. 45-5d.

FIG. 45-5. a: Extrinsic compression of the sigmoid resulting in lumen narrowing. In this case an enlarged left ovary (ovarian fibroid) compresses the anterior aspect of the mesenteric border (12 to 3 o'clock—see Chapter 39). **b:** Ischemic colitis with stricture. Colonoscopy was performed because of obstructive symptoms in a 70-year-old man 6 weeks after the onset of bloody diarrhea which resolved after 3 weeks. A stricture was found in the proximal descending colon with the surrounding mucosa somewhat erythematous but markedly friable (with considerable bleeding after a general attempt at traversing the stricture). The clinical picture and location suggest that the stricture resulted from focal severe injury to the bowel in the course of ischemic colitis. **c:** Anastomotic stricture of the rectosigmoid after resection of a carcinoma. The diameter of the lumen at this point is approximately 6 mm (two-thirds of the known open forceps width of 9 mm). This indicates that some narrowing has occurred, presumably from tension at the anastomosis (see Chapter 47). The short stricture length (<5 mm) and its symmetrical appearance argue against the diagnosis of recurrent carcinoma (Fig. 45-4d), although it cannot be excluded with absolute certainty. **d:** Lymphogranuloma venereum (LGV) with a mid-rectal stricture. Obstructive symptoms in a male homosexual prompted a fiberoptic examination of the rectum which disclosed this high-grade (diameter <5 mm) stricture 10 cm from the anus. A serum titer for LGV was 1:256 (normal is less than 1:132), indicating prior exposure to LGV in a patient with a typical location and appearance of an LVG stricture.

ifestation of a severe injury (see Chapter 44). Differentiation of a diverticular and ischemic stricture is based on whether the mucosal fold pattern is preserved, as in the case of the diverticular stricture (Fig. 45-3a), or obliterated, as occurs with ischemic injury (Fig. 45-5b). If this occurs along with ulceration set within the stricture in an elderly patient (over the age of 65) with a recent onset of symptoms suggestive of acute colitis (see Chapter 44), an ischemic etiology for the stricture is suggested (Fig. 45-5b).

Radiation Stricture

The history of irradiation in excess of 3,000 rads (see Chapter 44) with resulting focal narrowing, especially of the rectosigmoid, and obliteration of the mucosal fold pattern and telangiectasis causes one to suspect a radiation stricture even in the presence of scattered diverticula.

Postoperative Stricture

Patients with a history of surgery within the sigmoid may show narrowing at the anastomosis,[16] which in the presence of scattered diverticula could create a confusing picture (Fig. 45-5c). Adding further to the confusion in the face of diverticular disease is the patient in whom surgery was performed for malignancy, in which case three possibilities exist for the stricture: (a) a postoperative stricture (see Chapter 47); (b) a diverticular stricture; and (c) a malignant stricture from recurrent carcinoma (see Chapter 42). Colonoscopy is helpful in differentiating these possibilities from each other. In the case of postoperative changes, one expects to find some nodularity at the anastomosis (from interrupted suturing performed in its construction) but with intact mucosa around the narrowed segment, which is short (<2 cm), with a diameter between 5 and 10 mm (Fig. 45-5c). In the case of a diverticular stricture, the area of narrowing is generally longer than 2 cm, but as with the anastomotic stricture it has a luminal diameter of 5 to 10 mm. By contrast, recurrent carcinoma (Fig. 45-4b) is associated with an irregular, asymmetrical type of narrowing[17] (Fig. 45-4d). At the very least, any such asymmetrical type of narrowing should be regarded as an indeterminate appearance, which if occurring in the context of prior surgical resection of the malignancy should be regarded as highly suspicious[16] even if biopsies and/or brushings were negative[12] (Fig. 45-4d).

Lymphogranuloma Venereum

In lymphogranuloma venereum (LGV), caused by the *Chlamydia trachomatis* and being increasingly recognized among homosexuals,[18] stricture formation occurs in the mid-distal rectum within 3 to 5 cm of the anal verge.[17] Even when this extends into the proximal rectum or distal sigmoid, it is not likely to be confused with diverticular strictures which almost never involve the rectum. LGV should be suspected in any homosexual male with a stricture of the rectosigmoid that involves the rectum (Fig. 45-5d) and confirmed by a positive LGV serology (complement fixation titer >1:32).[18]

REFERENCES

1. Manousos, O. N., Truelove, S. C., and Lumsdon, K. (1967): Prevalence of colonic diverticulosis in the general population of the Oxford area. *Lancet,* 3:762–764.
2. Hughes, L. E. (1969): Post-mortem survey of diverticular disease of the colon. I. Diverticulosis and diverticulitis. *Gut,* 10:336–348.
3. Horner, J. L. (1958): Natural history of diverticulosis of the colon. *Am. J. Dig. Dis.,* 3:343–350.
4. Schnyder, P., Moss, A. A., Theoni, R. F., and Margulis, A. R. (1979): A double-blind study of radiologic accuracy in diverticulitis, diverticulosis, and carcinoma of the sigmoid. *J. Clin. Gastroenterol.,* 1:55–66.
5. Forde, K. A. (1977): Colonoscopy in complicated diverticular disease. *Gastrointest. Endosc.,* 23:192–193.

5a. Boulos, P. B., Karamanolis, D. G., Salmon, P. R., and Clark, C. G. (1984): Is colonoscopy necessary in diverticular disease? *Lancet,* 1:95–96.

6. Morson, B. C. (1975): Pathology of diverticular disease of the colon. *Clin. Gastroenterol.,* 4:37–42.
7. Almy, T. P., and Howell, D. A. (1980): Diverticular disease of the colon. *N. Engl. J. Med.,* 302:324–331.
8. Wallers, K. J. (1981): Giant diverticulum arising from the transverse colon in a patient with diverticulosis. *Br. J. Radiol.,* 54:683–684.
9. Roth, J. L. P. (1976): Complications of colonic diverticulitis. *Postgrad. Med.,* 60:115–124.
10. Forde, K. A., Lebwohl, O., and Segmon, W. B. (1980): Colonoscopy as an adjunctive technique in evaluating acquired colonic narrowing. *Surgery,* 87:243–247.
11. Rozen, P., Ratan, J., and Gilat, T. (1975): Colonoscopy in the differential diagnosis of colonic stricture: report of four cases. *Dis. Colon Rectum,* 18:425–429.
12. Aste, H., Pugliese, V., Munizzi, F., and Giacchero, A. (1983): Left-sided stenosing lesions in colonoscopy. *Gastrointest. Endosc.,* 29:18–20.
13. Winawer, S. J., Leidner, S. D., Hajdu, S. I., and Sherlock, P. (1978): Colonoscopic biopsy and cytology in the diagnosis of colon cancer. *Cancer,* 42:2849–2853.
14. Kobayashi, S., and Kasugai, T. (1978): Brushing cytology for diagnosis of gastric cancer involving the cardia or the lower esophagus. *Acta Cytol. (Baltimore),* 2:155–157.
15. Meyers, M. A., Alonzo, D. R., Morson, B. C., and Bartram, C. (1978): Pathogenesis of diverticulitis complicating granulomatous colitis. *Gastroenterology,* 74:24–31.
16. Marshak, R. H., Janowitz, H. D., and Present, D. H. (1970): Granulomatous colitis in association with diverticula. *N. Engl. J. Med.,* 283:1080–1084.

16a. Marshak, R. H., Lindner, A. E., and Maklansky, D. (1980): Paracolic fistulous tracts in diverticulitis and granulomatous colitis. *J.A.M.A.,* 243:1943–1946.

17. Gabrielsson, N., Granqvist, S., and Ohlsen, H. (1976): Recurrent carcinoma of the colon in the anastomosis diagnosed by roentgen examination and colonoscopy. *Endoscopy,* 8:47–57.
18. Levine, J. S., Smith, P. D., and Brugge, W. R. (1980): Chronic proctitis in male homosexuals due to lymphogranuloma venereum. *Gastroenterology,* 79:563–565.

46

COLONIC BLEEDING

Upper gastrointestinal (GI) bleeding is generally acute and of a magnitude and severity that requires hospitalization (see Chapter 32). Colonic bleeding, on the other hand, is more often of a chronic, intermittent nature. For the most part it is not immediately life-threatening, but prior to the widespread use of colonoscopy the danger had been from the high percentage of causative lesions that were missed using the then available diagnostic combination of proctoscopy and single-contrast barium studies. Since that time, colonoscopy has revealed that cancer may be expected in 10% of this group, adenomas in an additional 15%, and angiodysplasia in about 5%.[1-5] Colonoscopy therefore provides a diagnosis for one-third of patients with colonic bleeding for whom there might otherwise have been no explanation of their bleeding. In the case of cancer or angiodysplasia, the colonoscopic diagnosis may be life-saving.

A less common though more dramatic presentation is that of massive colonic bleeding that requires hospitalization. Prior to the advent of colonoscopy, such patients who had unrevealing proctoscopy, barium contrast studies, or even arteriography would have been simply transfused with a hope that their bleeding would stop and not recur after discharge. Unfortunately, in 20 to 30% the bleeding either continued or recurred. In many of these a resection of some or all of the colon was performed.[6] In these often elderly patients with cardiac and other major medical illnesses, the mortality of such empiric resections was high, approaching 10%,[6] and many who survived the surgery continued bleeding, especially if only a partial resection was performed.[6]

For a patient hospitalized now for colonic bleeding but whose bleeding stops, it has become routine to prepare such patients for colonoscopy in the standard fashion (see Chapter 39) in order to demonstrate the cause, similar to patients with chronic intermittent bleeding.[7] Even for patients whose active bleeding continues, colonoscopy has been reported as having a high diagnostic yield,[7] though this has not been our experience, where in this setting, it generally proves to be a futile exercise.

Our focus in this chapter, therefore, is on colonoscopy as a diagnostic tool for patients who are not actively bleeding. We consider the colonic appearances of such patients under two general headings: (a) nonvascular conditions, including neoplasms and diverticular bleeding; and (b) vascular conditions, with the major emphasis on colonic angiodysplasia.

NONVASCULAR CAUSES OF COLONIC BLEEDING

Neoplasms

In all reported series neoplasms (cancers and adenomas considered together) are the commonest lesions identified at colonoscopy in patients with colonic bleeding. These may be expected in up to 20 to 30% for both chronic intermittent[1-5] as well as acute bleeding.[7] They represent 60% or more of the lesions found in patients with chronic intermittent bleeding.[1,2] Significantly, cancers are found in about 10% (range 8 to 11%) of patients with chronic intermittent bleeding[1-5] as well as those with the acute type.[7]

Although the largest percentage of colonic neoplasms associated with bleeding are located in the rectosigmoid, at least 30% of the cancers are proximal to the sigmoid[8] and out of reach of the flexible (60 cm) sigmoidoscope. This makes total colonoscopy mandatory for any patient with colonic bleeding.

Appearance

Adenomas.

The adenomas which bleed tend to be large (Fig. 46-1a), 1 to 2+ cm.[5,6] Bleeding therefore may occur because the size of these polyps causes them to be repeatedly traumatized. In addition, the surface of a polyp which has bled is often quite friable (Fig. 46-1b), which predisposes to contact bleeding with the passage of stool (Fig. 46-1c), in contrast to smaller polyps (Fig. 46-1d). Occasionally, the preparation for the examination is vigorous enough to cause the polyp to begin to bleed (Fig. 46-1c), which facilitates their detection.

Carcinoma.

Carcinomas which are detected because of bleeding are generally of the polypoid type (Fig. 46-2a; see also Chapter 41). Many are found as focally invasive cancers in adenomas (Fig. 46-2b), which is the earliest type of colonic cancer that can be identified. These are almost always located in the sigmoid. Other colonic cancers associated with bleeding, especially those of the right colon (Fig. 46-2c), are discovered as ulcerated masses. In contrast to polypoid cancers of the sigmoid, many right-sided cancers that have this appearance (Fig. 46-2d) have already metastasized at the time they are detected, especially if the patient is symptomatic or there had been a delay in diagnosis from the onset of symptomless rectal bleeding.[8a] As a polypoid cancer of the left colon, the lesion may be visually indistinguishable from an adenoma (Fig. 46-2b), but more often its ulcerated, sharply angulated or rock-hard surface provides the examiner with some indication of its being malignant (Fig. 46-2d). As in the case of the adenoma, preparation for colonoscopy may induce bleeding from the carcinoma (Fig. 46-2c), which aids in its detection.

Inflammatory Bowel Disease

In patients with intermittent rectal bleeding who have negative or equivocal barium contrast studies and proctoscopy, 4 to 10% of the colonoscopic examinations performed reveal evidence of either ulcerative colitis or Crohn's disease.[1–5] Because rectal involvement in ulcerative colitis is usually striking and is expected to be readily diagnosed by proctoscopy, many of the cases which are initially diagnosed at colonoscopy are Crohn's disease, both because of its tendency for rectum sparing as well as its right-sided and segmental involvement, which may not be readily apparent on barium contrast examinations of the colon.

Appearance

The findings in patients with bleeding and inflammatory bowel disease do not differ from those in patients who present to colonoscopy for other reasons (see Chapter 43). In cases where colonoscopy is performed because of bleeding in ulcerative colitis, the picture of severe colitis (Fig. 46-3a) is observed with spontaneous bleeding from the mucosal surface (Fig. 46-3b). In the patient with Crohn's disease examined because of colonic bleeding, focal deep ulcerations are seen (Fig. 46-3c), especially at the anastomoses from prior surgery (Fig. 46-3d).

Ischemic Colitis

Approximately 1% of all patients who have colonoscopy because of rectal bleeding are found to have ischemic colitis[1,2]; however, for patients over the age of 65 the incidence may be higher, approaching 5%.[9] As we have noted elsewhere (see Chapter 44), these patients have had episodes of rectal bleeding, diarrhea, tenesmus, and fever that simulate inflammatory bowel disease, with similar colonoscopic and histologic appearances. Only the age of the patient (>65) and the rapid evolution of the episode toward healing are likely to suggest the correct diagnosis of ischemic colitis.[10]

Appearance

In patients with ischemic colitis who present with bleeding, one observes features of an acute stage (see Chapter 44); these include marked mucosal friability with spontaneous bleeding and intramucosal hemorrhage, evidenced by the presence of petechiae and ecchymoses (Fig. 46-4a).

Radiation Colitis

Among elderly patients (>65 years), up to 3%[9] have recurrent rectal bleeding secondary to irradiation, with the site of bleeding being the rectosigmoid. A history of pelvic irradiation for cervical or other gynecologic cancer in a patient with recurrent bleeding strongly suggests this diagnosis (see Chapter 44).

Appearance

Rectosigmoid narrowing associated with intense erythema and friability along with the presence of telangiectasis is the expected colonoscopic finding in patients with bleeding from this cause (Fig. 46-4b).[11]

Diverticular Disease

Diverticular disease accounts for an uncertain percentage of patients with colonic bleeding of both the acute and chronic-intermittent types. This is true for several reasons. First, diverticula are common in the general population over the age of 50 who are likely to bleed (see Chapter 45), occurring in upwards of one-third. Not surprisingly, diverticula are found in one-third or more of the patients who present with acute bleeding episodes[9] and in over half of the patients with chronic-intermittent bleeding in whom no lesion is found at colonoscopy (showing only diverticula).[2] Furthermore, if one were to require actual dem-

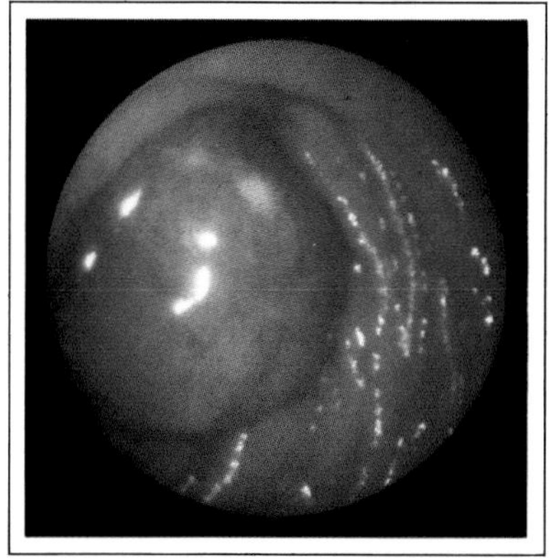

FIG. 46-1a.

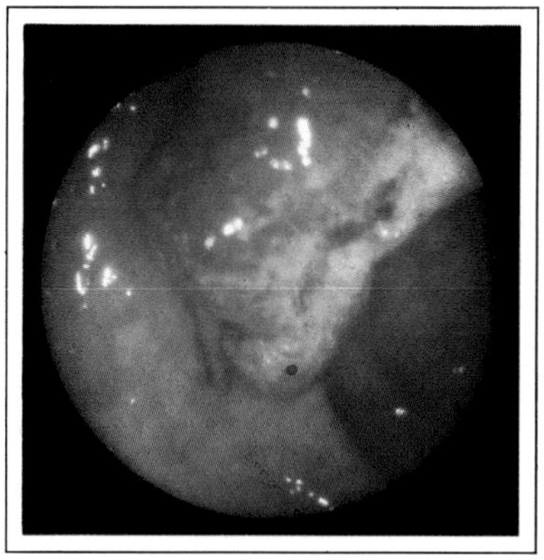

FIG. 46-1b.

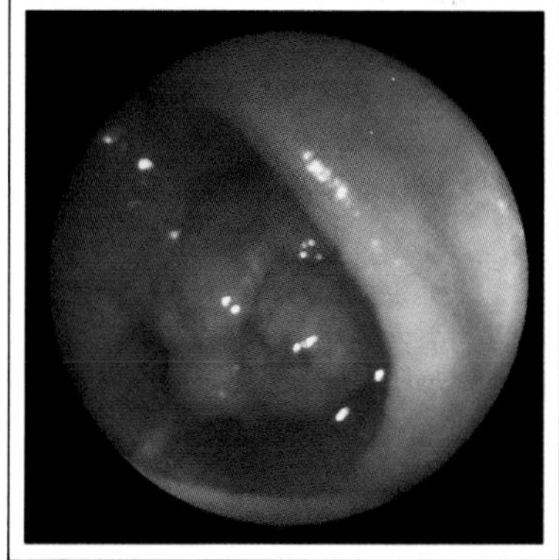

FIG. 46-1c.

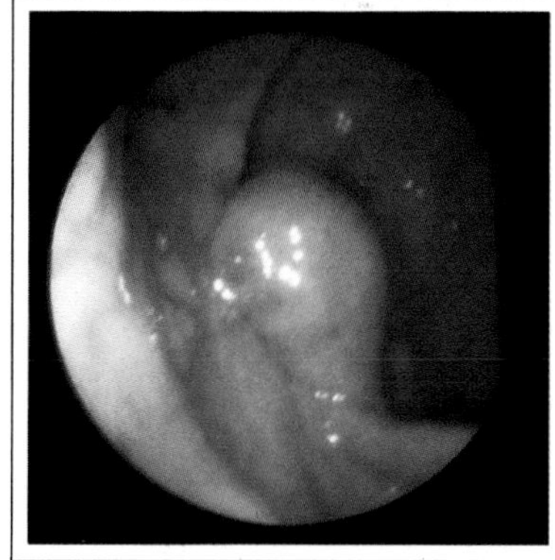

FIG. 46-1d.

FIG. 46-1. a: Large (1.5 cm) tubular adenoma of the sigmoid in a patient with intermittent rectal bleeding. Polyps of this size and location may bleed because they project into the lumen and are repeatedly traumatized by the passage of formed stool. **b:** Large (2.5 cm) villous adenoma of the sigmoid in a patient with intermittent rectal bleeding. The surface was erythematous and friable. In this polyp the size, location, and surface friability all contribute to its tendency to bleed. **c:** Large (1.5 cm) tubulovillous adenoma of the splenic flexure in a patient with one episode of rectal bleeding. The colonoscopic preparation itself has caused the friable surface of this polyp to bleed. **d:** Tubular adenoma (8 mm) of the sigmoid in a patient with a positive fecal occult blood test. A polyp of this size without evidence of surface friability may be considered an incidental finding. Polyps of this size might be expected in up to 10% of asymptomatic individuals over the age of 40.[23]

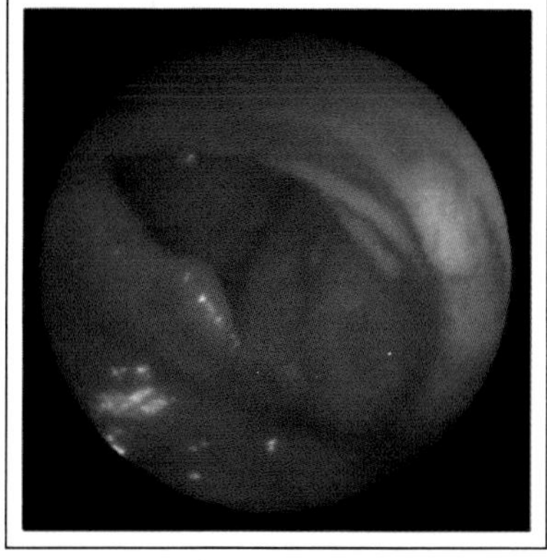

FIG. 46-2a.

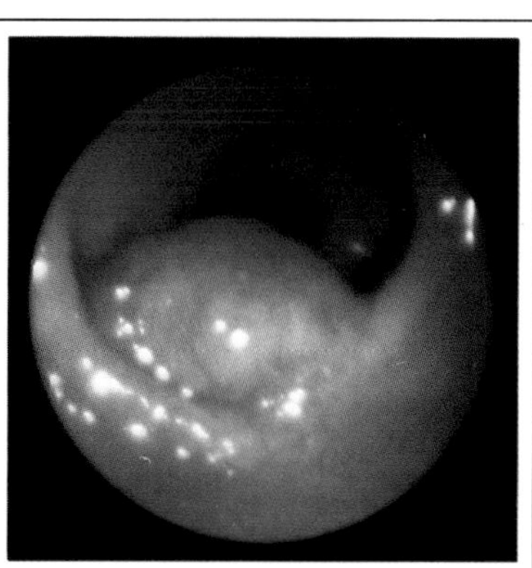

FIG. 46-2b.

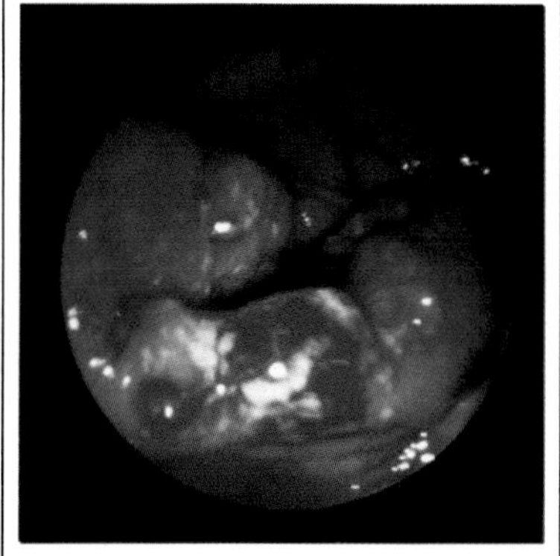

FIG. 46-2c.

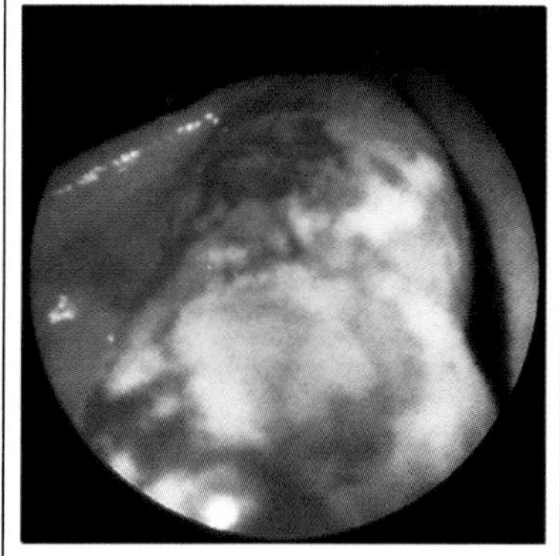

FIG. 46-2d.

FIG. 46-2. a: Polypoid carcinoma of the sigmoid in a patient presenting with several episodes of rectal bleeding and a negative single-contrast barium enema. As in the case of the adenoma, bleeding probably occurs because the friable surface is repeatedly traumatized with the passage of formed stool. Most carcinomas for which colonoscopy is performed because of bleeding are of the polypoid type and are located in the sigmoid.[3] **b:** Polypoid carcinoma of the sigmoid. The indication for colonoscopy was a positive test for fecal occult blood performed in an asymptomatic patient as part of a general physical examination. Repeated trauma to the surface by formed stool results in a positive test. The absence of obvious friability as well as the small size of the lesion may account for the absence of gross rectal bleeding. **c:** Cecal carcinoma in a patient with intermittent rectal bleeding and iron deficiency anemia. Up to one-third of carcinomas associated with rectal bleeding are right-sided,[6] making total colonoscopy rather than flexible sigmoidoscopy mandatory. Right-sided lesions, as in this case, are commonly advanced, i.e., a large mass with central deep ulcerations (see Chapter 42). In this case local as well as metastatic spread to the liver was found at surgery. **d:** Polypoid carcinoma of the ascending colon in an asymptomatic patient with a positive occult fecal blood test. Although most cancers found in such patients are in the sigmoid, some are right-sided lesions that require total colonoscopy. In this case the rock-hard surface and sharply angulated configuration suggested the correct diagnosis.

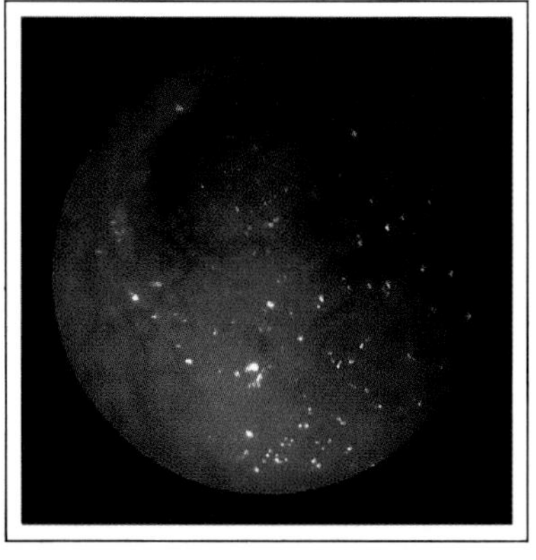

FIG. 46-3a.

FIG. 46-3b.

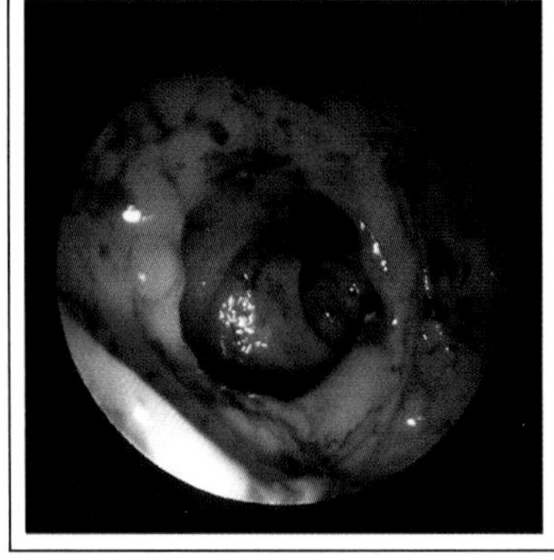

FIG. 46-3c.

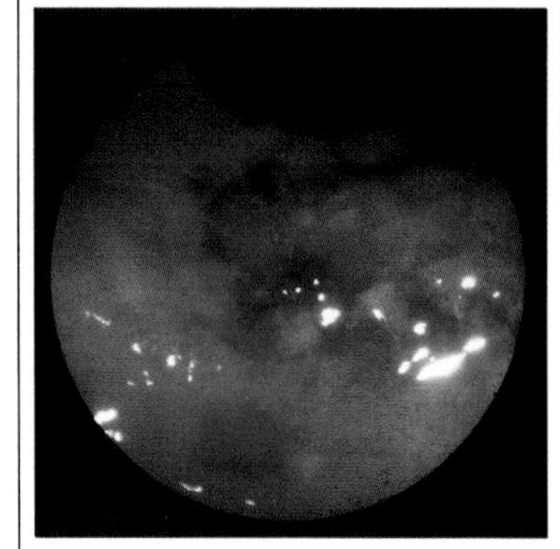

FIG. 46-3d.

FIG. 46-3. a: Ulcerative colitis, bleeding. Clinically significant bleeding is generally observed in severe colitis where blood exudes from large surface areas, particularly those of the descending and transverse colon. **b:** Ulcerative colitis, severe, associated with the clinical presentation of bleeding. Evidence of severe colitis is still present proximal to the transverse colon where active bleeding was observed (a) with a diffusely ulcerated, friable surface and a small amount of spontaneous bleeding. **c:** Crohn's colitis, bleeding. Bright red blood was observed from the 3 o'clock aspect of an ileocolic anastomosis in a patient whose estimated blood loss is 20 cc per day. The 5-mm depression from which the blood seems to emanate suggests the presence of a deep focal ulceration (confirmed at surgery). The dark material around the anastomosis is probably a mixture of iron (which the patient had been taking prior to examination) and old blood. **d:** Crohn's colitis, bleeding. An area of focal ulceration with clots in a patient with intermittent bleeding.

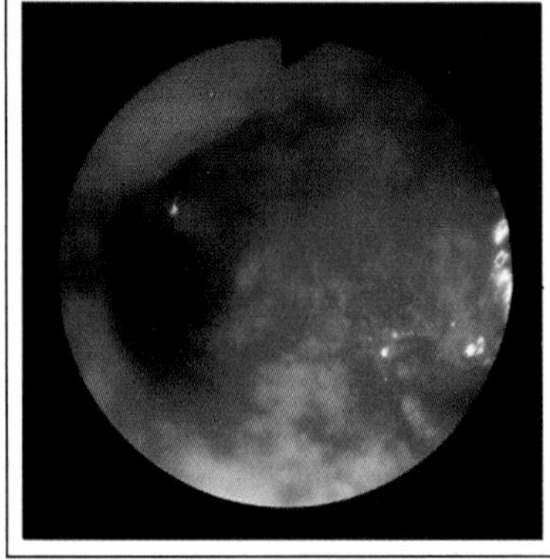

FIG. 46-4a.

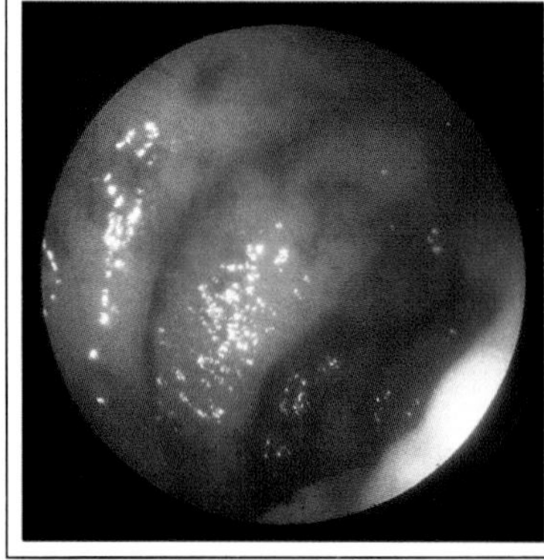

FIG. 46-4b.

FIG. 46-4. a: Ischemic colitis, bleeding. A focal area of narrowing and spontaneous bleeding at the rectosigmoid was noted with dusky mucosa elsewhere within the rectum. These changes, occurring in a patient with the recent onset of abdominal pain and bloody diarrhea, disappeared over the ensuing 3-week period. Rapid resolution (within 4 weeks) of an acute colitis in the absence of antibiotics or an infectious etiology favors a diagnosis of ischemic colitis. **b:** Radiation colitis, bleeding. Telangiectasia and thickening of the valvulae of the rectosigmoid were present in a patient with intermittent bleeding after receiving 4,500 rads to the pelvis for cervical carcinoma.

onstration of active bleeding from a diverticulum, either at colonoscopy or arteriography, to establish it as a cause of colonic bleeding, then one would be forced to consider diverticular bleeding rare—certainly for patients in whom colonoscopy was not performed emergently.[1] In one series of 250 patients who were examined for rectal bleeding but not emergently, diverticula were found in only 2 of 89 who had a definite diagnosis and in only 1% (2 of 215) for the group as a whole.[1] For hospitalized patients having colonoscopy because of acute bleeding, the percent having diverticular bleeding is higher, about 20%,[7] although proof of the actual bleeding site is not always possible in such patients, even among those who undergo surgery. Here the diagnosis of diverticular bleeding is based simply on the presence of diverticulosis and failure to identify other definite causes.[9] In one series where diverticular bleeding was thought to account for 43% of patients hospitalized because of colonic bleeding, in only one-fifth of these (8%) was a definite diagnosis established.[9] Still, the fact that diverticula appear in a high percentage of patients whose acute bleeding is otherwise unexplained[9] may indicate that they may also be a cause of chronic-intermittent bleeding in the patient in whom they are the only finding.[1] The fact that they are not generally observed to bleed may have resulted in diverticulosis being underestimated as a cause of chronic-intermittent colonic bleeding. Although it cannot be proved, one suspects that the thinness of the diverticular mucosal layer as well as its proximity to the penetrating nutrient artery could result in a more chronic-intermittent type of bleeding than is presently imagined, especially in the one-third of patients who are colonoscoped because of rectal bleeding where diverticula are the only finding.[2]

Pathogenesis of Diverticular Bleeding

As previously discussed (see Chapter 45), a diverticulum has a close anatomic relationship to the mucosal blood supply, forming at the site at which the penetrating nutrient artery runs. Many diverticula are found in association with circular muscle hypertrophy, noted both radiologically and at colonoscopy as enlarged valvulae. Measurements of intraluminal pressure in such cases show it to be raised. This increased intraluminal pressure may be transmitted through the wall of the diverticulum to the adjacent vessel, leading to eccentric, intimal thickening along with thinning of its medial wall. The distortion in the vessel wall is thought ultimately to weaken it and predispose it to rupture into the diverticulum, with resultant bleeding which is often massive.[12] Whether this process may also lead to smaller amounts of intermittent bleeding is often unknown, although certainly possible.

Location

Diverticular bleeding when massive is said to occur mainly on the right side; however, this impression is exclusively derived from arteriographic studies where extravasation of contrast material is demonstrated.[13] In other studies of surgically proven diverticular bleeding in patients with negative arteriograms, left-sided diverticula predominate.[9] As diverticular bleeding is demonstrated angiographically in only a small fraction of cases where it is the final diagnosis,[9] left-sided diverticula are probably commoner, although right-sided diverticula possibly tend to bleed more massively and so have a definitive arteriographic diagnosis before surgery. The occasional diverticula that we have observed to bleed at colonoscopy have been left-sided.

Appearance

Diverticular bleeding may be so brisk that the colonoscopist sees only blood (Fig. 46-5a). If he is fortunate enough to see the lumen, he may see blood welling up from the bleeding diverticulum which results in copious amounts of blood filling up the colon distal to this, whereas proximally there is little or no blood (Fig. 46-5b). Even if one did not see the bleeding diverticulum, localizing the site to the left colon would, in the face of diverticula but no other potential cause, cause the examiner to strongly suspect a diverticular origin.

Because of the reluctance of many examiners to attempt colonoscopy in the face of active bleeding, patients come to colonoscopy when the bleeding has stopped. In these cases only scattered, single or multiple diverticula are seen (Fig. 46-5c). With a patient who presents with colonic bleeding but no other apparent bleeding site and with no melena in the ileocecal area to cause one to suspect a bleeding site proximal to the colon (see below), the examiner suspects that the bleeding has a diverticular origin because of the prevalence of diverticula as a cause of colonic bleeding, which may approach 40% in patients over the age of 65.[9]

Other Nonvascular Causes

Colonic Causes

A variety of unusual causes of colonic bleeding accounts for less than 5% of patients with either acute[9] or chronic-intermittent bleeding.[1–5] Some were already considered under the heading "Unusual Causes of Colitis" (see Chapter 44), e.g., *Campylobacter*, antibiotic, and amebic colitis. Another rare cause is the colonic ulcer syndrome (see Chapter 47). Finally, some cases of massive, acute bleeding occur following colonoscopic polypectomy.

Small Intestinal Sites

Bleeding from small intestinal sites presents either as melena (Fig. 46-6a)[14] or as the maroon or bright red blood per rectum commonly associated with colonic bleeding.[15] In one series of 64 patients who were referred for colonoscopy because of acute rectal bleeding, 10% (7 of 64) of the bleeding originated in the small bowel or higher.[15] Small bowel bleeding sites from the terminal ileum may still be within reach of the colonoscope. These include ulcerating submucosal tumors (leiomyomas or carcinoids) or vascular causes (angiodysplasia or varices). In young patients (under 30), the bleeding may be from a Meckel's diverticulum. In cases where there are orthostatic blood pressure changes, the cause may be a duodenal bulb ulcer even if the nasogastric aspirate is negative for blood (see Chapter 38).

Appearance.

At colonoscopy for small intestinal bleeding, the commonest finding is melena throughout the colon (Fig. 46-6a). Although this often obscures colonic mucosa to a degree that a colonic lesion could be missed, the presence of this melena in the terminal ileum (Fig. 46-6b) is an important clue to its originating above the ileocecal valve. Because of the similarity in appearance between melena (Fig. 46-6b) and the presence of iron (Fig. 46-6c), which patients with chronic intermittent bleeding may have been

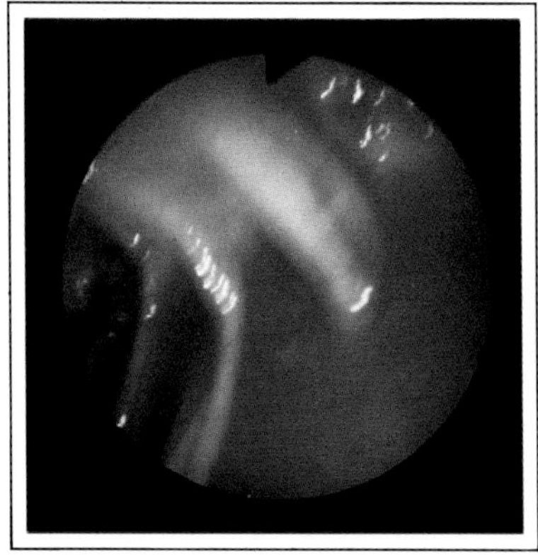

FIG. 46-5a.

FIG. 46-5b.

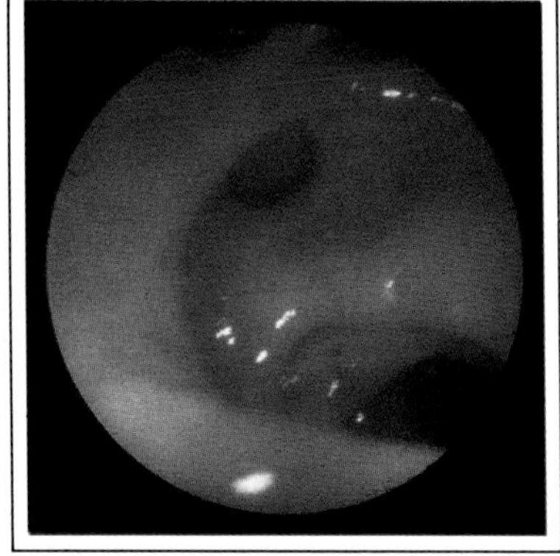

FIG. 46-5c.

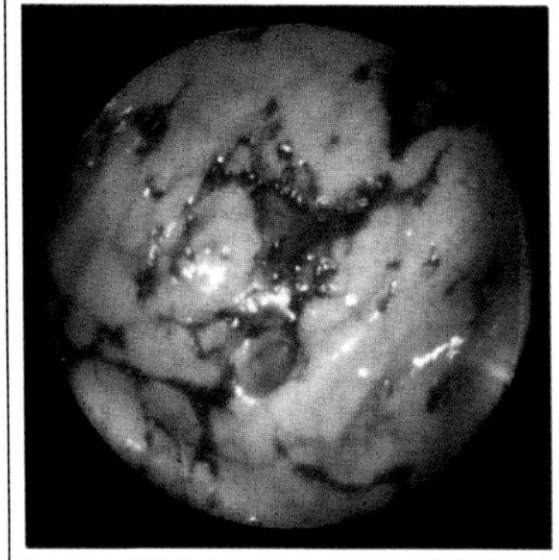

FIG. 46-6a.

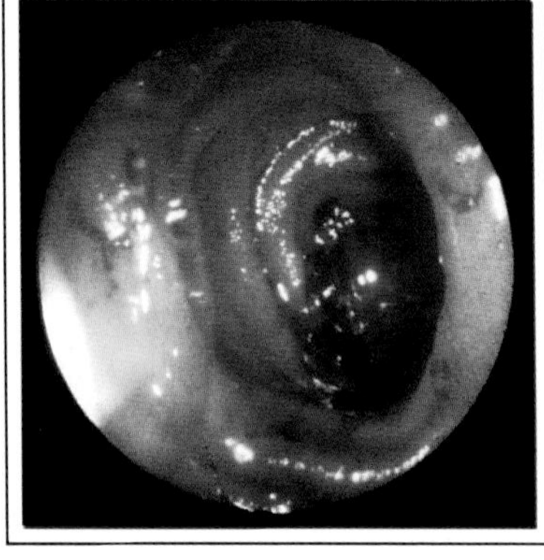

FIG. 46-6b.

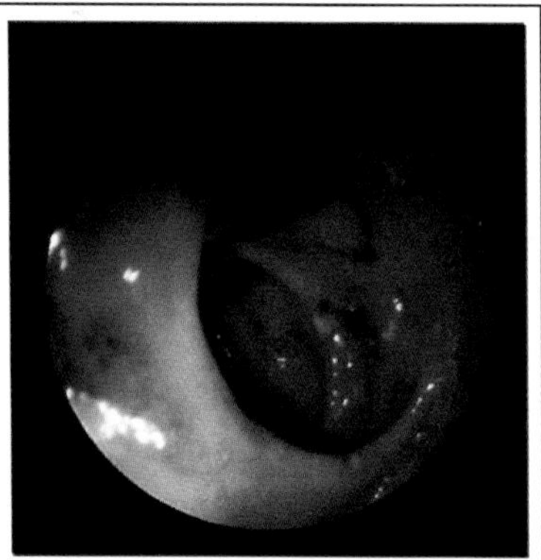

FIG. 46-6c.

FIG. 46-5. a: Diverticular bleeding, massive. Bright red blood could be seen welling up in the sigmoid in a patient with known diverticulosis which the blood completely obscures. In contrast to diverticular bleeding demonstrated by angiography,[12] at colonoscopy the bleeding is typically left-sided, with the proximal colon free of blood (b). **b:** Splenic flexure in a patient with massive diverticular bleeding from the sigmoid. In this case the splenic flexure is free of blood, indicating a distal site of bleeding. **c:** Sigmoid diverticular disease after recent bleeding. Only scattered diverticula were seen, with no other potential site of bleeding identified.

FIG. 46-6. a: Small intestinal bleeding, chronic. Examination of the colon revealed considerable amounts of melanotic material that was strongly guaiac-positive. **b:** Small intestinal bleeding. Intubation of the terminal ileum also showed melanotic material (seen in the distance). A definite bleeding site could not be identified, nor was one apparent on upper GI endoscopy. Surgical resection of 50 cm of terminal ileum and right colon failed to affect the bleeding diathesis, suggesting the possibility of single or multiple angiodysplasia lesions of the small bowel.[16] **c:** Iron within the terminal ileum simulating melena (b). Iron should be suspected where the melena has a greenish hue (best seen in this case at 7 o'clock) when intensely illuminated. In this case the melena was guaiac-negative, consistent with the presence of iron.

taking, one would wish to test the "melena" for blood; this can be done simply by aspirating a small quantity through a polyethylene cannula. Even if the site of bleeding cannot be more precisely identified because of the melena, as a result of the colonoscopy it is localized to the small bowel.

VASCULAR CAUSES OF COLONIC BLEEDING

With the advent of colonoscopy, it has been possible to visualize and often treat vascular lesions of the colon which hitherto could only be demonstrated angiographically or at surgery, but more often went undiagnosed. Colonoscopy has revealed that these vascular abnormalities, especially angiodysplasia, are an important cause of colonic bleeding, accounting for chronic-intermittent bleeding in up to 4% of patients overall and for up to 20% of major bleeding episodes in elderly patients (over the age of 65).[9]

Angiodysplasia

Even before colonoscopy became widely used, arteriography had already established angiodysplasia (also known as vascular ectasia, arteriovenous malformation, hemangiomas of the right colon, etc.)[16] as an important cause of both chronic-intermittent[16–18] and acute massive colonic bleeding.[9] The precise incidence of angiodysplasia as a cause of otherwise unexplained colonic bleeding has varied considerably. In angiographic studies performed on patients hospitalized for colonic bleeding, this has ranged between 12 and 70%,[16] with the actual figure probably closer to 20%.[9] The availability of colonoscopy has confirmed angiodysplasia as a significant cause of colonic bleeding, although with a low overall incidence of only 1%[1] to 8%,[7] even with acute colonic bleeding (8%).[7] Future studies are required to determine if the incidence at colonoscopy is higher (approaching 20%), as it is for patients over the age of 65 with bleeding who require hospitalization and who have arteriography.[9] Another subset of patients who may have a higher incidence of angiodysplasia are those with aortic stenosis.[16]

Pathogenesis

The origin of colonic angiodysplasia remains unsettled. It has been viewed as[16]: (a) congenital; (b) the result of mechanical factors; (c) an effect of hypoxemia; and (d) a degenerative change. Of these theories, the idea suggested by Boley et al.[17] that angiodysplasia is a result of degenerative vascular changes associated with aging seems best to account for this condition. According to this theory, the angiodysplasia lesion is the result of dilatation of normal capillary rings which surround the mucosal crypts, from partial obstruction of the submucosal veins which drain these rings at points where they pierce circular and longitudinal muscles. This obstruction, the result of hypertrophy of surrounding muscle fibers, causes the vein and associated capillary ring to become dilated and tortuous. Over time, other veins and venules draining into the obstructed veins become similarly involved, with the capillary ring finally becoming dilated, the precapillary sphincter incompetent, and an arteriovenous communication forming across the dilated ring.[17] In support of the concept that these lesions relate to aging, Boley et al. used a rubber injection technique to demonstrate angiodysplasia lesions in one-third of patients over the age of 50 (who had had a colectomy for reasons other than bleeding) which were identical to those in patients with bleeding. On the basis of this, he suggested that as many as one-third of middle-aged and elderly patients have the potential for colonic bleeding from angiodysplasia, although only a small percentage of these actually bleed. What may predispose patients with aortic stenosis and angiodysplasia lesions to bleed, Boley et al. suggested,[17] is an ischemic effect on the endothelial lining of the lesion,[17] the result of diminished cardiac output. Because of the larger diameter of the cecum and right colon (with greater amounts of tension on the colonic wall), most angiodysplasia lesions occur in these locations (with the colonic wall tension contributing to the partial obstruction of the submucosal veins); moreover, any angiodysplasia lesion present is prone to bleed with any alteration in cardiac output such as may occur with aortic stenosis.[17]

Location

In a review of all reported cases, in addition to 22 of their own, Meyer et al. found 77.5% of the 218 lesions reported up to 1978 to be in the cecum or right colon.[16] This represented 98% of all colonic sites.

Younger patients (under the age of 50) have a different distribution of intestinal angiodysplasia. In these cases the small bowel represents the site of 67% of the lesions, compared with only 18.8% of the group as a whole.[16]

Relation of Colonic to Gastric Angiodysplasia

Patients with one angiodysplasia lesion of the right colon may have a second.[18,19] When this occurs, the second lesion is generally elsewhere in the right colon and less often in the ileum; only rarely is the second site gastric. Therefore one does not expect to find gastric angiodysplasia (see Chapter 37) in patients with single or multiple colonic lesions. On the other hand, an uncertain but possibly significant percent of patients with gastric angiodysplasia (see Chapter 37) will have colonic lesions.[20] These should be sought by colonoscopy particularly in patients where some feature of the bleeding suggests it to be colonic, e.g., the passage of bright red blood or maroon colored stools, in addition to melena. In cases where patients do have multiple small (<5 mm) angiodysplasia lesions of the stomach, duodenum, and colon, one senses a similarity to patients with hereditary hemorrhagic telangiectasia (see below). However, it remains unsettled as to whether these patients without cutaneous telangiectasias have a *forme fruste* of hereditary hemorrhagic telangiectasia.[20]

Appearance

Two types of colonic lesion, based on size, are observed. These are: (a) small lesions (<5 mm in greatest dimension); and (b) large lesions (5 mm or more).

Small lesions.

Small lesions are observed as 2- to 5-mm single, flat, bright red spots (Fig. 46-7a) with round, uniform or slightly irregular margins (Fig. 46-7b). Tedesco et al.[19] found these to represent slightly more than half of the total (8 of 14) in their series, although Rogers found this size to represent less than half of the total at our institution.[18]

Large lesions.

Large lesions appear as raised, reddened areas with a maximum dimension exceeding 5 mm and a distinctly irregular margin, representing the communication of the lesion with the surrounding capillaries (Fig. 46-7c). Whereas Tedesco et al.[19] found these larger lesions to represent less than half of their total, they constituted more than half of the lesions found by Rogers, with one-third ranging in size between 9 and 15 mm.[18] Others have reported even larger lesions, of several centimeters.[16]

With the larger lesion, the patient generally has episodes of recurrent bleeding. In addition, one may find ulcerations from the lesion itself, possibly from ischemic necrosis (see above), which would be indicative of the proneness of the lesion to rebleed.

Number

Both Rogers[18] and Tedesco et al.[19] report the cases to be equally divided in regard to single and multiple lesions. Multiple lesions may be small and occur together (Fig. 46-8a) or be separated by considerable distances (Fig. 46-8b), although still distributed largely in the right or transverse colon (Fig. 46-8c). In about 10% the second area of involvement is the distal transverse colon or the descending colon. We have noted a distinctive appearance for multiple large angiodysplasia lesions where they appear in the same segment, being connected by small bridging capillaries (Fig. 46-8c).

Differentiation from Instrumental Artifacts

The irregular margin of a colonic angiodysplasia lesion resulting from its connection to the adjacent capillary bed (Fig. 46-7b) allows it to be distinguished from instrumental artifact, i.e., endoscope-induced intermucosal hemorrhage (Fig. 46-8d). In the latter case the margin is typically uniform. In some cases, however, it may be impossible to tell simply by appearance, as the margin of an instrumental artifact can be somewhat irregular. In these cases the location is crucial. The finding of a discrete red spot in the sigmoid, an uncommon location of angiodysplasia but a common one for an endoscope-induced traumatic artifact, argues for the latter. In this instance, one does not resort to endoscopic therapy but does wish to observe the red spot at a subsequent examination and treat it (see below) if it is present at that time.

Endoscopic Treatment and Biopsy

Treatment.

It has been possible to treat colonic angiodysplasia electrosurgically[18,21] using the Williams' biopsy forceps, which allows electrocoagulation of the lesion(s). For symptomatic patients with recurrent and symptomatic bleeding treatment has been effective, although several applications are necessary in up to 10%[21] especially for larger lesions (Fig. 46-9a), which are not entirely obliterated with just one treatment (Fig. 46-9c), and multiple lesions. Whether angiodysplasia discovered as an incidental finding should be treated is unsettled. The tendency of these lesions to bleed is variable (Fig. 46-7d). Even among the lesions which have already bled, a significant percentage do not rebleed. Tedesco et al. found that four of five untreated angiodysplasia lesions had no further bleeding over the next 8 to 13 months.[19] Meyer et al. noted recurrent bleeding in only 33%.[16] Furthermore, Boley et al. suggested that angiodysplasia lesions might actually be common in the middle-aged or elderly patient, occurring in 25% of the specimens injected by the silicon-rubber technique.[17] From colonoscopic series it has been found that even among patients with acute bleeding the incidence of angiodysplasia as a cause of bleeding appears to be less than 10%, which suggests that bleeding may never occur in more than half the cases where angiodysplasia lesions are present. The uncertain risk of bleeding when the lesion is discovered incidentally must be balanced against the small (1%) but definite possibility of gross hemorrhage after treatment (Fig. 46-9d).[21] It seems prudent to leave untreated small lesions in asymptomatic patients.

Biopsy.

Using the Williams' forceps it has been possible to biopsy angiodysplasia lesions. Histologically, one expects to find ectatic vessels within the mucosa distorting and compressing crypts (Fig. 46-10).[21] In addition, one may see communication of the angiodysplasia lesion with adjacent vessels. However, the classic histologic appearance is not always found in the specimen submitted to the pathologist, either because blood spills out into the lamina propria and obscures the angiodysplasia lesion or it collapses during the biopsy. In one series of 26 patients with a typical colonoscopic appearance and where adequate histologic material was submitted for 21, in only 11 were the above histologic criteria met.[21] In eight the diagnosis was established on the basis of both histologic and visual (photographic) appearance, whereas in two the histology did not support the diagnosis of angiodysplasia.[21] In about one-half of the cases, one must expect that the histology will not independently confirm the visual impression of angiodysplasia. However, it is unknown if such patients behave differently in terms of presentation or recurrence of bleeding. In the face of a typical appearance and location, one would be correct in regarding the lesion as angiodysplasia even if it were not supported histologically. One might still suspect the same rate of recurrent bleeding based on the size of the lesion even if the biopsy were nonspecific and would still recommend a second look within 6 months for any large lesion discovered because of prior colonic bleeding.

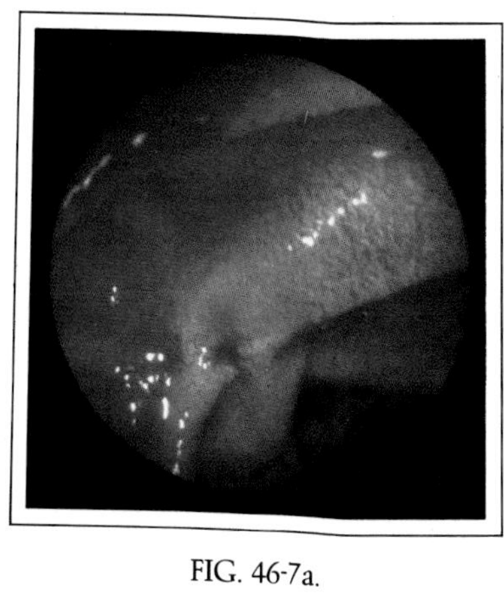

FIG. 46-7a.

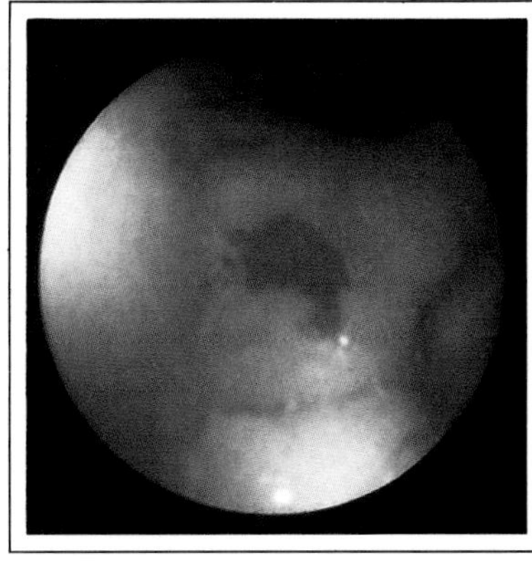

FIG. 46-7b.

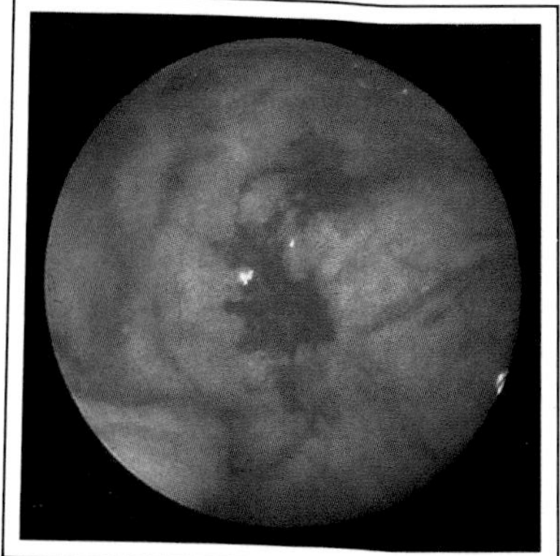

FIG. 46-7c.

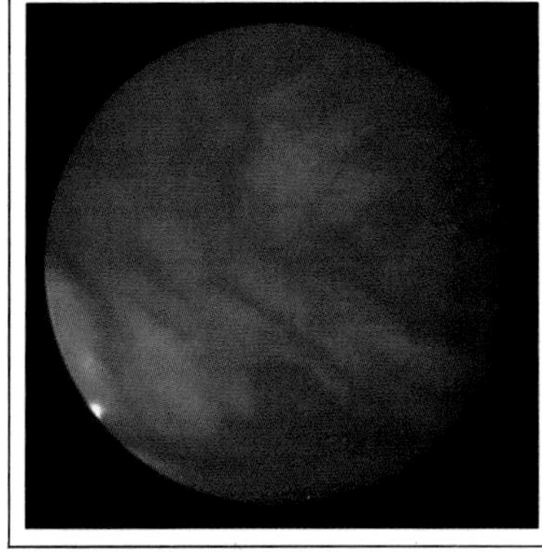

FIG. 46-7d.

FIG. 46-7. Colonic angiodysplasia. **a:** A small (3 mm) bright red lesion with an irregular margin, which is the result of typical spider-leg-like projections. This was found in a patient with several maroon stools and melena who required admission to the hospital for transfusion. Electrosurgical treatment (coagulation biopsy)[18] was applied, and no further episodes have occurred over a 3-year period. **b:** In the ascending colon. Note the large (6 mm) lesion in this patient with a single episode of bright red rectal bleeding. A separate small angiodysplasia lesion is seen just above the large lesion (toward 12 o'clock). **c:** In the cecum. A large (1.5 cm) lesion was observed that actually consisted of two smaller angiodysplasia lesions (5 to 6 mm) with interconnecting branches. Bleeding recurred 3 years after electrosurgical treatment (coagulation biopsy). **d:** In the ascending colon. A large (1.5 cm) lesion in a patient with one episode of melena. Electrosurgical treatment was not performed because of technical factors. However, no bleeding occurred over a follow-up period of 2 years, emphasizing the erratic nature of rebleeding from these lesions.

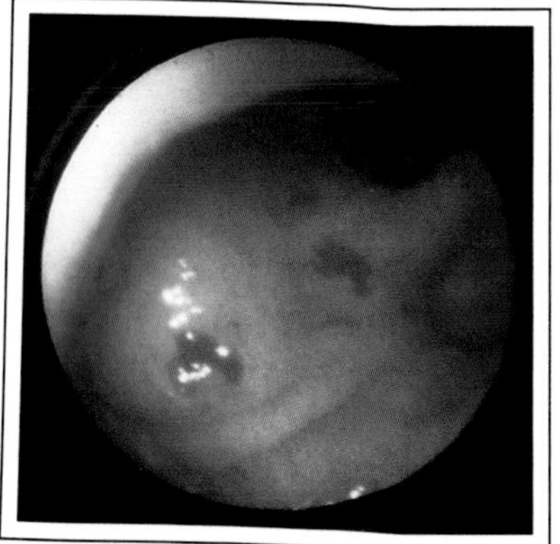

FIG. 46-8a.

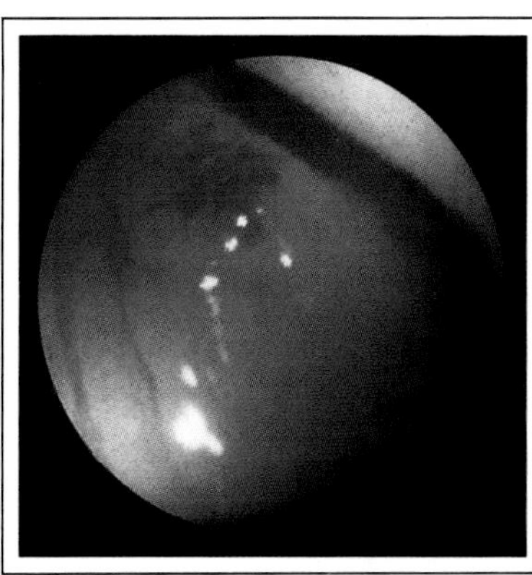

FIG. 46-8b.

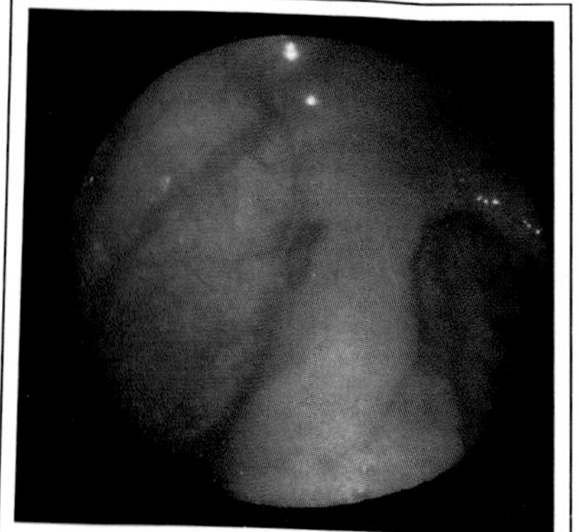

FIG. 46-8c.

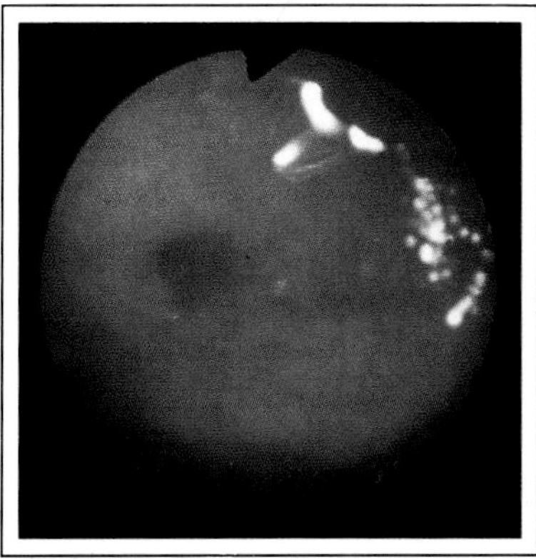

FIG. 46-8d.

FIG. 46-8. a: Colonic angiodysplasia in the cecum. Multiple small (2 to 4 mm) lesions, each with its own characteristically irregular margin. **b:** Colonic angiodysplasia in the right colon. This cecal lesion was one of the larger (5 mm) of several lesions (c) observed. **c:** Colonic angiodysplasia in the right colon. In addition to the one 5-mm lesion of the cecum (b), another small lesion (2 mm) was seen at the hepatic flexure at some distance from the large lesion (b). **d:** Endoscope trauma, artifact, in the sigmoid. A discrete zone of intramucosal hemorrhage induced by endoscope trauma has, on the whole, discrete regular margins as opposed to the spider-leg-like appearance (b). The location is also important. Endoscope artifacts are common in the sigmoid, whereas angiodysplasia is not.

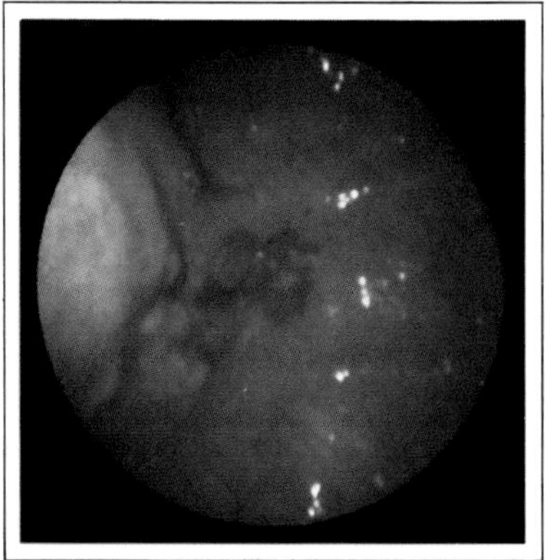

FIG. 46-9a.

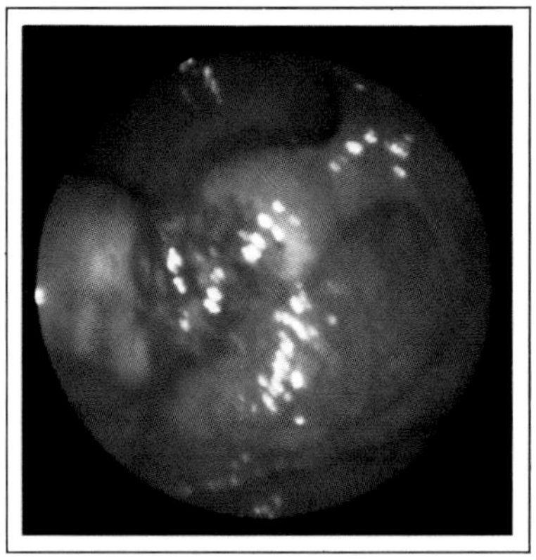

FIG. 46-9b.

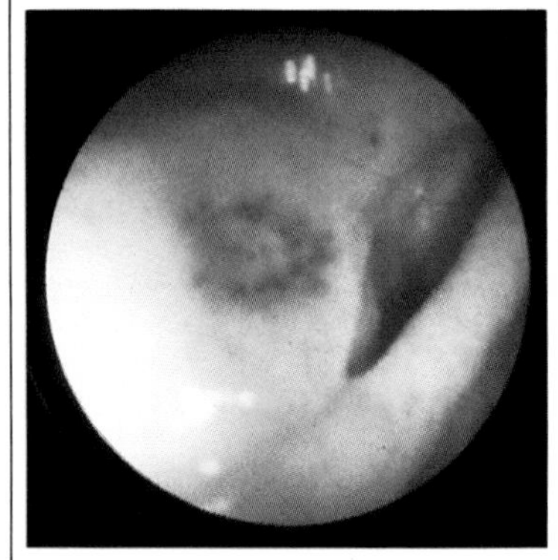

FIG. 46-9c.

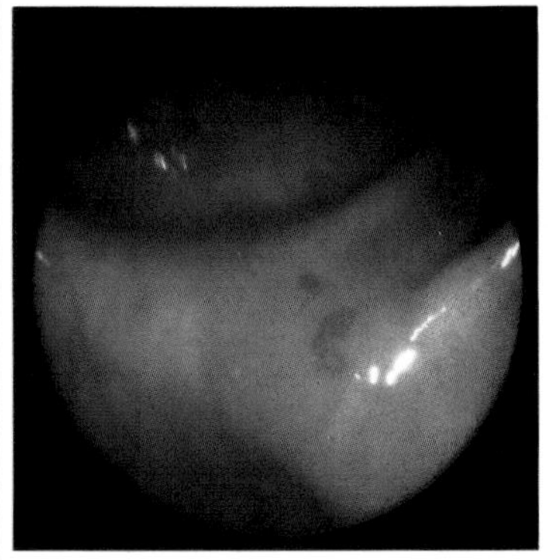

FIG. 46-9d.

FIG. 46-9. a: Colonic angiodysplasia in the cecum. Note this large (8 mm) bright red lesion with irregular margins in a patient presenting with recurrent episodes of rectal bleeding. Electrosurgical treatment was attempted at colonoscopy (b). **b:** Colonoscopic electrosurgical treatment (coagulation biopsy) with a Williams'-type forceps applied to the periphery of the angiodysplasia lesion in order to coagulate the lesion entirely. **c:** Colonic angiodysplasia, 3 months after electrosurgical treatment (b). Even though the lesion appeared completely obliterated at the time of treatment, some of its periphery was spared—enough to cause recurrent bleeding that required another electrosurgical treatment. **d:** Colonic angiodysplasia in the cecum. Although the patient was asymptomatic, electrosurgical treatment was performed [similar to the case in (b)], which resulted in massive bleeding 5 days later. Although the risk of bleeding after electrosurgical treatment of angiodysplasia is small (1%), it still seems to caution against prophylactic treatment in a patient whose angiodysplasia may never bleed on its own.

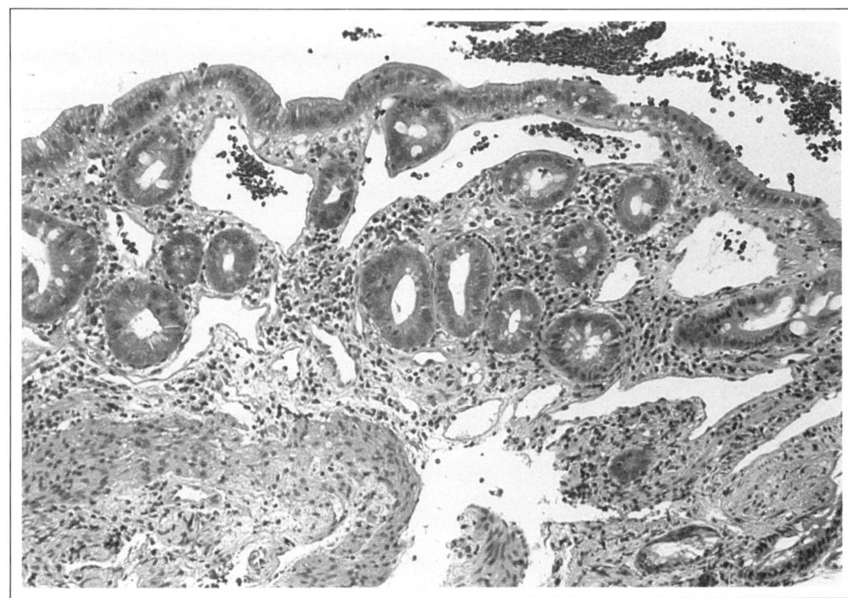

FIG. 46-10.

FIG. 46-10. Colonic angiodysplasia, histologic appearance. Ectatic thin-walled vessels occupy much of the lamina propria, displacing the adjacent crypts.

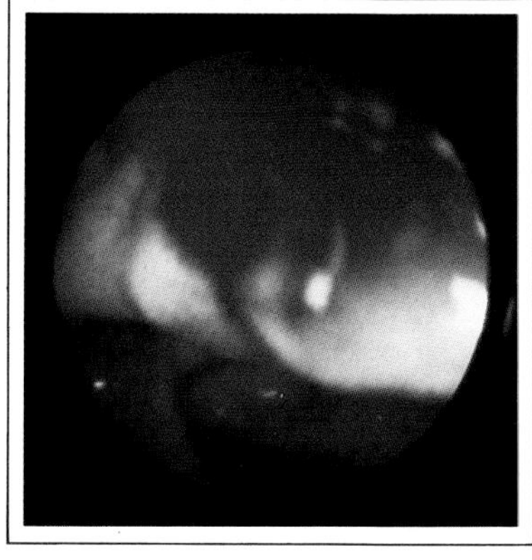

FIG. 46-11a.

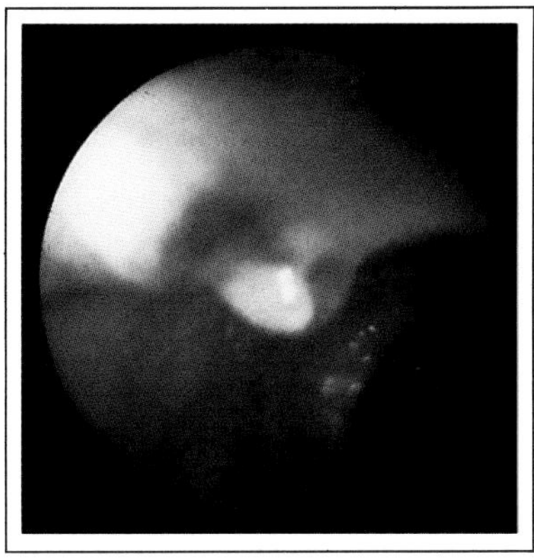

FIG. 46-11b.

FIG. 46-11. a: Hemorrhoidal bleeding, massive. Blood can be seen to ooze from the distal rectum just above the anorectal junction. Houston valves are seen in the distance. Although not substantiated in this case, massive hemorrhoidal bleeding always suggests underlying portal hypertension.[24] **b:** Internal hemorrhoid, 2 days after a bleeding episode (a). An adherent clot with granulation tissue is found over the hemorrhoid as evidence of its being the bleeding site. No other sites were identified in an examination to the terminal ileum.

Hemorrhoidal Bleeding

Patients with bleeding from internal or external hemorrhoids typically observe blood coating the stool or on toilet tissue. Such a history causes most physicians to perform a rigid examination of the anorectal area, which we find actually provides better visualization, especially if a short 3-cm anoscope is used. This might disclose anal fissures rather than hemorrhoids as the cause of the bleeding. If the examination is performed within several hours of the last passage of blood, the finding of stool within the rectal vault which is negative for occult blood supports the idea that the bleeding was from the anorectal area, especially given the typical history. Colonoscopy is still requested, however, because the physician wishes to be certain for patients over 40 that a colonic neoplasm (adenoma or cancer) is not the source of bleeding, especially where its presence may have been suggested on barium enema or because of a family history of cancer.[22] For any patient over 40 with rectal bleeding, fiberoptic sigmoidoscopy seems reasonable in that adenomas are found in at least 10% of even asymptomatic patients undergoing such an examination to 60 cm.[23] Whether total colonoscopy is performed in a patient with a history suggestive of only anorectal bleeding is a matter of individual judgment; however, most physicians would agree on the desirability of an examination of the sigmoid in its entirety.[23]

Massive Hemorrhoidal Bleeding

Rarely, hemorrhoidal bleeding is massive, requiring admission to the hospital. In these cases portal hypertension may be a contributing factor, with the hemorrhoids serving as a portosystemic collateral pathway.[24] Hemorrhoidal bleeding massive enough to require hospitalization and transfusion often occurs well up in the rectum and may reflux back into the sigmoid, so that on proctoscopic examination bleeding appears to be coming from above the rectum, thus prompting colonoscopy. In series where colonoscopy has been performed for acute rectal bleeding, hemorrhoids accounted for 1.6% (1 of 59) in one series[3] and 4% (1 of 25) in another.[7]

Appearance.

In patients with massive hemorrhoidal bleeding, one expects to find sizable quantities of blood and clots within the rectal vault (Fig. 46-11a). The blood may also be found in the sigmoid but usually not above it. With active bleeding it may be impossible to determine the bleeding site unless one sees blood oozing forth from the hemorrhoids with no other site of bleeding identified either within the rectum or above it. However, when the bleeding has ceased, one may observe stigmata of recent bleeding. In one case we observed, granulating areas (ulcerations) of the mucosa overlying the hemorrhoids were present, thus marking them as a likely site of bleeding (Fig. 46-11b).

Uncommon Vascular Causes

Colonic Varices

In rare cases portal hypertension leads to the formation of a collateral circulation that utilizes submucosal colonic veins and results in the formation of colonic varices.[25] At colonoscopy performed because of rectal bleeding, colonic varices may be expected in no more than 1 to 2% of cases, if that. Esophageal varices in these cases are not invariable, occurring in only half. The reason colonic varices form is uncertain, but previous abdominal surgery or injury with the formation of adhesions providing a vascular conduit to systemic veins may be a factor. Another may be the presence of congenital arteriovenous malformations which are enlarged with the development of portal hypertension associated with liver disease or simply alterations in mesenteric venous drainage secondary to a segmental resection as in one of our cases (Fig. 46-12a). Another extremely rare cause of colonic varices in a patient examined by us was the presence of pelvic and colonic lymphangiomatosis (see Chapter 47), which we suggested may have compressed the inferior mesenteric vein, resulting in the formation of rectal

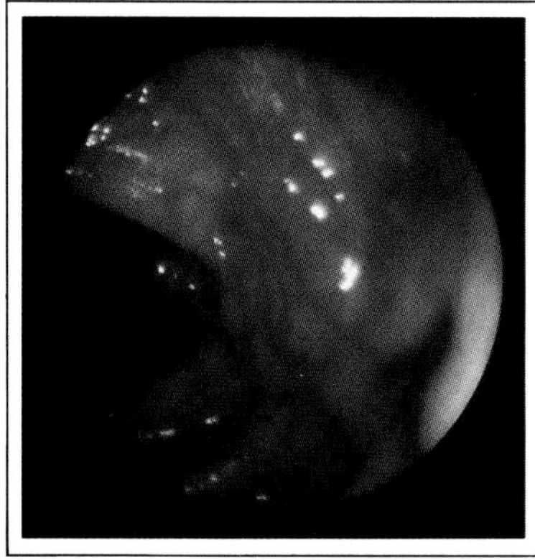

FIG. 46-12a.

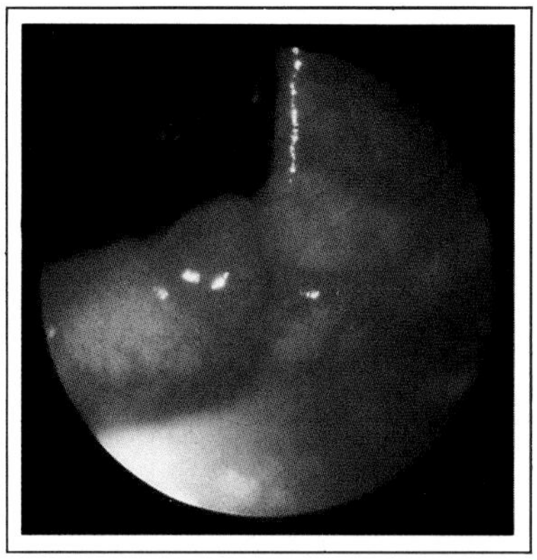

FIG. 46-12b.

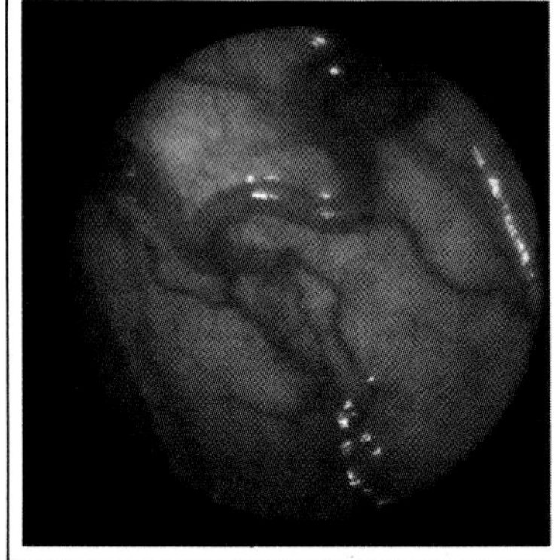

FIG. 46-12c.

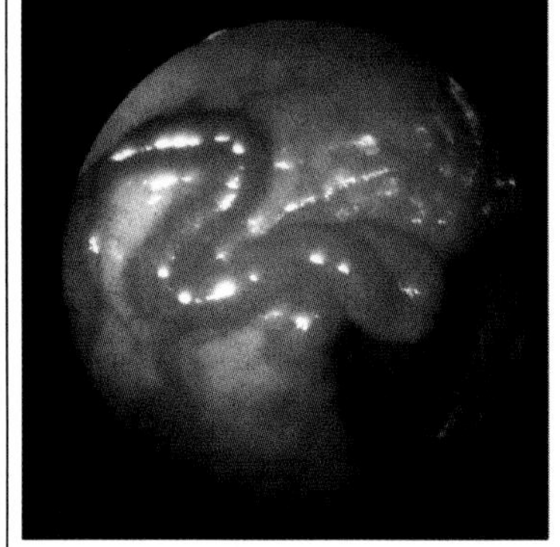

FIG. 46-12d.

FIG. 46-12. a: Colonic varices of the transverse colon. These were found in a 34-year-old women with several episodes of massive colonic bleeding, without liver disease but with a resection of the hepatic flexure 10 years previously for removal of a polyp. It was thought that this may have interfered with drainage of the mesenteric venous system, which opened up congenital arteriovenous communications. The varices have a characteristic gray-blue, serpiginous appearance and run perpendicular to the valvulae. **b:** Dilated colonic vein in the transverse colon, mistaken for a varix. Although similar in appearance to small varices (Fig. 46-11c), this vessel does not appear as part of a system as do varices (a). **c:** Small colonic varices of the rectosigmoid [same patient as in (a)]. This was seen as part of a system (d) where the varices enlarged as the examination proceeded more proximally (d). **d:** Colonic varices in the ascending colon [same case as in (a)]. The varices were at their maximum size in the right colon.

collaterals to drain into the vena cava by way of the inferior hemorrhoidal vein.[26]

Appearance.

Most colonic varices are left-sided, being located principally in the sigmoid and rectosigmoid area (Fig. 46-12a). These have a serpiginous gray-blue appearance, running perpendicular to the valvulae (Fig. 46-12a). In some cases they are large enough to simulate submucosal polypoid masses, although careful observation discloses these "masses" to be part of a system of varices. Another vascular structure from which they must be distinguished is the occasionally prominent submucosal colonic vein (Fig. 46-12b). This is possible only if the smaller vein-like varix (Fig. 46-12c) is followed proximally where it is seen to be part of a system of large varices (Fig. 46-12d).

Hereditary Hemorrhagic Telangiectasia

With colonoscopy it has now become possible to document colonic involvement in hereditary hemorrhagic telangiectasia,[27,28] which may occur in as many as 40% of patients with vascular abnormalities in the upper GI tract.[28] In one series colonoscopic evidence was found in two of five cases with lesions noted on upper GI endoscopy.[28]

Appearance.

Patients may be referred for colonoscopy because of episodic or continuous hematochezia.[27,28] In two such patients observed in our Unit, among seven in whom upper endoscopy had shown typical features of hereditary hemorrhagic telangiectasia (Fig. 46-13a), colonoscopy to the cecum was performed successfully. In one-third only a normal rectum and sigmoid were visualized. Of the two complete examinations, one showed scattered petechiae and telangiectasia of the rectosigmoid (Fig. 46-13b), whereas in the other case a 2-mm telangiectasia lesion of the ascending colon was observed (Fig. 46-13c). It seems from our experience and the limited experience of others[27,28] that there may be *two* patterns of colonic involvement—one in which multiple telangiectasia lesions are scattered in a discrete area (up to 5 cm of right colon)[27] and another in which there may be only one telangiectasia lesion of the right colon or several single lesions. It remains for future studies to determine if there is yet another group of patients with more diffuse colonic involvement than what has been reported to date.

Cavernous Hemangiomas

Colonic masses composed of vascular tissue are referred to as cavernous hemangiomas.[29,30] These are exceedingly

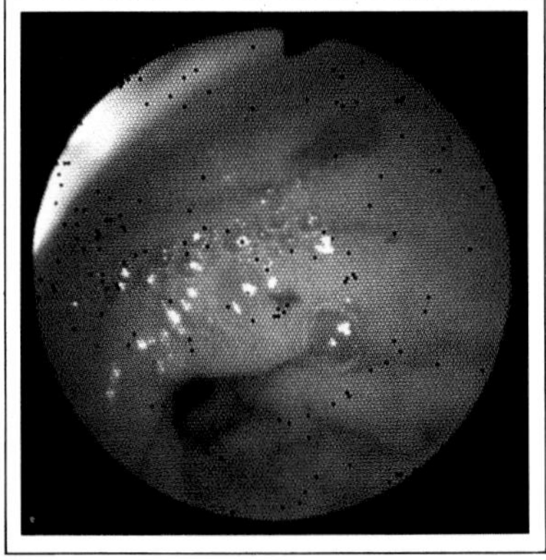

FIG. 46-13a.

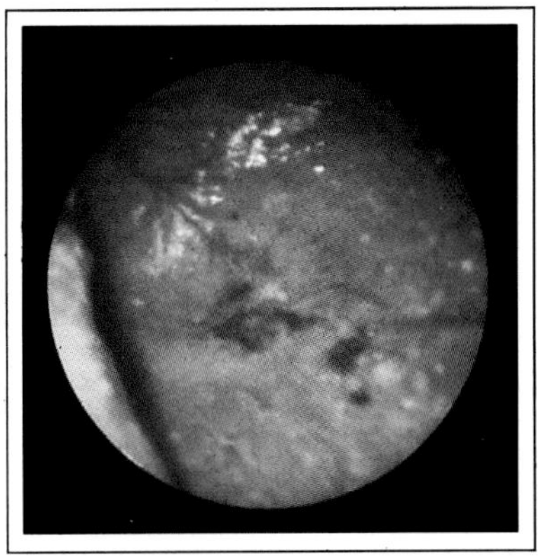

FIG. 46-13b.

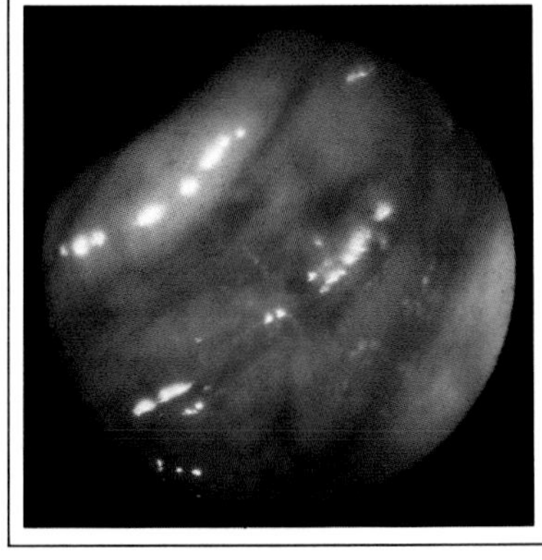

FIG. 46-13c.

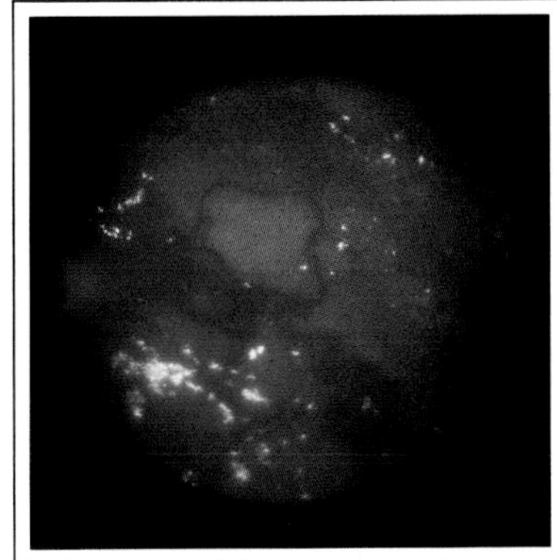

FIG. 46-14.

FIG. 46-13. Hereditary hemorrhagic telangiectasia (HHT). **a:** Involving the stomach. Typical (2 mm) cherry red spots in a patient with epistaxis, anemia, and hematochezia associated with colonic involvement (b). **b:** Involving the colon. This is part of a 3- to 6-cm area of ascending colon with multiple telangiectasias, similar to a case observed by Sogge et al.[27] **c:** Involving the colon. In this case only one colonic telangiectasia lesion was found in a patient with multiple gastric and duodenal lesions. This is similar to a case reported by Mayer and Hersh.[28]

FIG. 46-14. Cavernous hemangiomas, multiple phlebectasia lesions in a patient with Turner's syndrome (45 XO chromosome karyotype; short stature, webbed neck, and ovarian agenesis). In this view, two hemangiomas were seen as raised bluish vascular structures (at 9 and 5 o'clock) which appear to be interconnected, giving them a worm-like appearance. This has given rise to the term vermiform phlebectasia, which has been used to describe this appearance in Turner's syndrome.[34]

rare, with an incidence of 1 per 1,400 autopsied patients.[29] The masses themselves generally exceed 5 mm in both maximum dimension and height; these are not to be confused with flat angiodysplasia lesions, which are sometimes referred to as "hemangiomas of the cecum."[31] Cavernous hemangiomas are composed of large thin-walled dilated vessels with a supporting stroma.

The several subtypes of cavernous hemangioma include: (a) single or multiple, large (>5 mm) polypoid hemangiomas; (b) diffuse infiltrating hemangiomas; and (c) multiple, small (<5 mm) hemangiomas (phlebectasias).[30]

Location and appearance.

These lesions are most commonly located in the rectum or sigmoid.

1. *Polypoid type:* These appear as single or multiple, sessile, 5- to 10-mm strawberry-like lesions with a dark red or port-wine coloration.[31]
2. *Infiltrating type:* Large, diffusely infiltrating cavernous hemangiomas are found in the rectum. One suspects them in a patient with rectal bleeding and multiple phleboliths seen on plain abdominal radiographs.[33] In these cases the rectal lesions appear as ill-defined, bluish-red or dusky mass-like protrusions into the lumen.[32]
3. *Multiple phlebectasias:* These appear as smooth, focally dilated mucosal veins which are either diffuse or localized to a colonic segment. As an instance of a diffuse pattern, phlebectasias were observed by us in the setting of Turner's syndrome as a cause of recurrent hemorrhage (Fig. 46-14), similar to that reported by Frame et al.[34]

Endoscopic therapy.

Electrosurgical excision of cavernous hemangiomas of the polypoid has been reported.[32] These lesions were all under 1 cm, with most being 5 mm or less. However, the safety of endoscopic therapy for lesions of this size and larger is unknown.

Vasculitis of the Colon

The GI tract may be affected as one of multiple organs involved in systemic vasculitis. Systemic vasculitis is actually a collection of several disorders[35] in each of which there is vascular inflammation and necrosis. In the case of GI involvement, the commonest clinical presentation is that of ischemic bowel disease and perforation, which have been described for vasculitis associated with connective tissue disorders, e.g., rheumatoid arthritis or lupus erythematosus.[36] Gastrointestinal hemorrhage as melena or rectal bleeding has been reported in vasculitis associated with connective tissue disorders,[37] some cases of (nonspecific) vasculitis,[38] and the Henoch-Schönlein type vasculitis.[39] In

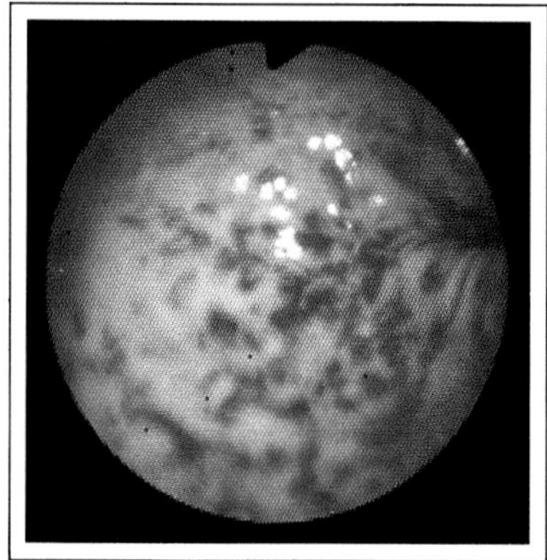

FIG. 46-15a.

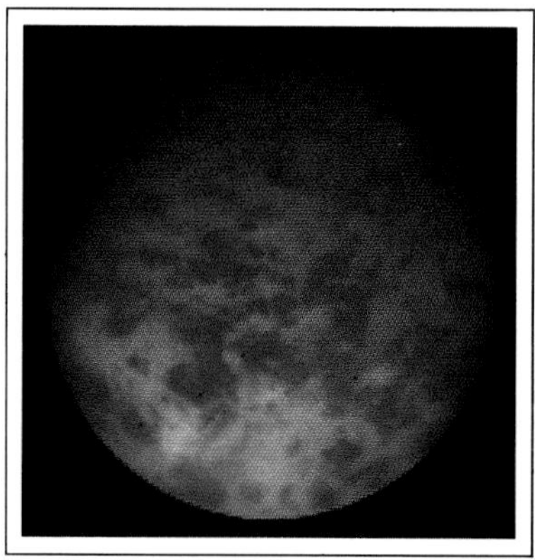

FIG. 46-15b.

FIG. 46-15. a: Colonic vasculitis, Henoch-Schönlein type. Note the multiple petechiae and small (3 to 5 mm) ecchymoses in a 10-cm segment of sigmoid. Biopsy from this area was consistent with acute vasculitis. **b:** Gastric mucosal involvement in a patient with Henoch-Schönlein type acute vasculitis. Petechiae and ecchymoses are seen in a 10-cm segment of the distal body and antrum, similar to that found in the sigmoid (a).

this type of vasculitis, which results from immune complex deposition of C3 and immunoglobulin A (IgA) in vessels of skin, kidney, and other organs (including the intestine), a high percentage of patients with GI involvement present with GI hemorrhage.

Appearance.

Colonoscopic findings have been reported in one case of vasculitis which occurred after trauma. In this case there was colonic involvement at 20 to 65 cm with "irregular, reddened areas with surrounding pale mucosa." Biopsies from these areas revealed evidence of acute vasculitis. A patient with Henoch-Schönlein vasculitis was examined in our Unit by colonoscopy and upper endoscopy because of lower GI bleeding. In the sigmoid (Fig. 46-15a) and the distal body of the stomach (Fig. 46-15b) there was a discrete 10-cm segment of involvement with multiple petechiae and ecchymoses. A biopsy of the colonic lesion was believed to be compatible with acute vasculitis, showing an infiltrate of neutrophils and eosinophils around the mucosal capillaries along with focal intramucosal hemorrhage.

REFERENCES

1. Teague, R. H., Thornton, J. R., Manning, A. P., and Salmon, P. R. (1978): Colonoscopy for investigation of unexplained rectal bleeding. *Lancet,* 1:1350–1351.
2. Tedesco, F. J., Waye, J. D., Raskin, J. B., Morris, S. J., and Greenwald, R. A. (1978): Colonoscopic evaluation of rectal bleeding: a study of 304 patients. *Ann. Intern. Med.,* 89:907–909.
3. Knoepp, L. F., and McCulloch, J. H. (1978): Colonoscopy in the diagnosis of unexplained rectal bleeding. *Dis. Colon Rectum,* 21:590–593.
4. Brand, E. J., Sullivan, B. H., Sivak, M. V., and Rankin, G. B. (1980): Colonoscopy in the diagnosis of unexplained rectal bleeding. *Ann. Surg.,* 192:111–113.
5. Knutson, C. O., and Max, M. H. (1980): Value of colonoscopy in patients with rectal blood loss unexplained by rigid proctosigmoidoscopy and barium contrast examinations. *Am. J. Surg.,* 139:84–87.
6. McGuire, H. H., and Haynes, B. W. (1972): Massive hemorrhage from diverticulosis of the colon: guidelines for therapy based on bleeding patterns observed in fifty cases. *Ann. Surg.,* 175:847–855.
7. Forde, K. A. (1981): Colonoscopy in acute rectal bleeding. *Gastrointest. Endosc.,* 27:219–220.
8. Tedesco, F. J., Waye, J. D., Avella, J. R., and Villalobos, M. M. (1980): Diagnostic implications of the spatial distribution of colonic mass lesions (polyps and cancers). *Gastrointest. Endosc.,* 26:95–97.

8a. Wright, H. K., and Higgins, E. F. (1982): Natural history of occult right colon cancer. *Am. J. Surg.,* 143:169–170.

9. Boley, S. J., Di Biase, A., Brandt, L. J., and Sammartino, R. J. (1979): Lower intestinal bleeding in the elderly. *Am. J. Surg.,* 137:57–64.
10. Scrowcroft, C. W., Sanowski, R. A., and Kozarek, R. A. (1981): Colonoscopy in ischemic colitis. *Gastrointest. Endosc.,* 27:156–161.
11. Reichelderfer, M., and Morrissey, J. F. (1980): Colonoscopy in radiation colitis. *Gastrointest. Endosc.,* 26:41–43.
12. Meyers, M. A., Alonso, D. R., Gray, G. F., and Baer, J. W. (1976): Pathogenesis of bleeding colonic diverticulosis. *Gastroenterology,* 71:577–583.
13. Casarella, W. J., Galloway, S. J., Taxin, R. N., Pollock, E. J., and Seaman, W. B. (1974): "Lower" gastrointestinal tract hemorrhage: new concepts based on arteriography. *Am. J. Roentgenol.,* 121:357–368.
14. Tedesco, F. J., Pickens, C. A., Griffin, J. W., Sivak, M. V., and Sullivan, B. H. (1981): Role of colonoscopy in patients with unexplained melena: analysis of 53 patients. *Gastrointest. Endosc.,* 27:221–224.
15. Farivar, M., and Perrotto, J. (1981): The efficacy of colonoscopy in acute renal bleeding. *Gastrointest. Endosc.,* 28:130.
16. Meyer, C. T., Troncale, F. J., Galloway, S., and Sheahan, D. G. (1981): Arteriovenous malformations of the bowel: an analysis of 22 cases and review of the literature. *Medicine,* 60:36–47.
17. Boley, S. J., Sammartino, R., Adams, A., Di Biase, A., Kleinhaus, S., and Sprayregen, S. (1977): The nature and etiology of vascular ectasias of the colon. *Gastroenterology,* 72:650–660.
18. Rogers, B. H. G. (1980): Endoscopic diagnosis and therapy of mucosal vascular abnormalities of the gastrointestinal tract occurring in elderly patients and associated with cardiac, vascular and pulmonary disease. *Gastrointest. Endosc.,* 26:134–138.
19. Tedesco, F. J., Griffin, J. W., and Khan, A. Q. (1980): Vascular ectasia of the colon: clinical, colonoscopic and radiographic features. *J. Clin. Gastroenterol.,* 2:233–238.
20. Weaver, G. A., Alpern, H. D., Davis, J. S., Ramsey, W. H., and Reichelderfer, M. (1979): Gastrointestinal angiodysplasia associated with aortic valve disease: part of a spectrum of angiodysplasia of the gut. *Gastroenterology,* 77:1–11.
21. Howard, O. M., Buchanan, J. D., and Hunt, R. H. (1982): Angiodysplasia of the colon: experience of 26 cases. *Lancet,* 2:16–19.
22. Winawer, S. J. (1980): Screening for colorectal cancer: an overview. *Cancer,* 45:1093–1098.
23. Meyer, C. T., McBride, W. J., Goldblatt, R. S., Borak, J., Marignani, P., Contino, C., and McCallum, R. W. (1979): Flexible fiberoptic sigmoidoscopy in asymptomatic and symptomatic patients: a comparative study. *Gastrointest. Endosc.,* 23:43.
24. Jacobs, D. M., Bubrick, M. P., Onstad, G. R., and Hitchcock, C. R. (1980): The relationship of hemorrhoids to portal hypertension. *Dis. Colon Rectum,* 23:567–569.
25. Patel, K. R., Wu, T. K., and Powers, S. R. (1979): Varices of the colon as a cause of gastrointestinal hemorrhage: report of a case and review of the literature. *Dis. Colon Rectum,* 22:321–323.

26. Blackstone, M. O., Rogers, B. H. G., and Baker, A. L. (1976): A cutaneous and pelvic lymphangioma with varices, lymphangiomas, and capillary hemangiomas of the rectosigmoid colon. *Gastrointest. Endosc.*, 23:39–41.

27. Sogge, M. R., Dale, J. A., and Butler, M. L. (1980): Detection of typical lesions of hereditary hemorrhagic telangiectasia by colonoscopy. *Gastrointest. Endosc.*, 22:52–53.

28. Mayer, I. E., and Hersh, T. (1981): Endoscopic diagnosis of hereditary hemorrhagic telangiectasia. *J. Clin. Gastroenterol.*, 3:361–365.

29. Allred, H. W., and Spencer, R. J. (1974): Hemangiomas of the colon, rectum and anus. *Mayo Clin. Proc.*, 49:739–741.

30. Head, H. D., Baker, J. Q., and Muir, R. W. (1973): Hemangiomas of the colon. *Am. J. Surg.*, 126:691–694.

31. Rogers, B. H. G., and Adler, F. (1976): Hemangiomas of the cecum: colonoscopic diagnosis and therapy. *Gastroenterology*, 71:1079–1082.

32. Hasegawa, K., Lee, W.-Y., Noguchi, T., Yaguchi, T., Sasaki, H., and Nagasako, K. (1981): Colonoscopic removal of hemangiomas. *Dis. Colon Rectum*, 24:85–89.

33. Parker, G. W., Murney, J. A., and Kenoyer, W. L. (1972): Cavernous hemangiomas of the rectum and rectosigmoid: a case report and review. *Dis. Colon Rectum*, 3:358–363.

34. Frame, B., Rao, D. S., Oharodnik, J. M., and Kwa, D. M. (1977): Gastrointestinal hemorrhage in Turner syndrome. *Arch. Intern. Med.*, 137:691–692.

35. Fauci, A. S., Haynes, B. F., and Katz, P. (1978): The spectrum of vasculitis: clinical, pathologic, immunologic, and therapeutic considerations. *Ann. Intern. Med.*, 89:660–676.

36. Finkbiner, R. B., and Decker, J. P. (1963): Ulceration and perforation of the intestine due to necrotizing arteriolitis. *N. Engl. J. Med.*, 268:14–18.

37. Shapeero, L. G., Meyers, A., Oberkircher, P. E., and Miller, W. T. (1974): Acute reversible lupus vasculitis of the gastrointestinal tract. *Radiology*, 112:569–574.

38. Korn, J. E., and Weaver, G. A. (1979): Vasculitis of the colon diagnosed by colonoscopy. *Gastrointest. Endosc.*, 25:156–158.

39. Morichau-Beauchant, M., Touchard, G., Maire, P., Briaud, M., Babin, P., Alcalay, D., and Matuchanski, C. (1982): Jejunal IgA and C3 deposition in adult Henoch-Schönlein purpura with severe intestinal manifestations. *Gastroenterology*, 82:1438–1442.

47

POSTSURGICAL APPEARANCES AND UNCOMMON COLONIC CONDITIONS

The colonoscopist must be prepared for a variety of postsurgical appearances and other less frequently observed conditions which are readily confused with those of common disorders. For example, variations in the overall shape of a colonic anastomosis may be mistaken for recurrent carcinoma or inflammatory bowel disease. Another confusing postsurgical condition is that of proctitis (and sigmoid colitis) in the "excluded" segment after diversion of the fecal stream because of obstruction, which can closely simulate inflammatory bowel disease. The endoscopic findings for "cathartic colon," an uncommon condition, may wrongly suggest to the examiner inflammatory bowel disease, especially in view of the strictures which may be found at the hepatic flexure and in the transverse colon. Conditions which are unusual outside of referral centers, e.g., the solitary rectal ulcer syndrome, other discrete colonic ulcers, colitis cystica profunda, and pneumatosis coli, can all easily be mistaken for either inflammatory bowel disease or neoplastic conditions if the correct diagnosis is not considered. It is our intent in this chapter to consider a variety of unusual conditions—all with potentially confusing appearances.

POSTSURGICAL APPEARANCES

Colonic Anastomosis

Approximately 3 to 5% of patients examined in our Unit have had previous segmental, or subtotal, colonic resections where the commonest indications for surgery were carcinoma or large (>3 cm) polyps, diverticular strictures, and Crohn's colitis. Of 1,000 patients examined in our Unit over a 3-year period, 55 (5.5%) had had previous surgery, with 30 operations being done for carcinoma or large polyps, 15 for Crohn's colitis, and 10 for diverticular disease or other conditions. The colonoscopist therefore needs to be aware of the range of appearances for an uncomplicated anastomosis which he may contrast with those of recurrent cancer (see Chapter 42) or Crohn's disease involving the anastomotic area (see Chapter 43).

Appearance

The anastomosis, whether ileocolic or colocolonic, is generally established with the use of interrupted sutures,[1] giving the anastomotic site the appearance of a rosette of somewhat nodular folds (Fig. 47-1a). A wide variation in the degree of nodularity may be expected, possibly because of individual differences among surgeons in creating the anastomosis. In some cases the nodular folds of the anastomosis exceed 5 mm, with the overlying mucosa appearing erythematous although with a soft and pliant character, and tenting well (see Chapter 40) when biopsied. Such an appearance, even with erythema and nodularity, is not evidence of Crohn's disease (see Chapter 43) or recurrent carcinoma (see Chapter 42).

In cases of surgery for Crohn's disease (see Chapter 43), the anastomoses are generally ileocolic, the terminal ileum being identified by the presence of ring-like Kerckring folds just beyond the anastomosis (Fig. 47-1b). Like the colocolonic anastomosis, there is much variation in its appearance. Features such as erythema and nodularity are nonspecific and should not be interpreted as evidence of recurrence in the absence of frank ulceration (see Chapter 43).

Suture Granuloma

The finding of an asymmetrical deformity at the anastomosis should cause the examiner to look carefully for the presence of retained suture material (Fig. 47-1c). A "mass" which forms around the suture results from the tissue reaction to retained suture material, which is further suggested by the finding of mucosal ulceration or acute

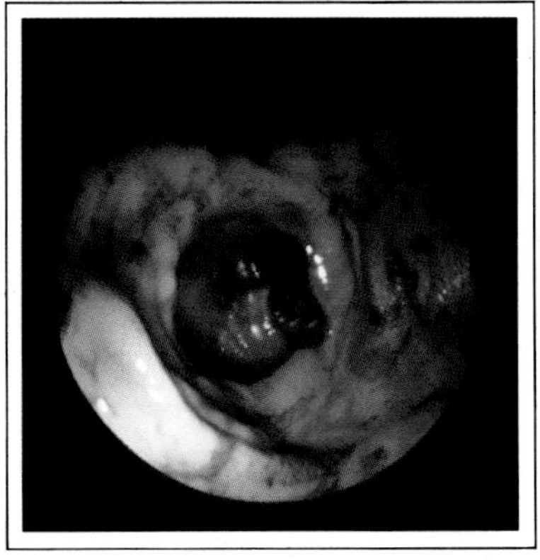

FIG. 47-1a.

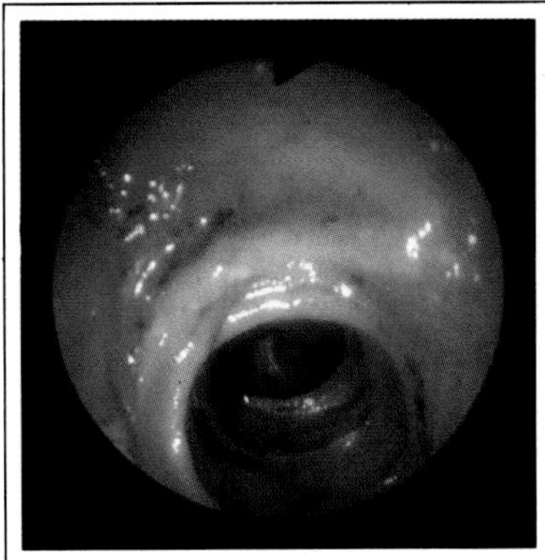

FIG. 47-1b.

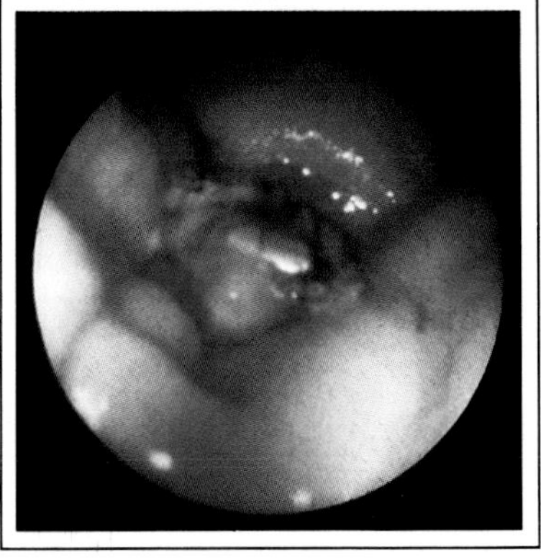

FIG. 47-1c.

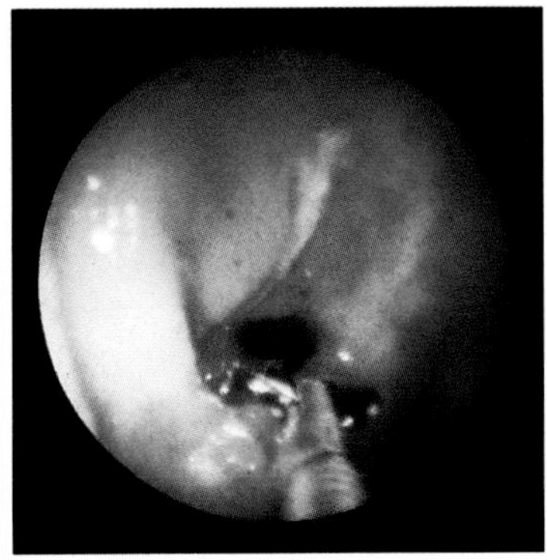

FIG. 47-1d.

FIG. 47-1. a: Ileocolic anastomosis. The ring-like deformity marking the anastomosis has a somewhat nodular appearance due to its being fashioned with interrupted sutures after resection of the terminal ileum and right colon because of Crohn's disease. The nodularity itself is not evidence of recurrence, but the finding of a discrete ulcer (marked by the depression in the 5 o'clock position) would be. Bleeding from the ulcer noted during the examination probably accounts for an iron deficiency anemia as well (as does the presence of dark staining, i.e., a combination of old blood and iron). **b:** Ileocolic anastomosis in the terminal ileum. Widely scattered short valvulae, located just beyond the ring-like deformity, and its rosette of nodular folds (a) denote the terminal ileum. **c:** Suture granuloma. At the anastomotic site, after resection for sigmoid carcinoma, an eccentric mass (in the 10 o'clock position) distorts the lumen, creating an asymmetrical radiographic appearance which raised the question of recurrence. The finding of a suture at colonoscopy within this mass suggested that it was a suture granuloma (ultimately proved at a second-look operation). **d:** Anastomotic stricture. The lumen is narrowed to approximately 5 mm (one-half the open width of the 9-mm forceps used to measure). Its appearance is symmetrical and the overlying mucosa intact, suggesting that the stricture is benign. Such strictures may form after a wide sigmoid and descending colon resection for sigmoid cancer with the resulting colorectal anastomosis under tension.

inflammatory exudate. This colonoscopic finding could explain the radiographic appearance of an asymmetrical mass deformity in a patient who has had prior surgery for malignancy,[2] although the finding does not exclude the possibility of residual or recurrent carcinoma.

Anastomotic Stricture

Some narrowing of the lumen at the site of an anastomosis is observed in the large majority of cases,[2] although the diameter still permits the colonoscope to be passed across easily. Significant narrowing of the anastomosis such that its diameter is less than 1 cm (Fig. 47-1d), resulting in an anastomotic stricture, is uncommon in the absence of residual carcinoma, diverticular disease, or Crohn's colitis. Of the 55 patients examined in our unit who had had previous surgery, only three had anastomotic strictures from the surgery itself rather than from the condition for which the surgery was performed.

Anastomotic strictures may occur in any location, although, as in our three cases, they tend to be found where there has been an extensive resection involving the entire sigmoid and a large part of descending colon so that there is a potential for the anastomosis to be placed under significant tension, a stimulus for submucosal fibrosis.[1] Because the surgery which has led to an anastomotic stricture is most commonly one for a sigmoid carcinoma, the anastomotic stricture appearance (Fig. 47-1d) immediately raises the question of recurrent carcinoma. The endoscopic appearance of a symmetrical stricture without rigidity, masses, or ulcerations favors the diagnosis of a benign anastomotic stricture rather than recurrent carcinoma,[2] although the latter can never be excluded with certainty even if biopsies and brushing cytology are negative.

Colostomy and Mucous Fistula

Colonic obstruction from cancer or diverticular disease may result in a colostomy being created to divert the colon proximal to the obstruction. This may be a "single-barreled" colostomy where only the proximal colon could be entered through the stoma, or it may be "double-barreled" where there is access through the stoma to both proximal and distal colon. With a single-barreled colostomy there may be a mucous fistula formed as a secondary stoma which allows for drainage of the colon distal to the colostomy but proximal to the obstruction.

In some cases, especially where the colostomy was performed as an emergency procedure, colonoscopy is requested for an examination of both the entire proximal colon and the site of obstruction. Although the obstruction may be reached via the rectum and assessed in the usual way (see

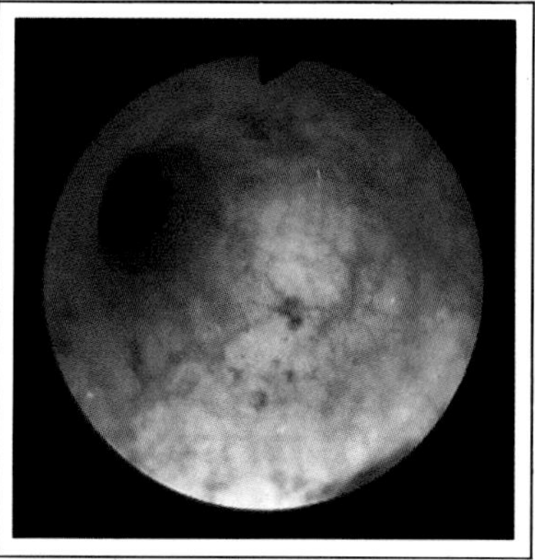

FIG. 47-2.

FIG. 47-2. Colitis, secondary to diversion of the fecal stream (disuse colitis). There is patchy erythema and blunting of the vascular pattern (with a decrease in apparent branching). Petechial hemorrhage was also noted as evidence of increased friability. These changes were seen throughout the diverted segments (rectum and sigmoid) in a patient who had surgery because of a diverticular stricture.

Chapter 45), it is generally desirable to attempt to reach the obstruction from above as well so as to give one the opportunity of determining its nature from observation, biopsy, and brushing of its proximal end. If one dilates a colostomy digitally, it is generally feasible to insert the standard colonoscope through. In the case of the mucous fistula, however, often the narrow-caliber (8 to 9 mm) pediatric-type endoscope must be used. Currently available narrow-caliber instruments with their larger biopsy channels allow sampling of a stricture with the standard colonoscopic biopsy forceps and cytology brushes.

Colitis Secondary to Diversion of the Fecal Stream

A nonspecific colitis has been observed in patients with an excluded rectum or rectosigmoid from the creation of a colostomy because of diverticular disease (obstruction, diverticulitis, or perforation) or fecal incontinence. It occurs in the excluded segment, and is generally seen as an incidental finding. Some patients, however, may have a bloody mucoid discharge which prompts examination of the segment. That the colitis completely resolves on reanastomosis suggests that some factor(s) in the fecal stream may be necessary for maintenance of an intact mucosa.[3]

Appearance

Erythema, a distorted vascular pattern, friability, granularity, and petechial hemorrhages (Fig. 47-2) have been reported to be the characteristic findings. In most cases the colitis occurs almost exclusively in the distal 2 to 3 cm of the rectum,[3] although the entire excluded segment may show similar changes. Neither the endoscopic appearance nor the histologic findings of acute and chronic inflammation, including crypt abscesses,[3] allow differentiation from inflammatory bowel disease, although the occurrence of these changes in an excluded segment should suggest to the examiner that these are secondary to diversion of the fecal stream.[3]

UNCOMMON COLONIC APPEARANCES

Colonic Appearances Secondary to Cathartics

Despite the fact that 15 to 30% of the population over the age of 60 take laxatives regularly,[4] the two laxative appearances, i.e., melanosis coli and laxative colon, are relatively rare, especially the latter. Out of 1,750 examinations performed over a 5-year period, we encountered only one case of cathartic colon and five of melanosis coli.

The laxatives commonly implicated in both conditions are the anthraquinones, which include cascara, senna, rhubarb, and other emodines where the active agent is hydroxyl methyl anthraquinone.[5,6] Other commonly used laxatives, e.g., phenolphthalein (Ex-Lax) and bisacodyl (Dulcolax), have been implicated as a cause of cathartic colon[6] but not of melanosis coli.

Melanosis Coli

Although melanosis coli is said to occur in 5% of patients having routine sigmoidoscopy,[5] we made this diagnosis at colonoscopy over a 5-year period in fewer than 0.5% (5 of 1,750 examinations). The origin of the appearance of melanosis coli is the deposition of pigment granules in submucosal macrophages.[7] The pigment itself disappears within a year after discontinuation of anthraquinone laxatives.[8] Histochemical studies have suggested the pigment to be a mixture of melanin and lipofuscin (lipo-melanin), which may originate from degenerating cellular organelles as a manifestation of anthraquinone-related cellular injury.[7]

Appearance.

One sees dark brown patches or streaks throughout the colon which appear to be interconnected in a reticulated pattern (Fig. 47-3a). Granularity and erythema are noted in cases where the melanosis coli is found as part of the cathartic colon (see below). In such cases the finding of melanosis coli is important as it indicates surreptitious laxative abuse in patients with symptoms who have a radiologic

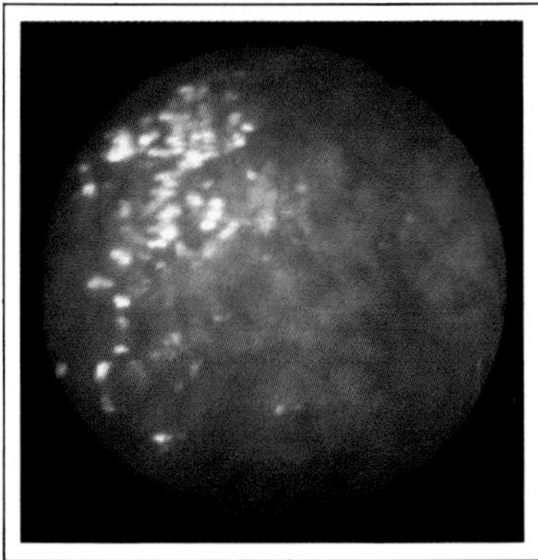

FIG. 47-3a.

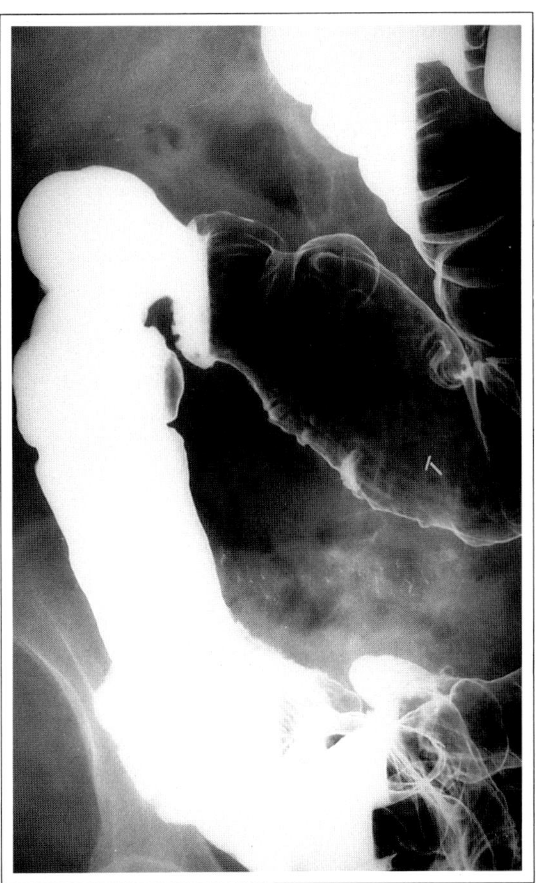

FIG. 47-3b.

FIG. 47-3. a: Melanosis coli in a patient with a cathartic colon. Focal discrete zones of brown pigmentation, which appear at points to be interconnected (reticulated), indicate the use of anthraquinone-type laxatives in a patient with diarrhea and a barium enema that showed a dilated, ahaustral right colon (b) suggestive of ulcerative colitis. **b:** Cathartic colon, radiographic appearance. The dilated, ahaustral appearance of the transverse and right colon is similar to that of ulcerative colitis. The striking melanosis coli found at endoscopy (a) was an important clue to surreptitious laxative abuse in this patient (ultimately proved by a room search).

appearance suggestive of ulcerative colitis (Fig. 47-3b). In cases where melanosis is suspected, a biopsy is obtained which reveals melanin pigment granules in large submucosal macrophages.

Cathartic Colon

With cathartic colon, an uncommon effect of long-term laxative usage, there are structural as well as mucosal changes. These are especially manifest on the right side radiographically with dilatation and loss of the expected haustral pattern.[6] In addition, there may be foreshortening and stricture formation, leading to an appearance that simulates ulcerative colitis (Fig. 47-3b). As in ulcerative colitis, the ileocecal valve may become patulous, and "backwash ileitis" can be observed.

The pathogenesis of colonic involvement in this condition is thought to result from accumulation of the anthraquinone within the muscle layer and myenteric plexuses leading to a loss of intrinsic innervation and atrophy of smooth muscle.[9] This has a structural effect, with the colon becoming dilated. Between areas of dilatation, one may note stricture formation, the result of focal muscle hypertrophy.[6] The origin of this change is uncertain, but it may be an ischemia-related mucosal injury that leads to an ulcerative colitis-like stricture composed of hypertrophic smooth muscle (see Chapter 43).

Colonoscopy may be requested in patients with cathartic colon because of the similarity of the radiographic appearance to that of ulcerative colitis (Fig. 47-3b). This is especially true if melanosis coli is not present at sigmoidoscopy and the patient denies laxative ingestion.

Appearance.

As the right colon is the principal area of involvement, one expects to find here a loss of the haustral pattern with dilatation. Often there is a patulous ileocecal valve. Melanosis, if present, is an indication of chronic laxative use and immediately causes the examiner to suspect a cathartic colon (Fig. 47-3a). Within the transverse colon there may be foreshortening and tubularization, as in ulcerative colitis, along with stricture formation which is usually at the hepatic flexure, mid-transverse colon, or descending colon. If the terminal ileum is entered, an appearance similar to that of ulcerative colitis backwash ileitis may be observed (see Chapter 48).

In cases where cathartic colon is suspected, biopsies showing melanosis are strong evidence in its favor. The absence of melanosis, however, does not exclude cathartic colon, as the destructive effects on the myenteric plexus could persist long after laxatives had been withdrawn, which would resolve the melanosis coli.[8] In such cases the biopsy may be indistinguishable from that of quiescent ulcerative colitis.[6]

Colonic Ulcer Syndromes

Three distinct colonic ulcer syndromes may be seen. One involves the rectum exclusively (the solitary rectal ulcer syndrome), and the two others involve the right and transverse colon. Of these two latter types, one is nonspecific, occurring in a variety of conditions, while the other is found in renal transplant recipients, often with cytomegalovirus infection.

Solitary Rectal Ulcer Syndrome

Although relatively uncommon, solitary rectal ulcer syndrome is encountered from time to time. During the past 5 years, we saw on the average one case per 750 examinations. In this condition there is repeated injury to a small area of rectum, generally along the anterior wall 5 to 10 cm from the anal verge. This is thought to occur as a result of excessive straining, which leads to repeated trauma in this area.[10,11] In addition, ischemic necrosis of the surface epithelium as well as repeated manual disimpaction or manipulation with solid objects may bear on the pathogenesis of this condition. However, for most patients the pathogenesis is thought to follow directly from the failure of the puborectalis muscle to relax during the act of defecation. This causes the patient to strain, and as a result there is a tendency toward prolapse of the rectal mucosa with repeated trauma, especially to its "lead point."

Patients with solitary rectal ulcer syndrome present with a history of constipation, tenesmus, a constant urge to defecate, and/or rectal bleeding. Barium enema may show rectal ulceration, narrowing, stricture formation, or inflammatory polyps.

Appearance.

Two types of appearance may be noted depending on the phase of the solitary rectal ulcer syndrome. These may be described as: (a) the preulceration phase; and (b) the ulcer state.

1. *Preulceration phase:* In these cases there may be a 3- to 5-cm area of heaped-up mucosa on the anterior wall (toward the 3 o'clock position—see Chapter 39) approximately 5 to 10 cm from the anal verge (Fig. 47-4a). The mucosa appears more erythematous than that which surrounds it, and petechial hemorrhages can be seen within this area. Biopsies taken from this mucosa show the characteristic appearance of smooth muscle and fibrosis (fibromuscular hyperplasia) within the lamina propria (Fig. 47-4d).[10] Evolution from this stage to that of frank ulceration (see below) has been observed.[11a]

2. *Ulcer state:* Ulcers of varying size (2 to 8 mm) are observed in this stage on the anterior wall 5 to 10 cm from the anal verge (Fig. 47-4b). The ulcers are punched-out with a well-demarcated edge and have surrounding, somewhat raised erythematous mucosa. In some cases the ulcerations take the form of inflammatory polyps (3 to 6 mm) with ulcerated tips (Fig. 47-5a), rather than punched-out ulcers, an appearance which suggests some mucosal degeneration in response to previous injury. The polyps may be set so close together as to suggest a single polypoid mass, e.g., a villous adenoma (Fig. 47-5b).

Biopsy.

The characteristic biopsy finding is fibromuscular hyperplasia within the lamina propria, presumably as a response to repeated trauma and prolapse (Fig. 47-4d). As the process continues, the muscle fibers actually extend to envelop the crypts, which may show regenerative changes, e.g., branching. Ultimately, there is a decreased number of crypts along with capillary dilatation and focal ulceration accompanying the macroscopic ulcers seen at colonoscopy.

Nonspecific Ulcers of the Colon

Much less common than even the solitary rectal ulcer syndrome are nonspecific ulcers which occur elsewhere in the colon, with fewer than 200 cases having been reported up to 1982.[12] Nonspecific ulcers of the colon are predominantly right-sided lesions (cecum and ascending colon), occurring in patients in their fourth to sixth decade. Because of the location of these ulcers, the typical presentation reported for about 50% of the cases is that of right-sided cramping abdominal pain and fever mimicking appendicitis.[12] Less often (in about 30%) the presentation is colonic bleeding, especially with left-sided ulcers.[12]

The cause of nonspecific ulcers of the colon is unknown, but a variety of conditions have been associated, including colonic stasis, foreign body trauma, infection, stress, ischemia,[12] and renal failure.[12a] The rapid healing of these ulcers which is sometimes observed argues against their being part of the spectrum of inflammatory bowel disease.[12] Colonoscopy, prompted by cramping abdominal pain or hematochezia, is effective in finding these ulcers and differentiating them from other conditions, specifically malignancy.[13]

Appearance.

These lesions have been reported as single or multiple (Fig. 47-6a) superficial ulcers that are sharply demarcated from the surrounding mucosa, which is either normal or

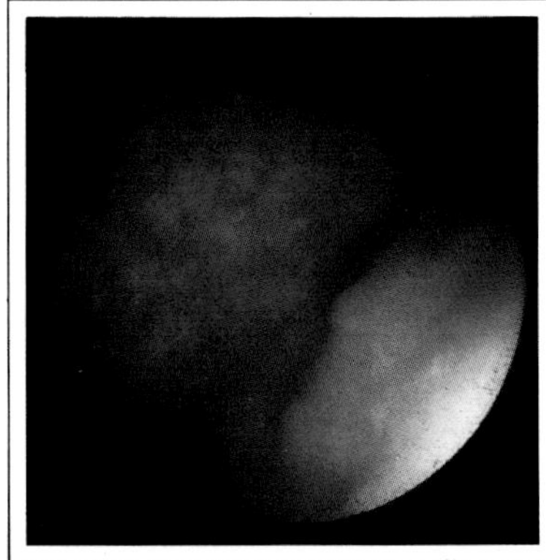

FIG. 47-4a.

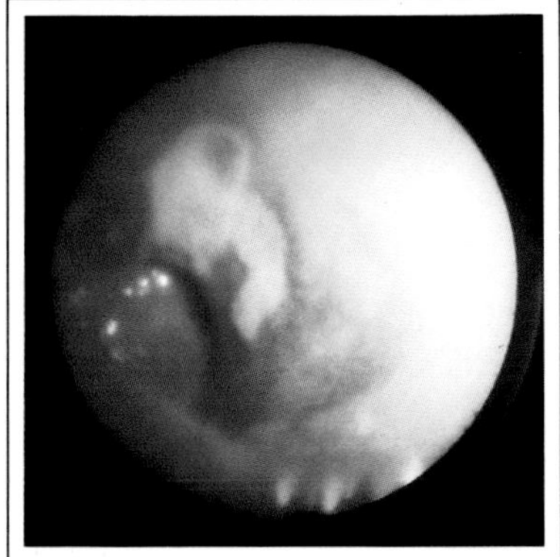

FIG. 47-4b.

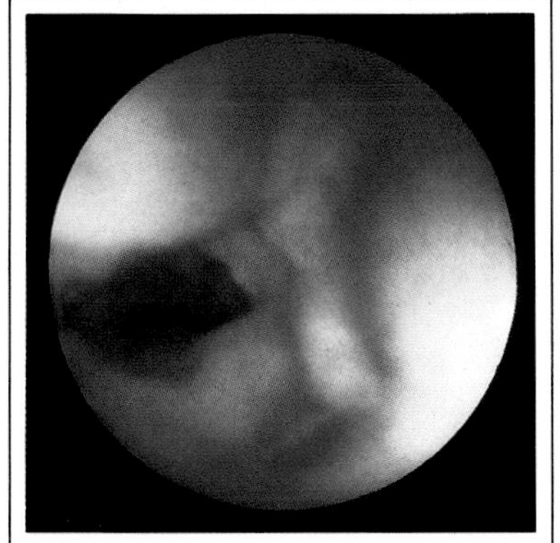

FIG. 47-4c.

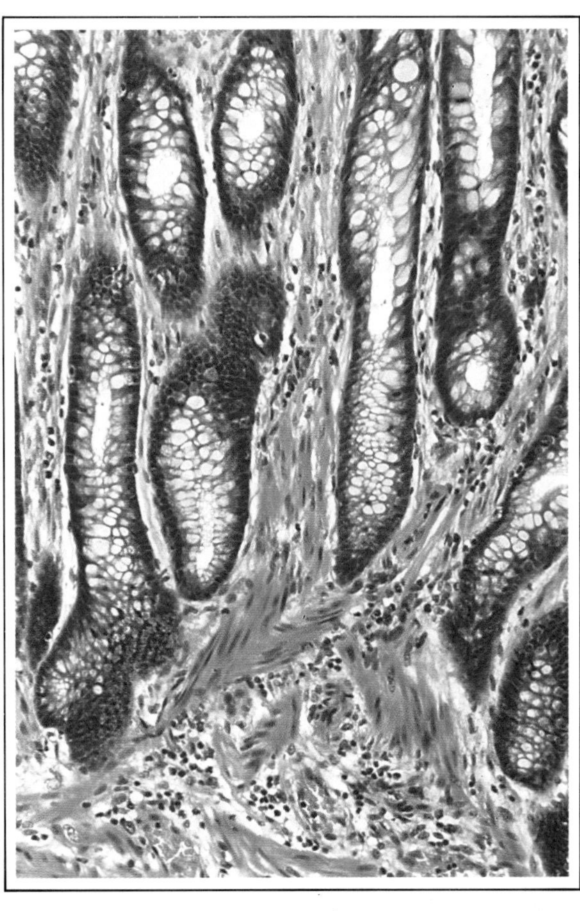

FIG. 47-4d.

FIG. 47-4. Solitary rectal ulcer syndrome. **a:** Preulcer stage. This is indicated by the presence of heaped-up mucosa found on the anterior wall (at 3 o'clock) within 10 cm of the anal verge. It is thought to occur because of repeated prolapse associated with failure of the levator ani to relax during the act of defecation. A biopsy of this redundant mucosa shows the histologic hallmark of solitary rectal ulcer syndrome, fibromuscular hyperplasia in the lamina propria (d). **b:** Ulcer stage. A discrete 5 × 8 mm punched-out ulcer was noted on the anterior (3 o'clock) wall in the proximal rectum. **c:** Ulcer stage. In the mid-rectum there is a large (1.5 × 0.75 cm) ulcer with adjacent narrowing of the lumen, presumably from scarification. The biopsy showed fibromuscular hyperplasia compatible with solitary rectal ulcer syndrome (d). **d:** Biopsy. This shows the characteristic appearance of fibroblasts (toward 12 o'clock) and muscle fibers (at 6 o'clock) within the lamina propria, encircling crypts.

shows some edema. Some ulcers are deeper (Fig. 47-6b), being associated with either a mass-like deformity or stricture formation (Fig. 47-6c). Except for their being confined to one segment of the colon, and in many cases being just a single ulcer, they are indistinguishable from the aphthous ulcers of Crohn's disease.

Colonic Ulcers in Renal Transplant Recipients

Colonic ulcers occurring in renal transplant patients often present as lower gastrointestinal (GI) bleeding,[13a] which could thus prompt colonoscopy, as in one case we personally observed. As in the case of nonspecific colonic ulcers (see above), those occurring in the transplant patients are typically right-sided, being for the most part cecal. They may be single, but more often number two to four. Those associated with lower GI bleeding range in size from 1–5 mm to 4 cm, generally with a maximum dimension of 2 cm.[13a]

The origin of cecal ulcers occurring in these patients is probably multifactorial. Evidence of cytomegalovirus (CMV) infection is frequently found in cecal ulcers that have been

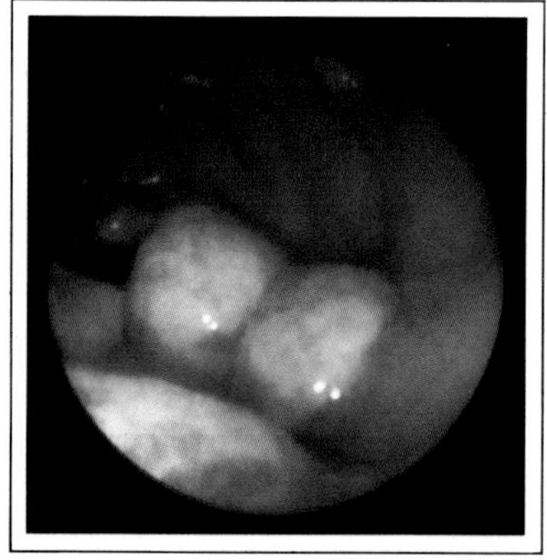

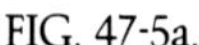

FIG. 47-5a.

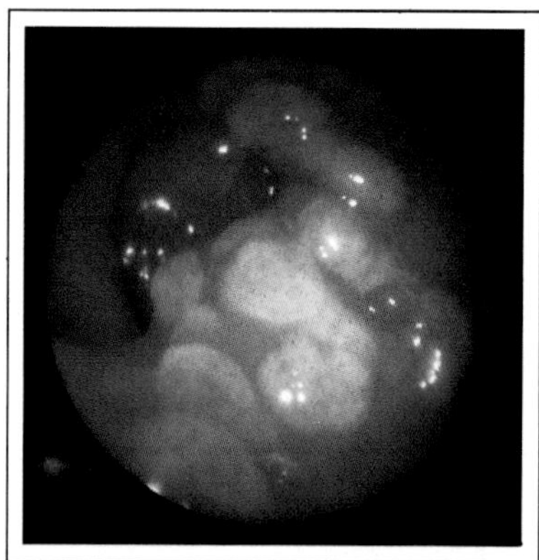

FIG. 47-5b.

FIG. 47-5. Solitary rectal ulcer syndrome. **a:** Ulcer stage with inflammatory polyps. Multiple 5- to 15-mm polypoid masses with ulcerated surfaces (composed of granulation tissue) are found rather than a discrete ulcer (Fig. 47-4b). **b:** Ulcer stage with polypoid masses. Rather than multiple discrete inflammatory polyps (a), these appear together as one large (1.5 × 2.5 cm) relatively discrete mass with nodules whose surfaces are composed of granulation tissue. In this case a large-particle biopsy showed superficial ulceration and fibromuscular hyperplasia of the lamina propria and muscularis mucosae. No submucosal mucin-containing cysts were observed, although the endoscopic appearance and the location (rectosigmoid) are indistinguishable from those of colitis cystica profunda.

FIG. 47-6a.

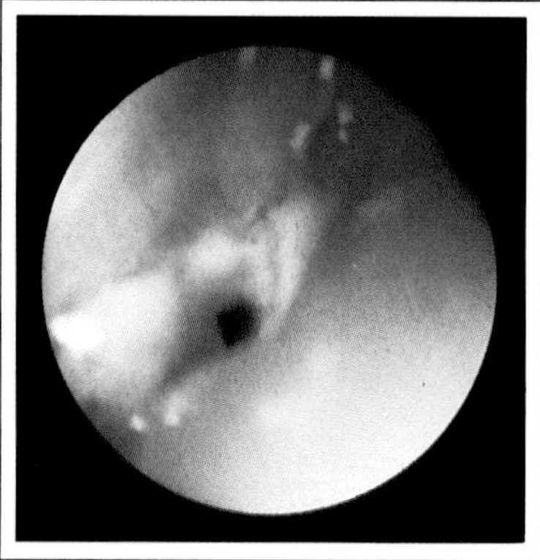

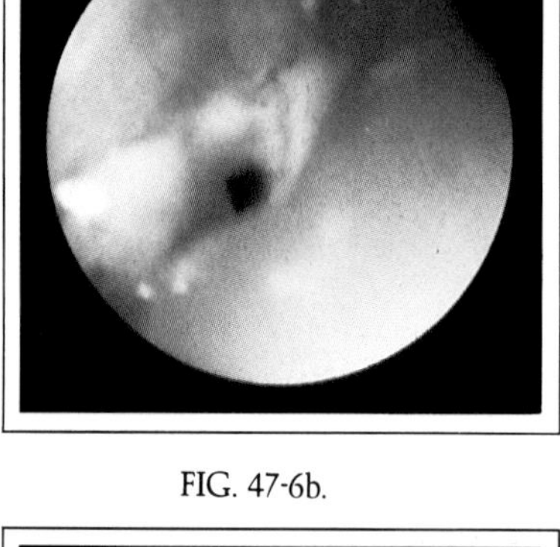

FIG. 47-6b.

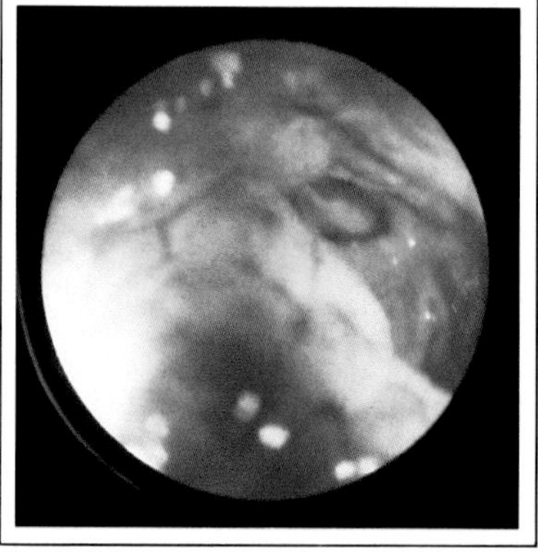

FIG. 47-6c.

FIG. 47-6. a: Nonspecific colonic ulcers in the ascending colon. Three discrete ulcers were found in an 80-year-old man with a history of hematochezia. The etiology for these ulcers is unknown. **b:** Nonspecific colonic ulcer of the sigmoid with stricture. A deep ulceration, in this case occurring in a patient with alcoholic pancreatitis and a pseudocyst, was associated with stricture formation. There was no communication between the pancreatic pseudocyst and the stricture at surgery, nor did the resected specimen show evidence of either inflammatory bowel disease or malignancy. This was therefore considered to be nonspecific colonic ulceration. **c:** Deep nonspecific colonic ulceration of the sigmoid associated with stricture formation (b).

associated with bleeding,[13a,13b] with CMV itself a cause of vasculitis,[13c] which may have been responsible both for the ulceration itself as well as its size and predisposition to bleed. Even in the absence of evidence of CMV, renal transplant recipients may develop colonic mucosal injury, secondary to ischemia.[13d] Ischemia, in conjunction with CMV vasculitis, could lead to worsening of the initial CMV injury.

Colitis Cystica Profunda

The nonneoplastic condition known as colitis cystica profunda is possibly related to the solitary rectal ulcer syndrome (see above). Although it is quite rare, it is important because of its resemblance to carcinoma, both radiographically and at colonoscopy.

The condition is characterized histologically by the presence of mucin-filled cysts in the submucosa.[14–16] These tend to be localized to the distal sigmoid and rectosigmoid junction. Although the etiology of these cysts is unknown, they are currently thought to result from invagination of colonic mucosa which occurs during the healing phase of solitary rectal ulcers. The invaginations which form around the margins of these ulcers then become closed off as the base of the ulcer itself becomes re-epithelialized.[10,14] As in the case of solitary rectal ulcers themselves, one may elicit a history of excessive straining. In addition, patients describe lower abdominal cramps, diarrhea, and tenesmus. In cases where a barium enema has been obtained, this may show a circumferential polypoid or ulcerating lesion which cannot be differentiated from carcinoma.[16]

Appearance

Although we ourselves have not observed a case, an endoscopic picture emerges from cases which have been reported of single or multiple nodules which on biopsy have a rubbery consistency with a slightly erythematous overlying mucosa.[14–16] The mucosa of these masses may be intact or superficially ulcerated, so that the appearance simulates quite closely that of the solitary rectal ulcer syndrome in which polypoid masses are present (Fig. 47-5b). The similarity in location and appearance suggests a common pathogenesis, as does the finding on biopsy, in both conditions, of an increased number of fibroblasts and smooth muscle fibers in the lamina propria extending up from the muscularis mucosae.[14]

Differentiation from Cancer

Although the presence of granular epithelium below the muscularis mucosae may raise the question of malignancy,[16] especially if the biopsy is fragmented or poorly oriented, there are no cytologic features of neoplasia, so the experienced pathologist is not likely to mistake this condition for mucinous (colloid) carcinoma.

Pneumatosis Coli

Pneumatosis coli, an unusual condition characterized by the presence of gas-filled cysts within the wall of the colon,[17,18] was encountered by us in only 2 of 1,900 examinations performed over a 7-year period. The origin of these cysts is unknown, although many theories have been proposed. Because many cases are associated with mechanical obstruction either from peptic ulcer disease, gastric cancer, or intestinal obstruction, the notion has arisen that the origin of these cysts is the dissection of gas from the gut lumen into the submucosa.[17] Other cases are associated with chronic obstructive pulmonary disease, which suggests a different origin, i.e., the rupture of alveoli with dissection of air into the mediastinum, then on to retroperitoneal tissues, the mesentery, and ultimately the intestinal submucosa.[17]

The symptoms associated with pneumatosis coli are nonspecific, e.g., alterations in bowel habits, hematochezia, and diarrhea. Such symptoms may prompt a barium enema, which shows filling defects (Fig. 47-7a) that if not observed in the wall of the colon could be mistaken for adenomas or even carcinoma.[18]

An even more worrisome presentation results from spontaneous rupture of the cysts into the peritoneum. If this should occur and a plain abdominal radiograph is obtained, the pneumoperitoneum observed may prompt emergency surgery with the mistaken diagnosis of intestinal perforation.[19]

The cysts of pneumatosis coli may be localized to one segment of the colon or occur throughout. Of interest are the patients with exclusive left-sided pneumatosis coli (involving the descending colon and sigmoid),[20] where there is a high incidence of underlying chronic obstructive pulmonary disease.

With the finding that the gas content of the cyst is largely nitrogen, management of patients with cysts producing obstructive symptoms has centered around the use of high-flow intermittent oxygen therapy to lower the nitrogen content of blood, thus favoring the resorption of nitrogen from the cysts.[21]

Appearance

The gas-filled cysts appear as submucosal polypoid masses ranging in size from 2 to 3 mm (Fig. 47-7b) to some well over 2 cm (Fig. 47-7d). These are soft and easily compressible, which suggests the correct diagnosis; however, because the overlying mucosa may show nonspecific erythema, these lesions may be mistaken for adenomas. Worse, because they potentially block the lumen and have an annular distribution, they may suggest carcinoma (Fig. 47-7c).

Forceps biopsy usually does not puncture the cysts, but a large-particle biopsy may, leading to a popping or hissing sound as the air is expelled and the cyst is seen to deflate. Histologically, the empty cyst is seen to be surrounded by large, multinucleated macrophages with a slight inflammatory exudate but preservation of the overlying mucosa.[21]

Fecaliths (Fecalomas) and Stercoral Ulcerations

Fecaliths (Fecalomas)

Patients with chronic constipation, especially those with diverticular strictures (see Chapter 45), may develop stone-like formations of fecal matter, i.e., fecaliths. These form because the increased contact time of stool with colonic mucosa, as it passes across an area of diverticular narrowing, allows for a loss of much of its water content so that it becomes rock-hard. Some fecaliths continue to enlarge, attaining the size of 2 cm or more in greatest diameter, and have been termed fecalomas.[22] We observed one such case which radiographically appeared as a smooth filling defect that resembled a large lipoma (Fig. 47-8a). The true nature of the filling defect was apparent at colonoscopy (Fig. 47-8b).

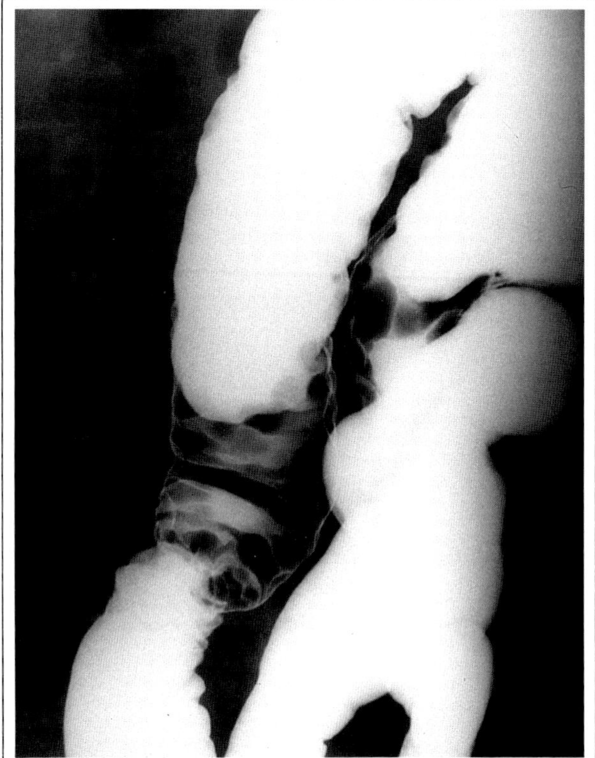

FIG. 47-7a.

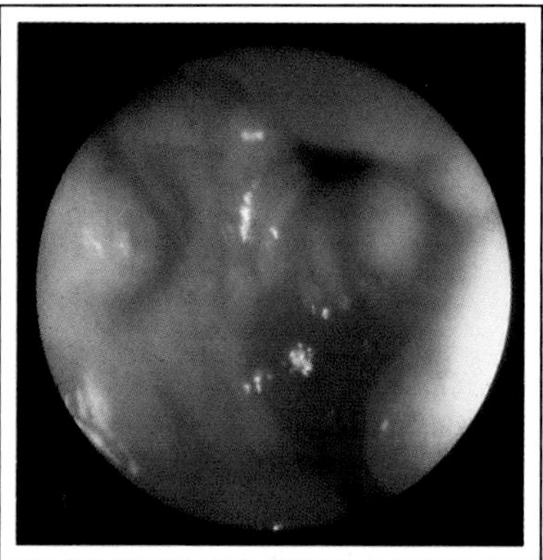

FIG. 47-7b.

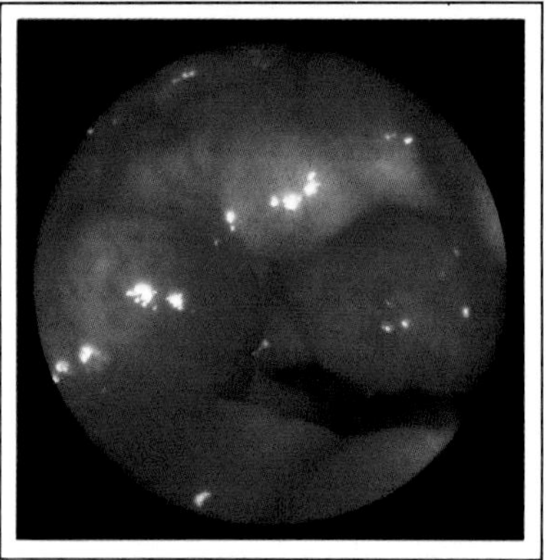

FIG. 47-7c.

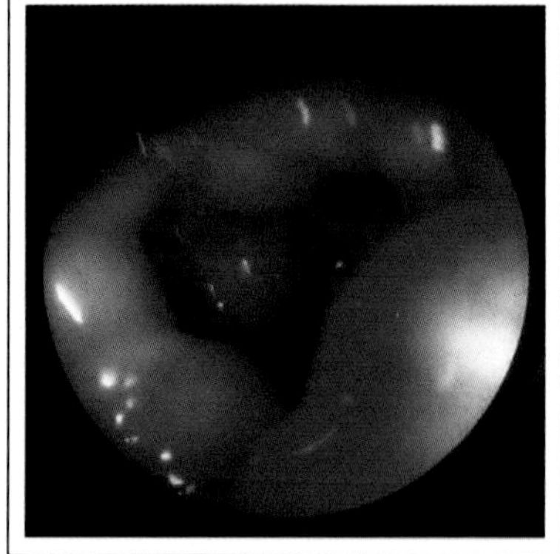

FIG. 47-7d.

FIG. 47-7. Pneumatosis coli. **a:** Radiographic (double-contrast) appearance. Multiple discrete filling defects (air densities) can be seen, especially within the wall. These project into the lumen and could be confused with inflammatory or neoplastic polyposis if submucosal cysts are not observed. **b:** Multiple discrete polypoid masses are observed, all with intact overlying mucosa in a patient having the radiographic appearance of pneumatosis coli (a). **c:** A cluster of submucosal cysts with slightly friable overlying mucosa simulates the appearance of an annular neoplasm, especially if the cysts are sizable. **d:** A large (2 cm) cyst was noted (in the 5 o'clock position) which was soft and easily compressible. In the context of other similar "masses," it suggests pneumatosis coli rather than a neoplastic polyposis syndrome (i.e., familial polyposis coli with malignant degeneration). Forceps biopsy had no effect on the polyp, but during the course of electrosurgical excision there was a popping sound as the nitrogen contained within the cyst was released.

Stercoral Ulceration

Pressure from the fecalith on the colonic mucosa may produce ulcerations from a combination of direct trauma and ischemic necrosis.[23,24] The distal colon is the most commonly affected site[23,24] with the appearance at colonoscopy of single (Fig. 47-8c) or multiple ulcerations.

Colonic Lymphoid Hyperplasia

The finding of multiple 1- to 2-mm, raised, pale areas throughout the colon which histologically proved to be lymphoid hyperplasia may be noted in both children[25] and adults.[26,27] Although possibly more common in children, in a practice which is largely confined to adults we observed only two cases out of 1,900 examinations performed over a 7-year period. In children, lymphoid hyperplasia is probably simply a variant from the normal amount of lymphatic tissue and not a harbinger of inflammatory bowel disease (Crohn's disease).[26] In adults it appears also simply as a variation in the amount of submucosal lymphatic tissue, although we observed one case of a patient with systemic sarcoid in which biopsy showed noncaseating (sarcoid type) granuloma. This case differed from other reported cases of

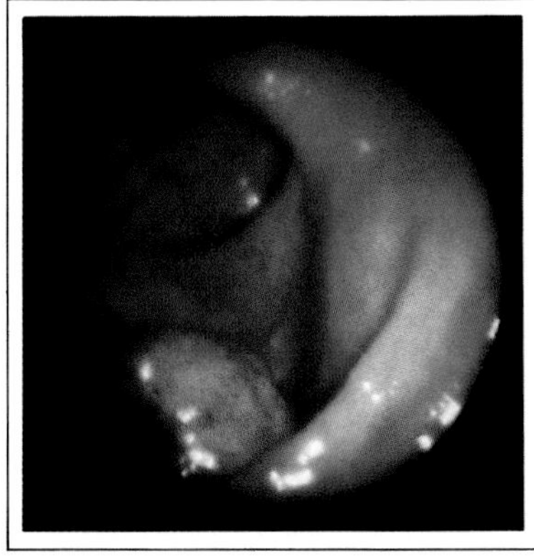

FIG. 47-8a.

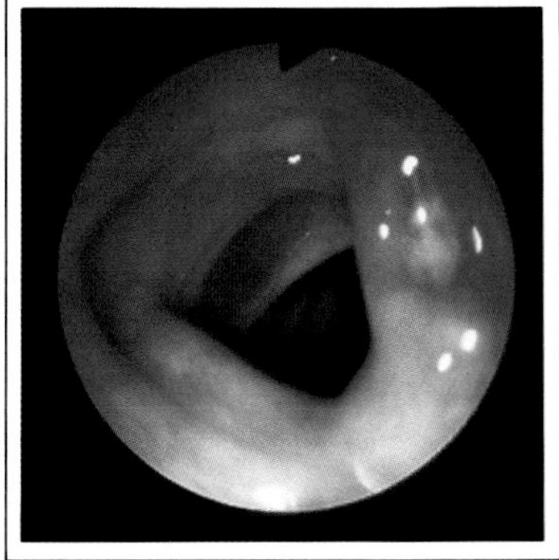

FIG. 47-8c.

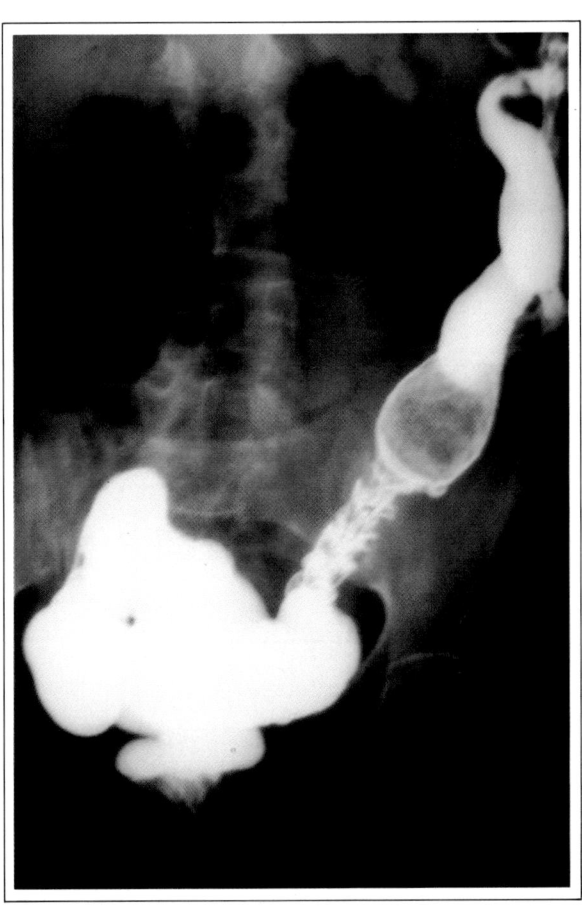

FIG. 47-8b.

FIG. 47-8. a: Fecaloma of the sigmoid colon. This 3-cm egg-shaped fecolith was found in a patient with symptoms of intermittent colonic obstruction. In this case the obstruction was due to the fecaloma periodically becoming lodged at the proximal end of an area of diverticular narrowing demonstrated radiographically (b). **b:** Fecaloma in the sigmoid, radiographic appearance. Because this large filling defect occupied a relatively fixed position at the proximal end of an area of diverticular narrowing, it was thought to represent a large lipoma. Its true nature was disclosed at colonoscopy. **c:** Stercoral ulceration in the sigmoid. A 5-mm ulcer was noted in the sigmoid of a patient with a long history of constipation. This single, discrete 5-mm ulcer may have been the result of trauma related to the hard consistency of stool found in constipated individuals.

sarcoid involving the rectum where the mucosa was either normal or showed nonspecific erythema and friability.[28]

Appearance

Colonoscopy performed in either children or adults with lymphoid hyperplasia shows a typical appearance of closely spaced, yellow-white, 1- to 2-mm raised areas (Fig. 47-9a) similar to nodular lymphoid hyperplasia of the duodenum (see Chapter 28). Biopsies taken from these show them to consist of simple lymphatic nodules (Peyer's patches).

Colonic Lymphangiomas

We have observed one case of colonic lymphangioma, an extremely benign tumor of the lymphatic system. As in our case, the condition usually presents during childhood[29] but can manifest for the first time in late adulthood.[30] The symptoms are nonspecific, including rectal pain, cramping, obstruction, and at least in one-third of the cases rectal bleeding.[29,30] In those cases where bleeding occurs, it can be the result of mucosal trauma from the presence of a submucosal tumor[31] or, as in the case we observed, from the formation of rectal varices secondary to compression of the inferior mesenteric vein by extraintestinal pelvic lymphangiomas.[32]

Appearance

In the case we observed, which presented with rectal bleeding, there were multiple, compressible submucosal masses in the distal rectum (Fig. 47-9b). Because of the presentation, biopsies were not taken although those obtained from similar lesions at other times showed multiple

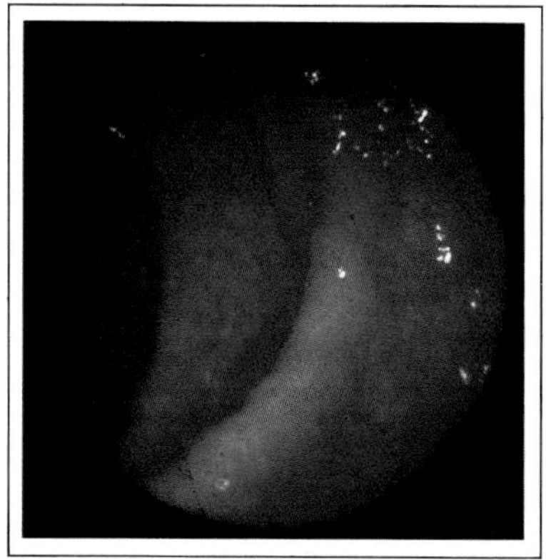

FIG. 47-9a.

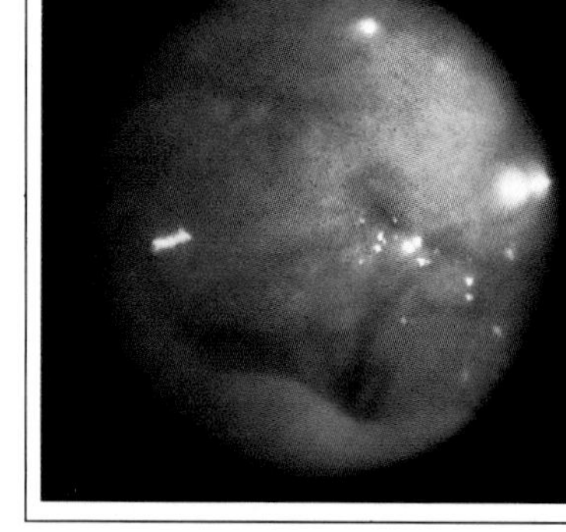

FIG. 47-9b.

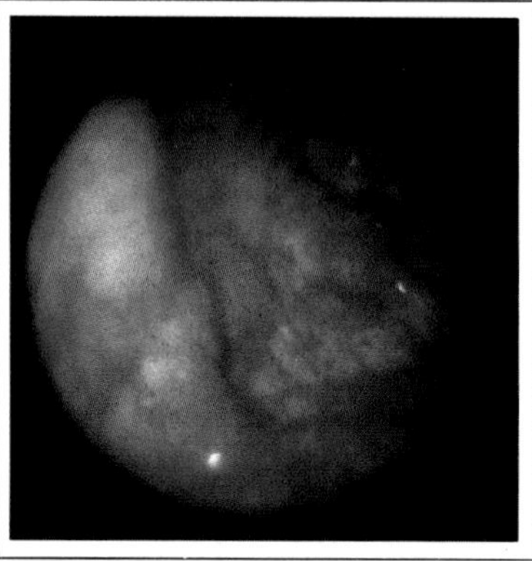

FIG. 47-9c.

FIG. 47-9. a: Lymphoid hyperplasia. Tiny mucosal excrescences are evident, especially along the peak of the intrahaustral fold, giving it a somewhat nodular appearance. In most individuals this has no significance, probably representing a nonspecific increase in submucosal lymphatic tissue (i.e., Peyer's patches). In this particular case, a patient with known pulmonary sarcoid, Langhans' giant cells were seen within the center of otherwise typical submucosal lymphoid nodules, which is suggestive of sarcoid. **b:** Lymphangiomas of the rectum, as submucosal masses. The masses themselves, ranging in size up to 2.5 to 3.5 cm, were soft and easily compressible. The overlying mucosa was intact but had a pale yellow coloration. Biopsies of similar lesions at other times showed changes suggestive of lymphangioma, i.e., cystic spaces separated by septae with lymphocytic infiltration. In addition to the lymphangiomas, rectal varices were observed (c). **c:** Rectal varices are seen with colonic lymphangiomas. These appear as interconnecting gray-blue vein-like elevations (best seen off the 9 and 12 o'clock positions). These were thought to result from compression of the inferior mesenteric vein by extraintestinal (pelvic) lymphangiomas.[32]

cystic spaces separated by septa with lymphocytic infiltration consistent with lymphangioma.[32] Two other vascular abnormalities were noted in our case, the first being the presence of capillary hemangiomas (angiodysplasia lesions) found between the lymphangioma masses. In addition, arteriographically proved rectal varices (Fig. 47-9c) were found and were thought to be secondary to inferior mesenteric vein compression by extraintestinal (pelvic) lymphangiomas.[32]

Colonic Volvulus

Colonic volvulus results from a segment of colon twisting around its mesenteric axis sufficient to produce obstruction. It represents the third commonest cause of colonic obstruction, accounting for 4 to 10% of the cases.[33,34] As it tends to occur in elderly patients, its mortality rate is high, between 8 and 20%,[35] especially in patients who develop intestinal perforation.[33,34]

Volvulus occurs when there is a freely movable, redundant segment of bowel located between two points of fixation, with the commonest locations in the colon being the sigmoid, accounting for 70%+, followed by the cecum, accounting for 15 to 30%.[34] In the case of the sigmoid, a volvulus forms as its redundant loop moves freely between the two fixed points, the retroperitoneal rectum and the descending colon.[33]

Patients with volvulus may present with intermittent cramping, nausea, vomiting, abdominal pain with progressive abdominal distention, and obstipation, with the latter being especially true for a sigmoid volvulus.[35] We have seen at the other extreme a cecal volvulus present with chronic diarrhea (4+ weeks) as a manifestation of intestinal hypersecretion secondary to incomplete obstruction.

Radiographic studies often suggest the diagnosis, especially a barium enema that shows a typical "bird beak" sign. Often the clinical suspicion prompts colonoscopy for both confirmation of the diagnosis and treatment through the evacuation of air and feces from the obstructed segment of colon.[36]

Appearance

In many cases the colonoscope may be advanced to the point of obstruction, where one sees a twisted appearance of the mucosa.[36] Liquid stool is seen in the vicinity. The mucosa is unremarkable or displays a dusky cyanosis with intermucosal hemorrhage. There is superimposed intestinal ischemia.

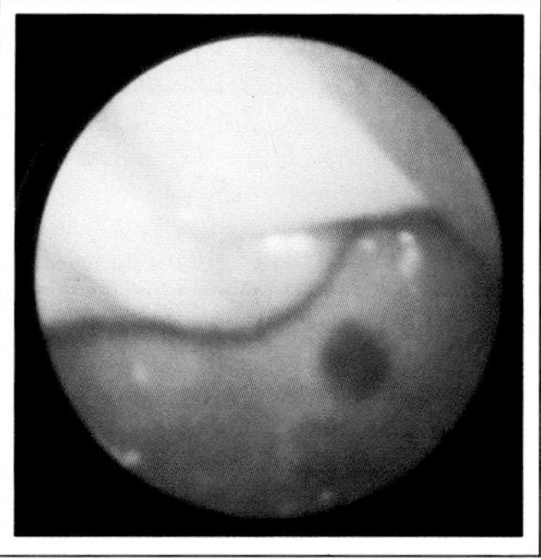

FIG. 47-10.

FIG. 47-10. Foreign body: Cantor tube in the cecum. The tube itself is seen just to the left of the prominent suction artifact (in the 4 o'clock position). The tip, which had migrated into the cecum, could not be retracted back into the terminal ileum and so had to be snared and withdrawn along with the colonoscope.

After recognition of the volvulus, the examiner attempts to enter the obstructed segment. This has proved to be feasible using the "slide by" technique (see Chapter 39) aided by the use of short bursts of air to inflate the obstructed segment.[36] Once inside, large amounts of air and liquid stool may be evacuated through the suction channel, which may bring about immediate detorsion of the volvulus.[36]

Even with successful colonoscopic treatment, surgery is still necessary because of the high recurrence rate without it, approaching 60%.[35] Prior decompression does appear to decrease the risk of surgery, with the mortality rate associated with surgery after detorsion reported to be less than 5%, contrasted with a rate in excess of 15% for patients who are still obstructed.[36]

Pseudo-obstruction of the Colon

Acute colonic distention unrelated to a mechanical cause such as a volvulus (see above) is quite rare.[37,38] It has been reported to occur in a variety of conditions, including systemic infections, chronic neurologic disorders such as parkinsonism, congestive heart failure, after fractures or other major trauma, after surgery, and with acute abdominal conditions such as pancreatitis and cholecystitis.[37,38] The administration of narcotics is common in patients who develop colonic pseudo-obstruction[38a] and may be a causative factor. It has also been reported after the use of phenothiazine and the alpha-adrenergic agonist (antihypertensive agent) clonidine.[38,39] It may be seen in connective tissue disorders, e.g., scleroderma, although usually with small bowel involvement as well.[38,39]

No unifying cause has been found to account for the impairment of colonic peristalsis in these patients which leads to the dilatation. What is common to these patients is their presentation of acute abdominal distention simulating mechanical obstruction, both in regard to the physical examination with preserved, sometimes hyperactive bowel sounds, as well as a plain abdominal radiograph showing dilatation often confined to the right side of the colon.

Where the diameter of the most dilated segment of colon is less than 10 cm, patients have been managed with nasogastric suction and a rectal "flatus tube."[37,38] Because of the fear of perforation, surgery for cecostomy may be a strong consideration for dilatation of more than 10 cm.[37]

In cases of pseudo-obstruction of the colon, especially where surgery is being considered, colonoscopy may be requested to confirm the diagnosis decompression alone[38a] as well as for placement of a drainage tube within the cecum.[40] In one series,[38a] colonoscopic decompression (without a drainage tube) was successful in 32 of 44 patients (73%).

Appearance

In the few cases where colonoscopy has been performed in patients with pseudo-obstruction, the most striking feature has been the marked dilatation, especially of the right colon, where the estimated diameter exceeds 15 cm. Along with this, nonspecific erythema has been observed.[40]

Foreign Bodies of the Colon

A variety of foreign bodies may be encountered. The commonest location for colonic foreign bodies is generally the rectum[41]; the objects here can be removed directly and so are not likely to prompt colonoscopy. Objects located above the rectum, however, can be reached[42] and removed endoscopically.[41,43] A variety of foreign bodies found at colonoscopy have been described, including toothpicks, chicken bones, and suture wire from previous surgery.[41-43] We ourselves have extracted a Cantor tube (Fig. 47-10) which had passed into the cecum and could not be removed from above. It was found in the cecum, snared, and withdrawn along with the colonoscope.

REFERENCES

1. Maingot, R. (1980): Resection and anastomosis of bowel. In: *Abdominal Operations,* edited by R. Maingot, pp. 2034–2065. Appleton-Century-Crofts, New York.

2. Gabrielsson, N., Granqvist, S., and Ohlsen, H. (1976): Recurrent carcinoma of the colon in the anastomosis diagnosed by roentgen examination and colonoscopy. ***Endoscopy,*** 8:47–52.
3. Glotzer, D. J., Glick, M. E., and Goldman, H. (1981): Proctitis and colitis following diversion of the fecal stream. ***Gastroenterology,*** 80:438–441.
4. Connell, A. M., Hilton, C., Irvine, G., Lennard-Jones, J. E., and Misiewicz, J. J. (1965): Variation in bowel habit in two population samples. *Br. Med. J.*, 2:1095–1099.
5. Earnest, D. L. (1978): Other diseases of the colon. In: ***Gastrointestinal Disease,*** edited by M. H. Sleisenger and J. S. Fordtram, pp. 1860–1864. Saunders, Philadelphia.
6. Urso, F. P., Urso, M. J., and Lee, C. H. (1975): The cathartic colon: pathological findings and radiogical/pathological correlation. ***Radiology,*** 116:557–559.
7. Ghadially, F. N., and Parry, E. W. (1966): An electronmicroscope and histochemical study of melanosis coli. *J. Pathol. Bacteriol.*, 92:313–317.
8. Speare, G. S. (1951): Melanosis coli. *Am. J. Surg.*, 82:631–637.
9. Smith, B. (1973): Pathologic changes in the colon produced by anthraquinone purgatives. *Dis. Colon Rectum,* 16:455–458.
10. Rutter, K. R. P., and Riddell, R. H. (1975): The solitary ulcer syndrome of the rectum. *Clin. Gastroenterol.*, 4:505–530.
11. Feczko, P. J., O'Connell, D. J., Riddell, R. H., and Frank, P. H. (1980): Solitary rectal ulcer syndrome: radiologic manifestations. *Am. J. Roentgenol.*, 135:499–506.
11a. Franzin, G., Dina, R., and Fratton, A. (1982): The evolution of the solitary ulcer syndrome of the rectum. An endoscopic and histopathologic study. ***Endoscopy,*** 14:131–134.
12. Ona, F. V., Allende, H. D., Vivenzio, R., Zaky, D., and Nadaraja, N. (1982): Diagnosis and management of nonspecific colon ulcer. *Arch. Surg.*, 117:888–894.
12a. Mills, B., Zuckerman, G., and Sicard, G. (1981): Discrete colon ulcers as a cause of lower gastrointestinal bleeding and perforation in end-stage renal disease. *Surgery,* 89:548–552.
13. Gardiner, G. A., and Bird, C. R. (1980): Nonspecific ulcers of the colon resembling annular carcinoma. ***Radiology,*** 137:331–334.
13a. Sutherland, D. E. R., Chan, F. Y., Foucar, E., Simmons, R. L., Howard, R. J., and Najarian, J. S. (1979): The bleeding cecal ulcer in transplant patients. ***Surgery,*** 86:386–398.
13b. Foucar, E., Mukai, K., Foucar, K., Sutherland, D. E. R., and Van Buren, C. T. (1981): Colon ulceration in lethal cytomegalovirus infection. *Am. J. Clin. Pathol.*, 76:788–801.
13c. Goodman, M. D., and Porter, D. D. (1973): Cytomegalovirus vasculitis with fatal colonic hemorrhage. *Arch. Pathol.*, 96:281–284.
13d. Margolis, D. M., Etheredge, E. E., Garza-Garza, R., Hruska, K., and Anderson, C. B. (1977): Ischemic bowel disease following bilateral nephrectomy or renal transplant. *Surgery,* 82:667–673.
14. Martin, J. K., Culp, C. E., and Weiland, L. H. (1980): Colitis cystica profunda. *Dis. Colon Rectum,* 23:488–491.
15. Tedesco, F. J., Sumner, H. W., and Kassens, W. D. (1976): Colitis cystica profunda. *Am. J. Gastroenterol.*, 65:339–343.
16. Nagasako, K., Nakae, Y., Kitao, Y., and Aoki, G. (1977): Colitis cystica profunda: report of a case in which differentiation from rectal cancer was difficult. *Dis. Colon Rectum,* 20:618–624.
17. Goodall, R. J. R. (1978): Pneumatosis coli: report of two cases. *Dis. Colon Rectum,* 21:61–65.
18. Born, A., Inouye, T., and Diamant, N. (1981): Pneumatosis coli: case report documenting time from x-ray appearance to onset of symptoms. *Dig. Dis. Sci.*, 26:855–859.
19. Mujahed, Z., and Evans, J. A. (1958): Gas cysts of the intestine (pneumatosis intestinalis). *Surg. Gynecol. Obstet.*, 107:151–160.
20. Grunberg, J. C., Grodsinsky, C., and Ponka, J. L. (1979): Pneumatosis intestinalis: a clinical classification. *Dis. Colon Rectum,* 22:5–9.
21. Holt, S., Gilmour, H. M., Buist, T. A. S., Marwick, K., and Heading, R. C. (1979): Highflow oxygen therapy for pneumatosis coli. *Gut,* 20:495–498.
22. Cid, A. A., Pietruk, T., Bidari, C. Z., and Ehrinpreis, M. N. (1981): Cecal fecaloma mimicking colonic neoplasm. *Dig. Dis. Sci.*, 26:1134–1137.
23. Shatila, A. H., and Ackerman, N. B. (1977): Stercoraceous ulcerations and perforations of the colon: report of cases and survey of the literature. *Dis. Colon Rectum,* 20:524–526.
24. Gekas, P., and Schuster, M. M. (1981): Stercoral perforation of the colon: case report and review of the literature. ***Gastroenterology,*** 80:1054–1058.
25. Riddlesberger, M. M., and Lebenthal, E. (1980): Nodular colonic mucosa of childhood: normal or pathologic? ***Gastroenterology,*** 79:265–270.
26. Kenney, P. J., Koehler, R. E., and Shackelford, G. D. (1982): The clinical significance of large lymphoid follicles of the colon. ***Radiology,*** 142:41–46.
27. Burbige, E. J., and Sobky, R. Z. F. (1977): Endoscopic appearance of colonic lymphoid nodules: a normal variant. ***Gastroenterology,*** 72:524–526.
28. Tobi, M., Korbrin, I., and Ariel, I. (1982): Rectal involvement in sarcoidosis. *Dis. Colon Rectum,* 25:491–493.
29. Harkins, G. A., and Sabiston, D. C. (1960): Lymphangiomas in infancy and childhood. *Surgery,* 47:811–817.
30. Beradi, R. S. (1974): Lymphangioma of the large intestine: report of a case and review of the literature. *Dis. Colon Rectum,* 17:265–272.
31. Kupic, E. A., and Eddy, W. M. (1973): Lymphangioma, a rare pelvic mass lesion. *Am. J. Roentgenol.*, 126:404–407.
32. Blackstone, M. O., Rogers, B. H. G., and Baker, A. L. (1975): A cutaneous and pelvic lymphangioma, with varices, lymphangiomas, and capillary hemangiomas of the rectosigmoid colon. *Gastrointest. Endosc.*, 23:39–41.
33. Avots-Avotins, K., and Waugh, D. E. (1982): Colon volvulus and the geriatric patient. *Surg. Clin. North Am.*, 62:249–260.
34. Grodsinsky, C., and Ponko, J. L. (1977): Volvulus of the colon. *Dis. Colon Rectum,* 20:314–324.
35. Siroospour, D., and Berardi, R. S. (1976): Volvulus of the sigmoid colon: a ten-year study. *Dis. Colon Rectum,* 19:535–541.
36. Sanner, C. J., and Saltzman, D. A. (1977): Detorsion of the sigmoid volvulus by colonoscopy. *Gastrointest. Endosc.*, 23:212–213.
37. Søreide, O., Bjerkeset, M. D., and Fossdal, J. E. (1977): Pseudoobstruction of the colon (Ogilvie's syndrome): a genuine clinical condition? Review of the literature (1948–1975) and report of five cases. *Dis. Colon Rectum,* 20:487–491.
38. Bachulis, B. L., and Smith, P. E. (1978): Pseudoobstruction of the colon. *Am. J. Surg.*, 136:66–72.
38a. Strodel, W. E., Nostrant, T. T., Eckhauser, F. E., and Dent, T. L. (1983): Therapeutic and diagnostic colonoscopy in nonobstructive colonic dilatation. *Ann. Surg.*, 197:416–421.
39. Schuffler, M. D., Rohrmann, C. A., Chaffee, R. G., Brand, D. L., Delaney, J. H., and Young, J. H. (1981): Chronic intestinal pseudoobstruction: a report of 27 cases and review of the literature. *Medicine,* 60:173–196.
40. Bernton, E., Myers, R., and Reyna, T. (1981): Pseudoobstruction of the colon: case report including a new endoscopic treatment. *Gastrointest. Endosc.*, 28:90–92.
41. Eftaiha, M., Hambrick, E., and Abcarian, H. (1977): Principles of management of colorectal foreign bodies. *Arch. Surg.*, 112:691–695.
42. Mapelli, P., Head, L. H., Conner, W. E., and Ferrante, W. E. (1980): Peforation of colon by ingested chicken bone diagnosed colonoscopically. *Gastrointest. Endosc.*, 26:20–21.
43. Oehler, J. R., Dent, T. L., Ibrahim, M. A. H., and Gracie, W. A. (1979): Endoscopic identification and removal of an unusual symptomatic colonic foreign body. *Dig. Dis. Sci.*, 24:236–239.

48

THE TERMINAL ILEUM—TECHNIQUE OF EXAMINATION, NORMAL APPEARANCE, AND FINDINGS WITH INFLAMMATORY BOWEL DISEASE, ILEOSTOMY, AND ILEAL TUMORS

TECHNIQUE OF EXAMINATION

A portion of terminal ileum can be examined as either part of the colonoscopic procedure[1–3] or, if an ileostomy is present, directly through its stoma.[4]

As Part of the Colonoscopic Examination

Locating the Ileocecal Valve

As already discussed (see Chapter 39, especially Fig. 39-16), the right colon may be entered by means of downward deflection with the hepatic flexure and mesenteric wall of the right colon observed in a 6 o'clock position. In this case, if the orientation is perfectly maintained throughout the intubation of the ascending colon and cecum, the posterior aspect of the mesenteric wall and the ileocecal valve are observed in the 3 to 6 o'clock positions (Fig. 48-1a). However, this orientation is generally not maintained because of the inherent tendency of the tip to rotate clockwise as the right colon is intubated so as to cause the 9 o'clock lens position to become aligned with the posterior aspect of the mesenteric wall (Fig. 48-1b) and ileocecal valve (see Fig. 39-19).

The cause of this clockwise rotation is unclear. One explanation is that it occurs because of the counterclockwise torque exerted on the shaft at the hepatic flexure as the more posterior right colon is intubated. With the tip already deflected downward, the torque starts it turning in a clockwise fashion. After complete intubation of the right colon, with more clockwise rotation and finally deflection of the tip, the ileocecal valve itself comes into view toward the 12 o'clock position (Fig. 48-1c), approximately 2 to 3 cm from the base of the cecum. Here the ileocecal valve is observed in its labial, papillary, or intermediate type configuration (see Chapter 39). With continued upward deflection of the tip, the ileocecal valve is observed toward the 6 to 9 o'clock position (Fig. 48-1c).

Intubation and Examination

With continued intubation and the tip in upward deflection "banking off" the base of the cecum, the orifice of the ileocecal valve begins to open (Fig. 48-1c). Once the orifice is observed to be open and in the 6 o'clock position (Fig. 48-1c), gentle downward deflection into the orifice and withdrawal (producing some paradoxical advancement) allows intubation of the terminal ileum.[1,2] Some use a biopsy forceps, which is first passed across the ileocecal valve as a guidewire to facilitate intubation[3]; however, most examiners do not find this necessary. Once the terminal ileum is intubated, it is possible to advance the endoscope and examine the mucosa for about 20 to 50 cm.[1]

Patients With an Ileostomy

In almost all cases the patient with an ileostomy can be examined endoscopically, often with a colonoscope of standard caliber (13 to 15 mm). In some cases, however, there is narrowing of the stomal lumen so that narrow-caliber (8 to 9 mm) pediatric-type endoscope is necessary.

The patient may be placed in the supine or right lateral recumbent position for the examination. After gentle dilatation of the stoma with the index or fifth finger,[4] the endoscope tip is introduced. Once the tip is below the skin the lumen is found by gentle air insufflation. The lumen then may be followed for approximately 30 to 50 cm, advancing by direct intubation and periodic withdrawal. If necessary, the tip position can be determined fluoroscopically.

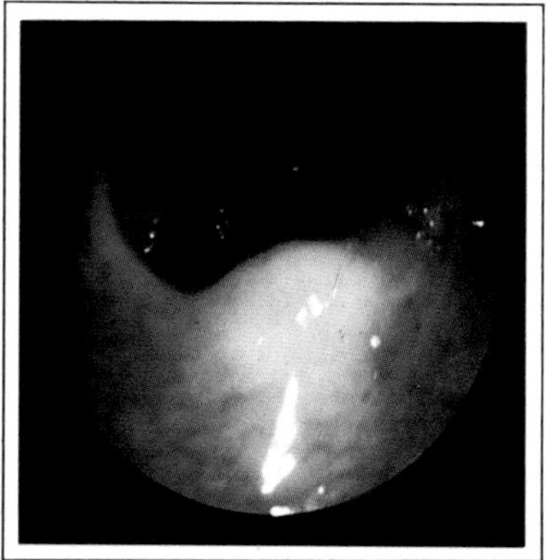

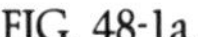
FIG. 48-1a.

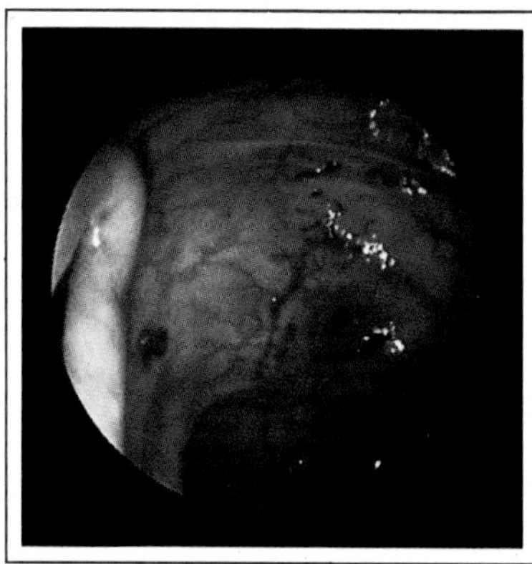
FIG. 48-1b.

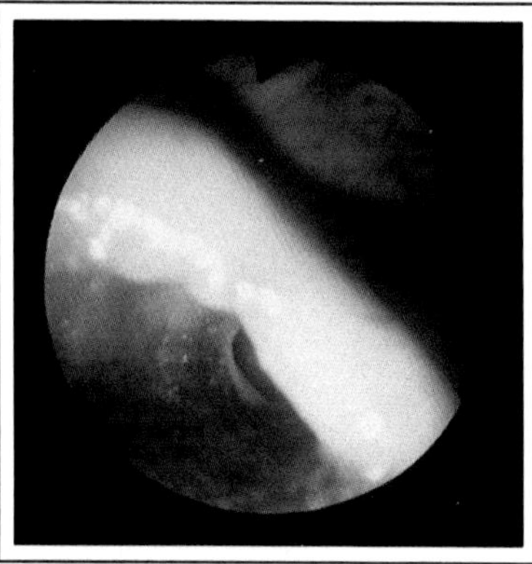
FIG. 48-1c.

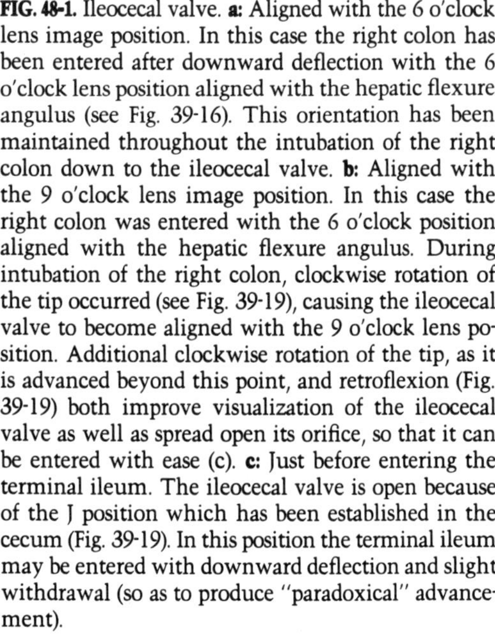
FIG. 48-1. Ileocecal valve. **a:** Aligned with the 6 o'clock lens image position. In this case the right colon has been entered after downward deflection with the 6 o'clock lens position aligned with the hepatic flexure angulus (see Fig. 39-16). This orientation has been maintained throughout the intubation of the right colon down to the ileocecal valve. **b:** Aligned with the 9 o'clock lens image position. In this case the right colon was entered with the 6 o'clock position aligned with the hepatic flexure angulus. During intubation of the right colon, clockwise rotation of the tip occurred (see Fig. 39-19), causing the ileocecal valve to become aligned with the 9 o'clock lens position. Additional clockwise rotation of the tip, as it is advanced beyond this point, and retroflexion (Fig. 39-19) both improve visualization of the ileocecal valve as well as spread open its orifice, so that it can be entered with ease (c). **c:** Just before entering the terminal ileum. The ileocecal valve is open because of the J position which has been established in the cecum (Fig. 39-19). In this position the terminal ileum may be entered with downward deflection and slight withdrawal (so as to produce "paradoxical" advancement).

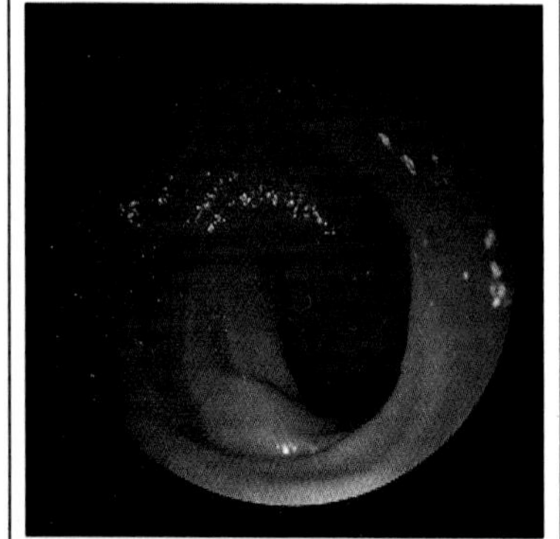
FIG. 48-2a.

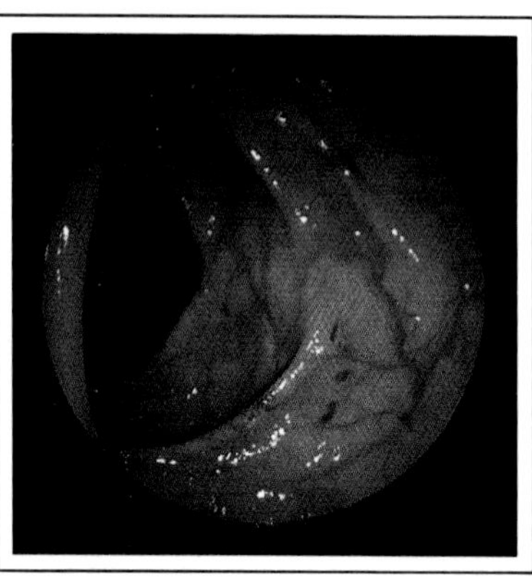
FIG. 48-2b.

FIG. 48-2. a: Terminal ileum, just beyond the ileocecal valve. The infrequent Kerckring folds and absent vascular pattern contrast with the ascending colon from which it has been entered (b). The ileal mucosa appears smooth, lacking the granularity of the duodenum at close range (compare with Fig. 24-10). **b:** Ascending colon, just proximal to the ileocecal valve. The prominent vascular pattern and broad interhaustral folds denote the right colon.

Shape

The terminal ileum has a relatively small-caliber (2 to 3 cm) lumen (Fig. 48-1a) with an indistinct or absent mucosal (Kerckring) fold pattern. This latter feature stands in contrast to the duodenum (see Chapter 24) and jejunum (observed as part of a gastrojejunostomy—see Chapter 19), both of which have prominent Kerckring folds. In cases where the terminal ileum has been entered from the ileocecal valve, its relatively foldless lumen (Fig. 48-2a) serves to distinguish it from the ascending colon (Fig. 48-2b) and cecum with their broad semilunar folds clearly in evidence.

Mucosal Features

Character

The character of the mucosa is variable, to a large extent depending on the age of the patient. In middle-aged and elderly patients, who lack prominent lymphoid follicles (see below), it may be smooth and glistening (Fig. 48-2a). Because of the shorter, less-prominent villi of the terminal ileum, the mucosa appears perfectly smooth, even viewed at close range (Fig. 48-2a), in contrast to the granularity of the duodenum that results from its taller, broader villi. In

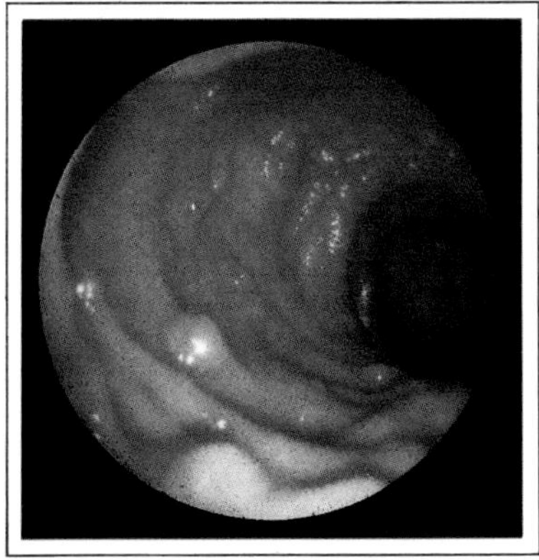

FIG. 48-3a.

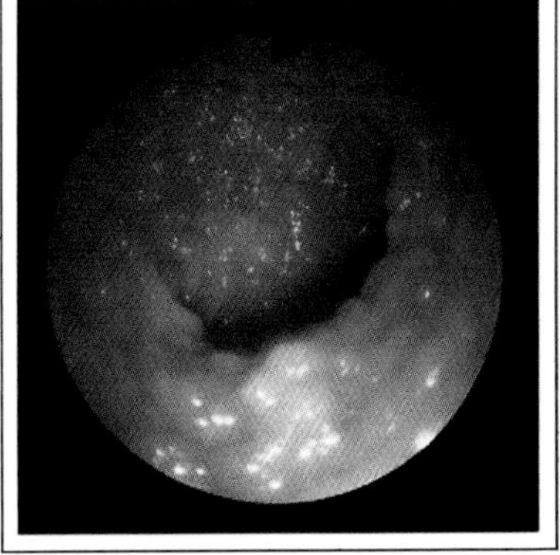

FIG. 48-3b.

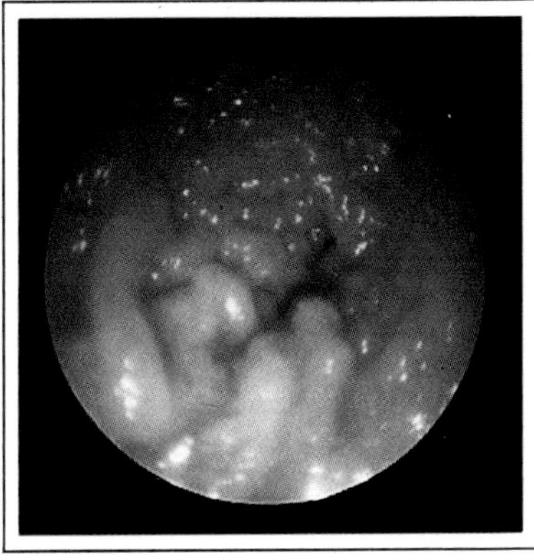

FIG. 48-3c.

FIG. 48-3. Lymphoid hyperplasia in the terminal ileum. **a:** Several tiny nodules (2 to 4 mm) were noted in the terminal ileum of this 19-year-old woman with intermittent abdominal pain. Biopsies showed lymphoid follicles, a normal finding. **b:** In this case the mucosa is carpeted by the presence of tiny (1 to 2 mm) nodules, giving it a granular appearance (contrast with Fig. 48-2a). Biopsies showed lymphoid follicles. **c:** The presence of tiny lymphoid nodules on the mucosal folds give them a corrugated, irregular appearance.

teenage patients and young adults, the mucosa may appear irregular due to the presence of prominent lymphoid follicles (see below).

Vascular Pattern

The vascular pattern is variable, although as in the duodenum the vascular pattern is generally indistinct or absent altogether (Fig. 48-2a).

Lymphoid Follicles

The lymphoid follicles are usually very prominent in patients under the age of 30 but are seen less often in older individuals.[1] When they are present, a spectrum of appearances may be observed, ranging from one or several large lymphoid follicles (Fig. 48-3a) to the mucosa being literally carpeted with tiny (1 to 3 mm) lymphoid nodules (Fig. 48-3b). As light is reflected more intensely from the tips of these nodules, one observes the mucosa to be granular with the light reflection breaking up into a myriad of dots (Fig. 48-3b). In addition, these nodules give the mucosal folds a corrugated appearance (Fig. 48-3c). In cases where the terminal ileum is not sufficiently insufflated, these may appear as nodular masses (Fig. 47-3c).

FINDINGS IN INFLAMMATORY BOWEL DISEASE

Ulcerative Colitis—"Backwash Ileitis"

It is our impression that backwash ileitis may be expected in up to 10% of the patients with ulcerative colitis, similar to its reported prevalence radiologically.[5] As is true when it is demonstrated radiographically, it occurs almost exclusively in patients with universal involvement, especially with tubularization and foreshortening of the right colon (see Chapter 43). The muscle hypertrophy within the wall of the colon which appears to underlie the structural changes within the right colon effaces the ileocecal valve, causing it to become patulous (Fig. 48-4a) and making it easily entered so that the involved mucosa of the terminal ileum can be examined.

Appearance

In cases where backwash ileitis has been suggested radiographically, there is tubularization of the terminal ileum with absent mucosal (Kerckring) folds. The mucosa may show some evidence of disease activity, e.g., patchy erythema. In rare cases more activity is present with evidence of acute inflammatory exudate (Fig. 48-4a), but discrete mucosal ulcerations are generally absent.[6]

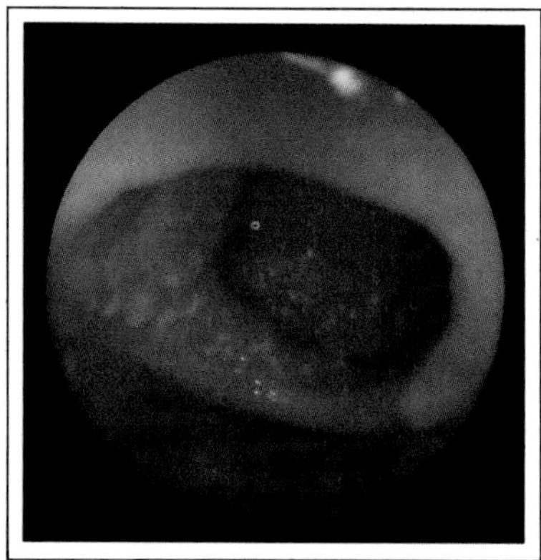

FIG. 48-4a.

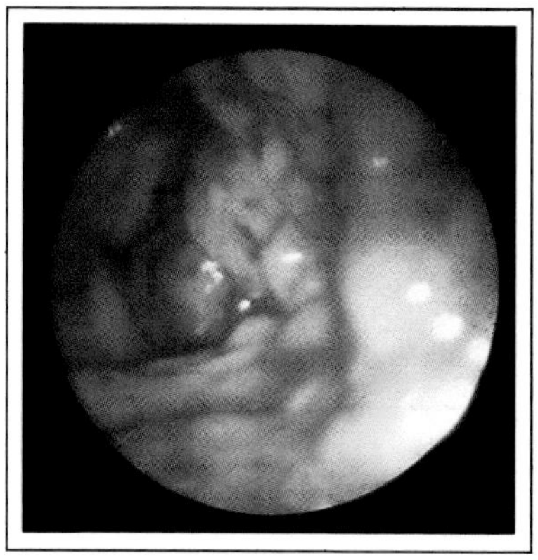

FIG. 48-4b.

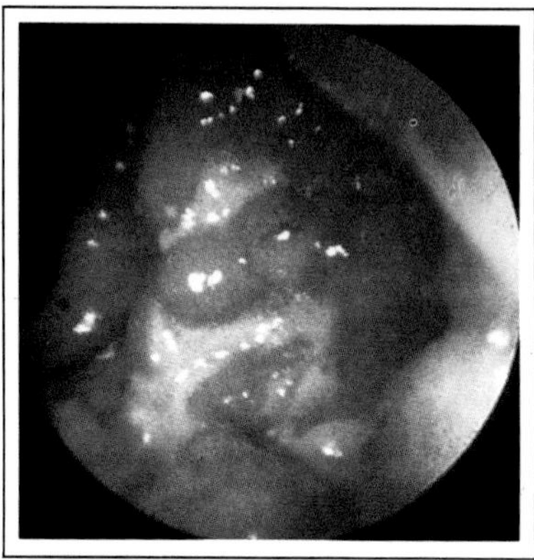

FIG. 48-4c.

FIG. 48-4. a: Backwash ileitis in a patient with long-standing ulcerative colitis. The ileocecal valve is extremely patulous, in contrast to its appearance in Crohn's disease (Fig. 48-4b). The ileal involvement consists of tiny ulcerations and a mucopurulent exudate that continues for about 20 cm. In most cases of backwash ileitis, the terminal ileum shows patchy or diffuse erythema rather than ulcerations. **b:** Crohn's colitis involving the cecum and ileocecal valve. Multiple inflammatory masses along with deep ulcerations are present. Because of these, the ileocecal valve could not be identified. **c:** Crohn's colitis with ileocecal involvement. Despite the ulcerations and apparent narrowing of the orifice, intubation of the terminal ileum was possible.

Crohn's Disease

It is more difficult to examine the terminal ileum in patients with Crohn's disease, as the ileocecal valve involvement, which may be expected in at least 50% of the cases,[7] characteristically produces ulceration and stenosis along with induration and edema (Fig. 48-4b), making it difficult if not impossible to enter. Unlike the ileocecal valve in ulcerative colitis, which is patulous and easily identified (Fig. 48-2a), in Crohn's disease this structure is closed, often tightly so, making it impossible to distinguish areas of activity (ulcerations and inflammatory masses) from the surrounding right colon.

Still, in occasional patients even with ileocecal valve involvement (Fig. 48-4c), it is possible to enter the terminal ileum and observe its appearance both in cases where no prior surgery has been performed as well as in those instances where the terminal ileum is observed following ileocecal resection to determine if the disease has recurred.

Unoperated Appearance

Even though the ileocecal valve is involved as part of Crohn's colitis, the terminal ileum may show only lymphoid follicles (Fig. 48-5a), which is an age-related normal variant (see above) and not a harbinger of future ileal disease. In at least half the cases,[7] when the ileocecal valve is involved there is both right colon and terminal ileal activity. One therefore expects to find evidence of activity in the form of focal ulcerations on entering the terminal ileum (Fig. 48-5b). These have a variable appearance, ranging from small (2 to 4 mm) superficial ulcerations (Fig. 48-5b) to large ulcers (up to 1 cm or more). Some of these large ulcers are associated with stricture formation (Fig. 48-5d). Between ulcerations there may be 5- to 10-cm skip areas, which themselves are indistinguishable from normal mucosa or show only slight enlargement of the Kerckring folds. These skip areas terminate with a resumption of activity (Fig. 48-6b) as evidenced by the presence of focal ulcerations.

Recurrent Crohn's Disease After Ileocolic Resection and Anastomosis

Most recurrences of Crohn's disease, especially those involving the terminal ileum, are found within 20 cm of the anastomosis, although not necessarily involving it.[8] Most often, ulcerations are seen just at and proximal to the anastomosis (Fig. 48-7a). When the terminal ileum is involved in a recurrence, the ulcer initially tends to be circumferential, on the ridges of the valvulae and sparing the mucosa in between (Fig. 48-7a). The ulcers tend to be superficial and have an aphthous appearance. Deeper ulcers

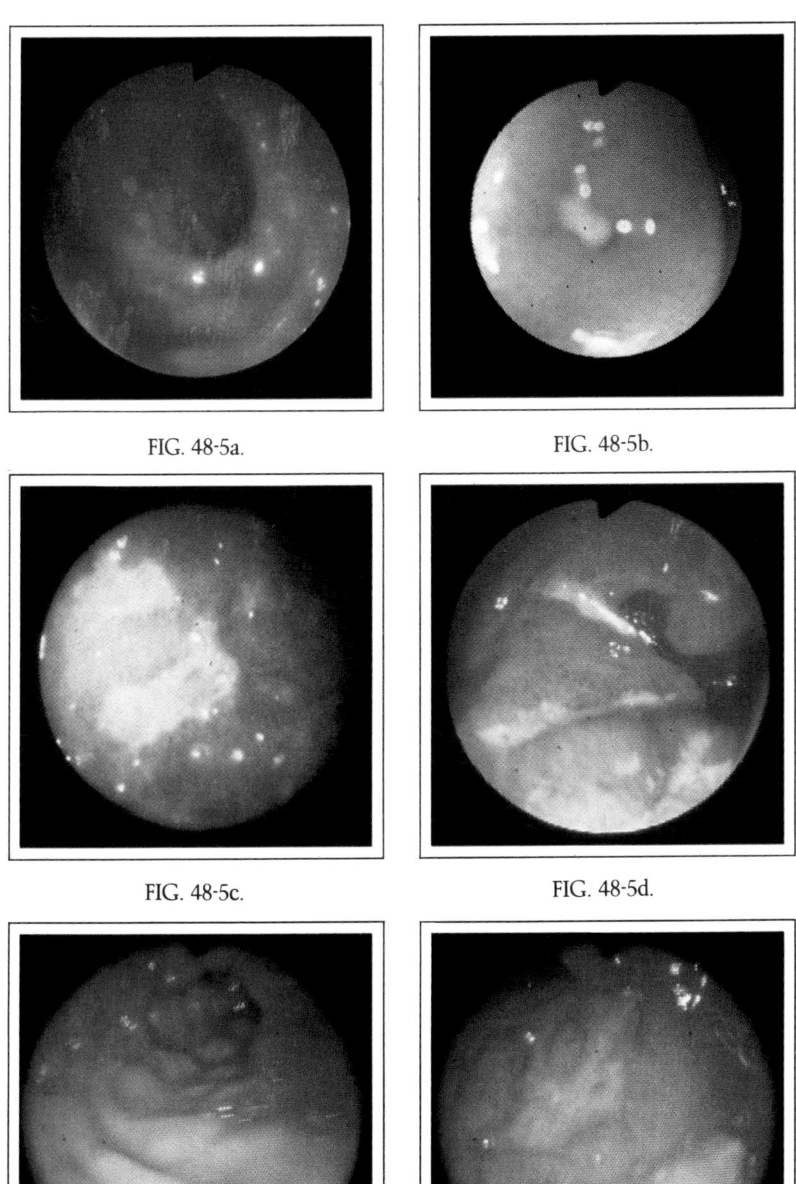

FIG. 48-5a. FIG. 48-5b. FIG. 48-5c. FIG. 48-5d. FIG. 48-6a. FIG. 48-6b.

FIG. 48-5. a: Lymphoid hyperplasia of the terminal ileum in a patient with Crohn's disease. This is an entirely nonspecific finding. **b:** Terminal ileum, Crohn's disease. The appearance of discrete, small (2 to 4 mm), slightly excavated aphthous ulcerations is the first definite indication of involvement. **c:** Terminal ileum, Crohn's disease. Multiple ulcers of various sizes (between 3 and 10 mm) are observed. The intervening mucosa is either normal or slightly erythematous. **d:** Terminal ileum, Crohn's disease with stricture. Ulcerations radiate out from within the stricture. In addition, a polyp of hyperplastic mucosa has formed between adjacent ulcerations.

FIG. 48-6. Terminal ileum, Crohn's disease. **a:** Skip area. The mucosa is entirely normal just proximal to a zone of activity (b). The skip area terminates abruptly into a zone of marked activity (b). **b:** Active. A skip area terminates abruptly into one of marked activity with large (1 to 1.5 cm) ulcers which run for approximately 5 to 10 cm.

are found on the anastomosis itself or just adjacent to it. Skip areas of 5 to 10 cm may be present between foci of activity (Fig. 48-7c). In some cases, especially at the anastomosis where there are deep ulcerations, there may be a cobblestone appearance because of adjacent zones of hyperplastic mucosa (Fig. 48-7d).

ILEOSTOMY

The patient with an ileostomy may be referred for endoscopy because of pain or ileostomy dysfunction, which may manifest as an output in excess of 1,500 to 2,000 cc per day. Such patients are referred for an endoscopic examination of the ileostomy stoma and adjacent small bowel, as are others with a history of intermittent ileostomy bleeding.

If the ileostomy was originally performed because of Crohn's colitis, the clinician suspects a recurrence at the ileostomy site.[8,9] In cases where the ileostomy followed a colectomy or either Crohn's disease or ulcerative colitis, he may suspect peristomal adhesions or nonspecific prestomal ileitis as the cause of ileostomy dysfunction.[9,10] In the case of patients with inflammatory bowel disease who have underlying cirrhosis, he may suspect the presence of ileal

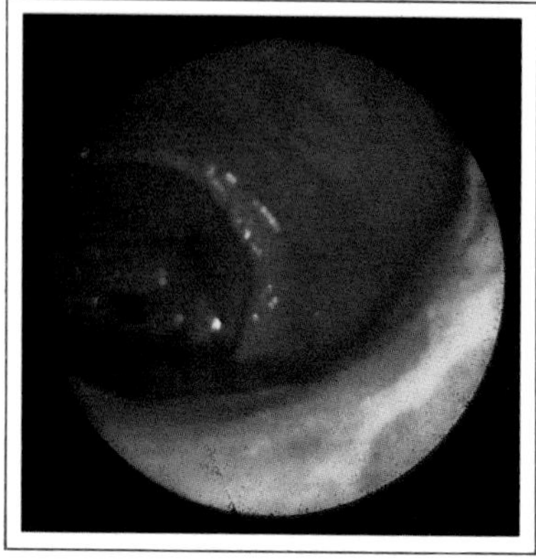

FIG. 48-7a.

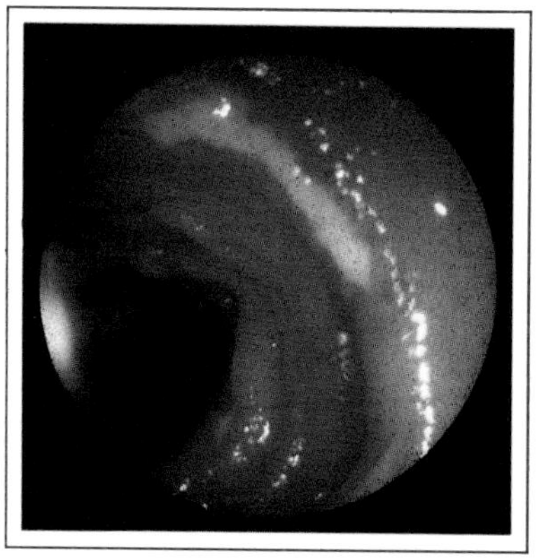

FIG. 48-7b.

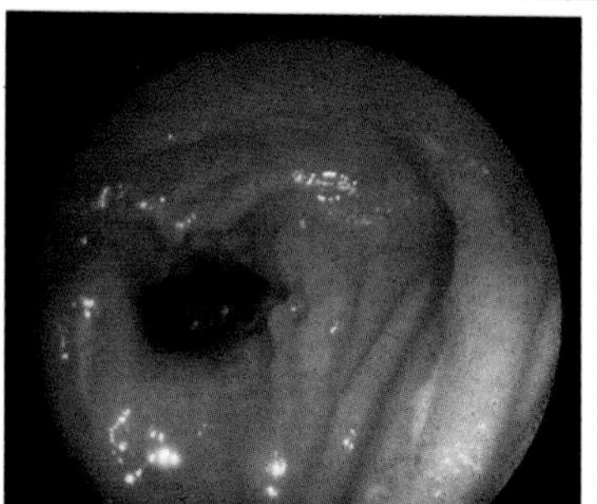

FIG. 48-7c.

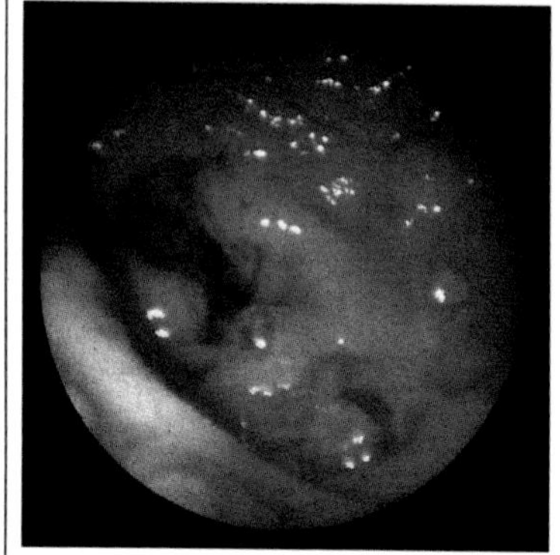

FIG. 48-7d.

FIG. 48-7. a: Ileocolic anastomosis after right hemicolectomy for Crohn's disease in a patient with symptoms that suggest recurrence. Extensive ulcerations are noted around the anastomosis (in the 3 and 6 o'clock positions) as well as more proximally (b). **b:** Terminal ileum with recurrent Crohn's disease above a similarly involved ileocolic anastomosis. Linear ulcerations are noted on the crests of the Kerckring folds, with the intervening mucosa either showing nonspecific erythema or being entirely skipped (c). **c:** Terminal ileum, recurrent Crohn's disease with a skip area. This segment, located just above one showing definite activity (b), is largely uninvolved except for tiny aphthous ulcers at 2 and 4 o'clock. Another segment of marked activity was noted proximal to this skip area. **d:** Nodular ileocolic anastomosis in a patient with recurrent Crohn's disease. Some of the nodules are polyps composed of hyperplastic mucosa which forms around the margin of ulcers as part of the cobblestone effect. The ulcers disappeared with treaatment, leaving only the nodular anastomosis.

varices as a cause of intermittent ileostomy bleeding. Finally, in patients who have had an ileostomy as part of an ileal conduit (ureteroileostomy) but who have developed new obstructive symptoms, endoscopy may be requested both for inspection of the conduit and its opening and for radiologic studies which can be performed as part of endoscopy.[11]

In the sections which follow, we consider some of the appearances for patients referred for an endoscopic examination of an ileostomy.

Normal Ileostomy Appearance

With a normal ileostomy appearance there is erythema as the stoma is entered; this is the result of the mucosa above the skin line flopping onto the lens and causing a "red-out" (Fig. 48-8a). It is generally a problem only above the level of the abdominal wall. Here it is difficult or impossible to keep the lumen insufflated and the mucosa off the lens. However, another reason for the erythematous appearance is that the mucosal vessels above the skin line tend to remain engorged, imparting a deep pink or reddish coloration to this mucosa. Below the abdominal wall the mucosa is easily observed, being either indistinguishable from normal (Fig. 48-8b), just slightly more erythematous especially in the adjacent 5 cm (Fig. 48-8c), or somewhat more pale.

Continent (Koch) Ileostomy Appearance

Although performed less often than a decade ago,[12] the examiner is still occasionally confronted by a patient who has had a continent (Koch) type ileostomy. This arrangement is essentially that of a pouch created by two adjacent loops of ileum which have been sewn together and around an intussuscepted portion of the terminal ileum (outflow tract) which ends at the ileostomy stoma. In contrast to the standard Brooke-type ileostomy, which continually drains into an appliance, as the internal pouch of a continent ileostomy fills it constricts the intussuscepted outflow tract so that it does not empty unless catheterized. As the continent ileostomy is not performed in patients with Crohn's colitis because of the risk of recurrence after this type of surgery, the principal indication for an endoscopic examination is incontinence and other symptoms of ileostomy dysfunction.

Appearance

We ourselves have no personal experience with a continent ileostomy. According to Waye et al.,[12] the method

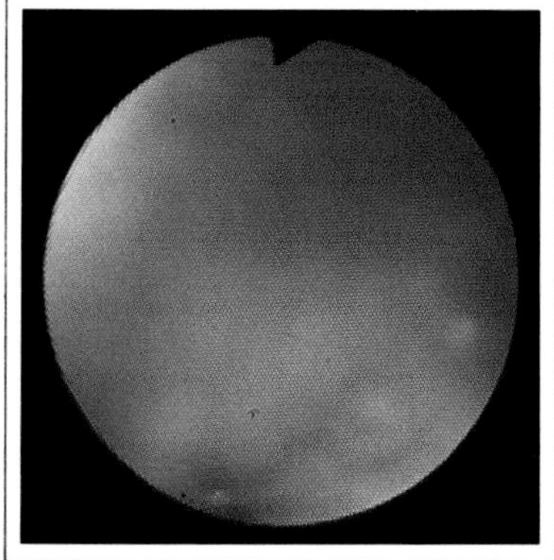

FIG. 48-8a.

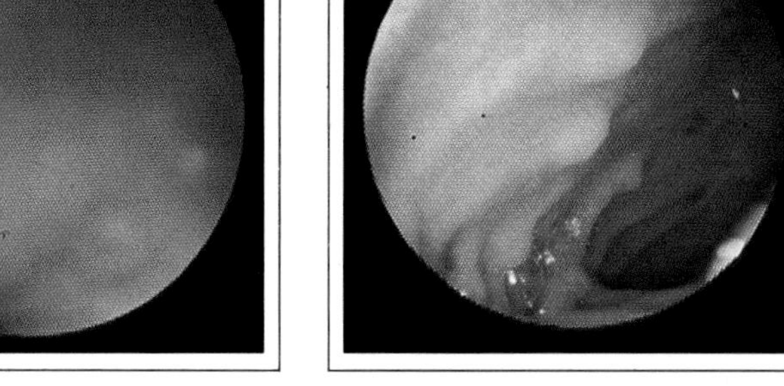

FIG. 48-8b.

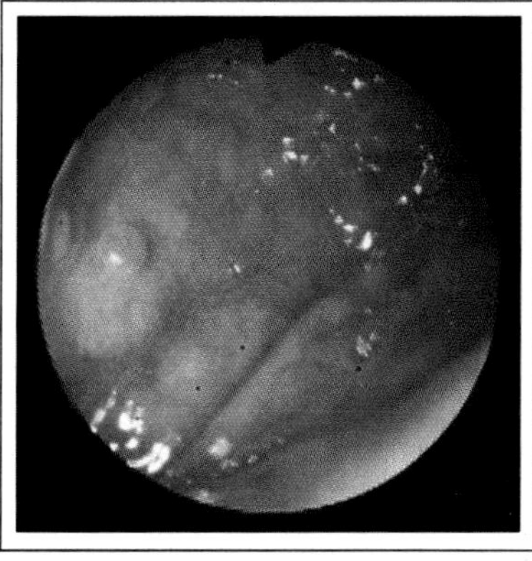

FIG. 48-8c.

FIG. 48-8. a: Ileostomy being entered. There is a "red-out" as the instrument is inserted through the stoma. Just beyond the abdominal wall, the mucosa has an entirely normal appearance. **b:** Terminal ileum, just beyond the ostomy orifice (a). The appearance is unremarkable except for the presence of lymphoid nodules, which are not a pathologic feature even in a patient who has had surgery for Crohn's disease. **c:** Terminal ileum showing nonspecific erythema just proximal to an ileostomy opening in a patient who had surgery for Crohn's disease and occasional cramping. This appearance itself does not imply recurrence.

of examination does not differ from that used for the standard Brooke-type ileostomy. The patient is examined in the supine position after digital examination of the stoma. As a retroflexed view of the outflow tract is desirable in all cases, the use of intermediate-caliber (10 to 11 mm) or pediatric-type instrument (8 to 9 mm) having the capability of 180° retroflexion is most desirable.

The instrument is introduced into the stoma, and the 5- to 6-cm outflow tract is intubated directly until the air-distended ileal pouch itself is entered. According to Waye et al.,[12] the pouch configuration is like that of the antrum of the stomach. There are no Kerckring folds, these having been lost within 1 month of its construction. Several long suture lines can be identified. The ileal inflow tract is located adjacent to the outflow tract, both of which are observed when the instrument is retroflexed by means of advancing the instrument within the pouch with the tip deflected maximally in the "up" position.[12] By observing the intussuscepted portion (outflow tract), Waye et al. were able to detect the absence of sliding, a finding which correctly indicated a loss of stability of the intussuscepted portion and a decrease in the completeness of its closure as the pouch filled. An appearance which indicated adhesions as the cause of incontinence was the finding of the nipple in a fixed position, which rendered it incapable of closing as the pouch filled. These problems as well as that of foreign bodies in the pouch can be treated endoscopically.[12]

Recurrent Crohn's Disease

At the time surgery is performed for Crohn's colitis, an ileostomy is fashioned from mucosa which is grossly and even histologically free of disease; however, recurrences are expected in 20% if the disease was confined to the colon and in 40% or more if small bowel was involved as well.[8] Abdominal pain, obstruction, high output, and ileostomy diarrhea all prompt an examination for a suspected recurrence.[13]

Appearance

The ileostomy stoma itself may be erythematous and indurated, a feature which should always cause the examiner to suspect recurrence. It will be apparent to the examiner that the orifice is narrowed and will admit only a 9-mm pediatric-type instrument. In addition to its narrow caliber, aphthous ulcers may be seen in the mucosa above the skin line, with deeper ulcerations just within (Fig. 48-9a). Some normal intervening mucosa may appear between deep ulcerations as skip areas (Fig. 48-9b) between focally

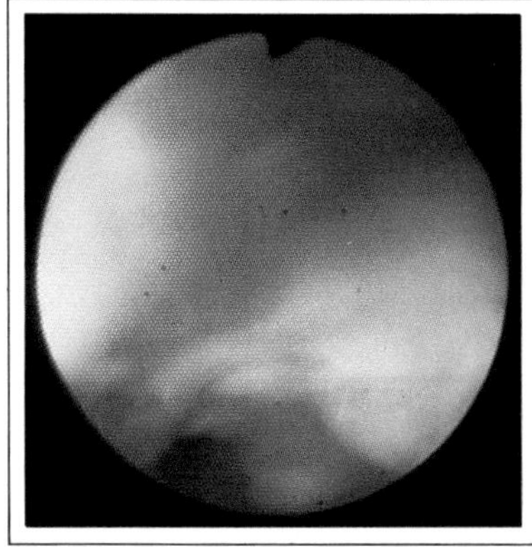

FIG. 48-9a.

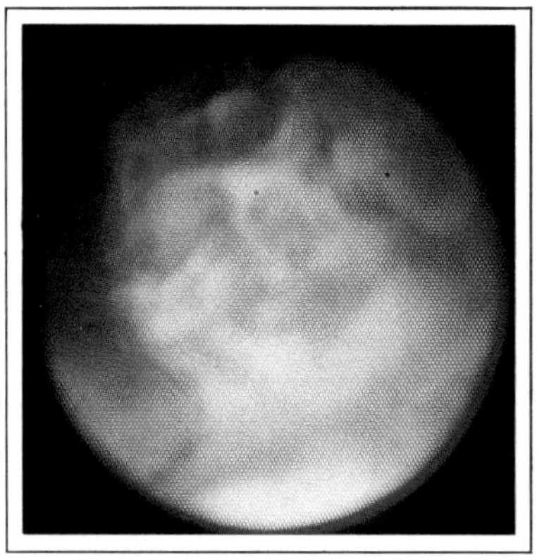

FIG. 48-9b.

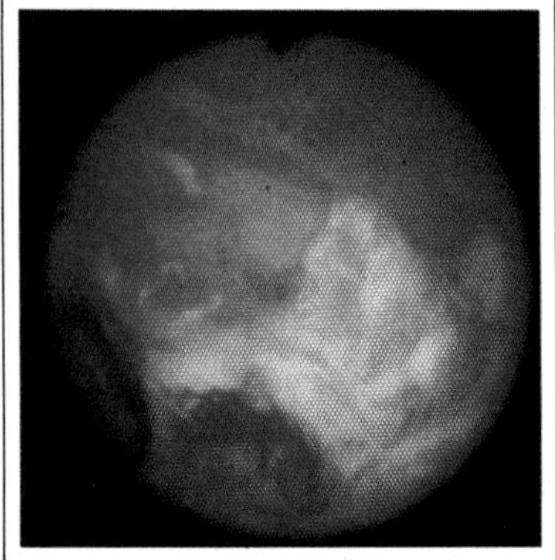

FIG. 48-9c.

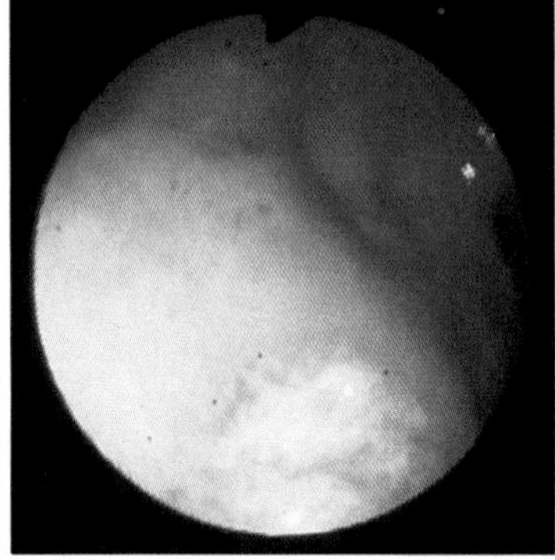

FIG. 48-10.

FIG. 48-9. Recurrent Crohn's disease. **a:** Affecting the ostomy orifice. Ulcerations are present on the outside of the ileostomy as well as just within it, even above the level of the abdominal wall. These were also noted to be present in the terminal ileum just proximal to the stoma (b). **b:** In the terminal ileum just proximal to a similarly involved ileostomy stoma. Extensive and deep ulcerations are seen along with skip areas (c), the typical appearance of Crohn's disease. **c:** In the terminal ileum just proximal to a skip area (in the 12 o'clock position).

FIG. 48-10. Prestomal ileitis, occurring 24 months after a colectomy for ulcerative colitis. Although the histology of the colectomy specimen was typical of ulcerative colitis, focal punched-out ulcerations indistinguishable from those of Crohn's disease were found just above the ileostomy, running for approximately 20 cm. In the resected specimen after ileostomy revision, focal ulcerations were found without other evidence of Crohn's disease, compatible with prestomal ileitis.[14]

set, deep ulcerations which may continue into the terminal ileum for 10 to 20 cm or more (Fig. 48-9c).

Prestomal Ileitis

For patients with prior colectomy for ulcerative colitis or other conditions who are examined because of symptoms suggestive of ileostomy dysfunction, evidence of prestomal ileitis may be observed as multiple, discrete ulcerations (Fig. 48-10) on a background of otherwise normal mucosa. Although the endoscopic picture may be indistinguishable from that of Crohn's disease involving the terminal ileum (Fig. 48-5c), including the presence of strictures (Fig. 48-5d), granulomas, the hallmark of Crohn's disease, are absent from both endoscopic biopsies and surgically resected specimens.[14] The etiology of prestomal ileitis is unknown, but some of the cases are undoubtedly associated with ileostomy obstruction, although obstruction does not always lead to the condition. Still, in a patient whose colectomy was performed for a condition other than Crohn's disease, the examiner may suspect prestomal ileitis when multiple discrete ulcerations are seen in association with a stoma which precludes the use of all but the narrowest-caliber (8 to 9 mm) instrument.

Peristomal Adhesions

Patients with adhesions have a history of episodic pain associated with high ileostomy diarrhea, suggesting periods of intermediate- to high-grade obstruction.[13] Conventional small bowel radiographic studies are often unrevealing, although retrograde injections may show kinking or acute angulation around the stoma just below the skin line (Fig. 48-11a).

Appearance

At endoscopy the acute angulation suspected in the retrograde barium study is reflected in an inability to intubate the ileostomy even with a narrow-caliber pediatric-type instrument much more than 2 to 3 cm below the abdominal wall. What mucosa can be observed has a normal appearance or shows only nonspecific erythema. The absence of ulcerations or histologic skip areas militate against the possibilities of both recurrent Crohn's disease and prestomal ileitis (see above).

The acute angulation present can be appreciated as a sharp change in the direction of the mucosa (Fig. 48-11b). Although this is evidence in support of the diagnosis of peristomal adhesions, it remains a nonspecific finding and is not conclusive. It should never be taken as an indication for surgery in the absence of other supporting radiologic

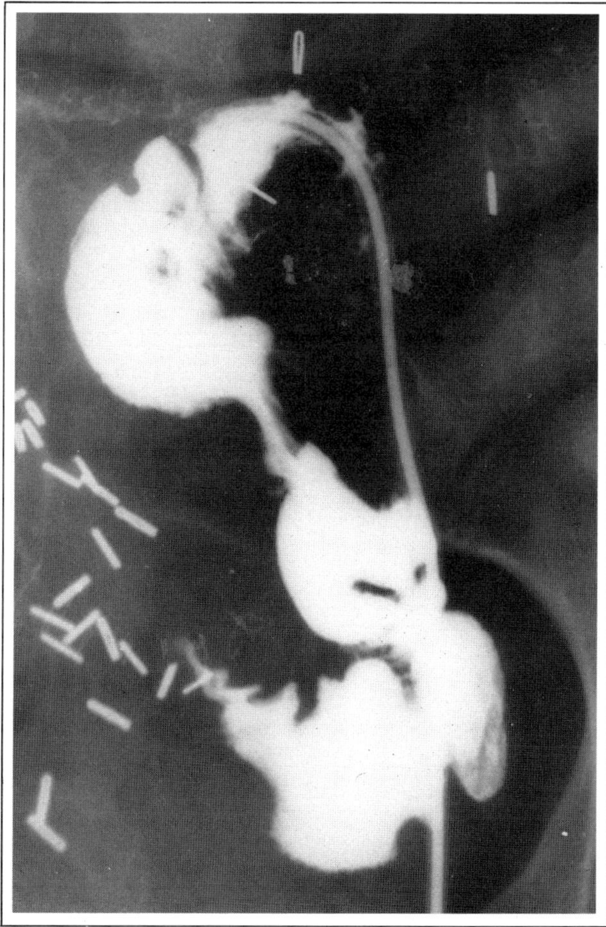

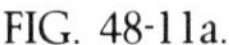

FIG. 48-11a.

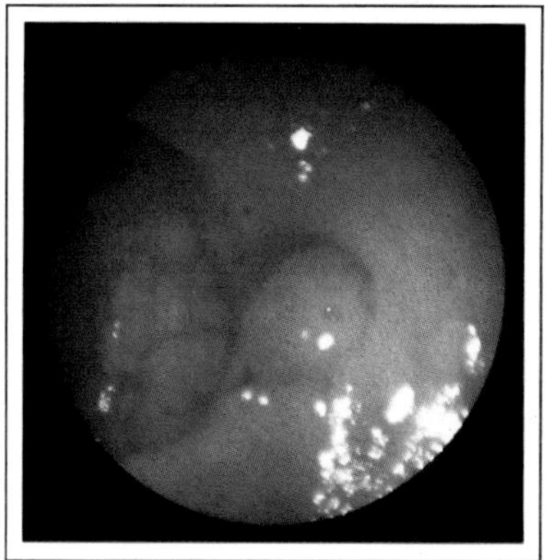

FIG. 48-11b.

FIG. 48-11. Ileostomy with peristomal adhesions. **a:** Demonstrated radiographically (surgically proved). In a patient with intermittent episodes of obstruction, a retrograde study through the stoma (*at top*) demonstrates kinking, focal dilatation, and sharp angulation of the terminal ileum, just proximal (at 5 cm) to the stoma. **b:** The lumen turns sharply toward the 9 o'clock position at a depth of 5 cm which proved impassable in a patient in whom peristomal adhesions were suggested radiographically (a). There was no evidence of recurrent Crohn's disease either endoscopically or at surgery.

evidence, e.g., a retrograde ileostomy barium study (Fig. 48-11a).

Ileostomy (Ileal) Varices

Patients with cirrhosis and portal hypertension who subsequently have an ileostomy may form portasystemic collaterals around the stoma and terminal ileum. These are thought to occur as the result of shunts which form across adhesions that connect the parietal surface of the mesenteric and posterior abdominal wall.[15] Whereas in most cases the ileostomy varices appear in patients who have had a colectomy for ulcerative colitis,[15] it may occur in patients with cirrhosis who have abdominoperineal resections for carcinoma[16] or ileal (ureterointestinal) conduits after cystectomy (see below).[17] The pattern of ileostomy bleeding is variable. It generally begins within 1 to 2 years of the creation of the ileostomy, although it may not appear for many years.[15] Once the bleeding commences, it is experienced as multiple painless episodes of hemorrhage into the ileostomy bag, often of a self-limited nature, being controlled by local measures. Recurrent bleeding, however, which is frequent and on occasion massive, prompts an endoscopic examination of the stoma and terminal ileum prior to the patient's being considered for angiography and ultimately shunt surgery.[15]

Appearance

Like duodenal varices (see Chapter 38), these may be seen as serpiginous submucosal gray-blue venous structures, generally 5 mm or more in diameter. They are situated between Kerckring folds, running obliquely or even perpendicular to these structures. Because Kerckring folds tend to be relatively thin and indistinct in the terminal ileum (Fig. 48-2a), the finding of prominent folds that have a diameter in excess of 5 mm in a patient with a compatible history should always make the examiner suspect ileal varices (Fig. 48-12a) and cause him to suggest arteriography for a definitive diagnosis (Fig. 48-12b).[15]

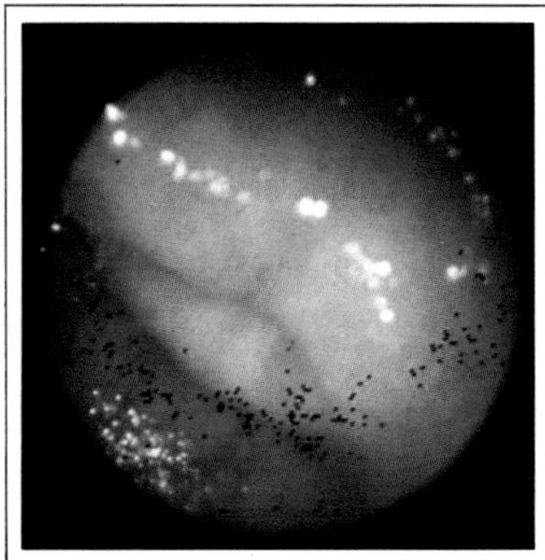

FIG. 48-12a.

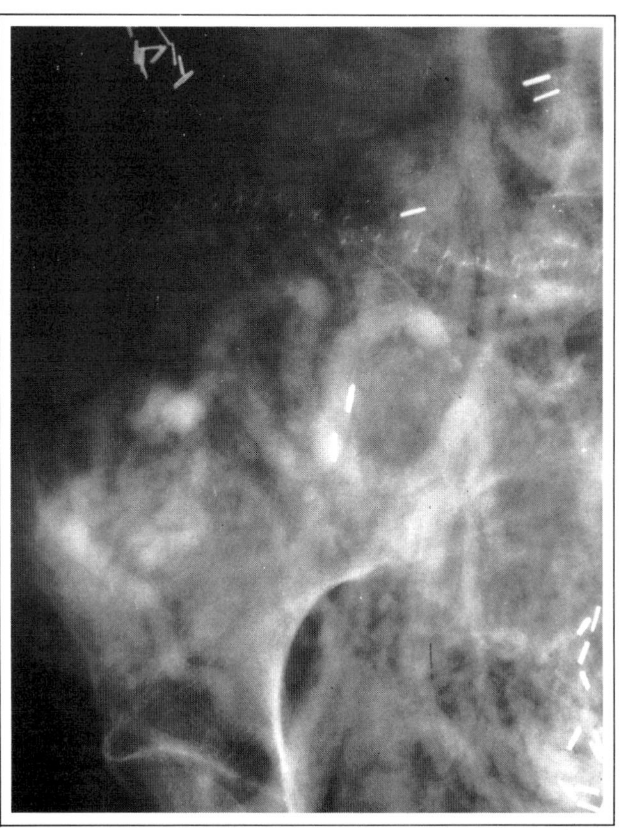

FIG. 48-12b.

FIG. 48-12. a: Ileostomy varices. In a patient with recurrent ileostomy bleeding and known postnecrotic cirrhosis, the appearance of an enlarged Kerckring fold, even if not obviously gray-blue and serpiginous, suggests this diagnosis and the need for an arteriogram (b). **b:** Ileal varices, demonstrated arteriographically. Prominent dilated ileal veins compatible with varices were seen throughout the terminal ileum and especially around the ostomy (*lower left*).

Ileostomy as Part of an Ileal (Ureterointestinal) Conduit

An ileostomy may have been created as part of an ileal conduit procedure for permanent urinary diversion. In these cases the bladder has been removed as part of radical pelvic surgery for malignancy or because it is nonfunctional.[11] The resulting blind loop of terminal ileum can be examined in the same manner as for any ileostomy. Generally, the narrowest-caliber endoscope (8 to 9 mm) is selected. It must be disinfected prior to the procedure but need not be gas-sterilized.[18] During the procedure Falkenstein et al. found it feasible to perform retrograde pyelography[11] once the ureteral orifices were identified. This is facilitated using an endoscope that has an elevating lever at its tip.[11]

Appearance

We have had no personal experience with the ileal conduit as described by Falkenstein et al.[11] They noted, however, that the mucosa of the ileal pouch was more friable in that petechial bleeding and mucosal abrasions were produced with minor endoscopic manipulations. These authors suggested that this could be due to mucosal villous atrophy reported for intestinal urinary conduits.[11] The ureteral anastomosis was described as a 1- to 2-mm outpouching from the intestinal wall or as "nippled structures, protruding into the intestinal lumen."[18] Recognition of these orifices was facilitated by the observation of urine bubbles at the anastomotic sites from the administered air used to distend the intestinal loop.

The principal pathologic feature within the ileal conduit is the presence of urinary calculi, reported to occur in 4 to 30%.[18] These may be removed endoscopically.[18]

ILEAL TUMORS

Although the ileum is the site of approximately 50% of benign small bowel tumors,[19] 50% of malignancies exclusive of carcinoma,[20,21] and 20% of carcinomas,[20,21] these are rarely found at colonoscopy. Over a 7-year period during which 2,500 examinations were performed, in only two were small bowel tumors found. The rarity of this finding is probably accounted for by: (a) the rarity of small bowel tumors themselves, being less than 1/100 as prevalent as colonic carcinomas in the general population[20]; (b) the fact that the terminal ileum is not routinely intubated at colonoscopy; and (c) the fact that tumors of the terminal ileum are not always within 30 to 50 cm of the ileocecal valve, the length of ileum which can generally be examined.

In cases where ileal tumors are present, the patients have been referred for colonoscopy because of abdominal pain,

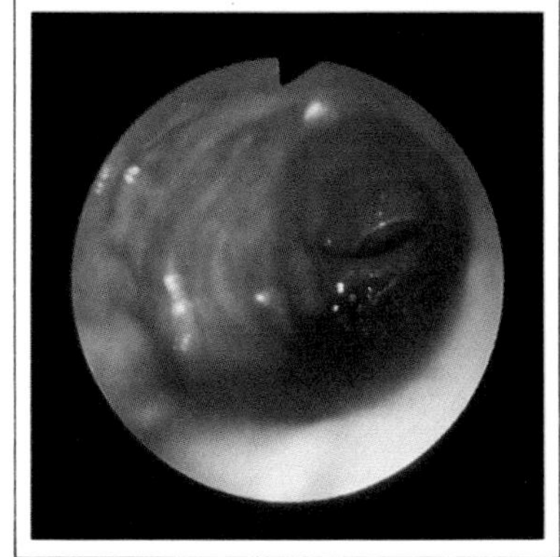

FIG. 48-13a.

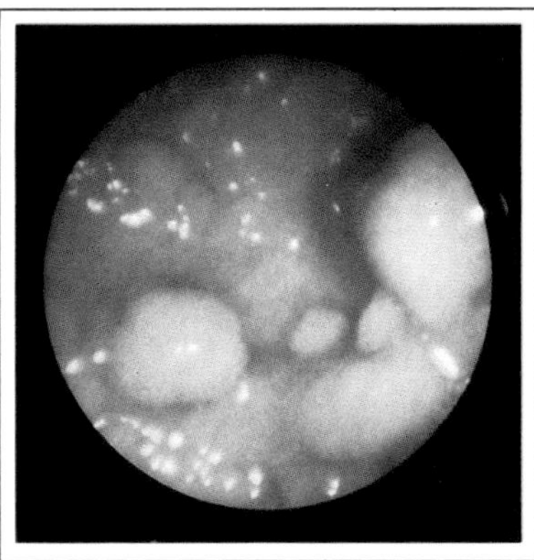

FIG. 48-13b.

FIG. 48-13. a: Ulcerated submucosal tumor of the terminal ileum. This 5-mm tumor is seen in the distance at the center of the field adjacent to a Kerckring fold. Its slightly ulcerated center suggests that it is a leiomyoma or a carcinoid. **b:** Multiple ileal polyps in a patient with known abdominal lymphoma (poorly differentiated type). Biopsy of these polyps showed lymphoma of the same cell type.

anemia, or lower gastrointestinal (GI) bleeding.[20] Others with previously diagnosed abdominal lymphoma are examined because of symptoms or radiologic findings which suggest ileal involvement.[22] Finally, an examination of the ileum may be sought in patients with carcinoid syndrome, as the ileum accounts for almost 25% of the GI sites for these tumors.[23]

Appearance

The findings in the two cases observed by us are perhaps representative of ileal tumors in the main. Most appear as single, discrete polypoid masses with intact or focally ulcerated overlying mucosa, suggesting that they have a submucosal origin (Fig. 48-13a), the commonest of these being lipomas,[19] leiomyomas,[19] fibromas,[19] and carcinoids.[20,21] The ileum is the least common site of small bowel carcinoma[21]; most are primary, although rarely one encounters metastasis to the ileum.[21] In either case one expects the finding of a nodular ulcerated mass. More often than carcinoma, the ileum is the site of a nonepithelial malignancy, e.g., leiomyosarcoma, which like carcinoma appears as a large nodular tumor mass.[20]

Multiple polyps of the terminal ileum (Fig. 48-13b) are almost always benign lymphoid follicles.[1] In patients with abdominal lymphoma, especially of the non-Hodgkin's type, biopsies of these polyps may show them to be lymphomatous, having a cell type identical to that found either in the abdomen or in peripheral lymph nodes.[22]

REFERENCES

1. Nagasako, K., and Takemoto, T. (1973): Endoscopy of the ileocecal area. *Gastroenterology,* 65:403–411.
2. Gaisford, W. D. (1974): Fiberendoscopy of the cecum and terminal ileum. *Gastrointest. Endosc.,* 21:13–17.
3. Gabrielsson, N., and Granqvist, S. (1977): A new technique for insertion of the colonoscope through the ileocecal valve. *Endoscopy,* 9:38–41.
4. Waye, J. D. (1976): Ileoscopy. I. Evaluation of ileostomy dysfunction. *Am. J. Gastroenterol.,* 65:360–361.
5. Marshak, R. H., and Lindner, A. E. (1980): Radiologic diagnosis of chronic ulcerative colitis and Crohn's disease. In: *Inflammatory Bowel Disease,* edited by J. B. Kirsner and R. G. Shortner, pp. 341–409. Lea & Febiger, New York.
6. Hogan, W. J., Hensley, G. T., and Geenen, J. E. (1980): Endoscopic evaluation of inflammatory bowel disease. *Med. Clin. North Am.,* 64:1083–1102.
7. Mekhjian, H., Switz, D. M., Melnyk, C. S., Rankin, G. B., and Brooks, R. K. (1979): Clinical features and natural history of Crohn's disease. *Gastroenterology,* 77:898–906.
8. Koch, T. R., Cave, D. R., Ford, H., and Kirsner, J. B. (1981): Crohn's ileitis and ileocolitis: a study of the anatomical distribution of recurrence. *Dig. Dis. Sci.,* 26:528–531.
9. Vender, R. J., Rickert, R. R., and Spiro, H. M. (1979): The outlook after total colectomy in patients with Crohn's colitis and ulcerative colitis. *J. Clin. Gastroenterol.,* 1:209–217.
10. Albechtsen, D., Bergan, A., Gjone, E., and Nygaard, K. (1981): Elective surgery for ulcerative colitis: colectomy in 158 patients. *Scand. J. Gastroenterol.,* 16:825–831.
11. Falkenstein, D. B., Reich, C. B., Golianbu, M. N., Warner, R. S., Morales, P. A., and Zimmon, D. S. (1975): Endoscopy of ureterointestinal conduits and retrograde pyelography. *Gastrointest. Endosc.,* 22:24–26.
12. Waye, J. D., Kreel, I., Bauer, J., and Gelernt, I. (1977): The continent ileostomy: diagnosis and treatment of problems by means of operative fiberoptic endoscopy. *Gastrointest. Endosc.,* 23:196–198.
13. Achkar, E. (1980): Ileostomy diarrhea. *Pract. Gastroenterol.,* 4(June):16–19.
14. Knill-Jones, R. P., Morson, B., and Williams, R. (1970): Prestomal ileitis: clinical and pathologic findings in five cases. *Q. J. Med.,* 39:287–297.
15. Ricci, R. L., Lee, K. R., and Greenberger, N. J. (1980): Chronic gastrointestinal bleeding from ileal varices after total proctocolectomy for ulcerative colitis: correction by mesocaval shunt. *Gastroenterology,* 78:1053–1058.
16. Goldstein, W. Z., Edoga, J., and Crystal, R. (1980): Management of colostomal hemorrhage resulting from portal hypertension. *Dis. Colon Rectum,* 23:86–90.
17. Eckhauser, F. E., Sonda, L. P., Strodel, W. E., Edgcomb, L. P., and Turcotte, J. G. (1980): Parastomal ileal conduit hemorrhage and portal hypertension. *Ann. Surg.,* 192:620–624.
18. Khera, D. C., and Sosa, F. (1980): Removal of a calculus from an ileal conduit with a fiber optic gastroscope. *Gastrointest. Endosc.,* 26:156–157.
19. Wilson, J. M., Melvin, D. B., Gray, G., and Thorbjarnarson, B. (1975): Benign small bowel tumor. *Ann. Surg.,* 181:247–250.
20. Norberg, K.-A., and Emas, S. (1981): Primary tumors of the small intestine. *Am. J. Surg.,* 142:569–573.
21. Kelsey, J. R. (1976): Small bowel tumors. In: *Gastroenterology,* Vol. 2, edited by H. L. Bockus, pp. 459–472. Saunders, Philadelphia.
22. Gray, G. M., Rosenberg, A., Cooper, A. D., Gregory, P. B., Stein, D. T., and Herzenberg, H. (1982): Lymphomas involving the gastrointestinal tract. *Gastroenterology,* 82:143–152.
23. Zakariai, Z. M., Quan, S. H. Q., and Hajdu, S. I. (1975): Carcinoid tumors of the gastrointestinal tract. *Cancer,* 35:588–591.

SUBJECT INDEX

K

L

M

R

S